INTRODUCTION TO RESPIRATORY CARE

Michael G. Levitzky, Ph.D.
Professor of Physiology
Louisiana State University Medical Center
New Orleans, Louisiana

Jimmy M. Cairo, Ph.D., R.R.T.
Associate Professor of Cardiopulmonary Science
Associate Professor of Physiology
Louisiana State University Medical Center;
Consultant, Pulmonary Diagnostic Laboratory
Children's Hospital of New Orleans
New Orleans, Louisiana

Stanley M. Hall, M.D., Ph.D.
Co-director, Department of Anesthesiology
Children's Hospital of New Orleans;
Clinical Assistant Professor of Anesthesiology, Physiology,
and Cardiopulmonary Science
Louisiana State University Medical Center;
Clinical Assistant Professor of Anesthesiology
Tulane University Medical Center;
Adjunct Assistant Professor of Nurse Anesthesiology
Xavier University of Louisiana
New Orleans, Louisiana

1990
W. B. SAUNDERS COMPANY
Harcourt Brace Jovanovich, Inc.
Philadelphia ■ London ■ Toronto ■ Montreal ■ Sydney ■ Tokyo

W. B. SAUNDERS COMPANY
Harcourt Brace Jovanovich, Inc.

The Curtis Center
Independence Square West
Philadelphia, PA 19106-3399

Library of Congress Cataloging-in-Publication Data

Levitzky, Michael G.
  Introduction to respiratory care / Michael G. Levitzky, Jimmy M. Cairo, Stanley M. Hall.
      p. cm.
   ISBN 0-7216-1090-0
    1. Cardiopulmonary system—Diseases. 2. Respiratory therapy.
  I. Cairo, Jimmy M. II. Hall, Stanley M. III. Title.
    [DNLM: 1. Heart Diseases—diagnosis. 2. Heart Diseases—therapy.
  3. Lung Diseases—diagnosis. 4. Lung Diseases—therapy.
  5. Respiratory Therapy.   WB 342 L6661]
   RC702.L48 1990
   616.1'2—dc20
   DNLM/DLC

Editor: Darlene Pedersen
Developmental Editor: Leslie E. Hoeltzel
Designer: Maureen Sweeney
Production Manager: Carolyn Naylor
Manuscript Editor: David Prout
Illustrator: Sharon Iwanczuk
Illustration Coordinator: Ceil Kunkle
Indexer: Ellen Murray

Introduction to Respiratory Care   ISBN 0-7216-1090-0

Copyright © 1990 by W. B. Saunders Company

All rights reserved. No part of this publication may be reproduced or transmitted in any form or by any means, electronic or mechanical, including photocopy, recording, or any information storage and retrieval system, without permission in writing from the publisher.

Printed in the United States of America.

Last digit is the print number: 9   8   7   6   5   4   3   2   1

To Our Families

ACKNOWLEDGMENTS

The authors would like to express their gratitude to the following people for providing inspiration and assistance in the preparation of this book: Baxter Venable; Charles Chapman; Dr. John J. Spitzer; L. Beatrice Abene; Betty Eckert; Gina Morris; Anna Cooks; Andrew Pellett; Dr. Joseph Smith; the Department of Respiratory Therapy of Children's Hospital of New Orleans; the faculty and students of the Department of Cardiopulmonary Science of LSUMC, particularly Dr. Raymond Edge and Terry Forrette; and our wives, Elizabeth Levitzky, Rhonda Cairo, and Ellen Hall.

PREFACE

To understand clinical respiratory care, one needs a solid background in the basic cardiopulmonary sciences. *Introduction to Respiratory Care* provides this foundation. The text is written in a manner that encourages self-sufficiency in the basic sciences *before* the student is introduced to clinical respiratory care areas, such as assessment of cardiopulmonary disease and therapeutic intervention. Thus, the student will find this textbook to be useful in one or more courses offered in respiratory care educational programs.

Each chapter contains *learning objectives* and a *chapter outline* on the chapter-opening page and a *bibliography* at the end of each chapter. Within chapters are descriptive diagrams, many of which are enhanced by a second color for instructive purposes and a clearer, quicker point of reference. There are also many useful tables that will serve as effective tools for retrieving information quickly.

Introduction to Respiratory Care is organized into three sections: Part I is the basic science part that includes an introductory chapter on physics and chemistry (Chapter 1). The remaining chapters in Part I emphasize cardiovascular physiology (Chapter 2), pulmonary physiology (Chapter 3), and pathophysiology (Chapter 5) as the basis for understanding clinical applications of respiratory care, thus encouraging the student to understand the rationale for making clinical decisions that involve diagnostic and therapeutic measures—in other words, *why* the therapist is doing what he or she is doing to the patient. Two useful inclusions in the basic science part are chapters on cardiopulmonary adjustments to stress (Chapter 4) and cardiopulmonary changes throughout life (Chapter 6).

The second part of *Introduction to Respiratory Care* assesses the patient for the presence of cardiopulmonary disease by such methods as history-taking and physical examination (Chapter 7), cardiovascular diagnostic tests (Chapter 8), pulmonary function tests (Chapter 9), blood gas analysis and determination of acid-base status (Chapter 10), exercise testing (Chapter 11), microbiology and clinical chemistry studies (Chapter 12), and radiologic procedures (Chapter 13). An integrated approach to patient assessment (perinatal, pediatric, and adult patients) is included in Chapter 14. In Part II, the student will learn *how* to measure cardiopulmonary function and *how* to interpret the data.

Part III of *Introduction to Respiratory Care* presents the most current therapeutic modalities used in the treatment of both acute and chronic cardiopulmonary disease. Included are chapters on pharmacology (Chapter 15), administration of oxygen and other therapeutic gases (Chapter 16), bronchopulmonary hygiene (Chapter 17), airway management (Chapter 18), and mechanical ventilation (Chapter 19). Emergency care, including cardiopulmonary resuscitation, and rehabilitation are discussed in Chapter 20.

Following Part III are appendices with tables of normal values for pulmonary function and laboratory tests, hemodynamic measurements, acid-base nomograms, and derivations of equations.

This core textbook is intended for entry-level students in certification programs and for those at the advanced-practitioner level in registry programs in respiratory care. It will serve the student well as solid preparation for the entry-level examination in respiratory care and for the written registry examination. Clinicians already practicing in the field will also find *Introduction to Respiratory Care* to be a useful reference.

MICHAEL G. LEVITZKY, PH.D.
JIMMY M. CAIRO, PH.D., R.R.T.
STANLEY M. HALL, M.D., PH.D.

CONTENTS

I
THE PHYSIOLOGIC BASIS OF RESPIRATORY CARE 1

1
BASIC PHYSICS AND CHEMISTRY 2

2
CARDIOVASCULAR ANATOMY AND PHYSIOLOGY 32

3
PULMONARY ANATOMY AND PHYSIOLOGY 86

4
CARDIOPULMONARY ADJUSTMENTS TO STRESS 156

5
PATHOPHYSIOLOGY OF CARDIOPULMONARY DISEASE 178

6
CARDIOPULMONARY CHANGES THROUGH LIFE 218

II
ASSESSMENT OF CARDIOPULMONARY DISEASE 247

7
HISTORY AND PHYSICAL EXAMINATION 248

8
CARDIOVASCULAR ASSESSMENT 270

9
PULMONARY ASSESSMENT 296

10
ANALYSIS OF BLOOD GASES AND ACID-BASE BALANCE 322

11
CLINICAL EXERCISE TESTING 342

12
CLINICAL CHEMISTRY AND MICROBIOLOGY 358

13
RADIOLOGY 376

14
INTEGRATED APPROACH TO PATIENT ASSESSMENT 398

III
TREATMENT OF CARDIOPULMONARY DISEASE 413

15
PHARMACOLOGY 414

16
ADMINISTRATION OF OXYGEN AND OTHER THERAPEUTIC GASES 440

17
BRONCHOPULMONARY HYGIENE 468

18
AIRWAY MANAGEMENT 486

19
MECHANICAL VENTILATION 512

20
INTEGRATED APPROACH TO PATIENT THERAPEUTICS 536

Appendix 1
PULMONARY TERMS AND SYMBOLS 555

Appendix 2
PREDICTION NOMOGRAM OF NORMAL VALUES FOR PULMONARY FUNCTION TESTING IN FEMALES AND MALES 565

Appendix 3
NORMAL CLINICAL LABORATORY VALUES 567

Appendix 4
NORMAL VALUES FOR CARDIAC PROFILES 568

Appendix 5
NOMOGRAM FOR CALCULATION OF BODY SURFACE AREA 569

INDEX 571

INTRODUCTION TO RESPIRATORY CARE

I
THE PHYSIOLOGIC BASIS OF RESPIRATORY CARE

OBJECTIVES

AFTER READING THIS CHAPTER, THE STUDENT WILL BE ABLE TO:

1. Describe the structure of the atom and relate it to the physical and chemical properties of matter.
2. Discuss chemical bonding.
3. Define the states of matter.
4. Define kinetic and potential energy.
5. Describe the kinetic theory of gases and the laws governing the behavior of gases.
6. Describe the properties of solutions, including equilibrium, vapor pressure, boiling point, and solubility.
7. Discuss the behavior of electrolytes and ions in solution.
8. Define acids, bases, and salts.
9. Describe the various methods for expressing the concentration of a solution.
10. Discuss chemical equilibria and the law of mass action.
11. Describe the structural properties of proteins, carbohydrates, lipids, and nucleic acids.
12. Describe the major metabolic pathways involved in energy production and utilization.

1
BASIC PHYSICS AND CHEMISTRY

CHAPTER OUTLINE

STRUCTURE OF THE ATOM
  Subatomic particles
  Energy sublevels
  Valence electrons
  Isotopes
  Periodic law
CHEMICAL BONDING
  Octet rule
  Ionic bonds
  Covalent bonds
  Ionization potentials and electronegativities
ENERGY AND MATTER
  Kinetic energy
  Potential energy
  States of matter
PROPERTIES OF GASES
  Boyle's law
  Charles' law
  Gay-Lussac's law
    Absolute temperature scale
  Dalton's law
  Avogadro's law
  Ideal gas equation
  Laws of diffusion
    Graham's law
    Henry's law
    Fick's law

PROPERTIES OF LIQUIDS AND SOLIDS
  Types of liquid mixtures
  Osmosis
  Ions and electrolytes
  Acids, bases, and salts
  pH
  Quantification of solutions
    Dilution methods
CHEMICAL REACTIONS
  Types of chemical reactions
  Factors influencing the rates of chemical reactions
  Chemical equilibria and the law of mass action
BIOCHEMICAL PROCESSES
  Proteins
  Carbohydrates
  Lipids
  Nucleic acids
CELLULAR METABOLISM AND ENERGY METABOLISM

Every student of respiratory care should have a working knowledge of physics and chemistry. The purpose of this chapter is to provide you with a basic understanding of the structure of matter and the physical laws that govern its behavior. Although this information may seem, at least initially, somewhat irrelevant to the practice of respiratory care, its importance in understanding topics such as acid-base balance, medical gas therapy, and metabolism cannot be overemphasized.

THE STRUCTURE OF THE ATOM

The Greek philosopher, Democritus (ca. 400 B.C.) is generally credited with introducing the concept that matter (which can be defined as anything having mass and occupying space) is composed of indestructible particles called *atoms*. These atoms (derived from the Greek word *atomos*, meaning indivisible) were considered to be the smallest unit into which any material could be divided yet retain its original identity. Although Democritus's idea was not accepted by many philosophers of his day, the notion of atomism persisted up to the early nineteenth century, when a more detailed explanation of the structure of matter was offered.

In 1808, John Dalton, an English school teacher and chemist, proposed a more precise definition of the indivisible building blocks of matter in what is now referred to as *Dalton's atomic theory*. Dalton stated that all matter is composed of *elements*, which in turn are composed of the indestructible particles proposed by Democritus. Dalton defined *elements* as substances containing only one type of atom (i.e., with the same mass and size) and *compounds* as combinations of atoms from more than one element. He also suggested that in any compound, the ratio of atoms of any two of the elements is either a whole number or a simple fraction.

Although Dalton's theory made no attempt to explain the structure and composition of atoms, it did provide scientists with a greater insight into the nature of matter. Furthermore, it should be emphasized that Dalton's theory marked the beginning of modern chemistry and formed the basis of the present concept of the atomic structure of matter.

Subatomic Particles

Toward the end of the nineteenth century, data began to accumulate that clearly demonstrated that atoms actually possess an internal structure; that is, they are made up of even smaller units, which are called *subatomic particles*. On the basis of data provided by scientists such as Rutherford, Thomson, Planck, Bohr, and Chadwick, the following facts emerged:

1. The atom is more or less spherical in shape with a diameter of about 1 angstrom (1×10^{-10} meters).

2. Atoms are composed of three major kinds of particles: *protons, neutrons,* and *electrons*.

3. At the center of each atom is a nucleus that contains positively charged protons and uncharged neutrons. The *atomic number* of an element is equal to the number of protons in the nucleus; the *atomic mass* is equal to the sum of protons and neutrons. (The term *atomic weight* is used interchangeably with atomic mass. Actually, the atomic weight of an element is the average relative weight of an element compared to some standard. Carbon, which has an atomic weight of 12, is now used as the standard.)

4. The number of negatively charged electrons (symbolized as z) within an atom is variable but approximately equal to the number of protons (symbolized by Z) present. In neutral atoms, the number of electrons equals the number of protons (or $Z = z$). If the number of electrons is greater than the number of protons present, a negatively charged ion or *anion* is formed (or $z > Z$). If the number of protons is greater than the number of electrons, a positively charged ion, or *cation*, is formed (or $Z > z$).

5. The electrons of an atom revolve around the nucleus in specified *energy shells,* which are arbitrarily labeled K, L, M, N, and so on, starting with the one closest to the nucleus (Fig. 1–1). The number of electrons that can be contained in an energy level is equal to $2n^2$. Thus, the K shell (the first energy level) can contain $2(1)^2$ or 2 electrons. The L shell can contain $2(2)^2$ or 8 electrons, M, $2(3)^2$ or 18, N, $2(4)^2$ or 32. The O shell has $2(4)^2$ or 32, P has $2(3)^2$ or 18, and Q has $2(1)^2$ or 2 electrons.

6. Each shell has a specific energy content, with the K shell (the one closest to the nucleus) having a lower energy value than those located at greater distances from the nucleus. Each electron can therefore have a certain energy content and occupy a specified region in the atom.

Energy Sublevels

Experimental data acquired during the last 50 years have shown that each energy shell within an

BASIC PHYSICS AND CHEMISTRY 5

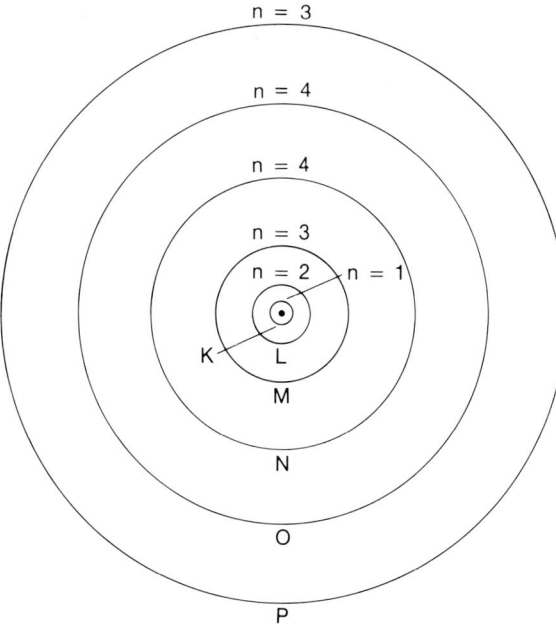

FIGURE 1–1. Bohr model of the atom.

atom (except the *K* shell) can be divided into energy sublevels. As Figure 1–2 shows, as one proceeds from the nucleus, each shell has one more subshell than the shell preceding it. The *K* shell is undivided; the *L* shell contains two subshells; the *M* shell has three subshells, and so on. These subshells are designated *s* for the lowest subshell in any energy level, *p* for the second lowest, *d* for the third, and *f* for the fourth. Thus, the *K* shell is simultaneously an *s* subshell; the *L* shell can contain *s* and *p* subshells; the *M* shell can contain *s*, *p*, and *d* subshells, and so on. The maximum number of electrons that each subshell can contain varies but in general is equal to $2(2n - 1)$, where *n* designates the subshell number (i.e., $s = 1$; $p = 2$; $d = 3$; $f = 4$).

Table 1–1 lists the first 18 elements in order of increasing atomic number. Note that the electronic configuration of each element can also be indicated in a shorthand form in which superscripts are used to designate the subshell population. For example, oxygen, which contains eight electrons, can be denoted as $1s^2\ 2s^2\ 2p^4$, which indicates there are two electrons in each of the *s* subshells ($1s$, $2s$), and four electrons in the $2p$ subshell.

Valence Electrons

The electrons in the outermost shell of an atom have the highest energy content for that atom. During chemical reactions, these are the electrons that participate directly in chemical bonding and are referred to as *valence electrons* (from the Latin *valentia*, meaning capacity). As discussed later in this chapter, the number of electrons present within the valence shell determines the bonding characteristics of an atom. Figure 1–3 illustrates a simple method for designating the valence of an electron (i.e., the *Lewis dot symbol*). These symbols show the valence electrons as dots surrounding the element and, therefore, represent the possibilities for bonding in an atom.

Isotopes

As stated previously, the mass of an atom is primarily determined by the number of protons and neutrons present within its nucleus. In 1932, James Chadwick showed that certain elements possess a heterogeneous group of constituent atoms called *isotopes*. Experimental evidence suggests that this heterogeneity results from the presence of additional neutrons in the nuclei of these atoms (Fig. 1–4). The atomic number is the same for each of an element's isotopes, but their atomic masses differ, which allows them to be used as markers or tracers. For example, there are three isotopes of hydrogen, each of which has an atomic number of

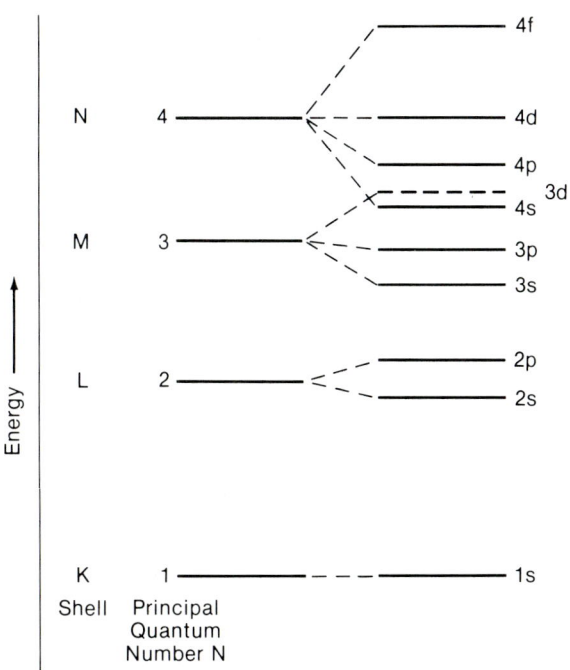

FIGURE 1–2. Diagram showing the relative energy levels of various electron subshells. (From Sienko, M. J., and Plane, R. A.: *Chemistry*, 4th ed. New York, McGraw-Hill, 1971, with permission.)

6 BASIC PHYSICS AND CHEMISTRY

TABLE 1–1. Electronic Configuration of the First 18 Elements in Order of Increasing Atomic Nuclei*

		1	2		3			4				5				6				7
Z	Element	s	s	p	s	p	d	s	p	d	f	s	p	d	f	s	p	d	f	s
1	H	1																		
2	He	2																		
3	Li	2	1																	
4	Be	2	2																	
5	B	2	2	1																
6	C	2	2	2																
7	N	2	2	3																
8	O	2	2	4																
9	F	2	2	5																
10	Ne	2	2	6																
11	Na	2	2	6	1															
12	Mg	2	2	6	2															
13	Al	2	2	6	2	1														
14	Si	2	2	6	2	2														
15	P	2	2	6	2	3														
16	S	2	2	6	2	4														
17	Cl	2	2	6	2	5														
18	Ar	2	2	6	2	6														

* Adapted with permission from Sienko, M., and Plane, R.: *Chemistry*, 4th ed. New York, McGraw-Hill, 1971.

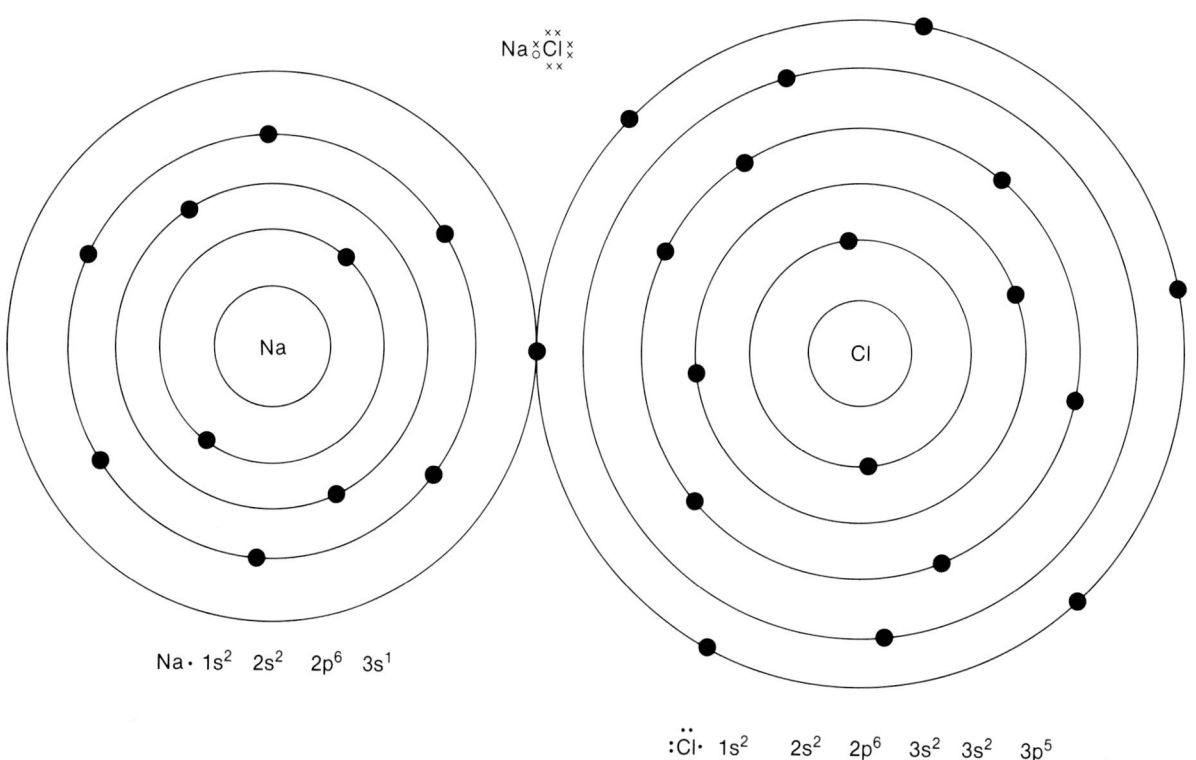

FIGURE 1–3. Lewis dot symbols for sodium chloride.

one. Hydrogen atoms that have one proton and no neutrons are designated as ^1_1H. Deuterium atoms have nuclei composed of one proton and one neutron; the atomic mass of a deuterium atom is 2 daltons. The symbol for deuterium is ^2_1H. Tritium atoms contain one proton and two neutrons, and the atomic mass of a tritium atom equals 3 daltons. ^3_1H is the symbol used to denote tritium.

Several elements have isotopes that contain unstable nuclei that undergo disintegration to emit particles or electromagnetic radiation spontaneously. These unstable isotopes are called radioactive and may occur naturally or be artificially produced by bombarding atomic nuclei with neutron "bullets" in atomic reactors. Elements with naturally occurring radioactive isotopes include uranium, radium, and thorium. Artificial radioactive elements can be produced from oxygen, phosphorus, iodine, and cobalt. As discussed later in this book, radioactive elements have important medical uses in both the diagnosis and treatment of various cardiopulmonary diseases.

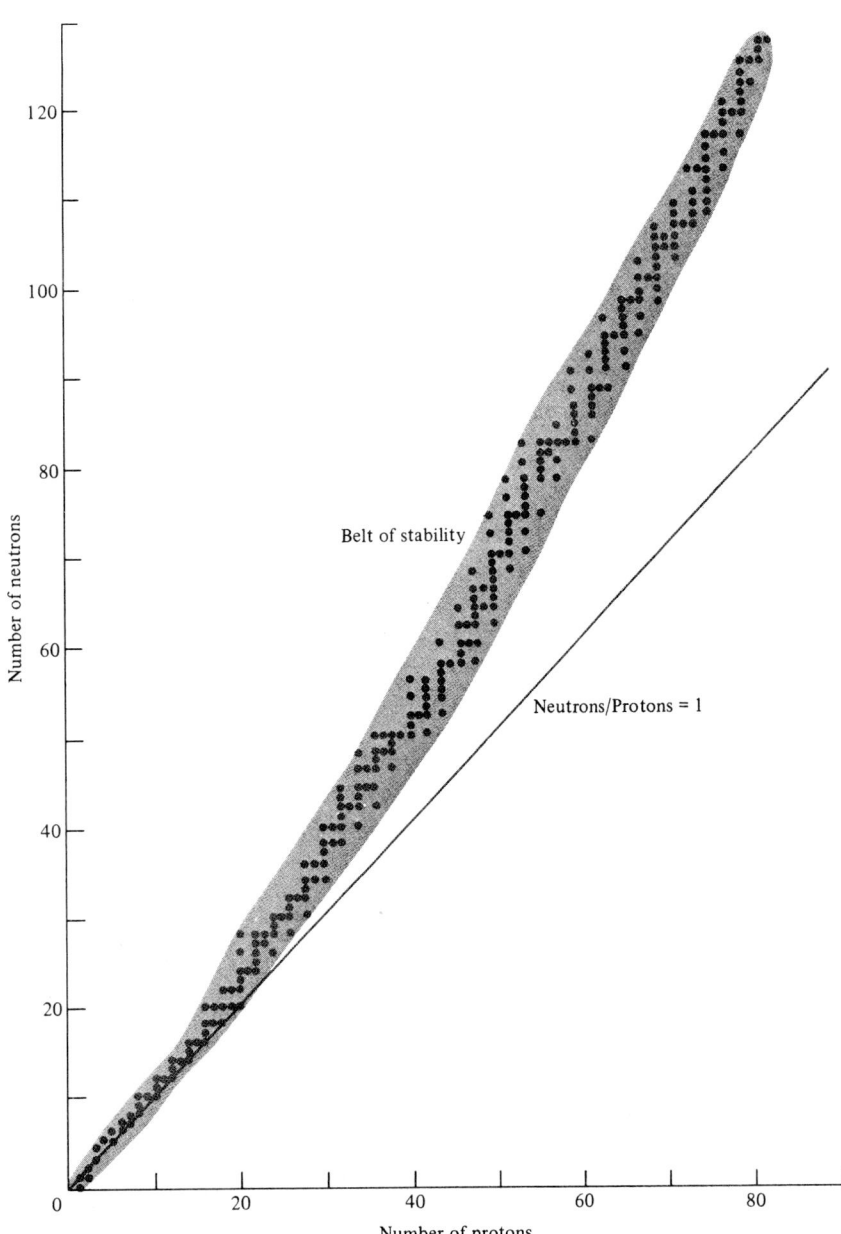

FIGURE 1–4. Proton-neutron distribution in stable nuclei. (From Chang, R.: *Chemistry*, 3rd ed. New York, Random House, 1988, with permission.)

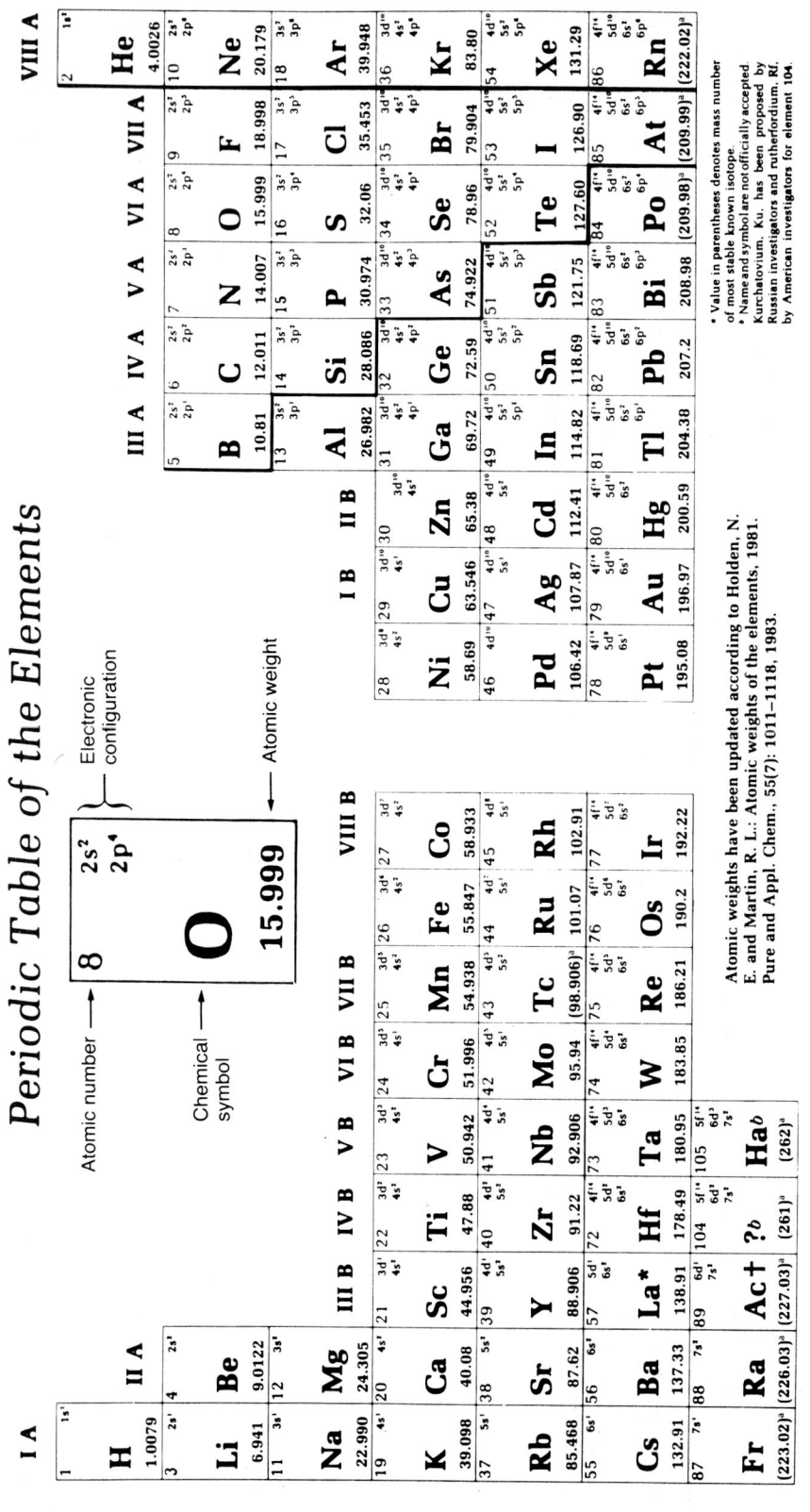

FIGURE 1–5. Periodic table of the elements. (From Tietz, N.W.: *Fundamentals of Clinical Chemistry.* 3rd ed. Philadelphia, W.B. Saunders, 1987.)

Periodic Law

As early as 1869, the Russian chemist Dmitry Mendeleyev proposed that when the chemical elements were arranged in order of increasing weights, similar chemical and physical properties would recur at regular intervals. This arrangement resulted in the statement of the *periodic law* and the construction of the *periodic table of the elements*. It has since been learned that the periodicity of the elements relates more closely to atomic number, so the present periodic table is based on this latter function rather than on atomic weight (Fig. 1–5). Each vertical column of elements is referred to as a *group* or *family*. Each horizontal row of the periodic table is called a *period*.

Group I elements have one valence electron and in general possess the properties of metals (i.e., soft, silvery-white in color, with a bright luster; hydrogen, which is a gas is an exception to this rule); Group VII elements have seven valence electrons and are nonmetals. These elements are often referred to as halogens (from the Greek *hals + gen*, meaning salt-former) because when they combine with metallic atoms (Group I elements) salts are formed. Groups II through VI have properties between those of Group I and Group VII elements. Group VIII elements have eight valence electrons and are considered to be chemically inert (i.e., do not combine with other elements to form compounds). These latter elements are referred to as the noble gases (from French word *noble*, meaning elite class). The two horizontal rows of elements located at the bottom of the periodic table are referred to as the *lanthanoid* and *actinoid* series of elements. Actually, cerium (Ce) should follow lanthanum (La), and thorium (Th) should come right after actinium (Ac). These two rows of elements are separated from the main body of the periodic table to maintain the symmetrical nature of the table.

CHEMICAL BONDING

Relatively few elements are found free within living organisms. Instead, most atoms are joined with other atoms to form more complex structures, such as ionic and molecular compounds. The symbols used to denote the elements are shown in Figure 1–5. To denote a compound, these symbols are combined into a chemical formula that shows the type and number of elements involved in the makeup.

Using the information already presented about electron configurations and the periodic table, we can now examine the two major types of chemical bonds: *ionic bonds*, in which electrons are transferred from one atom to another; and *covalent bonds*, in which electrons are shared between atoms.

Octet Rule

As stated earlier, elements containing eight electrons in their valence shell (i.e., the noble gases) have a particularly stable electronic configuration. Using this model, G. N. Lewis proposed that when two or more elements react, they tend to gain, lose, or share electrons so that the outermost energy level holds or shares four pairs of electrons (i.e., an octet). As the following discussion of chemical bonding shows, most elements obey the octet rule when forming compounds with other elements. (Note that hydrogen and helium have the $1s$ shell as their outermost energy level and therefore are stable with only two electrons, the maximum allowed in that orbital.)

Ionic Bonds

When sodium (Na, a Group I element containing one valence electron) reacts with chlorine (Cl, a Group VII element containing seven valence electrons), a lone electron from the sodium atom is transferred to the chlorine atom, resulting in the formation of a stable positive sodium ion and a negative chloride ion. The electrovalent attraction between these two elements, called an *ionic bond*, produces sodium chloride (NaCl).

Note that the formation of an ionic bond is favored by the reaction of an atom that has a low electron affinity (Group I) with an atom of high electron affinity (Group VII). In general, these ionic compounds resemble sodium chloride in being crystalline solids that dissolve in water to give solutions that can conduct an electrical current (*electrolytes*). The properties of salts are discussed in greater detail later in this chapter.

Covalent Bonds

Unlike the ionic bond, which results from the transfer of electrons from one atom to another, the *covalent bond* results from a sharing of electrons between two or more atoms. The simplest example of such an arrangement is demonstrated by the re-

BASIC PHYSICS AND CHEMISTRY

action of two hydrogen atoms to form molecular hydrogen. In this reaction, each hydrogen atom has one electron in its valence shell. When the two atoms combine, each atom can accommodate another electron in its unfilled valence shell. Neither atom gains complete possession of the two lone electrons, and a symmetric *nonpolar covalent* bond is formed between the two hydrogen atoms (Fig. 1–6).

Conversely, if the sharing of an electron between two atoms is not equal, a *polar covalent* bond is formed. Consider the reaction of hydrogen with chlorine to form hydrochloric acid (HCl). The molecule as a whole is neutral because it contains an equal number of positive and negative charges. However, because of the greater electron affinity of chlorine compared with that of hydrogen, the shared electron spends more time with the chlorine atom than the hydrogen atom. The separation of positive and negative charges within a molecule creates a *dipole*, which has magnetic properties when placed in an electric field and thus gives an experimental method for distinguishing polar from nonpolar molecules.

Note that more than one pair of electrons can be shared by two atoms to gain an octet. When two pairs of electrons are shared by two atoms, the result is a double covalent bond. For example, oxygen, which needs two electrons to fill its outer shell, can form a double bond with another oxygen, gaining its octet by sharing four electrons, as in molecular oxygen (O_2). Similarly, a triple covalent bond results when two atoms share three pairs of electrons, as in molecular nitrogen (N_2).

Ionization Potentials and Electronegativity

By measuring the energy required to remove an electron from an atom, the atom's ability to hold onto electrons, or its *ionization potential* (which is expressed in electron volts or kilogram calories per mole), can be described. Linus Pauling, in 1935, showed there is a close relationship between an atom's ionization potential and its ability to attract electrons, or its *electronegativity*. Thus, the greater the attraction of electrons that an atom has, the higher its ionization potential and associated electronegativity.

Figure 1–7 is a periodic table showing the electronegativities for each element except the noble gases. (Remember that these elements are chemically inert.) Note that electronegativities generally increase as you go across periods and down each group. The concept of electronegativity is useful when trying to decide whether a molecule is ionic or covalent in composition. Generally, if there are only slight differences in electronegativities of two elements joined in a chemical bond (i.e., less than 2), the chemical bond is considered to be a covalent bond; if the difference in electronegativities is greater than 2, an ionic bond is present.

ENERGY AND MATTER

Energy is the capacity to do work, where *work* means moving matter against a force. Quantifi-

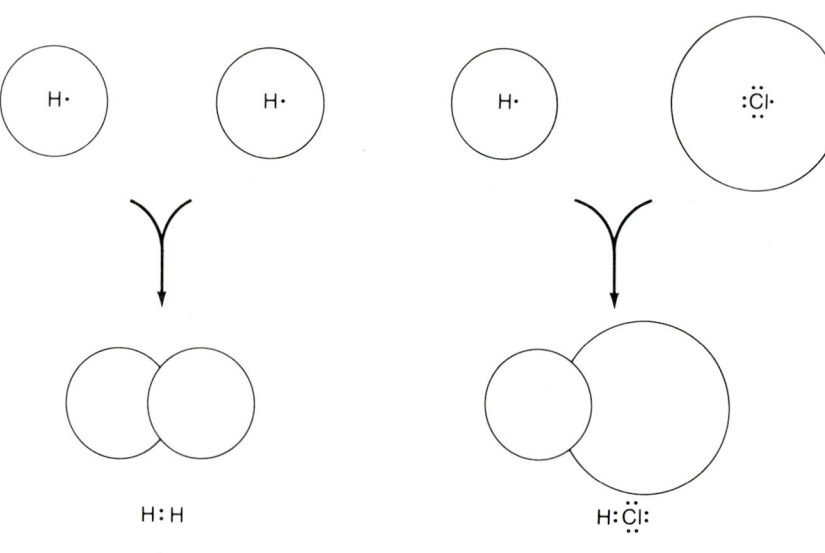

FIGURE 1–6. *A,* Nonpolar covalent bond. *B,* Polar covalent bond.

	1A	2A											3A	4A	5A	6A	7A	8A
	H 2.1																	
	Li 1.0	Be 1.5											B 2.0	C 2.5	N 3.0	O 3.5	F 4.0	
	Na 0.9	Mg 1.2	3B	4B	5B	6B	7B	⎯⎯ 8B ⎯⎯			1B	2B	Al 1.5	Si 1.8	P 2.1	S 2.5	Cl 3.0	
	K 0.8	Ca 1.0	Sc 1.3	Ti 1.5	V 1.6	Cr 1.6	Mn 1.5	Fe 1.8	Co 1.9	Ni 1.9	Cu 1.9	Zn 1.6	Ga 1.6	Ge 1.8	As 2.0	Se 2.4	Br 2.8	
	Rb 0.8	Sr 1.0	Y 1.2	Zr 1.4	Nb 1.6	Mo 1.8	Tc 1.9	Ru 2.2	Rh 2.2	Pd 2.2	Ag 1.9	Cd 1.7	In 1.7	Sn 1.8	Sb 1.9	Te 2.1	I 2.5	
	Cs 0.7	Ba 0.9	La-Lu 1.0-1.2	Hf 1.3	Ta 1.5	W 1.7	Re 1.9	Os 2.2	Ir 2.2	Pt 2.2	Au 2.4	Hg 1.9	Tl 1.8	Pb 1.9	Bi 1.9	Po 2.0	At 2.2	
	Fr 0.7	Ra 0.9																

Increasing electronegativity →
↑ Increasing electronegativity

FIGURE 1–7. The electronegativities of common elements. Note that the group VIII elements are not shown because they normally do not form compounds. (From Chang, R.: *Chemistry*, 3rd ed. New York, Random House, 1988, with permission.)

cation of the energy content of a system is therefore based on the amount of work that the system can do to accomplish a specified task. Table 1–2 lists several of the more common methods for expressing work and energy.

Since work is proportional to the force applied to an object to move it a specified distance, the total energy content of a system may be characterized as the energy it has by virtue of its motion plus the energy it possesses because of its position relative to other objects. The former type of energy is referred to as *kinetic energy*, whereas the latter is called *potential energy*.

Kinetic Energy

For any system in motion, its kinetic energy is expressed as the product of its mass and the square of the velocity at which it is traveling. More specifically, this relationship may be stated as:

$$\text{Kinetic energy} = \tfrac{1}{2} mv^2 *$$

where m equals mass and v equals velocity.

It should be evident from this equation that any factor that increases the internal molecular activity of a substance (e.g., increased temperature) also increases the kinetic energy content of that system.

Potential Energy

Any form of energy that is not kinetic is called potential energy. There are six forms of potential energy: mechanical, electrical, chemical, thermal, nuclear, and magnetic. The following are examples of each form of potential energy:

mechanical—coiled springs
electrical—charged capacitors
chemical—batteries
thermal—steam engines
nuclear—nuclear reactors
magnetic—transformers.

Remember that although energy can be neither created nor destroyed, it can be transformed from one form to another. This statement of the *law of conservation of energy* constitutes the basis of all physiochemical interactions.

TABLE 1–2. Methods for Expressing Work and Energy

1 electron volt (eV) = 1.6021×10^{-12} ergs
1 calorie (cal) = 4.1840×10^7 ergs
1 liter-atmosphere (L-atm) = 24.217 calories

---

*For objects moving faster than about a tenth of the speed of light, this formula is too inaccurate. We must rely instead on Einstein's relativistically derived equation, in which v is replaced with c (representing the speed of light), so that the equation then becomes $E = mc^2$.

12 BASIC PHYSICS AND CHEMISTRY

States of Matter

All matter, at least in principle, can exist in three states: (1) as a *gas*, (2) as a *liquid*, and (3) as a *solid*.

Gases are characterized by a random arrangement of constituent atoms or molecules, so they lack a specific shape and volume. When placed in a closed container, the gas particles arrange themselves so that they are equally dispersed throughout the entire volume provided.

Liquids have a slight degree of intermolecular attraction that gives them a greater amount of molecular order than is the case for gases. These attractive forces give liquids the ability to assume the shape of the container in which they are placed. Unlike gases, liquids do not expand to be dispersed equally in all parts of a container.

Solids have an inherently orderly association of constituent atoms, ions, and molecules that generally are resistant to change. At a given temperature, a solid has a fixed volume and density. Solids are generally classified as either amorphous (i.e., lacking a definite form) or crystalline in structure.

The following is a brief discussion of the physical laws that govern the behavior of gases, liquids, and solids. As you will see, the information contained in this discussion is the result of numerous experimental observations that have been made over the course of four centuries.

PROPERTIES OF GASES

In the practice of respiratory care, it is essential to have an understanding of the physical and chemical properties of gases. The foundation of this understanding is the *kinetic theory of gases*, which states that all gases are composed of molecules that are in continuous random motion. During random motion, these molecules collide with each other and with the walls of the vessel in which they are contained. These collisions exert pressure (which has the units of force/area) against the wall of the container. The collisions are totally elastic so that the gas molecules rebound with an energy equal to what they had before the collision. Thus, the pressure exerted by the gas is proportional to the frequency of collisions of particles with the container walls.

As we shall see, the kinetic theory can ultimately explain the behavior of gases in terms of expan-

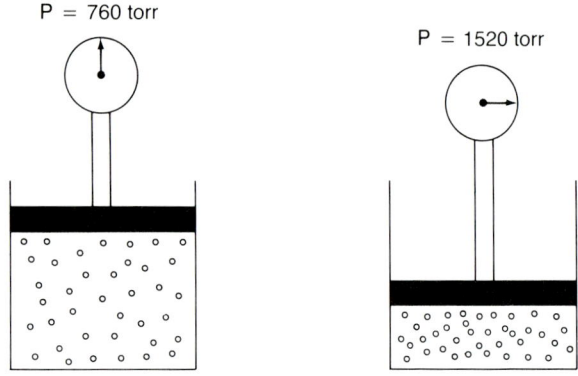

Constant temperature
FIGURE 1–8. Boyle's law.

sibility, compressibility, and diffusibility. Quantitative analysis is described using the gas laws.*

Boyle's Law

In 1662, Robert Boyle stated that if the temperature of a gas is kept constant, the volume that the gas occupies is inversely proportional to the gas pressure. If we designate pressure as P and volume as V, then this law can be symbolized as:

$$P \propto 1/V \quad \text{or}$$

$$P \times V = \text{a constant}$$

Boyle demonstrated the pressure-volume relationships of gases using an apparatus like the one shown in Figure 1–8. In this device, a known volume of gas is uniformly distributed in a closed container. Remember that the pressure a gas exerts depends on the frequency of collisions of its molecules with the walls of the vessel. As shown in Figure 1–8, at a container volume of 2 liters, the pressure is measured at 1 atmosphere (760 mmHg or 760 torr). When the volume is cut in half to 1 liter, the gas molecules are confined to a smaller space, and the probability of collisions increases, which results in an increase in pressure to 2 atmospheres (1520 mmHg or 1520 torr).

Although the individual values for pressure and volume can vary for a given sample of gas, if the amount of gas and the temperature do not change, then P times V is always equal to the same con-

---
* The gas laws describe the behavior of ideal gases rather than real gases. Although most real gases (such as hydrogen, oxygen, and nitrogen) obey these laws fairly well, certain gases (such as carbon dioxide) deviate considerably.

stant. Therefore, we can write,

$$P_1V_1 = \text{a constant} = P_2V_2 \quad or$$

$$P_1V_1 = P_2V_2$$

where P_1 and P_2 are the pressures at volumes V_1 and V_2, respectively. This expression of Boyle's law allows you to compare the pressure-volume characteristics of a gas under two different sets of conditions. We will discuss the application of Boyle's law throughout this book, as in describing mechanics of breathing, determination of lung volumes, and blood gas analysis.

Charles' Law

The pressure-volume relationships for gases expressed in Boyle's law depend on the temperature of the gas remaining constant. It would be appropriate to ask at this point, "How does changing the temperature of a gas affect the pressure-volume characteristics of the gas?" This question was answered in the late eighteenth century by Jacques Charles who found experimentally that if a gas is kept at a constant pressure, it expands when heated and contracts when cooled. Charles found that the increment of volume change is equal for each degree centigrade rise in temperature. In fact, he found that the increment of volume change is equal to 1/273 of the volume of the gas at 0°C.

The mathematical expression of Charles' law can therefore be stated as:

$$V \propto T \quad or$$

$$V/T = \text{a constant}$$

Figure 1–9 illustrates Charles' Law. If a gas is kept at a constant pressure of 1 atmosphere and the temperature of the gas is increased, the molecular activity of the gas increases and the volume of the gas expands.

Charles' law is used to calculate spirometric volume, as in volume corrections associated with environmental temperature changes. The mathematical expression used in these calculations is:

$$V_1/V_2 = T_1/T_2$$

where V_1 and V_2 represent the gas volumes at temperature T_1 and T_2.

Gay-Lussac's Law

Using the information gathered by Boyle and Charles, Joseph Louis Gay-Lussac proposed that

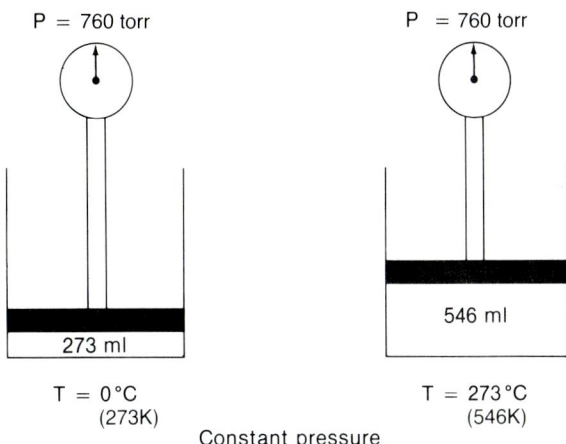

FIGURE 1–9. Charles' law.

the pressure exerted by a gas is directly related to its temperature if the volume of gas is kept constant, or

$$P \propto T$$

Rearranging this equation, the relationship becomes:

$$P/T = \text{a constant}$$

Figure 1–10 shows the effect of varying the temperature of a gas on the pressure exerted by a gas. As the temperature increases, the energy of the gas molecules increases and the movement of molecules increases. The gas molecules collide with the walls of the container more frequently, and the pressure exerted by the gas increases. This increase has been shown to be 1/273 of the pressure of the gas measured at 0°C for every 1°C rise in

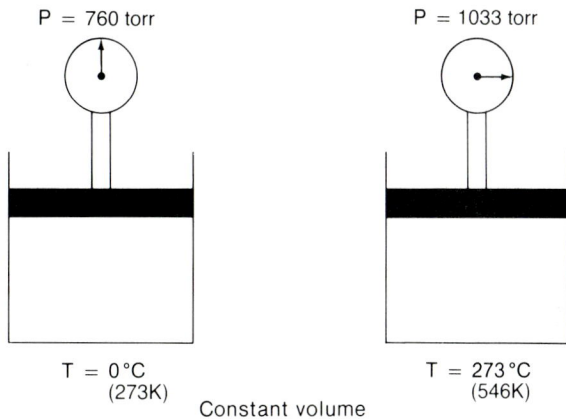

FIGURE 1–10. Gay-Lussac's law.

temperature. If the temperature of the gas decreases, the pressure falls by 1/273 of the gas volume at 0°C for every 1°C decrease.

The effect of temperature on gas pressure is of great importance when designing cylinders for storage of therapeutic gases. The mathematical form

$$P_1/P_2 = T_1/T_2$$

is used in the application of this law.

Absolute Temperature Scale

Using the experimental data of Charles and Gay-Lussac, Lord Kelvin in 1848 suggested that the temperature of −273°C was the lowest attainable temperature, and he called it *absolute zero*. With absolute zero as the starting point, he set up a temperature scale, now called the *Kelvin temperature scale*. In the Kelvin temperature scale, one degree Celsius is equal in magnitude to one kelvin (K). Note that the absolute temperature scale has no degree sign, so that 25 K is called 25 kelvins.

As Figure 1–11 shows, the only difference between the absolute temperature scale and the Celsius scale is that the zero position is shifted. The relationship between kelvins and degrees Celsius is:

$$T(K) = T(°C) + 273°C$$

With the development of the absolute temperature scale, we now express volume-temperature and pressure-temperature relationships for gases (i.e., Charles' and Gay-Lussac's laws, respectively) in terms of absolute temperature (K). Thus, in the case of Charles' law, if the pressure of a gas is kept constant, its volume varies directly with its absolute temperature; for Gay-Lussac's law, if the volume of a gas is kept constant, its pressure varies directly with its absolute temperature.

Dalton's Law

When a mixture of gases is confined in a closed container, the total pressure of the mixture is equal to the sum of the individual pressures exerted by the constituent gases. The individual pressures are called *partial pressures*, and they are symbolized as Px, where x denotes a particular gas (e.g., oxygen = O_2, nitrogen = N_2, carbon dioxide = CO_2). Dalton's law can therefore be written as:

$$P_T = P_1 + P_2 + P_3 + \text{etc.}$$

An analysis of atmospheric air can serve as an example of this relationship. It is known that dry atmospheric gas is composed primarily of nitrogen (~78%), oxygen (~20.9%), and carbon dioxide (~0.4%). According to Dalton's law, at a total barometric pressure of 760 torr, nitrogen would exert a partial pressure of 78/100 × 760 torr, or ~593 torr; oxygen would exert a partial pressure of 20.9/100 × 760 torr, or ~159 torr; carbon dioxide would exert a partial pressure of 0.04/100 × 760 torr, or ~0.3 torr.

As discussed later, applications of Dalton's law appear in calculations of alveolar gas concentra-

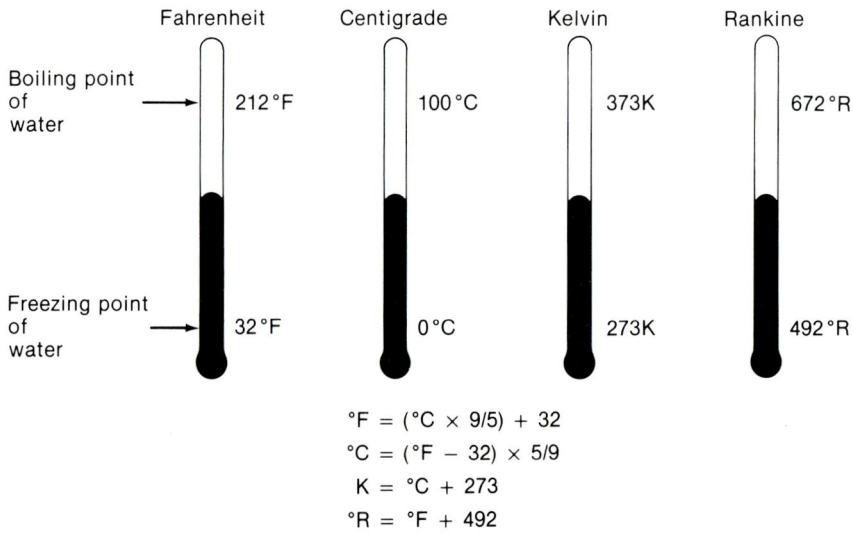

FIGURE 1–11. Four temperature scales.

tions as well as measurements of arterial blood gases.

Avogadro's Law

It can be shown empirically that equal volumes of gases at constant temperatures and pressures contain the same number of molecules. Amedeo Avogadro determined that for one gram molecular weight (or mol) of any gas, the volume occupied by the gas at 0°C and 1 atmosphere of pressure is 22.4 liters. The number of molecules in this mol volume was later shown to be equal to 6.02×10^{23} molecules, and subsequently called *Avogadro's number*. For example, one mol of nitrogen (or 28 g) occupies a volume of 22.4 liters and contains 6.02×10^{23} molecules when measured at 0°C (273 K) and 1 atmosphere.

Avogadro's law is used to calculate the density or mass of a gas per unit volume:

$$\frac{\text{molecular weight of gas}}{22.4 \text{ liters}} = \text{density in grams per liter}$$

Note that the equation can also be used to convert gas quantities expressed as mols (n) and volumes.

The *specific gravity* of a gas is defined as the ratio of a unit weight per volume of one gas to a comparable weight per volume of a standard gas, such as air. The specific gravities for several gases used in respiratory care and anesthesia are shown in Figure 1–12.

Ideal Gas Equation

The various gas laws discussed so far can be summarized as:

Boyle's law: $P \propto 1/V$ (at a constant n and T)
Charles' law: $V \propto T$ (at a constant n and P)
Gay-Lussac's law: $P \propto T$ (at a constant n and V)
Avogadro's law: $V \propto n$ (at a constant P and T)

If we combine these four equations to form a single equation:

$$V \propto nT/P$$

$$V = R\,nt/P$$

or

$$PV = nRT$$

where *n* equals the number of mols of gas present, R is a proportionality constant, called the gas constant (R is equal to 0.082 L atm/mol K), and T is the gas temperature in kelvins. The equation $PV = nRT$ describes the relationship among P, V, T, and n, and it is referred to as the *ideal gas equation*. As noted earlier, an ideal gas is a hypothetical gas whose pressure-volume-temperature behavior can be accounted for by the gas laws discussed. The molecules of an ideal gas do not attract or

FIGURE 1–12. Specific gravities for several gases that are used in respiratory care and anesthesia. The comparisons have been made with air at 25°C and 760 torr. (From Adriani, J.: *The Chemistry and Physics of Anesthesia*, 3rd ed. Springfield, IL, Charles C Thomas, 1979, with permission.)

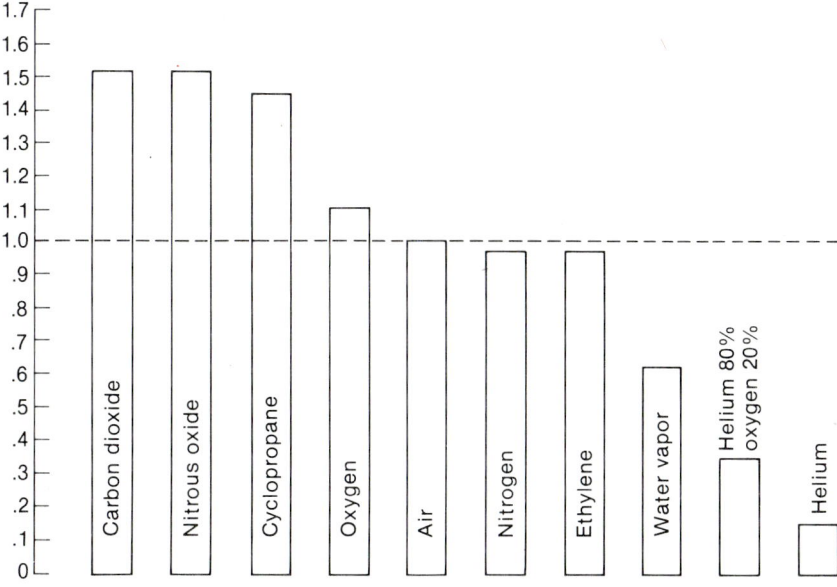

BASIC PHYSICS AND CHEMISTRY

repel each other, and their volume is negligible compared to the volume of the container. The behavior of real gases deviates from the gas laws in at least two ways: (1) when cooled, real gases liquefy and finally solidify because the molecules of the gas attract each other, and (2) at very high pressures, gas molecules of real gases cannot be compressed because the constituent molecules are pushed close together and resist compression.

Remember, however, that although there is no such thing as an ideal gas, the ideal gas equation can be safely applied to most real gases.

Laws of Diffusion

So far, we have discussed the behavior of gases in terms of their ability to expand and to be compressed. The third property that must be included in this analysis of the behavior of gases is *diffusibility*. Graham's, Henry's, and Fick's laws can describe this property of gases.

Graham's Law

According to the kinetic theory, when a gas is introduced into a container, its molecules distribute themselves evenly throughout the space provided. The net movement of gas molecules from an area of high concentration to an area of low concentration is called *diffusion*.

In 1832, Thomas Graham, a Scottish chemist, found that under the same conditions of temperature and pressure, the rates of diffusion of two gaseous substances are inversely proportional to the square root of their masses, or

$$r_1/r_2 = \sqrt{M_1/M_2}$$

where r_1 and r_2 represent diffusion rates, M_1 and M_2 are molar masses

If we consider that the mass of a gas is directly proportional to its density at a constant temperature and pressure, then

$$r_1/r_2 = \sqrt{d_1/d_2}$$

where d_1 and d_2 are the densities of the gases in question.

Henry's Law

When a gas is confined in a space adjacent to a liquid, a certain number of gas molecules dissolve in the liquid phase. William Henry found that at a specified temperature, the mass of a gas that dissolves in a given volume of liquid (with which it does not combine chemically) is directly proportional to the product of its partial pressure and its solubility coefficient. Thus, Henry's law may be stated as:

$$c \propto P \times S$$

where c is the molar concentration (in mol/L) of dissolved gas, P is the pressure (in atm) of gas over the liquid, and S is the solubility coefficient for the gas in that particular liquid (in L/atm or L/mmHg).

Note that the solubility of a gas in a particular liquid is equal to that volume of a gas, in liters, that will saturate 1 L of liquid at specified temperature and standard pressure (0°C, 1 atm of pressure). In respiratory physiology, we are primarily concerned with the solubility of oxygen and carbon dioxide in plasma at 37°C and atmospheric pressure (1 atm or 760 mmHg). Thus, oxygen has a solubility coefficient of 0.023 liter per liter of plasma (37°C, 1 atm) and that of carbon dioxide is 0.510 liter per liter of plasma (37°C, 1 atm).

Fick's Law

In the two preceding sections, the diffusion rate of a gas into another gas proved to be inversely proportional to the square root of its molecular weight (Graham's law), whereas the amount of a gas that dissolves in a liquid is directly related to its solubility coefficient and the partial pressure of the gas (Henry's law).

Throughout this book, we will be concerned with the diffusion of oxygen and carbon dioxide into and out of the respiratory and cardiovascular systems. Because biological systems contain semipermeable membranes (i.e., membranes not freely permeable to all components of a mixture), we must include this membrane factor when describing the movement of gases in biological systems ($\dot{V}$gas). Thus, Fick's law states that the flow of gas (per unit of time) into a membrane-bound fluid phase is directly proportional to the surface area available for diffusion, the partial pressure gradient between the two compartments, and the solubility of the gas. It is inversely proportional to the square root of the molecular weight of the gas and the thickness of the membrane. Fick's law may therefore be symbolized as:

$$\dot{V}\text{gas} \propto \frac{A \times S \times \Delta P}{\sqrt{M} \times T}$$

where A = surface area of the membrane
       S = solubility
       ΔP = partial pressure gradient across a semipermeable membrane
       M = molecular weight of the gas
       T = Thickness of the membrane.

Because the diffusivity of a gas equals its solubility divided by the square root of its molecular weight, or

$$D \propto S/\sqrt{M}$$

where D = diffusivity,
       S = solubility,
       M = molecular weight of the gas,

then Fick's law (Fig. 1–13) may be restated as:

$$\dot{V}_{gas} \propto \frac{A \times D \times \Delta P}{T}$$

This principle of diffusion will be discussed in more detail to explain cardiopulmonary physiology and pathology.

PROPERTIES OF LIQUIDS AND SOLIDS

Liquid mixtures may be divided into four types: solutions, suspensions, colloids, and emulsions. Although each of these has its own specific characteristics and uses, several properties are common to all liquids:

1. Molecules of liquids demonstrate a greater degree of intermolecular attraction than do the molecules of gases, and this greater attractiveness increases the tendency of liquids to coalesce and form clusters that settle at the bottom of a container.

2. Because liquids do not have an inherent shape, they assume the shape of the vessel in which they are placed.

3. The compressibility of liquids (as compared with that of gases) is negligible because of the decreased distance between molecules.

4. When placed in an open container, some of the liquid molecules leave the liquid phase to enter the gas phase above the liquid. This process of *evaporation* results from some of the liquid molecules achieving sufficient kinetic energy to overcome the attractive forces present in the liquid. (If heat is added to the liquid, the kinetic energy of the liquid increases, and more molecules enter the gas phase.)

5. If a liquid is placed in a closed container, molecules leaving the liquid phase to enter the gas phase reach an equilibrium with molecules of vapor reentering the liquid phase. This point is called the *vapor pressure*. Each liquid has a particular vapor pressure associated with a given temperature. Table 1–3 lists the vapor pressure-temperature relationships for water.

6. When the temperature of a liquid reaches the point at which the liquid's vapor pressure equals the total pressure of the gas phase above the liquid, the liquid boils. This temperature is therefore called the *boiling point* of a liquid. For water at 1 atmosphere of ambient pressure, the boiling point is 100°C. Decreasing the ambient pressure lowers the boiling point, whereas increasing the pressure raises the boiling point. Thus, at high altitudes (where the ambient pressure is decreased), water boils at a temperature well below 100°C; on the other hand, increasing the ambient pressure (as in a pressure cooker or autoclave) raises the boiling point.

Types of Liquid Mixtures

All liquid mixtures may be categorized into four types: *solutions, suspensions, colloids,* and *emulsions*.

Solutions may be defined as homogeneous mixtures of two or more substances. The liquid substance, which is in a higher proportion than any other constituent, is called the *solvent*. For aqueous solutions, water is the solvent. Those components remaining in the mixture are called *solutes*, and they are considered to be dissolved

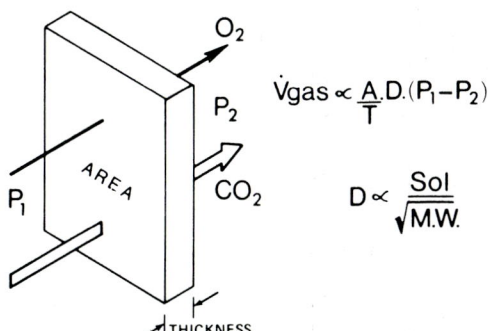

FIGURE 1–13. Fick's law of diffusion. (From West, J.B.: *Respiratory Physiology, The Essentials*. 3rd ed. Baltimore, Williams and Wilkins, 1985, p. 24, with permission.)

18 BASIC PHYSICS AND CHEMISTRY

TABLE 1–3. Temperature–Vapor Pressure Relationships for Water

Degrees Celsius	Vapor Pressure (mmHg)
0	4.58
10	9.21
11	9.84
12	10.52
13	11.23
14	11.99
15	12.79
16	13.63
17	14.53
18	15.48
19	16.48
20	17.54
21	18.65
22	19.83
23	21.07
24	22.38
25	23.76
26	25.21
27	26.74
28	28.35
29	30.04
30	31.82
31	33.70
32	35.66
33	37.73
34	39.90
35	42.18
36	44.56
37	47.07
38	49.70
39	52.44
40	55.32

in the solvent. The solubility of any material in a solvent depends on the nature of the molecules of the solute and solvent and on the temperature and pressure of the solution.

Suspensions are formed when insoluble particles are dispersed within a liquid. These mixtures are therefore heterogeneous in composition and appear opaque.

Colloids are similar to suspensions in that they contain particles dispersed in a liquid phase. However, colloid particles are much smaller than those in suspensions and thus offer a greater surface area. This increased surface area allows colloids to absorb other particles and thus serve both in a transport and storage capacity. When charged particles such as cations and anions are absorbed by colloids, the resulting colloids are considered to be electrically charged. Note that colloid suspensions include *gels* (characterized by a strong attraction between suspended particles and the liquid phase, e.g., gelatin in water, and are therefore semisolid) and *sols* (which have little attraction between the colloid particles and the liquid phase, e.g., starch in water, and therefore remain as liquids). Gels are considered to be *hydrophilic* (water-loving) and sols are said to be *hydrophobic* (water-hating) colloids.

Emulsions constitute the fourth group of liquid mixtures. They are formed when two immiscible liquids, such as oil and water, are mixed together. The oil forms droplets that appear to be suspended in the water. Depending on the stability of the droplets that are formed, emulsions may be classified as temporary or permanent.

Osmosis

Ordinarily, when a solute is placed in a liquid solvent, the solute molecules disperse throughout the solution so that the overall concentration of the solution is uniform. However, if two vessels containing different concentrations of solute molecules are separated by a membrane that is permeable only to the solvent particles and not to those of the solute (i.e., a semipermeable membrane), a new equilibrium volume for each vessel is established (Fig. 1–14). This process results from solvent molecules moving from the side with the lower concentration of solute to the side with the higher concentration of solute and is called *osmosis*. Note that the movement of solvent stops when the concentrations of the solutions in vessels A and B are nearly equal. (The movement of solvent across the membrane stops when the attractive force of the solute for the solvent is balanced by the hydrostatic pressure difference between the two vessels. The hydrostatic pressure gradient is increased owing to the increased weight of the column of solvent in vessel B compared with that of vessel A.) The pressure that holds back any further movement of solvent is called *osmotic pressure*.

Osmosis and osmotic pressure are critical in the maintenance of biological viability. We will consider phenomena that pertain to osmosis at various points in this book.

Ions and Electrolytes

In the previous section, we assumed that solute molecules retain their identity when dissolved in the liquid. There are, however, many solutions that are formed by the dissociation, or breaking apart, of solute molecules in a solvent. These dissociated particles usually carry an electrical

FIGURE 1–14. Osmotic pressure: *1*, The level of pure solvent is equal on both sides of the semipermeable membrane. *2*, During osmosis, the level of solvent on the right side of the semipermeable membrane rises as a result of the net flow of solvent from left to right. (o = solute.)

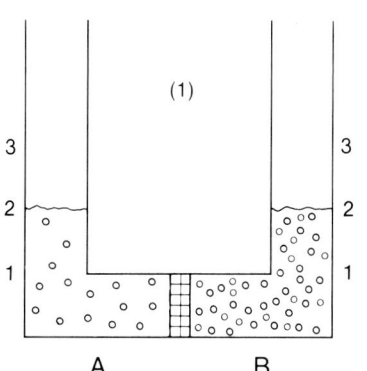
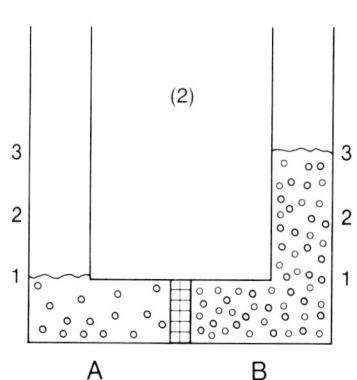

charge and are referred to as ions. Because these ions have an electric charge when they are placed in a liquid solution, they can conduct an electric current that can be measured by means of an ammeter (Fig. 1–15).

Solutions having this property of electrical conductivity are called *electrolytes*; solutions that do not form ions and cannot therefore carry an electric charge are referred to as *nonelectrolytes*.

Because the electrical conductivity of a solution is related to the number of ions present, electrolyte solutions can be characterized as strong or weak electrolytes, depending on the degree of dissociation that the solute undergoes. Table 1–4 lists several examples of each type of electrolyte solution.

Arrhenius summarized the behavior of electrolytes in solution by means of the *ionic theory*. This theory states:

1. When an electrolyte is dissolved in water, it dissociates into a fixed number of submolecular electrically charged particles called ions. The unit charge that an ion carries is called its valence (see the section on valence electrons).

2. If the original electrolyte is neutral, then it is considered to have a net charge of zero, and it dissociates into an equal number of positively and negatively charged ions.

3. When an electric charge is passed through an electrolyte solution, the positive ions, called cations, move toward the negative electrode (i.e., *cathode*) and negatively charged ions, called anions, move toward the positive electrode (i.e., *anode*).

4. Each ion in an electrolyte solution acts independently to affect the physical properties of the solution. The activity of each ion is equivalent to the activity of an uncharged (neutral) particle, so that if an electrolyte dissociates into two discrete particles (i.e., one positive and one negative, $NaCl \rightarrow Na^+ + Cl^-$), some of the properties of the solution, such as osmotic pressure, are affected twice as much as would be predicted from its molar concentration.

5. The extent of dissociation of an electrolyte in a solvent is influenced by the concentration of the electrolyte in the solution. For dilute aqueous solutions, a large number of water molecules are present compared with the number of solute molecules, and therefore, they can function to separate most of the constituent charges of the electrolyte on ionization. Conversely, in more concentrated solutions, the number of water molecules is closer to the number of solute molecules, and ionization is limited. (The ionic theory, there-

FIGURE 1–15. An ammeter.

TABLE 1–4. Strong Versus Weak Electrolytes

Strong ↑ A c i d s ↓ Weak		Weak ↑ B a s e s ↓ Strong
	HCl	Cl^-
	H_2SO_4	HSO_4^-
	HSO_4^-	$SO_4^=$
	$C_2H_3O_2^-H$	$C_2H_3O_2^-$
	H_2CO_3	HCO_3^-
	H_3O^+	OH^-

fore, can be used to explain the behavior of electrolytes in dilute solutions reasonably well; it does not, however, explain the behavior of electrolytes in concentrated solutions.)

Acids, Bases, and Salts

When discussing electrolyte solutions, we assume that only the solute dissociates into charged particles to conduct an electric current. For the purpose of explaining the properties of electrolytes, this is acceptable; however, it must be kept in mind that the solvent may also dissociate. In aqueous solutions, the electrolytic dissociation of water results in the formation of positive hydrogen ions (H^+, or protons) and negatively charged hydroxyl ions (OH^-). For pure water, the amount of hydrogen ions present after complete dissociation is 1×10^{-7} mol/L, or

$$H_2O \rightarrow H^+ + OH^-$$

Therefore, an equilibrium exists between the positively charged hydrogen ion concentration and the negatively charged hydroxyl ion concentration in pure water.

When certain substances are added to water, they can alter this equilibrium (i.e., increase the concentration of one species more than that of the other). For the purposes of this book, those substances that increase the concentration of hydrogen ions are called *acids*, and those that increase the concentration of negatively charged ions are called *bases*. This can be expressed more formally in the *Brönsted-Lowry* definition of acids and bases, which states that acids are substances that donate protons (H^+) and that bases are substances that accept protons.

pH

Because calculations involving concentrations such as 1×10^{-7} molar are cumbersome, Sorensen in 1909 introduced an abbreviated expression that he termed pH (for *power of hydrogen*). This value is equivalent to the negative logarithm to base 10 of the hydrogen ion concentration, or

$$pH = -\log [H^+]$$

Table 1–5 shows a comparison of hydrogen ion concentrations and their corresponding pH's. Note that metric prefixes may be substituted in place of scientific notation for another expression

TABLE 1–5. Relationship Between Hydrogen Ion Concentration and pH

Hydrogen Ion Concentration (nanomoles/L)	pH
1000	6.0
100	7.0
40	7.4
25	7.6
16	7.8
10	8.0
1	9.0

of hydrogen ion concentration (e.g., 1×10^{-3} M = 1 millimolar).

Quantification of Solutions

Besides expressing hydrogen ion concentration, solutions may be quantified in other ways. Table 1–6 lists several of the more commonly used conventions for expressing the activity of solute and solvent molecules in solutions.

Dilution Methods

Probably one of the most misunderstood calculations involving solutions is that for determining dilution. If we assume that the amount of solute in a solution remains constant, then increasing the amount of solvent in the solution will decrease the concentration of the solute:

$$\underset{\substack{\text{initial} \\ \text{volume} \\ \text{of solution}}}{V_1} \times \underset{\substack{\text{initial} \\ \text{concentration} \\ \text{of solute}}}{C_1} = \underset{\substack{\text{new} \\ \text{volume} \\ \text{of solution}}}{V_2} \times \underset{\substack{\text{new} \\ \text{concentration} \\ \text{of solute}}}{C_2}$$

In other words, because the concentration of solute (e.g., in mg/ml or g/L) times the volume of the solution (e.g., in ml or L) is equal to the total amount of solute in the solution (e.g., in mg or g), adding additional solvent decreases the concentration of the solute and increases the volume of the solution, but it doesn't change the total amount of solute.

Therefore, if the concentration of a given volume of solution is changed by the addition of more

BASIC PHYSICS AND CHEMISTRY

TABLE 1–6. Quantification of Solutions

Mole fraction

Mole fraction (XA) of component A of a solution is the ratio of the number of moles of A in the solution (nA) to the sum of the number of moles of all components of the solution.

$$XA = \frac{nA}{nA + nB + nC + \ldots}$$

Percentage by mass and volume

The percentage by mass of a solute to the mass of solution. The percentage by volume of a solute to the volume of solution.

$$\text{mass \%} = \frac{\text{mass of solute}}{\text{mass of solution}} \times 100$$

$$\text{volume \%} = \frac{\text{volume of solute}}{\text{volume of solution}} \times 100$$

Molarity

Molarity (M) of a solution is the number of moles (gram molecular weights) of solute per liter of solution.

$$M = \frac{\text{moles of solute}}{\text{liter of solution}}$$

Molality

Molality (m) of a solution is the number of moles of solute per kilogram of solvent.

$$m = \frac{\text{moles of solute}}{\text{kilograms of solvent}}$$

Normality

Normality (N) of a solution is the concentration of the solution expressed as equivalents per liter, where for example, one equivalent of acid generates one mol of hydrogen ions; one equivalent of base generates one mol of hydroxyl ions.

$$N = \frac{\text{equivalents}}{\text{liter of solution}}$$

Adapted from Goldwhite, H, and Spielman, J.: *College Chemistry*. San Diego, Harcourt Brace Jovanovich, 1984.

(liquid) solvent, then the new concentration can be calculated using this formula:

$$C_2 = V_1 C_1 / V_2$$

CHEMICAL REACTIONS

An understanding of the relationship between matter and energy is essential in discussions of biological processes. In a chemical reaction, the mass and energy of the substances undergoing change (reactants) equals the mass and energy of the products of the reaction. Restated as an equation, the expression reads:

$$\text{matter} + \text{energy} = \text{matter} + \text{energy}$$
$$\text{(reactants)} \qquad \text{(products)}$$

This relationship is known as the law of conservation of mass and energy, and it is the foundation of our understanding of chemical reactions.

Types of Chemical Reactions

All chemical reactions may be classified into four types: combination, decomposition, single displacement, and double displacement reactions (Table 1–7).

The study of chemical dynamics involves the characterization of rates and mechanisms of chemical reactions. Because of space limitations, our discussion is confined to those factors that influence the rates of reactions. We will not discuss reaction mechanisms. Information on reaction mechanisms can be found in several of the references listed at the end of this chapter.

Factors Influencing the Rates of Chemical Reactions

The rate of any chemical reaction is primarily influenced by four factors: (1) the nature of the re-

TABLE 1–7. Types of Chemical Reactions

Combination

Two or more substances combine to form a more complex substance:

$$Cu + Cl_2 \longrightarrow CuCl_2$$

Decomposition

A substance is broken down into two or more substances:

$$2KClO_3 + \text{Heat} \longrightarrow 2KCl + 3O_2$$

Single Displacement

An element replaces another element in a compound:

$$Mg + CuSO_4 \longrightarrow MgSO_4 + Cu$$

Double Displacement

Metal atoms or ions of two compounds exchange places:

$$NaCl + AgNO_3 \longrightarrow AgCl + NaNO_3$$

actions, (2) the concentration of the reactants, (3) the temperature at which the reaction is occurring, and (4) whether the reaction is mediated by a catalyst. We can qualitatively describe the influence of these four variables using the collision theory of chemical reactions.

According to this theory, the rate of a chemical reaction depends on the number of collisions occurring per second between reacting species and on the fraction of these collisions that are effective.

Because reactions differ as to the amount of energy that must be expended to allow two species to combine (i.e., the energy of activation of a reaction), we can say that the chemical nature of the reacting particles can influence the rate of reaction.

The concentration of reactants can affect the reaction rate because as the number of reactants is increased, the number of molecular collisions also increases (*law of mass action*).

Increasing the temperature at which a reaction is occurring increases the collision rate by increasing the average kinetic energy of the reactants. This kinetic energy increase causes reactant molecules to move faster and collide more frequently and more forcefully.

Catalysis is defined as a chemical reaction that is augmented by the addition of one or more agents (catalysts) that increase the number of effective collisions during a specified period. These catalysts are not used up during a chemical reaction but rather serve to help initiate or speed up the reactions that they affect. In biological systems, these catalysts are called *enzymes,* which are discussed in more detail later in this chapter.

Chemical Equilibria and the Law of Mass Action

We have stated that in a chemical reaction reactants are converted to products during a given period. If we look closely, however, we can see that in most reactions the concentration of reactants decreases to a point and then levels off before the reactants are completely utilized. The point at which the concentration of reactants, and therefore the products, do not change dramatically is referred to as a state of chemical equilibrium and may be symbolized as

$$A + B \rightleftharpoons C + D$$

Note that this state is achieved when products are converted to reactants at a rate that is comparable to the conversion of reactants to products. For a reaction involving w mols of A and x mols of B to produce y and z mols of C and D, respectively, the equilibrium state can be expressed as a ratio of products to reactants. Or, if:

$$wA + xB \rightleftharpoons yC + zD$$

then:

$$\frac{[C]^y[D]^z}{[A]^w[B]^x} = K$$

This fraction is called the *mass action equation*, and K is referred to as the equilibrium constant for the reaction. In the mass action equation, brackets are placed around the reactants and products to designate their concentrations in mols per liter. The number of mols of each species present (i.e., w, x, y, and z) represent the power to which each of these concentrations must be raised.

It should be evident that by quantifying the concentration of reactants and products and comparing them to the experimentally derived equilibrium constant, we can determine the probability that a reaction will occur in a particular direction. That is, if the actual ratio is greater than the K determined for a reaction, then the conversion of reactants to products is favored. Conversely, if the ratio is less than K, then the reaction of products to form reactants is favored.

The importance of chemical equilibria will become more obvious when we examine biological processes involving energy production and utilization as well as acid-base balance.

BIOCHEMICAL PROCESSES

Biochemistry can be simply defined as the chemistry of living organisms. More specifically, it can be defined as the study of the structure and composition of biologically active molecules and the reactions that these compounds undergo.

Of the 105 chemical elements that have been identified, only 11 elements are found in appreciable quantities within the human body and in most other organisms that have been studied (Table 1–8). Carbon, hydrogen, and oxygen are present in all of the compounds found in living organisms. Nitrogen, phosphorus, and sulfur are present in smaller quantities in living organisms but they play a major role in many biochemical processes. Sodium, potassium, calcium, and magnesium, often referred to as the *mineral elements*, are usually found either as ions or simple inorganic compounds.

BASIC PHYSICS AND CHEMISTRY

TABLE 1–8. Essential Elements in the Body

Symbol	Element
Major elements: 99.3% total atoms	
H (63%)	Hydrogen
O (26%)	Oxygen
C (9%)	Carbon
N (1%)	Nitrogen
Major minerals: 0.7% total atoms	
Ca	Calcium
P	Phosphorus
K	Potassium
S	Sulfur
Na	Sodium
Cl	Chlorine
Mg	Magnesium
Trace elements: less than 0.01% total atoms	
Fe	Iron
I	Iodine
Cu	Copper
Zn	Zinc
Mn	Manganese
Co	Cobalt
Cr	Chromium
Se	Selenium
Mo	Molybdenum
F	Fluorine
Sn	Tin
Si	Silicon
V	Vanadium

From Vander, A., Sherman, J., and Luciano, D.: *Human Physiology: The Mechanisms of Body Function*, 4th ed. New York, McGraw-Hill, 1985, with permission.

Water is by far the most abundant compound found in living organisms. In the human body, for example, it constitutes approximately 70% of the weight of muscles, 80% of the weight of blood, and 40% of the weight of bone. Its importance to biochemical processes can be summarized as follows:

1. Water is a chemical source of hydrogen and oxygen.
2. It is the medium in which materials are dispersed in the organization of protoplasm.
3. It is the medium in which soluble materials are absorbed from the environment.
4. It is the medium of transport of foods, minerals, and other vital substances in living systems.

In addition to water and mineral salts, there are four major types of compounds in the body: proteins, carbohydrates, lipids, and nucleic acids. These molecules not only make up the structure of the human body but also function in metabolism. *Metabolism* is used to describe the reactions that take place within the body. Metabolism is divided into *anabolism* or "building" reactions and *catabolism* or degradation reactions.

In the sections that follow, first the structure and composition of proteins, carbohydrates, lipids, and nucleic acids are discussed, followed by some of the major biochemical reactions that occur in the human body.

Proteins

The word *protein* is derived from the Greek word *prōtos*, which means of the first order of importance. This is an apt description of these molecules because they account for approximately 50% of the organic materials found in the human body and play a critical role in almost every physiologic process.

Proteins contain carbon, hydrogen, oxygen, nitrogen, and often sulfur. The elementary composition of proteins is very similar; approximate percentages for the various elements are C = 50%, H = 7%, O = 20%, and N = 16%. (Although these data provide little information about the structure of proteins, they do provide a useful method for determining the protein content of living matter and foodstuffs). Most proteins are very large molecules with molecular weights ranging from a few thousand to a million or more. Like most large molecules, proteins are formed by linking together a large number of small subunits. The basic subunit of proteins is the *amino acids*; thus, proteins are polymers of amino acids.

The general formula for naturally occurring amino acids may be represented as:

$$^+H_3N-\underset{\underset{R}{|}}{\overset{\overset{H}{|}}{C}}-COO^-$$

The proteins of living organisms are composed of 20 different amino acids. As Figure 1–16 shows, amino acids can be distinguished by the *R* side chains attached to a central carbon atom. Note that the side chains may be either nonpolar or polar.

In the formation of protein molecules, the carboxyl group of one amino acid is linked to the amino acid group of the next amino acid through a *peptide bond,* which is a type of bond that belongs to the general class of polar covalent bonds. The specific sequence of amino acids along a peptide chain constitutes the *primary* structure of the protein molecule. Higher levels of structure (i.e.,

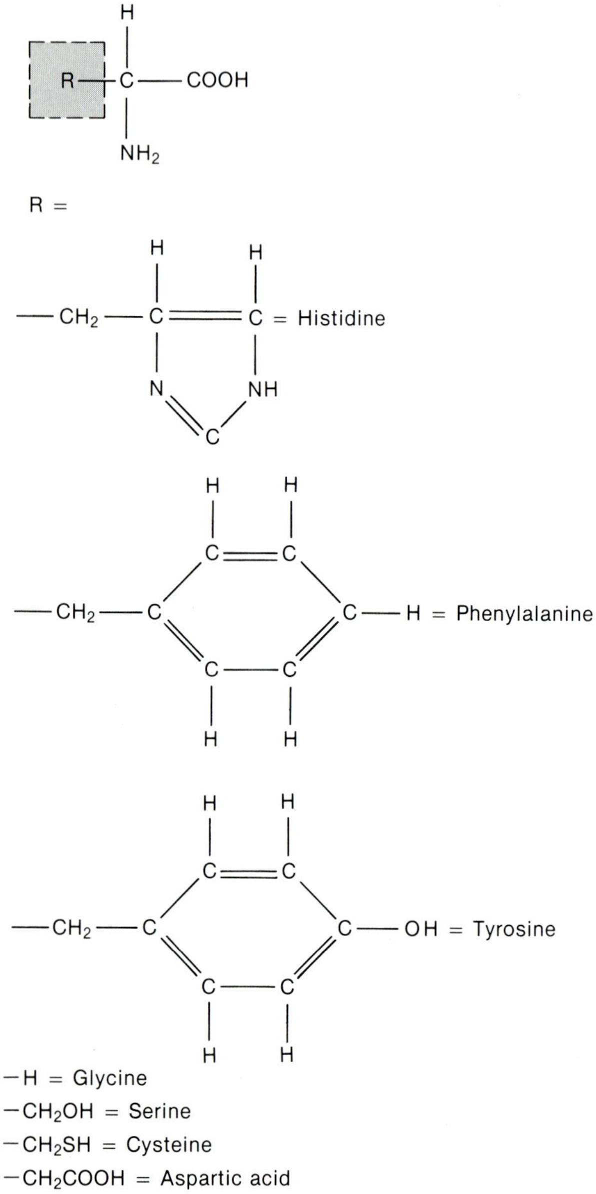

FIGURE 1-16. Structure of several common amino acids.

secondary, tertiary, and quaternary) relate to the extensive coiling and folding that occurs within and between protein molecules to give them a complex rigid structure. As Figure 1-17 shows, a variety of bonding forces contribute to the conformation of protein molecules.

Structurally, proteins are generally classified as *fibrous* or *globular*. *Fibrous* proteins are composed of individual, elongated, filamentous chains joined laterally by several types of cross-linkages to form a fairly stable, relatively insoluble structure. Typical examples include collagen and myosin. *Globular* proteins have an elliptical shape in which there is a considerable amount of folding of the long polypeptide chains. Biologically active molecules, such as hormones and antibodies, are common examples of globular proteins.

With regard to function, proteins can be grouped into at least seven categories: (1) structural proteins, (2) contractile proteins, (3) antibodies, (4) blood proteins, (5) hormones, (6) enzymes, and (7) nutrient proteins.

Carbohydrates

As their name implies, these compounds were originally thought to be "hydrates of carbon" because the ones first analyzed had the general formula $C_x(H_2O)_x$. However, as more information was reported, it became evident that the hydrogen and oxygen atoms of these molecules do not exhibit the properties of the water of hydration but rather are arranged in more complex organic functional groups, like aldehydes and ketones (Fig. 1-18). Biochemists now define carbohydrates as polyhydroxy aldehydes and ketones and their derivatives. Although carbohydrates constitute only 3% of the organic molecules found in the human body, they play a central role in the chemical reactions that provide cells with energy.

Carbohydrates may exist both as monomers and as polymers. The former types of molecules are called *monosaccharides* and the latter are referred to as *oligosaccharides* and *polysaccharides*. Monosaccharides contain a single chain of carbon atoms that can number between three and seven atoms. They are named by using a prefix that designates the number of carbon atoms followed by the suffix *-ose* (i.e., trioses contain three carbons, tetroses contain four carbons, pentoses contain five carbons, hexoses contain six carbons, and heptoses contain seven carbons). Monosaccharides that contain an aldehyde group are called *aldoses*, whereas those that contain a ketone group are called *ketoses*. In general, monosaccharides are crystalline solids that are sweet-tasting and readily soluble in water. The most important monosaccharide is glucose, a six-carbon molecule ($C_6H_{12}O_6$) often called "blood sugar."

Oligosaccharides and polysaccharides are carbohydrates that contain a variable number of monosaccharide subunits linked together through glycosidic bonds (Fig. 1-19). Oligosaccharides contain between two and 10 subunits linked together and therefore represent the simplest poly-

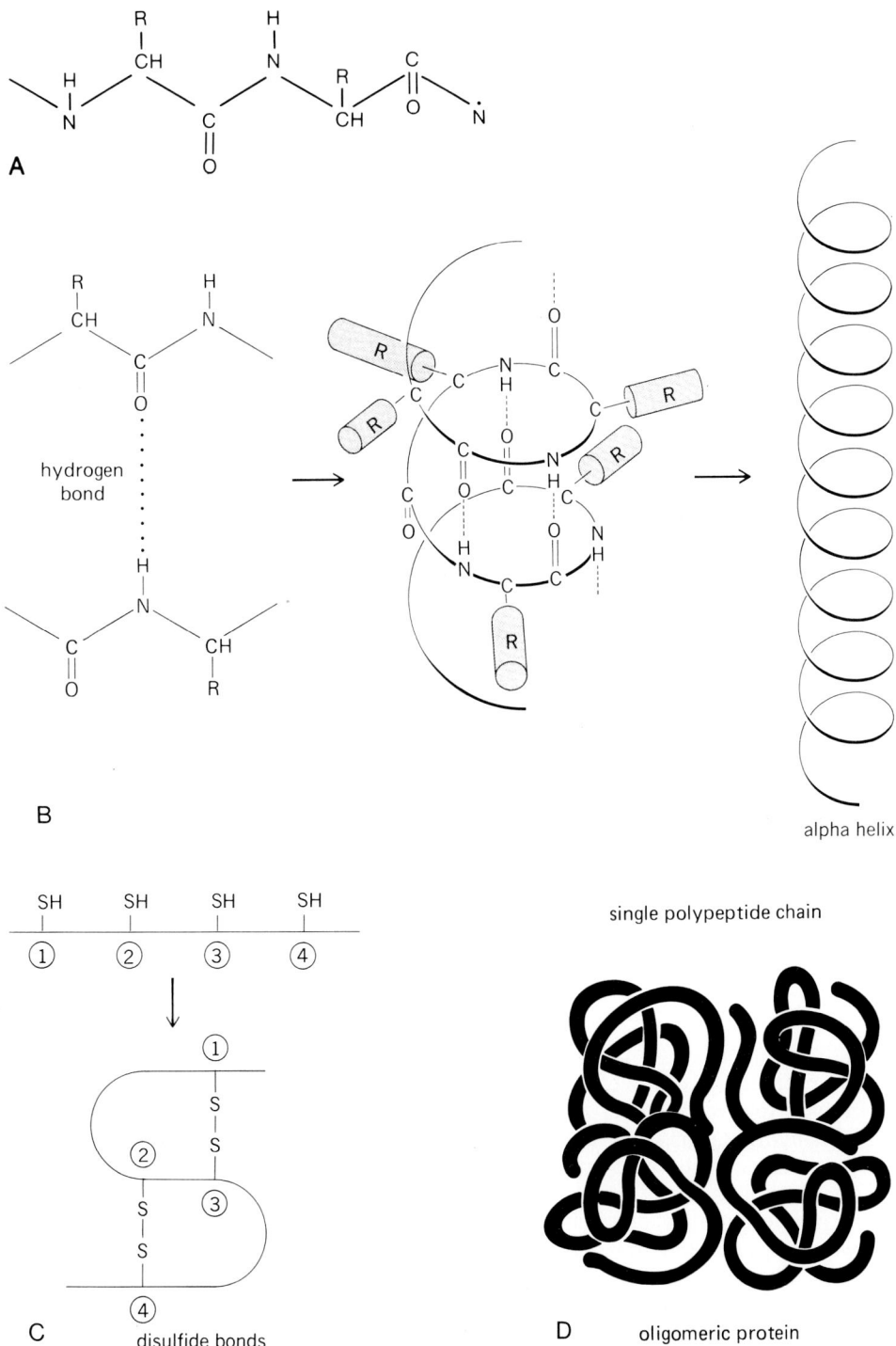

FIGURE 1–17. Structure of proteins. Proteins consist of a hierarchy of structure. *A, Primary structure* relates to the linear sequence of amino acids held together by *peptide bonds*. *B, Secondary structure* results from hydrogen bonds between amino acids forming regions of alpha-helical and random coil configurations. *C,* Additional bonds due to Van der Waal forces, disulfide linkages, and interaction between the protein molecule and surrounding water molecules constitute the *tertiary structure*. *D,* In proteins containing more than one polypeptide chain (i.e., oligomeric proteins), the fourth level or *quaternary structure* of proteins results when one or more chains are linked together. (Adapted with permission from Vander, A., Sherman, J., and Luciano, D.: *Human Physiology: The Mechanisms of Body Function,* 4th ed. New York, McGraw-Hill, 1985.)

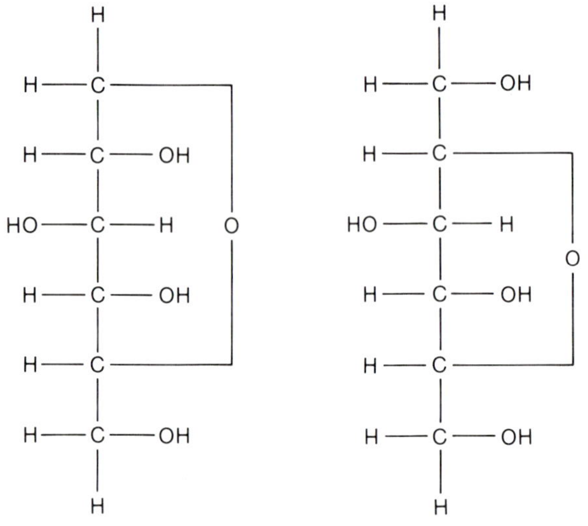

FIGURE 1–18. Examples of an aldose (glucose) and a ketose (fructose).

mers of carbohydrates, whereas polysaccharides are more complex molecules containing more than 10 monomers. Disaccharides, such as sucrose, lactose, and maltose, are the most common oligosaccharides, whereas starch and glycogen are the most important polysaccharides within biological systems (Fig. 1–20). Oligosaccharides are crystalline solids that are soluble in water, whereas polysaccharides generally are noncrystalline solids that are only slightly soluble in water.

Lipids

Lipids are a heterogeneous class of compounds that account for approximately 40% of the organic matter of the body. They are characterized as nonpolar hydrophobic hydrocarbons that have limited solubility in water and considerable solubility in organic solvents, such as alcohol, ether, or chloroform. Lipids are traditionally classified as *triglycerides, phospholipids,* and *steroids.* Other compounds that may be listed among lipids include the *carotenoids* and *vitamins A, D, E,* and *K.*

Triglycerides make up the majority of lipids in the human body, and it is these molecules that are generally referred to as fat. As Figure 1–21 shows, triglycerides are formed by linking together two types of molecules, glycerol and fatty acids. Glycerol is a three-carbon sugar alcohol, and fatty acids are long-chain hydrocarbons (typically 16 or 18 carbons long) with a carboxylic acid group (i.e., $-COOH$) at one end. When all of the carbons in a fatty acid are joined by single bonds, the fatty acid is said to be saturated. If the fatty acid contains double bonds, it is called an *unsaturated* fatty acid (if the fatty acid contains more than one double bond, then the fatty acid is said to be *polyunsaturated*). In general, animal fats contain high proportions of saturated fatty acids, whereas vegetable fats contain more polyunsaturated fatty acids.

Phospholipids have structures similar to triglycerides except that the third hydroxyl group of the glycerol moiety in phospholipids is attached to a phosphate group rather than to a fatty acid, as occurs in triglycerides. As Figure 1–22 shows, a small polar or ionized nitrogen compound is usually attached to the phosphate group. Note that both the phosphate and the nitrogen groups are electrically charged. These charged groups give the phospholipid a polar end in addition to the nonpolar end provided by the glycerol moiety; these molecules are therefore called *amphipathic*. The term *amphipathic* simply means that when phospholipids are mixed with water, they become organized into micelles, with their polar groups directed to the outside of the molecule toward the water molecules (i.e., *hydrophilic,* or water-loving) and their nonpolar groups directed to the interior of the molecule away from the water molecules (i.e., *hydrophobic,* or water-hating). It is this amphipathic behavior that makes phospholipids useful as constituents of cell membranes because they can serve as barriers to the indiscriminate exchange of compounds with the extracellular fluid surrounding cells.

The steroids constitute a group of cyclic compounds that resemble the structure shown in Figure 1–23. Although polar groups can be attached to the basic ring structure, they are usually not present in a large enough quantity to make steroids water-soluble; therefore, steroids are considered to be nonpolar compounds that are soluble in organic solvents. Examples of steroids include cholesterol, bile acids, adrenal corticosteroids, and male and female sex hormones (testosterone and estrogen, respectively). We will discuss the role of steroids in cardiopulmonary function later in this book.

Nucleic Acids

Although these molecules constitute only a small fraction of the organic material in the body, nucleic

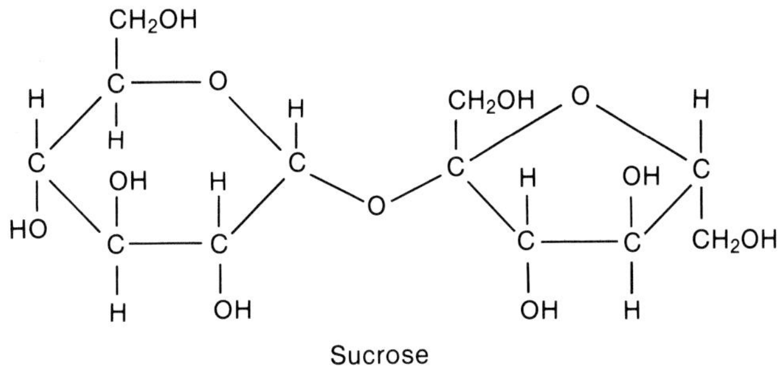

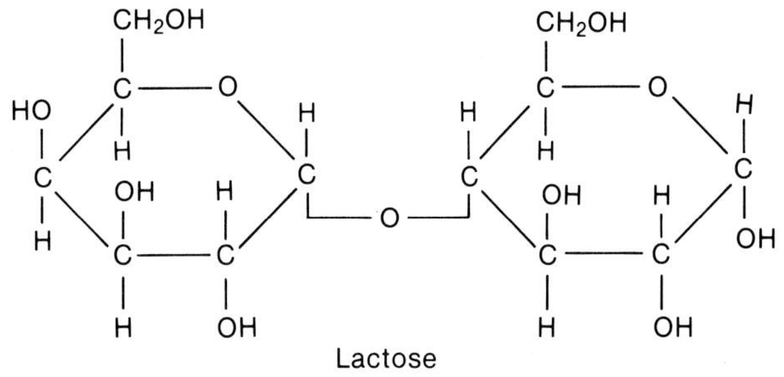

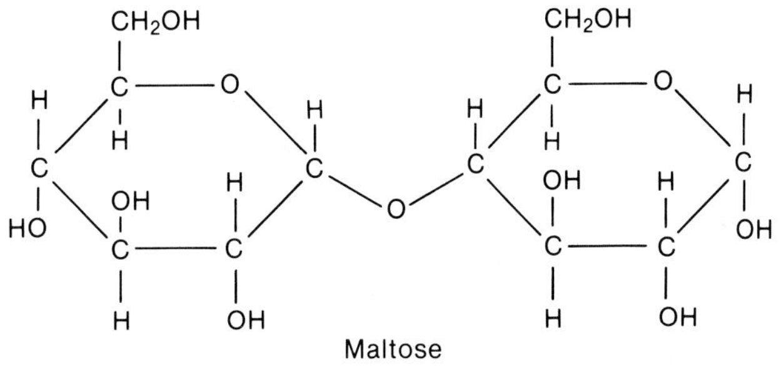

FIGURE 1–19. Common disaccharides. Note that two monosaccharides are joined by a glycosidic bond.

acids are essential to the maintenance of life because they are responsible for the storage of genetic information and its passage from cell to cell.

There are two types of nucleic acids: *deoxyribonucleic acid* (DNA) and *ribonucleic acid* (RNA). DNA molecules are responsible for storing genetic information in the form of repeating subunit structures, whereas RNA molecules are involved in the decoding of this information into instructions for linking together a specific sequence of amino acids required to synthesize a specific protein.

Both types of nucleic acids are polymers composed of a linear sequence of repeating subunits. Each subunit, which is known as a *nucleotide,* consists of a phosphate group, a sugar, and a hydrocarbon ring known as a base. The phosphate group is attached to the sugar moiety of the adjacent nucleotide to form a chain with the bases directed to the side of the phosphate-sugar backbone.

DNA contains the sugar deoxyribose and four different bases, which are usually grouped into two categories, *purines* or *pyrimidines*. As Figure 1–24 shows, the purine bases, which have two rings of carbon and nitrogen atoms linked together, include adenine and guanine. The pyrimidine bases have only one carbon-nitrogen ring and include thymine and cytosine.

The general structure of DNA is shown in Figure 1–25. Note that DNA consists of two chains of nucleotides coiled around each other in the form of a *double helix*. The formation of a double helical structure is possible because polar groups attached to the ring of a base on one chain form hydrogen bonds with polar groups attached to a base on a second chain. The location of the hydrogen bonds is such that adenine binds only with thymine and cytosine can bind only with guanine. Very simply stated, it is this specificity of base-pairing that provides the mechanism for duplicating and transferring genetic information.

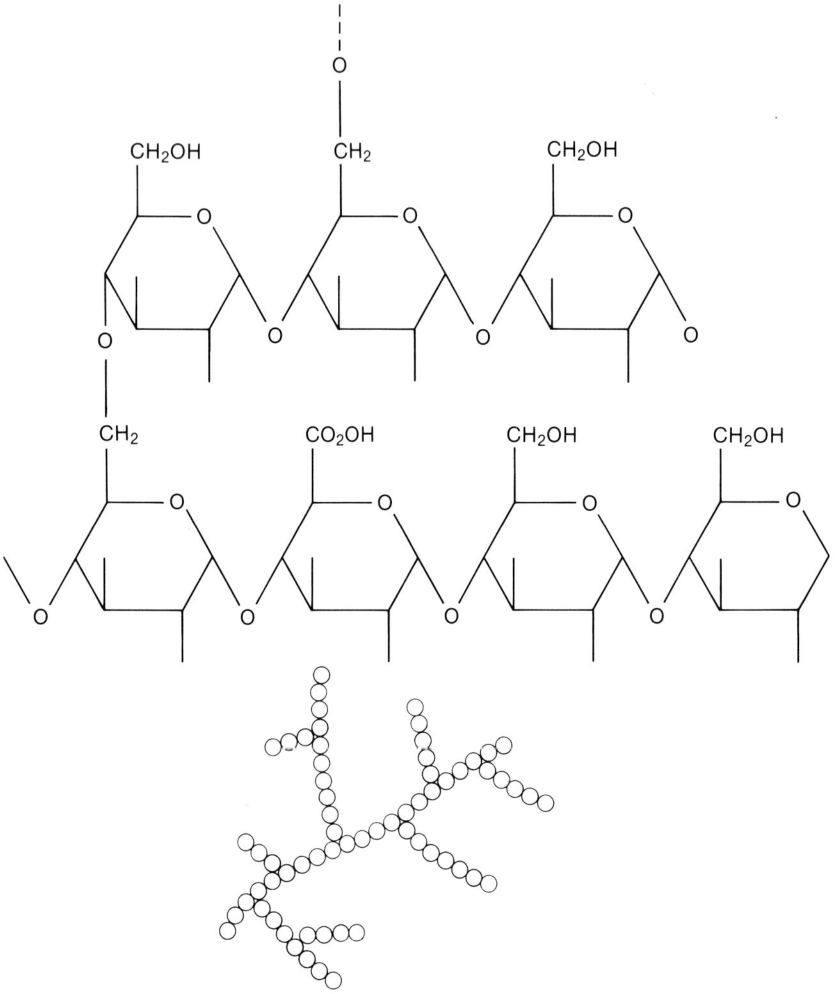

FIGURE 1-20. Structure of glycogen.

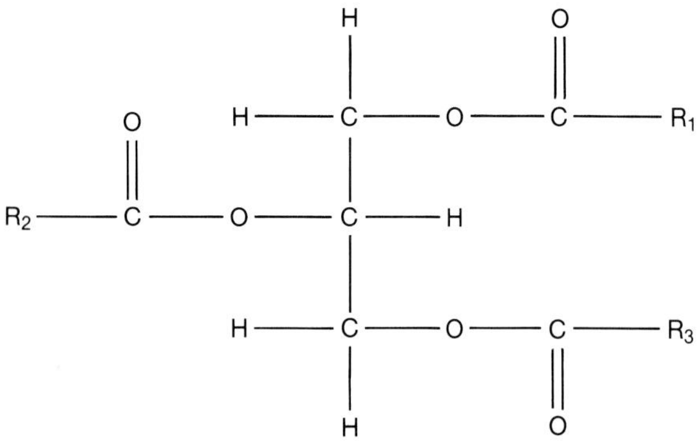

R_1, R_2, R_3 = Fatty acid residues

FIGURE 1-21. General structure of a triglyceride.

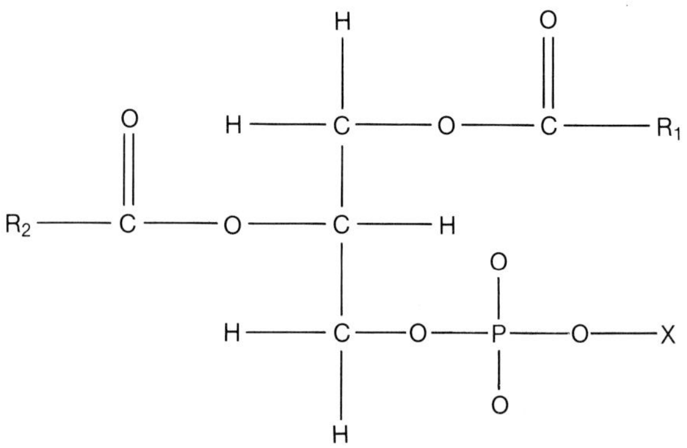

R = Fatty acid residues (hydrophobic)
X = Choline, inositol, etc. (hydrophilic)

FIGURE 1-22. General structure of a phospholipid.

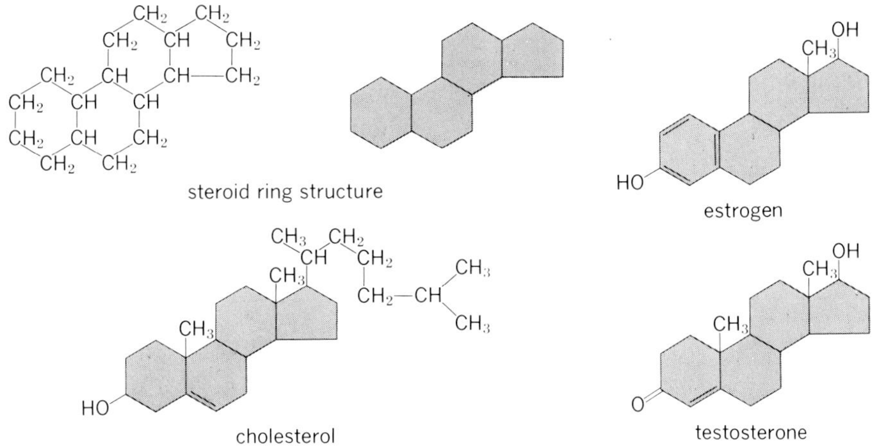

BASIC PHYSICS AND CHEMISTRY 29

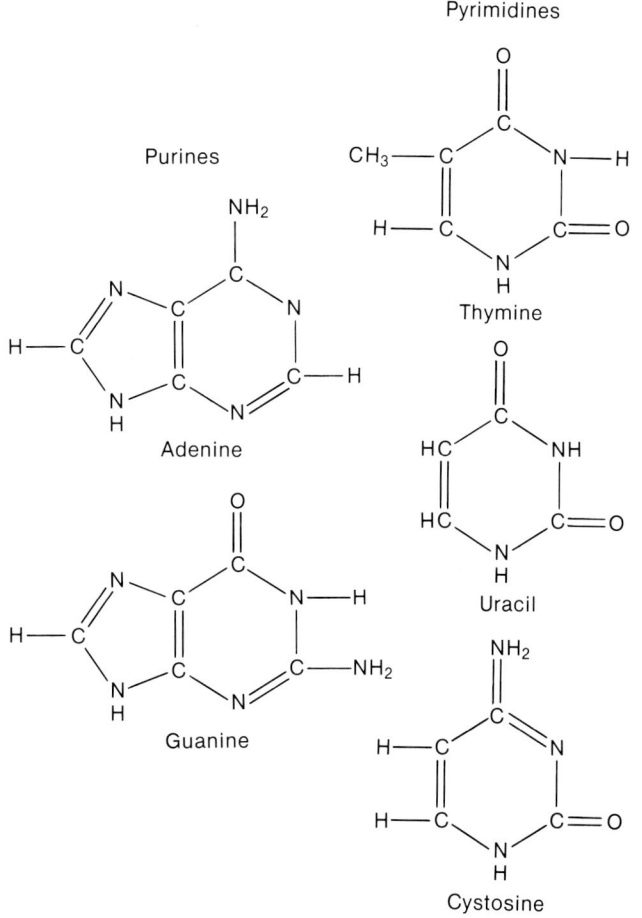

FIGURE 1–23. General structure of a steroid. (From Vander, A., Sherman, J., and Luciano, D.: *Human Physiology: The Mechanisms of Body Function,* 4th ed. New York, McGraw-Hill, 1985, with permission.)

FIGURE 1–24. Structures of purines and pyrimidines.

30 BASIC PHYSICS AND CHEMISTRY

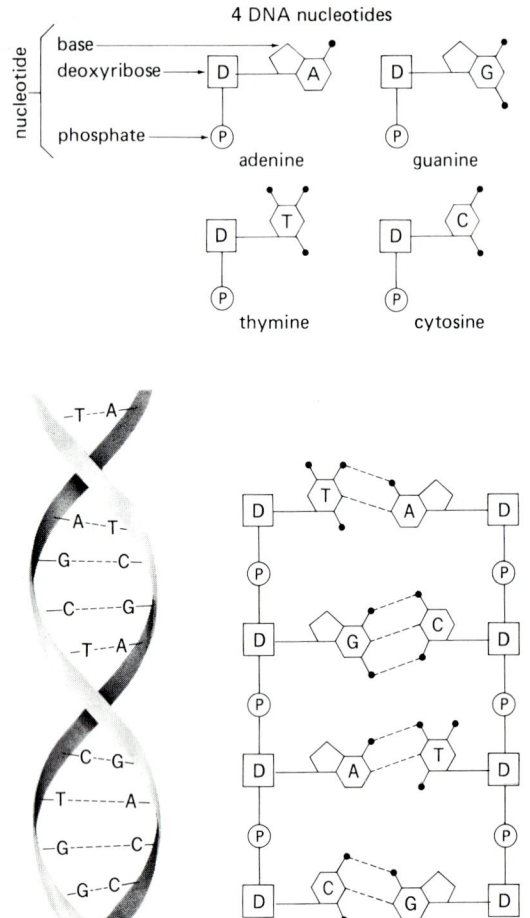

FIGURE 1-25. Deoxyribonucleic acid (DNA). (From Vander, A., Sherman, J., and Luciano, D.: *Human Physiology: The Mechanisms of Body Function*, 4th ed. New York, McGraw-Hill, 1985, with permission.)

The structure of RNA differs from that of DNA in several respects:
1. It contains the sugar ribose instead of deoxyribose.
2. The pyrimidine base thymine, which is present in DNA, is replaced by the base uracil.
3. RNA consists of a single chain of nucleotides rather than a double helix.

CELLULAR METABOLISM AND ENERGY PRODUCTION

So far, we have discussed only the structure and composition of the major biologically active compounds found in the human body. We now shift our attention to the breakdown of these compounds and the release of chemical energy. Carbohydrates, lipids, and proteins are the most important compounds involved in energy metabolism. Carbohydrates and lipids are considered to be the main source of energy production, whereas proteins serve as structural units and biological catalysts that speed the degradation (and also assimilation) of these former two molecules. Under normal conditions, proteins are not utilized as energy-yielding foodstuffs, however, in cases of protein excess and/or carbohydrate and lipid lack, proteins can be used as a source of energy.

Figure 1-26 illustrates the major biochemical pathways that are involved in energy metabolism. They include the *Embden-Meyerhof* (glycolytic) *pathway*, the *Krebs'* (tricarboxylic acid) *cycle*, and the *cytochrome electron transport chain*. For the

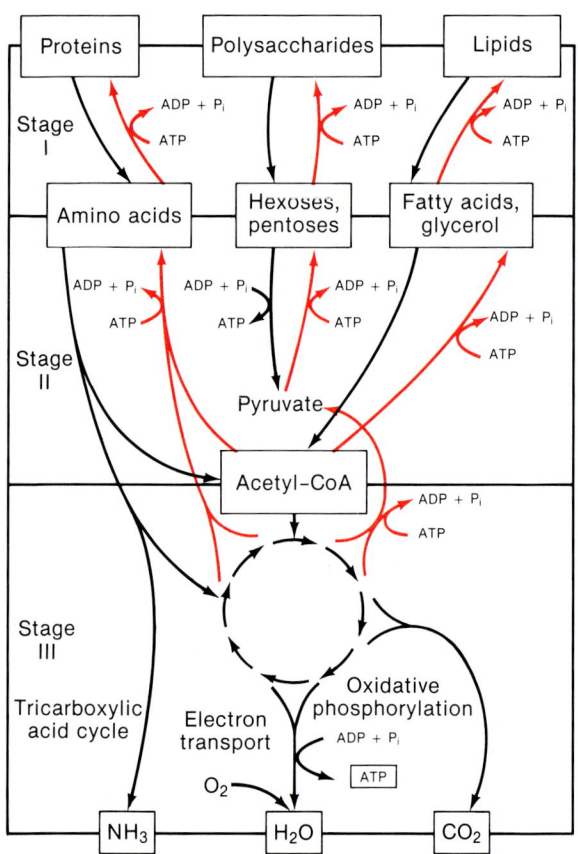

FIGURE 1-26. Major biochemical pathways. The catabolic pathways (black arrows) converge to form NH_3, H_2O, and CO_2. These processes result in the production of ATP. Anabolic pathways (red arrows) utilize ATP to yield macromolecules and other cell components. (Adapted from Lehninger, A.: *Biochemistry*, 2nd ed. New York, Worth Publishing, 1985.)

sake of simplicity, let's divide energy metabolism into three phases.

In phase 1, polysaccharides are hydrolyzed to monosaccharides, usually hexoses. Similarly, triglycerides, which make up the major fraction of the lipid food sources, are broken down to glycerol and fatty acids, while proteins are degraded to their component amino acids. Each of these processes is, for the most part, hydrolytic, and the energy released as these reactions occur is made available to the organism.

In phase 2, the monosaccharides, glycerol, fatty acids, and amino acids are further degraded to three compounds by processes that result in the formation of some energy-rich phosphate compounds. In glycolysis, the hexoses are converted to pyruvate and then to acetyl coenzyme A (CoA). Similarly, the long-chain fatty acids are oxidized to acetyl CoA while glycerol is converted to pyruvate and acetyl CoA by means of the glycolytic sequence. Amino acids yield either an intermediate of the tricarboxylic acid cycle (oxaloacetate or alpha-ketoglutarate) or acetyl CoA, which is in turn oxidized by means of the Krebs' cycle.

During phase 3, energy-rich adenosine triphosphate (ATP) is produced by oxidative phosphorylation by the cytochrome electron transport chain. Reducing equivalents generated in the Krebs' cycle are oxidized in the presence of oxygen to form ATP.

The energy derived from the above-mentioned reactions can be stored within the body or utilized by the organism to fuel activities, such as muscle contraction, repair of damaged cellular components, production of secretory products, and reproduction. As the following chapters show, the ability to maintain life depends not only on the availability of a sufficient amount of substrates but also on the efficiency with which an individual can assimilate and oxidize ingested food.

Bibliography

Baldwin, E.: *Dynamic Aspects of Biochemistry*, 5th ed. Cambridge, Cambridge University Press, 1967.
Best, W., and Taylor, J.: *The Living Body,* 4th ed. New York, Holt, Rinehart, and Winston, 1958.
Chang, R.: *Chemistry,* 3rd ed. New York, Random House, 1988.
Conn, E., and Stumpf, P.: *Outlines of Biochemistry,* 4th ed. New York, John Wiley and Sons, 1968.
Higgins, E.: *Physics*. New York, W.A. Benjamin, 1968.
Leicester, H., and Klickenstein, H.: *A Source Book in Chemistry: 1400–1900.* Cambridge, Mass., Harvard University Press, 1981.
Lehninger, A.: *Biochemistry,* 2nd ed. New York, W.A. Benjamin, 1974.
Martin, D., Mayes, P., and Rodwell, V.: *Harper's Review of Biochemistry,* 18th ed. Los Altos, Calif., Lange Medical Publications, 1981.
McGilvery, R.: *Biochemistry: A Functional Approach,* 2nd ed. Philadelphia, W.B. Saunders, 1979.
Moris, J.: *A Biologist's Physical Chemistry*. Reading, Mass., Addison-Wesley, 1968.
Pimentel, G., and Spratley, R.: *Understanding Chemistry*. San Francisco, Hoden-Day, 1971.
Segel, I.: *Biochemical Calculations*. New York, John Wiley and Sons, 1968.
Sienko, M., and Plane, R.: *Chemistry,* 4th ed. New York, McGraw-Hill, 1971.
Quagliana, J., and Vallarino, L.: *Chemistry,* 3rd ed. Englewood Cliffs, N.J., Prentice-Hall, 1969.
Vander, A., Sherman, J., and Luciano, D.: *Human Physiology: The Mechanisms of Body Function,* 4th ed. New York, McGraw-Hill, 1985.
West, J. B.: *Respiratory Physiology, The Essentials,* 3rd ed. Baltimore, Williams and Wilkins, 1985.

OBJECTIVES

AFTER READING THIS CHAPTER, THE STUDENT WILL BE ABLE TO:

1. State the two main functions of the cardiovascular system.
2. Describe the overall structure of the heart and cardiovascular system.
3. Relate myocardial cellular electrical activity to the electrocardiogram.
4. Describe ventricular function and distinguish between the length-tension relationship and alterations in contractility.
5. State the basic relationships that describe hemodynamics and use them to predict the physiologic consequences of alterations in the activity of the heart and blood vessels.
6. Discuss the autonomic, humoral, and local control of blood flow in the peripheral circulation.
7. Explain the factors that influence capillary fluid exchange.
8. Discuss the factors that determine cardiac output and venous return.
9. Summarize the major features of the special circulations.
10. Explain how central and local cardiovascular control mechanisms are integrated to regulate blood pressure, the distribution of blood flow, and blood volume.

2
CARDIOVASCULAR ANATOMY AND PHYSIOLOGY

CHAPTER OUTLINE

FUNCTIONS OF THE CARDIOVASCULAR SYSTEM
STRUCTURE OF THE CARDIOVASCULAR SYSTEM
  Components of Blood
    Plasma
    Blood Cells
  The Heart
  Systemic Circulation
  Pulmonary Circulation
  Lymphatic System
ELECTRICAL ACTIVITY OF THE HEART
  Resting Membrane Potential
  Excitability of Cells—Action Potential
    Cardiac Cell Action Potential
    Pacemaker Cell Action Potential
    Conduction Pathways of the Heart
  Electrocardiograms
    Vector Analysis
    Lead Systems
    The Normal Electrocardiogram
    Vectorcardiography
THE HEART AS A PUMP
  Myocardial Ultrastructure
  Excitation-Contraction Coupling
  Mechanism of Cardiac Contraction and Relaxation

The Cardiac Cycle
  Diastole
  Atrial Systole
  Ventricular Systole
  Heart Sounds
Ventricular Function
  Length-Tension Relationship
  Contractility
  Control of Cardiac Function
HEMODYNAMICS
  Pressure, Flow, and Resistance
  Determinants of Resistance—Poiseuille's Law
  Laminar and Turbulent Flow
  The Bernoulli Principle
  Laplace's Law
  Pulsatile Pressure and Flow
PERIPHERAL CIRCULATION AND THE CONTROL OF BLOOD FLOW
  Autonomic Control of Blood Flow
    Sympathetic Control of Blood Vessels
    Parasympathetic Control of Blood Vessels
  Humoral Control of Blood Flow
  Local Control of Blood Flow
MICROCIRCULATION AND CAPILLARY EXCHANGE
  Structure of the Microcirculation

Factors Influencing Filtration, Absorption, and
Capillary Exchange
  Diffusion
  Filtration and Absorption
  Edema
  Endocytosis
CARDIAC OUTPUT AND VENOUS RETURN
Determinants of Cardiac Output
  Heart Rate
  Stroke Volume
Determinants of Venous Return
  Vascular Tone, Capacitance, and Blood Volume
  Muscle Contraction and Venous Return
  The Thoracoabdominal Pump
THE SPECIAL CIRCULATIONS
Coronary Circulation
Cerebral Circulation
  Maintenance of Perfusion Pressure
  Neural Control of Cerebral Blood Flow
  Local Control of Cerebral Blood Flow
Renal Circulation
  Anatomy of the Renal Circulation
  Renal Blood Flow
  Control of Renal Circulation
Cutaneous Circulation
Splanchnic Circulation
  Gastrointestinal Circulation
  Hepatic Circulation
INTEGRATED CONTROL OF THE CARDIOVASCULAR SYSTEM
Control of Blood Pressure
  Cardiovascular Reflexes
Control of Blood Volume
Control of Blood Flow

FUNCTIONS OF THE CARDIOVASCULAR SYSTEM

The main function of the cardiovascular system is to provide a means of transportation for the cells of the body. The heart provides the energy for the movement of blood, which carries nutrients to and waste products from body tissues. The blood vessels branch many times, forming smaller and smaller vessels. The smallest of these, the thin-walled *capillaries*, are the site of exchange between the blood and body tissues (and in the case of pulmonary circulation, with the air spaces of the lung). The extremely large number of successive vessel branchings results in a tremendous number of capillaries, normally bringing every cell of the body into close proximity with the blood.

Oxygen, nutrients (such as proteins, amino acids, lipids, carbohydrates, and vitamins), hormones, and other material must pass through the capillary wall (the capillary *endothelium*), diffuse through the *interstitial fluid* that surrounds the cells, and either pass through the cell membrane into the interior of the cell or interact with receptors on the cell surface. Carbon dioxide, waste products of metabolism, and secretory products such as hormones, vasoactive substances, and stored nutrients released for use elsewhere in the body must follow the same route in the opposite direction.

The blood also contains many of the factors and specialized cells that help maintain the *constancy* of the body's internal environment (*homeostasis*) or that protect the body against foreign material and organisms. These maintenance and protective agents include buffers, clotting factors, and specialized blood cells, which can attack invading material and organisms in a variety of ways, including specific immunologic mechanisms.

STRUCTURE OF THE CARDIOVASCULAR SYSTEM

The general organization of the cardiovascular system is shown in Figure 2-1. Although anatomically the heart is a single organ, physiologically it acts as two pairs of pumps arranged in series. The right side of the heart consists of the *right atrium* and the *right ventricle*. The right atrium is a weak pumping chamber that pumps venous blood arriving from the body tissues via the *vena cavae* through the right atrioventricular valve (the *tricuspid valve*) into the stronger right ventricle (Fig. 2-2). The right ventricle pumps blood through the *pulmonic valve* into the pulmonary arteries. These branch many times, forming *lobar pulmonary arteries*, *arterioles*, and ultimately, the *pulmonary capillaries*, which pass between the air spaces (*alveoli*) of the lung. The alveoli and pulmonary cap-

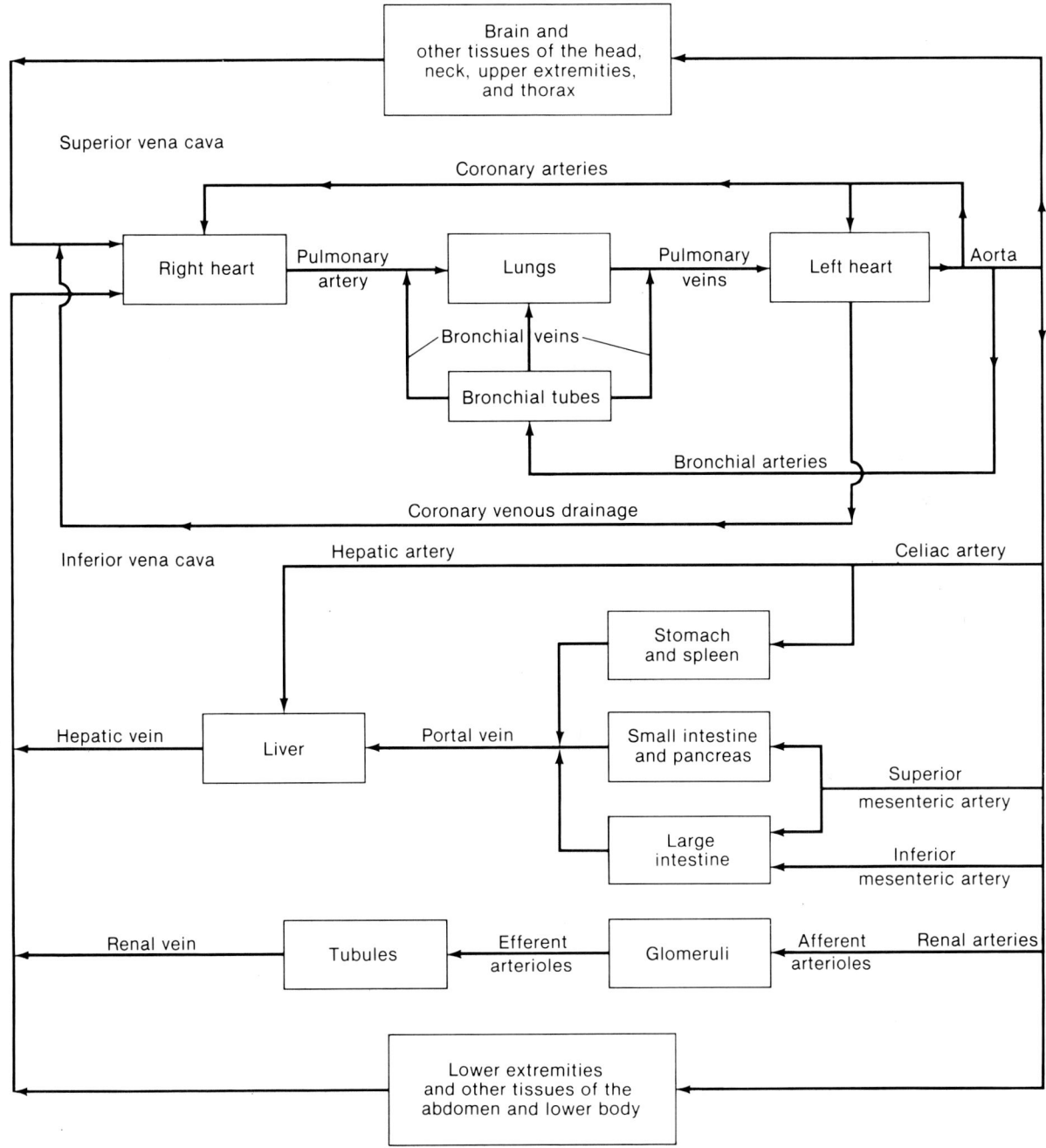

FIGURE 2–1. Diagram of the cardiovascular system.

illaries are the site of gas exchange between the body and external environment. The vessels distal to the pulmonary capillaries, which are called *venules,* merge to form *lobar veins,* which combine to form the four main *pulmonary veins.* The pulmonary veins carry blood to the left side of the heart.

The left side of the heart consists of the *left atrium* and the *left ventricle.* The left atrium pumps the blood returning from the lungs via the pulmonary veins through the left atrioventricular valve (the *mitral,* or *bicuspid,* valve) into the left ventricle. The left ventricle pumps blood through the *aortic valve* into the *aorta,* which branches into *arteries* that supply every organ of the body with

36 CARDIOVASCULAR ANATOMY AND PHYSIOLOGY

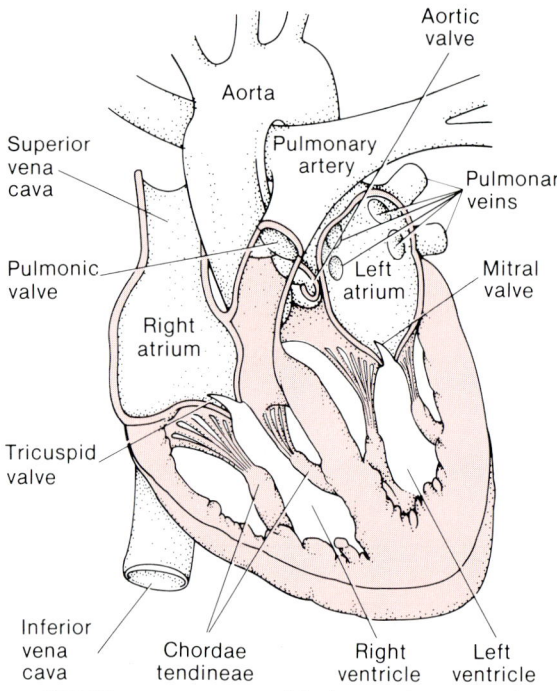

FIGURE 2–2. Anatomy of the heart and great vessels.

blood (see Fig. 2–1). The arteries divide into smaller vessels, the thick-walled *arterioles,* from which the capillaries orginate. The vessels distal to the capillaries, the venules, then form the larger veins, which ultimately combine to form the superior and inferior vena cavae.

Components of Blood

Blood is a suspension of different kinds of cells in an aqueous medium called *plasma.* The cellular constituents of blood can be separated easily from the plasma by centrifugation because the cells have a greater density. The cells, which are called the *formed elements,* are mainly red blood cells (erythrocytes) and normally constitute a little less than half of the total volume of blood. The ratio of the volume of the cells to the total volume of blood (expressed as a percentage) is called the *hematocrit.* The hematocrit is normally about 45% and is slightly higher in men (about 48%) than in women (about 42%). Approximately 1% of the total volume consists of white blood cells (leukocytes) and platelets. In centrifuged blood, these white cells form a layer called the *buffy coat,* which is found above the packed red blood cells, because their density falls between that of the red blood cells and plasma.

Plasma

Plasma is a clear, slightly yellow solution (it may appear cloudy after a fatty meal) that is about 90% water. Plasma contains a nearly incredible number of substances, including proteins, electrolytes, dissolved gases, foodstuffs and waste products of metabolism, hormones, clotting factors and vasoactive agents, and materials involved in immunologic reactions. Virtually anything transported to and from the body cells is carried in the blood, and most of it is carried in the plasma fraction. Note that the word *serum* refers to the fluid portion of blood obtained after coagulation has occurred, whereas plasma is the fluid portion of circulating blood.

Plasma Proteins. There are hundreds of kinds of proteins in plasma, and they constitute about 7% of its weight. The most abundant protein in plasma is *albumin,* which has several important functions. Albumin is synthesized in the liver and can bind reversibly to many substances that would be insoluble in plasma by themselves. It is therefore extremely important in the transport of many hormones and metabolic substrates and products. It also represents an emergency pool of protein substrate itself. Finally, as the main plasma protein, albumin is an important factor determining the movement of fluid across the walls of capillaries. Because the albumin molecule is just a little too large to fit easily through capillary pores, it exerts an osmotic influence on the aqueous portion of plasma and helps to prevent fluid from moving out of the capillaries. This effect is discussed later in this chapter.

Many other proteins act to bind and transport material that would otherwise be insoluble in plasma. For example, lipids, such as triglycerides, fatty acids, cholesterol, and phospholipids, are transported as lipoproteins. In other cases, specific proteins exist to transport metals, such as iron and copper, or specific hormones.

The second main group of plasma proteins comprises the various immunoglobulins, which are the antibodies that react with antigens in the body's immunologic defenses. Immunoglobulins are synthesized by plasma cells in the lymphoid organs. Another type of plasma protein, the complement group, also participates in immunologic reactions. Other plasma proteins include the clotting factors that participate in blood coagulation and enzymes.

Plasma Electrolytes. The plasma electrolytes are mainly inorganic ions. They maintain the osmolarity and pH of the blood within normal limits and therefore are of great importance in preserving the normal electrical and enzymatic activity of body cells. The main inorganic cation of plasma is sodium; others include potassium, calcium, and magnesium. The main inorganic anion of plasma is chloride. Other anions include bicarbonate, phosphate, sulfate, plasma proteins, and organic acids. The plasma electrolytes are discussed in Chapter 12 (see Fig. 12–2).

Other Plasma Components. Dissolved oxygen and carbon dioxide are carried in the plasma, although most of the oxygen carried by the blood is transported chemically bound to hemoglobin in the erythrocytes and most of the carbon dioxide is transported as bicarbonate. Foodstuffs and waste products of metabolism, such as glucose, amino acids, and urea, are also found in plasma.

Blood Cells

The cellular components of blood, sometimes called the *formed elements,* include erythrocytes, various kinds of leukocytes, and platelets. As noted in the section on hematocrit, the red cells are by far the most numerous.

Erythrocytes. There are normally about 5.2 million erythrocytes in one *microliter* (μl) of blood in men and a slightly lower number (4.8 million/μl) in women. The erythrocytes are biconcave discs that average about 8 μm in diameter and measure about 2 μm at their thickest part (see Fig. 3–6). The red blood cells therefore have a high surface area–to–volume ratio, which aids in the diffusion of oxygen and carbon dioxide into and out of the cell. Erythrocytes are deformable; that is, they can change their shape to help them get through small blood vessels. After passing through these vessels, they rapidly return to their normal biconcave shape. This is probably accomplished by contractile proteins in the cells. The red blood cells are surrounded by a cell membrane, but mature cells do not contain nuclei, mitochondria, ribosomes, or other organelles. However, the erythrocytes do have active metabolic processes and can consume oxygen themselves. Most of the energy required by the erythrocytes is supplied by the *anaerobic glycolysis pathway* (the Embden-Meyerhof pathway), which has two shunts. One of these, the *hexose monophosphate shunt,* is aerobic, and the other, the *2,3-DPG shunt,* is anaerobic. The average life span of an erythrocyte is about 120 days.

The main cellular component of the erythrocyte is hemoglobin, a conjugated protein with a molecular weight of about 64,500 daltons. As is well known, hemoglobin allows the cell to perform its main function, the transport of oxygen. In the next chapter, hemoglobin's importance in carbon dioxide transport and hydrogen ion buffering is explained.

Leukocytes. Normal whole blood contains between 4,000 and 10,000 leukocytes/μl. There are three groups of leukocytes: *granulocytes, monocytes,* and *lymphocytes.*

The granulocytes are further subgrouped into *neutrophils* (which are also called *polymorphonuclear leukocytes,* or "polys," because of the variable shapes of their segmented nuclei), *eosinophils,* and *basophils.* Granulocytes are usually about 12 to 15 μm in diameter and have multilobed nuclei. Neutrophils constitute between 40% and 75% of blood leukocytes, and they defend against bacterial infection by engulfing and ingesting bacteria. After this process, which is called *phagocytosis,* they are usually able to destroy the bacteria with lytic enzymes found in intracellular organelles known as lysosomes. Leukocytes also participate in inflammatory reactions, and so they gather at sites of tissue injury.

Eosinophils, which constitute only 1% to 6% of the blood leukocytes, usually appear to have bilobed nuclei. They are therefore less segmented than neutrophils, which may have five or more. Eosinophils seem to protect against parasites. They are known to increase in number when the body responds to abnormal endogenous or exogenous agents during an immunologic reaction. For example, the eosinophil count is elevated in persons suffering from allergies or asthma. Basophils, normally less than 1% of the white blood cell count, are similar to the *mast cells* found in other body tissues. They contain granules that may be filled with vasoactive substances stored for release into the blood, such as histamine or heparin (an anticoagulant). They may also participate in immunologic reactions.

Monocytes, normally 2% to 10% of the leukocytes, are the largest cells of the group, with average diameters of 15 to 20 μm. Monocytes usually have a large indented single nucleus and are similar to the *macrophages* found in other body tissues, including the lungs. Monocytes are also capable of phagocytosis and ingest microorganisms or injured cells. They may also participate in immunologic reactions by processing antigens so that the lymphocytes can produce specific antibodies to them.

Lymphocytes constitute 20% to 45% of white blood cells. They are a heterogeneous group of cells and range between 6 and 20 μm in diameter. One group of lymphocytes, the B cells, transform into *plasma cells* when they are stimulated by exposure to an antigen. Plasma cells synthesize the specific immunoglobulin antibodies. Another group, the T cells, participate in the delayed hypersensitivity reactions that do not depend on specific antibodies. A third group, the so-called *null cells,* do not seem similar to either T cells or B cells. Some of these cells (the killer cells) seem to be capable of destroying tissue cells that have been coated with antibody.

Platelets. Platelets are fragments of giant cells called *megakaryocytes,* which are found in the bone marrow. Platelets have no nuclei. They are important in the control of bleeding and blood clotting and also release vasoactive substances, such as thromboxane.

The Heart

The major structures of the heart can be seen in Figure 2–2. The two atria are separated from the more muscular ventricles by a fibrous ring that supports the four cardiac valves. These one-way valves consist of *cusps* composed of indistensible collagen covered by a layer of endocardium. The atrioventricular valves separate the atria from the ventricles. The left atrioventricular, or mitral, valve has two cusps and is often referred to as the bicuspid; the right atrioventricular valve has three and is often referred to as the tricuspid. The valve cusps are attached to the fibrous rings that separate the chambers. Their free edges are attached to projections of the ventricular myocardium called *papillary muscles* by endocardium-covered thread-like strands of collagen, called *chordae tendineae.* These strands keep the valves from *eversing* (that is, opening backward into the atria) and allowing regurgitation of blood into the atria during systole. The most striking feature about all four cardiac valves is how thin and delicate they appear. In a young healthy person, these thin membranous structures are translucent or nearly transparent.

The right atrium is a comparatively thin-walled muscular structure attached to the superior and inferior vena cavae. There is a rudimentary similunar valve separating the inferior vena cava from the right atrium; there is none at all between the superior vena cava and the right atrium. Another prominent feature of the right atrium is the coronary sinus, which returns venous blood from much of the heart muscle itself. It opens into the right atrium between the orifice of the inferior vena cava and the tricuspid valve. The right atrium contracts (*atrial systole*) during ventricular *diastole* (relaxation), keeping right atrial pressure above that in the right ventricle, thus helping continue the movement of venous blood through the tricuspid valve into the right ventricle.

The right ventricle is much more muscular than the right atrium. Part of its thick wall, the *ventricular septum,* is shared with the left ventricle. The remaining part, the "free wall," is much thinner than the left ventricle or septum in the adult, although it is much thicker than the walls of the atria. When the right ventricle contracts, the pressure inside it exceeds that in the right atrium, so the tricuspid valve closes, preventing backward flow into right atrium. As pressure inside the right ventricle increases above that in the pulmonary artery, the pulmonic valve opens, allowing blood to flow through the pulmonary arterial tree into the pulmonary capillaries.

Blood returns to the left atrium from the lungs via the four pulmonary veins. There are no valves between the pulmonary veins and the thin-walled left atrium. The inertia of the blood flowing in the vena cavae and pulmonary veins probably prevents much backward flow during atrial systole. The two atria are separated from each other by the atrial septum. Contraction of the left atrium helps keep left atrial pressure above that in the relaxed left ventricle, and blood continues to flow through the mitral valve into the left ventricle. When the left ventricle contracts, its pressure exceeds that in the left atrium, and the mitral valve closes. Like the tricuspid valve, the mitral valve is anchored to the papillary muscles by chordae tendineae. As left ventricular pressure continues to increase during ventricular systole, intraventricular pressure exceeds that in the aorta, and the aortic valve opens. The free wall of the left ventricle is as thick as the ventricular septum. The heart is located within an indistensible sac, the *pericardium,* which is lined with pericardial fluid. The pericardium helps prevent overdistention of the ventricles; the small volume of fluid acts as a lubricant.

The muscle of the heart is called the *myocardium.* The innermost portion of the myocardium is called the *endocardium,* and the outermost portion is called the *epicardium*.

Systemic Circulation

The aorta is thick-walled and elastic. It ascends upward as it leaves the left ventricle, then arches toward the left side of the body, and finally descends toward the lower extremities. The *coronary arteries* leave the aorta immediately distal to the aortic valve (Fig. 2–3). The blood supply to the upper limbs and head leaves the aorta at its arch via the *brachiocephalic (or innominate) artery,* which gives rise to the *right subclavian artery* and the *right common carotid artery,* and via the *left subclavian artery* and the *left common carotid artery.* The blood supply to the rib cage and intercostal muscles and the systemic arterial blood supply of the lungs leave the proximal part of the descending aorta via the *intercostal arteries* and the *bronchial arteries,* respectively.

The large systemic arterial vessels, such as the aorta and its major branches, have much more elastic tissue and collagen and fewer smooth muscle cells than smaller arteries and arterioles. The elastic tissue found in the aorta and the larger vessels allows them to stretch when the stroke volume is ejected into the proximal arterial tree during left ventricular systole. This tends to keep systemic arterial systolic blood pressure lower than it would be if these vessels were less distensible. During diastole, the potential energy stored in these expanded vessels maintains blood flow from the arterial tree. This maintains diastolic blood pressure and systemic capillary blood flow during diastole (Fig. 2–4).

The arterial tree terminates in the small muscular arterioles. The vascular smooth muscle of the arterioles is the main reason that they are the primary site of resistance to blood flow in the systemic circulation, as discussed in the hemodynamics section of this chapter. The smooth muscle fibers, which are arranged in a circular fashion around the vessels, are under both neural and humoral control. When they relax, the vessel dilates and its resistance to blood flow is decreased. When they contract, the vessel constricts and its resistance to blood flow is increased.

The arteriolar segment is the site of the greatest resistance to blood flow. As the arterial tree branches, the total cross-sectional area of the various segments of the systemic circulation increases dramatically, reaching its peak in the capillaries. It then decreases as veins merge to form larger vessels (Fig. 2–5). Because the total blood flow through the various segments is the same, as the total cross-sectional area increases, the linear velocity of blood flow decreases. Thus, the blood flows most slowly through the capillary segment. Figure 2–5 also shows that the largest fraction of the blood volume is normally found in the venous portion of the systemic circulation. Most of the decrease in blood pressure occurs in the arteriolar segment of the systemic circulation.

The microcirculation, consisting primarily of capillaries, is depicted in Figure 2–6. These vessels, which also include the *terminal arterioles, metarterioles,* and *postcapillary venules,* are less than 100 μ in diameter. The thin-walled capillaries, which contain no smooth muscle, originate from the metarterioles. Metarterioles, which do contain smooth muscle, can act as direct pathways between an arteriole and a venule. A small band of smooth muscle may be found at the origin of many capillaries. This is the *precapillary sphincter,* which can act to open or close off sections of capillary beds. They may be under both neural and *"local" control,* responding to alterations in the levels of oxygen, carbon dioxide, pH, metabolites, ions, and the temperature in their immediate environment by dilating or constricting. Some organs, such as the skin or portions of the gastrointestinal tract, may have *arteriovenous shunt*

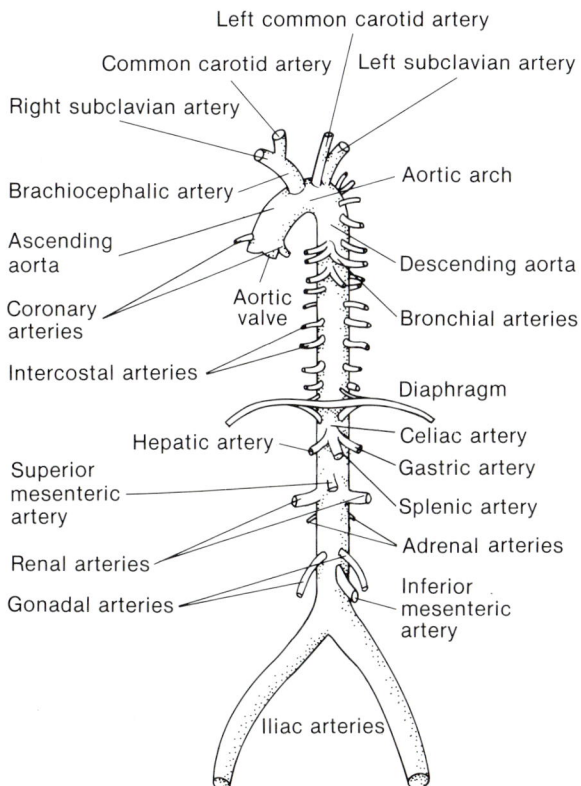

FIGURE 2–3. Major arterial branches of the aorta.

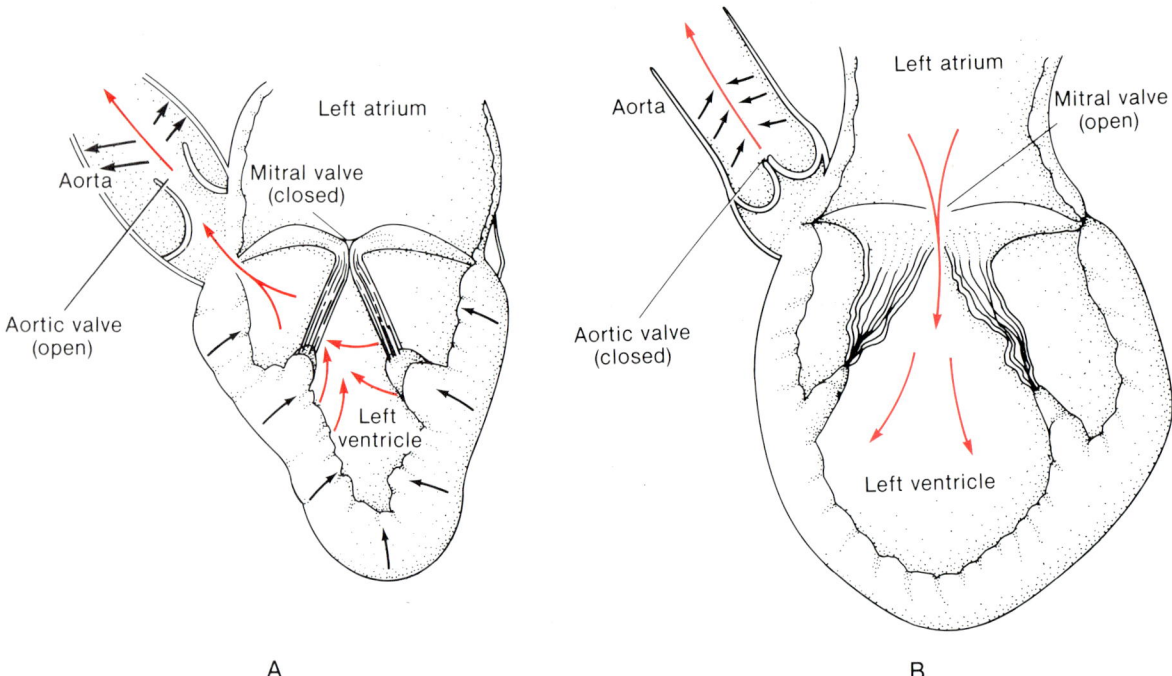

FIGURE 2–4. Reservoir action of the aorta during ventricular systole, allowing maintenance of blood flow and blood pressure during diastole. Red arrows indicate the direction of blood flow. *A*, Left ventricular systole; the small black arrows represent the force developed by the ventricular wall and by the lateral pressure of the blood against the aorta. *B*, Left ventricular diastole; the small black arrows represent the elastic recoil pressure developed by the aorta.

vessels, or a direct connection between an artery and vein (see Fig. 2–6). They can divert blood flow away from larger sections of the capillary bed.

The organization and structure of the capillary beds and the capillaries themselves vary considerably in different organs. Some organs, such as the liver, have capillaries with many pores called *fenestrations*. Others have capillaries with fewer fenestrations. These pores allow large molecules and substances that do not dissolve in the capillary wall (the capillary endothelium) to be exchanged between the cells of the tissue and the blood. Many small vesicles and granules may also be seen within the capillary walls. Large insoluble particles are transported through the capillary wall by a process called *endocytosis*, in which the cell membrane of the capillary surrounds the particles to form the vesicles used to transport them through the cell.

The capillaries, metarterioles, and shunt vessels all drain into venules. The venules are slightly larger in diameter than their corresponding arterioles, but they have much thinner walls (see Fig. 2–6). Because they have such thin walls, some material can probably be exchanged between the tissue cells and the blood in the venules. Venules and the larger veins that are formed by their convergence have smooth muscle that is under neural control (and possibly humoral as well).

There are usually *at least* two veins for every corresponding artery. Each vein usually has a greater internal diameter than its companion artery, and veins are also much easier to distend (at least at lower volumes) than are arteries. Thus, the total cross-sectional area of the veins is greater than that of the arteries (see Fig. 2–5). The volume of blood in the veins is therefore normally much greater than that in the arteries. Because of their capacity to "store" blood, the veins are often referred to as *capacitance vessels*. Similarly, the arterioles are frequently referred to as *resistance vessels*. Stimulation of the sympathetic innervation of the veins reduces their ability to store blood and may therefore help mobilize it into the arterial side of the systemic circulation when necessary.

The endothelial lining of the veins of the extremities periodically projects small, extremely delicate, crescent-shaped valves into the vessels. These one-way valves, which open toward the heart, allow blood to be returned to the heart, even

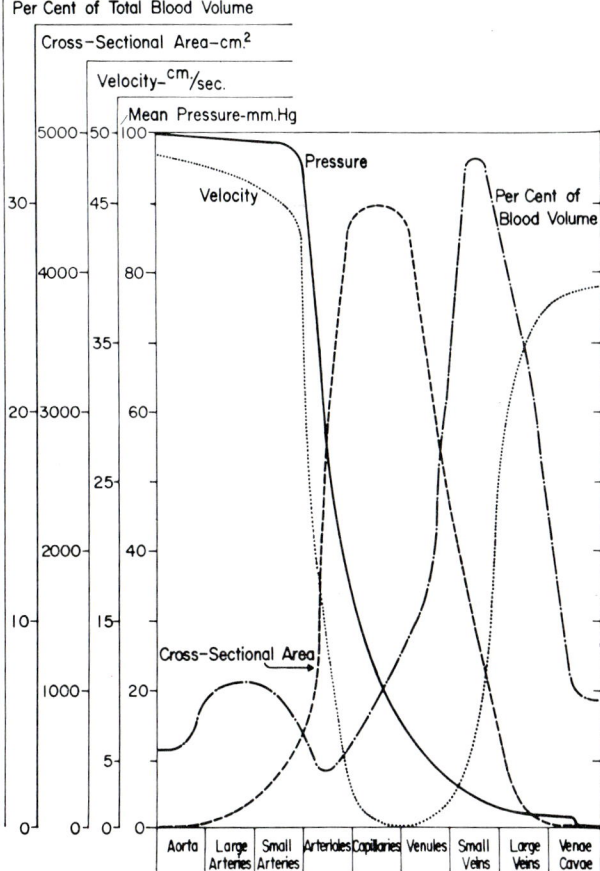

FIGURE 2–5 Alterations in pressure, linear velocity of blood flow, and total cross-sectional area, and the percent distribution of total blood volume in the various anatomic classes of blood vessels of the systemic circulation. (Reproduced by permission from: Berne, R.M., and Levy, M.N.: *Cardiovascular Physiology,* 4th ed. St. Louis, 1981, The C.V. Mosby Co.)

though there is not sufficient blood pressure in the veins to push the blood "uphill" to the heart. Blood cannot flow backward because the valves close, but if the vein is squeezed by the contraction of skeletal muscles, the valve closer to the heart will open, pushing blood toward the great veins and right atrium (Fig. 2–7). There are no valves in the veins of the thoracic, abdominal, or cerebral cavities.

Pulmonary Circulation

The pulmonary blood vessels have thinner walls, are generally shorter, and have larger lumens than the corresponding vessels in the systemic circulation. One very important difference between the systemic and pulmonary circulation is that the pulmonary vessels that correspond anatomically to the arterioles on the systemic side of the circulation have very little smooth muscle. As discussed in greater detail in Chapter 3, this arrangement has important physiologic consequences. One of the most obvious is that the pulmonary circulation offers much less resistance to blood flow than the systemic circulation. This results in a much lower pressure in the pulmonary artery than is normally seen in the aorta, even though the outputs of the left and right ventricles are nearly identical. There is some vascular smooth muscle in the small arteries of the pulmonary circulation that is innervated by the sympathetic nervous system and is also affected by local factors, which are discussed in Chapter 3.

The short vessels of the pulmonary arterial tree branch rapidly, ultimately forming as many as 280 billion pulmonary capillaries, which literally envelop the alveoli. Some researchers like to think of pulmonary capillary blood as flowing in sheets around the alveoli because there are so many capillaries per alveolus. The area of contact between the alveoli and the pulmonary capillaries is very great—about 60 to 80 m^2 in a normal adult. Thus,

42 CARDIOVASCULAR ANATOMY AND PHYSIOLOGY

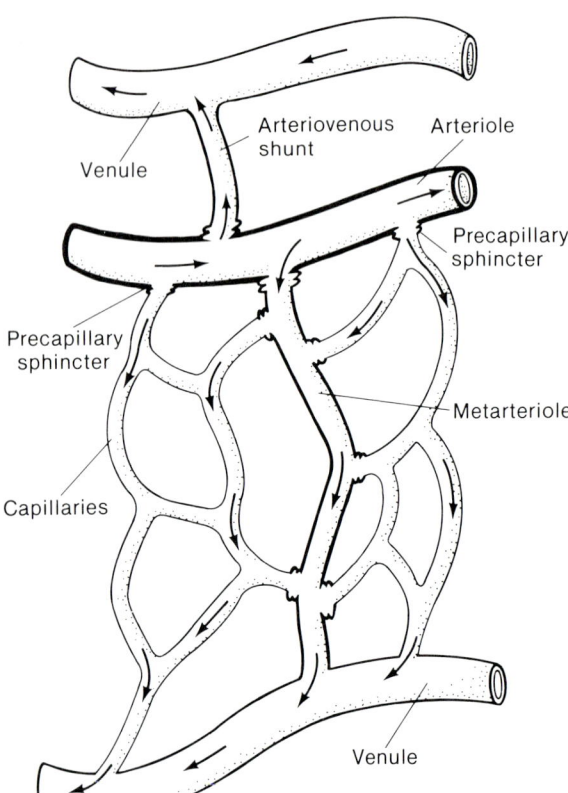

FIGURE 2–6. Major features of the microcirculation. Arrows denote direction of blood flow.

the lung is well designed for gas exchange between the alveoli and the pulmonary capillaries.

Lymphatic System

The lymphatic system has important transport and defense functions. As a transport system, it acts to return fluid and other materials that have moved out of the systemic and pulmonary circulations into the interstitial space to the systemic venous system. The lymph nodes serve as a means of defense against bacteria and other foreign material because they contain phagocytic cells and participate in immunologic reactions.

The lymphatics, which are frequently thought of as constituting a drainage system, begin with blind-ended vessels that are similar in structure to the systemic capillaries. Fluid and particles enter these vessels, which drain into larger vessels comparable to the systemic veins. The distribution and location of the larger lymphatic vessels is also similar to that of the systemic veins. The larger lymphatic vessels also have valves like those found in the systemic veins, so skeletal muscle contractions provide the main force for the movement of lymph. Lymph is returned to the circulation at the thoracic duct, the lymphatic duct, and the central veins.

ELECTRICAL ACTIVITY OF THE HEART

Contraction of cardiac muscle cells is initiated by their electrical excitation. The source of this excitation is provided by special cells of the heart that normally have the property of rhythmic spontaneous electrical activity. When these specialized cells discharge electrically, by a process called *depolarization* (discussed later), they usually cause the other electrically excitable cells of the heart to depolarize too. Therefore, the specialized cardiac cells that normally display the property of spontaneous rhythmic electrical excitation are called *pacemaker cells*. There are two aggregations of pacemaker cells in the heart, one in the *sinoatrial (SA) node* and the other in the *atrioventricular (AV) node*.

To understand the ability of cardiac cells (and nerve cells) to depolarize, we must first consider the charge difference found across the membrane of all living cells of the body. Because of the difference in the electrical charge between the fluid inside and outside of the cell membrane (intracellular versus interstitial fluid), the cells are said to be *polarized*. In electrically excitable cells, this polarization, which is measured in millivolts, is referred to as the *resting membrane potential*. When it is decreased or abolished, therefore, the cell is considered to be depolarized.

Resting Membrane Potential

The potential difference across the membrane of living cells is a result of several properties of the cell membrane itself. The first of these is the selective *permeability* of the cell membrane. The cell membrane is composed of phospholipids, so charged particles, such as ions, can only pass through its pores. Molecules too large to fit through the pores cannot pass through the cell membrane unless they are soluble in it and thus can be transported through the membrane in vesicles formed by endocytotic mechanisms. Many large molecules are therefore trapped inside the cell. Most of these have net negative charges, so they can be considered nondiffusible anions. There

CARDIOVASCULAR ANATOMY AND PHYSIOLOGY 43

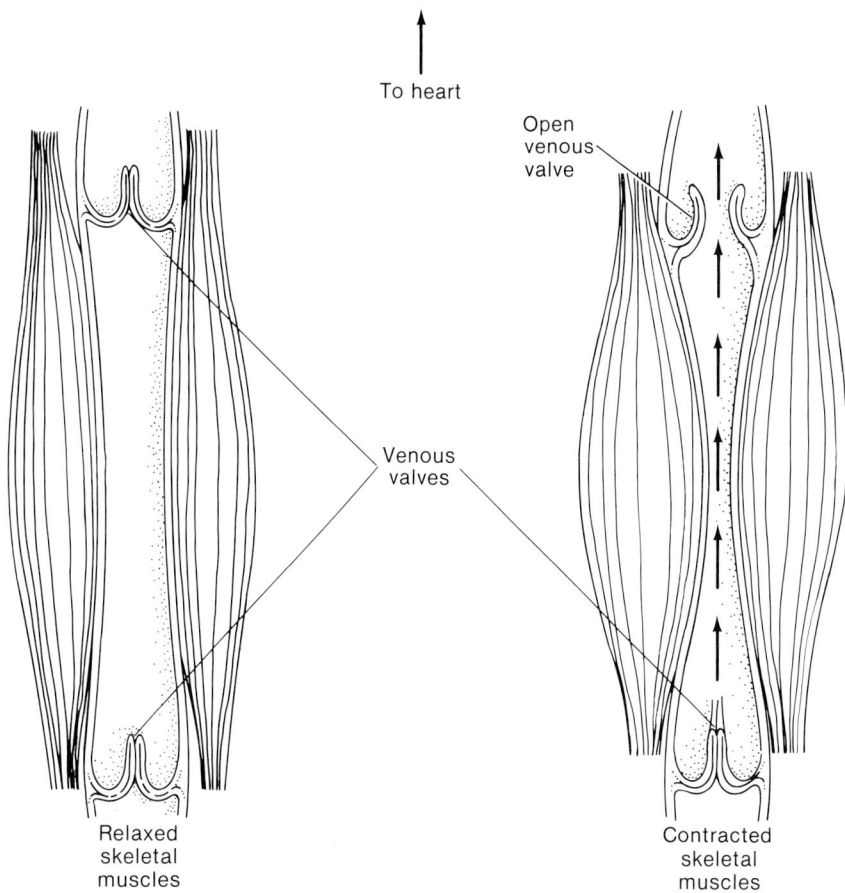

FIGURE 2–7. Muscle contraction causes small valves in veins of extremities to open, forcing blood toward the great veins and right atrium.

is a high concentration of potassium ions inside the cell and a high concentration of sodium ions outside the cell, but the resting cell membrane is much more permeable to potassium ions than the sodium or calcium ions found outside the cell. Therefore, the number of potassium ions leaking out of the cell is greater than the number of sodium or calcium ions leaking into the cell.

If the cell membrane were completely permeable to all ions, there would be no electrical potential difference across it. However, under resting conditions, the inside of the cell is negatively charged with regard to the outside because of the large nondiffusible anions inside the cell and the more frequent diffusion of positively charged potassium ions out of the cell than of sodium and calcium ions into the cell. This difference in diffusion occurs because the permeability of the cell membrane differs for the positively charged ions. In fact, potassium diffuses out of the cell only because of its higher concentration within the cell. This chemical force is opposed by electrical force, because the cell interior is negative relative to the interstitial fluid outside, and the positively charged potassium ions are therefore attracted to the net negative charges inside the cell. In contrast, sodium and calcium entry into the cell is favored by both chemical concentration (concentrations are greater outside the cell than inside) and electrical charge forces (attraction to the net negative charge of the cell interior). Regardless of the opposing electrical forces of potassium diffusion, the resting membrane is still more permeable to potassium ions, and the number of those ions leaving the cells is much greater than the number of sodium and calcium ions entering it.

The last factor that must be considered when discussing the resting membrane potential is the so-called *sodium-potassium pump*. This pump, which is really an enzyme, is located in the cell membrane. It acts to pump sodium out of the cell and potassium into it. Thus, the sodium and potassium that do leak through the cell membrane are "pumped" back to the other side. Without the pump, the cell would ultimately depolarize. The sodium-potassium pump carries sodium against an electrochemical gradient and potassium against a chemical gradient. Therefore, the pump requires energy in the form of ATP to perform its function. For this reason, the pump is frequently referred to as the *sodium-potassium ATPase*. The pump tends to move slightly more sodium ions out of the cell than it moves potassium ions into the cell, so it adds to the potential difference across the cell membrane. Figure 2–8 summarizes the factors contributing to the resting membrane potential.

Excitability of Cells—Action Potential

Virtually all living cells of the body have a resting potential. Cardiac cells, like nerve cells and other muscle cells, have the property of *excitability*, that is, they are able to depolarize rapidly and then repolarize in a process called an *action potential*. Because action potentials may be propagated, nerve cells can transmit information. Action potentials also initiate the contraction of muscle fibers.

Cardiac Cell Action Potential

Most of the excitable cardiac cells (*myocytes*), including the atrial and ventricular muscle cells and the specialized conducting cells such as the *Pur-kinje fibers*, have action potentials such as the one shown in Figure 2–9. The exceptions are the pacemaker cells of the SA and AV nodes, which we will discuss shortly. If an excitable cell is depolarized either by a propagated wave of excitation originally initiated by pacemaker cells or by artificial stimulation, it may reach a critical level called the *threshold* and thus result in action *potential*.

As Figure 2–9 shows, the cell membrane begins from its resting potential phase. The action potential begins when the cell membrane of an excitable cell is exposed to a depolarizing current. It begins with an extremely rapid depolarization of the myocyte (Phase 0 in Fig. 2–9). For a brief period called the "overshoot" (Phase 1 in Fig. 2–9), the inside of the cell is slightly positive with respect to the outside. During Phase 1, important changes occur in the permeability of the cell membrane of excitable cells when it is exposed to a depolarizing current. In some still unknown way, the membrane suddenly becomes extremely permeable to sodium. This process is referred to as *sodium activation* and can be compared to opening a gate or

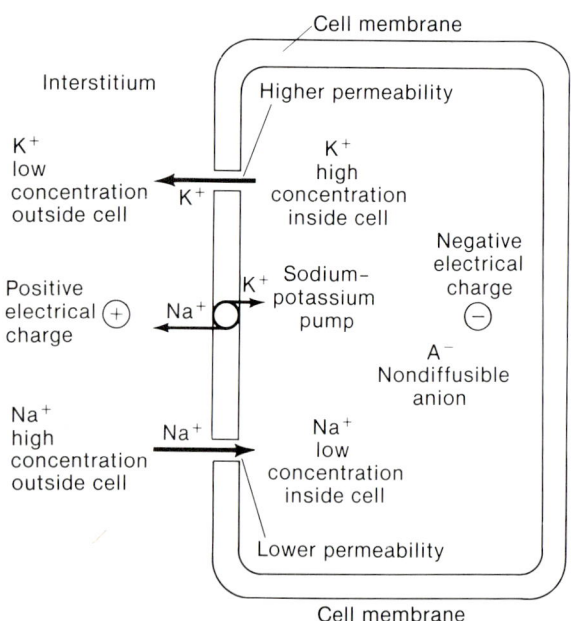

FIGURE 2–8. Diagram showing the factors that contribute to the membrane resting potential.

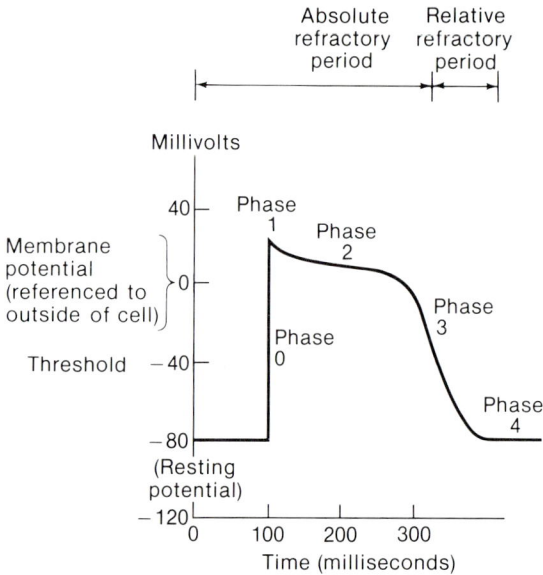

FIGURE 2–9. Duration and electrical voltage of each phase of the ventricular myocyte action potential. The initial segment is *Phase 0*, during which extremely rapid depolarization of the myocyte occurs (time is in milliseconds). *Phase 1* is the "overshoot," during which the inside of the cell becomes slightly positive in relation to the outside. During *Phase 2* there is slower entry of sodium and calcium ions into the cell (reflected by the long plateau period). *Phase 3* starts when the cell begins to repolarize and return to its negative resting potential (*Phase 4*). The inside of the cell is about 80 or 90 millivolts more negative than the outside.

channel to the sodium ions. Because the concentration of sodium ions outside the cell is much greater than inside the cell, as soon as the cell membrane becomes permeable to sodium ions, they rush into the cell. This movement of positive sodium ions into the interior of the cell depolarizes the cell and thus renders it briefly positive in relation to the outside of the cell.

Within a few milliseconds, this fast channel for sodium-ion entry begins to close. This closure is known as *sodium inactivation* and it occurs at the point labelled Phase 1 in Fig. 2–9. By this time, a second "slow" channel has opened, permitting a slower entry of sodium and calcium ions into the cell. This phase of increased permeability remains for a much longer period of time (reflected by the long plateau seen in Phase 2 of Fig. 2–9).

The beginning of Phase 3 occurs when the myocardial cell starts to repolarize and return toward the negative resting potential. This repolarization is caused by two factors: (1) the membrane becomes more permeable to potassium ions, allowing a greater number of these positively charged ions to move outside the cell, and (2) the inactivation of the slow channels for calcium and sodium ions. The increased efflux of positive potassium ions occurring at the same time as the decreased influx of sodium and calcium ions results in restoration of the negative resting membrane potential.

The entire period from the beginning of the action potential to the middle of Phase 3 is known as the *absolute refractory period*, when the myocyte *cannot* be depolarized again by any means. During the period from about the middle of Phase 3 to the beginning of Phase 4 (when the membrane has repolarized to its resting potential), the myocyte *can* again be depolarized but does not have an action potential of full amplitude, and hence is called the *relative refractory period*. During Phase 4 (and probably throughout the action potential as well) the sodium-potassium exchange pump restores potassium to the interior of the cell and removes sodium to the exterior.

Pacemaker Cell Action Potential

Pacemaker cells of the SA and AV nodes normally have action potentials different from those of the other excitable cells of the heart. The main differences are the spontaneous depolarization in Phase 4 and the lack of a long Phase 2 plateau (Fig. 2–10). In addition, the initial depolarization (Phase 0) and repolarization (Phase 3) are both slower. Figure 2–10 shows a transmembrane action potential from a pacemaker cell in the SA node. Note

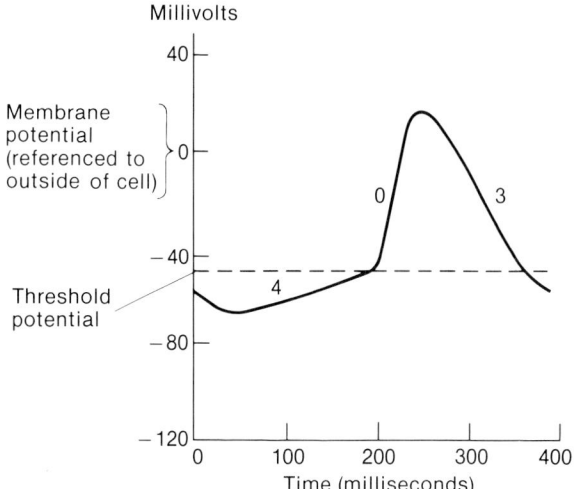

FIGURE 2–10. Action potential of an SA node pacemaker cell.

that the resting potential of pacemaker cells is not as negative as that seen in the other excitable cells of the heart. More important is the slow spontaneous depolarization that occurs during Phase 4. This slow depolarization ultimately causes the membrane potential to reach the threshold for depolarization, and the SA cell therefore has spontaneous action potentials. These spontaneous action potentials give the pacemaker cells their ability to set the heart rate because their depolarization is usually sufficient to cause some of the other cells of the heart to depolarize to their thresholds and, in turn, propagate action potentials to other cells.

The heart rate can be increased by anything that would increase the rate of spontaneous depolarization (that is, make the slope of Phase 4 steeper) or bring the resting membrane potential toward the threshold potential, either by lowering the threshold potential or depolarizing the resting potential toward the threshold. On the other hand, heart rate is decreased by anything that would decrease the rate of spontaneous Phase 4 depolarization, hyperpolarize the resting potential, or raise the threshold.

Normally, the heart rate is under the control of both divisions of the autonomic nervous system—the sympathetic and parasympathetic. *Norepinephrine*, the neurotransmitter released by the sympathetic innervation of the heart, mainly acts to increase heart rate by increasing the slope of the Phase 4 depolarization. *Epinephrine*, carried in the blood from the adrenal medulla, increases the heart rate the same way. *Acetylcholine*, the neurotransmitter released by the parasympathetic innervation of the heart, decreases the heart rate by hyperpolarizing the resting potential of the pacemaker cells and by decreasing the slope of the Phase 4 depolarization, both of which may occur by increased permeability to potassium ions. Because the pacemaker cells are usually *tonically* (continuously) influenced by both divisions of the autonomic nervous system, heart rate can be increased by increasing sympathetic stimulation and/or by withdrawing parasympathetic stimulation. Similarly, heart rate can be decreased by increasing parasympathetic activity and/or decreasing sympathetic tone.

The spontaneous depolarization of pacemaker cells could be accounted for by alterations in the permeability of their cell membranes to either sodium ions or potassium ions or both. As noted in the section on the cardiac cell action potential, during repolarization (Phase 3) the permeability to potassium ions is greatly increased, and the permeability to sodium and calcium ions is decreased to pre-excitation levels. Thus, more positively charged potassium ions are leaving the cell than positively charged sodium ions are entering it. The cardiac cell is therefore repolarizing, because the inside is becoming relatively more negative in relation to the outside. At this point, spontaneous depolarization could occur by either gradually *increasing* the permeability of the cell membrane to sodium ions, which would allow positive charges to enter the cell and depolarize it, or by gradually *decreasing* the permeability to potassium ions, which would slowly decrease the number of positively charged potassium ions leaving the cell while the rate of sodium ions entering it remained the same. In either case (or both), the pacemaker cell would depolarize gradually. Experiments have demonstrated that the latter mechanism, a gradual decrease in permeability to potassium ions while sodium ion permeability remains unchanged, is the source of the spontaneous depolarization seen in Phase 4 of the pacemaker cell action potential.

Conduction Pathways of the Heart

The SA node is normally the pacemaker of the heart because it has the highest rate of spontaneous depolarization, about 70 to 80 times per minute, if influences of the autonomic nervous system are removed. When one or more of the small round pacemaker cells of the SA node depolarize, their excitation spreads through the SA node, probably via specialized elongated conducting cells. Other cells within the node are brought to the threshold, and the entire node will likely depolarize. When myocardial cells other than those in the SA node (or AV node) act as a pacemaker, they are called *ectopic pacemakers*.

Once the SA node depolarizes, a wave of depolarization or excitation spreads over the right atrial muscle fibers by moving from fiber to fiber. A special high-speed conduction pathway called *Bachmann's bundle* (or the interatrial myocardial band) transmits the wave of excitation to the left atrium, where excitation of the left atrial muscle fibers also occurs by cell-to-cell conduction. The action potentials of atrial muscle fibers are similar to those of ventricular fibers, such as that shown in Figure 2–9, except that the Phase 2 plateau is shorter and less developed and repolarization takes longer.

Excitation of the SA node is transmitted to the AV node by three specialized high-speed conduction tracts, the *anterior, middle,* and *posterior internodal pathways*. The AV node is similar in structure to the SA node, consisting of round pacemaker cells and elongated conducting cells. The pacemaker cells of the AV node depolarize spontaneously and rhythmically, but usually at a slower rate than the SA node, about 40 to 60 times per minute. The action potentials of pacemaker cells in the AV node are similar to those in the SA node.

The region of the AV node closest to the nonspecialized atrial fibers is the site of a delay in conduction of excitation, which has important physiological consequences. This delay, which normally lasts at least 0.1 second, allows contraction of the atria to be completed before ventricular contraction is initiated. After this delay, the cells of the AV node depolarize, and the excitation spreads to the muscle cells of the ventricles via a specialized high-speed conduction system. The high-speed conduction system starts with the *bundle of His,* which then splits into the *left and right bundle branches* (Fig. 2–11). The bundle branches ultimately divide and subdivide into a complex network of specialized conducting fibers called *Purkinje fibers*. The high-speed conduction pathway cells, including the Purkinje fibers, also have the property of spontaneous rhythmicity, but they depolarize at a much slower rate, between 15 and 40 times per minute. Therefore, they do not normally serve as the pacemaker of the heart. The action potentials of Purkinje fibers are almost identical to those of ventricular muscle fibers, although they may show a slight Phase 4 depolarization.

The high-speed conduction system is located beneath the surface of the innermost layer of the

Electrocardiograms

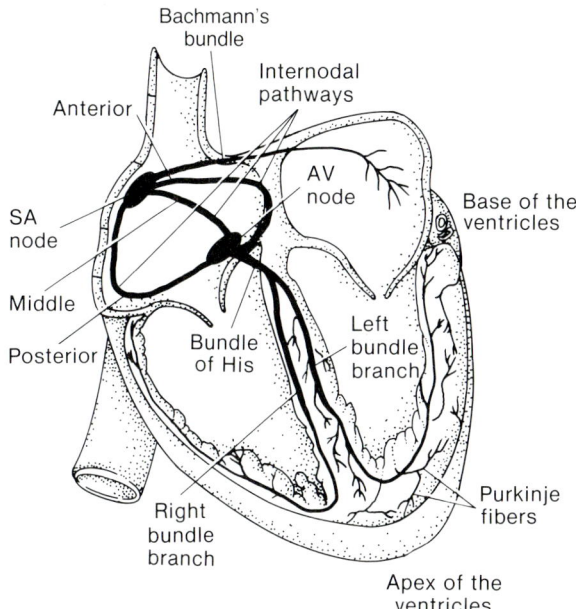

FIGURE 2–11. Conduction pathways of the heart.

heart muscle, the endocardium. Excitation of the ventricular muscle cells therefore occurs from the inner layers of myocardium to the outermost layer (the epicardium) by slower, cell-to-cell conduction. The events of the depolarization of the heart, including the velocity of the movement of excitation in the various portions of the conduction pathway, are summarized in Table 2–1.

Repolarization of the ventricles normally occurs from epicardium to endocardium, that is, in the opposite direction of depolarization. Repolarization of the ventricles also appears to usually begin in the apex of the heart and travel toward the base.

TABLE 2–1. Conduction Pathway of the Heart

Tissue	Spontaneous Rate of Depolarization	Conduction Velocity
SA node	70–80/min	0.05 m/sec
Atrial muscle cells	—	0.3–0.5 m/sec
Specialized atrial conduction fibers	—	0.9–1.8 m/sec
AV node	40–60/min	0.02–0.05 m/sec
Bundle of His and bundle branches	15–40/min	0.8–1.0 m/sec
Purkinje fibers	15–40/min	2.0–5.0 m/sec
Ventricular muscle cells	—	0.3–0.5 m/sec

Up to this point, we have really only considered the electrical activity of individual cardiac cells. The electrocardiogram (ECG or EKG), a record of the electrical activity of the entire heart, is usually obtained *noninvasively* (without surgery) by *electrodes* attached to a person's skin. These electrodes are connected to an electronic device, the *electrocardiograph*, which is essentially a very sensitive voltmeter. The electrodes are connected to the electronic circuitry of the electrocardiograph in such a way that one of the electrodes is always positive and one (or more) is either negative or neutral. The ECG obtained from any one electrode pair (or *lead*) gives information about electrical activity in one direction or dimension only, depending on the orientation of the lead used. Because the electrical activity of the heart actually occurs in a three-dimensional structure, it may be necessary to look at information obtained from several one-dimensional leads. This is the reason that the standard ECG has information from 12 different leads (see Fig. 8–7).

It is possible to record the electrical activity of the heart with electrodes placed on the limbs or chest for several reasons. First, the heart has a relatively large amount of electrically excitable tissue. Because the atrial fibers normally depolarize nearly simultaneously and the ventricular muscle fibers also normally depolarize nearly simultaneously, this activity occurs in groups. Second, the body is mainly an aqueous electrolyte solution, so some of the electrical activity is conducted throughout the entire body. The body is therefore termed a *volume conductor*. Finally, the ECG is extremely sensitive, measuring changes of electrical potentials of *millivolts*. Good contact must be made between the electrodes and the skin by using a highly conductive electrode paste.

The electrical activity measured by the ECG obviously is not directly comparable to that of the action potentials of *individual* cells. The ECG gives *summed* information from many cells at any instant, and the potential difference determined really shows the resolved *direction*, with respect to a particular frame of reference, of the movement of a wave of depolarization as it travels within the heart. The electrocardiograph machine is wired such that a wave of depolarization moving toward the positive electrode in any lead system gives an upward deflection on the recording paper or monitor. To understand the necessity for the various

48 CARDIOVASCULAR ANATOMY AND PHYSIOLOGY

lead systems, we must consider the depolarization of the heart in terms of *vectors*.

Vector Analysis

Vectors are linear representations of both magnitude and direction. They are frequently represented by arrows (Fig. 2–12A). The height or length of the arrow represents the magnitude of the vector, and the angle from the horizontal of the head and tail denotes its direction. Two or more vectors can be added, but because they have both magnitude and *direction,* their magnitudes can only be added as a simple sum when they are in the same or opposite direction (Fig. 2–12B). When they are not in the same or opposite direction, they must be added by graphic analysis (if drawn to scale) or by trigonometric or geometric means. For example, in Figure 2–12C, two vectors (labelled *a* and *b*) that are perpendicular to each other are added by graphic analysis to yield a third vector, labelled *c*. Vector *c* is of larger magnitude than either *a* or *b*, but it is smaller than the sum of the magnitudes of *a* plus *b*. The angle or direction of the resultant vector is dependent on the relative magnitudes of the two component vectors.

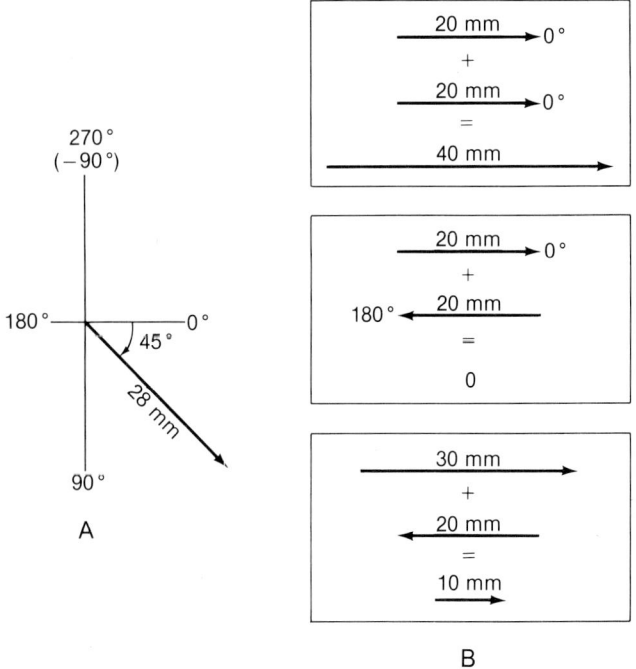

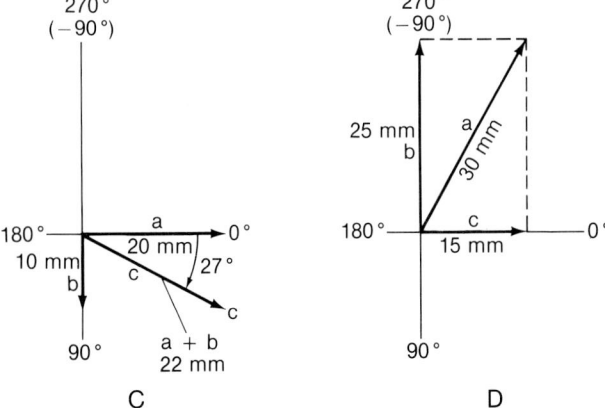

FIGURE 2–12. Vector analysis: A, Vectors have both magnitude and direction. B, Two vectors in the same or opposite direction add as a sum or difference of their magnitudes. C, Vectors A and B can be added graphically or trigonometrically to yield vector C. D, Vector A can be resolved into two vectors, one on the x-axis and one on the y-axis.

Conversely, a single vector can be *resolved* into component vectors. In Figure 2–12D, vector *a* is resolved into two component vectors, one labelled *b* along the y-axis and one labelled *c* along the x-axis. That is, vector *a*, which has a magnitude proportional to its length of 30 mm, can be thought of as representing a sum of one vector along the y-axis, with a magnitude proportional to its length of 25 mm, plus another along the x-axis, with a magnitude proportional to its length of 15 mm. When we look at the electrical activity of the heart by using a single-lead system, we are really resolving that portion of the three-dimensional depolarization of the heart into its component parallel to that particular lead system. We can therefore construct a three-dimensional picture of the heart's electrical activity by looking at information from several lead systems.

Lead Systems

The standard 12-lead ECG consists of the three *standard limb leads,* the three *augmented leads,* and the six *precordial* or *chest leads*. The standard limb leads plus the augmented leads are all in the frontal plane, whereas the precordial leads give information about electrical activity in the transverse plane.

Standard Limb Leads. The standard limb leads, designated leads I, II, and III, are depicted as an equilateral triangle (Einthoven's triangle) in Figure 2–13. They are *bipolar* leads—that is, one electrode is positive and the other is negative. In lead I, the left arm is positive and the right arm is negative. Because a wave of depolarization moving toward the positive electrode always gives an upward deflection on the electrocardiogram, electrical activity moving across the heart from right to left gives an upward deflection on the recording device for lead I; electrical activity moving from left to right gives a downward deflection. From the earlier discussion about resolving vectors into components, it should be clear that electrical activity moving from right to left gives the largest upward deflection in lead I; electrical activity moving from the head to the feet (or vice versa), that is, perpendicular to the lead, should give none at all.

In lead II, the left leg is positive and the right arm is negative. A wave of depolarization with components that can be resolved into primarily right-to-left and head-to-foot components should therefore give upward deflections. In lead III, the left leg is positive and the left arm is negative, so a wave of depolarization moving downward and to the right should give the largest upward deflection.

Augmented Leads. The augmented leads are arranged such that each one of the three limb electrodes may be made the positive electrode and the other two taken together are zero. Therefore, the augmented leads are *unipolar* leads. As shown in the triangle in Figure 2–13B, in lead aV_R, the right arm is positive, and the left arm and leg taken together are zero. In lead aV_L, the left arm is positive, and the right arm and left leg taken together are zero. In lead aV_F, the left leg is positive, and the two arm electrodes taken together are zero. It should be evident by now that a wave of depolarization moving in the direction from the head to the left leg should give the largest upward deflection in lead aV_F and give small downward deflections in leads aV_L and aV_R. Note that the same four electrodes (the left and right arms and the left and right legs) are used in both the standard and augmented leads. The right leg lead is used as a ground. It is the internal circuitry of the electrocardiograph that is switched as one changes between leads.

Precordial Leads. The precordial leads, or chest leads V_1 to V_6, are arranged around the chest (Fig. 2–13C and D). In actual use, a single *exploring electrode* is usually moved to each of the standard positions. The three limb leads taken together are the zero reference, which is called the *central terminal*. The precordial leads are therefore unipolar, like the augmented leads. The arrangement of the precordial leads gives information in the transverse plane (Fig. 2–13D).

Leads other than the standard 12 leads may be used in certain circumstances. For example, the MCL_1 *lead* is often used in emergency and critical care situations. In this lead, the negative electrode is placed near the left shoulder, usually under the outer third of the left clavicle; the positive lead is placed near the right nipple; and the ground is usually placed below the right pectoral muscle.

The Normal Electrocardiogram

The main features—or *waves, complexes,* and *intervals*—of a normal ECG taken from lead II are shown in Figure 2–14. Certain conventions are followed so that unless there is information to the contrary, all ECGs are standardized. Paper moves from right to left at 25 mm per second, which is equal to 1,500 mm per minute. ECG paper is ruled in millimeters, with heavy lines at every fifth millimeter. Therefore, time is on the x-axis, with each millimeter representing 0.04 second and 0.2 sec-

50 CARDIOVASCULAR ANATOMY AND PHYSIOLOGY

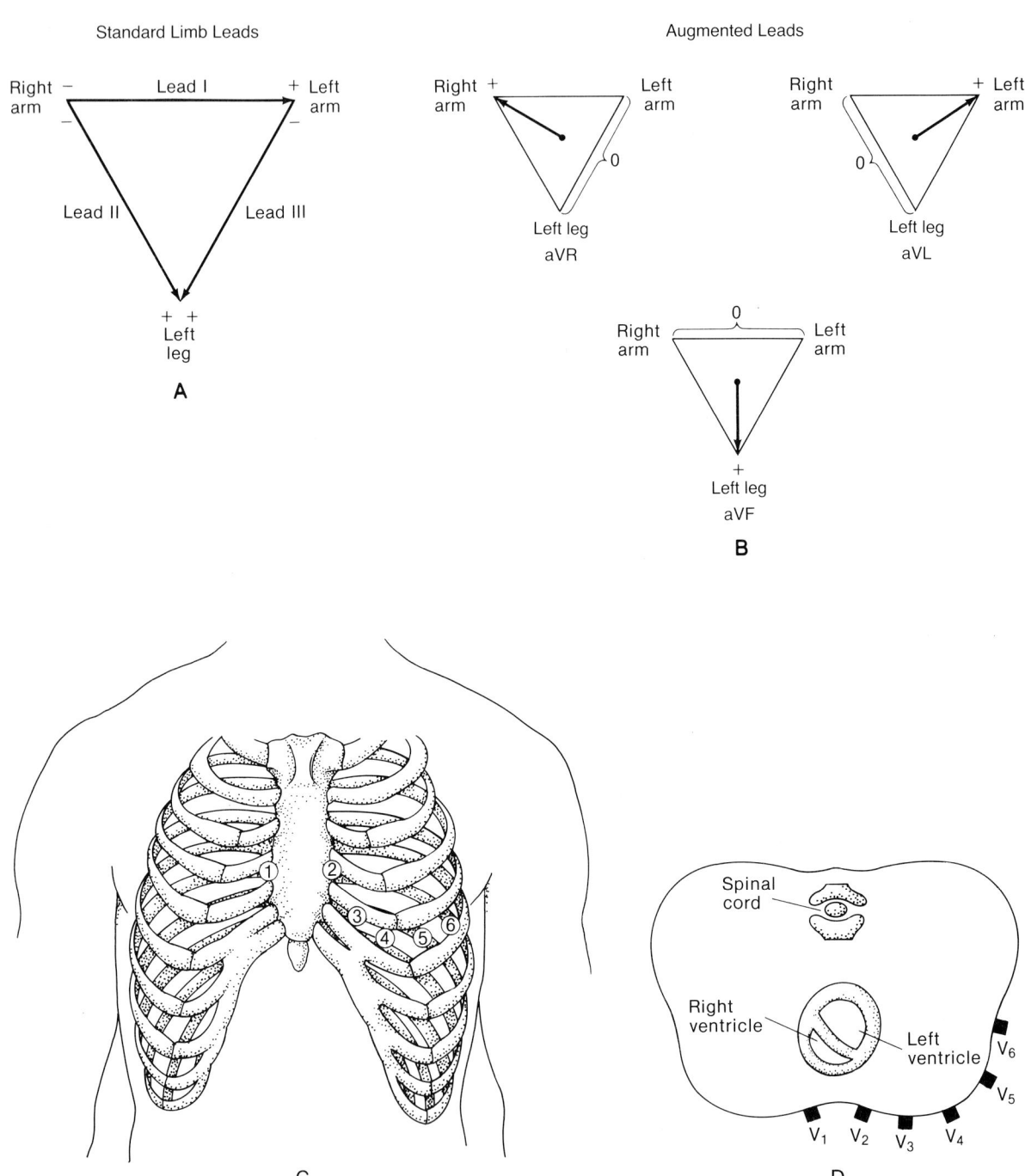

FIGURE 2–13. Electrocardiographic lead systems: *A*, The standard limb leads. Arrows show equivalent vectors. *B*, The augmented leads. Arrows show equivalent vectors. *C*, Placement of the precordial electrodes. *D*, Transverse section of the thorax showing placement of the precordial electrodes.

ond between each pair of heavy vertical lines. Marks are often seen at 75 mm intervals along the top of the strip, which are therefore 3 seconds apart. ECGs are also calibrated so that 10 mm on the y-axis is equal to one millivolt (mV). Therefore, each millimeter on the y-axis is equal to 0.1 mV.

P Wave. The P wave represents the depolarization of the atria. As already discussed, atrial depolarization normally begins in the SA node and travels from right to left as well as toward the AV node. The P wave is therefore prominent and upward in leads I, II, aV_F, and V_1 to V_6, and is usually inverted in lead aV_R.

P-R Interval. The P-R interval starts at the beginning of the P wave and ends at the beginning of the QRS complex. It therefore represents the time from the beginning of atrial depolarization, normally initiated in the SA node, to the beginning of the QRS complex, which is initiated in the AV node. The P-R interval therefore normally includes the 0.1 second delay that occurs in the AV node and allows atrial contraction to contribute to ventricular filling. All or part of the delay occurs after the entire atrial muscle mass has depolarized completely, so the *P-R segment* (between the end of the P wave and the beginning of the QRS complex) is on the line of zero potential, which is called the *isoelectric line.* Blocks in conduction through the AV node, which is discussed in greater detail in Chapter 8, may result in either a prolonged P-R interval or P waves not followed by QRS complexes. These are called *first-, second-,* and *third-degree AV block.*

QRS Complex. The QRS complex represents depolarization of the ventricles. The *Q wave* is defined as a downward deflection that precedes the upward deflection or *R wave. S waves* are downward deflections following the R wave. The QRS complex is normally sharply defined with no jagged edges. The *QRS duration* is usually rather short; that is, under normal circumstances the entire mass of ventricular muscle depolarizes rapidly because of the high-speed conduction system consisting of the bundle of His, left and right bundle branches, and the Purkinje fibers. Long QRS durations with abnormal-appearing QRS complexes indicate either blocks in the high-speed conduction pathway or ventricular muscle cell to muscle cell conduction caused by initiation of ventricular depolarization by an ectopic focus. The QRS complex is normally upright in leads I and II, aV_L, and V_5 and V_6. It is usually inverted in leads aV_R and V_1. This is because the resolved vector of ventricular depolarization, which is called the *mean electrical axis,* moves downward and to the left in the frontal plane and from right to left and usually slightly ventrally in the transverse plane (Fig. 2–15). The mean electrical axis begins at the AV node, then travels down the septum via the bundle

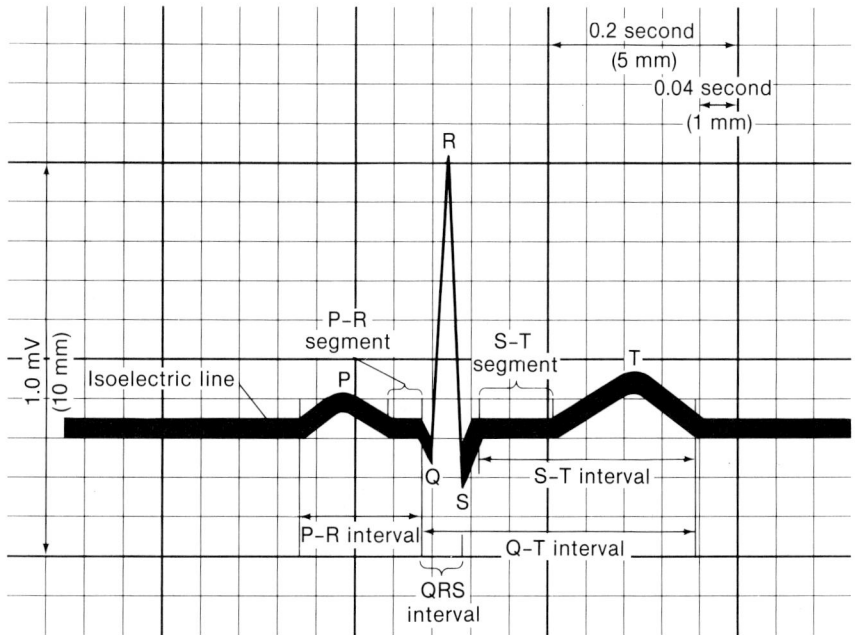

FIGURE 2–14. A normal electrocardiogram.

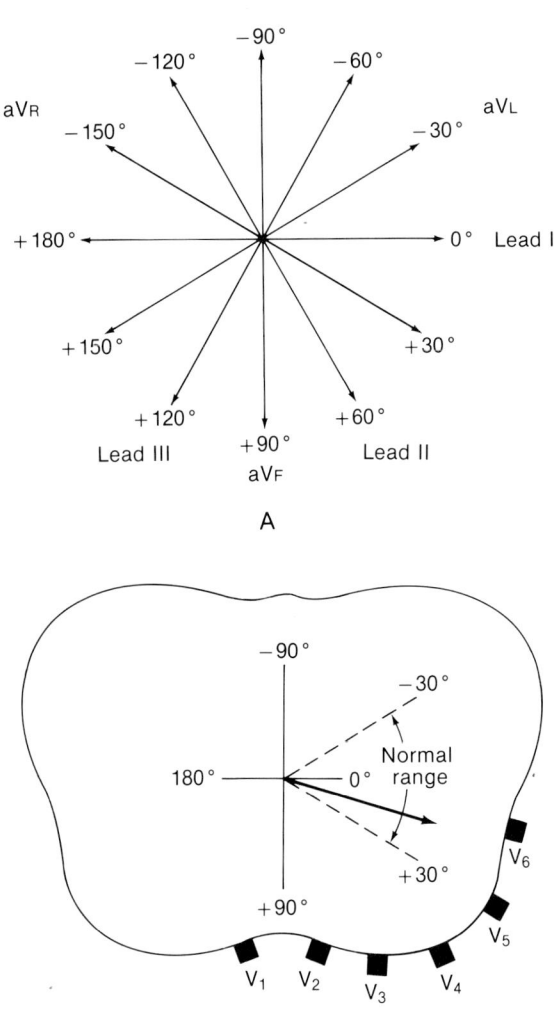
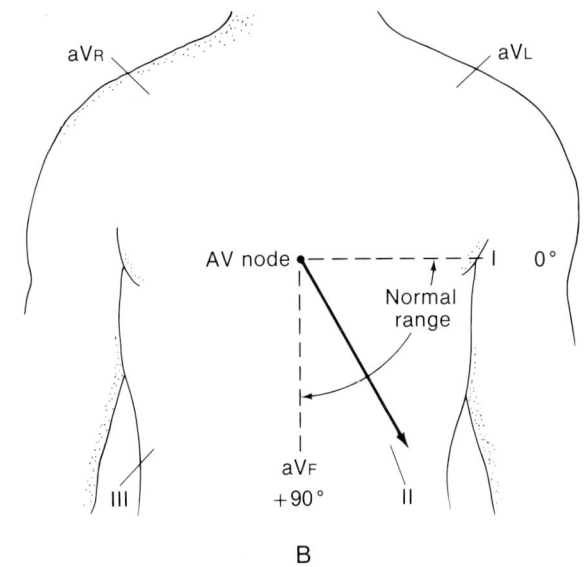

FIGURE 2–15. The mean electrical axis: *A,* The six frontal lead systems plotted together. *B,* The normal frontal mean electrical axis and its normal range. *C,* The normal transverse mean electrical axis and its normal range.

of His and the left and right bundle branches. The ventricular septum usually depolarizes from the left to the right, which gives the small Q wave usually seen in lead I. The apex and bases of the ventricles are then rapidly depolarized as the depolarization moves through the Purkinje fibers and finally by cell-to-cell conduction.

The mean electrical axis moves from right to left because of the leftward orientation of the heart in the chest, and because there is more electrically excitable tissue in the left ventricle than the right. Remember that as the ventricles depolarize, electrical activities of equal magnitude but moving in opposite directions cancel each other out and contribute nothing to the mean electrical axis.

The interval (in millimeters) between successive QRS complexes, which is usually referred to as the R-R interval, can be divided into the paper speed of 1,500 mm/minute to calculate the heart rate. However, this rate is not always the same as that determined by palpating the pulse because ventricular depolarization may not result in sufficient force development to open the aortic valve at high heart rates or in some disease states.

S-T Segment. The ventricles normally depolarize completely within a very short time, as noted in the discussion of the QRS duration. Once the ventricles are completely depolarized, there is no further ventricular electrical activity until repolarization starts with the beginning of the T wave. The ventricles stay completely depolarized for a substantial interval, as noted in the discussion of the long Phase 2 plateau in the section on ventricular action potentials. Thus, the S-T segment is usually fairly long, and it also falls on the isoelectric line. S-T segments above or below the isoelectric line may be seen during myocardial injury as a result of "currents of injury" caused by ions moving into and out of injured cardiac cells, as discussed in greater detail in Chapters 5 and 8.

T Wave. The T wave represents ventricular repolarization. It is usually upright if the QRS complex is upright. At first, this may seem odd because repolarization is the electrical opposite of depolarization, but as noted before, repolarization usually occurs in the opposite *direction* of depolarization. Repolarization is energy dependent and mainly a function of the movement of potassium ions. Any situation compromising the energy state of the heart, such as *ischemia* (reduced blood flow), or altering the potassium ion balance of the body, results in altered T waves. Atrial repolarization is not usually visible in the electrocardiogram because it does not involve much electrical activity and because it normally occurs during ventricular depolarization. Electrical evidence of atrial repolarization is therefore usually obscured by the QRS complex.

Vectorcardiography

As already noted, the instantaneously resolved electrical vector of both the atria and ventricles changes through the course of atrial and ventricular depolarization. Vectorcardiography gives *two-dimensional* information of the electrical excitation of the heart by tracing the changes in the orientation of the resolved electrical vector with time in the frontal, sagittal, and transverse planes. This is done simultaneously using combinations of leads that give two-dimensional information. For example, the frontal plane vectorcardiogram is obtained as a loop displayed on an x-y oscilloscope connected to lead I for the x-axis (right arm to left arm) and lead aV_F for the y-axis (head to foot).

THE HEART AS A PUMP

The process that converts the electrical activity of the cardiac cell action potential to the mechanical force of muscle contraction is called *excitation-contraction coupling*. To understand excitation-contraction coupling as it occurs in the heart we must briefly discuss the ultrastructure of the myocardial cell.

Myocardial Ultrastructure

Myocardial cells are composed of bundles of muscle fibers that are, in turn, composed of subunits arranged in a highly organized fashion. This organization gives cardiac muscle (and skeletal muscle) its characteristic *striated,* or striped, appearance. Junctions of cardiac cells are specially adapted for transmission of electrical excitation from cell to cell. These low-resistance connections between cells are called *intercalated discs*.

The cell membrane of the myocardial cell, which is called the *sarcolemma,* is also specially adapted (Fig. 2–16). Each sarcolemma surrounds numerous *mitochondria* (the main site of energy conversion to produce ATP), a centrally located *nucleus*, and bundles of muscle fibers. The muscle fibers consist of smaller units called *myofibrils* (Fig. 2–17). Myofibrils are composed of the *contractile proteins*, which are capable of causing the cardiac muscle to contract. The contractile proteins are arranged in a repeating pattern to form subunits of the myofibrils called *sarcomeres*.

Each sarcomere consists of two major types: the thin filaments, *actin,* and the thick filaments, *myosin*. The actin and myosin filaments overlap in some regions of the sarcomere, and the degree of overlap is related to the extent of muscle contraction.

The regions of overlap between the actin and myosin filaments are generally accepted as the site of the contraction mechanism. These *crossbridges* are believed to break apart and then form new bonds during contraction, allowing the actin filaments to slide between the myosin filaments. When the muscle contracts, sarcomeres get smaller as the filaments slide together.

The exact mechanism by which the *sliding filament theory* can account for the development of muscular force is not completely worked out, but one well-accepted hypothesis is summarized in Figure 2–18. It is well established that the thin filaments are constructed of several subunits, the major component of which is actin. Actin molecules, represented by the open circles, are arranged in two intertwined chains. Two chains of *tropomyosin,* with periodic *troponin* molecules, appear to be wrapped around the double actin chains. Each tropomyosin molecule appears to cover about seven actin molecules. The troponin molecules appear to be the site of action of calcium ions, which play a major role in the excitation-contraction coupling of cardiac muscle.

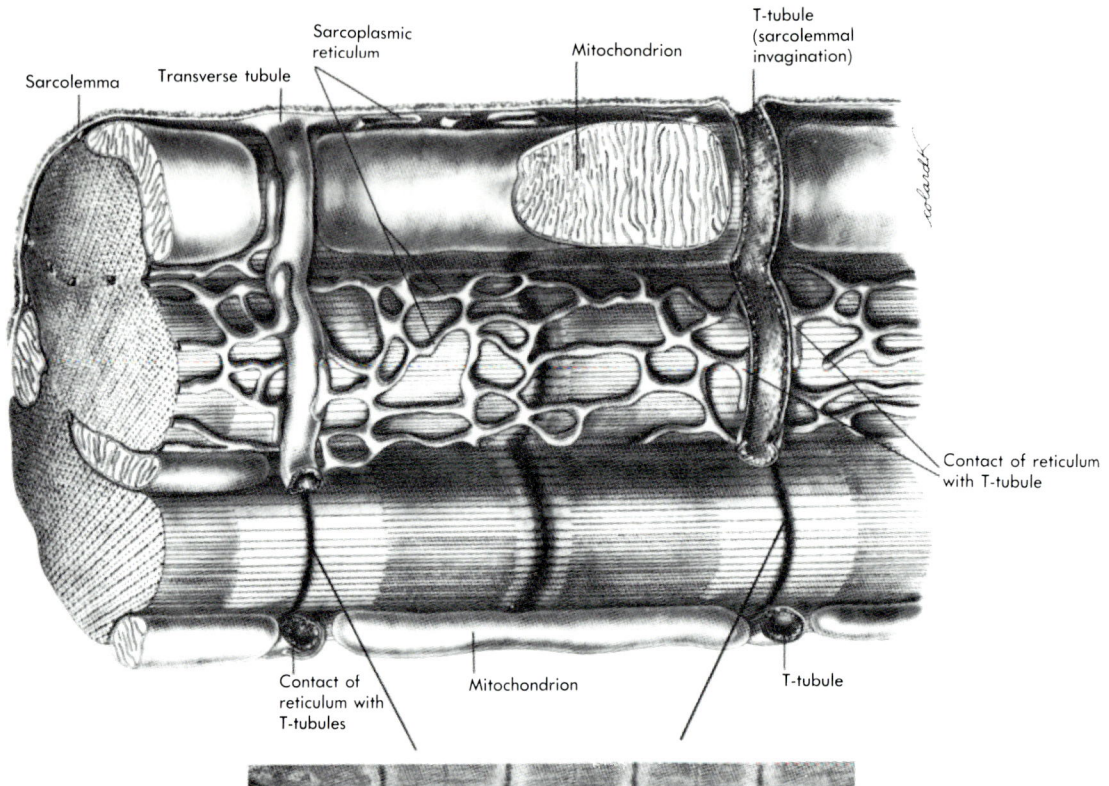

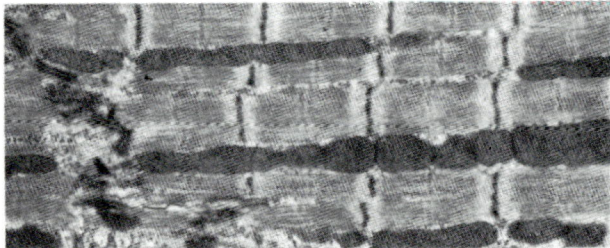

FIGURE 2–16. Detailed structure of the cardiac muscle. (From Rushmer, R.F.: *Cardiovascular Dynamics,* 4th ed. Philadelphia, W.B. Saunders, 1976, with permission.)

Excitation-Contraction Coupling

The process that converts the electrical activity of the cardiac cell action potential to the mechanical force of muscle contraction is called excitation-contraction coupling. When a wave of depolarization sweeps over the myocardium, the sarcolemma of each myocyte in the heart is depolarized because of both the specialized conduction pathways of the heart and the low electrical resistance to cell-to-cell conduction. As discussed in the section on ventricular cell action potentials, depolarization of the cardiac myocyte cell membrane increases its permeability to sodium and calcium ions, which then enter the cell from the interstitium. Figure 2–16 shows that the sarcolemma of cardiac myocytes is highly organized, with deep invaginations into the fibrils. These invaginations are called *transverse tubules,* or simply *T-tubules,* and their lumens are continuous with the interstitial fluid. When the sarcolemma is depolarized, the T-tubules also depolarize and become more permeable to calcium ions, thus allowing calcium ions to enter the myofibrils.

Also shown in Figure 2–16 is a network of intracellular organelles called the *sarcoplasmic reticulum*. The sarcoplasmic reticulum does not appear to be continuous with the sarcolemma or the T-tubule system, but it does appear to make close contact with the T-tubule system at the blind sacs shown in the figure. The sarcoplasmic reticulum is the major intracellular site of storage and reuptake of calcium ions. When the T-tubules depolarize, the sarcoplasmic reticulum depolarizes too, and it releases calcium ions into the interior of the myofibrils.

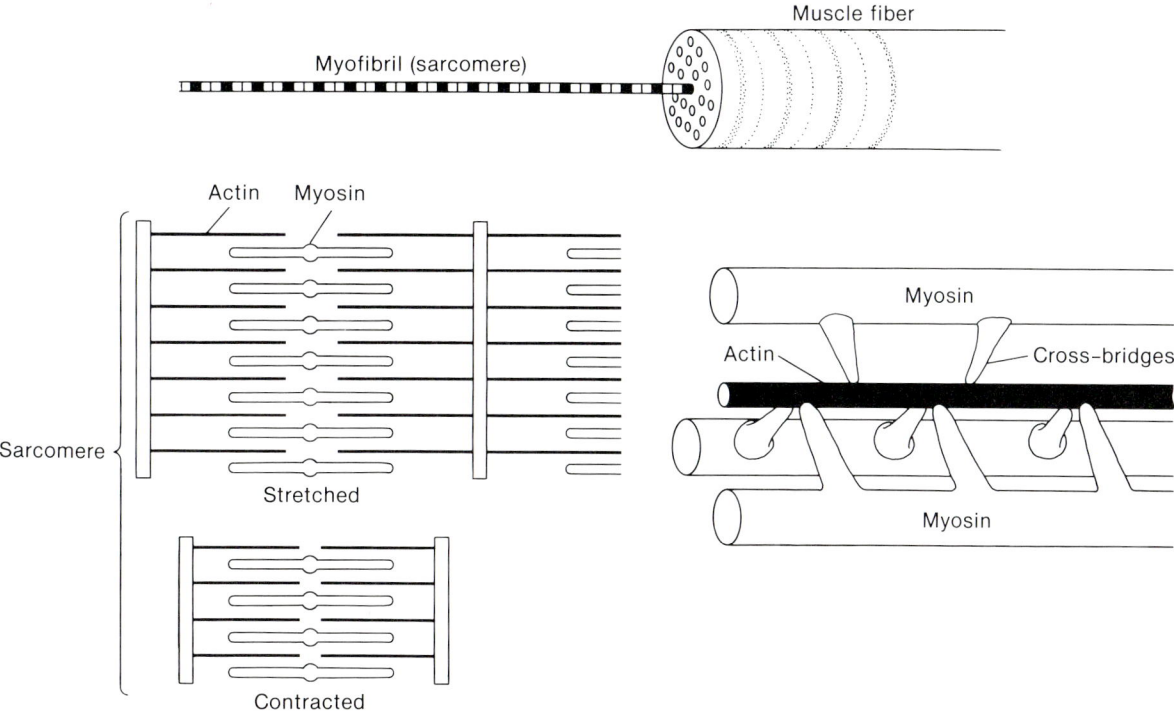

FIGURE 2–17. Diagram of the cardiac muscle contraction mechanism. The muscle fiber is composed of myofibrils. The myofibrils are constructed of actin (thin filaments) and myosin (thick filaments), which are arranged so that the actin filaments slide between the myosin filaments, as shown in the lower portion of the figure. The actin and myosin filaments form, break, and reform cross-bridges to generate contractile force. (Adapted from Rushmer, R.F.: *Cardiovascular Dynamics,* 4th ed. Philadelphia, W.B. Saunders, 1976, with permission.)

Mechanism of Cardiac Contraction and Relaxation

Cross-bridges occur in regions of overlap between the actin and myosin filaments and are presumed to be the site of the contraction mechanism. The calcium ions released from the T-tubules and sarcoplasmic reticulum bind to the troponin molecules of the actin filaments (see Fig. 2–18). The binding of calcium ions to the troponin triggers the sliding of the thin filaments by causing conformational changes in the contractile proteins that

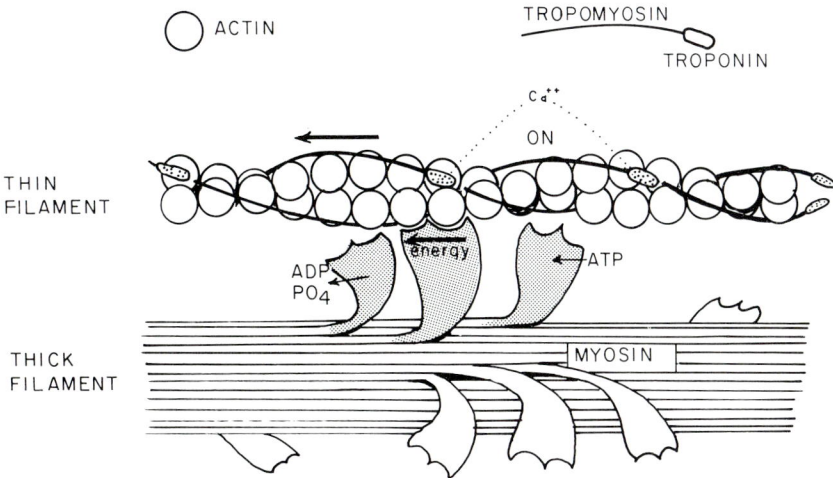

FIGURE 2–18. Diagram of the cardiac muscle contraction mechanism. Calcium ions released from the sarcoplasmic reticulum and T-tubules bind with troponin and activate the formation of cross-bridges between the thin filaments and thick filaments. (From Rushmer, R.F.: *Cardiovascular Dynamics,* 4th ed. Philadelphia, W.B. Saunders, 1976, with permission.)

allow cross-bridges to be broken and to form again. The cross-bridges are thought to attach to the actin molecules, rotate or swivel, and then break again. This process is repeated many times, thus sliding the thin filaments along the myosin filaments and causing the muscle to contract. The energy necessary for this process is supplied by the hydrolysis of ATP, converting it to ADP and an inorganic phosphate, as shown in Figure 2–18.

Relaxation of cardiac muscle occurs when calcium ions are returned to the sarcoplasmic reticulum, T-tubules, or the outside of the cell. This is accomplished against a concentration gradient and therefore requires an energy-dependent active pump. Again, the energy is supplied by the hydrolysis of ATP.

The Cardiac Cycle

Having discussed the electrical and mechanical activity of the heart, as well as the structure of the cardiovascular system, we can now look at the sequence of events in the cardiac cycle shown in Figure 2–19. Although the figure is based on the data from an experiment done on an anesthetized dog, except for the values for volume and blood flow, the data are similar to values obtained from humans.

The cardiac cycle is divided into two phases, systole and diastole. Systole is the time during which blood is ejected from the ventricles; during diastole, the ventricles relax and fill with blood.

The top panel of Figure 2–19 shows the time course of the changes in pressures that were measured in the aorta, left ventricle, and left atrium during a complete cycle of the heart at a resting heart rate. The next panel shows the *phasic* (that is, instantaneous rather than mean) blood flow through the root of the aorta as it was measured by using an electromagnetic flow probe implanted around the root of the aorta. The third panel shows the changes in left ventricular volume through the course of the cardiac cycle, and the fourth panel shows a phonocardiographic record of the heart sounds. The bottom panel shows the electrocardiogram, which provides us with a convenient time reference. Note the time scale on the x-axis. The entire cycle takes about 0.8 second, corresponding to a heart rate of about 75/minute.

Diastole

The events of the cardiac cycle are normally initiated with the spontaneous depolarization of the

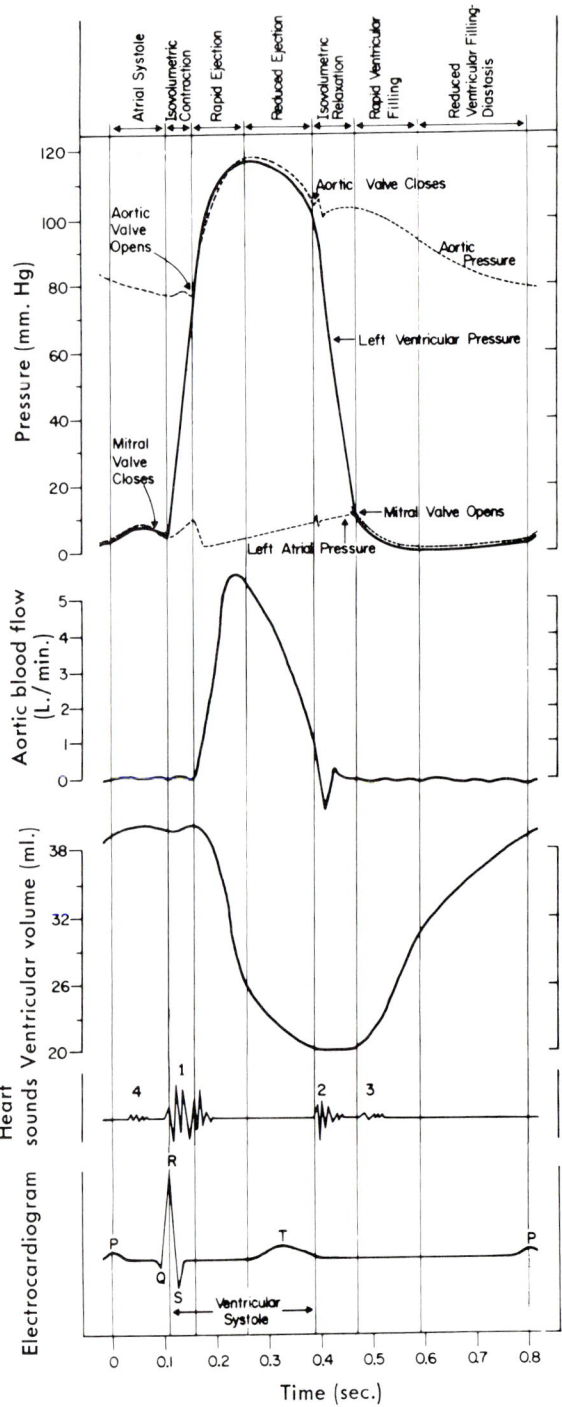

FIGURE 2–19. The cardiac cycle. Shown are the aortic, left ventricular, and left atrial pressures; aortic blood flow; left ventricular volume; a phonocardiograph of heart sounds; and the electrocardiogram. (Reproduced by permission from: Berne, R.M., and Levy, M.N.: *Cardiovascular Physiology*, 4th ed. St. Louis, 1981, The C.V. Mosby Co.)

SA node. Before the SA node causes atrial depolarization, resulting in the appearance of the P wave in the ECG, the entire heart is relaxed.

During diastole, the pressure in the aorta is much greater than the pressure in the left ventricle, as can be seen at right in the figure. The left ventricle is normally very compliant when the muscle fibers are not contracting, and even though there is a large volume of blood in the ventricle at the end of diastole, the left ventricular end-diastolic pressure is nearly zero (see Fig. 2–19). On the other hand, aortic diastolic pressure is much higher, about 80 mmHg, because blood ejected into the arterial tree during left ventricular contraction (*systole*) flows through the resistance vessels slowly. The greater the arteriolar tone, the more slowly the blood flows into the capillary beds. A second factor maintaining aortic diastolic pressure higher than left ventricular diastolic pressure is the elastic recoil of the aorta and large arterial vessels (see Fig. 2–4). Because the aortic pressure is higher than left ventricular pressure during diastole, the aortic valve remains closed. There is little or no aortic blood flow indicated in the figure at the end of diastole. This is in part due to the placement of the flow probe around the most proximal part of the aorta.

Left atrial pressure is slightly higher than left ventricular pressure during diastole, so the mitral valve remains open. The left ventricle fills continuously through diastole (because blood flows continuously from the pulmonary veins), even before atrial contraction. In fact, atrial contraction is probably normally responsible for less than 25% of left ventricular filling. Most of the increase in ventricular volume occurs during early diastole (labelled "rapid ventricular filling" in Fig. 2–19). Much less ventricular filling occurs in late diastole (labelled "reduced ventricular filling" or "diastasis" in Fig. 2–19).

Systemic venous return to the right atrium and ventricle is continuous during diastole. The right atrial pressure is slightly higher than right ventricular pressure during diastole, so the right atrioventricular valve also remains open.

Atrial Systole

As already noted, atrial contraction is normally initiated by the spontaneous depolarization of the SA node. This results in a wave of depolarization spreading over the atria, which is reflected in the P wave of the ECG. After a delay of a few hundredths of a second, the atria contract, causing a slight increase in both atrial and ventricular pressures lasting about 0.1 second. Although there are no valves between the atria and the pulmonary veins and vena cavae, inertia of the returning blood probably prevents blood from being pumped backward into the veins. Note the very small increase in left ventricular volume caused by left atrial contraction.

As atrial relaxation begins, the atrial pressure falls. As soon as left ventricular pressure exceeds left atrial pressure, the mitral valve closes. This may occur merely as a result of atrial relaxation ("presystolic shutting" in Fig. 2–19), or more commonly, it occurs during the onset of ventricular systole, when ventricular pressure is rising rapidly ("isovolumetric contraction").

Ventricular Systole

After the aforementioned conduction delay of about 0.1 second, the AV node depolarizes. Depolarization is then conducted to all parts of both ventricles via the high-speed conduction pathway consisting of the bundle of His, the left and the right bundle branches, and the Purkinje fibers. Mechanical contraction of the ventricles begins very shortly after the onset of depolarization (the QRS complex), and the ventricles continue to contract until repolarization (the T wave) is essentially complete. The Q-T interval is often thought of as representing "electrical systole of the ventricles."

As the ventricular muscles contract, the tension they develop causes a rapid rise in ventricular pressure. The mitral valve closes (if there is no presystolic shutting) as left ventricular pressure exceeds left atrial pressure. The aortic valve remains closed until left ventricular pressure exceeds aortic pressure. Thus, there is a brief period of approximately 0.02 to 0.06 second during which the ventricular muscle fibers are contracting without any change in ventricular volume. This is referred to as *isovolumetric contraction* in Figure 2–19. The situation in the right ventricle is similar. There is a slight increase in left atrial pressure during left ventricular isovolumetric contraction as the mitral valve bulges into the atrium.

The aortic valve then opens, as left ventricular pressure exceeds aortic pressure. During the initial period, there is a great deal of blood flowing from the left ventricle, as indicated in the aortic blood flow trace. As right ventricular pressure exceeds pulmonary artery pressure, the pulmonary valve opens, so blood is also flowing rapidly into the pulmonary artery. This period is called the *rapid ejection phase*. Note the rapid decrease in ventricular volume during this phase. The rapid increase in aortic pressure is transmitted through the entire arterial tree (up to the arterioles) as the *pulse wave*.

The ventricular muscle begins to relax with the onset of repolarization, as indicated by the T-wave of the electrocardiogram. As it relaxes, both ventricular and aortic pressures fall. As indicated in the figure, this is a time of *reduced ejection*. During rapid rejection, left ventricular pressure is slightly higher than aortic pressure; during reduced ejection, aortic pressure may be slightly higher than left ventricular pressure. However, blood continues to flow from the ventricle into the aorta because of its momentum.

As ventricular relaxation continues, left ventricular pressure falls well below aortic pressure. Because the mitral valve remains closed until left ventricular pressure falls below left atrial pressure, this is a period referred to as *isovolumetric relaxation*. The same situation exists in the right ventricle.

When the pressure gradient between the left ventricle and the aorta reverses during isovolumetric relaxation, the aortic valve closes, and there is a very brief period in which aortic blood flow is reversed (see Fig. 2–19). This coincides with a dip (the *dicrotic notch,* or *incisura*) seen in the aortic pressure trace, as the aortic valve leaflets bulge backward into the left ventricle. This brief reversal of flow and pressure in the aorta is enhanced by the reflection of the pulse waves off the indistensible arterioles. The pulse waves therefore are transmitted all the way down the arterial tree to the arterioles and are then partly reflected back toward the heart. The brief period of retrograde (backward) flow in the aorta and the incisura in the aortic pressure trace therefore occur because of the simultaneous fall of left ventricular pressure below aortic pressure and the coincident arrival of the reflected pressure wave.

As blood continues to return from the systemic and pulmonary veins, the atria fill and atrial pressure rises, as seen throughout the ventricular ejection phases and isovolumetric relaxation phase in Figure 2–19. As the ventricular pressure continues to fall, left atrial pressure soon exceeds left ventricular pressure, and the mitral valve opens. The same situation is occurring in the right ventricle, so the tricuspid valve also opens. As soon as the mitral valve opens, there is a period of *rapid ventricular filling,* as can be seen in the ventricular volume trace in the figure. This is followed by a phase of *reduced ventricular filling,* or *diastasis*. During diastasis, aortic pressure continues to fall as blood flows through the arterioles and out of the arterial tree into the capillary beds. At this point, the cardiac cycle has been completed. Remember that this entire process takes less than one second and may take much less time at higher heart rates.

Heart Sounds

Heart sounds are produced by vibrations in the heart muscle, valves, blood vessels, or the blood itself. Heart sounds have important diagnostic uses. They may be heard with a stethoscope or amplified electronically and displayed graphically with a phonocardiograph (see Fig. 2–19).

The first heart sound, S_1, probably originates with vibrations from the contracting heart muscle and with the closure of the atrioventricular valves and the opening of the semilunar valves (the aortic and pulmonary valves). The second sound, S_2, represents closure of the semilunar valves and the reversal of blood flow in the aorta. The third heart sound, S_3, is usually only heard in children and is probably related to the rapid inflow of blood into the ventricles. The fourth heart sound, S_4, is rarely audible and is related to atrial contraction. Heart *murmurs* are abnormal audible vibrations caused by turbulent blood flow in pathologic states such as valvular *stenosis* (valvular narrowing). Some of the conditions associated with heart murmurs are discussed in Chapter 5.

Ventricular Function

In our discussion of the cardiac cycle, we saw that the left and right ventricles provide the force for the movement of blood flow through the systemic and pulmonary circulations, respectively. In order to understand the physiology and pathophysiology of the cardiovascular system, we must therefore discuss the factors that can determine or modify the function of the ventricles. Most of the work done on the determinants of cardiac function has been concerned with left ventricular performance, because the left ventricle must develop higher pressures than the right ventricle and because problems in left ventricular function occur more frequently and are usually more dramatic than those of right ventricular function. While focusing on left ventricular function, we will assume that the same factors also affect right ventricular function in a similar manner.

Length-Tension Relationship

The force developed by the contraction of cardiac muscle is dependent on the *length* of the muscle before it contracts from depolarization and subsequent excitation-contraction coupling. As can be seen in Figure 2–20, as initial fiber length increases, the force developed during ventricular *systole* (measured as *peak systolic wall tension* or *intraventricular systolic pressure*) increases. Note that there is a range of optimal fiber lengths, above which further increases in length result in decreased force development. The cardiac muscle length-tension relationship is frequently referred to as the *Frank-Starling relationship,* after the two physiologists credited with its discovery. It is also called *Starling's Law of the Heart*. Skeletal muscle shows a similar length-tension relationship.

Figure 2–20 distinguishes the effects of increased fiber length on both *active* ventricular tension development and *passive* ventricular tension development. The relaxed left ventricle is a distensible vessel, so stretching the ventricular fibers by increasing the volume of blood in the ventricle during diastole results in increased wall tension, which can be measured as an increased left ventricular diastolic pressure. This is passive tension development, caused by the elastic recoil of the relaxed ventricular muscle fibers and other structural components. As already noted, the ventricles are quite compliant during diastole, so diastolic ventricular pressure hardly increases until ventricular volume becomes very large. Note that compliance is equal to the change in volume divided by the change in pressure, and it is the *inverse* of elastic recoil.

The relationship between resting ventricular muscle fiber length, which we have now related to left ventricular end-diastolic pressure, and the active tension developed during ventricular contraction can be explained in terms of the sliding filament hypothesis already discussed in this chapter. If we assume that the tension developed by cardiac muscle is a function of the number of *cross-bridges* formed, broken, and then reformed between actin and myosin molecules, as shown in Figures 2–17 and 2–18, then it is easy to see how the initial length of cardiac muscle can affect its active tension development. The greatest tension development should occur at the range of resting fiber lengths that allows the formation of the most cross-bridges between actin and myosin.

The Frank-Starling relationship represents an intrinsic mechanism for the adjustment of the output of the ventricles in situations in which venous return to the heart is changing, or those in which the pressure the ventricles must work against is changing. For example, if pulmonary venous return to the left heart were to increase suddenly, we would expect an increase in left ventricular end-diastolic volume (and pressure too). This increase in what is frequently referred to as the *preload* of the ventricle should result in an increase in systolic force development by the ventricle and therefore result in an increase in the volume the ventricle ejects into the aorta on the next contraction. The volume per beat ejected by the left ventricle into the aorta (or by the right ventricle into the pulmonary artery) is called the *stroke volume*. The stroke volume increases in this situation only if the ventricle is operating at an initial volume that has its sarcomere length below the optimal range. Thus, the Frank-Starling relationship shows how the heart can increase its output to match increased venous return without any extrinsic influences, such as those of the autonomic nervous system.

If the pressure the ventricle must pump the blood out against were to increase, the length-tension relationship of cardiac muscle would allow for an increased force of contraction to meet the increased work load on the ventricle. The pressure the left ventricle pumps out against, which is often called the *afterload,* is the blood pressure in the aorta. When the left ventricle begins to contract, it must exceed aortic diastolic pressure to open the aortic valve, as in Figure 2–19. It must continue to exceed aortic pressure throughout the rapid ejection phase and it is nearly the same as aortic pressure until the aortic valve closes again. Therefore, the mean aortic blood pressure can be considered the afterload, and the work the left ventricle must do with each beat, which is called the

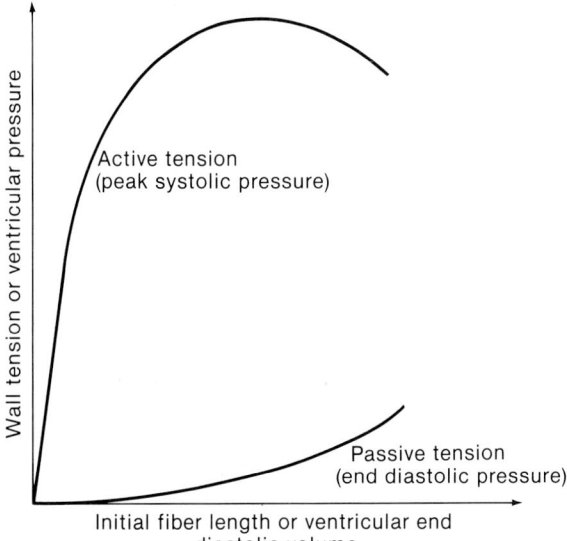

FIGURE 2–20. The length-tension relationship for cardiac muscle. Upper trace: active tension; lower trace: passive tension.

stroke work, is calculated by multiplying the stroke volume times the mean aortic blood pressure (or mean arterial blood pressure).

The afterload of the left ventricle increases if the resistance to blood flow offered by the blood vessels of the systemic circulation increases. This resistance, which can be described as the systemic vascular resistance, will be defined more precisely later in this chapter.

If the afterload were to increase suddenly, the work the ventricle must do to pump the same stroke volume would also increase. If the left ventricle performed only its normal amount of stroke work on the first beat after the increase in afterload, then the stroke volume pumped out on that first beat would be less than normal. If it started at a normal left ventricular end-diastolic volume and pumped out a smaller stroke volume than normal, the volume remaining in the ventricle at the end of systole, which is called the *residual volume,* would increase. Starting at a higher *residual volume* and assuming a normal venous return from the pulmonary circulation, we can predict that the left ventricular end-diastolic volume before the second beat would be increased. Therefore, the second contraction following the increase in afterload should generate a greater force of contraction to adjust to the increased workload. Thus, within a few beats of the heart, the length-tension relationship can compensate for the increased afterload, if the ventricle starts at a resting sarcomere length below the optimal range.

Contractility

Although increased resting fiber length causes an increase in the force of contraction generated by the ventricles, this does not represent an increase in *contractility,* as it is conventionally defined. An increase in contractility is defined as an increase in the active tension developed by heart muscle *at a given fiber length.* In the Frank-Starling mechanism, the increase in tension development occurs because the initial resting length of the sarcomere has increased. Strictly speaking, an increase in contractility (also known as a *positive inotropic effect*) occurs only when an increase in tension development is seen at the *same* (or even shorter) initial resting fiber length. This can be seen in Figure 2–21, in which a family of "Starling curves" is shown. Each of the curves represents a different level of contractility. Increased contractility occurs in response to increased release of norepinephrine by the sympathetic postganglionic fibers, which innervate the heart, or in response to epinephrine released by the adrenal medulla or in-

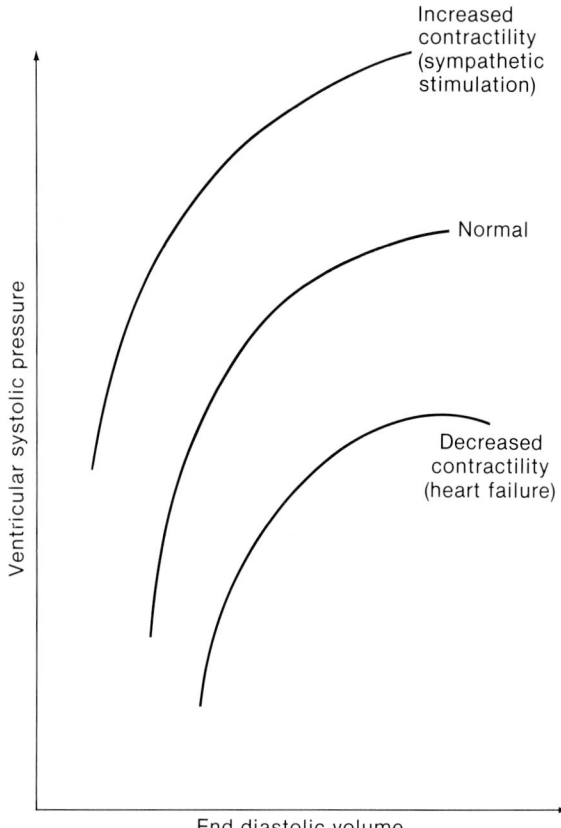

FIGURE 2–21. Representative ventricular function curves for normal, increased, and decreased contractility.

jected by a physician, or injected digitalis. Decreased contractility (*negative inotropic effect*) occurs when the ventricles fail as a result of poor perfusion (*ischemia*) or destruction of myocardium secondary to ischemia (*infarction*) or in response to adverse effects of drugs, toxins, or poisons.

Other indices of myocardial contractility include the maximal velocity of fiber shortening (V_{max}), which increases with increased contractility, and the *rate of change,* or slope of left ventricular pressure development (dP/dt), which also increases with increased contractility. The effect of alterations of contractility on dP/dt is shown in Figure 2–22. Another index of contractility that is used clinically is the *ejection fraction.* The ejection fraction is defined as the ratio of the stroke volume to the left ventricular end diastolic volume. The ejection fraction increases with increased contractility.

Control of Cardiac Function

We have now seen that the function of the heart is under both intrinsic and extrinsic regulation.

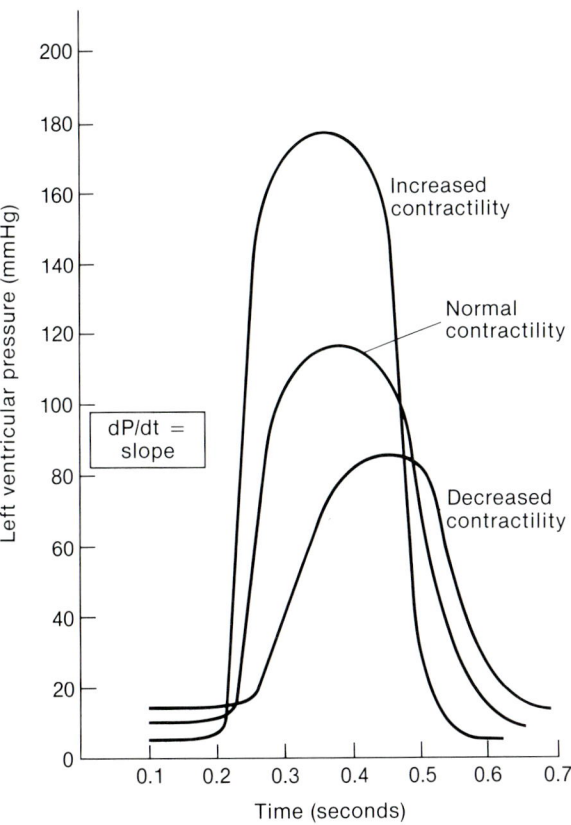

FIGURE 2–22. Left ventricular pressure curves showing the effect of increased and decreased contractility on dP/dt. (Adapted from Berne, R.M., and Levy, M.N.: *Cardiovascular Physiology*, 4th ed. St. Louis, 1981, The C.V. Mosby Co., with permission.)

The length-tension relationship represents one type of intrinsic control of cardiac function. There are other less important mechanisms of intrinsic control of the heart, including responses to increased venous return, increased afterload, and increased heart rate, which can be demonstrated in isolated hearts or papillary muscles, even though they remain *at the same fiber lengths*. These are examples of *homeometric autoregulation* of the heart because they occur at the same fiber length. The Frank-Starling mechanism represents *heterometric autoregulation* because it involves different fiber lengths. Homeometric mechanisms of myocardial autoregulation probably involve alterations in the ability of calcium ions to move into the myocardial cell interior.

In most cases, however, it is the extrinsic control of the heart that is the more important regulator of cardiac function. The autonomic nervous system acts as the final common pathway for many integrated responses of the cardiovascular system (such as in exercise) or for reflexes arising in the cardiovascular system itself or elsewhere in the body. These are discussed later in this chapter and include the *baroreceptor* and *chemoreceptor* reflexes.

The sympathetic nervous system influences both the rate of spontaneous depolarization of the pacemaker cells and the contractility of the heart. Stimulation of the sympathetic postganglionic fibers innervating the heart causes the release of norepinephrine and therefore increases the slope of the Phase 4 depolarization of SA node pacemaker cells (see Fig. 2–10) and those of the AV node as well, thus increasing the heart rate. In addition, the norepinephrine released by the sympathetic postganglionic fibers increases the contractility of the ventricles (as well as the atria) by increasing the permeability of the cell membranes to calcium ions. Catecholamines, such as norepinephrine and epinephrine, also increase the speed of conduction of electrical excitation in the heart and make all cardiac muscle cells more electrically excitable, which may lead to ectopic pacemakers.

The parasympathetic postganglionic fibers of the vagus release acetylcholine, which primarily acts to decrease heart rate by hyperpolarizing the pacemaker cells and decreasing the slope of their spontaneous depolarization. As already noted, this occurs by increasing their permeability to potassium ions. The acetylcholine released by vagal stimulation also decreases the conduction speed of electrical excitation, especially through the AV node. It also decreases the contractility of the atria and, to a lesser extent, the ventricles. Finally, we should note again that the heart is normally under both sympathetic and parasympathetic tone, so that alterations in cardiac function may be brought about by changes in the activity of either or both branches of the autonomic nervous system.

HEMODYNAMICS

The study of blood flow in blood vessels is called hemodynamics. Up to this point, only heart function has been discussed, and we must now consider the function of the blood vessels in greater detail. But before doing so, we must consider some basic concepts concerned with the behavior of fluids in general and blood in particular.

Pressure, Flow, and Resistance

The relationship of pressure, flow, and resistance for a simple liquid (such as water) flowing steadily (i.e., nonpulsatile flow) in *laminar* fashion through rigid unbranched cylindrical tubing is known as

Poiseuille's Law and may be written as:

$$P_1 - P_2 = \dot{Q} \times R \quad \text{or} \quad \Delta P = \dot{Q} \times R$$

where P_1 is the pressure at the beginning of the tube; P_2 is the pressure at the end of the tube; $\dot{Q}$ is the flow (the dot represents *per time*); and R is the resistance to flow offered by the tube. (Laminar flow is discussed in a later section.)

The centimeter-gram-second (cgs) units for measuring pressure are those of force per unit area, that is, dynes/cm^2. For flow, they are cm^3/second (or per minute); and for resistance, they are dyne seconds/cm^5. Clinically, the units used most frequently for the measurement of pressure are mmHg (millimeters of mercury or torr, after Torricelli, the inventor of the barometer). Millimeters of mercury can be used to express pressure because the pressure at the bottom of a column of a liquid is equal to the density of the liquid times the height of the column times gravity:

$$P = \rho \times h \times g$$

where P is pressure; ρ is the density of the liquid; h is the height of the column; and g is gravity. A column of mercury is used when high pressures are anticipated because mercury is the most dense liquid at room temperature. When lower pressures are anticipated, for example, in studies of respiratory system pressures, a column of water is used. Mercury is 13.6 times as dense as water, so a much smaller column can be used; on the other hand, a column of water expands the scale and improves the resolution of measurement of low pressures. One mmHg equals 1,333 dynes/cm^2. Pressures are also frequently expressed in units called *kilopascals* (kPa). One kPa equals 7.5 mmHg.

Unless specified otherwise, the reference for zero pressure is atmospheric pressure. When blood pressures are being measured, the zero pressure reference level is atmospheric pressure at the level of the heart (usually, the atria). We can now see the importance of this zero reference level: when we say that arterial blood pressure is 120/80 (systolic over diastolic), it is with reference to atmospheric pressure at the level of the heart. It should now be obvious that the arterial blood pressure in the feet of a standing person with a normal blood pressure is much greater than 120/80 because the blood in the arteries (and veins) form a column with a height equal to the vertical distance between the atria and the feet. Thus, the pressure measured in the arteries of the feet might be 210/170. Similarly blood pressure decreases as one moves above the heart, so cerebral arterial pressure might be only about 80/40. These differences are abolished if the person changes to the supine position, because the long "columns" of blood are no longer present.

Although we have stated that the cgs unit for measuring blood flow is cm^3/second, cm^3/minute or ml/minute or L/minute are used more conventionally. The usual units for resistance are therefore:

$$R = \Delta P/\dot{Q} = \text{mmHg/L/minute}$$

The unit mmHg/L/minute can be converted to dyne-second/cm^5 by multiplying by 80.

Thus, the total resistance to blood flow offered by the vessels of the systemic circulation is approximately equal to the difference of the mean aortic blood pressure minus the right atrial pressure divided by cardiac output. This is called the *systemic vascular resistance* (SVR) or *total peripheral resistance* (TPR).

The relationship $\Delta P = \dot{Q} \times R$ is analogous to Ohm's Law for electricity:

$$E = I \times R$$

or voltage equals current times resistance. The addition of resistances is also similar to the addition of electrical resistances. Resistances arranged in *series* (that is, those that all the fluid must move through successively) add directly. Resistances arranged in *parallel* (that is, those that the liquid can go through one of several branches) add as reciprocals:

For resistances in series:

$$R_T = R_1 + R_2 + R_3 + \cdots$$

That is, the total resistance (R_T) is equal to the sum of the individual resistances.

For resistances in parallel:

$$1/R_T = 1/R_1 + 1/R_2 + 1/R_3 + \cdots$$

That is, one over the total resistance (R_T) is equal to the sum of the reciprocals of the individual resistances.

This is an important concept to understand. For example, if we have four tubes, each with a resistance of 1 dyne-second/cm^5, and they are arranged *in series*, the total resistance offered by the four tubes is equal to 4 dyne-seconds/cm^5. On the other hand, if they are arranged *in parallel*, the total resistance (R_T) equals:

$1/R_T$ = 1/1 dyne-second/cm^5

   + 1/1 dyne-second/cm^5

   + 1/1 dyne-second/cm^5

   + 1/1 dyne-second/cm^5

$1/R_T$ = 4/1 dyne-second/cm^5

R_T = 1/4 dyne-second/cm^5

Determinants of Resistance—Poiseuille's Law

In 1846, the French physician Poiseuille summarized the results of experiments he had done on liquids, such as water, flowing steadily through unbranched rigid glass tubes, with the formula $\Delta P = \dot{Q} \times R$. He found that the factors that determine resistance in this situation could be expressed as:

$$R = \frac{8\eta l}{\pi r^4}$$

where η is the viscosity of the liquid; l is the length of the tube; and r is the radius of the tube. The resistance the tube offers to the flow of the liquid is directly proportional to the viscosity of the liquid and the length of the tube. The more viscous (defined later) the liquid, the greater the pressure gradient necessary to cause it to flow at a given rate through a given tube. The fact that the resistance is directly proportional to the length of the tube should be no surprise at this point because we can think of the length of the tube as comprising a number of smaller segments arranged in series. If we add more segments, we are adding more resistances in series, and the total resistance as well as the pressure gradient between the two ends of the tube should increase proportionately (Fig. 2–23). The viscosity of blood is dependent upon the hematocrit. At high hematocrits, blood becomes more viscous.

The most surprising part of the equation is that the resistance to flow is inversely proportional to the radius of the tube *to the fourth power*. This means that small changes in the radius of the tube have profound effects on the resistance to flow. If the radius of the tube is doubled, the resistance it offers to flow decreases to 1/16 of the original figure:

$R \propto 1/r^4$; if $r = 1$, then $R = 1$

$R \propto 1/(2)^4$; if $r = 2$, then $R = 1/16$

On the other hand, if r is cut in half, then the resistance the tube offers to flow increases to sixteen times the original resistance:

$R \propto 1/(\frac{1}{2})^4$; if $r = \frac{1}{2}$, then $R = 16$

As we will see, the influence of small changes in the radius of blood vessels on resistance gives the cardiovascular system a great deal of control over the distribution of blood flow. Small increases in the radii of blood vessels supplying body tissues that have increased metabolic demand can send much more blood to these areas at the same arterial blood pressure. Conversely, small decreases in the radii of blood vessels supplying nonessential tissues can divert blood flow away from these areas to more critical vascular beds in order to help maintain arterial blood pressure without compromising the perfusion of such organs as the heart and brain.

Another way of looking at the relationship $\Delta P = \dot{Q} \times R$ is to consider what would happen to the pressure gradient (or pressure drop) from one end of the tube to the other if the resistance were to change in a situation in which constant flow is maintained. If the resistance to flow increases because the radius decreases or the length increases, the pressure gradient increases—more of the pressure is dissipated or "used up" by the increased resistance, so the difference between the pressure at the beginning of the tube and that at the end of the tube increases. Conversely, if the resistance to flow decreases, the pressure gradient decreases, and the downstream pressure is higher and closer to the upstream pressure.

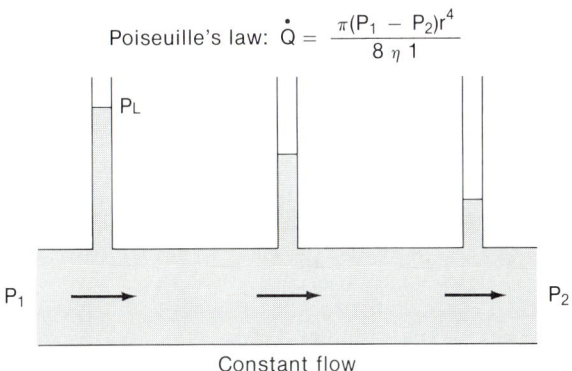

FIGURE 2–23. Poiseuille's law: Note that the lateral pressure P_L falls with length as a result of the effects of resistance.

Laminar and Turbulent Flow

At the beginning of the section on hemodynamics we stated that the relationship $\Delta P = \dot{Q} \times R$ is true only for laminar flow. *Laminar* (or streamline) *flow* consists of a number of concentrically arranged cylinders of fluid flowing at different rates. As Figure 2–24 shows, this telescope-like arrangement is such that the cylinder closest to the vessel wall has the slowest velocity, a result of frictional forces with the wall. The pathway in the center of the vessel has the highest velocity. We can now define *viscosity* as the ratio of stress to the velocity gradient. The stress is the pressure gradient, and the velocity gradient is the difference in velocity from one concentric layer to the next.

During *turbulent flow*, this orderly concentric flow pattern breaks down, and many eddy currents and vortices form (see Fig. 2–24). More important, the relationship between the pressure difference, flow, and resistance changes. The pressure difference required to generate the flow is proportional to the flow *squared*. Flow changes from laminar to turbulent when *Reynold's number* is exceeded. Reynold's number is determined by the density of the fluid, ρ, times the velocity of the fluid, v, times the diameter of the tube, D, and the viscosity of the fluid, η:

$$\text{Reynold's number} = \frac{\rho \times v \times D}{\eta}$$

Turbulent flow is said to occur when Reynold's number exceeds about 2,000. Unlike laminar flow, which is mainly dependent on the viscosity of the fluid, turbulent flow is mainly dependent on the density of the fluid. *Transitional flow* is a mixture of laminar and turbulent flow, which may occur at valves and branch points.

If one listens with a stethoscope over an area containing a major blood vessel that has turbulent blood flow, characteristic sounds called *murmurs*, or *bruits*, are heard.

The Bernoulli Principle

As already noted, at a constant flow rate, if the cross-sectional area of the vessel through which a fluid is flowing increases, the linear velocity of the fluid decreases. Linear velocity, in cm/seconds, equals flow, in cm³/seconds, divided by the cross-sectional area, in cm². Conversely, if the cross-sectional area decreases, then the linear velocity of flow increases. If the tube that a fluid is flowing through narrows, therefore, the linear velocity of the fluid flowing through the tube increases. The *kinetic energy* of the fluid moving through the tube is equal to ½ ρv^2, where ρ is the density of the fluid, and v is the linear velocity. Thus, if the linear velocity of the fluid increases at the narrow point, then the kinetic energy of the fluid increases.

The Bernoulli principle states that the *total energy* at the narrow point must be equal to the total energy at the larger diameter portion, if the energy used to overcome viscous forces and resistance is ignored (Fig. 2–25). If this is the case, then the *potential energy* of the system, which can be measured as the *lateral pressure* (the pressure pushing radially in the tube), should be decreased at the narrow point because the kinetic energy has increased.

We can measure the total pressure in a vessel by inserting a catheter so that the open end faces the direction of flow. The catheter contains a column of fluid (usually saline), which is connected to either a transducer or a column of mercury. In either case, flow in the portion of the stream impinging on the open end of the catheter falls to virtually zero, so all of the kinetic energy is converted to pressure energy.

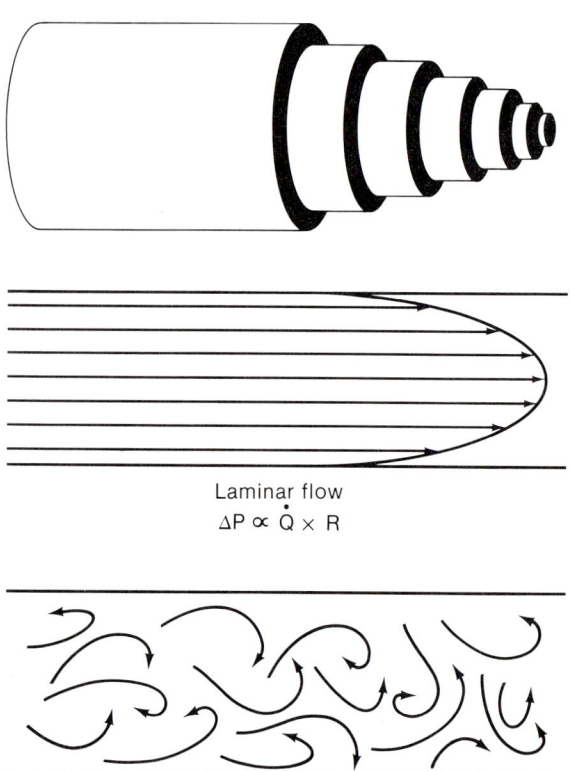

FIGURE 2–24. Diagram of laminar and turbulent flow. Laminar flow is represented by telescoped layers of cylinders. Those closest to the center of the cylinder have the greatest linear velocity. In turbulent flow, the orderly flow pattern is broken down.

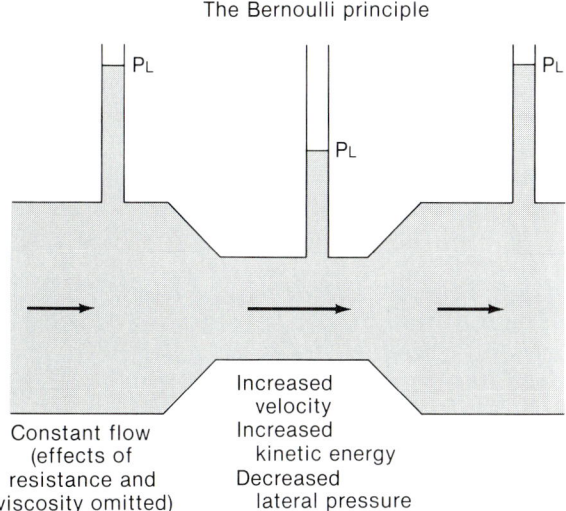

FIGURE 2–25. The Bernoulli principle: As the tube narrows, the linear velocity of flow and the kinetic energy increase. Because the total energy is the same (if we ignore energy lost to frictional forces as resistance and viscosity), lateral pressure decreases.

Laplace's Law

Up to this point, we have considered flow through rigid, indistensible tubes. The blood vessels, like the heart, are distensible and have elastic recoil. Elasticity, the inverse of compliance, is the physical property of a solid that causes it to return to its original shape and size after it has been deformed.

The relationship among the pressure, wall tension, and radius of an elastic cylinder was derived by the French physicist and mathematician Laplace around the beginning of the nineteenth century:

$$T = P \times r$$

where T is the circumferential wall tension; r is the radius of the cylinder; and P is the net pressure inside the cylinder (Fig. 2–26).

The net pressure inside the cylinder is called the *transmural pressure gradient*. It is (by convention) the pressure inside the vessel, P_i, minus the pressure outside the vessel, P_o. The concept of transmural pressure is extremely important to understanding both cardiovascular and pulmonary physiology. When the transmural pressure gradient increases, distensible vessels (blood vessels, alveoli, or airways) are stretched; their radii increase as does their elastic recoil or wall tension. When the transmural pressure gradient decreases, the vessels become smaller. Negative transmural

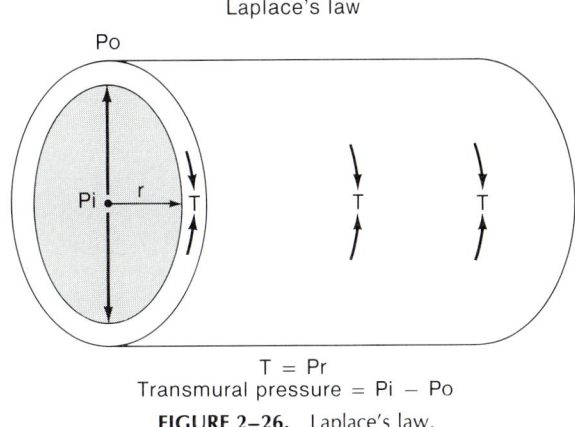

$T = Pr$
Transmural pressure $= P_i - P_o$
FIGURE 2–26. Laplace's law.

pressure gradients (outside pressure greater than inside pressure) may result in the collapse of vessels.

Pulsatile Pressure and Flow

Thus far in our discussion of hemodynamics, we have considered blood pressure and blood flow as if they were steady or nonpulsatile. However, we know from our discussion of the cardiac cycle that, at least on the arterial side of the systemic circulation, both arterial blood pressure and blood flow are pulsatile. Chapter 3 shows that, in the pulmonary circulation, blood flow may even be pulsatile in the pulmonary capillaries.

One effect of the pulsatility of the vascular system is that the Poiseuille relationship is only an approximation during pulsatile flow. Resistance is a meaningful term only during steady flow; during pulsatile flow, the capacitance of the large vessels, reflected pressure waves, and other factors must be considered. The term *vascular impedance* is used to denote the forces opposing pulsatile flow.

In the arteries, both pressure and flow are pulsatile. The pressure pulses are transmitted down the arterial tree much faster than the blood is flowing. The highly resistant and relatively indistensible arterioles reflect much of the pressure pulse back toward the heart and also damp out nearly all of the flow pulsatility. Thus, the blood flow and pressure in the systemic capillaries and veins are nonpulsatile.

The difference between the systolic arterial pressure and the diastolic arterial pressure is called the *pulse pressure,* which is the pressure felt when a person palpates the arterial pulse in a peripheral artery, such as the radial artery. A *sphygmomanometer* must be used to actually determine the systolic and diastolic arterial pressure, as discussed in Chapter 8.

The systolic arterial pressure is mainly determined by the magnitude of the stroke volume, the contractility of the left ventricle, and the capacitance or compliance of the proximal arterial tree, especially the aorta. Large stroke volumes, increased contractility, and decreased compliance of the aorta all lead to a greater pulse pressure and thus increase the systolic pressure more than the diastolic pressure.

The diastolic pressure is mainly determined by the resistance of the arterioles, the heart rate, and the reservoir function of the aorta. When the arteriolar resistance is high, blood runs out into the capillaries slowly and diastolic pressure stays high. Blood stored by the capacitant aorta during systole is released during diastole (see Fig. 2–4). This also helps keep diastolic pressure high. High heart rates prevent diastolic pressures from falling too far during diastole.

PERIPHERAL CIRCULATION AND THE CONTROL OF BLOOD FLOW

Now that we have discussed the physical factors that influence blood flow, we can begin to consider the control of the peripheral circulation and the distribution of the cardiac output. Like the heart, the activity of the peripheral blood vessels is influenced by the autonomic nervous system, humoral factors, and local factors.

Autonomic Control of Blood Flow

Both the sympathetic and parasympathetic divisions of the autonomic nervous system may alter the activity of blood vessels. Some blood vessels are innervated by both sympathetic and parasympathetic fibers; others are influenced by only one or the other. Another consideration is the relative importance of the autonomic nervous system in determining the blood flow to a particular vascular bed. In some organs, the extrinsic neural control predominates over local autoregulatory mechanisms; in others, local control predominates.

Sympathetic Control of Blood Vessels

The main integrating site for the sympathetic control of the circulation is located in the medulla oblongata, in an area referred to as the *vasomotor center*. There appear to be two anatomically diffuse but functionally integrated areas. The *pressor area*, which is thought to act via fibers that release norepinephrine to stimulate sympathetic preganglionic neurons, causes constriction of the arteriolar resistance vessels and the venous capacitance vessels. These adrenergic neurons are also responsible for increasing heart rate and myocardial contractility. The *depressor area*, which is thought to act via fibers that release serotonin (5-hydroxytryptamine), inhibits the activity of the pressor area. Thus, stimulation of the pressor area results in an increase in blood pressure (and may also increase cardiac output); stimulation of the depressor area results in a decrease in blood pressure.

As Figure 2–27 shows, sympathetic pressor and depressor fibers emanating from the brain stem travel down the spinal cord to terminate on the sympathetic preganglionic fibers located in different levels of the spinal cord from T-1 to L-2 or L-3 (T = thoracic and L = lumbar spine). The preganglionic myelinated fibers travel a short distance to the sympathetic ganglia, where they synapse with postganglionic fibers. The neurotransmitter in the sympathetic ganglia is acetylcholine. Unmyelinated postganglionic neurons then travel to the blood vessels, heart, and other effector organs, such as gastrointestinal smooth muscles and sweat glands. Almost all sympathetic postganglionic fibers release norepinephrine. There are, however, some sympathetic postganglionic fibers that release acetylcholine. Each sympathetic preganglionic fiber may innervate several postganglionic fibers.

The influence of the sympathetic nervous system on any vascular bed is dependent on the density of the sympathetic innervation of the blood vessels of that organ and on the types and number of *receptors* for the neurotransmitter released by the postganglionic fibers.

The arteriolar resistance vessels of most organs and the splanchnic and cutaneous veins are very densely innervated, and when the sympathetic postganglionic fibers to these vessels are stimulated, they constrict. This results in an increased resistance to blood flow in those organs in which the arterioles constrict, and a decreased storage or pooling of blood in the constricted veins. Therefore, blood is mobilized to help increase the car-

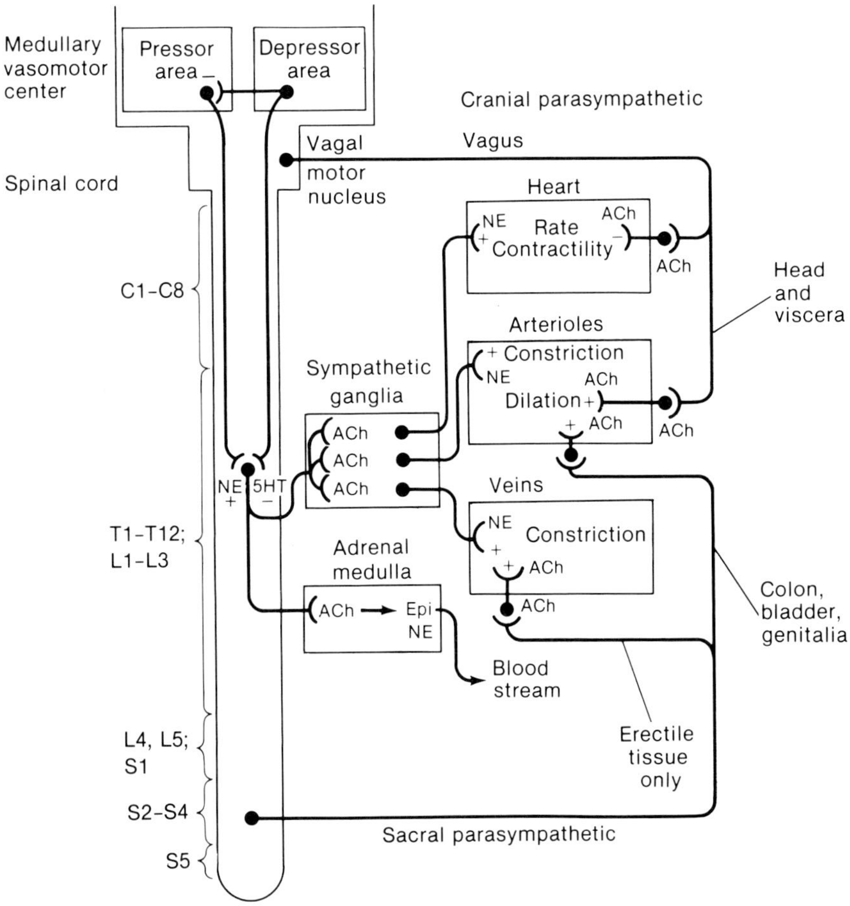

FIGURE 2–27. Autonomic control of the circulation: Note that the transmitter in both sympathetic and parasympathetic ganglia is acetylcholine (ACh). Sympathetic preganglionic fibers are stimulated by norepinephrine (NE) and inhibited by serotonin (5HT). Sympathetic ganglia are located farther away from the effectors than the parasympathetic ganglia, which are located close to the effector organs. Sympathetic postganglionic fibers release norepinephrine; parasympathetic postganglionic fibers release acetylcholine. The adrenal medulla acts as a sympathetic postganglionic fiber, with acetylcholine causing the release of epinephrine (Epi) and norepinephrine into the blood stream.

diac output, resistance is increased to help maintain or elevate arterial blood pressure, and blood flow is diverted away from the strongly innervated vessels to other vascular beds in which local control predominates. On the other hand, the sympathetic innervation of the coronary and cerebral blood vessels, the veins draining skeletal muscle, large conduit vessels, and the pulmonary vasculature are much less dense. In these vascular beds, local control or passive mechanical factors play a much greater role in the regulation of blood flow.

Sympathetic Adrenergic Receptors

Adrenergic receptors were originally classified into two types, *alpha* and *beta receptors*. Stimulation of alpha receptors causes constriction of the resistance and capacitance vessels in the organs in which they predominate. Stimulation of beta receptors increases heart rate and myocardial contractility and may dilate resistance vessels in the coronary circulation, in the skeletal muscles, and in the splanchnic circulation. Beta receptors are further subdivided into $beta_1$ receptors, which are responsible for increased heart rate and myocardial contractility; and $beta_2$ receptors, which cause dilation of skeletal, coronary, and splanchnic arterioles; systemic veins; and bronchiolar smooth muscle. Norepinephrine released from sympathetic postganglionic fibers or injected intravenously stimulates alpha receptors and cardiac $beta_1$ receptors, but it has greater alpha effects than $beta_2$ effects on vascular smooth muscle. Norepinephrine normally increases the vascular resistance of all systemic vessels, except for the cerebral and coronary vessels. Coronary vessels, which are strong *metabolic autoregulators* (discussed later), dilate in response to the increased metabolic activity caused by norepinephrine's positive chronotropic (increased heart rate) and inotropic effects. Norepinephrine released from the fibers innervating the bronchioles stimulates beta$_2$ receptors to cause bronchodilation, as discussed in Chapter 3.

Epinephrine is released into the blood stream by the adrenal medulla in response to stimulation of its sympathetic preganglionic fibers (see Fig. 2–27). Epinephrine released by the adrenal medulla or injected intravenously stimulates cardiac beta$_1$ receptors to cause positive chronotropic and inotropic effects, stimulates alpha receptors in most vascular beds to cause constriction of arterioles and veins, and dilates coronary, skeletal muscle, and liver resistance vessels by stimulating beta$_2$ receptors. After binding with receptors, norepinephrine and epinephrine released by sympathetic postganglionic fibers is either taken back into the postglanglionic nerve terminals ("reuptake") or destroyed enzymatically by monamine oxidase or catechol-0-methyl transferase.

Sympathetic Cholinergic Fibers

As already noted, there are fibers that originate anatomically from the sympathetic chain ganglia, yet release acetylcholine from their postganglionic fibers. These *sympathetic cholinergic fibers* can cause active dilation—that is, they do not simply decrease the adrenergically mediated constrictor tone, but they cause dilation independently. The sympathetic cholinergic fibers originate in the cerebral cortex, synapse in the hypothalamus, and descend into the spinal cord without passing through the medullary cardiovascular centers. These fibers innervate sweat glands (which have indirect effects on blood flow) and have also been shown to innervate blood vessels in the skeletal muscle of dogs and cats.

Controversy exists about whether sympathetic cholinergic fibers play a role in skeletal muscle blood flow in humans, but they could be involved in increasing blood flow to skeletal muscle as a person *anticipates* exercise. However, although human skeletal muscle does have beta$_2$ receptors and may also have these sympathetic cholinergic fibers, the major cause of increased skeletal muscle blood flow during exercise is metabolic autoregulation, as discussed in a later section of this chapter. Another possible manifestation of sympathetic cholinergic stimulation in humans may be seen in the increased blood flow to skeletal muscle that occurs during emotional stress. Sympathetic cholinergics may also be involved in blushing, but this seems more likely to be a result of profound sympathetically mediated vasodilation or venoconstriction. Pharmacologic modification of the sympathetic control of the cardiovascular system is discussed in Chapter 15.

Parasympathetic Control of Blood Vessels

Efferent fibers of the parasympathetic nervous system originate in two sites, the *cranial* and *sacral* divisions. The origin of the cranial division is the nucleus of the vagus in the medulla oblongata. It gives rise to preganglionic fibers that synapse with their postganglionic fibers near the atria, ventricles, and pacemakers of the heart. The neurotransmitter in the parasympathetic ganglionic synapse is acetylcholine, as was the case for sympathetic ganglia. As already discussed, these postglanglionic parasympathetic fibers release acetylcholine and inhibit the heart rate and myocardial contractility. Cranial parasympathetic fibers also innervate the blood vessels of the head and viscera, including the heart, gastrointestinal tract, and the lungs. Stimulation of the parasympathetic innervation of blood vessels causes vasodilation. As was the case for the cardioinhibitory fibers, acetylcholine is released in the ganglia by the preganglionic fibers and also at the vessels by the postganglionic fibers. Parasympathetic ganglia are usually located close to the effector organs, as opposed to those of the sympathetic nervous system, which are located in the sympathetic chain ganglia along the spinal cord and must send long postganglionic fibers to the effector organs.

The sacral preganglionic fibers arise from the spinal cord segments S-2 to S-4. They also synapse with their postganglionic fibers near the effector organs. Again, acetylcholine is the mediator both in the ganglia and at the effector organ. The sacral division of the parasympathetic nervous system innervates the blood vessels of the colon, bladder, and genitals and causes vasodilation. Each preganglionic fiber of the parasympathetic nervous system may synapse with many postglanglionic fibers. Blood vessels of skeletal muscle and skin do not have any parasympathetic innervation. There is no parasympathetic, cholinergic innervation of systemic veins, except for those in erectile tissues, such as the penis, in which it causes vasoconstriction. After it is released from its receptors, acetylcholine is broken down into choline and acetate by the enzyme acetylcholinesterase, which is found in high concentration in tissues with cholinergic innervation. Pharmacologic modifications of the parasympathetic control of the cardiovascular system are discussed in Chapter 15.

Humoral Control of Blood Flow

Many vasoactive substances are produced in one or more sites in the body, released into the blood stream, and then carried in the blood to act either locally, at another site, or generally within the cardiovascular system. Such blood-borne substances include epinephrine and norepinephrine (already discussed), angiotensin, vasopressin, bradykinin, prostaglandins, and histamine.

Epinephrine and Norepinephrine. When the adrenal gland is stimulated, both epinephrine and norepinephrine are released into its venous drainage. Much more epinephrine is released than norepinephrine; the ratio is about 4:1. The adrenal medulla releases small fluctuating amounts of epinephrine and norepinephrine under normal circumstances, but during severe physiologic stress, such as hemorrhage or heart failure, it may release very large quantities. Of course, in such a situation, sympathetic postganglionic nerve activity is also greatly increased. We have already discussed the effects of injected epinephrine, including increased heart rate, contractility, and excitability (which may lead to arrhythmias); constriction of most systemic arterioles; dilation of arterioles in the skeletal muscle and liver; constriction of systemic veins; coronary vasodilation; bronchodilation; and increased lipolysis in adipose tissue and glycogenolysis in liver and skeletal muscle. Epinephrine released from the adrenal medulla has similar effects.

Angiotensin. The terminal portion of the afferent arterioles of the glomeruli of the kidney consists of highly specialized secretory cells called the *juxtaglomerular apparatus*. When these cells are stimulated by decreased blood flow causing decreased blood pressure in the arterioles (the "renal baroreceptor"), or by decreases in the amount of sodium passing by the *macula densa* (a specialized portion of the distal tubules of the nephron), or by increased renal sympathetic nerve activity, they release the proteolytic enzyme *renin* from their secretory granules. Renin acts on a circulating plasma protein, the alpha$_2$-globulin *angiotensinogen*, to split off the vasoactive decapeptide *angiotensin I*. Angiotensin I is further modified by a converting enzyme into the more vasoactive octapeptide *angiotensin II* as it passes through the lungs.

Angiotensin I and II are very potent arteriolar constrictors and also cause a somewhat weaker venoconstriction. Angiotensin also acts by enhancing the response of the arterioles to norepinephrine and also generally increases sympathetic activity. Angiotensin stimulates the formation of the hormone *aldosterone,* which increases the reabsorption of sodium (in exchange for potassium) by the renal tubules. Finally, angiotensin stimulates thirst.

Vasopressin. Vasopressin is also known as *antidiuretic hormone* (ADH). It is formed by the supraoptic and paraventricular nuclei of the hypothalamus and travels to the posterior pituitary gland, where it is released into the blood. The main function of vasopressin is to act on the kidney, where it prevents water excretion and helps to concentrate the urine. Patients unable to produce normal levels of ADH suffer from *diabetes insipidus,* a disease characterized by the production of very large volumes of dilute urine. However, vasopressin is also a very powerful arteriolar constrictor and may play a role in the regulation of the peripheral vasculature. In normal circumstances, it is present in the blood in such tiny concentrations that it seems unlikely to be involved in the control of the cardiovascular system. However, in states of stress, such as hemorrhage, vasopressin levels are greatly elevated, and it may be an important means of maintaining blood pressure. Positive pressure ventilation increases ADH secretion, probably by decreasing the activity of stretch receptors in the atria that are believed to help control ADH release.

Bradykinin. Stimulation of sweat glands by sympathetic cholinergic fibers causes the formation and release of *kinins,* which are locally vasoactive substances. The enzyme *kallikrein* acts on a circulating alpha$_2$-globulin *kininogen* to form the decapeptide *kallidin* (lysin bradykinin). Kallidin is further acted upon by proteolytic enzymes in the plasma and tissues to form a smaller polypeptide, *bradykinin.* Bradykinin is a vasodilator that increases capillary permeability, resulting in extravasation of fluid.

Serotonin. Serotonin (or 5-hydroxytryptamine) is present in high concentrations in platelets and chromaffin tissue in the gastrointestinal tract. When it is released, it may cause constriction or dilation, depending on which vascular bed is involved and the prevailing local conditions. It helps mediate the vasoconstriction that occurs following the disruption of blood vessels. In the blood supply of the brain, it may act to cause vasospasms involved in migraine headaches. In the gastrointestinal tract, serotonin dilates arterioles, increases capillary permeability, and constricts venules and veins.

Histamine. Histamine can be found in virtually all blood vessels. Much of it is stored in *mast cells*. Histamine is released when tissues are injured. It acts to relax arteriolar smooth muscle, causing vasodilation; increase capillary permeability; and constrict veins. These combine to greatly increase the extravasation of fluid. Histamine's role in normal physiology is not clear, but it is certainly involved in allergic reactions, anaphylaxis, and the formation of blisters and welts.

Prostaglandins. All cell membranes contain the long-chain fatty acid *arachidonic acid*. Arachidonic acid may be transformed into a labile group of compounds called *endoperoxides* by enzymes called cyclo-oxygenases. From this intermediate stage, the endoperoxides may be converted into *prostacyclin, prostaglandins,* and *thromboxane*. These all appear to act locally. Prostacyclin inhibits platelet aggregation and is a vasodilator. Thus, it normally helps to inhibit the cascade of events that occurs in response to vascular injury. There are many different prostaglandins—in general, E-series prostaglandins are vasodilators, and F-series prostaglandins cause vasoconstriction. Positive pressure ventilation apparently causes release of vasodilator prostaglandins from the pulmonary circulation that may lead to systemic hypotension. Many prostaglandins are nearly completely removed from the circulation in only one pass through the lungs. Thromboxane induces platelet aggregation and causes vasoconstriction. It is therefore a major component of the response to vascular injury.

The effects of several humoral agents on the control of blood flow are summarized in Table 2–2.

TABLE 2–2. Humoral Control of Blood Flow

Factor	Effect
Epinephrine	Constriction of most systemic arterioles and systemic veins; dilation of arterioles in liver and skeletal muscle.
Angiotensin I and II	Constriction of systemic arterioles.
Vasopressin	Constriction of systemic arterioles.
Bradykinin	Dilation of systemic arterioles; increased capillary permeability.
Serotonin	Dilation or constriction of systemic arterioles, depending on vascular bed.
Histamine	Dilation of systemic arterioles; constriction of systemic veins; increased capillary permeability.
Prostaglandins	Dilation or constriction of arterioles, depending on the particular prostaglandin and the vascular bed.

Local Control of Blood Flow

Several organs have the ability to participate in the regulation of their own blood flow. That is, they possess a mechanism by which they can alter their own vascular resistance in order to increase their perfusion to meet increased metabolic demand for oxygen and nutrients. Vascular beds possessing this ability to *autoregulate* their blood flow can usually be demonstrated to maintain relatively constant steady state blood flow in the face of fairly large alterations in their perfusion pressure. Thus, as the perfusion pressure of an isolated organ capable of autoregulation and performing constant metabolic work is increased, it increases its vascular resistance to keep blood flow constant.

Similarly, if its perfusion pressure is decreased, it decreases its resistance by vasodilating in order to maintain constant perfusion. Of course, this ability to adjust vascular resistance to meet changes in metabolic demand or perfusion pressure can compensate for only a limited range of alterations.

The ability to autoregulate varies considerably from organ to organ. The coronary and cerebral circulations show the greatest ability to autoregulate; skeletal muscle is also notable for vasodilating in response to increased metabolic demands during exercise. Other tissues, such as the skin, show little ability to adjust their blood flow intrinsically. The resistance of these vascular beds is almost entirely under the extrinsic control of the autonomic nervous system. Finally, some organs, such as those of the gastrointestinal tract, show a balance between intrinsic and extrinsic mechanisms of blood flow regulation.

Several hypotheses have been proposed to explain the intrinsic ability of vascular beds to match their perfusion to altered metabolic demands and their ability to maintain blood flow in response to altered perfusion pressures. The most plausible of these is called *metabolic autoregulation*. If an end-product or by-product of the steady state metabolism of a tissue has the ability to cause arteriolar dilation when it diffuses near the resistance vessels, then it is easy to envision how blood flow can be matched to metabolic demand. If cellular metabolism is increased, then more vasodilator metabolites are released. This causes a vasodilation and increased blood flow to the tissue. If blood flow to the tissue is increased without a change in metabolism, for example, by increasing perfusion pressure, then the vasodilator metabolites are washed out of the tissue faster, and the resistance vessels are less dilated. If perfusion pressure is decreased, then the vasodilator metabolites accumulate more rapidly, and the resistance vessels dilate to increase perfusion. This is especially true if the vasodilator metabolites include some products of *anaerobic metabolism*. Thus, if the oxygen supply were decreased because of decreased blood flow, then there would be increased anaerobic metabolism, resulting in increased production of vasodilator metabolites.

This can be demonstrated by briefly occluding the blood supply to a vascular bed capable of autoregulation. For example, if a branch of one of the coronary arteries is occluded for about ten seconds and then released, there is a brief period of *increased* blood flow (greater than that before the occlusion), which is called a *reactive hyperemia*. The reactive hyperemia appears to make up for the period of no perfusion because the vasodilator metabolites that accumulated dilate the arterioles. When perfusion is restored to its original level, blood flow is increased because of the reduced vascular resistance.

Many substances or situations have been proposed as the mediator of metabolic autoregulation, including reduced oxygen supply, decreased tissue Po_2, increased Pco_2, increased interstitial fluid osmolarity, and increases in the concentration of lactic acid, hydrogen ions, potassium ions, inorganic phosphate ions, prostaglandins, and adenosine (a breakdown product of ATP). Quite possibly, there is more than one mediator or different mediators in different tissues.

Other mechanisms proposed to explain the constancy of steady state blood flow with changing perfusion pressure include the myogenic and the tissue-pressure hypotheses. Vascular smooth muscle contracts in response to stretch. According to the *myogenic hypothesis,* increased perfusion pressure initially stretches resistance vessels (probably the precapillary sphincters), causing them to contract and thus increasing vascular resistance. Reduced perfusion pressure causes them to relax, thus decreasing the resistance to blood flow. The *tissue pressure hypothesis* is based on the concept that increased perfusion pressure leads to increased movement of fluid from the intravascular space to the interstitium. Fluid buildup compresses the blood vessels, increasing their resistance to blood flow. Decreased perfusion pressure should have the opposite effect. The problem with the myogenic and tissue pressure hypotheses is that they do not really link blood flow to metabolism.

MICROCIRCULATION AND CAPILLARY EXCHANGE

Capillaries are the site of the main function of the cardiopulmonary system, which is the exchange of respiratory gases, nutrients, waste products, and other material. This exchange occurs between the cells of the body and the blood for the systemic capillaries, and between the blood and the external environment for the pulmonary capillaries.

Structure of the Microcirculation

We have already discussed the main structural features of the systemic microcirculation (see Fig. 2–6). (The pulmonary capillaries are discussed in Chapter 3).

There is a tremendous number of capillaries in the systemic circulation—at least hundreds of billions, probably trillions. The estimated total cross-sectional area of all of the systemic capillaries (note that they are mainly arranged in parallel) taken together is about 2,500 to 5,000 cm^2 (see Fig. 2–5). Although the systemic capillaries receive the entire cardiac output, the linear velocity of the blood flowing through them is very slow. Furthermore, as already indicated, the average diameter of erythrocytes (8 μ) is approximately the same or slightly greater than the internal diameter of capillaries, making it necessary for the erythrocytes to actively alter their shapes in order to pass through. The slow movement of blood through capillaries aids in the processes involved in the exchange between the blood and body tissues.

The number of capillaries per volume of body tissue, which is called the *capillary density*, varies considerably from organ to organ. In metabolically active tissues such as the heart, the capillary density is high; in less active tissues such as the skin, the capillary density is low. As already noted, the structure of capillaries also varies considerably from organ to organ. Capillaries with no known spaces or gaps between or within their endothelial cells are called *continuous*. Continuous capillaries are found in such tissues as fat and muscle. Some capillaries, such as those in parts of the kidney or intestine, have small openings or gaps called *fenestrae*. *Discontinuous* capillaries have large gaps between their endothelial cells. These gaps, which may be referred to as *sinusoids*, are found in the capillaries of the liver, spleen, and bone marrow.

At any instant, only a small fraction of all the systemic capillaries is open and perfused, depending on both the type and activity of the organ involved: Some vascular beds, such as those in skeletal muscles, show a great increase in the number of capillaries perfused during increased activity.

Factors Influencing Filtration, Absorption, and Capillary Exchange

The main mechanisms of capillary exchange are diffusion, filtration and absorption, and endocytosis. Most substances move through the capillaries by diffusion.

Diffusion

Diffusion is the *net* movement of a substance from a region of high concentration of that substance to a region of lower concentration. Fick's law for diffusion, given in Chapter 1, can be stated as follows for capillary exchange:

$$\dot{N} = DA\, dc/dx$$

where $\dot{N}$ is the quantity of a substance moved per unit of time (the dot over the N means "per time"). D is the diffusivity, which is directly proportional to the solubility and permeability of a particular substance in the plasma, capillary endothelium, interstitium, and cell membrane of the tissue cell; it is inversely proportional to the square root of the molecular weight or density of the substance. A is the area of the diffusion pathway, which is dependent on how many capillaries are being perfused. Finally, dc/dx is the concentration gradient (per distance) of the substance across the barrier.

For diffusion of a substance to occur across the capillary endothelium, the substance must be either soluble in the endothelial wall or able to pass through pores in the capillaries.

Filtration and Absorption

The movement of water or other liquids through the capillary wall and into the interstitium is called *filtration*. The movement of liquids from the interstitium into the capillaries is called *absorption*. The direction and magnitude of the movement of these liquids are determined by a number of physical factors, including how permeable the capillary is to the liquid and how easily solute particles (such as proteins) can pass through the membrane; the hydrostatic pressure inside and outside the capillary; and the osmotic pressure of solute particles inside and outside the capillary.

Small particles, such as sodium ions, potassium ions, hydrogen ions, chloride ions, and bicarbonate ions, pass through pores in most capillaries very easily, so they do not exert an osmotic pressure across the capillary wall. This is in contrast to the situation across the plasma membrane of *cells*, which are much less permeable to these ions.

Larger particles, such as proteins, do not pass through capillary pores easily, so they do exert an osmotic pressure. Thus, for cells, it is the ions that have an osmotic effect; for capillaries, it is mainly the proteins. The osmotic effect of proteins across capillary walls is called the *colloid osmotic* (or *oncotic*) *pressure*.

If we think about the factors that determine liquid movement through the capillary walls, we can group them into those that tend to push or pull the liquid out of the capillary, those that push or pull liquid into the capillary, and those that quantify how easily liquid and large solute particles pass through the capillary wall. Capillary hydrostatic pressure tends to push liquid out of the capillary, but the pressure in the interstitium tends to oppose this by pushing liquid back in. Plasma colloid osmotic pressure tends to pull liquid into the capillary, but the interstitial fluid colloid osmotic pressure pulls liquid out of the capillary. The relationship of these factors can be formally stated by the equation known as the Starling hypothesis:

$$\dot{Q}_f = K_f[(P_c - P_{is}) - \sigma(\pi pl - \pi is)]$$

where $\dot{Q}_f$ is the *net* flow of liquid per time. K_f is the capillary filtration coefficient, which describes the permeability characteristics of the membrane to the liquid. P_c is the capillary hydrostatic pressure. P_{is} is the hydrostatic pressure of the interstitial fluid. σ is the reflection coefficient, which describes the ability of the capillary endothelium to prevent solute particles from leaving the capillary. πpl is the colloid osmotic (oncotic) pressure of the plasma. πis is the colloid osmotic pressure of the interstitial fluid.

If $\dot{Q}_f$ is positive, liquid leaves the capillary, which is called *filtration*. If $\dot{Q}_f$ is negative, liquid enters the capillary from the surrounding interstitium, which is called *absorption*.

The Capillary Filtration Coefficient. The capillary filtration coefficient, K_f, varies from tissue to tissue, depending on whether the capillary endothelium is continuous or discontinuous, the size and number of pores present, and the number of capillaries open and perfused. Capillary injury caused by toxins or burns increases the capillary filtration coefficient by destroying endothelial integrity. Therefore, more liquid tends to leave the vessels. Capillary *recruitment,* that is, an increased number of perfused capillaries, also increases the capillary filtration coefficient.

Capillary Hydrostatic Pressure. The capillary hydrostatic pressure, P_c, is determined by several factors. The pressure on the arterial side is dependent on systemic arterial pressure and, therefore, the factors that influence cardiac output and systemic vascular resistance.

Generally speaking, if systemic vascular resistance increases, the arterial pressure increases, so we would expect capillary hydrostatic pressure to increase. However, if we consider an individual arteriole supplying a particular capillary bed at a constant mean arterial blood pressure, the greater its resistance to blood flow, the greater is the pressure drop across the arteriole, and the *lower* is the capillary hydrostatic pressure. Similarly, if its precapillary sphincter constricts, hydrostatic pressure inside the capillary falls. On the other hand, if venous pressure increases, or if the veins distal to the capillary constrict, then capillary hydrostatic pressure increases. Capillary hydrostatic pressure pushes liquid *out* of the capillaries. Capillary hydrostatic pressure falls along the course of the capillary because liquid leaves the vessel and because of the pressure drop itself. Because the oncotic pressure is fairly constant along the capillary, we usually think of every capillary as having some filtration at the arterial end and absorption at the venous end.

Interstitial Hydrostatic Pressure. In theory, the interstitial hydrostatic pressure should oppose the filtration of liquid out of the capillaries. In fact, this is the basis of the *tissue pressure hypothesis* of local control of blood flow, as discussed in a previous section of this chapter. However, the effect of the interstitial fluid pressure on capillary fluid dynamics has received a great deal of attention in recent years because studies have determined the interstitial hydrostatic pressure to be *negative* in many tissues, instead of slightly positive as was thought previously. No doubt, in some states, such as *edema* (discussed later), or in some regions of the body, such as those in which interstitial fluid collects because of gravity, the interstitial fluid pressure may be positive and oppose extravasation of liquid. On the other hand, in tissues with negative interstitial fluid hydrostatic pressure, filtration is enhanced by the interstitial hydrostatic pressure.

One major determinant of the interstitial hydrostatic pressure in a vascular bed is its lymphatic drainage. Under normal circumstances, the lymphatic drainage is sufficient to keep up with tissue filtration, so interstitial pressure stays negative or low, and liquid does not collect in the interstitium. If liquid leaves the capillaries faster than the lymphatic system can remove it from the interstitium or if the lymphatic drainage has been interfered with, liquid collects in the interstitium, a condition called *edema*.

The Reflection Coefficient, σ, depends on various solutes in the plasma and the relative porosity of the particular capillary bed. A σ of one means that the solute cannot get through the capillary endothelium at all. A σ of zero means that it is freely permeable.

The Plasma Oncotic Pressure is the osmotic pressure generated by the plasma proteins that cannot get through the capillary endothelium. As already noted, this is not really the same as the osmotic pressure we discussed with reference to cell membranes because the ions responsible for that osmotic pressure (i.e., sodium and potassium) easily pass through *capillaries* and exert no osmotic pressure across the capillary wall. Albumin is the plasma protein found in greatest concentration, and its reflection coefficient is almost equal to one; globulins are even larger molecules. The plasma oncotic or osmotic pressure is normally about 25 mmHg. That is, it exerts a force of 25 mmHg, tending to keep liquid in the capillary or pull it in from the interstitium. A decrease in the concentration of plasma proteins decreases the colloid osmotic pressure and may lead to edema.

Interstitial Oncotic Pressure. Under normal circumstances, a few albumin molecules pass through the capillary pores of some vascular beds, and they may exert a small oncotic pressure. Pathologic states leading to more extravasation of protein may increase this factor favoring filtration.

Edema

Normally, the factors listed in the Starling equation are nearly balanced, with a tendency for filtration to occur in most vascular beds. The liquid leaving the capillaries enters the lymphatics and is subsequently returned to the circulation. Edema tends to occur, either in the systemic circulation or in the lungs, when these factors are altered and no longer in balance. Pulmonary interstitial edema interferes with gas diffusion in the lungs; alveolar edema is life-threatening. (Pulmonary edema is discussed in Chapter 3.) Edema may occur locally or generally within the systemic circulation.

Edema fluid usually collects in gravity-dependent regions, such as the feet. Edema fluid in the abdominal cavity is a cause of *ascites*, a general term indicating an accumulation of serous fluid in the abdomen.

In summary, factors tending to cause edema in the systemic circulation include:

- Anything causing increased capillary hydrostatic pressure, such as hypertension, right ventricular failure, or pathologic states causing venous occlusion.
- Reduced capillary oncotic pressure caused by dilution (as in blood loss followed with saline infusions), hepatic or renal disorders, or protein starvation.
- Decreased capillary integrity (that is, increased permeability) caused by toxins, burns, or shock.
- Lymphatic insufficiency, as caused by tumors obstructing lymphatic drainage.

Endocytosis

Endocytosis is a process that capillaries use to move substances that cannot pass through pores or dissolve in the capillary endothelial wall. These are usually large lipid-insoluble molecules. This is apparently accomplished by pinching off a portion of cell membrane to form a vesicle that completely surrounds the substance that is to be moved by endocytosis. The vesicle then moves through the capillary endothelial wall, attaches to the cell membrane on the other side of the endothelial cell, and releases the material to the other side of the capillary wall.

CARDIAC OUTPUT AND VENOUS RETURN

Except for the briefest periods, cardiac output must be matched to the venous return of the heart. If left ventricular output is unable to keep up with the return of blood from the systemic veins, blood accumulates in the pulmonary circulation. Such is the case in left ventricular failure, a state in which pulmonary vascular congestion frequently leads to decreased lung compliance, pulmonary interstitial edema, and occasionally alveolar edema, as well as decreased left ventricular output and decreased arterial blood pressure. Right ventricular failure may lead to systemic venous distention, peripheral edema, especially in the lower extremities, decreased pulmonary perfusion, and decreased ventricular output, leading to a fall in arterial blood pressure.

If venous return is not sufficient to meet the demand for an increased cardiac output, arterial blood pressure falls. For example, during exercise, the increased metabolic activity of the skeletal muscles results in vasodilation, mainly mediated by metabolic autoregulation. As systemic vascular resistance falls, arterial blood pressure also falls unless cardiac output increases to meet it, as can be seen from the formula:

$$\Delta P = \dot{Q} \times R, \quad \text{or}$$
$$MABP - RAP = CO \times SVR$$

where *MABP* is mean arterial blood pressure. *RAP* is right atrial pressure, that is, the downstream pressure for the left side of the circulation (right atrial pressure is approximately equal to central venous pressure [CVP], the pressure in the thoracic vena cavae). *CO* is cardiac output. *SVR* is systemic vascular resistance (or total peripheral resistance).

The cardiac output is the product of the heart rate (HR) and the stroke volume (SV):

$$CO = HR \times SV$$

If venous return does not keep up with the output of the two ventricles, the stroke volume falls. Increasing heart rate in a situation in which there is a fixed inadequate venous return would only decrease cardiac output because of decreased time for ventricular filling leading to smaller stroke volumes, according to Starling's law of the heart.

Determinants of Cardiac Output

As we have just noted, cardiac output is the product of the heart rate and the stroke volume.

Heart Rate

The heart rate is normally a result of the intrinsic rhymicity of the sinoatrial node as it is modified by the sympathetic and parasympathetic divisions of the autonomic nervous system and by humoral factors, such as circulating epinephrine. These influences on the heart rate are parts of reflexes and integrated cardiovascular responses that are discussed in the final section of this chapter.

The heart rate is usually under the tonic influence of both the sympathetic and parasympathetic systems. As we have seen, the heart rate can be increased by withdrawal of parasympathetic tone as well as by increasing sympathetic tone. Conversely, heart rate can be decreased by increasing cardiac vagal activity as well as by decreasing sympathetic activity.

Stroke Volume

The stroke volume is mainly determined by three factors: the *preload*, the *contractility* of the ventricle, and the *afterload*. The main determinant of left ventricular preload (defined as the left ventricular end-diastolic volume) is the flow of blood from the pulmonary veins and left atrium. Thus, *venous return from the systemic and pulmonary veins is a major determinant of stroke volume and, therefore, cardiac output*. According to Starling's law of the heart (the length-tension relationship of cardiac muscle), within limits, stroke volume increases with increased preload. We have also referred to this as heterometric autoregulation of the heart. As already pointed out, the heart rate may have an indirect effect on stroke volume if at high heart rates there is insufficient time for left ventricular filling.

Increases in contractility normally increase the stroke volume. We have defined an increase in contractility (a positive inotropic effect) as an increase in *stroke work* at the same or decreased ventricular end-diastolic volume. This is therefore homeometric regulation of the heart. Left ventricular stroke work is equal to the product of the stroke volume and the difference between the mean aortic blood pressure and the left ventricular end-diastolic pressure; right ventricular stroke work is equal to the product of the stroke volume and the difference between the mean pulmonary artery pressure and the right ventricular end-diastolic pressure. Increased contractility may be affected by increased cardiac sympathetic activity and, to a lesser extent, by decreased cardiac vagal tone. Autonomic nervous system mediated increases in contractility and increases in heart rate, therefore, almost always occur simultaneously.

The afterload has an indirect effect on the stroke volume. We have defined the afterload as the mean arterial blood pressure for the left ventricle and mean pulmonary artery pressure for the right ventricle. If the afterload increases, the heart must develop additional wall tension in order to generate the pressure gradient necessary to cause blood to flow from the left ventricle into the aorta. Therefore, stroke volume is decreased unless contractility increases accordingly.

Determinants of Venous Return

The main determinants of venous return are venomotor tone and its effect on the capacitance of the veins, the blood volume, the effects of muscle contraction on venous return, and the so-called thoracoabdominal pumping mechanism. The effects of arteriolar constriction on peripheral resistance also influence venous return.

Vascular Tone, Capacitance, and Blood Volume

Venous return to the right atrium is dependent on the pressure gradient between the veins and the right atrium. Of course, the pressures in the veins vary widely, for anatomic and physiologic reasons and because of the hydrostatic effects of gravity. For this reason, we usually think of venous pressure in terms of the pressure in the vena cavae, which is called *central venous pressure*.

Capacitance is related to pressure by the following formula:

$$C = \Delta V / \Delta P$$

where C is capacitance, V is volume, and P is pressure.

We can therefore think of the central venous pressure as resulting from the interaction of the capacitance of the veins and the volume of blood in them:

$$P = V/C$$

Stimulation of the sympathetic innervation of the veins or increased levels of humoral sympathetic mediators cause an increase in venomotor tone that results in a *decrease* in the capacitance of the veins. If the volume of blood in the veins remains about the same, central venous pressure increases and the pressure gradient for venous return also increases.

The capacitance of the veins is about 20 times that of the arteries. The main consequence of this is that most of the total blood volume is located in the veins (see Fig. 2–5). If the blood volume is increased, as from a blood transfusion, then venous pressure increases (if capacitance is unchanged), and the pressure gradient for venous return also increases, resulting in increased venous return. If the blood volume is decreased, as from hemorrhage or dehydration, then venous pressure decreases, resulting in decreased venous return.

Changes in arteriolar tone can affect venous pressure in two ways. Arteriolar constriction decreases the capacitance of the systemic arterial circulation and therefore changes the ratio of the capacitances of the veins and arteries. As the arteries become less capacitant, blood would be expected to shift into the veins and thereby increase venous pressure. However, this is not the case—vasoconstriction *decreases* venous pressure, most likely because there is very little blood in the arterial tree to be shifted into the veins. Instead, venous pressure *decreases,* probably because of the increased pressure drop resulting from the increased arteriolar resistance. Capillary hydrostatic pressure decreases, as does central venous pressure. Vasodilation decreases the pressure drop and therefore increases capillary hydrostatic and central venous pressure.

Muscle Contraction and Venous Return

We have already discussed the role of muscle contraction on venous return at the beginning of this chapter. As shown in Figure 2-7, valves in the veins of the extremities confer unidirectional flow on venous blood. When skeletal muscle in the extremities contracts, the veins in the area are squeezed. Blood cannot flow backwards because the valve closes, but it can flow toward the heart.

The Thoracoabdominal Pump

As discussed in Chapter 3, normal inspiration occurs by contracting the inspiratory muscles, especially the diaphragm, to increase the volume of the thoracic cavity. As the volume of the thoracic cavity increases, the intrathoracic pressure outside the lungs, which is called the *intrapleural pressure,* becomes more negative (with respect to the atmospheric pressure). As the pressure outside the vena cavae and right atrium becomes more negative, their *transmural pressure gradients* (inside pressure minus outside pressure) increase, and the atria and veins distend (Fig. 2-28). As they distend, their capacitance increases and the pressure inside decreases. At the same time, the downward movement of the diaphragm *increases* abdominal pressure and therefore increases the pressure outside the veins of the gastrointestinal tract. This increased pressure is transmitted to the blood in the veins. Thus, *inspiration results in increased pressure in the veins of the abdomen and decreased pressure in the central veins and the right atrium.* Taken together, this represents an increased pressure gradient for venous return, especially from the abdominal viscera.

During a *forced expiration,* intrapleural pressure becomes positive and may reach high levels. This impedes venous return and may even collapse the great veins. Positive pressure ventilation, for example, with a mechanical ventilator, also increases intrapleural pressure and impedes venous return. This can decrease the cardiac output, as described in Chapter 19.

THE SPECIAL CIRCULATIONS

The circulations of the various organs differ with respect to their anatomy and physiology. These

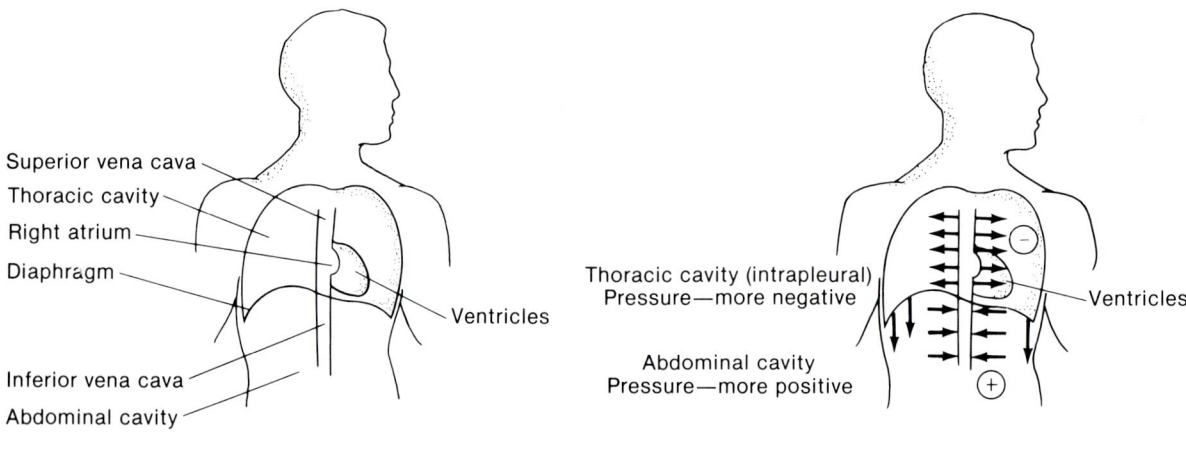

FIGURE 2-28. The effects of respiration on venous return (the "thoracoabdominal pump"). Inspiration increases abdominal pressure while causing intrapleural pressure to become more negative, thus increasing the gradient for venous return of blood pooled in the abdominal viscera.

differences are a reflection of the function of the organs themselves. In this regard, virtually every organ has a special circulation. In this chapter, we will briefly discuss those circulations with interesting and important characteristics. We have already discussed some of the characteristics of blood flow to skeletal muscle; pulmonary blood flow is discussed in Chapter 3.

Coronary Circulation

The heart is the organ responsible for the perfusion of the entire body, including itself. The coronary circulation must be able to supply the heart muscle with sufficient blood flow to meet its own metabolic needs; otherwise, cardiac output falls and systemic and pulmonary perfusion may be inadequate to supply the body's needs. The oxygen supply of the ventricles is especially critical. The heart, which must work constantly, has one of the highest metabolic demands per weight of tissue in the body, even when a person is at rest. Furthermore, it is an aerobic organ. The *oxygen content* of the venous blood draining the left ventricle is normally the lowest in the body. Looking at this another way, the left ventricular *arteriovenous oxygen difference* is the highest in the body. This nearly maximal oxygen extraction results in low coronary sinus P_{O_2} and oxygen content, even at rest. During times of increased myocardial metabolic demand, the only available way to increase the myocardial oxygen supply is to increase coronary blood flow, as can be seen by the following relationship:

$$\dot{V}_{O_2} = \dot{Q} \times (C_{aO_2} - C_{\bar{v}O_2})$$

where $\dot{V}_{O_2}$ is oxygen consumption (ml O_2/minute); $\dot{Q}$ is blood flow (ml blood/minute); and ($C_{aO_2} - C_{\bar{v}O_2}$) is the arteriovenous oxygen content difference (ml O_2/100 ml blood)

The factors that influence coronary blood flow include mechanical factors and the perfusion pressure, the heart rate, neural and humoral effects, and metabolic factors. Of these, metabolic effects are usually the most important.

Mechanical Factors and Perfusion Pressure. As already noted, the heart must generate its own perfusion pressure. The coronary arteries arise from the aorta, just distal to the aortic valve, so the upstream pressure for coronary blood flow is aortic pressure. Unlike the other systemic vascular beds, most of the left ventricular perfusion occurs during *diastole*. This is a result of the effect of left ventricular contraction on its own perfusion. As the myocardium contracts, the blood vessels coursing from the epicardium to the endocardium (that is, running perpendicular to the contraction of the heart walls) are compressed. This *extravascular compression* restricts coronary blood flow during systole, especially in the endocardium of the left ventricle. The effect is not as pronounced in the right ventricle. During diastole, the ventricular muscle is relaxed, and blood flow is greatly increased, especially in the endocardium, because of metabolic vasodilation.

Heart Rate. Increasing the heart rate has two effects on coronary perfusion. Less time is spent in diastole, which tends to decrease coronary perfusion. However, this is overridden by the increased work and metabolic demand causing metabolic vasodilation and increased coronary perfusion.

Neural and Humoral Factors. Although direct effects of the sympathetic and parasympathetic nervous systems can be demonstrated under careful experimental conditions, the most important effects of the autonomic nervous system on coronary blood flow are metabolic. Sympathetic stimulation increases both heart rate and contractility, thus increasing the myocardial metabolic demand and blood flow. Parasympathetic stimulation decreases heart rate, contractility, metabolic demand, and therefore blood flow.

Metabolic Factors. Coronary blood flow is very closely matched to myocardial metabolic demand. Increased cardiac work causes an increase in coronary perfusion. Similarly, hypoxemia (low arterial P_{O_2}) also causes increased coronary blood flow. The mediator or mediators of this metabolic control of coronary blood flow have not been completely established, but *adenosine*, a breakdown product of ATP, is considered a likely candidate by many experts.

Cerebral Circulation

Blood flow to the brain is critical for the maintenance of consciousness and cortical function; blood flow to the brain stem is necessary for the maintenance of life itself, because breathing is initiated in the medulla oblongata, as discussed in Chapter 3. Our main considerations of the cerebral circulation include the importance of maintaining perfusion pressure, such as the effect of the indistensibility of the skull, and neural and local control of cerebral blood flow. The capillaries of the cerebral circulation are very continuous and impermeable to almost anything that is not lipid-soluble. This is the anatomic basis of the *blood-brain barrier*.

Maintenance of Perfusion Pressure

The blood supply of the brain comes from the two internal carotid arteries and the two vertebral arteries. The vertebral arteries join to form the basilar artery, which forms the *circle of Willis* with branches of the internal carotids. This junction of the main arteries supplying the blood flow of the brain adds a safety factor of collateral flow to cerebral perfusion in case one of these vessels is partly occluded.

The heart and peripheral vasculature must maintain sufficient arterial blood pressure to pump blood "uphill" to the brain when a person is standing or seated upright. If sufficient blood pressure is not maintained, the person feels dizzy and loses consciousness, unless a reflex increase in blood pressure occurs. A lack of cerebral perfusion for only a few minutes may result in irreversible brain damage. As discussed shortly, arterial blood pressure is normally maintained by the *baroreceptor reflex*.

In the adult, the brain is enclosed in a rigid indistensible structure, the cranial vault. Increases in intracranial pressure (as from elevated cerebrospinal fluid pressure, growing tumors, edema secondary to trauma, or intracranial hemorrhage) compress cerebral blood vessels and increase the resistance to blood flow in the cerebral vasculature. If arterial blood pressure does not increase accordingly, effective cerebral perfusion pressure, which in this case is approximately equal to cerebral arterial blood pressure minus intracranial pressure, is decreased and cerebral blood flow is impaired. A reflex called the *Cushing response*, which is apparently initiated by ischemia of the medullary cardiovascular centers, or specialized pressure receptors, usually causes an increase in systemic arterial pressure in response to elevated intracranial pressure. This helps to maintain the cerebral perfusion pressure.

Neural Control of Cerebral Blood Flow

Although the cerebral blood vessels receive some innervation from both the sympathetic and parasympathetic nervous systems, neural factors are probably unimportant in the regulation of cerebral blood flow. Local factors appear to be much more important in the control of cerebral perfusion, especially in diverting blood flow to active areas of the brain.

Local Control of Cerebral Blood Flow

Cerebral blood vessels dilate in response to elevated carbon dioxide; increased concentrations of hydrogen ions, potassium ions, and adenosine; and decreased oxygen. Each of these factors may be involved in the local metabolic control of blood flow (autoregulation) to the brain. It is likely that the carbon dioxide response occurs by increasing the hydrogen ion concentration around cerebral arterioles. Thus, acute hyperventilation (increasing alveolar ventilation and decreasing arterial carbon dioxide) can decrease cerebral blood flow; acute hypoventilation (which increases arterial carbon dioxide and decreases arterial P_{O_2}) can increase cerebral perfusion. Elevated systemic arterial carbon dioxide levels can also abolish metabolic autoregulatory control of cerebral perfusion.

In summary, cerebral blood flow, like coronary blood flow, is normally almost entirely under local metabolic control.

Renal Circulation

The complex anatomy of the renal circulation reflects the complicated functions of the kidney (Fig. 2–29). These include water and electrolyte balance, blood volume and blood pressure regulation, and acid-base balance.

Anatomy of the Renal Circulation

The renal arteries branch into the interlobar arteries, which course radially from the hilus of the kidney, to form the arcuate arteries. These travel in the border zone between the renal cortex and medulla to give rise to the interlobular branches. The interlobular arteries branch to form the *afferent arterioles*. These vessels are called afferent arterioles because they are the arterioles proximal to the first of two renal capillary beds that are arranged in series. The first of these capillary beds comprises the highly adapted *glomeruli*, which act to filter blood cells and protein from the renal tubular fluid that is treated by the kidney. There are about one million glomeruli in each kidney. Each glomerulus is enveloped by *Bowman's capsule*, which acts to collect the fluid filtered from the blood in the glomerulus. Bowman's capsule is the

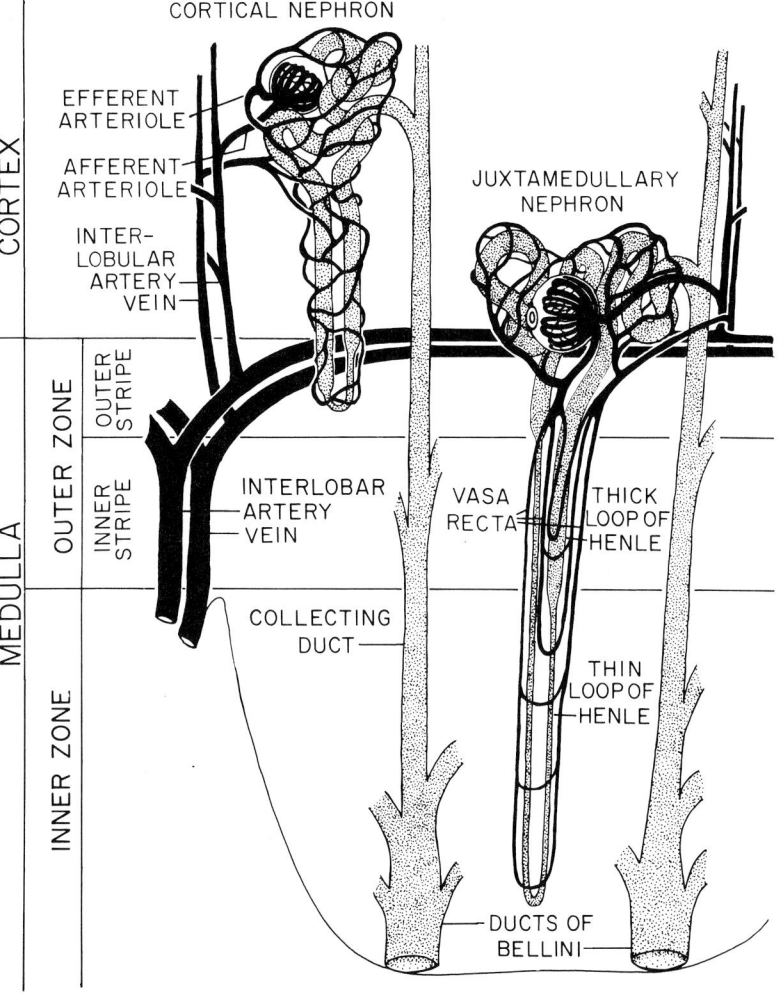

FIGURE 2-29. Diagram of the renal circulation. (Reproduced with permission from Pitts, R.F.: *Physiology of the Kidney and Body Fluids,* 3rd ed. Copyright © 1974 by Year Book Medical Publishers, Inc., Chicago.)

origin of the renal tubule and contains the initial renal tubular fluid. The filtered erythrocytes and proteins therefore remain in the blood vessels, while the filtrate enters the renal tubule.

The vessel carrying *blood* from the renal tubule is also called an arteriole. This *efferent arteriole* gives rise to a second capillary bed, the *peritubular capillaries*. These capillaries surround the renal tubules of the cortex and allow the exchange of ions, water, and other material between the renal tubular fluid and the circulation. Most of the renal tubules are located in the cortex (*cortical nephrons*) and penetrate only a short distance into the renal medulla. However, about 10% of the nephrons send long projections, called the *loops of Henle,* deep into the renal medulla. These nephrons, which are specially adapted for concentrating the urine (that is, retaining body water), are called the *juxtamedullary nephrons*. The efferent arterioles of the juxtamedullary nephrons give rise to specially adapted capillaries called *vasa recta,* which follow the loops of Henle. The venous drainage of the kidney generally follows the arterial supply (see Fig. 2–29).

Renal Blood Flow

The kidneys receive a very large portion of the cardiac output, about 20%. Although the kidneys have one of the highest metabolic rates in the body, the high blood flow is only partly explained by its metabolic demand. This can be seen by its relatively low oxygen extraction and its relatively high renal venous oxygen content. Renal blood flow may be as much as 10 times that necessary to satisfy its metabolic demand. Obviously, this overperfusion enables the kidneys to treat large volumes of blood at a time.

There is little pressure drop on the arterial side of the renal circulation until the afferent arterioles are reached. Even the afferent arterioles normally offer comparatively low resistance to blood flow, so the pressure in the glomerular capillaries is normally high, about 50 or 60 mmHg. From what we have learned about the Starling hypothesis of capillary dynamics, we can see that this high glomerular capillary hydrostatic pressure favors filtration of large quantities of fluid in Bowman's capsules and renal tubules. Normally, about 20% of the plasma fluid leaves the glomerular capillaries and enters the tubules to form the tubular fluid. This is called the *glomerular filtration rate* (GFR) and is normally about 125 ml/minute. The high glomerular capillary hydrostatic pressure is also maintained by the high resistance of the efferent arterioles. This high resistance results in a large pressure drop, so the peritubular capillary hydrostatic pressure is low, only about 10 to 20 mmHg. This low capillary hydrostatic pressure favors reabsorption of fluid.

Control of the Renal Circulation

Both local autoregulatory factors and neural factors contribute to the regulation of the renal circulation. As already noted, the kidneys play a role in the regulation of systemic blood pressure and blood volume, so the kidneys can indirectly alter their own perfusion via the systemic circulation.

Steady state renal blood flow stays virtually constant over a range of perfusion pressures between 80 and 180 mmHg in the isolated perfused kidney, thus demonstrating the ability of the kidneys to autoregulate. There are large transient changes in renal blood flow with changes in perfusion pressure, but as pressure is decreased, the renal vascular resistance decreases, and as pressure is increased, the vessels constrict. The mediator of this local renal autoregulatory mechanism is not known.

The renal vasculature has extensive sympathetic innervation, and stimulation of these nerves may result in constriction of the afferent and efferent arterioles, and possibly even the vasa recta. This allows renal blood flow to be diverted elsewhere during stresses on the cardiac output, such as hemorrhage, in order to perfuse more critically important vascular beds and maintain arterial blood pressure. A second consequence of this is that it decreases the excretion of sodium chloride and water and helps maintain body fluids and blood volume.

The renal arterioles are also very sensitive to angiotensin, which causes vasoconstriction. The events that lead to the activation of the renin-angiotensin system begin in the kidney, so this may represent a feedback mechanism. Many prostaglandins are released within the kidney, and they may play a role in local intrarenal regulation of blood flow.

Cutaneous Circulation

The metabolic requirements of the skin are relatively modest, and local metabolic control of cutaneous blood flow is not usually a major factor in its regulation. The main function of the cutaneous circulation is its role in the regulation of body temperature. Temperature changes at the skin surface and at sensors of internal body temperature located in the hypothalamus are the most important influences on cutaneous blood flow.

There are two types of resistance vessels in the skin—arterioles, similar to those found in other vascular beds, and *arteriovenous anastomoses*. The conventional arterioles have sympathetic innervation and also can demonstrate local autoregulation, although this may be myogenic rather than metabolic. The sympathetic innervation of the conventional arterioles causes constriction, and it is much more important than local factors in the control of arteriolar resistance. Both norepinephrine and epinephrine released or injected into the cutaneous circulation cause constriction of these arterioles. Stimulation of the sympathetic cholinergic innervation of the cutaneous sweat glands indirectly causes vasodilation by releasing bradykinin, as noted earlier.

Arteriovenous anastomoses are located primarily in the fingertips, palms, toes, soles, ears, nose, and lips. These anastomoses have thick muscular walls and are richly innervated with sympathetic nerve fibers. They can be stimulated by their sympathetic innervation or humoral epinephrine to constrict until they are completely shut. They do not exhibit basal tone (vascular tone in the absence of innervation) or autoregulation of blood flow. The regulation of the resistance of the arteriovenous anastomoses is therefore primarily under control of the hypothalamic thermoregulatory nuclei and reflexes from higher centers. Thus, blood flow can be diverted away from the cutaneous circulation, when necessary, to maintain blood pressure.

Exposure to cold causes a generalized constriction of cutaneous arterioles, arteriovenous anastomoses, and veins. This constriction diverts the warm blood away from the skin, a site of temperature loss, and sends it to the rest of the body. This is most pronounced in the hands and feet. There is also a direct cutaneous response to local cold temperatures that results in constriction of both types of cutaneous arterioles and the veins. However, this local response is only maintained for a few minutes and is then followed by vasodilation. Similarly, increased core temperature sensed at the hypothalamic thermoregulatory site causes a generalized vasodilation of both types of arterioles as well as capacitance vessels in order to bring heat to the body surface to help dissipate it. This vasodilation is enhanced by the activity of sweat glands. Thus, during exercise in a warm environment, cutaneous blood flow may increase tremendously because of the increased body temperature caused by skeletal muscle contraction. Local heating seems to bring about both a direct local vaso- and venodilation, for which nerves are apparently not required, and may also elicit a generalized reflex dilation in other parts of the body. However, the local heating may simply result in warmer blood reaching the hypothalamic thermoregulatory centers.

Splanchnic Circulation

The splanchnic circulation comprises the vasculature of the gastrointestinal tract, liver, spleen and pancreas. It receives about 30% of the cardiac output. In this section, the gastrointestinal and hepatic circulations are briefly discussed.

Gastrointestinal Circulation

The blood supply of the gastrointestinal tract comes from three large arteries: the celiac, superior mesenteric, and inferior mesenteric arteries (see Fig. 2–3). The intestinal circulation is mainly innervated by the sympathetic nervous system. Because alpha receptors predominate, sympathetic stimulation causes arteriolar and precapillary vasoconstriction as well as constriction of the capacitance vessels. Beta receptors, which cause dilation, are also present, but can only be demonstrated with pure beta receptor agonists. During generalized sympathetic activity (for example, after hemorrhage), blood flow to the gastrointestinal tract is greatly decreased by sympathetically mediated vasoconstriction. Blood flow is diverted to other vascular beds, such as the heart and brain. Sympathetically mediated constriction of splanchnic veins also releases pooled blood into the general circulation by decreasing their capacitance. The gastrointestinal vascular bed can exhibit autoregulation, but it does not appear to be as important a mechanism as it is in the cerebral and coronary circulations. Gastrointestinal vascular autoregulation seems to be predominantly metabolic, although the myogenic mechanism may also play a role. Foodstuffs in the gastrointestinal organs cause local increases in blood flow. This hyperemia may result from distention, hyperosmolarity, or the release of gastrointestinal hormones, such as cholecystokinin or gastrin.

Hepatic Circulation

The liver itself receives about 25% of the cardiac output, which comes from two sources, the portal vein and the hepatic artery. Portal venous blood, which contains the venous drainage of the gastrointestinal circulation, constitutes about three fourths of the blood flow to the liver (see Fig. 2–1). Because it is venous blood, low in oxygen, it supplies only about one fourth of the oxygen supply of the liver. The other one fourth of the blood supply of the liver comes from the hepatic artery and accounts for three fourths of its oxygen supply.

The smallest branches of the hepatic artery and the portal vein come together in the hepatic acini (the functional units of the liver) to terminate in the *hepatic sinusoids*. These discontinuous capillaries of the liver are structurally adapted for the exchange of material. The venous drainage of hepatic sinusoids ultimately forms the hepatic veins.

The mean blood pressure in the portal vein is normally only about 10 mmHg. Hepatic arterial pressure is about 90 mmHg, but the blood pressure in the hepatic sinusoids is only about 8 to 10 mmHg, or 2 to 3 mmHg higher than the pressure in the hepatic veins and inferior vena cava. Thus, the hepatic arteriolar resistance is normally quite high because the pressure drop between the artery and the sinusoids is so great. There is also hardly any resistance between the great veins and the hepatic sinusoids, so when central venous pressure rises, as it does in congestive heart failure, the elevated pressure is transmitted to the hepatic sinusoids.

The portal venous vascular bed does not appear to autoregulate; the hepatic arterial system does show some autoregulation, but it is weak. There is a weak reciprocal relationship between blood flow in the hepatic arterial system and that in the portal venous system, so that when one is decreased, the other increases. This compensation, however, is not usually complete. The sympathetic innervation of the hepatic arterioles and portal vein can cause a constriction in both, but the sympathetic effects on the hepatic capacitance vessels may be more important because the liver normally contains about 15% of the total body blood volume. Under sympathetic constriction, about half of this can be released into the general circulation.

INTEGRATED CONTROL OF THE CARDIOVASCULAR SYSTEM

At this point, we are ready to consider the integrated control of the cardiovascular system. This can be seen in the multifactorial control of blood pressure, blood volume, and overall control of blood flow, that is, the distribution of the cardiac output. We will discuss the integrated control of the cardiovascular system again in Chapter 4, when the cardiopulmonary responses to stress are described.

Control of Blood Pressure

A number of physiologic responses and reflexes are involved in the control of arterial blood pressure. These include both short-term (minutes or hours) and long-term (weeks or months) mechanisms. Many of the long-term mechanisms of the control of blood pressure work by adjusting the blood volume, so those responses are discussed in the next section.

Cardiovascular Reflexes

The most important short-term regulator of arterial blood pressure is the systemic arterial baroreceptor reflex. The baroreceptors are thought of as pressure receptors (*baro-* means pressure or weight). This is not quite correct because the receptors really respond to being *stretched*, rather than absolute pressure changes. However, under most circumstances, increased arterial pressure results in increased stretch of these receptors.

The baroreceptors are located in the carotid sinuses of the internal carotid arteries, just distal to the bifurcation of the common carotid arteries, and in the arch of the aorta. The location of these receptors makes sense: The carotid sinus receptors are located high in the neck and can give the central cardiovascular controller an indication as to whether perfusion pressure is sufficient to bring blood to the brain; the aortic receptors are in a position to give information on the mechanical performance of the heart.

Afferent information from the baroreceptors is carried to the cardiovascular centers in the medulla via the glossopharyngeal nerve from the carotid sinus baroreceptors and via the vagus nerve from the aortic arch baroreceptors. The receptors increase their discharge rate with increased stretch and, therefore, increased blood pressure. They decrease their discharge rate when blood pressure falls. In fact, they do not fire when blood pressure falls below about 60 mmHg. Some fibers do not depolarize at all or only discharge during systole at normal blood pressures but may be "recruited" when pressure is increased. Many fibers also respond more to *changes* in pressure than to steady state pressure. Increased baroreceptor activity resulting from increased blood pressure inhibits the cardioexcitatory center and the pressor area of the vasomotor center and stimulates the cardioinhibitory center and depressor area. Thus, the response to increased blood pressure is decreased heart rate, contractility, and systemic vascular resistance and even decreased venomotor tone. These responses decrease the cardiac output and the vascular resistance, resulting in a return to decreased arterial blood pressure. Decreased baroreceptor activity resulting from decreased arterial blood pressure removes the inhibition from the cardioexcitatory center and the pressor area of the vasomotor center and inhibits the cardioinhibitory center and depressor area. This results in increased heart rate, contractility, systemic vascular resistance, and venomotor tone, all leading to increased arterial blood pressure. Because the baroreceptors do not fire below arterial pressures of about 60 mmHg, the response does not increase at lower pressures. It takes only a few *seconds* for the baroreceptor reflex to become operational.

There are many other stretch receptors located throughout the cardiopulmonary system that can influence blood pressure and cardiac output. These *cardiopulmonary reflexes* include receptors in the atria and vena cavae, the ventricles, the pulmonary vasculature, and the airways of the lung. The different pathways of these responses all involve the vagus nerve.

Receptors in the atria and vena cavae have effects on heart rate and blood volume. Increased stretch of these receptors, especially those in the atria, usually results in an increased heart rate by increased central blood volume. This is called the *Bainbridge reflex*. Stretch of these receptors also results in increased urine flow, which decreases the blood volume. This may occur by release of a hormone called *atrial natriuretic factor* or by inhibition of the release of antidiuretic hormone from the posterior pituitary gland and decreased renin release. There may also be reflex sympathetic effects on renal blood flow.

Ventricular receptors, when stretched, result in bradycardia and vasodilation, which decreases cardiac work. Receptors in the pulmonary vessels, located close to the capillaries (the juxtapulmonary, or "J," receptors), respond to stretch caused by pulmonary vascular congestion and cause tachycardia, rapid shallow breathing, and dyspnea (difficulty breathing). Stretching the small airways of the lung by large inflations results in tachycardia and sometimes vasodilation. This lung-inflation reflex and the response of the "J" receptors are discussed in more detail in Chapter 3. Other receptors in the heart and lungs with vagal afferent pathways seem to tonically inhibit the heart rate and blood pressure.

The arterial chemoreceptors, discussed in greater detail in Chapter 3, have both direct and indirect effects on the cardiovascular system. The receptors are located in the carotid bodies, which are near the carotid sinuses, and in the aortic bodies, which are in the arch of the aorta. They respond to decreased arterial P_{O_2}, increased arterial P_{CO_2}, and increased arterial hydrogen ion concentration. Their afferent pathways are the glossopharyngeal and vagus nerves. The direct effect of arterial chemoreceptor stimulation on the cardiovascular system is bradycardia and vasoconstriction. However, *chemoreceptor stimulation has the main effect of increasing the depth and rate of breathing*. The increased heart rate of the lung inflation reflex, therefore, usually overrides the direct bradycardia effect, unless ventilation is clinically or experimentally controlled. Thus, arterial chemoreceptor stimulation usually results in an increased heart rate and blood pressure.

Moderate levels of pain and exposure to cold usually result in increased blood pressure, secondary to increased sympathetic stimulation. Pain also usually increases heart rate. However, intense pain usually causes bradycardia and hypotension.

Responses from higher centers also have effects on arterial blood pressure. Areas in the hypothalamus that coordinate the response to exercise, the defense reaction, and other responses can increase heart rate and contractility and cause vaso- and venoconstriction. One dramatic effect on blood pressure is the CNS ischemia response, or the response of the brain to very poor perfusion or hypoxia, as in hemorrhagic hypotension. The response is probably initiated by hypoxia of the medullary cardiovascular centers themselves, secondary to arterial blood pressures below 50 to 70 mmHg. The response is a profound generalized vasoconstriction and increased sympathetic activity to the heart. (Parasympathetic activity may also be increased but is overridden.) The CNS ischemia response is usually accompanied by a series of deep gasping breaths. It may be related to the Cushing response, which was discussed in the section on cerebral circulation.

If the afferent fibers from the systemic arterial baroreceptors of dogs are transected experimentally, the animals undergo a period of hypertension and tachycardia that lasts for a week or two. Following this period, the mean arterial blood pressure of these animals returns to normal, although it fluctuates much more in response to perturbations and takes longer to recover. The hypertension is exactly what we would expect, based on our understanding of the systemic arterial baroreceptors. As far as the medullary cardiovascular centers are concerned, arterial blood pressure is zero—or at least below 60 mmHg. The pressor area of the vasomotor center and cardioexcitatory center are not inhibited by impulses from the baroreceptors, and blood pressure is increased. However, the fact that pressure ultimately returns to normal indicates that the long-term regulators of blood pressure override the lack of baroreceptor input. As noted in the introduction to this section, the long-term regulation of blood pressure is mainly mediated by control of blood volume, which is itself related to urine output.

Control of Blood Volume

The control of blood volume is mainly a function of the kidney, with an important role also played by the intake of water and elecrolytes. Renal control of fluid and electrolyte balance is a subject too large to address in this book, but several renal mechanisms of volume control can be reviewed.

The first of these is the effect of arterial blood pressure (and the sodium in the plasma) on the renin-angiotensin system. If renal perfusion pressure is decreased because of decreased blood pressure, the juxtaglomerular cells of the kidney release more renin. This results in conversion of angiotensinogen to angiotensin I and, subsequently, conversion of angiotensin I to angiotensin II in the lungs. Angiotensin II directly causes a vasoconstriction, enhances sympathetic activity, stimulates the thirst mechanism, and causes more aldosterone to be released. Aldosterone acts on the kidney to cause sodium and water retention. This causes an increase in extracellular fluid volume and blood volume. Decreased blood volume is also sensed by the low-pressure baroreceptors—the atrial and venous stretch receptors discussed in the previous section. Decreased stretch of these receptors results in decreased release of atrial nutriuretic factor and increased release of antidiuretic hormone. It may also increase renin release. Finally, decreased renal perfusion pressure decreases the glomerular filtration rate and therefore decreases renal sodium and water output. Increases in arterial blood pressure act to suppress renin release, resulting in decreased angiotensin and aldosterone levels; increases in blood volume suppress antidiuretic hormone release and increase release of atrial natriuretic factor. Renal mechanisms of blood volume and long-term blood pressure control are frequently a causative factor in arterial hypertension and may lead to complications in congestive heart failure.

The kidney also participates in the regulation of the erythrocyte levels of the blood. Chronic hypoxia is sensed by the kidney, resulting in the release of *erythropoietin*. Erythropoietin stimulates the production and maturation of red blood cells, increasing the red cell volume, hematocrit, and hemoglobin concentration of the blood.

Other factors that may be involved in the long-term regulation of blood pressure and blood volume include sympathetic influences from the medulla and higher centers, alterations in the basal tone of arterioles, changes in vascular distensibility, and autoregulation of vascular beds.

Control of Blood Flow

The distribution of the cardiac output is determined by the interplay between the central and local regulatory mechanisms we have described in this chapter. Centrally mediated vascular mechanisms predominate in some vascular beds, such as the cutaneous circulation; local regulatory mechanisms predominate in other organs, such as the heart and brain. In other organs, blood flow is determined by the balance between neural and local mechanisms. In Chapter 4, we will see examples of alterations in the balance of central and local regulatory mechanisms in response to stresses like exercise and hemorrhage.

Bibliography

Berne, R.M., and Levy, M.N.: The Cardiovascular System. In Berne, R.M., and Levy, M.N. (eds.): *Physiology,* 2nd ed. St. Louis, C.V. Mosby, 1988, pp 395–572.

Berne, R.M., and Levy, M.N.: *Cardiovascular Physiology,* 5th ed. St. Louis, C.V. Mosby, 1986.

Cohn, F.: *Clinical Cardiovascular Physiology.* Philadelphia, W.B. Saunders, 1985.

Conley, C.L.: The Blood. In Mountcastle, V.B. (ed.): *Medical Physiology,* 14th ed. St. Louis, C.V. Mosby, 1980, pp 1126–1136.

Green, J.F.: *Fundamental Cardiovascular and Pulmonary Physiology,* 2nd ed. Philadelphia, Lea and Febiger, 1987, pp 3–17.

Guyton, A.C.: *Textbook of Medical Physiology,* 7th ed. Philadelphia, W.B. Saunders, 1986, pp 41–86, 149–346.

Little, R.C.: *Physiology of the Heart and Circulation,* 3rd ed. Chicago, Year Book Medical Publishers, 1985.

Milnor, W.R.: *Hemodynamics.* Baltimore, Williams and Wilkins, 1982, pp 11–48.

Mohrman, D.E., and Heller, L.J.: *Cardiovascular Physiology,* 2nd ed. New York, McGraw-Hill, 1986.

Rapaport, S.I.: Blood and Lymph. In West, J.B. (ed.): *Best and Taylor's Physiological Basis of Medical Practice,* 11th ed. Baltimore, Williams and Wilkins, 1985, pp 334–436.

Ratnoff, O.D.: Blood. In Berne, R.M., and Levy, M.N. (eds.): *Physiology,* 2nd ed. St. Louis, C.V. Mosby, 1988, pp 359–391.

Shepherd, J.T., and Vanhoutte, P.M.: *The Human Cardiovascular System: Facts and Concepts.* New York, Raven Press, 1979.

Smith, J.J., and Kampine, J.P.: *Circulatory Physiology—The Essentials,* 2nd ed. Baltimore, Williams and Wilkins, 1984.

Vander, A.J.: *Renal Physiology,* 3rd ed. New York, McGraw-Hill, 1985, pp 70–85, 111–142.

OBJECTIVES

AFTER READING THIS CHAPTER, THE STUDENT WILL BE ABLE TO:

1. State the functions of the respiratory system.
2. Describe the structure of the respiratory system.
3. Discuss the mechanics of breathing, including the pressure-flow and pressure-volume relationships of the lung and chest wall as well as the determinants of airways resistance.
4. List and define the standard lung volumes and capacities, and define the anatomic, alveolar, and physiologic dead spaces.
5. Predict the effects of changes in alveolar ventilation on alveolar and arterial oxygen and carbon dioxide levels.
6. Present the major aspects of the pulmonary circulation, and compare and contrast them with those of the systemic circulation.
7. Explain the concept of matching ventilation and perfusion in the lungs and how to predict the effects of ventilation-perfusion mismatch.
8. Describe regional differences in ventilation, perfusion, and ventilation-perfusion ratios in the lung and how to predict the effects of these differences on regional gas exchange in the lung.
9. Summarize the main features of the diffusion and transport of oxygen and carbon dioxide in the cardiopulmonary system.
10. Define and categorize the types of acidosis and alkalosis, discuss the physiologic compensatory mechanisms for these conditions, and use this information in the interpretation of blood gas data.
11. Discuss the generation of the spontaneous initiation and rhythmicity of breathing and present the neural and chemical stimuli that can modify the pattern of breathing.
12. List the nonrespiratory functions of the lung, including its defense mechanisms and metabolic functions.

3
PULMONARY ANATOMY AND PHYSIOLOGY

CHAPTER OUTLINE

FUNCTIONS OF THE RESPIRATORY SYSTEM
  Gas Exchange
  Other Functions
STRUCTURE OF THE RESPIRATORY SYSTEM
  Upper Airways
    Pharynx
    Larynx
  Tracheobronchial Tree
    Structure of the Airways
  Pulmonary Parenchyma
  Blood Supply of the Lungs
  Alveolar-Capillary Unit
  Chest Wall and Muscles of Respiration
  Central Nervous System
MECHANICS OF BREATHING
  Pressure-Flow Relationships in Breathing
  Pressure-Volume Relationships and
    Compliance
    Elastic Recoil of the Lung
    Surface Tension in the Alveoli
    Mechanical Interdependence of the Lung
      and Chest Wall
  Airways Resistance
    Laminar and Turbulent Flow
    Determinants of Airways Resistance
  The Work of Breathing

ALVEOLAR VENTILATION
  Lung Volumes
  Anatomic Dead Space
  Physiologic Dead Space
  Effects of Alveolar Ventilation on Oxygen and
    Carbon Dioxide Levels
    Partial Pressures of Respiratory Gases
    Alveolar Ventilation and Carbon Dioxide
    Alveolar Ventilation and Oxygen
  Regional Distribution of Alveolar Ventilation
BLOOD SUPPLY OF THE LUNGS
  Bronchial Circulation
  Pulmonary Circulation
    Determinants of Pulmonary Vascular
      Resistance
VENTILATION-PERFUSION RELATIONSHIPS
  Importance of Matching Ventilation and
    Perfusion
  Consequences of $\dot{V}_A/\dot{Q}c$ Mismatch
  Regional $\dot{V}/\dot{Q}$ in the Lung
DIFFUSION OF GASES
  Fick's Law for Diffusion
  Perfusion Limitation of Gas Transfer
  Diffusion Limitation of Gas Transfer
  Diffusion of Oxygen
  Diffusion of Carbon Dioxide

OXYGEN AND CARBON DIOXIDE TRANSPORT
  Transport of Oxygen in the Blood
    Physically Dissolved
    Chemically Combined with Hemoglobin
    Oxyhemoglobin Dissociation Curve
    Loading Oxygen in the Lung
    Unloading Oxygen at the Tissues
    Influences on the Oxyhemoglobin Dissociation Curve
    Other Factors Affecting Oxygen Transport
  Transport of Carbon Dioxide in the Blood
    Physically Dissolved
    As Carbamino Compounds
    As Bicarbonate
    Carbon Dioxide Dissociation Curve
ACID-BASE PHYSIOLOGY
  Acids, Bases, and Buffers
    Sources of Acids in the Body
  Buffers in the Human Body
  Acidosis
  Alkalosis
  Respiratory Compensatory Mechanisms
  Renal Compensatory Mechanisms
CONTROL OF BREATHING
  Generation of Spontaneous Respiratory Rhythmicity
  Medullary and Pontine Respiratory Centers
  Spinal Pathways
  Reflex Mechanisms of Respiratory Control
  Influences of Higher Centers
  Chemical Control of Breathing
    Response to Carbon Dioxide
    Peripheral and Central Chemoreceptors
    Response to Hydrogen Ions
    Response to Hypoxia
NONRESPIRATORY FUNCTIONS OF THE RESPIRATORY SYSTEM
  Pulmonary Defense Mechanisms
  Nonrespiratory Functions of the Pulmonary Circulation
  Metabolic Functions of the Lung

FUNCTIONS OF THE RESPIRATORY SYSTEM

Oxygen must be continuously available to most of the cells of the body in order for them to produce energy and function normally. Carbon dioxide, a by-product of this aerobic metabolism, must be removed from the metabolizing cells. In addition to this, hydrogen ions are produced as a result of several metabolic pathways, and the respiratory system assists in their removal. The respiratory system, then, has to take oxygen from the atmosphere, supply it to the cells, and remove from the body the carbon dioxide and hydrogen ions produced by cellular metabolism. Other functions of the respiratory system include acid-base balance, phonation, pulmonary defense and metabolism, and the handling of bioactive materials.

Gas Exchange

The exchange of metabolically produced carbon dioxide for atmospheric oxygen occurs in the lungs. The respiratory muscles generate the forces that cause fresh air, containing oxygen, to be inspired through the conducting airways into the lungs. These muscles act on commands initiated by the respiratory center in the central nervous system. At the same time, the right ventricle pumps venous blood returning from the various body tissues and containing elevated levels of carbon dioxide and lower levels of oxygen into the lungs. In the pulmonary capillaries, carbon dioxide is exchanged for oxygen. The blood leaving the lungs, having a high oxygen content and a decreased carbon dioxide content, is distributed to the tissues of the body by the left side of the cardiovascular system. Gas that has a high concentration of carbon dioxide is expelled from the body during expiration.

Other Functions

Acid-Base Balance. In the body, increased concentrations of carbon dioxide lead to increased hydrogen ion concentrations because of these reactions:

$$CO_2 + H_2O \overset{1}{\rightleftharpoons} H_2CO_3 \overset{2}{\rightleftharpoons} H^+ + HCO_3^-$$

In the first of these reactions (labelled 1), carbon dioxide combines with water to form carbonic acid. In the second (labelled 2), the carbonic acid dissociates, forming a hydrogen ion and a bicarbonate ion.

Note that these reactions, which can be referred to together as the carbonic acid reaction, are both reversible. The respiratory system can therefore participate in acid-base balance by removing hydrogen ions in the form of CO_2 from the body. The central nervous system has sensors for the CO_2 and hydrogen ion levels in the arterial blood and in the cerebrospinal fluid, which send information to the controllers of breathing.

Phonation. The sounds produced by the movement of air over the vocal cords is called phonation. Speech, singing, and other sounds are produced by the action of the central nervous system controllers on the muscles of respiration, causing air to flow over the vibrating vocal cords. Phonation will not be discussed in detail in this book.

Pulmonary Defense Mechanisms. Each breath brings into the lungs a small sample of the local atmospheric environment. This sample may include microorganisms, dust, particles of silica or asbestos, toxic gases, smoke (cigarette and other types), and other pollutants. Furthermore, the temperature and humidity of the local atmosphere can vary greatly.

Pulmonary Metabolism and the Handling of Bioactive Materials. To supply energy and nutrients for their own maintenance, the cells of the lung must metabolize substrate. Some specialized pulmonary cells produce substances necessary for normal pulmonary function. Furthermore, the pulmonary vascular endothelium contains many enzymes that can metabolize or modify naturally occurring vasoactive substances found in venous blood.

STRUCTURE OF THE RESPIRATORY SYSTEM

The respiratory system comprises the lungs, conducting airways, parts of the central nervous system concerned with the control of the muscles of respiration, and the chest wall. The chest wall consists of the muscles of respiration, including the diaphragm and intercostal muscles as well as the rib cage. The abdominal muscles also function as part of the respiratory system, as discussed later.

Upper Airways

Air enters the respiratory system through the nose or mouth. Air entering through the nose is filtered, heated to body temperature, and humidified as it passes through the nose and nasal turbinates. Air breathed through the nose enters the airways via the nasopharynx; air breathed through the mouth enters via the oropharynx. Passing next through the glottis and larynx, air then enters the tracheobronchial tree. The upper airways are shown in Figure 3–1. They consist of the conducting airways (including the external nose), the nasal passages, the pharynx from the nose to the esophagus, the mouth, and the larynx as well as the paranasal sinuses and eustachian tubes.

Pharynx

The *nose* is normally the main entrance route for air entering the lungs, because of the additional pulmonary defense mechanisms offered by the nasal airways. These mechanisms, which were noted above, are discussed in detail at the end of this chapter. The two *nostrils* are the entrance point of the *anterior nares,* which are the beginning of the nasal passages. The anterior nares extend back to the beginning of the ciliated mucosa at the anterior ends of the *nasal septum* and *nasal turbinates,* which are shown in cross section in the inset of Figure 3–1. This anterior portion of the nasal passage normally has the smallest total cross-sectional area of any portion of the respiratory tract.

The main nasal passage, including the nasal turbinates and the septum, extends posteriorly about 6 to 8 cm and has a much larger cross-sectional area because of the configuration of the nasal turbinates. The nasal turbinates themselves present a very large surface area, yet air passing by the turbinates is forced to flow in narrow streams. Both of these effects are a result of the folding of the turbinates (as shown in the inset), and they are important in the pulmonary defense mechanisms discussed at the end of this chapter. The mucosa lining this region is ciliated, highly vascular (a source of nosebleeds, or *epistaxis*), and rich in mucus-secreting glands and goblet cells. The upper portion of this region contains branches of the olfactory nerve, which are the receptors responsible for the sense of smell.

The end of the septum marks the beginning of the *nasopharynx,* at which point the airway is no longer split in two. The nasal passages open into the nasopharynx via the *choana,* or *internal nares.* At the nasopharynx, which is about 12 to 14 cm from the nostrils, the lining mucosa makes a transition to a flatter unciliated cell type, which continues downward to the larynx. The exceptions to

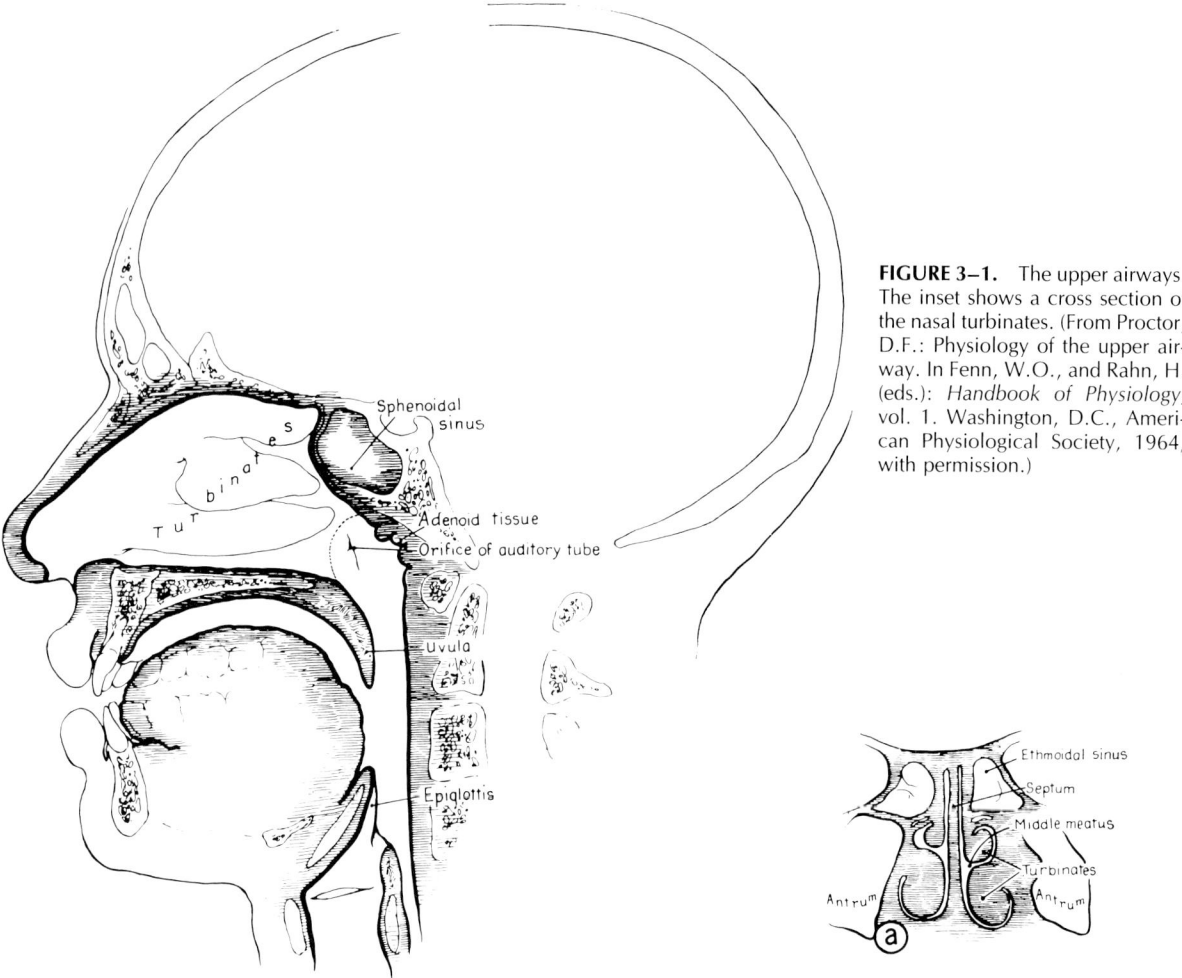

FIGURE 3–1. The upper airways. The inset shows a cross section of the nasal turbinates. (From Proctor, D.F.: Physiology of the upper airway. In Fenn, W.O., and Rahn, H. (eds.): *Handbook of Physiology*, vol. 1. Washington, D.C., American Physiological Society, 1964, with permission.)

this are the partially ciliated tonsil and adenoid tissue, which participate in pulmonary defense mechanisms. The eustachian tubes, which connect to the ears, enter the nasopharynx on its lateral walls. The nasopharynx extends downward to the end of the soft palate, where it terminates and joins with the *oropharynx.*

The oropharynx begins at the back end of the soft palate and extends downward to the level of the base of the tongue and the upper border of the epiglottis. It contains two masses of lymphoid tissue called the *palatine tonsils,* which are located in its lateral walls. These tonsils sometimes become chronically inflamed during childhood. The *laryngopharynx,* which is also referred to as the *hypopharynx,* begins at the uppermost portion of the epiglottis and continues to the lowermost portion of the larynx, the *cricoid cartilage.* The laryngopharynx is a common site of obstruction by foreign bodies and may also be obstructed by the tongue in comatose states.

The *accessory air spaces* or *paranasal sinuses* are a group of air spaces in the facial bones. They are lined with ciliated, mucus-secreting cells, as are the eustachian tubes. The paranasal sinuses and eustachian tubes are normally open to the nasopharynx, and their cilia clear surface fluid into the nasopharynx. This communication with the nasopharynx is also necessary for sinus and middle-ear pressure equalization with the external environment when ambient pressure changes. This is well known to those who suffer from sinus headaches as well as divers and air travelers.

Starting with the nasopharynx, the shape and diameter of the airway are normally a function of the state of contraction of the muscles controlling the pharynx, larynx, tongue, and soft palate. Relaxation of these muscles during sleep is the main cause of episodes of upper airway obstruction, resulting in snoring and even in *obstructive sleep apnea*. As already noted, inflammation of the lymphoid tissue of the tonsils and adenoids, tumors, and foreign objects caught in the throat may also obstruct this airway.

Larynx

The larynx consists of a group of cartilages, muscles, and ligaments serving at least three major functions (Fig. 3–2). The first of these is to keep the airway open during breathing; the second is to act as a valve to separate the airway from the digestive tract during swallowing; the third is phonation. The cricoid cartilage (Fig. 3–2B–D) is the only laryngeal cartilage that forms a complete ring, and it acts as the foundation of the larynx. The cricoid cartilage is attached at its posterior lateral surfaces to the *thyroid cartilage* (Adam's apple). The cricothyroid joint allows the thyroid cartilage to move both up and down and backward and forward. The *epiglottis* attaches to the inner surface of the anterior portion of the thyroid cartilage and extends upward to the base of the tongue. The two *arytenoid cartilages* are seated on the upper surface of the posterior portion of the cricoid cartilage, and the cricoarytenoid joints permit movement in the lateral plane as well as rotation in a plane extending across the airway. The true *vocal cords* extend from the anterior processes of the arytenoids to the thyroid cartilage. Above the true vocal cords are the false vocal cords, which are folds of mucous membranes that play no known role in vocalization. Beneath the larynx, the first ring of the trachea is attached to the thyroid cartilage by a ligament. The laryngeal cartilages are also attached to each other by ligaments, and the thyroid cartilage is attached to the *hyoid bone* above it by another ligament. Most of the larynx is lined with a mucus-secreting epithelium, except for part of the epiglottis, which has a ciliated lining.

The larynx is mainly suspended by the so-called strap muscles of the anterior portion of the neck (also called the *infrahyoid muscles* and consisting of the omohyoid, sternohyoid, sternothyroid, and thyrohyoid muscles) and the pharyngeal constrictor muscles, which hold the posterior portion of the larynx against the vertebral column, except when they relax during swallowing. The extrinsic and intrinsic laryngeal muscles are important during breathing, swallowing, and phonation. During swallowing, the vocal cords are pulled together, or *adducted*, and the larynx is raised and tilted backward to close the *glottis*, the vocal opening

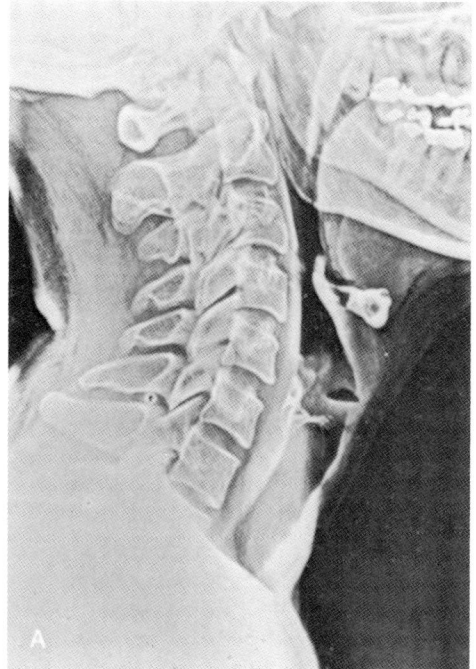 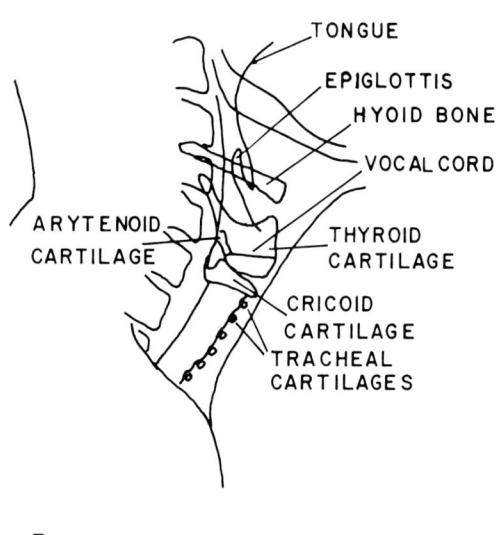

FIGURE 3–2. *A*, Xeroradiograph of the laryngotracheal airway. *B*, Diagram identifying key structures. (From Proctor, D.F.: The upper airways. *American Review of Respiratory Disease* 115:316, 1977, with permission.)

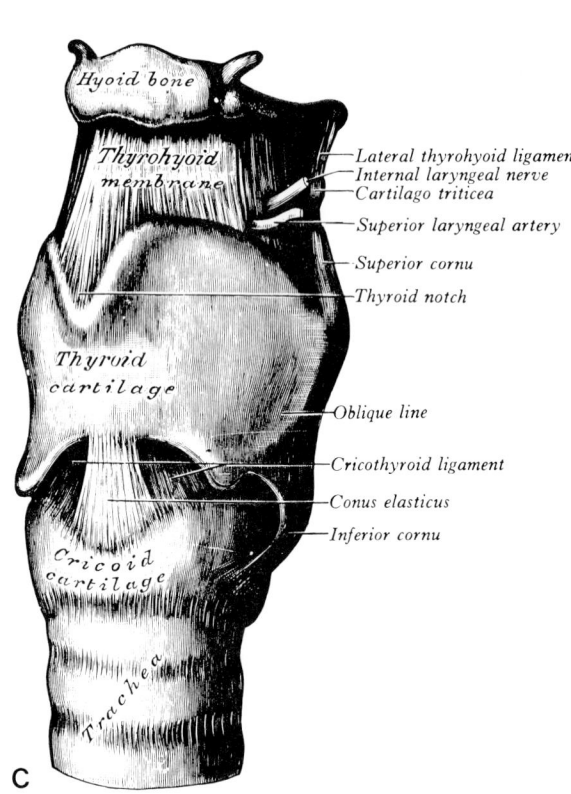

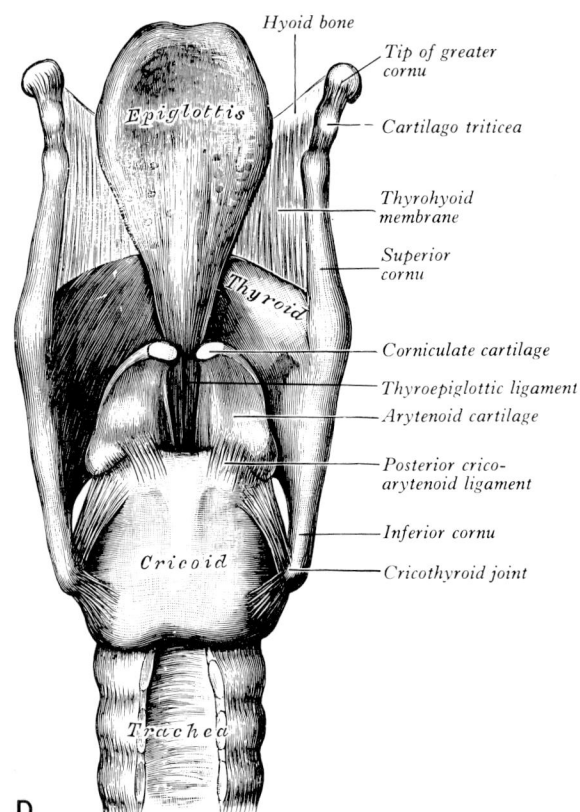

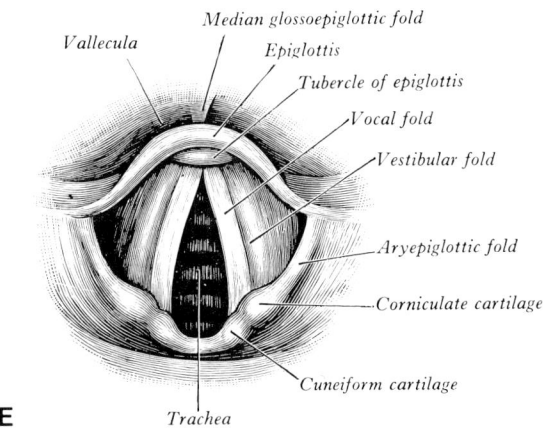

FIGURE 3–2 Continued C, The ligaments of the larynx, anterolateral aspect. D, The ligaments of the larynx, posterior aspect. E, The interior of the larynx as seen through a laryngoscope. (From Williams, P.L., and Warwick, R.: Gray's Anatomy, 36th British ed. New York, Churchill Livingstone, 1980, with permission.)

of the larynx (Fig. 3–2E). Thus, the airway is closed during swallowing. The epiglottis does not close the glottis, and it does not appear to be essential for swallowing. During breathing, the vocal cords are pulled apart, or *abducted,* posteriorly, and the glottis is opened. The triangular glottic opening parts slightly during inspiration and closes slightly during expiration. In phonation, the partly relaxed glottic closure produces the voice.

The intrinsic laryngeal musculature responsible for closing the glottis is innervated by the recurrent laryngeal nerve with the exception of the cricothyroid muscle, which is supplied by the superior laryngeal nerve. Both of these nerves are branches of the vagus. The larynx is discussed in greater detail in Chapter 18.

Tracheobronchial Tree

After passing through the nose or mouth, pharynx, and larynx, air enters the *tracheobronchial tree.* Starting with the trachea, the air may pass through as few as 10 or as many as 23 *generations,* or branchings, on its way to the alveoli. The branchings of the tracheobronchial tree and the nomenclature of the branches are shown in Figure 3–3. Alveolar gas exchange units are denoted by the U-shaped sacs.

The first 16 generations of airways, the *conducting zone,* do not bring inspired air in contact with mixed venous blood and thus are anatomically incapable of gas exchange. They constitute the *anatomic dead space.* Alveoli start to appear at the 17th through 19th generations, in the respiratory bronchioles, which are called the *transitional zone.* The 20th to 23rd generations are lined with alveoli. The *alveolar ducts* and *alveolar sacs,* referred to as the *respiratory zone,* terminate the tracheobronchial tree.

The many branchings of the airways result in a great total cross-sectional area of the distal portions of the tracheobronchial tree, even though the diameters of the individual airways are quite small.

Structure of the Airways

The airways vary considerably in their structure, depending on their location in the tracheobronchial tree. The trachea is a fibromuscular tube consisting of C-shaped rings of cartilage completed at the back by smooth muscle. The cartilage of the large bronchi is semicircular, like that of the trachea, but as the bronchi enter the lungs, the cartilage rings disappear and are replaced by irregularly shaped cartilage plates. The plates completely surround the bronchi and give the intrapulmonary bronchi their cylindrical shape. The plates also help support the larger airways but diminish progressively in the smaller distal airways, disappearing completely in airways about 1 mm in diameter. By definition, airways with no cartilage are termed *bronchioles.* Because the bronchioles and alveolar ducts contain no cartilaginous support, they are likely to collapse when compressed and expand when their transmural pressure gradient increases. This tendency is partly opposed by the attachment of the alveolar septa to their walls (see Figs. 3–6 and 3–17). As the cartilage plates become irregularly distributed around the tube, the muscular layer, which is intermingled with elastic fibers, completely surrounds the bronchus. As the bronchioles proceed toward the alveoli, the muscle layer becomes thinner, although smooth muscle fibers can even be found in the walls of the alveolar ducts. Bronchiolar smooth muscle is innervated by the autonomic nervous system. The parasympathetic innervation causes constriction and the sympathetic innervation causes dilation. The outermost layer of the bronchial wall is surrounded by dense connective tissue with many elastic fibers.

The entire respiratory tract—except for part of the pharynx, larynx, anterior third of the nose, and terminal respiratory units distal to the respiratory bronchioles—is lined with ciliated cells interspersed with mucus-secreting goblet cells and other secretory cells. In the bronchioles, the goblet cells become less frequent and are replaced by another type of secretory cell, the Clara cell. The ciliated epithelium, along with the mucus secreted

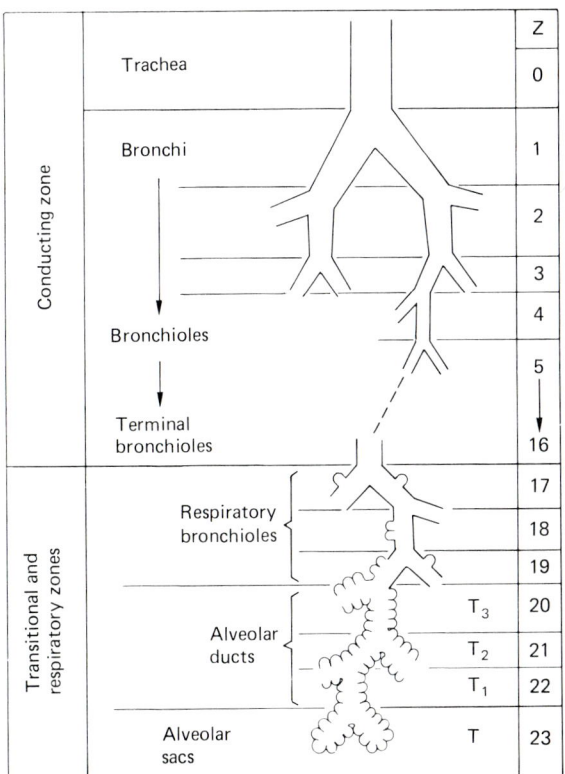

FIGURE 3–3. Diagram of airway branching in the human lung. (From Weibel, E.R.: *Morphometry of the Human Lungs.* Berlin, Springer Verlag, 1963, with permission.)

by glands along the airways and goblet cells and the secretory products of Clara cells, constitutes an important mechanism for the protection of the lung, called the *mucociliary escalator*.

The lung is supported within the chest by the *hilus*, which is the point where the airways and blood vessels enter the lungs from the *mediastinum*, and by the *pulmonary ligament*, an attachment between the *visceral pleura* (the outside surface of the lung) and the *mediastinal pleura* (the outside surface of the mediastinum). The mediastinum is the portion of the thorax that lies between the right and left pleural sacs and isolates the two lungs from each other. It contains the heart and major blood vessels. The normally expanded lung completely fills the pleural cavity spaces not occupied by the other contents of the mediastinum. The *parietal pleura* lines the inside of most of the chest wall.

The structure and nomenclature of the two lungs follow the divisions of the tracheobronchial tree. The *left and right main-stem bronchi* give rise to the left and right lungs. The right main bronchus is a shorter, straighter, and more vertically oriented branch of the trachea, so aspirated material passes more frequently into the right airway than the left. The right main bronchus divides into three branches, the *right upper lobar bronchus*, the *right middle lobar bronchus*, and the *right lower lobar bronchus*. These give rise to the *right upper, middle,* and *lower lobes*, respectively. The left main-stem bronchus is longer than the right because it must pass under the arch of the aorta. It divides into only two branches, the *left upper and lower lobar bronchi*. These give rise to the *left upper and lower lobes*.

The lobar bronchi each branch to form *segmental bronchi*, which give rise to subdivisions of the lobes, called *lung segments* or *bronchopulmonary segments*. These are shown and named in Figure 3–4 and are discussed in greater detail in Chapter 17 in connection with postural lung drainage. The segmental bronchi divide and branch to form *bronchioles*, then *terminal bronchioles*, and finally *respiratory bronchioles* (see Fig. 3–3). The portion of lung supplied by a primary respiratory bronchiole is called an *acinus*. Three to five terminal bronchioles may be separated from other similar units by connective tissue septa to form an anatomic unit called a *lobule*, which is not really defined in terms of the branching of the tracheobronchial tree. The acinus comprises the primary respiratory bronchiole and its branches (usually three generations), which branch to form the alveolar ducts and alveolar sacs. The alveoli of the respiratory bronchioles, alveolar ducts, and alveolar sacs, along with the pulmonary capillaries supplying them with mixed venous blood, constitute the *pulmonary parenchyma*.

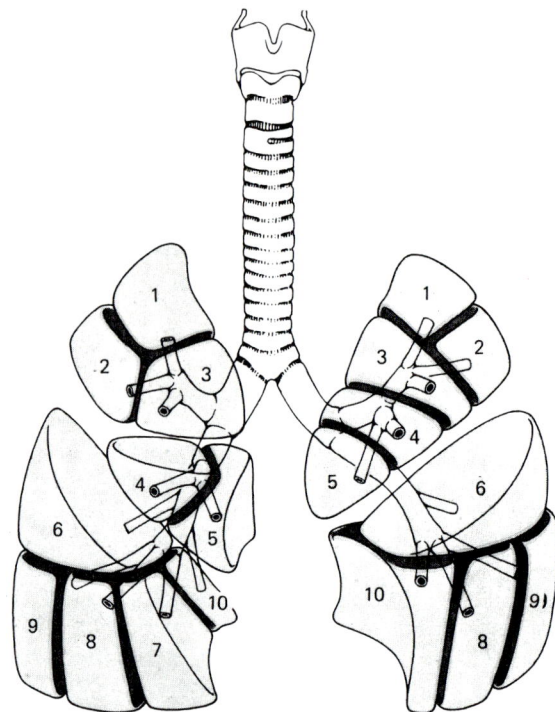

FIGURE 3–4. Bronchopulmonary segments of the human lung. *Left and right upper lobes:* (1) Apical, (2) posterior, (3) anterior, (4) superior lingular, (5) inferior lingular segments. *Right middle lobe:* (4) Lateral, (5) medial segments. *Lower Lobes:* (6) Superior (apical), (7) medial-basal, (8) anterior-basal, (9) lateral-basal, (10) posterior-basal. There is no medial-basal lobe in the left lung. (From Weibel, E.R.: Design and structure of the human lung. In Fishman, A.P. (ed.): *Pulmonary Diseases and Disorders*, vol. 1. New York, McGraw-Hill, 1980, with permission.)

Pulmonary Parenchyma

The parenchyma of a tissue can be defined as the cells that give it its function, as delineated from those cells and structural aspects that merely support the tissue. The pulmonary parenchyma consists mainly of alveolar epithelial cells and pulmonary capillary endothelial cells.

The alveolar surface is composed mainly of a single layer of flat epithelial cells called *type I alveolar cells,* or type I pneumocytes. Type I cells are the cells through which the gas exchange between the alveoli and pulmonary capillaries takes place, and they constitute as much as 97% of the alveolar lining. Their very thin cytoplasm extends over large areas, and they have small nuclei. They contain few organelles other than pinocytotic vesicles. Interspersed among the predominant type I cells are larger cuboidal *type II alveolar cells,* or type II pneumocytes. They are packed with organelles and special *lamellar bodies,* or layered granules, which are believed to contain concentrated stored material that is released onto the alveolar surface to form the alveolar surface film. This surface film has important physiologic consequences, which are discussed later in this chapter. A third cell type, the free-ranging phagocytic *alveolar macrophage,* is found in varying numbers in the extracellular lining of the alveolar surface. These cells patrol the alveolar surface and phagocytize inspired particles, such as bacteria. The function of the alveolar macrophages is discussed in the section on nonrespiratory functions of the lung.

The pulmonary capillary endothelial cells are also flat epithelial-type cells formed in a single layer. They usually have broad cytoplasmic extensions with small flat nuclei, as was the case with type I alveolar cells. They also have few subcellular organelles—only a few small mitochondria, and a poorly developed secretory apparatus. They do contain many pinocytotic vesicles. The pulmonary capillary endothelium is usually continuous and has no fenestra. A pulmonary capillary endothelial cell and part of a type I alveolar cell are shown in Figure 3–5.

The endothelium of small pulmonary arteries and veins is thicker than that of the capillaries, and it contains many subcellular organelles of various kinds. These cells appear to be much more active metabolically than are the capillary endothelial cells, and they are probably the site of many of the nonrespiratory metabolic activities of the lung.

The barrier to gas exchange between the alveoli and pulmonary capillaries can also be seen in Figure 3–5. It consists of the alveolar epithelium, the capillary endothelium, and the interstitial space between them. Gases must also pass through the fluid lining the alveolar surface (not visible in the figure), the plasma in the capillary, and the erythrocyte cell membrane. The barrier to diffusion is about ½ μm thick. Gas exchange by diffusion is discussed later in this chapter.

Blood Supply of the Lungs

The lungs receive blood flow from two sources, the bronchial and pulmonary circulations. The bronchial circulation arises variably from the aorta and supplies lung tissue down to the level of the terminal bronchioles with oxygen and nutrients. The pulmonary circulation brings the entire venous drainage of the body to the lungs via the pulmonary artery so that gas exchange with the alveoli can take place. The pulmonary circulation supplies lung tissue distal to the terminal bronchioles with nutrients. This tissue, which begins with the respiratory bronchioles, probably receives its oxygen directly from alveolar air.

The course and branching pattern of the pulmonary arterial supply follows that of the airways (and runs along with them) out to the smallest branches. The veins usually lie in the boundaries between two or three acinar units and therefore drain several at once.

The pulmonary vessels, especially those on the arterial side, generally have much thinner walls and contain much less vascular smooth muscle than do corresponding vessels in the systemic circulation. As shown later in this chapter, this has important physiologic consequences. The vessels are also generally shorter, because they have to travel only to the upper and lower reaches of the lungs.

The pulmonary arteries divide more frequently than do the bronchi, and it appears that there are some 28 generations of pulmonary arterial branching instead of 23. The walls of the major pulmonary vessels close to the heart have layers of elastic fibers interconnected with smooth muscle fibers, a structure similar to that of the aorta. This pattern is seen in vessels down to those about 1 mm in diameter. Branches of the pulmonary circulation smaller than 1 mm in diameter are mainly composed of smooth muscle. It appears that the tone of the smooth muscle of the larger vessels mainly determines their distensibility, whereas that of the small vessels alters their resistance. Vessels exactly corresponding to systemic arterioles are not easy to demonstrate in the pulmonary circulation, although branches from about 100 μm to about 20 or 40 μm in diameter do have single layers of smooth muscle. The pulmonary veins are similar to the systemic veins of the upper parts of the body.

Alveolar-Capillary Unit

The functional unit of the lung is the alveolus and its capillaries. It is the site of gas exchange between the alveolar air and the blood. There are said to be approximately 300 million alveoli in the normal adult lung. As Figure 3–6 shows, each al-

96 PULMONARY ANATOMY AND PHYSIOLOGY

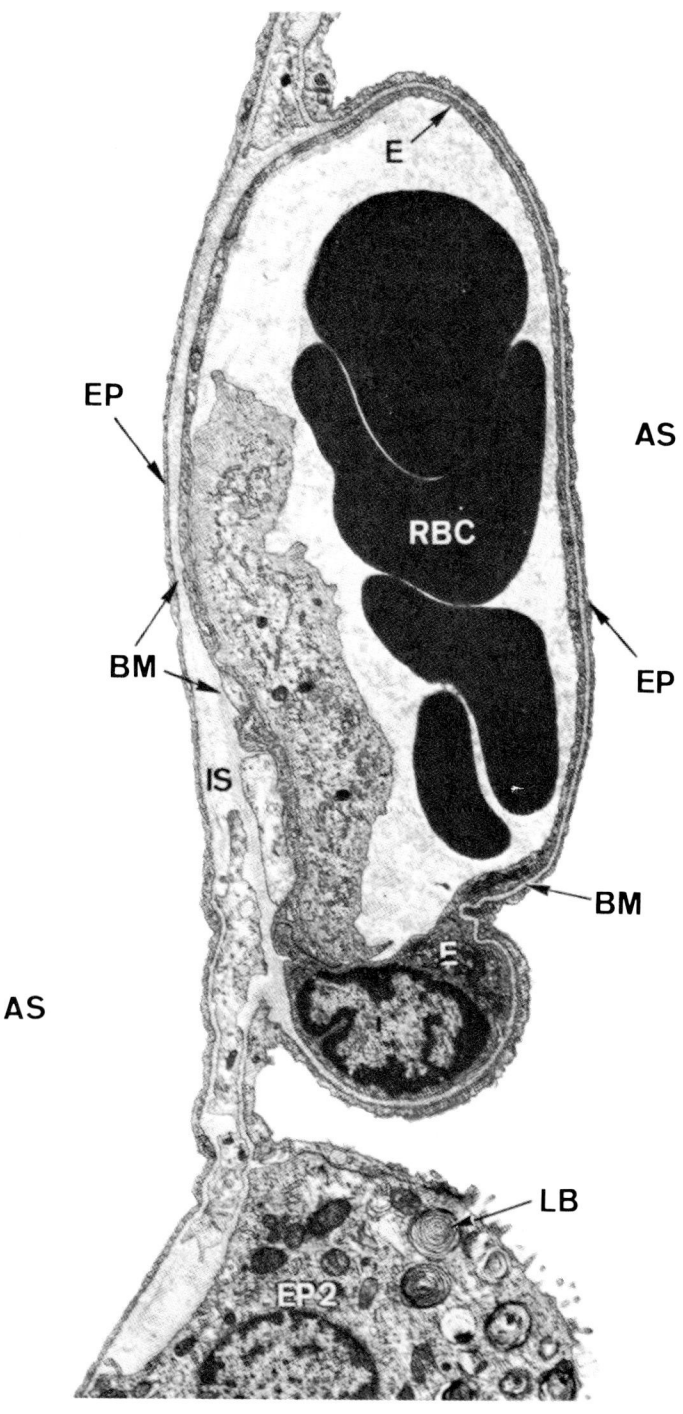

FIGURE 3–5. Transmission electron micrograph of a transverse section through a pulmonary capillary. AS = alveolar air space; EP = epithelium of a type I alveolar cell; IS = interstitial space; E = capillary endothelium; BM = basement membrane; RBC = red blood cell. Magnification ×11,500; electron micrograph by Dr. E.R. Weibel. (From Murray, J.F.: *The Normal Lung*, 2nd ed. Philadelphia, W.B. Saunders, 1986, with permission.)

veolus is literally enveloped in pulmonary capillaries. Estimates of the number of pulmonary capillaries are on the order of 280 *billion*, which works out to about 1,000 capillaries per alveolus. Although not all of the capillaries of the lung are normally perfused with mixed venous blood, estimates of the potential surface area of contact between the alveolar air and pulmonary capillary blood range from 50 to 100 m^2. This huge surface area combined with a small distance for gases to travel makes the lung well-suited for gas diffusion.

Alveoli average about 250 μm in diameter at the

normal resting lung volume. As the figure shows, the alveolar septa, which surround the alveolar air spaces, appear to be almost entirely constructed of pulmonary capillaries covered by the cytoplasm of the thin type I alveolar cells. Erythrocytes can be seen inside the pulmonary capillaries. Elastic and connective tissue fibers, not visible in the figure, are interlaced between the capillaries in the alveolar septa. Also shown in this figure are the *pores of Kohn* or interalveolar communications, which may be important in *collateral ventilation*— that is, ventilation by the same duct of two adjacent alveoli normally supplied by different alveolar ducts. This can occur if the duct to the other alveolus has been occluded. The *canals of Lambert* also provide collateral ventilation.

Chest Wall and Muscles of Respiration

The muscles of respiration and the chest wall are essential components of the respiratory system.

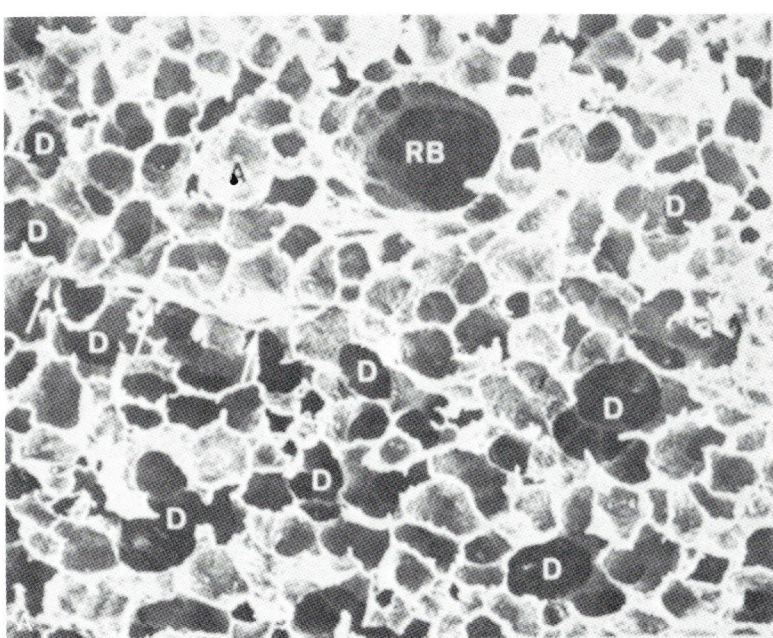
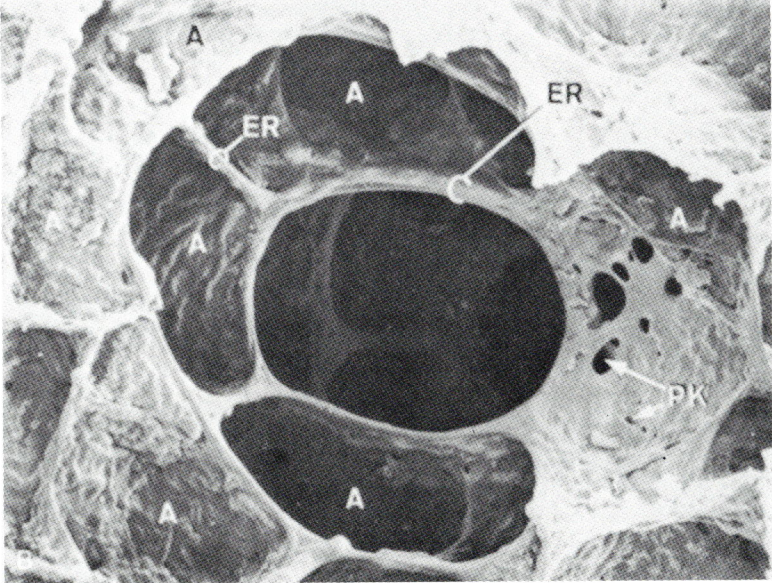

FIGURE 3–6. Scanning electron micrographs of human lung parenchyma: *A*, Respiratory bronchiole ×55. *B*, Alveolar duct ×235.

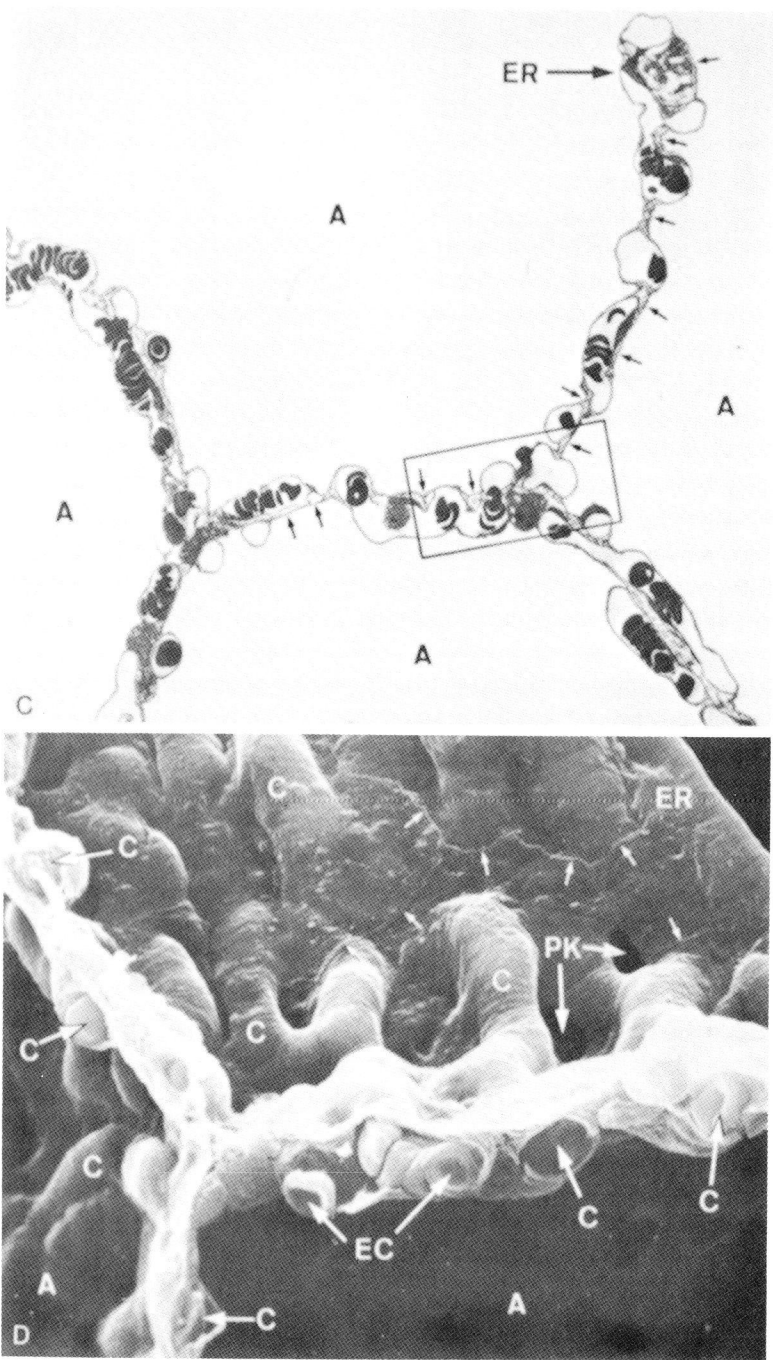

FIGURE 3–6 Continued C, Electron micrographs of interalveolar septa with capillaries: Transmission electron micrograph ×595. D, Scanning electron micrograph ×900. (A = alveolus; D = alveolar duct; RB = respiratory bronchiole; ER = entrance ring of alveolus; PK = pore of Kohn; C = capillary; EC = erythrocyte.) (From Gehr, P., Bachofen, M., and Weibel, E.R.: The normal human lung: Ultrastructure and morphometric estimation of diffusion capacity. *Respiration Physiology* 32:121, 1978, with permission.)

The lungs cannot inflate themselves—the force of this inflation must be supplied by the muscles of respiration. As we will see shortly, the chest wall must be intact and able to expand if air is to enter the alveoli.

Figure 3–7 shows the primary components of the chest wall. These include the rib cage; the external and internal intercostal muscles and the diaphragm, which are the main muscles of respiration; and the lining of the chest wall, the visceral and parietal pleura. Other muscles of respiration include the abdominal muscles, chiefly the rectus

PULMONARY ANATOMY AND PHYSIOLOGY 99

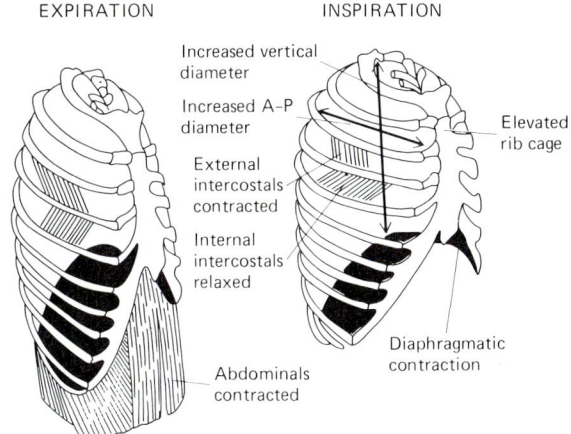

FIGURE 3–7. The chest wall and the muscles of breathing. (From Guyton, A.: *Textbook of Medical Physiology*, 7th ed. Philadelphia, W.B. Saunders, 1986, with permission.)

abdominis; the parasternal intercartilaginous muscles; and the accessory muscles of inspiration, the sternocleidomastoid and scalene muscles.

Central Nervous System

The final component of the respiratory system to be considered is the central nervous system. The impulse for each breath is originated in the brain, and this message is carried to the respiratory muscles via the spinal cord and nerves innervating the respiratory muscles. Thus, the muscles of respiration, unlike cardiac muscles, do not contract spontaneously.

Spontaneous automatic breathing is generated by groups of neurons located in the medulla. This medullary respiratory center, which is located close to the cardiovascular center, is also the final integration point for influences from higher brain centers, such as those concerned with voluntary breathing and speech; information from arterial chemoreceptors and those in the cerebrospinal fluid; and afferent information from neural receptors in the airways, joints and muscles, skin, and elsewhere in the body. Structural aspects of the control of breathing are discussed later in this chapter.

MECHANICS OF BREATHING

Air, like other fluids, moves from a region of higher pressure to one of lower pressure. Therefore, for air to be moved into or out of the lungs, a pressure difference between the atmosphere and the alveoli must be established. If there is no pressure gradient, no air flow occurs. The generation of this pressure gradient and the forces involved in moving the air and the lungs and chest wall are called the mechanics of breathing.

Air is normally moved from the atmosphere into the alveoli by causing alveolar pressure to fall below atmospheric pressure. Because atmospheric pressure is conventionally referred to as 0 cmH_2O in discussions of pulmonary physiology (measurements in cmH_2O are used instead of mmHg because the pressures are generally lower than those encountered in cardiovascular physiology), lowering alveolar pressure below atmospheric pressure is referred to as *negative-pressure breathing*. In the practice of respiratory therapy and anesthesia, it is frequently necessary to deliver air or other gas mixtures to the alveoli by raising the pressure at the nose and mouth above alveolar pressure. Such *positive-pressure breathing* is used on patients unable to generate a sufficient pressure gradient between the atmosphere and alveoli to move air through the airways. Expiration occurs when alveolar pressure exceeds atmospheric pressure by an amount sufficient to overcome the resistance to air flow offered by the conducting airways.

Pressure-Flow Relationships in Breathing

Alveoli are not capable of expanding themselves. They expand passively in response to an increased distending pressure (that is, an increased transmural pressure gradient) across the alveolar wall. This is accomplished by contraction of the muscles of inspiration, which increases the *volume* of the sealed thoracic cavity. According to Boyle's Law, this decreases the *pressure* outside of the lungs (the intrapleural pressure, or more correctly, *pleural surface pressure*), thus increasing the distending force exerted on the very distensible or *compliant* alveoli.

The intrapleural pressure is normally slightly negative with respect to atmospheric pressure, even when no respiratory muscles are contracting. This pressure is usually about -3 to -5 cmH_2O at the end of a normal expiration (when all of the respiratory muscles are relaxed), because of the mechanical interaction between the lung and chest wall. As we will see later in this chapter, the lung and chest wall are recoiling in opposite directions at the end of a normal expiration. The lung is tending to *decrease* its volume because of the *inward* elastic recoil of its distended alveolar septa; the chest wall is tending to *increase* its volume because of its *outward* elastic recoil. The chest wall is therefore acting to hold the alveoli open in opposition to their elastic recoil. Similarly, the lung is acting, by its inward elastic recoil, to hold the chest wall in.

The tiny fluid-filled space between the outside of the lung and the inside of the chest wall (between the visceral and parietal pleura) is therefore caught between these two opposing forces. This creates a slight partial vacuum and is thus responsible for the negative intrapleural pressure. There is normally no gas in the intrapleural space, which is about 5 to 10 μm thick, with a *total* volume of lining liquid estimated to be only 2 ml. Thus the outside of the lung is virtually sealed to the inside of the chest wall by the pleural liquid.

The events involved in breathing are summarized in Figure 3–8 and Table 3–1. Inspiration is initiated in the brain, either in conscious centers or automatically in the medullary respiratory center. Stimulation of the nerves innervating the inspiratory muscles causes them to contract. The main inspiratory muscles are the diaphragm and external intercostal muscles. The accessory muscles of inspiration are called into play during exercise, sneezing, and other situations requiring deep inspirations.

The diaphragm, which is a large dome-shaped muscle about 250 cm^2 in surface area, is innervated by the two phrenic nerves, which leave the spinal cord at the third through the fifth cervical segments. When the diaphragm contracts, its dome descends into the abdominal cavity, elongating the thorax. Because it is inserted into the lower rib margins, the lower ribs are also elevated during deep diaphragmatic contractions. The diaphragm is the primary muscle of inspiration, and it is responsible for about two thirds of the air that enters the lungs during normal quiet breathing (which is called *eupnea*).

The external intercostals (and parasternal intercartilaginous muscles) raise and enlarge the rib cage when they are stimulated to contract. This action increases the anteroposterior dimension of the chest as the ribs rotate upward about their axes and also increases the transverse dimension of the lower portion of the chest. These muscles are innervated by the intercostal nerves leaving the spinal cord at the first through the 11th thoracic segments.

Initially, before any air flow occurs, the pressure

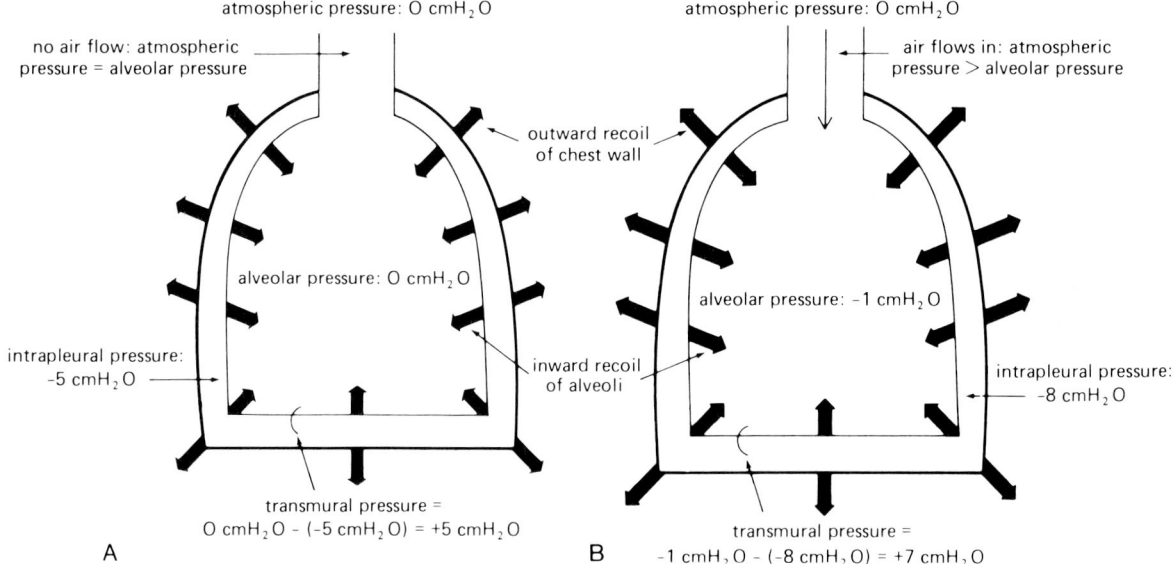

FIGURE 3–8. The interaction of the lung and chest wall: *A,* At end-expiration the muscles of respiration are relaxed. The inward elastic recoil of the lung is balanced by the outward elastic recoil of the chest wall. Intrapleural pressue is −5 cmH$_2$O; alveolar pressure is 0. The transmural pressure gradient across the alveolus is therefore 0 cmH$_2$O −(−5 cmH$_2$O) or 5 cmH$_2$O. Since alveolar pressure is equal to atmospheric pressure, no air flow occurs. *B,* During inspiration, contraction of the muscles of inspiration causes intrapleural pressure to become more negative. The transmural pressure gradient increases, and the alveoli are distended, decreasing alveolar pressure below atmospheric pressure, which causes air to flow into the alveoli. (From Levitzky, M.G.: *Pulmonary Physiology,* 2nd ed. New York, McGraw-Hill, 1986, with permission.)

PULMONARY ANATOMY AND PHYSIOLOGY

TABLE 3–1. Events Involved in a Normal Tidal Breath

Inspiration
1. Brain initiates inspiratory effort.
2. Nerves carry the inspiratory command to the inspiratory muscles.
3. Diaphragm (and/or external intercostal muscles) contracts.
4. Thoracic volume increases as the chest wall expands.*
5. Intrapleural pressure becomes more negative.
6. Alveolar transmural pressure increases.
7. Alveoli expand (according to their individual compliance curves) in response to the increased transmural pressure gradient. This increases alveolar elastic recoil.
8. Alveolar pressure falls below atmospheric pressure as the alveolar volume increases, thus establishing a pressure gradient for air flow.
9. Air flows into the alveoli until alveolar pressure equilibrates with atmospheric pressure.

Expiration (passive)
1. Brain ceases inspiratory command.
2. Inspiratory muscles relax.
3. Thoracic volume decreases, causing intrapleural pressure to become less negative and decreasing the alveolar transmural pressure gradient.†
4. Decreased alveolar transmural pressure gradient allows the increased alveolar elastic recoil to return the alveoli to their preinspiratory volumes.
5. Decreased alveolar volume increases alveolar pressure above atmospheric pressure, thus establishing a pressure gradient for air flow.
6. Air flows out of the alveoli until alveolar pressure equilibrates with atmospheric pressure.

* Note that Nos. 4 to 8 occur simultaneously.
† Note that Nos. 3 to 5 occur simultaneously.

inside the alveoli is the same as atmospheric pressure, that is, 0 cmH$_2$O. As the inspiratory muscles contract, expanding the thoracic volume and increasing the outward stress on the lung, the intrapleural pressure becomes *more negative*. Therefore, the transmural pressure gradient tending to distend the alveolar wall increases, and the alveoli enlarge passively, lowering alveolar pressure and establishing the pressure gradient for air flow into the lung. In reality, only a small number of alveoli are directly exposed to the intrapleural surface pressure, and it is difficult to see how alveoli located centrally in the lung could be expanded by a more negative intrapleural pressure. Careful analysis has shown, however, that the distending pressure of the alveoli at the pleural surface is transmitted through the alveolar walls to more centrally located alveoli. This structural *interdependence* of alveolar units is demonstrated in Figure 3–9.

As the air flows into the alveoli, alveolar pressure returns to 0 cmH$_2$O, and air flow into the lung ceases. When the inspiratory effort ends and the muscles relax, the intrapleural pressure becomes less negative, and the elastic recoil of the alveolar walls, which is increased at the higher lung volume, compresses the alveolar gas. This raises alveolar pressure, according to Boyle's Law, above atmospheric pressure so that air flows out of the lung until an alveolar pressure of 0 cmH$_2$O is restored.

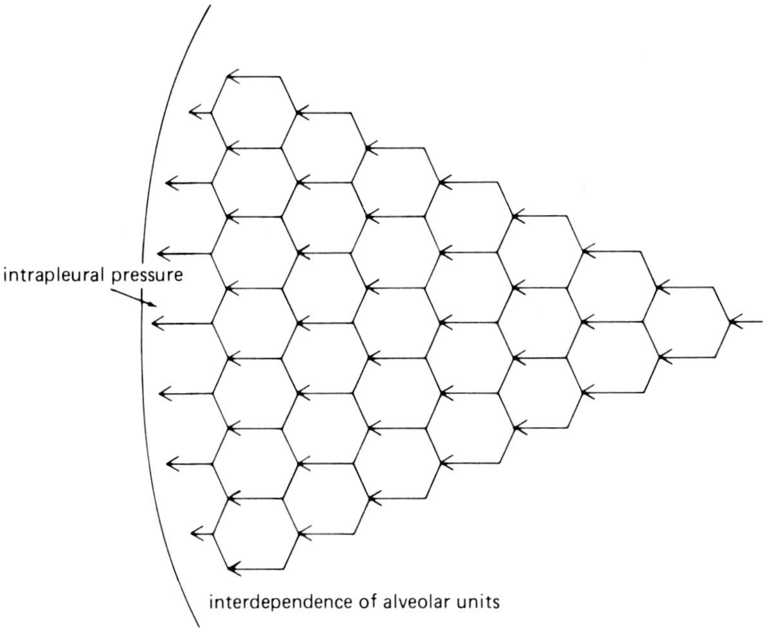

FIGURE 3–9. Structural interdependence of alveolar units. The pressure gradient across the outermost alveoli is transmitted mechanically through the lung via the alveolar septa. (From Levitzky, M.G.: *Pulmonary Physiology*, 2nd ed. New York, McGraw-Hill, 1986, with permission.)

In other words, expiration is *passive* during normal quiet breathing, and it is not necessary for any respiratory muscles to contract. As the inspiratory muscles relax, the increased elastic recoil of the distended alveoli is sufficient to decrease the alveolar volume and raise alveolar pressure above atmospheric pressure.

Active expiration occurs during exercise, speech, singing, and the expiratory phase of coughing or sneezing and in pathologic states, such as chronic bronchitis. The muscles of expiration are the muscles of the abdominal wall, including the rectus abdominis, external and internal oblique muscles, and transversus abdominis, and the internal intercostal muscles.

Abdominal Muscles. When the abdominal muscles contract, they compress the abdominal contents against the relaxed diaphragm, forcing it upward into the thoracic cavity. They also help to depress the lower ribs and pull down the anterior part of the lower chest. The abdominal muscles are innervated by the lower six thoracic and first lumbar spinal nerves.

Internal Intercostal Muscles. Contraction of the internal intercostal muscles depresses the rib cage downward in a manner opposite to the actions of the external intercostals.

Contraction of the expiratory muscles to cause a forced expiration results in *positive* intrapleural pressures. This may compress small airways and greatly increase the resistance to air flow. This important effect is discussed later in this chapter.

Pressure-Volume Relationships and Compliance

One way to look at the pressure-volume relationships of the lung is to remove the lungs from an animal and then graph the changes in volume that occur for each change in *transpulmonary pressure* the lungs are subjected to. That is how Figure 3–10 was obtained. The transpulmonary pressure is equal to the pressure in the trachea minus the intrapleural pressure. Thus, it is the pressure difference across the *whole lung*. The pressure in the alveoli, however, is the same as the pressure in the airways at the beginning and end of each normal breath; that is, end-expiratory or end-inspiratory alveolar pressure is 0 cmH$_2$O. Therefore, under static conditions, the transpulmonary pressure and the alveolar transmural pressure or alveolar distending pressure are equivalent terms.

Figure 3–10 shows that as the transpulmonary pressure increases, the lung volume increases.

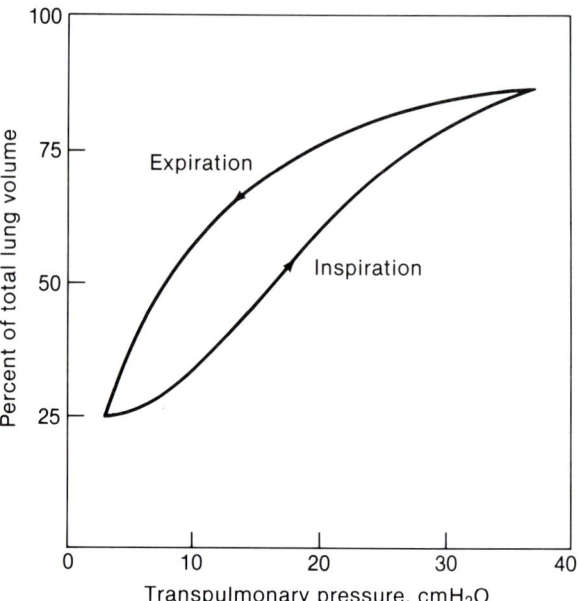

FIGURE 3–10. Pressure-volume curve for isolated lungs.

This relationship is not a straight line because the lung is composed of living tissue. Although at low lung volumes the lung distends easily, at high lung volumes the elastic tissue components of alveolar walls have already been stretched out and large increases in transpulmonary pressure only yield small increases in volume.

Elastic Recoil of the Lung

The slope between two points on a pressure-volume curve, like the one in Figure 3–10, is called the *compliance*. Compliance is therefore defined as the change in volume divided by the change in pressure. Compliance is the *inverse* of elasticity or elastic recoil. Compliance denotes the ease with which something can be stretched or distorted; elasticity refers to the tendency for something to oppose stretch or distortion as well as its ability to return to its original configuration after the distorting force is removed. As noted in the previous paragraph, the lungs are more compliant at lower volumes and less compliant at higher volumes. A curve like the one in Figure 3–10 is the same whether the lungs are inflated with positive pressure (by forcing air into the trachea) or with negative pressure (by suspending the lung except for the trachea in a closed chamber and pumping out the air around the lung). So, when the lung alone is considered, only the transpulmonary pressure is important, not how the transpulmonary pressure is generated. This is not the case if the chest wall is included because in a normal negative-pressure breath the chest wall *generates* the negative pressure, whereas in a positive-pressure breath the chest wall elastic recoil may act to oppose inflation. Note that the pressure-volume curve for inflation and the curve for deflation differ, as shown by the arrows in Figure 3–10. Such a difference is called *hysteresis*. Finally, it is helpful to think of each alveolus as having its own pressure-volume curve like the one in Figure 3–10.

The compliances of the lung and chest wall provide very useful information for the clinical evaluation of a patient's respiratory system, because many diseases or pathologic states affect either the compliance of the lung or chest wall or both. The clinical assessment of lung and chest wall compliance is discussed in greater detail in Chapter 9. Pathologic conditions that decrease lung compliance shift the pulmonary pressure-volume curve to the right. In such conditions as pulmonary fibrosis, pneumothorax, or lung collapse, greater transpulmonary pressures must be generated during inspiration to move the same volume of air. Decreased compliance of the *chest wall* may be caused by obesity or musculoskeletal deformities, and that effect also increases the work of breathing.

Surface Tension in the Alveoli

Thus far, we have discussed elastic recoil of the lungs as though it is due to only the elastic properties of the pulmonary parenchyma itself. There is another component of the elastic recoil of the lung, however, besides the constituents of the lung tissue, which is the *surface tension* at the air-liquid interface in the alveoli.

Surface tension forces occur whenever a gas and a liquid or two different immiscible liquids come in contact with one another. They are generated by the cohesive forces between the molecules of the liquid. These cohesive forces balance each other within the liquid phase but are unopposed at the surface of the liquid. This imbalance therefore causes an inward force. Surface tension is what causes water to bead and form droplets.

The role of surface tension forces in the elastic recoil of the lung can be demonstrated in an experiment, such as the one shown in Figure 3–11, which was performed on an excised lung in a manner similar to that employed in Figure 3–10. At the right side of the figure, the lung is inflated with air so that an air-liquid interface is present in the lung and surface tension forces contribute to the elastic recoil of the lung. Then, all of the gas is removed from the lung, and it is inflated again, this time with saline instead of air, as shown at the left. In this situation of no gas-liquid interface, surface tension forces are absent. The elastic recoil results only from the elastic recoil of the lung itself. Note that there is no hysteresis with saline inflation. Whatever causes the hysteresis appears to be related to surface tension in the lung.

The demonstration of the large role of surface tension forces in the recoil pressure of the lung led to consideration of how surface tension affects the alveoli. If the alveolus is considered to be a sphere, as in Figure 3–12, then the relationship between the pressure inside the alveolus and the wall tension of the alveolus is given by Laplace's Law:

$$T \propto \frac{Pr}{2}$$

where T is the tension in dynes/cm, P is the pres-

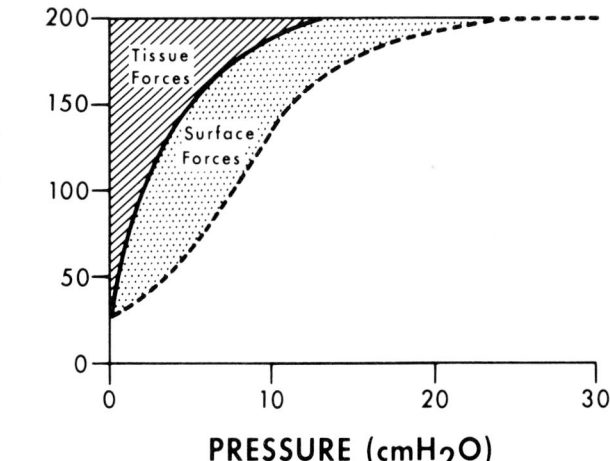

FIGURE 3–11. Separation of the normal pressure-volume curve of excised lungs into tissue recoil forces and surface tension forces. (From Murray, J.F.: *The Normal Lung*, 2nd ed. Philadelphia, W.B. Saunders, 1986, with permission.)

104 PULMONARY ANATOMY AND PHYSIOLOGY

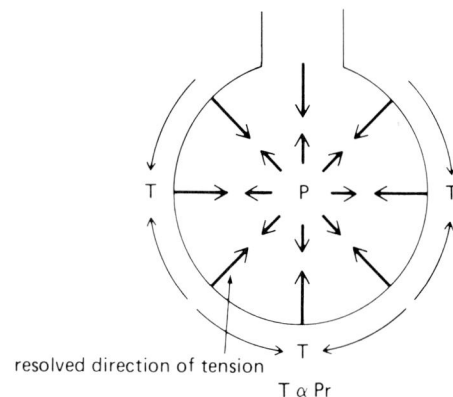

FIGURE 3–12. Relationship between the pressure inside a distensible sphere such as an alveolus and its wall tension. (From Levitzky, M.G.: *Pulmonary Physiology*, 2nd ed. New York, McGraw-Hill, 1986, with permission.)

sure in dynes/cm^2, and r is the radius of the sphere in cm.

The surface tension of most liquids (such as water) is constant and not dependent on the surface area of the air-liquid interface. Consider what this would mean in the lung, where alveoli of different sizes are connected to each other by common airways and collateral ventilation pathways. If we imagine two alveoli of different sizes connected by a common airway, as shown in Figure 3–13, and that the surface tension of the two alveoli is equal, then according to Laplace's Law the pressure in the smaller alveolus must be greater than that in the larger alveolus. Therefore, the smaller alveolus would empty into the larger alveolus.

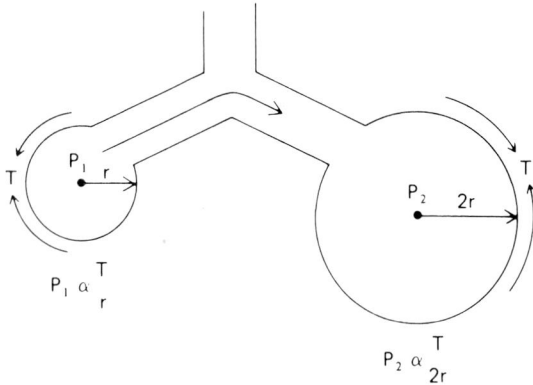

FIGURE 3–13. Diagram of two alveoli of different sizes connected to a common airway. If the surface tension is the same in both alveoli, then the smaller alveolus will have a higher pressure and will empty into the larger alveolus. (From Levitzky, M.G.: *Pulmonary Physiology*, 2nd ed. New York, McGraw-Hill, 1986, with permission.)

Thus, if the lung were composed of interconnected alveoli of different sizes (which it is) with a *constant surface tension* at the air-liquid interface, we would expect it to be inherently unstable, with a tendency for smaller alveoli to collapse into larger ones. Normally, this is not the case. This is fortunate because collapsed alveoli require very high distending pressures to reopen, partly because of the cohesive forces at the liquid-liquid interface. At least two additional factors contribute to the stability of the alveoli: a substance called *pulmonary surfactant* and the *structural interdependence of the alveoli.* (Collateral ventilation may also contribute to the stability of alveoli.)

The results of a series of experiments done to determine the surface tension properties of the lung lining liquid are shown in Figure 3–14. Various liquids were placed in a trough that had one moveable wall. Therefore, the size of the trough, and thus the size of the air-liquid interface, could be altered. Surface tension was measured by determining the downward pull on a thin strip of metal suspended from a force transducer so that it partly entered the liquid phase.

The surface tension properties of water, water after the addition of detergent, blood serum, and lung extract are plotted with respect to the relative surface area of the trough. Water has a relatively

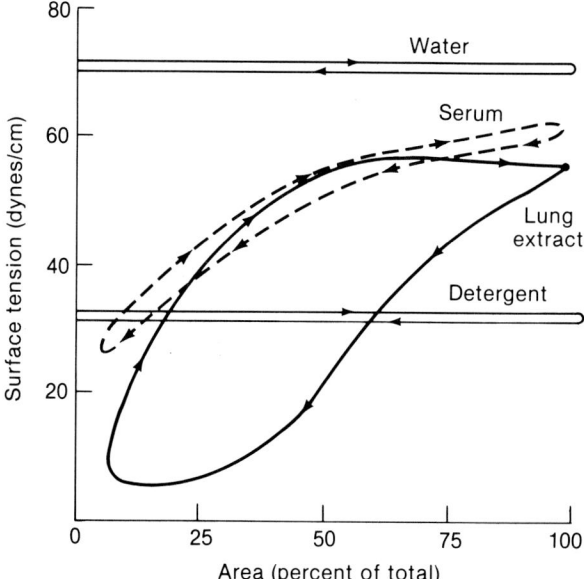

FIGURE 3–14. Diagram of surface tension-area relationships of water, water with detergent, serum, and lung extract. (Adapted from Clements, J.A., and Tierney D.F.: Alveolar instability associated with altered surface tension. In Fenn, W.O., and Rahn, H. (eds.): *Handbook of Physiology*, vol. 2. Washington, D.C., American Physiological Society, 1965, with permission.)

high surface tension, about 72 dynes/cm, and it is completely independent of surface area. Adding detergent to the water decreases the surface tension, but it is still independent of surface area. Blood serum has a surface tension lower than that of water, and to a small extent, its surface tension is dependent on surface area because its surface tension is somewhat lower at smaller relative areas. Lung extract, which was obtained by washing the liquid film that lines the alveoli out with saline, displays both low overall surface tension and a great deal of area dependence. At high surface areas its surface tension is about 45 dynes/cm. At low surface areas, the surface tension falls to nearly 0 dynes/cm. Futhermore, the lung extract also displays a great deal of hysteresis.

We can therefore conclude that the alveoli are lined with a liquid that lowers the component of their elastic recoil owing to surface tension, even at high lung volumes. This increases the compliance of the lungs and thus decreases the work of breathing on inspiration. Because the surface tension is decreased at relatively low areas, it is likely that the surface tension of different-sized alveoli is *not constant* but rather that smaller alveoli have lower surface tensions. This helps to equalize alveolar pressures throughout the lung (so the end-expiratory pressure of all the alveoli is 0 cmH$_2$O), and it also helps to stabilize alveoli. Finally, the hysteresis seen in lung pressure-volume curves seems to be a property of the fluid lining the alveoli.

The surface active component of the lung extract is called *pulmonary surfactant*. It is a complex of different phospholipids, with dipalmitoyl lecithin constituting the largest fraction. It is manufactured by type II alveolar epithelial cells, as we noted earlier in this chapter. Pulmonary surfactant appears to be continuously produced in and in some way destroyed or used up in the lung. The clinical consequences of a lack of functional pulmonary surfactant can be seen in several conditions, including Adult Respiratory Distress Syndrome (discussed in Chapter 5) and Infant Respiratory Distress Syndrome (discussed in Chapter 6).

In summary, pulmonary surfactant helps to lower the work of inspiration by lowering the surface tension of the alveoli, which reduces the elastic recoil of the lung and makes the lung more compliant. Surfactant also helps stabilize the alveoli by decreasing the surface tension of smaller alveoli, thus equalizing the pressure inside alveoli of different sizes.

The second factor tending to stabilize alveoli is their *mechanical interdependence*. If an alveolus were to begin to collapse, it would increase the stresses on the walls of the alveoli adjacent to it, which would tend to hold it open. This would oppose a tendency for isolated alveoli suffering from a relative lack of pulmonary surfactant to collapse spontaneously. Conversely, if a whole subdivision of the lung (such as a lobule) has collapsed, the first alveolus reinflated helps to pull other alveoli open by its mechanical interdependence with them.

Mechanical Interdependence of the Lung and Chest Wall

We discussed the interaction between the lung and chest wall earlier in this chapter. The inward elastic recoil of the lung opposes the outward elastic recoil of the chest wall and vice versa. If the integrity of the lung-chest wall system is disturbed by opening the chest wall, as by a surgical incision or a knife wound, the inward elastic recoil of the lung can no longer be opposed by the outward recoil of the chest wall, and their interdependence ceases. Lung volume decreases, and alveoli have a much greater tendency to collapse. As air moves in through the wound, intrapleural pressure equalizes with atmospheric pressure and abolishes the transpulmonary pressure gradient. At this point, nothing is tending to hold the alveoli open in opposition to their elastic recoil, which is causing them to collapse. Similarly, the chest wall tends to expand because its outward recoil is no longer opposed by the inward recoil of the lung.

When the lung-chest wall system is intact and the respiratory muscles are relaxed, the volume of gas left in the lungs is determined by the balance of these two forces. The volume of gas in the lungs at the end of a normal expiration is known as the *functional residual capacity* (FRC). For any given situation, the FRC is the lung volume at which the outward recoil of the chest wall is equal to the inward recoil of the lungs. The relationship between lung elastic recoil and chest wall elastic recoil is illustrated in static (or relaxation) pressure-volume curves (Fig. 3–15).

When a relaxation pressure-volume curve is obtained, subjects breathe air from a spirometer so that lung volumes can be measured. Intrapleural pressure is measured with an esophageal balloon; pressure is also measured at the subject's nose or mouth. Subjects are instructed to breathe air into or from the spirometer and then suddenly relax their respiratory muscles at the same time a stopcock in the airway is turned to occlude airflow. The stopcock is positioned in the airway just distal

106 PULMONARY ANATOMY AND PHYSIOLOGY

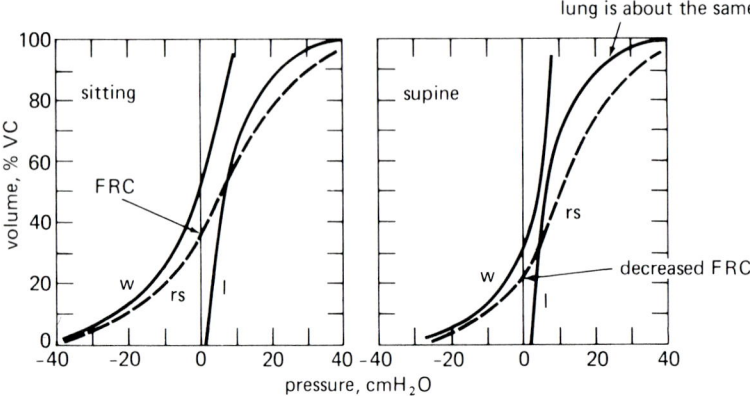

FIGURE 3–15. Static volume-pressure curves of the lung, chest wall, and total system in the sitting and supine positions. (Adapted from Agostoni, E.: Mechanics of the pleural space. *Physiological Reviews* 52:63, 1972, with permission.)

to the mouth, so the pressure measured at the mouth represents the total recoil pressure of the lungs and the chest wall. It is also equal to alveolar pressure because no airflow is occurring. This total recoil pressure is labelled *rs* (respiratory system) in the figure. The individual recoil pressures of the lung and chest wall can be calculated because the intrapleural pressure is known. Lung recoil pressure is labelled *l* on the graph; chest wall recoil pressure is labelled *w*. The graph on the left was made from data obtained when subjects were sitting up; the graph on the right was made from data obtained when subjects were lying on their backs.

The graphs show that the pressure measured at the mouth (line *rs*) is equal to 0 cmH$_2$O at the point at which lung recoil pressure is equal and opposite to chest wall recoil pressure. Therefore, alveolar pressure is also 0 cmH$_2$O. The lung volume at this point is the subject's FRC.

As the subject increases his or her lung volume, the total system recoil pressure becomes positive because of two factors: the increased inward recoil of the lung and the decreased outward recoil of the chest wall. In fact, at high lung volumes, the recoil pressure of the chest wall is also positive. This is because at high lung volumes, above about 75% of the *total lung capacity* (TLC), where line *w* crosses the zero pressure line, the chest wall also has inward elastic recoil. In other words, if one could imagine a relaxed, intact chest wall with no lungs in it, its resting volume would be about 75% of the volume of the chest wall when the lungs are maximally (voluntarily) expanded. At chest wall volumes below about 75% of the TLC, the chest wall elastic recoil is outward; at chest wall volumes above 75% of the TLC, the recoil is inward. Therefore, at high lung volumes, the mouth pressure is highly positive because both lung and chest wall elastic recoil is inward. At low lung volumes (below the FRC), the relaxation pressure measured at the mouth is negative because the outward recoil of the chest wall is now greater than the reduced inward recoil of the lungs.

The point of this discussion can be seen in the right-hand graph, in which the subject is supine. The elastic recoil curve for the lung is relatively unchanged, but the recoil curves for the chest wall and respiratory system are shifted to the right. This is because of the effect of gravity on the mechanics of the chest wall, especially the diaphragm. When a person is standing or sitting, the contents of the abdomen are being pulled away from the diaphragm by gravity. When the same person lies down, the abdominal contents are pushing inward against the relaxed diaphragm. This occurrence decreases the overall outward recoil of the chest wall and shifts the chest wall elastic recoil curve to the right. The respiratory system curve is the sum of the lung and chest wall curves, so it is also shifted to the right.

The lung volume at which the outward recoil of the chest wall is equal to the inward recoil of the lung (FRC) is much lower in the supine position, as can be seen by the point where the *rs* line crosses the zero recoil pressure line. Studies have shown that the FRC decreases by about one liter (or about one third) when a person changes from the standing or sitting position to the supine position.

Airways Resistance

We have seen that one major portion of the work of breathing is to overcome the elastic recoil of the lungs and chest wall. From our discussions of the generation of the pressure gradient between the alveoli and atmosphere and the work of the heart in Chapter 2, it should be obvious that the other major component of the work of breathing is to overcome the resistance to air flow offered by the conducting airways. There are a few other factors involved in the work of breathing, including the inertia of the system, which is usually negligible, and the pulmonary tissue resistance. Pulmonary tissue resistance is caused by the friction encountered as the lung tissues move against each other as the lung expands. The airways resistance plus pulmonary tissue resistance is often referred to as *pulmonary resistance*. Pulmonary tissue resistance normally contributes about 20% of the pulmonary resistance, with airways resistance responsible for the other 80%.

Laminar and Turbulent Flow

As stated in Chapter 2, the relationship for pressure, flow, and resistance is:

$$\text{Pressure difference} = \text{flow} \times \text{resistance}$$

The symbol $\dot{V}$ is used to denote air flow, so:

$$\Delta P = \dot{V} \times R \quad \text{or}$$

$$R = \frac{\Delta P \, (cmH_2O)}{\dot{V} \, (L/sec)}$$

Thus, the units of airways resistance are usually $cmH_2O/L/sec$. As noted in the section on vascular resistance in Chapter 2, resistances in series add directly; resistances in parallel add as reciprocals.

Air flow, like blood flow, can occur as laminar, turbulent, or transitional (a mixture of laminar and turbulent) flow. As Figure 2–24 showed, during laminar flow:

$$\Delta P \propto \dot{V} \times R_1$$

and follows Poiseuille's Law, but during turbulent flow:

$$\Delta P \propto \dot{V}^2 \times R_2$$

As also noted in Chapter 2, laminar flow changes to turbulent flow when a Reynold's number of about 2,000 is exceeded. One important difference between laminar air flow and turbulent air flow is that during turbulent flow, the resistance term R_2 is influenced more by the gas *density;* during laminar flow, the resistance term R_1 is influenced more by the *viscosity* of the gas.

According to the formula for Reynold's number, turbulent flow tends to occur if the linear velocity of air flow is high, if gas density is high, and/or if the tube radius is large. True laminar flow probably only occurs in the smallest airways, where the linear velocity of air flow is extremely low. Linear velocity (cm/sec) is equal to the flow (cm^3/sec) divided by the cross-sectional area. The total cross-sectional area of the smallest airways is very large, so the linear velocity of air flow is very low. The air flow in the trachea and larger airways is either turbulent or transitional.

Determinants of Airways Resistance

About 25% to 40% of the total resistance to air flow is located in the upper airways: the nose, nasal turbinates, oropharynx, nasopharynx, and larynx. Resistance is greater when one breathes through the nose rather than the mouth.

In the tracheobronchial tree, the component with the highest individual resistance is obviously the smallest airway, which has the smallest radius. However, because the smallest airways are all arranged in parallel, their resistances add as reciprocals. Thus, the total resistance to air flow offered by the millions of airways is extremely low during normal, quiet breathing. Under normal circumstances, therefore, the greatest resistance to air flow resides in the medium-sized bronchi.

Bronchial Tone

The smooth muscle of the airways from the trachea down to the alveolar ducts is under the control of efferent fibers of the autonomic nervous system. Stimulation of the cholinergic *parasympathetic* postganglionic fibers causes constriction of bronchial smooth muscle as well as increased glandular mucus secretion. The preganglionic fibers travel in the vagus. Stimulation of the adrenergic *sympathetic* fibers causes dilation of bronchial and bronchiolar smooth muscle as well as inhibiting glandular secretion. This dilation of the airway smooth muscle is mediated by $beta_2$ receptors, which predominate in the airways. Selective stimulation of the alpha receptors with pharmacologic agents causes bronchoconstriction.

Inhalation of chemical irritants, smoke, or dust, as well as stimulation of the arterial chemoreceptors and other stimuli such as histamine, cause *reflex constriction* of the airways. Decreased CO_2 in the branches of the conducting system causes a *local* constriction of the smooth muscle of the nearby airways. This may help to balance ventilation and perfusion after a pulmonary embolus. Increased CO_2 causes a local dilation of the small airways.

Lung Volume

Airways resistance decreases at higher lung volumes, as shown in Figure 3–16. Even more striking

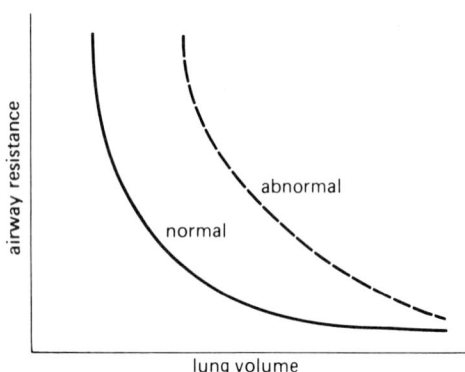

FIGURE 3–16. Relationship between lung volume and airways resistance. Total lung capacity is at right; residual volume is at left. Solid line represents normal lung; dashed line, abnormal (emphysematous) lung. (Reprinted by permission of *The Western Journal of Medicine* [formerly *California Medicine*], Murray, J.F., Greenspan, R.H., Gold, W.M., and Cohen, A.B.: Early diagnosis of chronic obstructive lung disease, 116:43, 1972.)

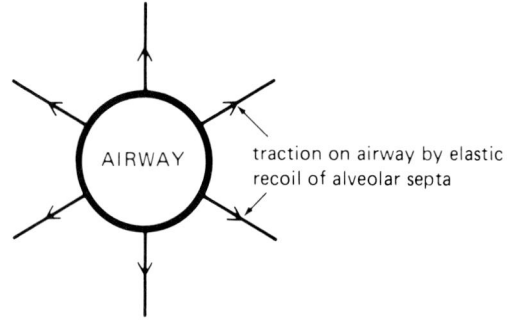

FIGURE 3–17. Representation of "traction" of the alveolar septa on small distensible airways. (From Levitzky, M.G.: *Pulmonary Physiology*, 2nd ed. New York, McGraw-Hill, 1986, with permission.)

is the effect of low lung volumes on airways resistance: At low lung volumes, airways resistance increases dramatically. This relationship is still true in an emphysematous lung, but the resistance is higher at all lung volumes and is especially higher at very low lung volumes. The pathophysiology of emphysema and other obstructive lung diseases is discussed in Chapter 5.

There are two explanations for the relationship between lung volume and airways resistance. They both involve the distensibility and compressibility of the smaller airways, which, as already noted, have little or no cartilaginous support. One is the transmural pressure gradient; the other is the role of alveolar septal attachments to the small airways.

Let's look first at the decreased airways resistance seen at high lung volumes. To increase lung volume, a person breathing normally takes a deep breath, that is, he or she makes a strong inspiratory effort. This effort causes intrapleural pressure to become much more negative than the −7 or −10 cmH$_2$O seen in a normal quiet breath. The transmural pressure gradient across the wall of the airways exposed to intrapleural pressure becomes much more positive and the small airways are distended.

A second reason for the decreased airways resistance seen at higher lung volumes is the so-called traction on small airways. As Figure 3–17 shows, the small airways traveling through the lung form attachments to alveolar septa. As the alveoli expand during the course of deep inspiration, the elastic recoil in their walls increases. This elastic recoil is transmitted to the attachments at the airway, pulling it open.

Airways resistance is extremely high at low lung volumes (see Fig. 3–16). To achieve low lung volumes, a person must make a forced expiratory effort by contracting the muscles of expiration, mainly the abdominal and internal intercostal muscles. This effort generates *positive* intrapleural pressure, which can be as high as 100 cmH$_2$O during a maximal forced expiratory effort. (Maximal inspiratory intrapleural pressures can be as low as −80 cmH$_2$O.) The effect of this high positive intrapleural pressure on the transmural pressure gradient during a forced expiration can be seen at the right in Figure 3–18, a schematic of a single alveolus and airway.

Dynamic Compression

In Figure 3–18, the muscles of expiration are generating a positive intrapleural pressure of +25 cmH$_2$O. Pressure in the alveolus is higher than intrapleural pressure because of the alveolar elastic recoil pressure of +10 cmH$_2$O, which gives an alveolar pressure of +35 cmH$_2$O. Note that the alveolar pressure is always greater than the intrapleural pressure because the *alveolar pressure is equal to the intrapleural pressure plus the alveolar elastic recoil pressure*.

The alveolar elastic recoil pressure decreases at lower lung volumes because the alveoli are not as distended. In the figure, a gradient has been established from the alveolar pressure of +35 cmH$_2$O to the atmospheric pressure of 0 cmH$_2$O. If the airways were rigid and incompressible, this large expiratory pressure gradient would generate very high rates of air flow. However, the airways are not uniformly rigid, and the smallest airways,

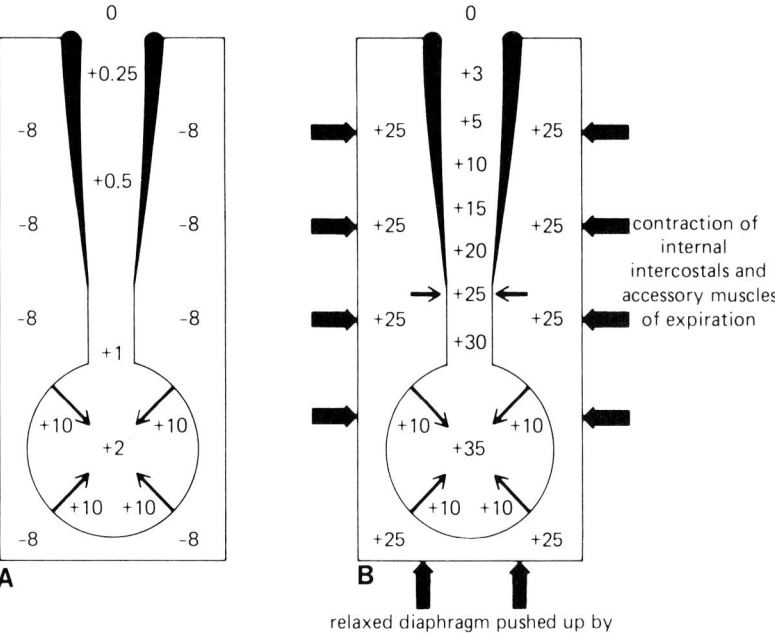

FIGURE 3–18. Dynamic compression of airways and the equal pressure point hypothesis during a forced expiration. A, Passive (eupneic) expiration. B, Forced expiration. See text for complete description. (From Levitzky, M.G.: *Pulmonary Physiology*, 2nd ed. New York, McGraw-Hill, 1986, with permission.)

which have no cartilaginous support, may be compressed or even collapsed. Whether or not they collapse depends on the transmural pressure gradient of the smallest airways and how much support they receive from alveolar septa.

The situation during a normal *passive* expiration at the same lung volume (note the same alveolar recoil pressure) is shown at the left in Figure 3–18. The transmural pressure gradient across the smallest airway is $+1$ cmH_2O $-(-8)$ cmH_2O = $+9$ cmH_2O, tending to hold the airway open. During the *forced expiration* at right, the transmural pressure gradient is 30 cmH_2O $-$ 25 cmH_2O or only 5 cmH_2O holding the airway open. The airway is likely to be slightly compressed, and its resistance to air flow is greater than that during passive expiration. This increased resistance during a forced expiration is called *dynamic compression* of airways.

One way of looking at dynamic compression is the *equal pressure point hypothesis*. According to this hypothesis, at any instant during a forced expiration, there must be a point along the airway where the pressure inside the airway is just equal to the pressure outside the airway. At that point, the transmural pressure gradient is zero (note the arrows in Fig. 3–18). Above that point, the transmural pressure gradient is *negative*: The pressure outside the airway is greater than the pressure inside it, and the airway collapses if cartilaginous support or alveolar septal traction is insufficient to keep it open.

As the forced expiratory effort continues, the equal pressure point is likely to *move down the airway* from larger to smaller airways because, as the muscular effort of expiration increases, intrapleural pressure increases and because, as lung volume decreases, alveolar elastic recoil pressure decreases. As the equal pressure point moves down the airway, dynamic compression increases and airways ultimately begin to collapse. This airway closure can only be demonstrated at especially low lung volumes in healthy subjects, but the *closing volume* may occur at higher lung volumes in patients with emphysema or elderly subjects, as discussed in Chapters 5 and 6, respectively. The closing volume test is discussed in Chapter 9.

It is important to consider the pressure gradient for air flow during dynamic compression. During a passive expiration, the pressure gradient for air flow (the ΔP in $\Delta P = \dot{V}R$) is simply alveolar pressure minus atmospheric pressure. But if dynamic compression occurs, the effective pressure gradient is alveolar pressure minus *intrapleural pressure*, because intrapleural pressure is higher than atmospheric pressure and because intrapleural pressure can exert its effects on the compressible portion of the airways. We have already seen that the alveolar pressure minus the intrapleural pressure is the alveolar elastic recoil pressure. Thus, as lung volume decreases, alveolar elastic recoil decreases, and the driving pressure for forced expiratory air flow decreases.

One way to demonstrate the interaction of the dynamic compression of airways and the lung volume is the *isovolumetric pressure-flow curve*. These curves, which are not used in clinical assessment because the data are tedious to work up, are obtained by having a subject make repeated forced expiratory maneuvers with different degrees of effort. Intrapleural pressures are estimated from those obtained from a balloon in the thoracic portion of the esophagus, lung volumes are determined with a spirometer, and air flow rates are determined by using a pneumotachograph. The pressure-flow relationship for each of the expiratory maneuvers of various efforts is plotted on a curve for a *particular lung volume*. For example, the middle curve of Figure 3–19 was constructed by determining the intrapleural pressure and air flow for each expiratory maneuver at the instant the subject's lung volume passed through 50% of vital capacity. *Vital capacity* (VC) is defined as the maximum volume of air that can be exhaled following a maximal inspiratory effort. It is defined more precisely in the next section.

Figure 3–19 demonstrates the effects of dynamic compression of the airways. The middle curve represents pressure-flow relationships at a single lung volume (50% of the vital capacity). The alveolar elastic recoil is therefore constant for this curve. Increasing the expiratory effort increases air flow up to a point. Beyond that point, generating more positive intrapleural pressure does not increase air flow: Air flow becomes *effort-independent*. Airways resistance must be increasing with increasing expiratory effort. The air flow has become independent of effort because of greater dynamic compression with more positive intrapleural pressures. The equal pressure point has moved to compressible small airways and is fixed there. Note that, even at lower lung volumes (25% *VC*) at which there is less alveolar elastic recoil, this occurs with lower maximal air flow rates. At high lung volumes (75% VC), air flow increases steadily with increasing effort. It is entirely *effort-dependent* because alveolar elastic recoil pressure is high and because highly positive intrapleural pressures cannot be attained at such high lung volumes (if the glottis is open). The concepts of dynamic compression and effort independence can also be seen in *flow-volume curves*, which are discussed in Chapter 9.

The Work of Breathing

We can summarize the main points of the mechanics of breathing by considering the *work of*

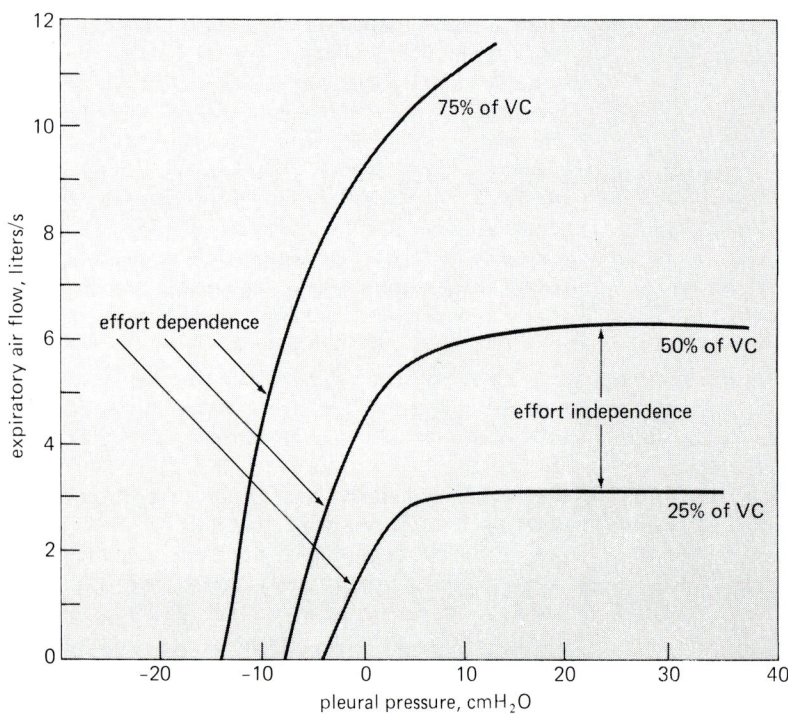

FIGURE 3–19. Isovolumetric pressure-flow curves at three different lung volumes: 75%, 50%, and 25% of the vital capacity. (Adapted from Hyatt, R.E.: Dynamic lung volumes. In Fenn, W.O., and Rahn, H. (eds.): *Handbook of Physiology*, vol. 2. Washington, D.C., American Physiological Society, 1965, with permission.)

breathing. In physics, this work can be defined as the pressure change times the volume change. The volume change is the volume of air moved into and out of the lung, the *tidal volume*. The pressure change is the change in transpulmonary pressure necessary to overcome the *elastic* work of breathing and the *resistive* work of breathing.

The elastic work of breathing is the work done to overcome the elastic recoil of the chest wall and the pulmonary parenchyma and to overcome the surface tension of the alveoli. The resistive work of breathing is the work done to overcome the tissue resistance and airways resistance. Normally, most of the resistive work is that done to overcome airways resistance. The resistive work of breathing can be extremely great during a forced expiration, when dynamic compression occurs. This is especially true in patients who already have elevated resistance during normal quiet breathing.

Patients with restrictive lung diseases have to expend much effort to inhale deeply, and even the work of generating normal inspirations is greatly increased. As a result, they usually breathe at higher rates with smaller tidal volumes. Patients with obstructive lung diseases usually breathe at lower rates and deeper tidal volumes. The mechanisms by which the respiratory controller makes these adjustments is not completely understood.

The oxygen cost of normal quiet (eupneic) breathing is usually less than 5% of the total body oxygen uptake. This percentage can increase to as much as 30% in healthy subjects during maximal exercise. In patients with obstructive lung disease, however, the work of breathing can be the factor that limits exercise.

ALVEOLAR VENTILATION

Alveolar ventilation is defined as the volume of fresh air entering the alveoli per minute. A similar volume of alveolar air must leave the body per minute, but the two volumes are not usually exactly equal. This is because not every molecule of oxygen used by the body results in a molecule of CO_2 released by the body, and because of the heating and humidification of inspired air.

Lung Volumes

The volume of gas in the lungs at any instant depends on the mechanics of the lungs and chest wall and the activity of the respiratory muscles. Standardization of the conditions under which lung volumes are measured allows comparisons to be made between subjects or patients. Because the size of a person's lungs depends on height and weight or body surface area as well as his or her age and sex, the lung volumes for a patient are usually compared to data from a table of predicted lung volumes matched to age, sex, and body size. The lung volumes are normally expressed at body temperature, ambient pressure, and saturated with water vapor (BTPS).

There are four basic standard lung *volumes* and four standard lung *capacities,* which are combinations of the standard lung volumes. These are shown in Figure 3–20.

Tidal Volume. The tidal volume (TV, or V_T) is the volume of air coming into or out of the nose or mouth per breath. It is determined by the activity of the respiratory control centers in the brain as they cause the contraction of respiratory muscles and by the mechanics of the lung and chest wall. During normal quiet breathing (eupnea), the tidal volume of a 70 kg adult is about 500 ml per breath, but this volume can be greatly increased, for example, during exercise.

Residual Volume. The residual volume (RV) is the volume of gas left in the lungs after a maximal forced expiration. It is determined by the force generated by the muscles of expiration acting in concert with the inward elastic recoil of the lungs to oppose the outward elastic recoil of the chest wall. Dynamic compression of the airways during the forced expiratory effort may also be an important determinant of the residual volume as airway collapse occurs, thus trapping gas in the alveoli. The residual volume of a healthy 70 kg adult is about 1.5 L, but it can be much greater in obstructive lung disease, such as emphysema.

Expiratory Reserve Volume. The expiratory reserve volume (ERV) is the volume of gas expelled from the lungs during a maximal forced expiration that *starts* at the end of a normal tidal expiration. It is therefore determined by the difference between the functional residual capacity and the residual volume. The expiratory reserve volume is about 1.5 L in a healthy 70 kg adult.

Inspiratory Reserve Volume. The inspiratory reserve volume (IRV) is the volume of gas inhaled into the lungs during a maximal forced inspiration that starts at the end of a normal tidal inspiration. It is determined by the strength of contraction of the inspiratory muscles, the inward elastic recoil of the lung and chest wall, and the starting point, which is the functional residual capacity plus the tidal volume. The inspiratory reserve volume of a normal 70 kg adult is about 2.5 L.

Functional Residual Capacity. The functional residual capacity (FRC) is the volume of gas re-

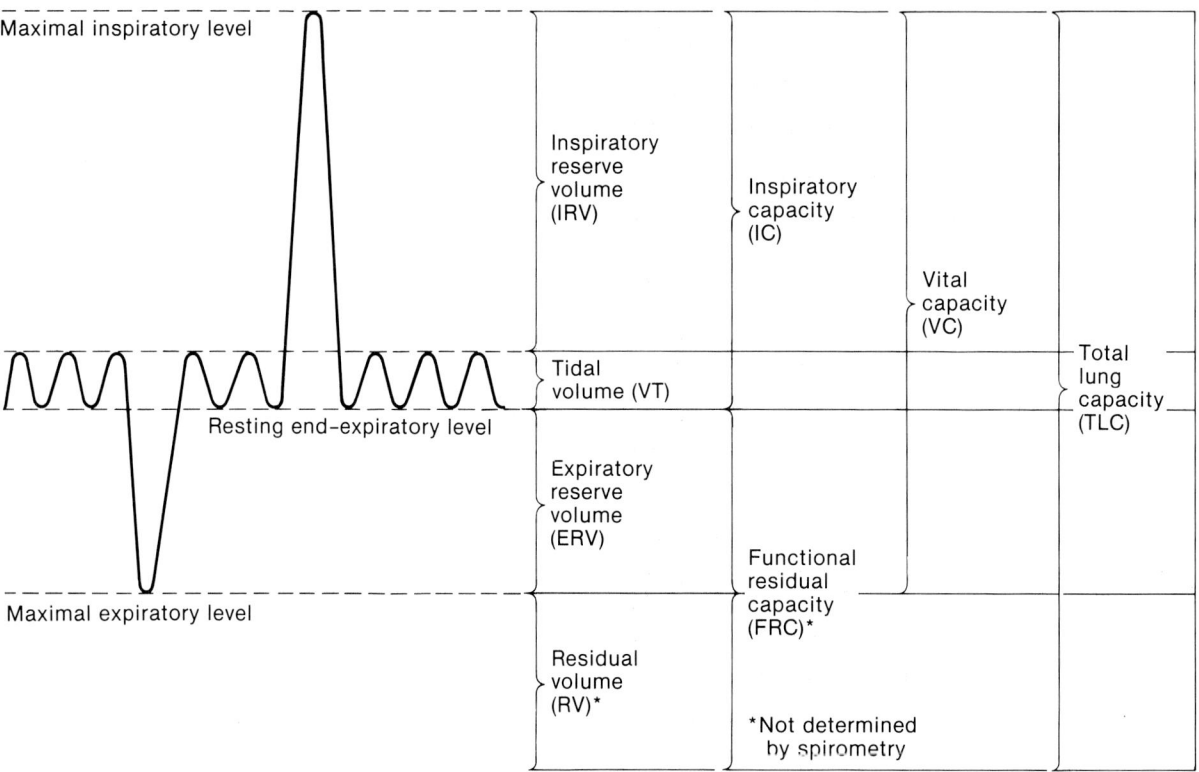

FIGURE 3-20. The standard lung volumes and capacities.

maining in the lungs at the end of a normal tidal expiration. Because no muscles of respiration are contracting at this time, it represents the balance point between the inward elastic recoil of the lungs and the outward elastic recoil of the chest wall, as discussed earlier. The FRC, as seen in Figure 3-20, consists of the residual volume plus the expiratory reserve volume. It is therefore about 3 L in a healthy 70 kg adult.

Inspiratory Capacity. The inspiratory capacity (IC) is the volume of air inhaled into the lungs during a maximal inspiratory effort that begins at the end of a normal tidal expiration (the FRC). It is therefore equal to the tidal volume plus the inspiratory reserve volume (see Fig. 3-20). The inspiratory capacity of a normal 70 kg adult is about 3 L.

Total Lung Capacity. The total lung capacity (TLC) is the volume of air in the lungs after a maximal inspiratory effort. It is determined by the strength of contraction of the inspiratory muscles and the inward elastic recoil of the lungs and chest wall. The total lung capacity consists of all four lung volumes: the residual volume plus the tidal volume plus the inspiratory and expiratory reserve volumes. It is about 6 L in the healthy 70 kg adult.

Vital Capacity. The vital capacity (VC) is the volume of air expelled from the lungs during a maximal forced expiration starting after a maximal forced inspiration. The vital capacity is therefore equal to the total lung capacity minus the residual volume, or about 4.5 L in a healthy 70 kg adult. The vital capacity is also equal to the sum of the tidal volume and the inspiratory and expiratory reserve volumes. It is determined by the same factors that determine total lung capacity and residual volume.

Measurement of the lung volumes is important clinically because many pathologic states can alter specific lung volumes or their relationships to each other (see Chapter 9). Lung volumes can also change for normal physiologic reasons. Changing from a standing to a supine posture decreases the functional residual capacity because gravity is no longer pulling the abdominal contents away from the diaphragm. This decreases the outward elastic recoil of the chest wall, as noted earlier. If the functional residual capacity is decreased, then the expiratory reserve volume also decreases, and the inspiratory reserve volume increases. The vital capacity may decrease slightly because some of the venous blood that collects in the lower extremities and abdomen when a person is standing returns to the thoracic cavity when he or she lies down.

Anatomic Dead Space

The volume of air entering and leaving the nose or mouth per minute, the *minute volume,* is not equal to the volume of air entering and leaving the alveoli per minute. *Alveolar ventilation* is *less* than the minute volume because the last part of each inspiration remains in the conducting airways and does not reach the alveoli. Similarly, the last part of each expiration remains in the conducting airways and is not expelled from the body. No gas exchange occurs in the conducting airways for anatomic reasons: The walls of the conducting airways are too thick for much diffusion to take place; mixed venous blood does not come into contact with the air. The conducting airways are therefore referred to as the *anatomic dead space*.

The relationship between the tidal volume (V_T) breathed in and out through the nose or mouth, the dead space volume (V_D), and the volume of gas entering and leaving the alveoli per breath (V_A) is:

$$V_T = V_D + V_A$$

or

$$V_A = V_T - V_D$$

Thus, if a person with an anatomic dead space of 150 ml has a tidal volume of 500 ml per breath, only 350 ml of gas enters and leaves the alveoli per breath.

Multiplying both sides of the above equation by the breathing frequency (n) in breaths per minute:

$$n(V_A) = n(V_T) - n(V_D)$$

$$\dot{V}_A = \dot{V}_E - \dot{V}_D$$

The alveolar ventilation ($\dot{V}_A$) in liters per minute is equal to the minute volume ($\dot{V}_E$) minus the volume wasted ventilating the dead space per minute ($\dot{V}_D$).

The dots over the V's indicate *per minute*. The symbol $\dot{V}_E$ is used because expired gas is usually collected. Thus, in the example above, if the breathing frequency (n) is 15 breaths/min, then

5250 ml/min = 7500 ml/min
alveolar ventilation   minute ventilation
                      − 2250 ml/min
                         dead space ventilation

Alveolar ventilation cannot be measured directly but must be determined from the tidal volume, breathing frequency, and dead space ventilation. The anatomic dead space in a normal person is usually about 1 ml/kg. The measurement of the anatomic dead space is discussed in Chapter 9.

Physiologic Dead Space

There is another kind of wasted ventilation that may occur in the lung—the ventilation of unperfused alveoli. Alveoli that are ventilated but not perfused are called *alveolar dead space*. They contribute nothing to gas exchange, although it is not because they are *anatomically* unable to participate in gas exchange. Alveolar dead space may occur distal to portions of the pulmonary circulation that have become occluded by blood clots (pulmonary emboli) or if right ventricular output is unable to perfuse upper regions of the lungs. Normal young healthy adults usually do not have any alveolar dead space.

The *Bohr equation* is used to determine the alveolar dead space *plus* the anatomic dead space. This is called the *physiologic dead space*:

Physiologic dead space = Anatomic dead space
                       + Alveolar dead space

The Bohr equation is based on the concept that air expired from alveoli that are both ventilated and perfused with mixed venous blood contributes carbon dioxide to the mixed expired air. On the other hand, air coming from anatomic or alveolar dead space has received no carbon dioxide from the mixed venous blood and is expired with only the tiny amount of carbon dioxide found in the inspired air. The Bohr equation is discussed in greater detail in Chapter 9.

Effects of Alveolar Ventilation on Oxygen and Carbon Dioxide Levels

The levels of oxygen and carbon dioxide in the alveolar gas are determined by the alveolar ventilation, the fractional concentrations of oxygen and carbon dioxide breathed, the oxygen consumption ($\dot{V}_{O_2}$) of the body, the carbon dioxide production of the body ($\dot{V}_{CO_2}$), and the flow of mixed venous blood to the lungs. Each tidal breath brings about 350 ml of fresh air, about 21% of which is oxygen, into the 3 L of gas already in the lungs (the FRC) and removes about 350 ml of air, about 5% or 6% of which is carbon dioxide. Meanwhile, about 250 ml of carbon dioxide diffuses from the pulmonary capillary blood into the alveoli and about 300 ml of oxygen diffuses from the alveolar air into the pulmonary capillary blood each minute.

Partial Pressures of Respiratory Gases

According to Dalton's Law, in a gas mixture, the pressure exerted by each individual gas in a space is independent of the pressures of other gases in the mixture. The partial pressure of a particular gas is therefore equal to its fractional concentration times the total pressure of all the gases in the mixture.

Oxygen constitutes 20.93% of dry atmospheric air. At a standard barometric pressure of 760 mmHg,

$$P_{O_2} = 0.2093 \times 760 \text{ torr} = 159 \text{ torr}$$

(The units of pressure are expressed as torr in honor of Torricelli, the inventor of the barometer.) Carbon dioxide constitutes only about 0.04% of dry atmospheric air, so

$$P_{CO_2} = 0.0004 \times 760 \text{ torr} = 0.3 \text{ torr}$$

Dry Atmospheric Gas at Standard Barometric Pressure

P_{O_2} = 159.0 torr
P_{CO_2} = 0.3 torr
P_{N_2} = 600.6 torr

As air is inspired through the upper airways, it is heated and humidified. The partial pressure of water vapor is a relatively constant 47 torr at body temperature. Therefore, humidification (that is, saturating it with water vapor) of a liter of dry gas *in a container* at 760 torr would increase its total pressure to 807 torr (760 + 47 torr). In the body, the gas simply expands, according to Boyle's Law so that we can think of the 1L of gas at 760 torr as *diluted* by the added water vapor. The P_{O_2} of inspired air (saturated with water vapor at a standard barometric pressure) then is equal to 0.2093 (760 − 47) torr, or 149 torr. The P_{CO_2} of inspired air is 0.0004 (760 − 47) torr, or 0.29 torr, which can be rounded off to 0.3 torr.

Inspired Gas at Standard Barometric Pressure

P_{IO_2} = 149.0 torr
P_{ICO_2} = 0.3 torr
P_{IN_2} = 564.0 torr
P_{IH_2O} = 47.0 torr

The partial pressures of oxygen and carbon dioxide in the alveolar air are determined by the alveolar ventilation, inspired P_{O_2} and P_{CO_2}, the oxygen uptake, and the carbon dioxide delivery to the lungs. Mixed venous blood, with a carbon dioxide partial pressure of 45 or 46 torr and an oxygen partial pressure of 40 torr, is continuously entering the pulmonary capillaries. As discussed later, alveolar ventilation is normally regulated by the respiratory control center in the brain to keep mean arterial and alveolar P_{CO_2} at about 40 torr. Mean alveolar P_{O_2} is about 104 torr.

Alveolar Gas at Standard Barometric Pressure

P_{AO_2} = 104 torr
P_{ACO_2} = 40 torr
P_{AN_2} = 569 torr
P_{AH_2O} = 47 torr

Alveolar P_{O_2} increases by 2 to 4 torr with each normal tidal inspiration and falls slowly until the next inspiration. Similarly, the alveolar P_{CO_2} falls 2 to 4 torr with each inspiration and increases slowly until the next inspiration. Expired air is a mixture of about 350 ml of alveolar air and 150 ml of air from the dead space. Therefore, the P_{O_2} of mixed expired air is higher than alveolar P_{O_2} and less than the inspired P_{O_2}, or about 120 torr. Similarly, the P_{CO_2} of mixed expired air is much higher than the inspired P_{CO_2} but lower than the alveolar P_{CO_2}, or about 27 torr.

Mixed Expired Air at Standard Barometric Pressure

P_{EO_2} = 120 torr
P_{ECO_2} = 27 torr
P_{EN_2} = 566 torr
P_{EH_2O} = 47 torr

Alveolar Ventilation and Carbon Dioxide

The concentration of carbon dioxide in alveolar gas, as already discussed, depends on the alveolar ventilation and the rate of carbon dioxide production by the body (and its delivery to the lungs in the mixed venous blood). The volume of carbon dioxide *expired* per unit of time ($\dot{V}_{ECO_2}$) is equal to the alveolar ventilation ($\dot{V}_A$) times the alveolar fractional concentration of carbon dioxide

(F_{ACO_2}). Remember that no carbon dioxide comes from the dead space.

$$\dot{V}_{ECO_2} = \dot{V}_A \times F_{ACO_2}$$

Similarly, the fractional concentration of carbon dioxide in the alveoli is directly proportional to the carbon dioxide production by the body ($\dot{V}_{CO_2}$) and is inversely proportional to the alveolar ventilation:

$$F_{ACO_2} \propto \frac{\dot{V}_{CO_2}}{\dot{V}_A}$$

Because:

$$F_{ACO_2} \times (760 - 47) = P_{ACO_2}$$

then:

$$P_{ACO_2} \propto \frac{\dot{V}_{CO_2}}{\dot{V}_A}$$

In healthy persons, alveolar P_{CO_2} is in equilibrium with arterial P_{CO_2} (P_{aCO_2}). Thus, if alveolar ventilation is doubled (and carbon dioxide production is unchanged), the alveolar and arterial P_{CO_2} are reduced by one half. If alveolar ventilation is cut in half, then alveolar and arterial P_{CO_2} double.

Alveolar Ventilation and Oxygen

As alveolar ventilation increases, the alveolar P_{O_2} should also increase. However, doubling alveolar ventilation cannot double P_{AO_2} in a person whose alveolar P_{O_2} is already 104 torr because the highest P_{AO_2} one can achieve (breathing air at sea level) is the inspired P_{O_2} of about 149 torr. The alveolar P_{O_2} can be calculated from the *alveolar air equation*. (The derivation of this formula is outside of the scope of this book.)

$$P_{AO_2} = P_{IO_2} - \frac{P_{ACO_2}}{R} + F$$

where R is the respiratory exchange ratio ($R = \dot{V}_{CO_2}/\dot{V}_{O_2}$) and F is a correction factor.

As alveolar ventilation increases, the alveolar P_{CO_2} decreases, bringing the alveolar P_{O_2} closer to the inspired P_{O_2}.

Regional Distribution of Alveolar Ventilation

Although it may seem reasonable to assume that the alveolar ventilation is distributed fairly evenly to all alveoli throughout the lungs, this is not the case. Studies done on normal subjects seated in the upright position and breathing from the FRC have shown that alveoli in the lower regions of the lungs receive more ventilation per unit volume than those in the upper regions of the lung. (This difference can be seen in the line for ventilation in Fig. 3–26.)

If a similar study is done on a subject lying on his or her side, the regional differences in ventilation between the *anatomic* upper and lower regions of the lung disappear, although relative ventilation of the lower lung is better than that of the upper lung. The regional differences in ventilation thus seem to be influenced by gravity, with the lower regions of the lung (the *dependent* regions) relatively better ventilated than the higher regions (the *nondependent* regions).

The most likely explanation for this regional difference of alveolar ventilation is based on regional differences in the intrapleural pressure and the pressure-volume curves of individual alveoli. Earlier in this chapter, the intrapleural surface pressure was discussed as if it were uniform throughout the thorax. Precise measurements of intrapleural surface pressures of intact chests in the upright position have shown that this is not the case: The intrapleural surface pressure is *less negative* in the lower gravity-dependent regions of the thorax than in the upper nondependent regions. A gradient of the intrapleural surface pressure exists such that, for every centimeter of vertical displacement down the lung (from nondependent to dependent regions), the intrapleural surface pressure increases by about $+0.2$ to $+0.3$ cmH$_2$O. This gradient is apparently caused by gravity and by mechanical interactions between the lung and the chest wall.

The influence of this gradient of intrapleural surface pressure on regional alveolar ventilation can be explained by predicting its effect on the transpulmonary pressure in upper and lower regions of the lung. Because the alveolar pressure is zero throughout the lung at the FRC and intrapleural pressure is *more negative in upper regions* of the lung than in lower regions, the alveolar distending pressure (alveolar minus intrapleural) is greater in upper regions of the lung. The alveoli in upper regions are subjected to greater distending pressures than those in more dependent regions, so they have greater *volumes* than the alveoli in more dependent regions.

We can see how this difference in alveolar volume results in a difference in ventilation between alveoli located in upper and lower regions of the lung by taking another look at the pressure-volume curve for the whole lung (see Figure 3–10). We can imagine each alveolus as having its own pressure-volume curve like the one shown in the figure.

An alveolus in the upper part of the lung has a greater transpulmonary pressure and therefore is at a larger volume than an alveolus in the lower part of the lung. At the functional residual capacity, therefore, an alveolus in the upper part of the lung is on a flatter portion of its alveolar pressure-volume curve (that is, it is *less compliant*) than an alveolus in the lower region. An alveolus in a lower lung region is on a steeper portion of its pressure-volume curve, so any change in the transpulmonary pressure during a normal respiratory cycle causes a greater *change in volume* in the alveolus in the lower region. Because the alveoli in the lower parts of the lung have a greater change in volume per inspiration and per expiration, they are better *ventilated* than those alveoli in nondependent regions (during eupneic breathing from the FRC).

A second effect of the intrapleural pressure gradient in a person standing or seated upright is on regional static lung volume. At the functional residual capacity, most of the alveolar air is in upper regions of the lung, because those alveoli have larger volumes. Most of the expiratory reserve volume is also in upper portions of the lung. On the other hand, most of the inspiratory reserve volume and inspiratory capacity are in lower regions of the lung.

In summary, most of the air inspired during a tidal breath begun at the functional residual capacity enters the alveoli in lower regions of the lung. However, if a slow inspiration is begun at the *residual volume,* the initial part of the breath enters the upper alveoli, and alveoli in lower regions begin to fill later in the breath. Of course, this is also a result of the intrapleural pressure gradient. During a forced expiration to the residual volume, alveoli in lower lung regions, which start at a lower volume than alveoli in upper lung regions, initially empty more rapidly. As positive intrapleural pressures are generated, small airways in lower regions of the lung are much more likely to be the first to collapse as a result of dynamic compression. This is because intrapleural pressure is slightly more positive in lower regions of the thorax and because the smaller alveoli in lower lung regions have less elastic recoil, so they offer less alveolar septal traction to hold the small airways open.

Therefore, at the beginning of an inspiration from the residual volume, airways in the lowest regions of the lung may still be collapsed and require large transpulmonary pressures to open. At the same time, alveoli in upper lung regions, which are at a lower volume than they would be at the functional residual capacity, are now on the steep portion of their pressure-volume curves. Thus, they are more compliant at the residual volume than they are at the functional residual capacity, and they receive more of the air initially inspired in the breath. It is also important to note that most of the residual volume is located in upper alveoli.

The lung volume at which airways begin to close is called the *closing capacity* or *closing volume*. The determination of the closing volume is discussed in Chapter 9.

BLOOD SUPPLY OF THE LUNGS

As already noted, the lung receives blood flow from both the bronchial and pulmonary circulations. *Bronchial blood flow* is only a small portion of the output of the left ventricle. *Pulmonary blood flow* constitutes the entire output of the right ventricle, supplying the lung with mixed venous blood draining all of the tissues of the body. It is this blood that undergoes gas exchange with the alveolar air in the pulmonary capillaries. The right and left ventricles are arranged in series, so pulmonary blood flow is about equal to 100% of the output of the left ventricle. That is, pulmonary blood flow is equal to the cardiac output—normally about 3.5 L per minute per square meter of body surface area at rest.

Bronchial Circulation

The bronchial arteries arise variably from the aorta. The blood flow in the bronchial circulation constitutes about 2% of the output of the left ventricle. Blood pressure in the bronchial arteries is the same as that in the other systemic arteries.

Although some of the bronchial venous blood enters the *azygos vein,* a substantial portion of bronchial venous blood enters the *pulmonary veins*. Because the blood in the pulmonary veins has undergone gas exchange with the alveolar air (that is, the pulmonary veins contain "arterial" blood), the bronchial venous blood that mixes with the pulmonary venous blood is part of the normal anatomic right-to-left *shunt,* which is discussed later. Anastomoses, or connections, between some bronchial capillaries and pulmonary capillaries and between bronchial arteries and branches of the pulmonary artery have also been demonstrated. These connections are probably not open in a normal healthy person but may open in pathologic states, when either bronchial or pulmonary blood flow to a portion of lung is occluded. For example, if pulmonary blood flow to an area of the lung is blocked by a pulmonary embolus, bronchial blood flow to that area increases.

Pulmonary Circulation

At any instant, there is about 250 to 300 ml of blood per square meter of body surface area in the pulmonary circulation. About 60 to 70 ml/m^2 is contained in the pulmonary capillaries. It takes a red blood cell an average of 4 to 5 seconds to travel through the pulmonary circulation at resting cardiac outputs; about 0.75 to 1.2 seconds of that time is spent in pulmonary capillaries. In traveling through the lung, an erythrocyte passes through a number of successive pulmonary capillaries. Gas exchange starts to occur in smaller pulmonary arterial vessels, which are not truly capillaries by histologic standards. These arterial segments and successive capillaries may be thought of as *functional pulmonary capillaries*. Usually, when we refer to pulmonary capillaries, we mean functional pulmonary capillaries rather than anatomic capillaries.

The alveoli are completely enveloped in pulmonary capillaries. The capillaries are so near to each other that some investigators have described pulmonary capillary blood flow as resembling blood flowing through two parallel sheets of endothelium held together by occasional connective tissue supports.

Determinants of Pulmonary Vascular Resistance

As already noted, there is much less vascular smooth muscle in the vessel walls of the pulmonary arterial tree, and there are no highly muscular vessels that correspond to the systemic arterioles. The thin walls and small amount of smooth muscle of the pulmonary arteries have important physiologic consequences. The pulmonary vessels offer much less resistance to blood flow and are also much more *distensible* than systemic arterial vessels. These factors lead to much lower intravascular pressures than those found in the systemic arteries. The lower intravascular pressures make the pulmonary arterial vessels much more compressible than systemic arterial vessels. Because the pulmonary vessels are distensible and compressible and because they are situated in the thorax and subject to alveolar and intrapleural pressures (which can change greatly during inspiratory or forced expiratory efforts), factors other than the tone of the pulmonary vascular smooth muscle have profound effects on the pulmonary vascular resistance. These include gravity, body position, lung volume, alveolar and intrapleural pressure, right ventricular output, and pulmonary arterial and left atrial pressure.

Calculation of Pulmonary Vascular Resistance

According to Poiseuille's Law:

$$R = (P_1 - P_2)/\dot{Q}$$

where P_1 is the pressure at the beginning of the tube, P_2 is the pressure at the end of the tube, $\dot{Q}$ equals the flow, and R is the resistance.

For the pulmonary circulation, then

$$PVR = \frac{MPAP - MLAP}{PBF}$$

That is, the pulmonary vascular resistance (PVR) is equal to the mean pulmonary artery pressure (MPAP) minus the left atrial pressure (MLAP), with the result divided by pulmonary blood flow (PBF) or cardiac output. The measurement of pulmonary blood flow (cardiac output) is discussed in Chapter 8.

This formula is only an approximation under the most optimal circumstances, because of these factors: Blood is not a Newtonian fluid, pulmonary blood flow is *pulsatile* (and may also be turbulent), the pulmonary circulation is distensible and *compressible,* and the pulmonary circulation is an extremely complex branching structure. Furthermore, as discussed later, the mean left atrial pressure may not always be the appropriate downstream pressure to use in the calculation of pulmonary vascular resistance.

The right and left circulations are in series, so the outputs of the right and left ventricles must be about equal to each other over the long run. (If they are not, blood and edema fluid build up in the lungs or periphery.) If the two outputs are equal and the measured pressure drop across the systemic circulation and the pulmonary circulation are about 98 mmHg and 10 mmHg, respectively (Fig. 3–21), then the pulmonary vascular resistance must be about $\frac{1}{10}$ that of the systemic vascular resistance. This low resistance to blood flow offered by the pulmonary circulation is due to its *structural* aspects, as already discussed.

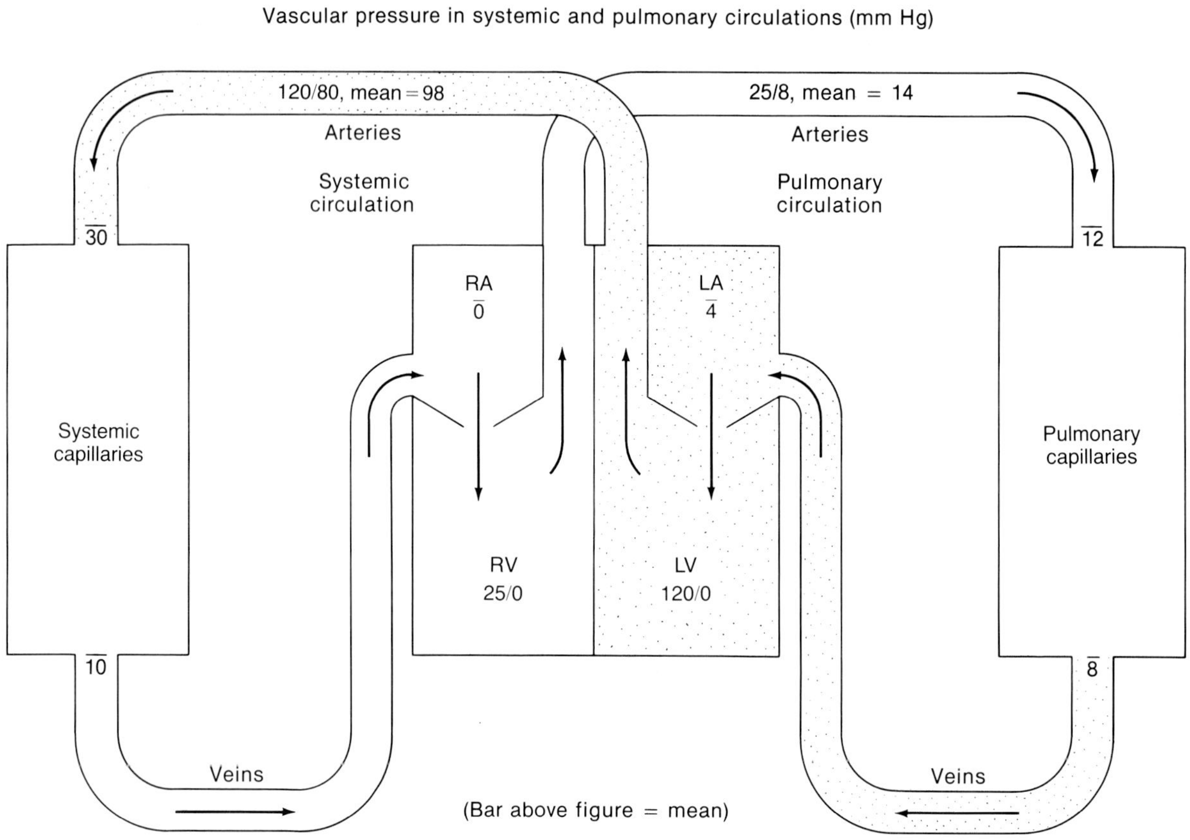

118 PULMONARY ANATOMY AND PHYSIOLOGY

Vascular pressure in systemic and pulmonary circulations (mm Hg)

FIGURE 3–21. Comparison of the pulmonary and systemic circulations.

Distribution of Pulmonary Vascular Resistance

As can be seen by looking at the pressure drop across the three major components of the pulmonary circulation, the resistance to blood flow at the FRC is fairly evenly distributed among the pulmonary arteries, capillaries, and veins. About one third of the resistance to blood flow is located in the pulmonary arteries, another third is located in the pulmonary capillaries, and about one third is located in the pulmonary veins. This is in contrast to the systemic circulation, in which about 70% of the resistance to blood flow is located in the muscular systemic arterioles.

Lung Volume

In considering the effects of lung volume on pulmonary vascular resistance, we must think in terms of two different groups of vessels: those exposed to alveolar pressure (*alveolar vessels,* mainly pulmonary capillaries) and those not exposed to alveolar pressure (*extra-alveolar vessels*). As lung volume increases during a normal negative-pressure inspiration, the alveoli increase in volume. As they expand, the vessels interposed between them, mainly pulmonary capillaries, are compressed. At high lung volumes, the resistance to blood flow offered by the alveolar vessels increases; at low lung volumes, the resistance to blood flow offered by the alveolar vessels decreases. These effects can be seen in the alveolar curve in Figure 3–22.

One component of the *extra-alveolar* vessels, the larger arteries and veins, is exposed to the intrapleural pressure. As lung volume is increased by making intrapleural pressure more negative, their transmural pressure gradient increases, and they distend. Another factor tending to decrease the resistance to blood flow offered by the extra-alveolar vessels at higher lung volumes is radial traction by the connective tissue and alveolar septa holding the larger vessels in place in the lung. Thus, at high lung volumes (attained by normal negative-pressure breathing), the resistance to blood flow offered by the extra-alveolar vessels decreases, as shown in Figure 3–22. During a forced expiration to low lung volumes, however, intrapleural pressure becomes strongly positive. The resistance to blood flow offered by the extra-alveolar vessels increases greatly, as seen at left in the figure.

Because the alveolar and extra-alveolar vessels may be thought of as two groups of resistances in series with each other, the resistances of those two groups of vessels are additive at any lung volume. Thus, the effect of changes in lung volume on the *total* pulmonary vascular resistance gives the U-shaped curve seen in Figure 3–22. Pulmonary vascular resistance is lowest near the functional residual capacity and increases at both high and low lung volumes.

A second type of extra-alveolar vessel is the so-called corner vessel or extra-alveolar capillary (Fig. 3–23). Although these vessels are found between alveoli, their locations at junctions of alveolar septa give them different mechanical properties, as the figure shows. Expansion of the alveoli during inspiration increases the wall tension of the alveolar septa, and the corner vessels are distended, whereas the alveolar capillaries are compressed.

During *mechanical* positive-pressure ventilation, intrapleural pressure is *positive* during *inspiration*. In this case, both the alveolar and extra-alveolar vessels should be compressed as lung volume increases (radial traction may oppose this in the extra-alveolar vessels), and the resistance to blood flow offered by both alveolar and extra-alveolar vessels increases during lung inflation. Positive intrapleural pressures may also compress the vena cavae and other intrathoracic vessels and, therefore, may decrease cardiac output. The physiologic effects of mechanical ventilation are discussed in Chapter 19.

Recruitment and Distensibility

During exercise, cardiac output can increase four- to five-fold without a correspondingly great increase in mean pulmonary artery pressure. Although the mean pulmonary artery pressure does increase, the increase is only a few mmHg, even if cardiac output has doubled or tripled. The pressure drop across the pulmonary circulation is proportional to the cardiac output times the pulmonary vascular resistance (that is, $\Delta P = \dot{Q} \times R$), so a decrease in pulmonary vascular resistance must have occurred.

This fall in pulmonary vascular resistance is *passive*—that is, not resulting from changes in the tone of pulmonary vascular smooth muscle caused by neural mechanisms or humoral agents. In fact,

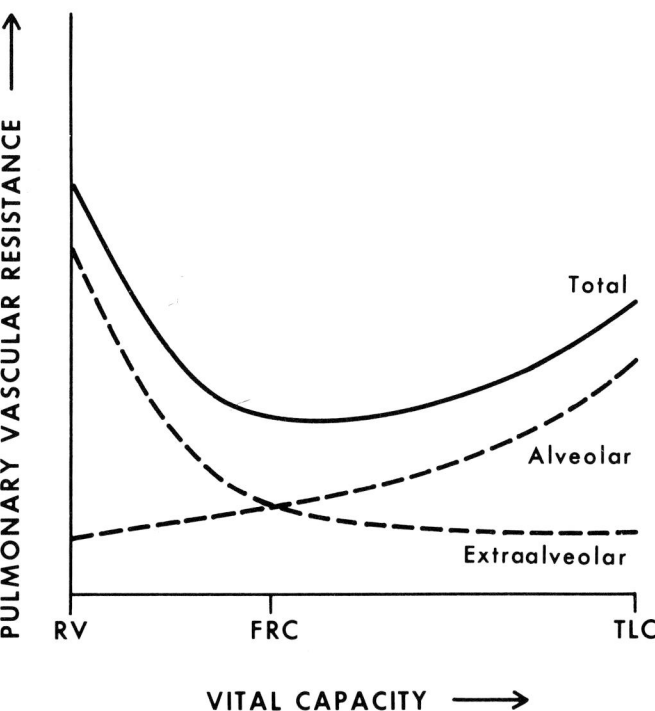

FIGURE 3–22. The effects of lung volume on pulmonary vascular resistance. PVR is lowest near the FRC and increases at both high and low lung volumes because of the combined effects on the alveolar and extra-alveolar vessels. To achieve low lung volumes, *positive* intrapleural pressures must be generated, which compresses the extra-alveolar vessels, as seen at left in the figure. (Adapted from Murray, J.F.: *The Normal Lung*, 2nd ed. Philadelphia, W.B. Saunders, 1986, with permission.)

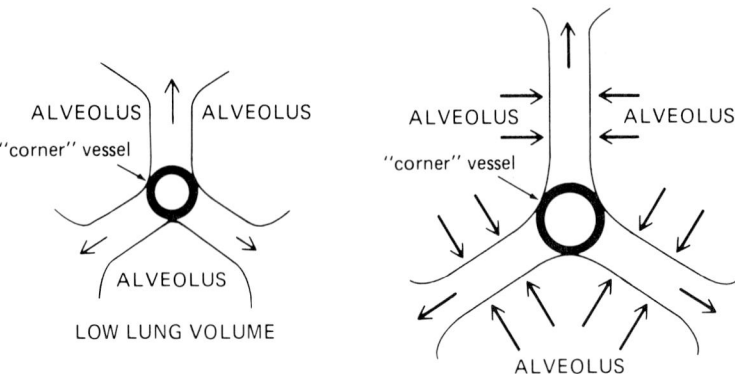

FIGURE 3–23. Diagram of the extra-alveolar corner vessels located at junctions of alveolar septa. Expansion of the alveoli causes radial traction on the corner vessels and expands them. The alveolar vessels are compressed at high lung volumes. (From Levitzky, M.G.: *Pulmonary Physiology,* 2nd ed. New York, McGraw-Hill, 1986, with permission.)

a decrease in pulmonary vascular resistance in response to increased blood flow or an increase in perfusion pressure can be demonstrated in an isolated perfused lung. Two different mechanisms can explain this decrease in pulmonary vascular resistance in response to elevated blood flow and perfusion pressure: *recruitment* and *distention.*

Not all of the pulmonary capillaries are perfused at resting cardiac outputs. Some are not perfused as a result of hydrostatic effects, which are discussed later. Others may be unperfused because they have a relatively high *critical opening pressure.* That is, these vessels, because of their high vascular smooth muscle tone, require a higher perfusion pressure than that solely needed to overcome hydrostatic forces. The critical opening pressures for pulmonary blood vessels are not likely to be very great because they have so little smooth muscle. As discussed later, elevated alveolar pressure can also increase the critical opening pressure.

As blood flow increases, the mean pulmonary artery pressure also increases, thus helping to overcome hydrostatic forces and exceed the critical opening pressure in vessels with high vascular tone. These changes cause new parallel pathways for blood flow to open, thus decreasing the pulmonary vascular resistance. The opening of these new pathways is called *recruitment.* It is important to know that as the cardiac output or pulmonary artery pressure decreases, a *derecruitment* of pulmonary capillaries can result. Obviously, recruiting more pulmonary capillaries allows these vessels to participate in gas exchange. On the other hand, derecruiting pulmonary capillaries decreases the ability of the lung to function as a gas exchange unit.

Pulmonary vascular distensibility has already been reviewed. As perfusion pressure increases, the lateral pressure component increases, thus increasing the transmural pressure gradient of the pulmonary vessels and causing their *distention.* As the vessels distend, their radii increase, which decreases their resistance to blood flow.

Is it recruitment or distention that causes the decreased pulmonary vascular resistance seen with elevated right ventricular output or perfusion pressure? Probably both do. It is likely that recruitment of pulmonary capillaries occurs at lower pulmonary vascular pressures and distention at higher pressures.

Control of Pulmonary Vascular Smooth Muscle

Pulmonary vascular smooth muscle responds to *neural* and *humoral* influences. Both produce active changes in pulmonary vascular resistance, in contrast to the passive factors discussed previously. We will consider another passive factor, *gravity,* shortly.

The pulmonary vasculature receives its innervation from sympathetic and parasympathetic fibers. That innervation is relatively sparse compared to the innervation of systemic vessels, with the larger elastic vessels receiving relatively more innervation and the smaller muscular vessels less. Vessels smaller than 30 μ in diameter apparently have no innervation, and intrapulmonary veins and venules have little if any.

What happens when the sympathetic innervation of the pulmonary vasculature is stimulated? The findings are somewhat controversial. Some investigators have shown that the pulmonary vascular resistance increases when the sympathetic innervation of the pulmonary vasculature is stimulated, whereas others have found that *distensibility* decreases but the calculated pulmonary vascular resistance remains unchanged. If the parasympathetic innervation of the pulmonary vessels is stimulated, vasodilation generally results, although the physiologic importance of this response is not known.

When injected into the pulmonary circulation, the catecholamines epinephrine and norepinephrine increase pulmonary vascular resistance. Pulmonary vascular constrictors include serotonin, histamine (found in the lung mast cells and appears to be mainly a venoconstrictor), some prostaglandins (such as $PGF_{2\alpha}$, PGE_2, and thromboxane), and some prostaglandin precursors and breakdown products. Alveolar hypoxia and hypercapnia, which can also cause pulmonary vascular constriction, are discussed later. Pulmonary vasodilators include acetylcholine, the beta adrenergic agonist isoproterenol, and certain prostaglandins, such as PGE_1 and prostacyclin.

Regional Distribution of Pulmonary Blood Flow

Determinations of the regional distribution of pulmonary blood flow have shown that *gravity* is one of the most important passive factors affecting local pulmonary vascular resistance and regional pulmonary blood flow. The interaction of gravity and extravascular pressures may profoundly influence the relative perfusion of different areas of the lung.

If the vertical distribution of pulmonary blood flow is determined, a pattern like that shown for the perfusion line in Figure 3–26 is seen. There is more blood flow per unit volume to lower regions of the lung than to upper regions of the lung.

If a person lies down, this pattern of regional perfusion changes so that perfusion to the *anatomically* upper and lower portions of the lung is approximately distributed evenly, but blood flow per unit volume remains greater in the more gravity-dependent regions of the lung. If, for example, the person were to lie down on his left side, blood flow per unit volume would be greater to the left lung than to the right. Exercise, by increasing the cardiac output, increases the blood flow per unit volume to all regions of the lung, but the perfusion gradient persists so that, in more gravity-dependent regions of the lung, the blood flow per unit volume remains relatively greater.

The cause of this gradient of regional perfusion of the lung is *gravity*. As already discussed, the pressure at the bottom of a column of a liquid is proportional to the product of the column's height, the liquid's density, and the force of gravity. Thus, in more gravity-dependent portions of the lung, the intravascular pressures exceed those in upper regions. Because those pressures are greater in the more gravity-dependent regions of the lung, the *resistance to blood flow is less* in lower lung regions because of *recruitment* or *distention* of vessels there. Thus, both gravity and the peculiar characteristics of the pulmonary circulation cause the increased blood flow to more dependent regions of the lung. The same hydrostatic effects occur to an even greater extent in the left side of the circulation, but the thick walls of the systemic arteries are not affected by the higher intravascular pressures.

Experiments done on excised, perfused animal lungs have shown the same gradient of increased perfusion per unit volume from the top to the bottom of the lung. When the pump outputs were low, so that the pulmonary artery pressure was low, the uppermost regions of the lung received no blood flow. Perfusion of the lung ceased at the point at which alveolar pressure (P_A) was just equal to pulmonary arterial pressure (P_a). Above this point, where alveolar pressure exceeded pulmonary arterial pressure, no perfusion occurred because the transmural pressure gradient across capillary walls was negative. Below this point, perfusion per unit volume increased with increased distance down the lung.

Thus, under circumstances in which alveolar pressure is higher than pulmonary artery pressure in the upper parts of the lung, no blood flow occurs in that region. This is referred to as Zone 1 (Fig. 3–24). If it is ventilated, it is *alveolar dead space*, because it is ventilated but not perfused. During normal quiet breathing in a person with a normal cardiac output, pulmonary artery pressure, even in the uppermost regions of the lung, is higher than alveolar pressure, so there is no Zone 1.

The lower portion of the lung in Figure 3–24 is said to be in Zone 3. In that region, the pulmonary artery pressure and pulmonary vein pressure (P_v) both exceed alveolar pressure. The driving pressure for blood flow through the lung in that region is simply pulmonary artery pressure minus pulmonary vein pressure. Note that this driving pressure remains constant as one moves further down the lung in Zone 3 because the hydrostatic pressure effects are the same for both the arteries and the veins.

The middle portion of the lung in Figure 3–24 is in Zone 2, in which pulmonary artery pressure exceeds alveolar pressure, so blood does flow. Nevertheless, because alveolar pressure is greater than pulmonary vein pressure, the *effective* driving

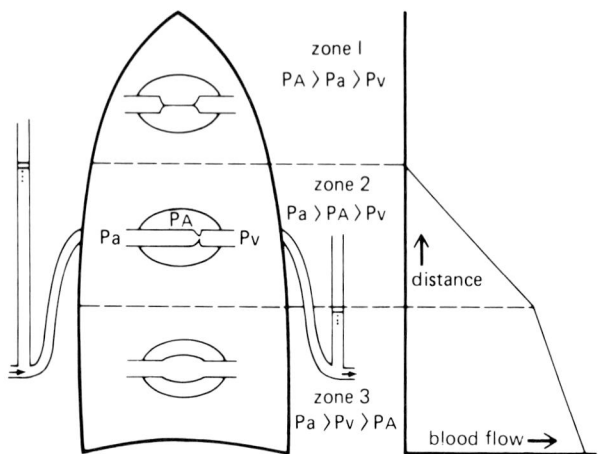

FIGURE 3–24. The zones of the lung: The effects of gravity and alveolar pressure on the perfusion of the lung. (From West, J.B., Dollery, C.T., and Naimark, A.: Distribution of blood flow in isolated lung; relation to vascular and alveolar pressure. *Journal of Applied Physiology* 19:713–724, 1964, with permission.)

pressure for blood flow is pulmonary artery pressure minus alveolar pressure. Notice that, in Zone 2 (at right in Fig. 3–24), the increase in blood flow per unit of distance down the lung is greater than in Zone 3. This difference occurs because the upstream driving pressure, the pulmonary artery pressure, increases according to the hydrostatic pressure increase, but the effective downstream pressure, alveolar pressure, is constant throughout the lung at any instant.

To summarize then, in Zone 1:

$$P_A > P_a > P_v$$

and blood does not flow (except perhaps in corner vessels, such as those in Fig. 3–23, which are not exposed to alveolar pressure).

In Zone 2:

$$P_a > P_A > P_v$$

and the effective driving pressure for blood flow is $P_a - P_A$.

In Zone 3:

$$P_a > P_v > P_A$$

and the driving pressure for blood flow is $P_a - P_v$.

It is important to realize that the boundaries between the zones depend on physiologic conditions—they are not fixed anatomic landmarks. During the course of each breath, alveolar pressure changes. During eupneic breathing, these changes amount to only a few cmH$_2$O, but they may be much greater during speech, exercise, or positive pressure ventilation. Similarly, after a hemorrhage or during general anesthesia, pulmonary blood flow and pulmonary artery pressure are low and Zone 1 conditions are also likely. Changes in body position alter the orientation of the zones with regard to the anatomic locations in the lung, but the same relationships exist with regard to gravity and alveolar pressure.

Hypoxic Pulmonary Vasoconstriction

Alveolar hypoxia or atelectasis causes an active vasoconstriction in the pulmonary circulation. The site of vascular smooth muscle constriction appears to be in the arterial (precapillary) vessels close to the alveoli. The mechanism of the hypoxic pulmonary vasoconstriction is not completely understood. The response occurs locally, that is, only in the area of the alveolar hypoxia. Connections to the central nervous system are not necessary. Hypoxia may act directly on the vascular smooth muscle or may cause the release of a vasoactive substance from the pulmonary parenchyma or mast cells in the area.

The function of pulmonary vasoconstriction in localized hypoxia is fairly obvious. If part of the lung becomes hypoxic because airways are obstructed, or if localized atelectasis occurs, any mixed venous blood flowing to that area undergoes little or no gas exchange and mixes with blood draining well-ventilated areas of the lung as it enters the left atrium. Such mixing lowers the overall arterial P$_{O_2}$ and may even increase the arterial P$_{CO_2}$. The hypoxic pulmonary vasoconstriction diverts mixed venous blood flow away from poorly ventilated areas of the lung by locally increasing the vascular resistance; therefore, it shifts blood flow to better-ventilated parts of the lung.

The hypoxic pulmonary vasoconstriction, however, is not a very strong response, which is not surprising because pulmonary arteries have so little smooth muscle. Very high pulmonary artery pressures can interfere with hypoxic pulmonary vasoconstriction, as can other physiologic disturbances, such as alkalosis.

Alveolar hypercapnia (high carbon dioxide) also causes pulmonary vasoconstriction. Whether this occurs by the same mechanism as the hypoxic pulmonary vasoconstriction is not clear.

Pulmonary Edema

Pulmonary edema, the extravascular accumulation of fluid in the lung, may be caused by one or more physiologic abnormalities. The result is inevitably impaired gas transfer. As the fluid accumulates, first in the interstitium and later in alveoli, diffusion of gases, particularly oxygen, decreases.

We have already discussed the Starling equation in Chapter 2. Factors that may predispose to pulmonary edema are summarized in Table 3–2.

Pulmonary capillary hydrostatic pressure is estimated to be about 7 to 12 mmHg under normal conditions. Although some investigators believe that the pulmonary interstitial hydrostatic pressure is slightly positive, many recent studies have determined it to be negative, in the range of -5 to -7 mmHg. This seems reasonable in light of the normally negative intrapleural pressure, which may be transmitted through much of the pulmonary interstitium.

VENTILATION-PERFUSION RELATIONSHIPS

Alveolar ventilation brings inspired gas with a P_{O_2} of about 150 mmHg and a P_{CO_2} of about 0.3 mmHg into the alveoli. At the same time, the right ventricle pumps mixed venous blood with a P_{O_2} of about 40 mmHg and a P_{CO_2} of about 45 mmHg into the pulmonary capillaries. Oxygen diffuses from the alveoli into the pulmonary capillaries at the same time that carbon dioxide diffuses from the pulmonary capillaries. The P_{O_2} and P_{CO_2} of an alveolar-capillary unit are *determined* by the relative ventilation and perfusion of that unit. Increasing the ventilation relative to the perfusion increases the P_{O_2} and decreases the P_{CO_2} of that alveolus. Increasing the perfusion relative to the ventilation decreases the P_{O_2} and increases the P_{CO_2} of that alveolus.

Importance of Matching Ventilation and Perfusion

Alveolar ventilation ($\dot{V}_A$) is normally about 4 to 6 L of air per minute, and pulmonary capillary blood flow ($\dot{Q}c$) has a similar range, so the ratio of ventilation to perfusion for the whole lung is about 0.8 to 1.2. However, ventilation and perfusion must be matched on the *alveolar-capillary level*. The $\dot{V}_A/\dot{Q}c$ for the whole lung is really of interest only as an approximation of the situation in all the alveolar-capillary units of the lung.

Clearly, alveoli that are ventilated but not perfused constitute alveolar dead space and contribute nothing to gas exchange in the lung. Similarly, alveoli that are perfused but not ventilated, constitute an *intrapulmonary shunt* and return mixed venous blood to the systemic circulation. These two situations are the extreme cases for ventilation-perfusion ratios—infinite $\dot{V}_A/\dot{Q}c$ and zero $\dot{V}_A/\dot{Q}c$, respectively (Fig. 3–25).

Consequences of $\dot{V}_A/\dot{Q}c$ Mismatch

Alveolar-capillary unit *A* in Figure 3–25 has a normal ventilation-perfusion ratio. Inspired air enter-

TABLE 3–2. Factors Predisposing to Pulmonary Edema

Factor in Starling Equation	Clinical Problems
Increased capillary permeability (K_f; σ)	Adult respiratory distress syndrome
	Oxygen toxicity
	Inhaled or circulating toxins
Increased capillary hydrostatic pressure (Pc)	Increased left atrial pressure resulting from left ventricular infarction or mitral stenosis
	Overadministration of intravenous fluids
Decreased interstitial hydrostatic pressure (Pis)	Too rapid evacuation of pneumothorax or hemothorax
Decreased colloid osmotic pressure (πpl)	Protein starvation
	Dilution of blood proteins by intravenous solutions
	Renal problems resulting in urinary protein loss (proteinuria)
Other Etiologies	**Clinical Problems**
Insufficient pulmonary lymphatic drainage	Tumors
	Interstitial fibrosing diseases
Unknown etiology	High-altitude pulmonary edema
	Pulmonary edema after head injury (neurogenic pulmonary edema)
	Drug overdose

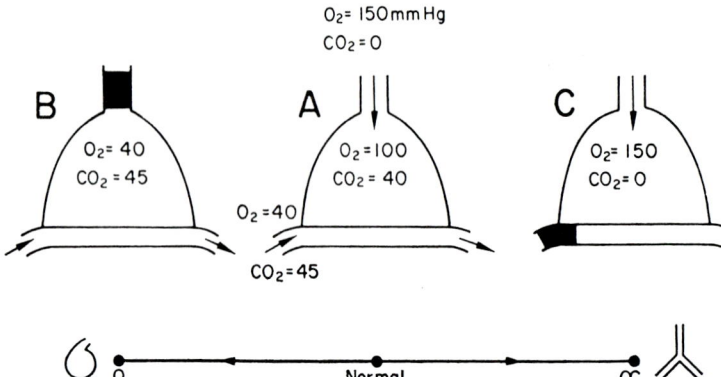

FIGURE 3–25. The effect of changes in the ventilation-perfusion ratio on the alveolar P_{O_2} and P_{CO_2}. *A*, Normal $\dot{V}_A/\dot{Q}c$. *B*, $\dot{V}_A/\dot{Q}c = 0$. *C*, $\dot{V}_A/\dot{Q}c$ is infinite. (From West, J.B.: *Ventilation/Blood Flow and Gas Exchange,* 4th ed. Oxford, Blackwell Scientific Publications, 1985, with permission.)

ing the alveolus has a P_{O_2} of about 150 torr and a P_{CO_2} of nearly 0 torr. Mixed venous blood entering the pulmonary capillary has a P_{O_2} of about 40 torr and a P_{CO_2} of about 45 torr. This results in an alveolar P_{O_2} of about 100 torr and an alveolar P_{CO_2} of 40 torr. The partial pressure gradient for oxygen diffusion is thus about 100 − 40, or 60 torr; the partial pressure gradient for carbon dioxide is about 45 − 40, or 5 torr.

The airway supplying unit *B* has become completely occluded. Its $\dot{V}_A/\dot{Q}c$ is zero. In time, the air trapped in the alveolus equilibrates by diffusion with the gas dissolved in the mixed venous blood entering the alveolar-capillary unit. (If the blockage persists, the alveolus will likely collapse.) No gas can be exchanged, and any blood perfusing this alveolus is the same at exit as at entry. Unit *B*, therefore, acts as a right-to-left shunt.

A pulmonary embolus blocks the blood flow to unit *C*, which is therefore completely unperfused. The unit has an infinite $\dot{V}_A/\dot{Q}c$. Because no oxygen can diffuse from the alveolus into pulmonary capillary blood, and no carbon dioxide can enter the alveolus from the blood, the P_{O_2} of the alveolus is about 150 torr, and its P_{CO_2} is about zero. Thus, the gas composition of this unperfused alveolus is the same as that of inspired air. Unit *C* is alveolar dead space. If unit *C* were unperfused because its alveolar pressure exceeded its precapillary pressure (instead of as the result of an embolus), it would also correspond to part of Zone 1.

As already noted, units *B* and *C* represent the two extremes of a *continuum* of ventilation-perfusion ratios. The ventilation-perfusion ratio of a particular alveolar-capillary unit can fall anywhere along this continuum, as Figure 3–25 shows. The alveolar P_{O_2} and P_{CO_2} of such units, therefore, fall between the two extremes shown in the figure: Units with *low* ventilation-perfusion ratios have relatively low P_{O_2}'s and high P_{CO_2}'s; units with *high* ventilation-perfusion ratios have relatively high P_{O_2}'s and low P_{CO_2}'s.

Regional $\dot{V}/\dot{Q}$ in the Lung

We have already discussed the regional differences in ventilation and pulmonary blood flow in this chapter. During normal ventilation from the functional residual capacity in a person in an upright posture, lower regions of the lung are better ventilated than the upper lung regions, as shown by the *ventilation* line in Figure 3–26. The lower regions of the lung also receive more blood flow per unit volume than the upper lung regions, as is shown by the *blood flow* line in Figure 3–26.

Figure 3–26 also shows that the gradient of perfusion from the bottom to the top of the lung exceeds the gradient of ventilation. Because of this, the *ventilation-perfusion ratio* calculated at various points is relatively low in more gravity-dependent regions and higher in upper regions of the lung. In fact, if pulmonary perfusion pressure is low, for example, from hemorrhage, and/or if alveolar pressure is high, from positive-pressure ventilation with positive end-expiratory pressure, then there may be areas of Zone 1 in the upper parts of the lung with infinite ventilation-perfusion ratios.

The effects of regional differences in $\dot{V}_A/\dot{Q}c$ on the alveolar P_{O_2} and P_{CO_2} can be estimated by looking at Figures 3–25 and 3–26. Under normal circumstances, the blood in the pulmonary capillaries equilibrates with the alveolar P_{O_2} (P_AO_2) and P_{CO_2} (P_ACO_2), so blood in the pulmonary venule draining an alveolar-capillary unit has the same P_{O_2} and P_{CO_2} as the alveolus.

The lower regions of the lung receive both better

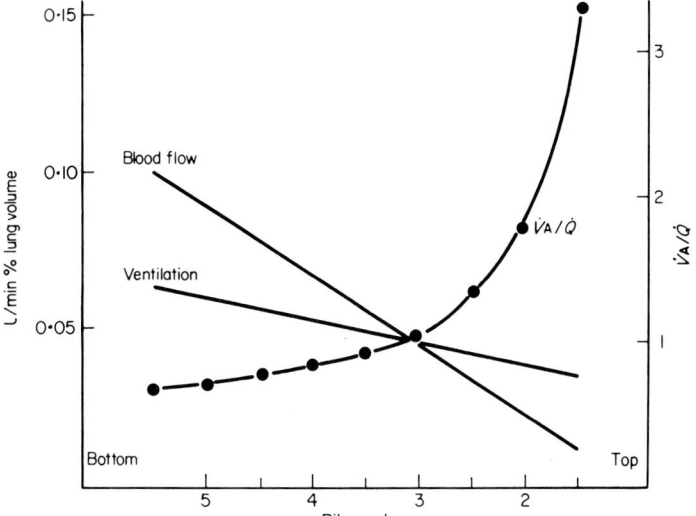

FIGURE 3–26. Regional differences in ventilation, perfusion and ventilation-perfusion ratios of the normal upright lung. (From West, J.B.: *Ventilation/Blood Flow and Gas Exchange,* 4th ed. Oxford, Blackwell Scientific Publications, 1985, with permission.)

ventilation and better perfusion than upper regions of the lung. However, as can be seen in Figure 3–26, the perfusion gradient is more severe than the ventilation gradient, so the ventilation-perfusion ratio is much higher in upper regions than lower regions. As a result, the alveolar P_{O_2} is higher and the alveolar P_{CO_2} is lower in upper regions than in lower regions. This means that the oxygen *content* of blood draining the upper regions is higher, and the carbon dioxide content is lower than those of the blood draining the lower regions. *Contents* are based, however, on milliliters of blood (see the section on gas transport by the blood later in this chapter), and there is much less blood flow to upper lung regions than lower regions. Therefore, even though the uppermost lung regions have the highest $\dot{V}_A/\dot{Q}c$'s and P_{O_2}'s and the lowest P_{CO_2}'s, there is more *gas exchange* in the more basal sections.

DIFFUSION OF GASES

Diffusion of a gas occurs when there is a net movement of molecules from an area in which that particular gas exerts a high partial pressure to an area in which it exerts a lower partial pressure. Movement by diffusion, therefore, differs from the movement of gases through the conducting airways, which occurs by bulk flow (mass movement or convection). During bulk flow, gas movement results from differences in *total* pressure, and molecules of different gases move together along the total pressure gradient.

During diffusion, gas movement occurs in both directions, but because of its greater number of molecules per unit volume, the area of higher partial pressure has proportionately more random departures. The *net* movement of gas, therefore, depends on the partial pressure difference between the two areas. Diffusion is dependent on temperature because random molecular movement increases at higher temperatures. In a static situation, diffusion continues until no partial pressure differences exist. In the lungs, oxygen and carbon dioxide continuously enter and leave the alveoli, so such an equilibrium is never reached.

Fick's Law for Diffusion

By the time inspired air reaches the alveoli, the linear velocity of bulk flow decreases to zero. This decrease results mainly from the tremendous increase in the total cross-sectional area of the branching conducting airways, respiratory bronchioles, and alveolar ducts. As noted in Chapter 2, as the total cross-sectional area increases, the linear velocity decreases:

Flow (cm^3/sec) = Cross-sectional area (cm^2) × Linear velocity (cm/sec)

In the alveoli, oxygen then moves through the gas phase according to its own partial pressure gradient. The distance from the alveolar duct to the alveolar-capillary interface is probably less than 1 mm. In the alveolar gas phase, diffusion occurs very rapidly and is believed to be greatly assisted by the pulsations of the heart and blood flow that are transmitted to the alveoli and increase molecular motion.

Oxygen then diffuses through the alveolar-capillary interface. It must first, therefore, move from the gas phase to the liquid phase, according to *Henry's Law* (see Chapter 1), which states that the amount of a gas absorbed by a liquid with which it does not combine chemically is directly proportional to the partial pressure of the gas and the solubility of the gas in the liquid. Oxygen must dissolve in and diffuse through the thin layer of pulmonary surfactant, the alveolar epithelium, the interstitium, and the capillary endothelium. It must then diffuse through the plasma, where some remains dissolved but most diffuses through the erythrocyte cell membrane and combines with hemoglobin.

The blood then, by bulk flow, carries the oxygen out of the lung and distributes it to the other tissues of the body. At the tissues, oxygen diffuses from the red blood cell through the cell membrane, plasma, capillary endothelium, interstitium, tissue cell membrane, and cell interior into the mitochondrial membrane. For carbon dioxide, the process is almost exactly reversed.

Factors that determine the rate of diffusion of a gas through the alveolar-capillary barrier are described by Fick's law for diffusion, which was discussed in Chapter 1:

$$\dot{V}_{gas} = \frac{A \times D \times (P_1 - P_2)}{T}$$

where $\dot{V}_{gas}$ is the volume of gas diffusing through the tissue barrier per unit of time (ml/min); A is the surface area of the barrier available for diffusion; D is the diffusion coefficient, or diffusivity, for the particular gas in the barrier; T is the thickness of the barrier, or the diffusion distance; and $P_1 - P_2$ is the partial pressure difference of the gas across the barrier.

Thus, the volume of gas moving across the alveolar-capillary barrier per unit of time is directly proportional to the surface area of the barrier, the diffusivity, and the difference in concentration between the two sides, but it is inversely proportional to the barrier thickness.

The surface area of the blood-gas barrier is believed to be at least 70 m² in a healthy average-sized adult at rest. That is, about 70 m² of the *potential* surface area is both ventilated and perfused at rest. If more capillaries are recruited, the surface area available for diffusion increases; if venous return falls, capillaries may be derecruited, and the surface area available for diffusion may decrease.

The thickness of the alveolar-capillary diffusion barrier is only about 0.2 to 0.5 μ. This barrier thickness can increase in interstitial fibrosis or interstitial edema, thus interfering with diffusion.

As stated in Chapter 1, the diffusivity, or diffusion constant, for a gas is directly proportional to the solubility of the gas in the diffusion barrier and inversely proportional to the square root of the density of the gas:

$$D \propto \frac{\text{Solubility}}{\sqrt{\text{M.W.}}}$$

The diffusivity is inversely proportional to the square root of the molecular weight of the gas because, at the same temperature, different gases with equal numbers of molecules in equal volumes have the same molecular energy. Therefore, light molecules travel faster, have more frequent collisions, and diffuse more rapidly.

Because carbon dioxide is more dense than oxygen, it diffuses only 0.85 times as fast as oxygen as it moves through the gas phase in the alveoli. In the alveolar-capillary barrier, however, the relative *solubilities* of oxygen and carbon dioxide must also be considered. In the liquid phase, the solubility of carbon dioxide is about 24 times that of oxygen, so carbon dioxide diffuses about 0.85 × 24, or about *20 times* more rapidly than does oxygen through the alveolar-capillary barrier. Thus, in situations of diffusion impairment, patients develop problems in oxygen diffusion through the alveolar-capillary barrier before carbon dioxide retention.

Perfusion Limitation of Gas Transfer

The partial pressures of a gas in the mixed venous blood and in the blood as it travels through the pulmonary capillary are important factors in determining the rate of diffusion of a gas. This is because they, along with the alveolar partial pressures, constitute the pressure gradient for gas diffusion.

At resting cardiac outputs, a red blood cell, along with the plasma surrounding it, spends an average of about 0.75 to 1.20 seconds inside a functional pulmonary capillary. If the partial pressure of a gas in the blood traveling through a pulmonary capillary equilibrates with the alveolar partial pressure before the blood has finished moving through the capillary, no further gas exchange takes place for that blood. This is because, when the partial pressures equilibrate, there is no longer a pressure gradient for diffusion, and according to Fick's equation, diffusion falls to zero. Of course, new mixed venous blood just entering the capillary at the arterial end is not equilibrated with the alveolar partial pressure, so gas exchange occurs at the arterial end. To increase the gas exchange in that alveolar-capillary unit, the rate of blood flow through the capillary must be increased to get unequilibrated blood exposed to the alveolar gas partial pressure. This is therefore called *perfusion* limitation of diffusion.

Nitrous oxide, a gas used in anesthesia, normally shows perfusion limitation of diffusion. It is so soluble in the alveolar-capillary barrier that its pulmonary capillary partial pressure equilibrates with the alveolar partial pressure within about 0.10 seconds. The remaining time that the equilibrated blood spends in the pulmonary capillary results in no further gas exchange. The only way to increase the rate of nitrous oxide uptake by the blood in that pulmonary capillary is to increase the velocity of blood flow through the vessel. Nitrous oxide uptake is therefore perfusion-limited. As discussed shortly, under normal circumstances, the diffusion of both oxygen and carbon dioxide in the lung is also perfusion-limited.

It is important to realize that increasing cardiac output normally increases gas diffusion in the lung by another mechanism, besides increasing the velocity of blood flow through the pulmonary capillaries and decreasing perfusion limitation of gas transfer. As discussed earlier, increasing the cardiac output recruits more pulmonary capillaries. This increases the *surface area* for diffusion, so it increases the rate of gas diffusion by a mechanism other than maintaining the partial pressure gradient term in the Fick equation.

Diffusion Limitation of Gas Transfer

The transfer of carbon monoxide from an alveolus into pulmonary capillary blood is not perfusion limited because, in a normal person, equilibration between the alveolar and pulmonary capillary partial pressures of carbon monoxide does not take place within the amount of time the blood spends in the pulmonary capillary. The partial pressure of carbon monoxide in the pulmonary capillary blood stays very close to zero because unlike nitrous oxide, which does not bind to hemoglobin, carbon monoxide combines *chemically* with the hemoglobin inside the erythrocytes. In fact, the affinity of carbon monoxide for hemoglobin is more than 200 times that of oxygen. The carbon monoxide that chemically combines with hemoglobin does not contribute to the partial pressure of carbon monoxide in the blood. Therefore, the partial pressure of carbon monoxide in the pulmonary capillary blood does not approach the partial pressure of carbon monoxide in the alveoli while the blood is exposed to the alveolar carbon monoxide. The partial pressure gradient across the alveolar-capillary barrier for carbon monoxide is thus well-maintained for the entire time the blood spends in the pulmonary capillary, and the diffusion of carbon monoxide is limited only by its diffusivity in the barrier, the surface area, and thickness of the barrier. Carbon monoxide transfer from the alveolus to the pulmonary capillary blood is therefore *diffusion*-limited rather than perfusion-limited. As shown in Chapter 9, carbon monoxide is used (in very low nonlethal concentrations, of course) for this reason to test the diffusion characteristics of the alveolar-capillary barrier.

Diffusion of Oxygen

The time course for oxygen transfer is shown in Figure 3–27A. The P_{O_2} in the mixed venous blood is 40 torr, as shown at the left at time zero, when the mixed venous blood first enters the functional pulmonary capillary. The P_{O_2} in the alveolus is 100 torr. The P_{O_2} of the blood in the pulmonary capillary rises fairly rapidly and equilibrates with the alveolar P_{O_2} within about 0.25 seconds, or about one third of the time the blood is in the pulmonary capillary at normal resting cardiac outputs.

Oxygen moves easily through the alveolar-capillary barrier and into the red blood cells, where it rapidly combines chemically with hemoglobin (although not as fast as carbon monoxide does). The oxygen chemically combined with hemoglobin does not contribute to the P_{O_2} of the plasma in the pulmonary capillary. Therefore, the partial pressure gradient across the alveolar-capillary barrier is initially well-maintained, and the diffusion of oxygen occurs.

The chemical combination of oxygen and hemoglobin, however, occurs rapidly (within hundredths of a second), and at the normal alveolar P_{O_2}, the hemoglobin very quickly becomes nearly saturated with oxygen, as discussed shortly. As this happens, the partial pressure of oxygen in the

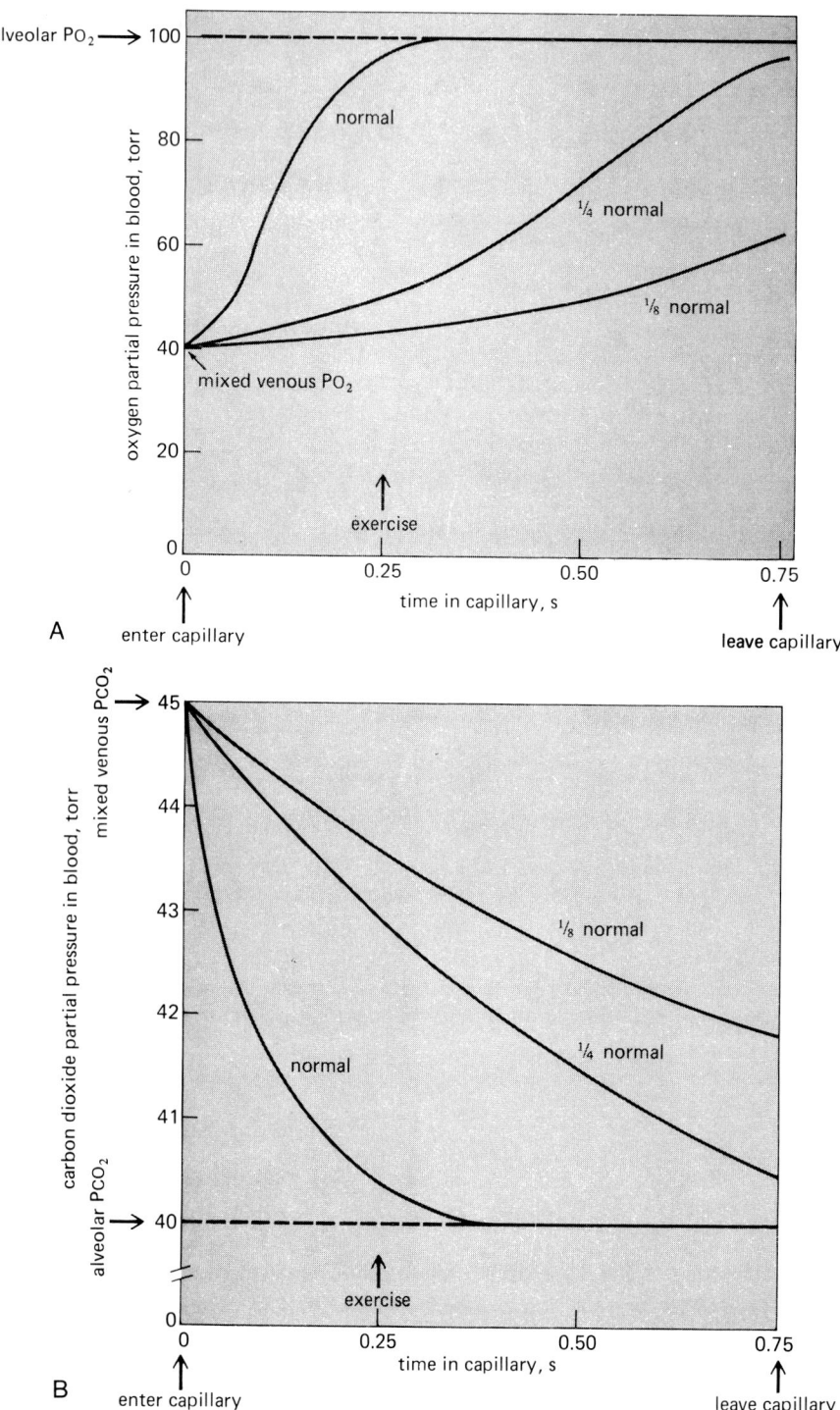

FIGURE 3–27. *A,* Calculated changes in the partial pressure of oxygen as blood passes through a pulmonary capillary. The alveolar P_{O_2} of about 100 torr is denoted by the dotted line. Patterns for normal and abnormal diffusion through the alveolar-capillary barrier are shown. Note that the partial pressure of oxygen normally equilibrates rapidly with the alveolar P_{O_2}. *B,* Calculated changes in the partial pressure of carbon dioxide as blood passes through a pulmonary capillary. The mixed venous P_{CO_2} is about 45 torr. The alveolar P_{CO_2} is indicated by the dotted line. Patterns for normal and abnormal diffusion through the alveolar-capillary barrier are shown. Note that the partial pressure of CO_2 in the pulmonary capillary blood normally equilibrates rapidly with the alveolar P_{CO_2}. (Adapted from Wagner, P.D., and West, J.B.: Effects of diffusion impairment on O_2 and CO_2 time courses in pulmonary capillaries. *Journal of Applied Physiology* 33:62–71, 1972, with permission.)

blood rises rapidly to that in the alveolus, and from that point, oxygen can no longer transfer from the alveolus to the equilibrated blood. Under a normal alveolar P_{O_2} and a normal resting cardiac output, therefore, oxygen transfer from alveolus to pulmonary capillary is perfusion-limited.

During exercise, the movement of blood through the pulmonary capillary is much more rapid than at resting cardiac outputs. In fact, during severe exercise blood may stay in the functional pulmonary capillary an average of only about 0.25 seconds, as indicated by the figure. The rate of oxygen transfer into the blood per unit of time increases greatly because little or no perfusion limitation of oxygen transfer occurs. (Indeed, the blood that stays in the capillary *less* than the average may be subjected to diffusion limitation of oxygen transfer.) Note that *total* oxygen transfer also increases during exercise because of recruitment of previously unperfused capillaries, which increases the surface area for diffusion, and also because of better matching of ventilation and perfusion. A person with an abnormal alveolar-capillary barrier due to a fibrotic thickening or interstitial edema may approach diffusion limitation of oxygen transfer at rest and may have a serious diffusion limitation of oxygen transfer during strenuous exercise, as can be seen in the middle curve in the figure. A person with an extremely abnormal alveolar-capillary barrier might have diffusion limitation of oxygen transfer even at rest, as seen at the right in the figure. Emphysema can also cause diffusion limitation of oxygen transfer during exercise, because the destruction of alveolar septa decreases the surface area for diffusion, as will be discussed in Chapter 5.

Diffusion of Carbon Dioxide

Figure 3-27B shows the time course of carbon dioxide transfer from the pulmonary capillary blood to the alveolus. In a normal person having a mixed venous partial pressure of carbon dioxide of 45 torr and an alveolar partial pressure of carbon dioxide of 40 torr, an equilibrium is reached in about 0.25 seconds, or about the same time as that for oxygen. This may seem surprising, since the diffusivity of carbon dioxide is about 20 times that of oxygen, but the partial pressure gradient is normally only about 5 torr for carbon dioxide, whereas it is about 60 torr for oxygen. Carbon dioxide transfer is also normally *perfusion-limited*, as shown in the figure; it may be diffusion-limited in a person with an abnormal alveolar-capillary barrier.

OXYGEN AND CARBON DIOXIDE TRANSPORT

The final step in the exchange of gases between the external environment and the tissues is the transport of oxygen and carbon dioxide to and from the lung by the blood. The heart provides the energy for the movement of blood, which occurs by bulk flow.

Transport of Oxygen in the Blood

The blood carries oxygen both physically dissolved in the blood and chemically bound to the hemoglobin in red blood cells. Normally, much more oxygen is transported in combination with hemoglobin than physically dissolved in the blood. Without hemoglobin, the cardiovascular system could not transport sufficient oxygen to meet tissue demands.

Physically Dissolved

The solubility of oxygen in plasma is such that at a temperature of 37°C, 1 ml of plasma contains 0.00003 ml of oxygen per torr P_{O_2}. This corresponds to Henry's Law, as discussed in Chapter 1. Oxygen dissolves in the fluid inside the red blood cells in about the same amount, so *whole blood* contains a similar amount of dissolved oxygen per milliliter.

Blood oxygen content is conventionally expressed in milliliters of oxygen per 100 ml of blood (called *volumes percent*), so there is 0.003 ml of oxygen per torr P_{O_2} physically dissolved in 100 ml of whole blood. Thus, at an arterial P_{O_2} of 100 torr, there is only 0.3 ml of oxygen transported physically dissolved in 100 ml of blood. It is easy to see that to supply the 250 to 300 ml of oxygen consumed per minute by the body at rest, the cardiac output would have to be very high, even if all of the physically dissolved oxygen were extracted by the tissues:

0.3 ml O_2/100 ml of blood = 3 ml O_2/liter of blood

300 ml O_2/min ÷ 3 ml O_2/liter of blood = 100 L of blood/min

130 PULMONARY ANATOMY AND PHYSIOLOGY

Thus, the cardiac output would have to be 20 times normal (or four times maximal) to just supply the oxygen consumed *at rest,* if oxygen were only transported physically dissolved in blood. During severe exercise, oxygen consumption can increase to as much as 4 L/min, in which case cardiac output would have to exceed 1,000 L/min to meet this demand.

Chemically Combined with Hemoglobin

Hemoglobin is a complex molecule with a molecular weight of about 65,000 daltons. The protein portion (globin) consists of four linked polypeptide chains, each of which is attached to a protoporphyrin (heme) group. Each heme group consists of four symmetrically arranged pyrrole groups with a ferrous (Fe^{++}) iron atom at its center. The iron atom is bound to each of the pyrrole groups and to one of the four polypeptide chains. A sixth binding site on the ferrous iron atom can bind with oxygen (or carbon monoxide). Therefore, *each* of the four polypeptide chains is able to bind an oxygen (or carbon monoxide) molecule to the iron atom in its own heme group. Thus, the tetrameric hemoglobin molecule can combine chemically with four oxygen molecules.

Hemoglobin rapidly combines *reversibly* with oxygen. The reversibility of the reaction allows oxygen to be released to the tissues. The reaction is extremely fast, with a half-time of 0.01 seconds or less. Each gram of hemoglobin can theoretically combine with about 1.39 ml of oxygen under optimal conditions but normally some hemoglobin may be in forms that cannot bind oxygen, such as methemoglobin (the iron atom is in the ferric [Fe^{+++}] state) or combined with carbon monoxide. For this reason, the oxygen-carrying *capacity* of hemoglobin is conventionally considered to be 1.34 ml of oxygen per gram of hemoglobin. That is, each gram of hemoglobin, when *fully saturated* with oxygen, binds 1.34 ml of oxygen.

The reaction of hemoglobin and oxygen is conventionally written:

$$Hb + O_2 \rightleftharpoons HbO_2$$
$$\text{deoxyhemoglobin} \quad \text{oxyhemoglobin}$$

The equilibrium point of the reversible reaction of hemoglobin and oxygen depends on how much oxygen the hemoglobin in blood is exposed to. This exposure corresponds directly to the P_{O_2} in the plasma under the conditions in the body. Thus, the P_{O_2} of the plasma *determines* the amount of oxygen that binds to the hemoglobin in the red blood cells.

One way to express the proportion of hemoglobin that is bound to oxygen is as *percent saturation* (SaO_2). This is equal to the amount of oxygen in the blood (minus that part physically dissolved), divided by the oxygen-carrying capacity of the hemoglobin in the blood, times 100%:

% Hb saturation
$$= \frac{O_2 \text{ content of hemoglobin}}{O_2 \text{ capacity of Hb}} \times 100\%$$

Note that a person's oxygen-carrying *capacity* depends on the amount of hemoglobin in that person's blood. The blood oxygen *content* also depends on the amount of hemoglobin present (as well as on the P_{O_2}). Both content and capacity are expressed as milliliters of oxygen per 100 ml of blood. The percent hemoglobin saturation, on the other hand, expresses only a percentage and not an amount or volume of oxygen. Therefore, percent saturation is not interchangeable with oxygen content. For example, two patients may have the same arterial P_{O_2} and the same percent hemoglobin saturation, but if one has a lower blood hemoglobin concentration because of anemia, he or she also has a lower blood oxygen content.

Oxyhemoglobin Dissociation Curve

The relationship between the P_{O_2} of the plasma and the percent of hemoglobin saturation is demonstrated by the *oxyhemoglobin dissociation curve* (Fig. 3–28).

The oxyhemoglobin dissociation curve is a way of expressing how the availability of one reactant, oxygen (expressed as the P_{O_2} of the plasma), affects the reversible chemical reaction of oxygen and hemoglobin. The product, oxyhemoglobin, is expressed as percent saturation—really a percent of the maximum for any given amount of hemoglobin.

Figure 3–28 shows that the relationship between P_{O_2} and HbO_2 is not linear; it is an S-shaped curve, steep at lower P_{O_2}'s and nearly flat when the P_{O_2} is above 70 torr. The reason that the curve is not linear is that it is actually a plot of four successive reactions, as each of the four hemoglobin subunits combines with a molecule of oxygen.

Loading Oxygen in the Lung

Mixed venous blood entering the pulmonary capillaries normally has a P_{O_2} of about 40 torr. As

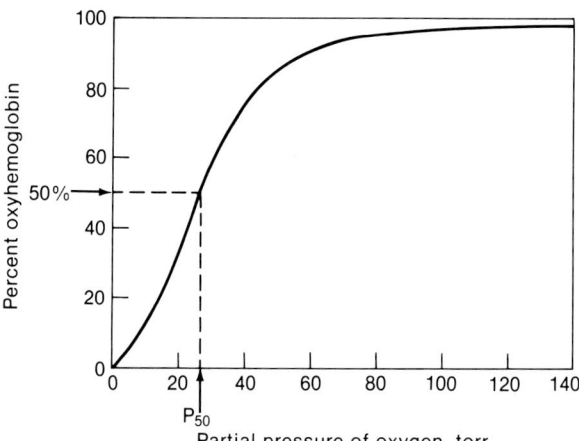

FIGURE 3–28. A typical "normal" adult oxyhemoglobin dissociation curve for blood at a pH of 7.40, a P_{CO_2} of 40 torr, and at 37°C. The P_{50} is the partial pressure of oxygen at which hemoglobin is 50% saturated with oxygen.

Figure 3–28 shows, at a P_{O_2} of 40 torr, hemoglobin is about 75% saturated with oxygen. If we assume the blood hemoglobin concentration to be 15 g of hemoglobin per 100 ml of blood, this corresponds to 15.08 ml of oxygen per 100 ml of blood *bound to hemoglobin* plus an additional 0.12 ml of oxygen per 100 ml of blood *physically dissolved;* then the *total oxygen content* is about 15.20 ml of oxygen per 100 ml of blood:

Oxygen carrying *capacity* is determined:

$$\frac{15 \text{ g Hb}}{100 \text{ ml blood}} \times \frac{1.34 \text{ ml O}_2}{\text{gram Hb}} = \frac{20.1 \text{ ml O}_2}{100 \text{ ml blood}}$$

Oxygen *bound to hemoglobin* at a P_{O_2} of 40 torr (at 37°C and pH of 7.4) is determined:

$$\underset{\text{capacity}}{\frac{20.1 \text{ ml O}_2}{100 \text{ ml blood}}} \times \underset{\text{\% of saturation}}{75\%} = \underset{\text{content}}{\frac{15.08 \text{ ml O}_2}{100 \text{ ml blood}}}$$

Oxygen physically dissolved at a P_{O_2} of 40 torr is determined:

$$\frac{0.003 \text{ ml O}_2}{100 \text{ ml blood}} \times 40 \text{ torr} = \frac{0.12 \text{ ml O}_2}{100 \text{ ml blood}}$$

Total blood oxygen content at a P_{O_2} of 40 torr (37°C and pH of 7.4) is determined:

$$\underset{\text{bound to Hb}}{\frac{15.08 \text{ ml O}_2}{100 \text{ ml blood}}} + \underset{\text{physically dissolved}}{\frac{0.12 \text{ ml O}_2}{100 \text{ ml blood}}} = \underset{\text{total}}{\frac{15.20 \text{ ml O}_2}{100 \text{ ml blood}}}$$

As the blood passes through the pulmonary capillaries, it equilibrates with the alveolar P_{O_2} of about 100 torr. At a P_{O_2} of 100 torr, hemoglobin is about 97.4% saturated with oxygen (see Fig. 3–28). This corresponds to 19.58 ml of oxygen per 100 ml of blood bound to hemoglobin plus 0.3 ml of oxygen per 100 ml of blood physically dissolved or a *total oxygen content* of 19.88 ml of oxygen per 100 ml of blood:

Oxygen *bound to hemoglobin* at a P_{O_2} of 100 torr (at 37°C and pH of 7.4) is determined:

$$\underset{\text{capacity}}{\frac{20.1 \text{ ml O}_2}{100 \text{ ml blood}}} \times \underset{\text{\% of saturation}}{97.4\%} = \underset{\text{content}}{\frac{19.58 \text{ ml O}_2}{100 \text{ ml blood}}}$$

Oxygen physically dissolved at a P_{O_2} of 100 torr is determined:

$$\frac{0.003 \text{ ml O}_2}{100 \text{ ml blood}} \times 100 \text{ torr} = \frac{0.3 \text{ ml O}_2}{100 \text{ ml blood}}$$

Total blood oxygen content at a P_{O_2} of 100 torr (37°C and pH of 7.4) is determined:

$$\underset{\text{bound to Hb}}{\frac{19.58 \text{ ml O}_2}{100 \text{ ml blood}}} + \underset{\text{physically dissolved}}{\frac{0.3 \text{ ml O}_2}{100 \text{ ml blood}}} = \underset{\text{total}}{\frac{19.88 \text{ ml O}_2}{100 \text{ ml blood}}}$$

Thus, in passing through the lungs, each 100 ml of blood has loaded (19.88 − 15.20) or 4.68 ml of oxygen. Assuming a cardiac output of 5.5 L/min, this means that about 257 ml of oxygen is loaded into the blood per minute:

$$\frac{5.5 \text{ L blood}}{\text{min}} \times \frac{46.8 \text{ ml O}_2}{\text{L blood}} = \frac{257 \text{ ml O}_2}{\text{min}}$$

Note that the oxyhemoglobin dissociation curve is relatively flat at P_{O_2}'s greater than about 70 torr. This is important physiologically, because it means that the oxygen content of blood decreases only slightly if it is equilibrated with a P_{O_2} of 70 torr instead of 100 torr. Similarly, because hemoglobin is about 97.4% saturated at a P_{O_2} of 100 torr, raising the alveolar P_{O_2} above 100 torr can load little additional oxygen onto hemoglobin. Hemoglobin is fully saturated with oxygen at a P_{O_2} of about 250 torr.

Unloading Oxygen at the Tissues

As blood passes from the arteries into the systemic capillaries, it is exposed to lower P_{O_2}'s, and oxygen is released by the hemoglobin. The P_{O_2} in the capillaries varies from tissue to tissue, being very low in some (e.g., the myocardium) and relatively higher in others (e.g., the kidney). As Figure 3–28 shows, the oxyhemoglobin dissociation curve is rather steep in the range of 10 to 40 torr. This means that small decreases in P_{O_2} can result in a substantial further dissociation of oxygen and hemoglobin, unloading more oxygen for use by the tissues.

Influences on the Oxyhemoglobin Dissociation Curve

The unloading of oxygen at the tissues is also facilitated by other physiologic factors that can *alter the shape and position* of the oxyhemoglobin dissociation curve. These factors include the pH, P_{CO_2}, and temperature of the blood, and the concentration of 2,3-diphosphoglycerate (2,3-DPG) in the red blood cells.

Figure 3–29 shows the influence of temperature, pH, P_{CO_2}, and the concentration of 2,3-DPG on the oxyhemoglobin dissociation curve. Elevated temperature, low pH, high P_{CO_2}, and elevated levels of 2,3-DPG all shift the oxyhemoglobin dissociation curve to the right. That is, for any particular P_{O_2}, less oxygen is chemically combined with he-

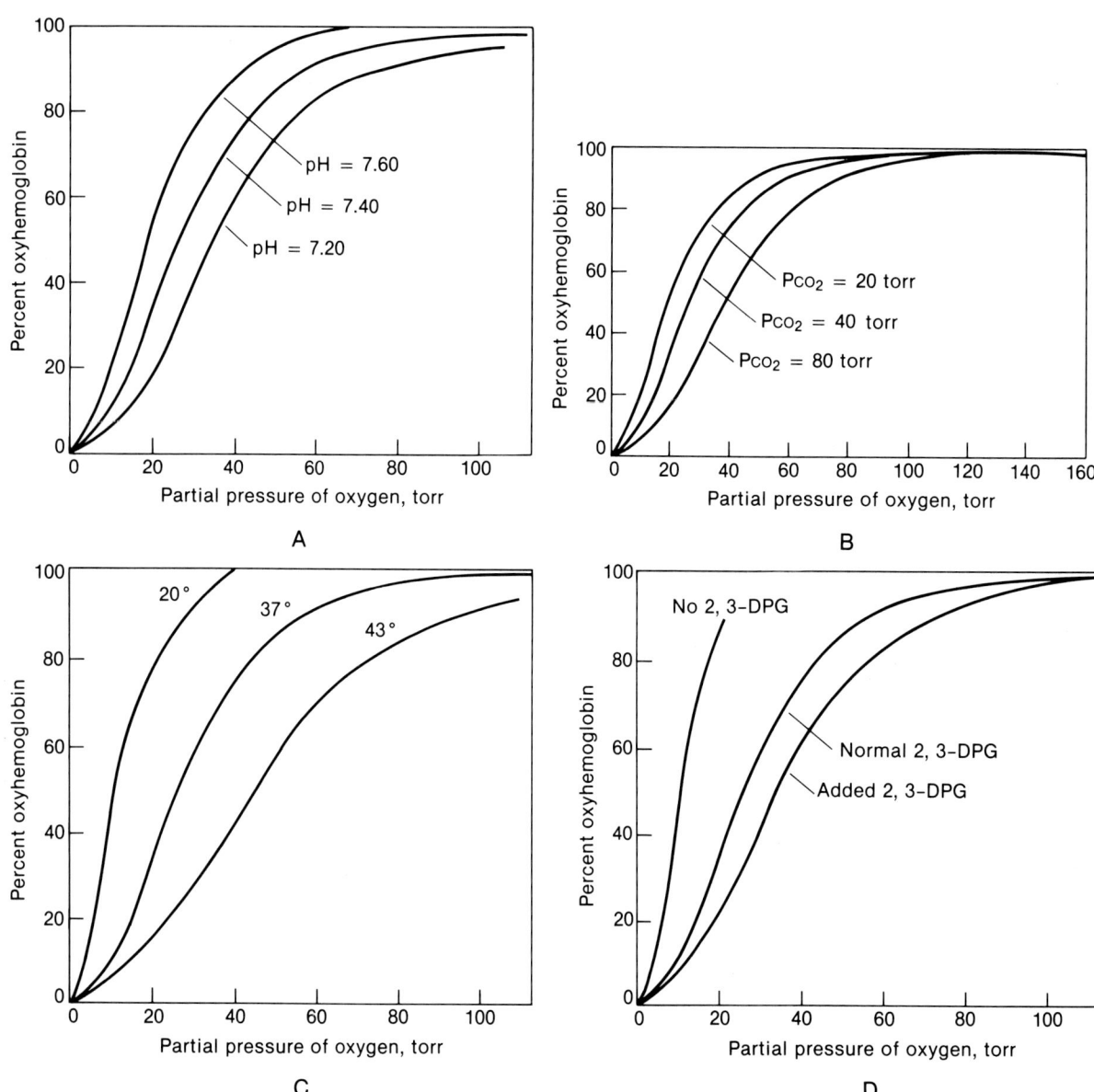

FIGURE 3–29. The effects of pH (*A*), P_{CO_2} (*B*), temperature (*C*), and 2,3-DPG (*D*) on the oxyhemoglobin dissociation curve.

moglobin at higher temperatures, lower pH's, higher P_{CO_2}'s, and elevated levels of 2,3-DPG. The influence of pH (and P_{CO_2}) on the oxyhemoglobin dissociation curve, referred to as the Bohr effect, is discussed later.

High temperatures shift the curve to the right; low temperatures shift it to the left. At extremely low blood temperatures, hemoglobin has such high affinity for oxygen that it does not release it even at very low P_{O_2}'s. Note that oxygen is more soluble in water or plasma at lower temperatures than at normal body temperature. At 20°C, about 50% more oxygen dissolves in plasma. Produced by red blood cells during anaerobic glycolysis, 2,3-DPG is normally present in fairly high concentrations within those cells. Higher concentrations of 2,3-DPG shift the oxyhemoglobin dissociation curve to the right (see Fig. 3–29). More 2,3-DPG is produced during chronic hypoxia, thereby shifting the dissociation curve to the right and allowing more oxygen to be released from hemoglobin at a particular P_{O_2}. Very low levels of 2,3-DPG shift the curve far to the left, as shown in the figure. This shift means that blood deficient in 2,3-DPG does not unload much oxygen except at very low P_{O_2}'s. Blood stored in blood banks may be deficient in 2,3-DPG unless steps are taken to restore it.

The physiologic consequences of the effects on the oxyhemoglobin dissociation curve shown in Figure 3–29 make sense if we think of the situation in a metabolically active tissue like skeletal muscle during exercise. The muscle releases carbon dioxide as the end product of aerobic metabolism and hydrogen ions as an end product of anaerobic metabolism (lactic acid). The temperature increases because heat is released as a result of the inefficiency of energy utilization in the process of muscle contraction. Because low pH, high P_{CO_2}, and higher temperature shift the oxyhemoglobin dissociation curve to the right, they all can help to unload oxygen from hemoglobin at the tissues.

The hemoglobin in blood draining metabolically active tissues has been exposed to conditions quite different from the situation depicted in Figure 3–28, which was for blood with a pH of 7.4 and a P_{CO_2} of 40 torr at a temperature of 37°C. Mixed venous blood has a lower pH and higher P_{CO_2} and may even have a higher temperature and 2,3-DPG concentration than arterial blood. Thus the oxyhemoglobin dissociation curve is shifted to the right for venous blood. As the venous blood returns to the lung and carbon dioxide leaves the blood (which increases the pH), the affinity of hemoglobin for oxygen increases as the curve shifts back to the left.

The effects of pH, P_{CO_2}, and temperature shown in Figure 3–28 are all more pronounced at lower P_{O_2}'s than at higher P_{O_2}'s. That is, their enhancement of the unloading of oxygen at the tissues is more profound than their interference with its loading at the lungs.

The P_{50}, shown in Figure 3–28, is a convenient term for discussing shifts in the oxyhemoglobin dissociation curve. The P_{50} is the P_{O_2} at which 50% of the hemoglobin in the blood is deoxyhemoglobin and 50% is oxyhemoglobin. At a temperature of 37°C, a pH of 7.4, and a P_{CO_2} of 40 torr, normal human blood has a P_{50} of 26 or 27 torr. If the oxyhemoglobin dissociation curve is shifted to the right, the P_{50} increases; if it is shifted to the left, the P_{50} decreases.

Other Factors Affecting Oxygen Transport

Anemia, carbon monoxide poisoning, methemoglobinemia, and abnormal levels of hemoglobin can all affect oxygen transport adversely. Most forms of anemia do not affect the oxyhemoglobin dissociation curve if the association of oxygen and hemoglobin are expressed as percent saturation. For example, anemia secondary to blood loss does not affect the combination of oxygen and hemoglobin for the remaining erythrocytes. It is the *amount* of functional hemoglobin, and therefore, the oxygen carrying *capacity* that decreases, not the percent saturation or even the arterial P_{O_2}. The arterial *content* of oxygen is also decreased.

Carbon monoxide has a much greater affinity for hemoglobin than oxygen, as already discussed. Because oxygen cannot be bound to iron atoms already combined with carbon monoxide, the latter can effectively block the combination of oxygen with hemoglobin. Carbon monoxide has a second deleterious effect: it shifts the oxyhemoglobin dissociation curve to the left. Thus, carbon monoxide can both prevent the loading of oxygen into the blood in the lungs as well as interfere with the unloading of oxygen at the tissues. Carbon monoxide is especially dangerous because it is colorless, odorless, and tasteless. It does not elicit any reflex increase in ventilation or protective reflex, such as coughing or sneezing. Its effects are cumulative because hemoglobin has such a high affinity for carbon monoxide.

A normal healthy adult who smokes and lives in an urban area has small amounts of carboxyhemoglobin in his or her blood. A nonsmoker living in a rural area may have only about 1% carboxyhemoglobin; a heavy smoker living in an urban area may have 5% to 8% carboxyhemoglobin in his or her blood.

Methemoglobin—hemoglobin with its iron in the ferric (Fe^{+++}) state—can be caused by nitrite poisoning or toxic reactions to oxidant drugs. It is also a congenital aberration in patients with hemoglobin M. In the Fe^{+++} state, iron atoms do not combine with oxygen.

Abnormal hemoglobins may have affinities for oxygen different from that of normal adult hemoglobin A. The best known of the abnormal hemoglobins, hemoglobin S, is reponsible for sickle cell anemia. When in the deoxyhemoglobin state, hemoglobin S is not very soluble in the intracellular fluid of erythrocytes. At low P_{O_2}'s, it may crystallize within the red blood cells. This crystallization changes the shape of the erythrocyte from the normal biconcave disc to a crescent or sickle shape. Sickle cells are more fragile than normal red blood cells, and they also have a greater tendency to adhere to each other. This adherence increases blood viscosity and may also cause thrombosis and blood vessel blockage.

Other abnormal hemoglobins, which like hemoglobin S are usually of genetic origin, may have either increased or decreased affinities for oxygen. These include Hb Seattle and Hb Kansas (decreased affinity) and Hb Rainier (increased affinity).

Transport of Carbon Dioxide in the Blood

The blood carries carbon dioxide in physical solution, chemically combined to amino acids in blood proteins, and as bicarbonate ions. A resting 70 kg person produces about 200 to 250 ml of carbon dioxide each minute as a result of metabolism, and the venous blood must carry the carbon dioxide to the lung for removal from the body. With the heart pumping blood at 5 L/min, each 100 ml passing through the lungs must unload 4 to 5 ml of carbon dioxide.

Physically Dissolved

Carbon dioxide is about 20 times more soluble in plasma (and inside the erythrocytes) than oxygen. About 5% to 10% of the total carbon dioxide transported by the blood is carried in physical solution. At an arterial P_{CO_2} of 40 torr, the total CO_2 content of whole blood is about 48 ml of CO_2 per 100 ml (Fig. 3–30). About 2 to 4 ml of CO_2 per 100 ml of arterial blood is carried physically dissolved, or about 5% to 10% of the total. At a venous P_{CO_2} of 45 torr, about 2.7 ml of CO_2 is physically dissolved in the mixed venous blood. The total carbon dioxide content of venous blood is about 52.5 ml of

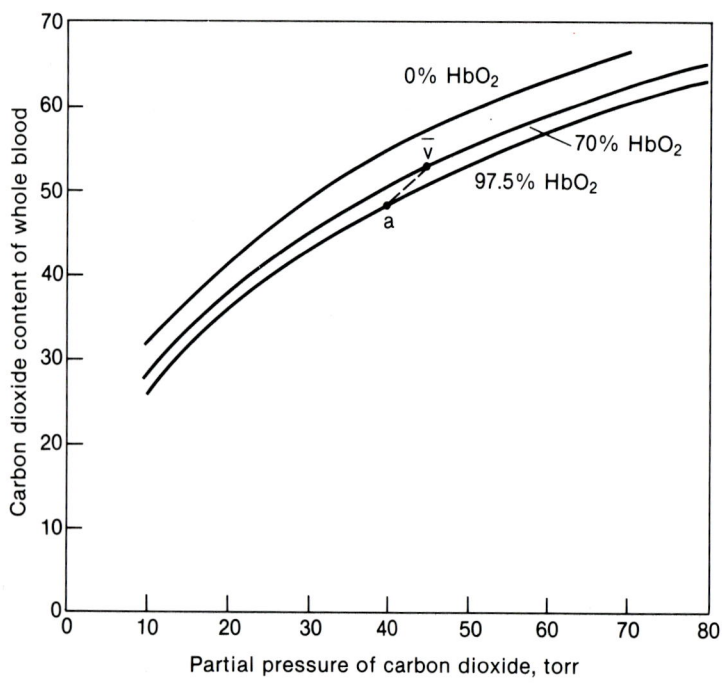

FIGURE 3–30. Carbon dioxide dissociation curves for whole blood (37°C) at different oxyhemoglobin saturations. Note that the ordinate is whole blood CO_2 content in milliliters of CO_2 per 100 ml of blood.

CO_2 per 100 ml of blood, so a little more than 5% of the total CO_2 content of venous blood is in physical solution.

As Carbamino Compounds

Carbon dioxide can combine chemically with the terminal amine groups in blood proteins to form *carbamino compounds*:

$$R-N\begin{matrix}H\\ \\H\end{matrix} + CO_2 \rightleftharpoons R-N\begin{matrix}H\\ \\COO^-\end{matrix} + H^+$$

terminal amine group   carbamino compound

The reaction occurs rapidly; no enzymes are required.

Because hemoglobin is the protein found in greatest concentration in the blood, most of the carbon dioxide carried in this manner is bound to the amino acids of hemoglobin. Deoxyhemoglobin can bind more carbon dioxide as carbamino groups than can oxyhemoglobin. Therefore, as the venous blood enters the lung and the hemoglobin combines with oxygen, carbon dioxide is released from its terminal amine groups. About 5% to 10% of the blood's total carbon dioxide content is in the form of carbamino compounds.

As Bicarbonate

The remaining 80% to 90% of the carbon dioxide in the blood is carried as bicarbonate ions. The following reaction shows how this occurs:

$$CO_2 + H_2O \xrightleftharpoons[]{\text{Carbonic anhydrase}} H_2CO_3 \rightleftharpoons H^+ + HCO_3^-$$

Carbon dioxide forms carbonic acid by combining with water. It can then dissociate into a hydrogen ion and a bicarbonate ion.

Little carbonic acid is formed by the association of water and carbon dioxide without the presence of carbonic anhydrase, an enzyme present in the erythrocytes, because the reaction occurs so slowly. Carbonic anhydrase makes the reaction proceed about 13,000 times faster. Hemoglobin also plays a critical role in the transport of carbon dioxide as bicarbonate because it can accept the hydrogen ion liberated by the dissociation of carbonic acid and thereby allows the reaction to continue. This is discussed in greater detail later.

Carbon Dioxide Dissociation Curve

The carbon dioxide dissociation curve for whole blood depicted in Figure 3–30 (note that the Y-axis is CO_2 content) shows that, within the normal physiologic range of P_{CO_2}'s, the curve is nearly a straight line. If plotted on axes similar to those for oxygen content, the carbon dioxide dissociation curve for whole blood is steeper than the oxygen dissociation curve for whole blood. That is, the change in carbon dioxide content per torr change in P_{CO_2} is greater than the change in oxygen content per torr change in P_{O_2}.

The carbon dioxide dissociation curve for whole blood shifts to the right when blood contains mainly oxyhemoglobin; it shifts to the left when blood contains mainly deoxyhemoglobin. This is known as the *Haldane effect*. The Haldane effect allows the blood to load more carbon dioxide at the tissues, where more deoxyhemoglobin is present, and unload more carbon dioxide in the lungs, where more oxyhemoglobin is present.

The Bohr and Haldane effects are both mainly explained by the fact that *deoxyhemoglobin is a weaker acid than oxyhemoglobin*. That is, deoxyhemoglobin more readily accepts the hydrogen ion liberated by the dissociation of carbonic acid, thus permitting more carbon dioxide to be carried in the form of bicarbonate ions. This increased transport of carbon dioxide is referred to as the isohydric shift. On the other hand, the association of hydrogen ions with the amino acids of hemoglobin lowers the affinity of hemoglobin for oxygen, thereby shifting the oxyhemoglobin dissociation curve to the right at low pH's or high P_{CO_2}'s. The following equation shows these actions:

$$H^+Hb + O_2 \rightleftharpoons H^+ + HbO_2$$

These effects of oxygen and carbon dioxide transport can be seen in Figure 3–31.

At the tissues, the P_{O_2} is low and the P_{CO_2} is high. Carbon dioxide dissolves in the plasma, and some of it then diffuses into the erythrocytes. Some of this carbon dioxide dissolves in the cytosol, some forms carbamino compounds with hemoglobin, and some is hydrated by carbonic anhydrase to form carbonic acid. At low P_{O_2}'s, the erythrocytes contain substantial amounts of deoxyhemoglobin, which is able to accept the hydrogen ion liberated by the dissociation of carbonic acid. Because bicarbonate ions diffuse out of the erythrocyte through the cell membrane much more readily than do hydrogen ions, an electrical imbalance within the cell should occur. How-

136 PULMONARY ANATOMY AND PHYSIOLOGY

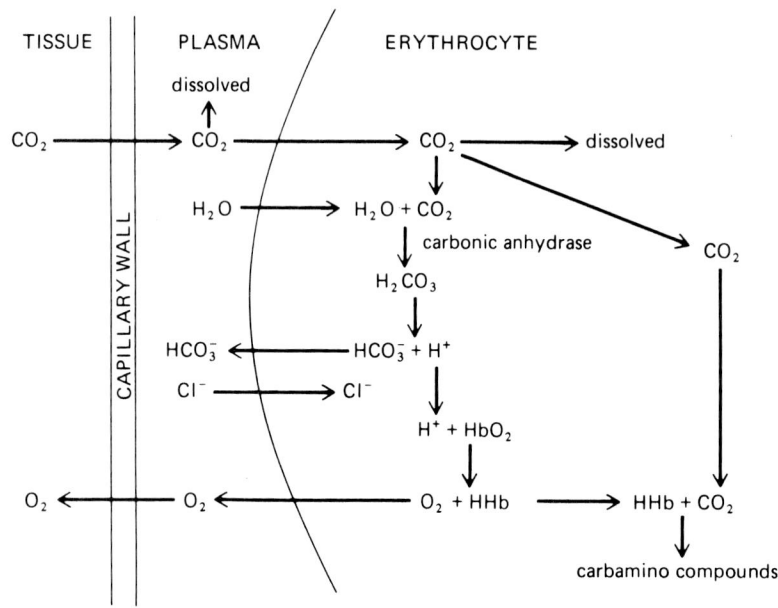

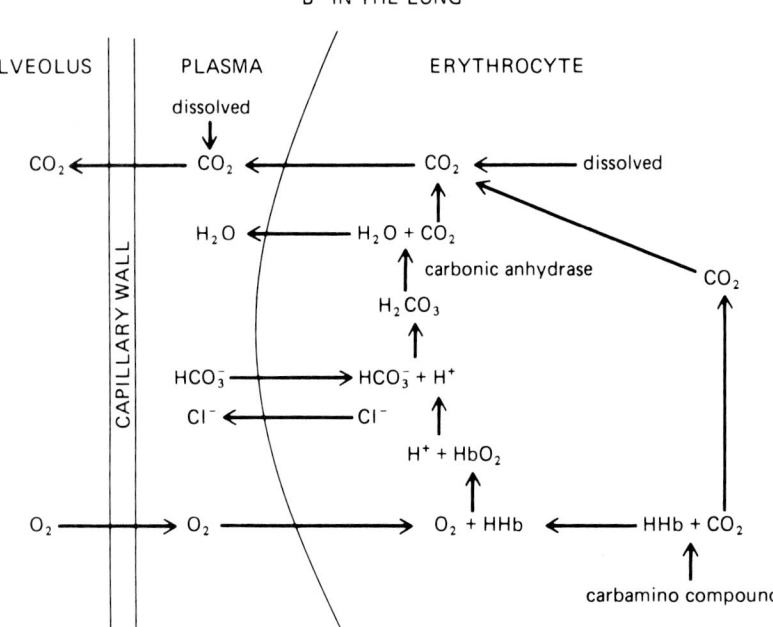

FIGURE 3–31. Representation of uptake and release of carbon dioxide and oxygen at the tissues (A) and in the lung (B). Note that negligible amounts of CO_2 can form carbamino compounds with blood proteins other than hemoglobin and may also be hydrated in trivial amounts in the plasma to form carbonic acid and then bicarbonate (not shown in diagram). (From Levitzky, M.G.: *Pulmonary Physiology*, 2nd ed. New York, McGraw-Hill, 1986, with permission.)

ever, electrical neutrality is maintained by the diffusion of chloride ions into the cell to match the movement of bicarbonate ions out of the cell. This is called the chloride shift. To maintain the osmotic equilibrium, small amounts of water also move into the cell.

At the lung, the P_{O_2} is high and the P_{CO_2} is low. As oxygen combines with hemoglobin, the hydrogen ions that had been absorbed when the hemoglobin was in the deoxyhemoglobin state are released. They combine with bicarbonate ions to form carbonic acid. The acid, in turn, breaks down into carbon dioxide and water. Coincidentally, carbon dioxide is also released from the carbamino compounds, the formation of which is less favorable at high P_{O_2}'s. Carbon dioxide then diffuses out of the erythrocytes and plasma and into the alveoli. A chloride shift also occurs in a direction opposite to that in the tissues to maintain electrical neutrality.

ACID-BASE PHYSIOLOGY

The respiratory system plays an important role in the balance of acids and bases in the body. It works with the kidneys and the buffer systems of the body to keep the pH of the blood and other body tissues within limits that allow them to function normally. Hydrogen ions are the most reactive cations normally found in body fluids, and they interact with negatively charged regions of other molecules such as proteins. These interactions with proteins can alter their structural conformations and, in doing so, alter their behavior. We have already seen an example of the effect of pH on the oxyhemoglobin dissociation curve. The effects of large alterations in hydrogen-ion concentration on the activity of enzymes alter the metabolic functions of all body tissues.

Acids, Bases, and Buffers

In Chapter 1, an *acid* was defined as a substance that can donate a hydrogen ion (a proton) to another substance, and a *base* as a substance that can accept a hydrogen ion from another substance. Note that a *strong acid* is one that is wholly or almost wholly dissociated into hydrogen ions and its corresponding, or *conjugate,* base in dilute aqueous solution; a *weak acid* is only slightly ionized in aqueous solution. In general, a strong acid has a weak conjugate base and a weak acid, a strong conjugate base. Do not confuse the *strength* of an acid or a base with its *concentration.*

A *buffer* is a mixture of substances dissolved in water or another medium, usually a combination of a weak acid and its conjugate base, that can resist changes in hydrogen-ion concentration when strong acids or bases are added. That is, when a strong acid or base is added to a buffer system, the changes in hydrogen-ion concentration are much smaller than those that would occur if the same amount of acid or base were added to pure water or another nonbuffer solution.

The *activity* of the hydrogen ions in a solution determines the acidity of the solution. The hydrogen-ion activity, denoted by the symbol αH^+, is closely related to the concentration of hydrogen ions ($[H^+]$) in a solution. In extremely dilute solutions, the hydrogen-ion activity equals the hydrogen-ion concentration; in highly concentrated solutions, the activity is less than the concentration. In blood, the hydrogen-ion concentration is low enough that the hydrogen-ion activity may be considered to be equal to the hydrogen ion concentration.

The hydrogen-ion activity of pure water is about 1.0×10^{-7} mols per liter. By convention, solutions with hydrogen-ion activities above 10^{-7} mols per liter are considered to be *acid;* those with hydrogen-ion activities below 10^{-7} are considered to be *alkaline.*

The pH of a solution is the negative logarithm of its hydrogen-ion activity. Therefore:

$$pH = -\log(\alpha H^+)$$

In the blood, the hydrogen-ion activity is approximately equal to the hydrogen-ion concentration. Thus:

$$pH = -\log[H^+]$$

The pH of arterial blood is normally close to 7.40, with the normal range considered to be about 7.35 to 7.45. An *increase* in pH from 7.40 to 7.70 represents a *decrease* in hydrogen-ion concentration. Table 3–3 shows the corresponding decreases in hydrogen-ion concentration as the pH increases from 6.90 to 7.80. As can be seen from the table, the increase of only 0.3 pH units indicates that hydrogen-ion concentration was cut in *half.*

Sources of Acids in the Body

The main source of acids in the body are the metabolic waste products of substances ingested as foodstuffs. Most hydrogen ions derive from carbonic acid, which in turn is produced by the combination of carbon dioxide with water. The carbon dioxide is produced as one of the end products of the oxidation of glucose and fatty acids during aerobic metabolism. In the lungs, hydrogen ions released from hemoglobin combine with bicarbonate, forming carbonic acid. The carbonic acid dis-

TABLE 3–3. Hydrogen-Ion Concentrations at Various pH's

pH	Hydrogen-Ion Concentration in Nanomols (10^{-9} mol/L)
6.90	126
7.00	100
7.10	79
7.20	63
7.30	50
7.40	40
7.50	32
7.60	25
7.70	20
7.80	16

sociates into water and carbon dioxide, which diffuses into the alveoli and is ultimately expired. Carbonic acid is therefore said to be a *volatile acid*, because it can be converted into a gas and removed from the body by the lungs. Great amounts of carbonic acid can be converted to carbon dioxide in the lungs, and the carbon dioxide is then removed by alveolar ventilation: Under normal circumstances about 24,000 mEq of carbonic acid is removed via the lungs daily.

A much smaller amount of *fixed* or *nonvolatile acids* is also normally produced during the metabolic breakdown of food. The fixed acids produced by the body include the following: sulfuric acid, which originates from the oxidation of sulfur-containing amino acids such as cysteine; phosphoric acid, produced from the oxidation of phospholipids and phosphoproteins; hydrochloric acid, produced during the conversion of ingested ammonium chloride to urea and by other reactions; and lactic acid, produced from the anaerobic metabolism of glucose. Lactic acid is sometimes converted to carbon dioxide and therefore is not always a fixed acid. Other fixed acids may be ingested accidentally or formed in abnormally large quantities by disease processes (e.g., the acetoacetic and butyric acid formed during diabetic ketoacidosis). About 50 mEq of fixed acids is normally removed from the body daily. This removal is done primarily by the kidneys, as discussed later.

Buffers in the Human Body

The body has various substances that can act as buffers in the physiologic pH range. These include bicarbonate, phosphate, and proteins.

An acid, HA, can dissociate into a hydrogen ion, H^+, and its base, A^-.

$$HA \rightleftharpoons H^+ + A^-$$

According to the law of mass action, the relationship between the undissociated acid and the proton and the base at equilibrium can be stated as follows:

$$\frac{[H^+][A^-]}{[HA]} = K'$$

That is, the product of the concentrations of hydrogen ion and base divided by the concentration of the acid is equal to a constant, K', the *dissociation constant*. This equation can be rearranged to read:

$$[H^+] = K' \frac{[HA]}{[A^-]}$$

After taking the logarithm of both sides:

$$\log[H^+] = \log K' + \log \frac{[HA]}{[A^-]}$$

Multiplying both sides by -1:

$$-\log[H^+] = -\log K' + \log \frac{[A^-]}{[HA]}$$

$$pH = pK' + \log \frac{[A^-]}{[HA]}$$

This is the *Henderson-Hasselbalch equation*.

The buffer capacity of a buffer pair is greatest at or near the pK' of the weak acid. When the concentrations of HA and A^- are equal, the pH of a solution is equal to its pK'.

As already stated, the human body has a number of buffers and buffer pairs. All the buffer pairs in a homogeneous solution are in equilibrium with the same hydrogen-ion concentration. For this reason, all the buffer pairs in the plasma behave similarly, with the relative concentrations of their undissociated acids and their bases determined by their respective pK's.

The *bicarbonate buffer system* consists of the buffer pair of the weak acid carbonic acid and its conjugate base, bicarbonate. As already stated, in the body:

$$CO_2 \text{ (gas phase)} \rightleftharpoons CO_2 \text{ (dissolved in the aqueous phase)} + H_2O \xrightleftharpoons[]{\text{Carbonic anhydrase}} H_2CO_3 = H^+ + HCO_3^-$$

The ability of the bicarbonate system to act as a buffer of fixed acids in the body is almost entirely due to the ability of the lungs to remove carbon dioxide from the body.

At a temperature of 38°C, about 0.03 millimols of carbon dioxide per torr P_{CO_2} dissolves in a liter of plasma. Therefore, the carbon dioxide *dissolved* in the plasma, expressed as millimols per liter, is equal to $0.03 \times P_{CO_2}$. At body temperature in plasma, the equilibrium of the second part of the series of equations (see above) is far to the left, and consequently, about 1,000 times as much carbon dioxide is physically dissolved in the plasma as there is in the form of carbonic acid. However, the dissolved carbon dioxide is in *equilibrium* with the carbonic acid, and therefore, in the Henderson-Hasselbalch equation for the bicarbonate system, *both* the dissolved carbon dioxide and the carbonic acid are considered to be the undissociated HA:

$$pH = pK' + \log \frac{[HCO_3^-]p}{[CO_2 + H_2CO_3]}$$

Because the concentration of carbonic acid is negligible, the equation becomes:

$$pH = pK' + \log \frac{[HCO_3^-]p}{0.03 \times P_{CO_2}}$$

The pK' of this system at physiologic pH's and at 38°C is 6.1. Therefore, at an arterial pH of 7.40 and an arterial P_{CO_2} of 40 torr:

$$7.40 = 6.1 + \log \frac{[HCO_3^-]p}{1.2 \text{ mM/L}}$$

Thus the arterial plasma bicarbonate concentration is normally about 24 millimols per liter, because the logarithm of 20 is equal to 1.3.

Note that the term *total carbon dioxide* is used to refer to the dissolved carbon dioxide (including carbonic acid) *plus* the carbon dioxide present as bicarbonate.

The *pH-bicarbonate diagram* shows a useful way to indicate the interrelationships between the variables of pH, P_{CO_2}, and bicarbonate concentration of the plasma, as expressed by the Henderson-Hasselbalch equation (Fig. 3–32).

In Figure 3–32, pH is on the abscissa, and the plasma bicarbonate concentration in millimols per liter, on the ordinate. For each value of pH and bicarbonate ion concentration, the graph shows a single corresponding P_{CO_2}. Conversely, for a given pH and P_{CO_2}, only one bicarbonate ion concen-

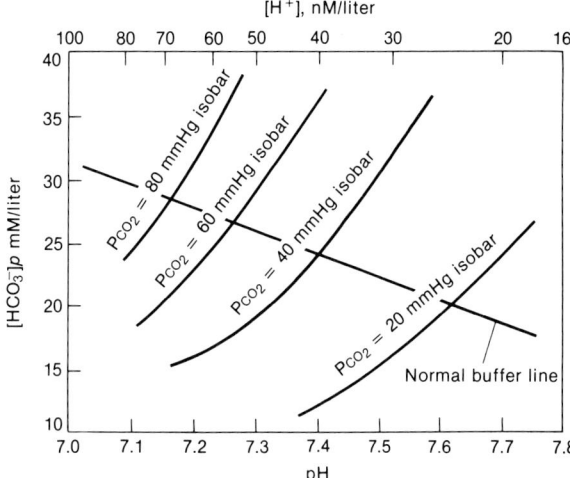

FIGURE 3–32. The pH-bicarbonate diagram with P_{CO_2} isobars. Note the hydrogen ion concentration in nanomols per liter at the top of the figure corresponding to the pH on the abscissa. (Reprinted from *The ABC of Acid-Base Chemistry*, 6th ed., 1974, revised, by H.W. Davenport by permission of the University of Chicago Press.)

tration will satisfy the Henderson-Hasselbalch equation. If the P_{CO_2} remains constant (for example at 40 torr) but the pH varies, an *isobar* line connecting the resulting points can be constructed. The representative isobars shown in the figure indicate the potential alterations of acid-base status when alveolar ventilation increases or decreases. If all else remains constant, hypoventilation leads to acidosis; hyperventilation leads to alkalosis.

The bicarbonate buffer system is a poor buffer for carbonic acid. Hemoglobin makes blood a much better buffer because, as carbon dioxide is added to whole blood, the hydrogen ions formed by the dissociation of carbonic acid are buffered by hemoglobin. Most of the bicarbonate ions formed by this dissociation can therefore diffuse into the plasma. The buffer value of plasma containing hemoglobin is four to five times that of plasma separated from erythrocytes.

The *phosphate buffer system* consists chiefly of the buffer pair of dihydrogenphosphate ($H_2PO_4^-$) and monohydrogenphosphate ($HPO_4^=$) anions:

$$H_2PO_4^- \rightleftharpoons H^+ + HPO_4^=$$

The pK' of the acid form is 6.8; in pH's ranging near 7.0, therefore, the acid form can readily release a proton, and the base form can accept a proton. Many organic phosphates in the body also have a pK' within ±0.5 pH units of 7.0, and those compounds also act as buffers. The organic phosphates include such compounds as glucose-1-phosphate and ATP.

Although several potential buffering groups are found on *proteins*, only one large category has a pK′ in the pH range of the blood: the imidazole groups in the histidine residues of the peptide chains. The pK′ of various histidine residues on the different *plasma proteins* ranges from about 5.5 to about 8.5, thus providing a broad spectrum of buffer pairs. The most preponderant protein in the blood is *hemoglobin*. As already noted, deoxyhemoglobin is a weaker acid than oxyhemoglobin. Thus, as oxygen is released from hemoglobin in the tissue capillaries, the imidazole groups remove hydrogen ions from the erythrocyte interior, allowing more carbon dioxide to be carried as bicarbonate. This process is reversed in the lungs.

The volume of the interstitial compartment is much larger than that of the plasma, so the interstitial fluid may play an important role in buffering changes in hydrogen ion concentration. The bicarbonate buffer system is the major buffer in the *interstitial fluid,* including the lymph. The phosphate buffer pair is also present in the interstitial fluid.

The extracellular portion of *bone* contains large deposits of calcium and phosphate salts. In an adult, bone salts can buffer hydrogen ions in chronic acidosis. This chronic buffering of hydrogen ions by the bone salts may result in demineralization of the bone.

In most cells, the *intracellular proteins and organic phosphates* can buffer both fixed acids and carbonic acid. This buffering is also largely a function of the histidine groups on the proteins and of phosphate groups on such compounds as ATP and glucose-1-phosphate.

Acidosis

Acid-base disorders can be categorized into four major groups: respiratory acidosis, metabolic acidosis, respiratory alkalosis, and metabolic alkalosis. These primary acid-base disorders may occur singly (simple) or in combination (mixed) or be altered by compensatory mechanisms.

Respiratory Acidosis. The arterial P_{CO_2} is normally kept at or near 40 torr (the normal range is considered 35 to 45 torr) by the mechanisms that regulate breathing. Any short-term alterations (i.e., those that occur without renal compensation, as discussed later in this section) in alveolar ventilation that result in an increase in alveolar, and therefore arterial, P_{CO_2} tend to lower the arterial pH, resulting in respiratory *acidosis*. This process can be seen by looking at the $P_{CO_2} = 60$ torr and $P_{CO_2} = 80$ torr isobars in Figures 3–32 and 3–33. The exact arterial pH at any Pa_{CO_2} depends on the bicarbonate and other buffers in the blood. Pure changes in arterial P_{CO_2} caused by changes in ventilation travel along the normal in vivo buffer line, as shown in the figure. Note that the more buffers *other than* bicarbonate present, the steeper the slope of the normal in vivo buffer line. Nonbicarbonate buffers can take up hydrogen ions liberated by the dissociation of carbonic acid, thus liberating bicarbonate ions. Pure uncompensated respiratory acidosis resulting from *hypoventilation* would correspond with point C on Figure 3–33: at the in-

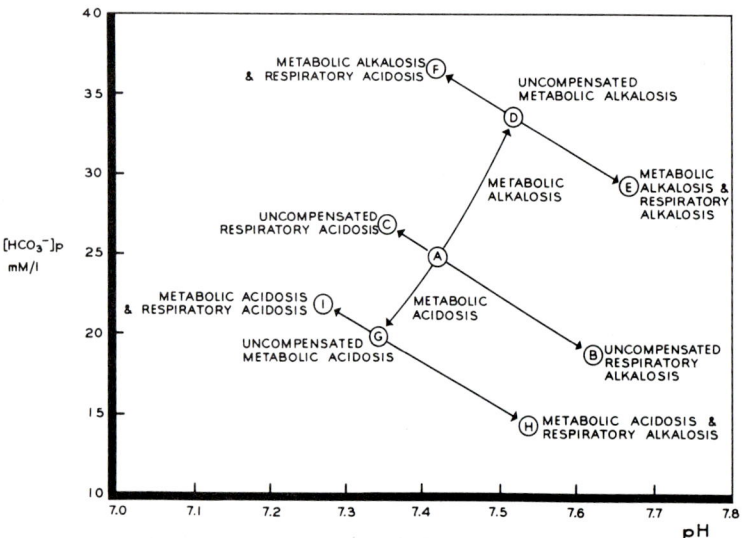

FIGURE 3–33. Acid-base paths in vivo. (Reprinted from *The ABC of Acid-Base Chemistry*, 6th ed., 1974, revised, by H.W. Davenport by permission of the University of Chicago Press.)

tersection of an elevated P_{CO_2} isobar and the normal buffer line.

In respiratory acidosis, the bicarbonate–to–carbon dioxide ratio decreases. Yet, as seen at point C in Figure 3–33, in uncompensated primary (simple) respiratory acidosis, the absolute plasma bicarbonate concentration does increase slightly because some of the hydrogen ions liberated by the dissociation of carbonic acid are buffered by nonbicarbonate compounds.

Metabolic Acidosis. This condition should more properly be referred to as nonrespiratory acidosis; metabolic acidosis does not always involve aberrations in metabolism. Causes of this condition include: ingestion, infusion, or production of a fixed acid; decreased excretion of hydrogen ions by the kidneys; the movement of hydrogen ions from inside to outside the cell; and the loss of bicarbonate or other bases from the extracellular compartment. As Figure 3–33 shows, primary uncompensated metabolic acidosis results in a downward movement along the $P_{CO_2} = 40$ torr isobar to point G. When a net loss of buffer occurs, a new blood buffer line becomes established, one lower than and parallel to the normal blood buffer line. P_{CO_2} does not change, but the hydrogen-ion concentration increases, and the ratio of bicarbonate concentration to carbon dioxide decreases.

Alkalosis

Respiratory Alkalosis. If alveolar ventilation exceeds that needed to keep pace with body carbon dioxide production, alveolar and arterial P_{CO_2} levels fall below 35 torr. Such *hyperventilation* results in respiratory alkalosis. As was true with primary respiratory acidosis and as seen at point B in Figure 3–33, uncompensated primary respiratory alkalosis results in movement to a lower P_{CO_2} isobar along the normal buffer line. The decreased $PaCO_2$ shifts to the left the equilibrium of the series of reactions describing carbon dioxide hydration and carbonic acid dissociation. This shift results in a decreased arterial hydrogen-ion concentration, elevates the pH, and lowers plasma bicarbonate concentration. The bicarbonate–to–carbon dioxide ratio increases.

Metabolic Alkalosis. Metabolic, or nonrespiratory, alkalosis occurs when loss of fixed acids from the body is excessive or when the ingestion, infusion, or reabsorption of bases (e.g., bicarbonate) by the kidneys is abnormally high. Figure 3–33 shows that primary uncompensated metabolic alkalosis moves up the $P_{CO_2} = 40$ torr isobar to point D. Thus, a net gain of buffer establishes a new blood buffer line higher than and parallel to the normal one. P_{CO_2} is unchanged, hydrogen-ion concentration is decreased, and the ratio of bicarbonate concentration to carbon dioxide is increased. The causes of acid-base imbalances are summarized in Table 3–4.

Respiratory Compensatory Mechanisms

The respiratory system can compensate for metabolic acidosis or metabolic alkalosis by altering alveolar ventilation. As discussed previously, if carbon dioxide production is constant, the alveolar P_{CO_2} is almost inversely proportional to the alveolar ventilation. In *metabolic acidosis*, the elevated blood hydrogen-ion concentration stimulates chemoreceptors that, in turn, increase alveolar ventilation, thereby decreasing arterial P_{CO_2}. This effect increases the arterial pH, returning it toward normal.

These events are shown in Figure 3–33. Point G represents uncompensated metabolic acidosis. As the respiratory apparatus compensates for the metabolic acidosis by increased ventilation, the arterial P_{CO_2} level declines. The point representing blood pH_a, $PaCO_2$, and bicarbonate concentration would then move a short distance along the lower-than-normal buffer line (from point G toward point H) until a new lower $PaCO_2$ is reached. This action returns the arterial pH *toward* normal; complete compensation does not usually occur. The respiratory compensation for metabolic acidosis usually occurs almost simultaneously with the development of the acidosis, so that the point takes an intermediate pathway between lines A-G and G-H.

The respiratory system compensates for *metabolic alkalosis* by decreasing alveolar ventilation, thus raising $PaCO_2$. This decreases arterial pH toward the normal level, as Figure 3–33 shows. Point D represents uncompensated metabolic alkalosis; respiratory compensation would shift the blood pH_a, $PaCO_2$, and bicarbonate concentration point a short distance along the new higher-than-normal blood buffer line toward point F. Again, the compensation occurs as the alkalosis develops, with the point moving along an intermediate course.

The *cause* of *respiratory acidosis* or *respiratory alkalosis* is a dysfunction in the ventilatory control mechanism or in the breathing apparatus itself. In these conditions, therefore, compensation for acidosis or alkalosis must come from outside the res-

TABLE 3–4. Causes of Simple Acid-Base Imbalances

Condition	pH	P_{CO_2}	$[HCO_3^-]$	$\dfrac{[HCO_3^-]}{P_{CO_2}}$	Causes
Respiratory acidosis	⇓	⇑	↑	↓	Hypoventilation: respiratory center depression, obstructive disease, restrictive disease, obliteration of lung tissue, respiratory muscle paralysis or dysfunction.
Respiratory alkalosis	⇑	⇓	↓	↑	Hyperventilation: CNS disorders; psychological causes; drugs, toxins, hormones, and pathogens; fever; hypoxemia; mechanical overventilation; low F_{IO_2}; altitude.
Metabolic acidosis	⇓	↔	⇓	⇓	Metabolic production of fixed acids: diabetic ketoacidosis and lactic acid production. Ingestion or infusion of fixed acids. Loss of bicarbonate: diarrhea and renal dysfunction. Inability to excrete hydrogen ions: renal dysfunction.
Metabolic alkalosis	⇑	↔	⇑	⇑	Loss of hydrogen ions: vomiting. Ingestion or infusion of bicarbonate or other bases: antacids. Drug and hormone therapy: diuretics and steroids. Potassium depletion.

piratory system. The respiratory compensatory mechanism can operate rapidly (within minutes) to partially correct metabolic acidosis or alkalosis.

Renal Compensatory Mechanisms

The kidneys can compensate for *respiratory acidosis* and *metabolic acidosis* of nonrenal origin by excreting fixed acids and by retaining filtered bicarbonate. The renal tubular cells normally secrete hydrogen ions into the tubular fluid by the generation of hydrogen ions and bicarbonate ions from the dissociation of carbonic acid from within the cell. As shown in the upper panel of Figure 3–34, carbonic acid is formed by the hydration of carbon dioxide via the carbonic anhydrase reaction. Carbon dioxide may be produced metabolically by the tubular cell itself or be carried dissolved into the tubular fluid after production elsewhere in the body. The hydrogen ion generated by this process is carried into the tubular lumen, and the bicarbonate ion is reabsorbed into the peritubular capillary. Electrical neutrality is maintained by the exchange of sodium ions for hydrogen ions in the tubular fluid. An interrelationship also exists between renal potassium ion secretion and renal hydrogen ion secretion: when the secretion of one of these ions increases, secretion of the other decreases. For this reason, disturbances in acid-base balance are usually associated with changes in potassium-ion balance and vice versa. The hydrogen ion secreted into the tubular lumen is buffered by tubular bicarbonate, phosphate, or the small quantities of other buffers found in the tubular fluid.

When a hydrogen ion combines with a tubular bicarbonate ion, forming carbonic acid, it may be converted to carbon dioxide by the carbonic anhydrase in the cell membrane of the proximal tubular cell. The bicarbonate ion that is reabsorbed into the peritubular capillary is the one formed in the tubular cell. About 90% of all filtered bicarbonate ions are reabsorbed in the proximal tubule, either by *direct transport* from the tubular fluid or by the carbonic acid mechanism.

The remaining 10% of bicarbonate ions are either reabsorbed by this mechanism in the distal tubules and collecting duct or in the process of titration of tubular *phosphate ions*, as shown in the middle panel of Figure 3–34, or by the generation of *ammonium ions*, as shown in the bottom panel of that figure. In each mechanism, a bicarbonate ion is returned to the peritubular capillary.

In renal cells, ammonia (NH_3) is actively formed by the deamination of amino acids. The ammonia

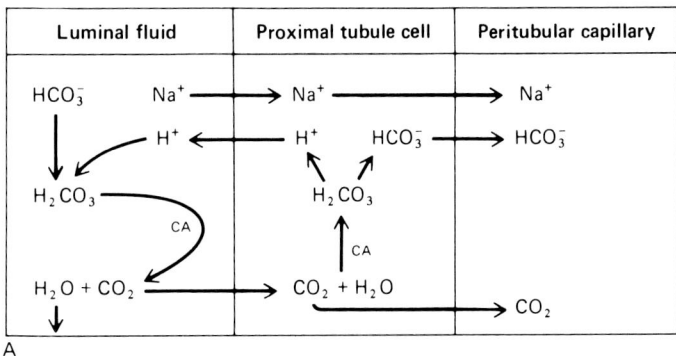

FIGURE 3–34. Representation of renal fixed acid excretion and bicarbonate retention. (From Levitzky, M.G.: *Pulmonary Physiology*, 2nd ed. New York, McGraw-Hill, 1986, with permission.)

then diffuses into the tubular lumen and combines with a hydrogen ion, forming ammonium (NH_4^+) ions. Ammonium ions do not readily diffuse back into the renal tubular cells, and they are highly soluble in tubular fluid; furthermore, ammonium is a weak acid at tubular fluid pH's. The pK of the system is about 9.3.

Normally, the kidneys secrete about 50 mEq of hydrogen ions and reabsorb about 50 mEq of bicarbonate each day. This secretion-reabsorption process can increase during acidosis to a point at which the urine becomes acidified to pH's as low as 4 or 5. This level of acidity is about 800 times greater than that of normal plasma.

The kidneys can compensate for *respiratory alkalosis* or *metabolic alkalosis* of nonrenal origin by decreasing hydrogen-ion excretion and by decreasing the retention of filtered bicarbonate. The kidney tends to reabsorb almost all of the filtered bicarbonate until the plasma bicarbonate concentration reaches about 27 or 28 mEq/L (normally the level is about 24 mEq/L). Above that threshold, plasma bicarbonate is excreted. Renal compensatory mechanisms for acid-base disturbances work much more slowly than do respiratory compensatory mechanisms. For example the renal compensatory responses to sustained respiratory acidosis or alkalosis may take 3 to 6 days.

CONTROL OF BREATHING

Breathing is initiated in the central nervous system. Neurons in the brain stem *automatically* generate a cycle of inspiration and expiration. In eupneic states, breathing occurs without a conscious initiation of inspiration and expiration. This spontaneously generated cycle of inspiration and expiration can be modified, altered, or even temporarily suppressed by reflexes, or by higher centers in the brain.

The respiratory centers in the brain stem control breathing via a *final common pathway* consisting of the spinal cord, the innervation of the muscles of respiration (such as the phrenic nerves), and the muscles of respiration themselves. The *interval* between successive groups of discharges of the respiratory neurons determines the breathing frequency. The frequency and duration of neural discharges to each respiratory muscle fiber and the number of respiratory muscle fibers and types of muscles activated determine the tidal volume.

Generation of Spontaneous Respiratory Rhythmicity

The centers controlling breathing are found in the reticular formation of the medulla, beneath the floor of the fourth ventricle. If the brain stem of an anesthetized animal is cut *above* this area, as shown in the transection labelled III in Figure 3–35, a pattern of inspiration and expiration continues, even if all other nerves leading to this area, including the vagi, are also cut. If the brain stem is cut *below* this area, as seen in transection IV, breathing stops. This area is known as the *medullary center* (or medullary respiratory center).

The medullary respiratory center consists of two dense bilateral aggregations of respiratory neurons known as the *dorsal respiratory groups* (DRG) and the *ventral respiratory groups* (VRG). Inspiratory and expiratory neurons are anatomically intermingled to a greater or lesser extent within these areas.

The dorsal respiratory groups consist mainly of *inspiratory cells*, which project their fibers primarily to the contralateral spinal cord and innervate inspiratory muscles. They probably serve as the chief initiators of the activity of the phrenic nerves and are therefore responsible for maintaining the activity of the diaphragm. Although the dorsal respiratory group neurons send collateral fibers to neurons in the ventral respiratory groups, the latter does not send collateral fibers to the dorsal respiratory groups.

The dorsal respiratory groups are located in the neuroanatomic structures called the nuclei of the tractus solitarius, which are the primary projection sites of afferent fibers of the ninth cranial nerve (the glossopharyngeal) and the tenth cranial nerve (the vagus). These nerves carry information about the arterial P_{O_2}, P_{CO_2}, and pH from the carotid and aortic arterial chemoreceptors, and information about the systemic arterial blood pressure from the carotid and aortic baroreceptors. In addition, the vagus carries information from stretch receptors and other sensors in the lungs that may also profoundly influence the control of breathing. The location of the dorsal respiratory groups within the nuclei of the tractus solitarius suggests that that group may be the site of integration of various inputs that can reflexively alter the spontaneous pattern of inspiration and expiration.

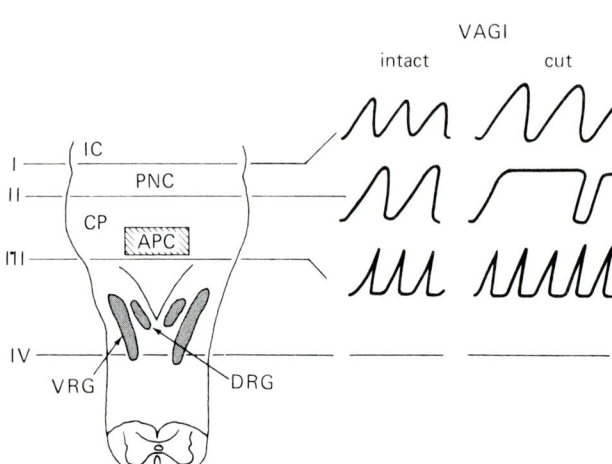

FIGURE 3–35. The effects of transections at different levels of the brain stem on the ventilatory pattern of anesthetized animals. *At left* is a diagram of the dorsal surface of the lower brain stem. *At right* is a diagram of the breathing patterns (inspiration is upward) corresponding to the transections with the vagus nerves intact or transected. (DRG = dorsal respiratory group; VRG = ventral respiratory group; APC = apneustic center; PNC = pneumotaxic center; IC = inferior colliculus; CP = cerebellar peduncle.) (From Berger, A.J., Mitchell, R.A. and Severinghaus, J.W.: Regulation of respiration. Reprinted by permission of the *New England Journal of Medicine* 297:139, 1977.)

The dorsal respiratory groups have two populations of inspiratory neurons. One population, called the *I alpha cells,* is inhibited by lung inflation; the second population, the *I beta cells,* is excited by lung inflation. These cells may play an important role in the Hering-Breuer reflexes described later.

The ventral respiratory group neurons include both inspiratory and expiratory cells. The major function of these cells is to drive either spinal respiratory neurons, innervating mainly the intercostal and abdominal muscles, or the auxiliary muscles of respiration innervated by the vagus nerves. Because the dorsal respiratory groups send fibers to the ventral respiratory groups, but not vice versa, the dorsal respiratory groups may drive the ventral respiratory groups, but reciprocal inhibition between the two groups is unlikely. The ventral respiratory groups do not appear to be an initial processing site for sensory information.

The exact mechanism by which the spontaneous rhythmicity of breathing is generated is as yet unknown. It now seems that cells in or near to the dorsal respiratory groups act as pacemakers themselves and that their activity is modulated by information received from afferent nerves and higher brain centers.

Medullary and Pontine Respiratory Centers

If the brain stem is transected in the pons at the level denoted by the line labelled II in Figure 3–35 and if the vagus nerves have also been transected, a breathing pattern called *apneusis* results. Apneustic breathing is characterized by prolonged inspiratory efforts interrupted by occasional expirations. Afferent information reaching this *apneustic center* (labelled APC) via the vagus nerves must be important in preventing apneusis because apneusis does not occur if the vagus nerves are left intact, as shown in the figure.

Apneusis probably involves a sustained discharge of medullary inspiratory neurons. Investigators believe that the apneustic center may be the site of the normal "inspiratory cut-off switch," that is, the site of projection of various types of afferent information that can *terminate inspiration.* Apneusis results from the inactivation of the inspiratory cut-off mechanism. The specific group of neurons that functions as the apneustic center has not been identified.

If the brain stem is transected immediately below the inferior colliculus, as indicated by line I in Figure 3–35, the balance between inspiration and expiration remains essentially normal—even if the vagus nerves are transected. A group of respiratory neurons known as the *pneumotaxic center* (labelled PNC), therefore, acts to modulate the response of the apneustic center. These cells probably function to fine-tune the breathing pattern. Pulmonary inflation afferent information can inhibit the activity of the pneumotaxic center, which in turn may modulate the threshold for lung inflation–elicited inspiratory cut-off. The pneumotaxic center may also modulate the respiratory control system's response to other stimuli, such as hypercapnia or hypoxia.

Spinal Pathways

Axons from the dorsal respiratory groups, ventral respiratory groups, cortex, and other supraspinal sites project to the spinal white matter to affect the action of the phrenic, intercostal, and abdominal muscles of respiration. At the level of these spinal respiratory motor neurons, there is integration of descending influences as well as the presence of local spinal reflexes. In the spinal cord, ascending pathways carrying information from pain, touch, and temperature receptors as well as from proprioceptors can also affect breathing, as discussed in the next section. Inspiratory and expiratory fibers are apparently separated in the spinal cord.

Reflex Mechanisms of Respiratory Control

A great number of sensors in the lungs, cardiovascular system, muscles and tendons, and skin and viscera can affect the control of breathing by eliciting reflex changes. Stimulation of the pulmonary stretch receptors can elicit three respiratory reflexes: the Hering-Breuer inflation reflex, the Hering-Breuer deflation reflex, and the paradoxical reflex of Head.

Hering-Breuer Inflation Reflex. In 1868, Breuer and Hering reported that a maintained inflation of the lungs of anesthetized animals decreased the frequency of the inspiratory effort or caused a transient apnea. The sensors are *stretch receptors* within the smooth muscle of large and small airways. The afferent pathway consists of fibers in the vagus; as mentioned previously, these fibers apparently enter the brain stem and lead to the nucleus of the tractus solitarius and the pneumotaxic center. The efferent branch of the reflex causes bronchodilation as well as the apnea of slowing of ventilatory frequency (resulting from an increase in expiration time). Lung inflation can also cause reflex effects in the cardiovascular system: Moderate lung inflations increase the heart rate and may cause a slight vasoconstriction; large inflations may decrease the heart rate and systemic vascular resistance.

The Hering-Breuer inflation reflex was originally believed to act tonically to limit the tidal volume because vagotomized, anesthetized animals breathe much more deeply and at a lower rate than they do before their vagus nerves are transected. However, more recent studies done on conscious adult humans have shown that the threshold of the Hering-Breuer inflation reflex occurs at tidal volumes greater than 800 to 1,000 ml. The Hering-Breuer inflation reflex may help to minimize the work of breathing by inhibiting large tidal volumes and may prevent overdistention of the alveoli at high lung volumes. The reflex may also be important in the control of breathing in infants.

Hering-Breuer Deflation Reflex. Breuer and Hering also noted that abrupt *deflation* of the lungs increases the ventilatory rate. This increased rate could be a result of *decreased* stretch receptor activity, the stimulation of as yet unknown receptors in the lungs, or the stimulation of other pulmonary receptors, such as the irritant receptors and "J" receptors, which are discussed shortly. The afferent pathway is the vagus and the effect is hyperpnea. The deflation reflex may be responsible for the increased ventilation elicited when the lungs are deflated abnormally, as in pneumothorax, or it may play a role in the periodic spontaneous deep breaths (sighs) that help to prevent atelectasis. These sighs, which occur occasionally and irregularly during normal, quiet breathing, consist of a slow deep inspiration (larger than a normal tidal volume) followed by a slow expiration. This response may be important because patients maintained on mechanical ventilators must be given deep breaths periodically or they develop diffuse atelectasis, which may lead to arterial hypoxemia.

The Paradoxical Reflex of Head. In 1889, Henry Head experimented with the Hering-Breuer inflation reflex. Instead of transecting the vagus nerves, however, he blocked their function by cooling them to 0°C. As he rewarmed the vagus nerves, he noted that in a selective *partial* block of those nerves, lung inflation resulted in further deep inspiration—instead of the apnea expected when the vagus nerves were fully functional. The receptors for this paradoxical reflex are in the lungs, but their location is not known precisely. This reflex may also be involved in the sigh response. Some investigators have suggested that the reflex is involved in generating the first breath of the newborn baby.

Respiratory Irritant Receptors. If the airways (and possibly the alveoli) are irritated mechanically or chemically, a reflex cough or sneeze, hyperpnea, bronchoconstriction, and increased blood pressure can result. The receptors for these responses are found in the nasal mucosa, upper airways, and tracheobronchial tree and perhaps in the alveoli themselves. The vagus nerves provide the afferent pathways for all but the nasal mucosa receptors, which send information centrally by means of the trigeminal and olfactory tracts. Receptors in the airways also respond to changes in temperature, causing reflex alterations in blood flow to the airways. These receptors may be responsible for bronchospasm during exercise in cold air.

Pulmonary Vascular Reflexes. Pulmonary embolism causes rapid shallow breathing; pulmonary vascular congestion causes hyperpnea. Injection of some drugs or chemicals into the pulmonary circulation may result in apnea. The receptors that initiate these responses are believed to be in the walls of the pulmonary capillaries; therefore, they are named "J" (for juxtapulmonary-capillary) receptors. They are stimulated by pulmonary vascular congestion or an increase in pulmonary interstitial fluid volume. Furthermore, they might also be the cause of the *dyspnea* (difficult or labored breathing) that occurs during the pulmonary vascular congestion and edema secondary to left ventricular failure or even the dyspnea that healthy persons have as the result of exercise. The slow-conducting nonmyelinated vagal fibers provide the afferent pathways for these reflexes.

Arterial Chemoreceptors. The arterial chemoreceptors are discussed in greater detail later, but as already noted in Chapter 2, the arterial chemoreceptors respond to decreased P_{O_2}, increased P_{CO_2}, and low pH. Hering's nerve, a branch of the glossopharyngeal nerve, is the afferent pathway from the carotid body; the vagus is the afferent pathway from the aortic body. Stimulation of the arterial chemoreceptors results in reflex hyperpnea, bronchoconstriction, and increased blood pressure. As noted in Chapter 2, the *direct* effect of arterial chemoreceptor stimulation is a decrease in heart rate; however, this decreased rate is usually masked by an increase in heart rate that is secondary to the increase in lung inflation.

Arterial Baroreceptors. The influence of the arterial baroreceptors on the control of ventilation is minor. Hering's nerve and the glossopharyngeal nerve are the afferent pathways for the carotid baroreceptors; the vagus nerve is the afferent pathway for the aortic baroreceptors. Elevated blood pressure stimulates the arterial baroreceptors, resulting in apnea and bronchodilation.

Muscle and Tendon Receptors (Proprioceptors). Ventilation can be increased by stimulation of receptors in the muscles, tendons, and joints. Among these receptors are those in the muscles of respiration (e.g., muscle spindles) and rib cage as well as other skeletal muscles, joints, and tendons. The receptors may be important in compensating for elevated work loads and may help to minimize the work of breathing. They may also participate in increasing ventilation during exercise. Afferent information ascends to the respiratory centers via the spinal cord.

Pain Receptors. Somatic pain generally causes hyperpnea; visceral pain generally causes apnea or decreased ventilation. Physicians occasionally pinch patients whose breathing is depressed to increase ventilation via the ventilatory response to somatic pain.

Influences of Higher Centers

The spontaneous rhythmicity generated by the medullary respiratory center can be altered and even completely suppressed (for short periods). A person can voluntarily hyperventilate or hold his or her breath for several minutes. During speech, singing, or playing a wind instrument, higher brain centers automatically modify the normal cycle of inspiration and expiration.

Chemical Control of Breathing

Changes in the P_{O_2}, P_{CO_2}, and pH of the body usually result in adjustments of alveolar ventilation designed to return these variables to their normal levels. Chemoreceptors alter their activity when their own local chemical environment changes. They can therefore supply the central respiratory controller with the information necessary to properly adjust alveolar ventilation and to change the whole-body P_{O_2}, P_{CO_2}, and pH. The respiratory control system, therefore, acts as a *negative feedback system*.

Response to Carbon Dioxide

The arterial and cerebrospinal fluid partial pressures of carbon dioxide are probably the most important inputs to the central respiratory controller in establishing the breath-to-breath ventilatory rate and tidal volume. Elevated carbon dioxide levels are an extremely strong stimulus to ventilation. Only voluntary hyperventilation and exercise produce greater minute ventilations. The respiratory system normally regulates the arterial P_{CO_2} very precisely: during exercise, metabolic carbon dioxide production may be increased by a factor of 10, yet the arterial P_{CO_2} usually changes less than 1 torr.

Elevated levels of carbon dioxide in the inspired air (the $F_{I}CO_2$) generally increase alveolar ventilation. The greatest response is seen with about 5% to 10% carbon dioxide in the inspired gas, which corresponds to alveolar P_{CO_2}'s between about 40 and 70 torr. Above 10% to 15% carbon dioxide in inspired air, little further increase occurs in alveolar ventilation. Very high arterial P_{CO_2}'s (70 to 80 torr) may directly produce respiratory depression if they are encountered acutely. Patients with hypercapnia resulting from chronic obstructive lung disease have secondary acid-base changes (renal and cerebrospinal fluid bicarbonate retention) and may have relatively normal arterial pH's and ventilation, as discussed in Chapter 5. Acutely encountered high carbon dioxide levels may result in dyspnea, severe headaches (partly from cerebral vasodilation), faintness, dulling of the consciousness, muscular rigidity, tremors, and ultimately convulsions.

Figure 3–36 shows the ventilatory response of a normal conscious person to physiologic levels of carbon dioxide. Inspired concentrations of carbon dioxide or metabolically produced carbon dioxide resulting in alveolar (and arterial) P_{CO_2}'s in the range of 38 to 50 torr increase alveolar ventilation linearly. The slope is rather steep; it varies from person to person, with young healthy adults having a slope of 2 to 5 L/min/torr P_{ACO_2} (mean = 2.0 to 2.5 L/min/torr P_{ACO_2}).

Hypoxemia potentiates the ventilatory response to carbon dioxide, as shown in Figure 3–36. At lower arterial P_{O_2}'s (e.g., 35 and 50 torr) the response curve shifts to the left and the slope becomes steeper. That is, for any particular arterial P_{CO_2}, the ventilatory response becomes greater as the arterial P_{O_2} decreases. This increased ventilatory response may be an effect of the hypoxia at the chemoreceptor itself, or changes in the central acid-base status secondary to the hypoxia.

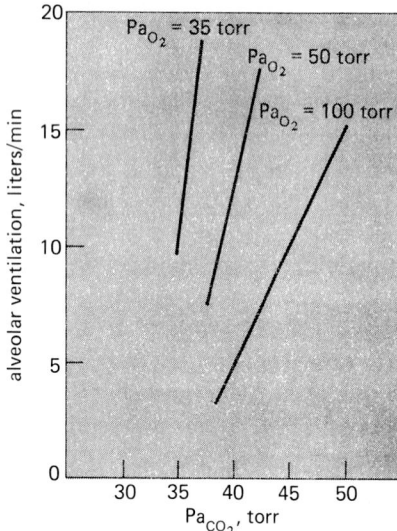

FIGURE 3–36. Diagram of ventilatory CO_2 response curves at three different levels of arterial P_{O_2}. (From Levitzky, M.G.: *Pulmonary Physiology,* 2nd ed. New York, McGraw-Hill, 1986 with permission.)

Other factors affecting the carbon dioxide response curve are shown in Figure 3–37. Sleep shifts the curve slightly to the right. The arterial P_{CO_2} normally increases about 5 to 6 torr during slow-wave sleep. A depressed or abnormal response to carbon dioxide during sleep may be involved in *central sleep apnea.* During sleep apnea, abnormally long periods (as much as 1 to 2 minutes) may occur between breaths. In *obstructive sleep apnea,* the central respiratory controller's response to carbon dioxide may be normal, but obstruction of the upper airway occurs. In central sleep apnea, the defect is in the chemoreceptors or in the central respiratory controller itself. Central sleep apnea may be an important etiologic factor in *sudden infant death syndrome* (SIDS), and it is also seen in adults, although rarely.

Narcotics and anesthetics may profoundly depress the ventilatory response to carbon dioxide. Respiratory depression is the most common cause of death in cases of overdoses of opiate alkaloids and their derivatives as well as barbiturates and most anesthetics. The hypoxic drive may be solely responsible for maintaining spontaneous breathing in patients with a depressed response to carbon dioxide. Administration of high F_{IO_2}'s without ventilatory support may cease the spontaneous breathing of these patients. Endorphins (naturally-occurring opiate-like substances found in the brain) probably also depress the response to carbon dioxide. Chronic obstructive lung diseases depress the ventilatory response to hypercapnia, partly as a result of central acid-base changes and partly because the work of breathing may be so great that ventilation cannot be increased. Metabolic acidosis displaces the carbon dioxide response curve to the left, indicating that for any particular $PaCO_2$ ventilation is increased during metabolic acidosis.

As already noted, the respiratory control system is a negative feedback system. The response to carbon dioxide exemplifies this fact. Increased *metabolic production* of carbon dioxide increases the carbon dioxide carried to the lung. If alveolar

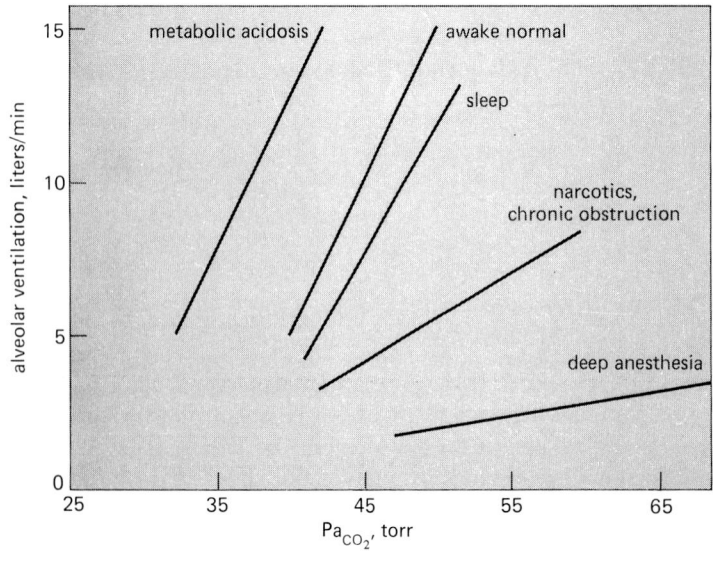

FIGURE 3–37. Diagram of the effects of sleep, narcotics, chronic obstructive pulmonary disease, deep anesthesia, and metabolic acidosis on the ventilatory response to carbon dioxide. (From Levitzky, M.G.: *Pulmonary Physiology,* 2nd ed. New York, McGraw-Hill, 1986, with permission.)

ventilation does not change immediately, the alveolar P_{CO_2} increases, resulting in increased arterial and cerebrospinal fluid P_{CO_2}. The increased arterial and cerebrospinal fluid (CSF) P_{CO_2}'s stimulate ventilation resulting in increased pulmonary carbon dioxide removal and decreased alveolar, arterial, and CSF P_{CO_2}'s.

Peripheral and Central Chemoreceptors

The *arterial chemoreceptors* (or peripheral chemoreceptors) alter their firing rate in response to changes in the gas composition and hydrogen-ion concentration of the *arterial blood*. Increased arterial P_{CO_2} or decreased arterial pH and P_{O_2} stimulate the peripheral chemoreceptors. The impulse traffic in the afferent fibers from the arterial chemoreceptors is considerable at normal levels of arterial P_{O_2}, P_{CO_2}, and pH. The response of the receptors is sufficiently rapid and sensitive that they can relay information about breath-to-breath changes in the arterial blood composition to the medullary respiratory center. Single afferent fibers respond to changes in all three stimuli, but it is not clear whether there are individual sensors for each. The carotid bodies apparently exert a much greater influence on the respiratory controller than the aortic bodies, especially with respect to decreased P_{O_2} and pH; the aortic bodies may exert a greater influence on the cardiovascular system.

The arterial chemoreceptors increase their activity *nearly linearly* with the arterial P_{CO_2} throughout the range of 20 to 60 torr. The linear response of the arterial chemoreceptors to $PaCO_2$ is partly reflected in the CO_2 response curves (see Figs. 3–36 and 3–37).

The exact mechanism by which the chemoreceptors work remains uncertain. Chemoreceptors have a complicated ultrastructure, including several types of so-called glomus cells having many nerve fibers in close proximity. Whether the glomus cells or the fiber endings act as the chemosensitive element is unclear. A great amount of blood flows through the carotid body; the arteriovenous oxygen difference is extremely small (about 0.5 ml O_2/100 ml blood) despite the fact that it has one of the highest metabolic rates in the body. Certain drugs and enzyme poisons that block the formation of ATP stimulate the carotid body. For example, both cyanide and dinitrophenol directly stimulate the carotid body; this action may relate to the mechanism of the stimulatory effect of hypoxia on the arterial chemoreceptors.

Although the *central chemoreceptors* are in contact with CSF, they are not directly exposed to the arterial blood. The blood-brain barrier separates CSF from the arterial blood. Carbon dioxide easily diffuses through the blood-brain barrier, but hydrogen ions and bicarbonate ions do not. Because of this diffusibility difference, alterations in the arterial P_{CO_2} are rapidly transmitted to CSF, taking only about 1 to 2 minutes. Changes in arterial pH that do not result from changes in P_{CO_2} take considerably longer to affect the CSF. In fact, in some circumstances, CSF may undergo changes in hydrogen-ion concentration *opposite* to those in the blood, as discussed shortly.

The composition of CSF is considerably different from that of the blood. The pH of CSF is normally about 7.32, compared to the pH of 7.40 of arterial blood. The bicarbonate-ion concentration is similar to that of the arterial blood, but the P_{CO_2} of CSF is about 50 torr. The higher CSF P_{CO_2} is partly a result of the diffusion of metabolically produced carbon dioxide from cerebral tissue.

In CSF, the concentration of proteins is only in the range of 15 to 45 *milligrams*/100 ml, whereas in the *plasma* it normally ranges from 6.6 to 8.6 *grams*/100 ml. This figure does not even include the hemoglobin in the red blood cells. Therefore, the only buffer of consequence in CSF is bicarbonate. Arterial hypercapnia or metabolic acidosis in the brain thus leads to greater changes in hydrogen-ion concentration in CSF than in the arterial blood.

The central chemoreceptors respond to local increases in hydrogen-ion concentration and/or P_{CO_2}. They are not stimulated by hypoxia and may even be depressed by it. The central chemoreceptors are situated ventrolaterally at or just beneath the surface of the medulla. Increases in their activity are thought to stimulate the medullary respiratory neurons in a manner similar to that of the peripheral chemoreceptors.

The relative contribution of the peripheral and central chemoreceptors in the ventilatory response to increased carbon dioxide levels is somewhat controversial. Experimental animals from which the fibers leading from the arterial chemoreceptors have been cut, or patients from whom carotid bodies have been removed, show about 80% to 90% of the normal total *steady state* response to increased inspired carbon dioxide concentrations delivered in hyperoxic gas mixtures. This finding shows that the peripheral chemoreceptors contribute only about 10% to 20% of the steady state response to hypercapnia. Other studies done on normoxic men show that up to one third or one half of the *transient* response can come from the arterial chemoreceptors when the arterial P_{CO_2} changes rapidly. That is, although the central chemoreceptors may be almost solely responsible for determining the resting ventilatory level or the long-term response to carbon dioxide inhalation, the peripheral chemoreceptors may be more important in short-term responses to carbon dioxide.

Response to Hydrogen Ions

Changes in hydrogen-ion concentration over the range of 20 to 60 nanoequivalents per liter produce linear increases in ventilation. A metabolic acidosis that originates outside the brain results in hyperpnea coming almost exclusively from the peripheral chemoreceptors. Because hydrogen ions cross the blood-brain barrier so slowly, the central chemoreceptors are not affected at first. As acidotic stimulation of the peripheral chemoreceptors occurs, alveolar ventilation increases and the arterial P_{CO_2} falls. Because the CSF P_{CO_2} is in a kind of equilibrium with the arterial P_{CO_2}, carbon dioxide diffuses out of CSF and the CSF pH increases. Stimulation of the central chemoreceptor therefore decreases. If the situation persists (for hours or days), the bicarbonate concentration of CSF slowly declines, returning the pH of the cerebrospinal fluid toward normal (7.32). Investigators do not agree on how this occurs. The mechanism may be the slow diffusion of bicarbonate ions across the blood-brain barrier, the active transport of bicarbonate ions out of the CSF, or decreased *formation* of bicarbonate ions by carbonic anhydrase during formation of CSF. The bicarbonate concentration in the cerebrospinal fluid in patients having chronic respiratory acidosis (as in chronic obstructive lung disease) may be increased by similar mechanisms, because the pH of the cerebrospinal fluid is nearly normal.

Response to Hypoxia

The ventilatory response to hypoxia arises solely from the peripheral chemoreceptors. In this response, the carotid bodies are much more important than the aortic bodies, which cannot sustain the ventilatory response to hypoxia by themselves. When no peripheral chemoreceptors are present, increasing degrees of hypoxia result in a progressive *depression* of the central respiratory controller. Therefore, when the peripheral chemoreceptors are intact, their excitation of the central respiratory controller must offset the direct depressant effect of hypoxia.

Figure 3-38 shows the response of the respiratory system to hypoxia. At a normal arterial P_{CO_2} of about 38 to 40 torr, little increase in ventilation occurs until the arterial P_{O_2} falls below about 50 to 60 torr. Note that the response to hypoxemia is potentiated at higher arterial P_{CO_2}'s.

Studies have shown that the respiratory response to hypoxia relates to the change in P_{O_2} rather than the change in *oxygen content*. In a person who has anemia (without acidosis), therefore, the condition does not stimulate ventilation in as much as the arterial P_{O_2} is normal and the arterial chemoreceptors are not stimulated.

Hypoxia alone, by stimulating alveolar ventilation, causes the arterial P_{CO_2} to decrease, which in turn, may lead to respiratory alkalosis, as discussed in Chapter 4.

NONRESPIRATORY FUNCTIONS OF THE RESPIRATORY SYSTEM

The nonrespiratory functions of the respiratory system include its own defense against inhaled particulate matter; the storage and filtration of blood for the systemic circulation; the conversion, me-

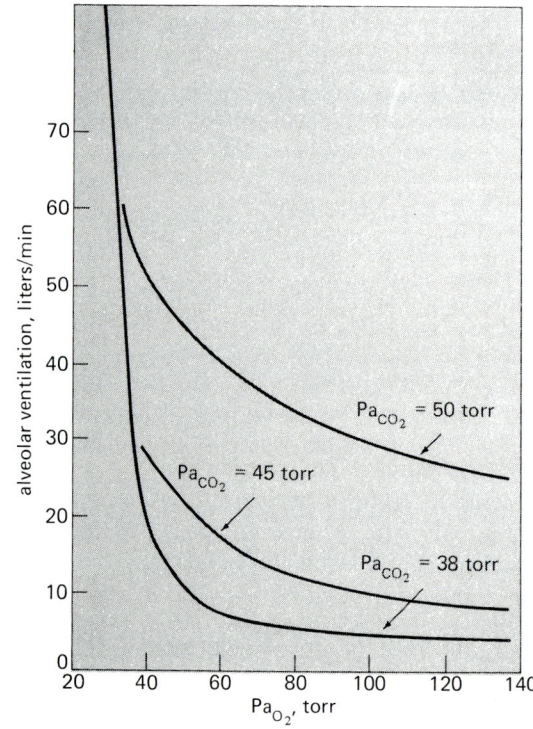

FIGURE 3-38. Diagram of the ventilatory response to hypoxia at three different arterial P_{CO_2} levels. (From Levitzky, M.G.: *Pulmonary Physiology*, 2nd ed. New York, McGraw-Hill, 1986, with permission.)

tabolism, and release of vasoactive agents in the blood; and the formation and release of substances used in the alveoli, airways, or systemic circulation.

Pulmonary Defense Mechanisms

Inspired air may contain dust, pollen, ash and other products of combustion, microorganisms, particulate material, hazardous chemicals, and toxic gases. Each day, a person brings 8,000 to 10,000 L of air through the airways, and about two thirds of that reaches the delicate alveolar surfaces.

"Air Conditioning." The temperature and humidity of the ambient air vary widely, so some protection must be given to the alveoli against the cold and in order to keep them from drying out. The mucosa lining the nose, the nasal turbinates, and the oropharynx and nasopharynx have a large surface area and a rich blood supply. The surface area of the nasal turbinates (see Fig. 3–1) is said to be about 160 cm^2. As inhaled air passes over these surfaces, it is warmed to body temperature and humidified, especially if breathing is done through the nose.

Olfaction. Because the olfactory receptors are positioned in the posterior nasal cavity and not in the trachea or alveoli, a person can *sniff* to try to detect gases or other material in the air that may be hazardous. This quick, shallow inhalation through the nose brings gases into contact with the olfactory sensors without inspiring the gases into the lung.

Filtration and Removal of Inspired Particles. The filtration system works better if one is breathing through the nose. Air moving through the nose is first filtered by passing through the nasal hairs, or *vibrissae*. This action stops most particles larger than 10 to 15 μm in diameter from moving farther toward the lung. Most particles greater than 10 μm in diameter are caught in the large surface area of the nasal septum and turbinates. The direction of the inspired air stream changes abruptly at the nasopharynx, and most particles of about 10 μm in diameter, because of their inertia, land on the back wall of the pharynx. The tonsils and adenoids, located near this impaction site, provide immunologic defense against biologically active material filtered at that point. Air entering the trachea usually has few particles larger than 10 μm, and most of these impact at the carina or within the bronchi.

Most particles in the size range of 2 to 5 μm settle out by gravity in the smaller airways, where the linear velocity is extremely low. Thus, impaction or sedimentation remove most of the particles between 2 to 10 μm in diameter, which become trapped in the mucus lining the upper airways, trachea, bronchi, and bronchioles. Smaller particles and all foreign gases enter the alveolar ducts and alveoli. Some smaller particles (0.1 μm and smaller) are deposited by virtue of Brownian motion; other particles, between 0.1 and 0.5 μm in diameter, generally remain suspended as aerosols, and about 80% of them are exhaled.

Filtered material trapped in the mucus lining of the respiratory tract can be removed in several ways, including the *mucociliary escalator* and reflex coughing or sneezing.

As noted earlier, a mucus-covered, ciliated epithelium lines the entire respiratory tract, from the upper airways to the terminal bronchioles. The only exceptions are parts of the pharynx and the anterior third of the nasal cavity. The mucus is produced by the goblet cells and mucus-secreting glands of the airways. In pathologic states, such as chronic bronchitis, the number of goblet cells may increase and the mucous glands may hypertrophy, causing mucous gland secretion and mucus viscosity to increase considerably.

The cilia lining the airways beat in such a way that the mucus covering them is always pushed up the airway, away from the alveoli and toward the pharynx. Several studies have shown that cigarette smoking inhibits or impairs ciliary function.

The mucociliary escalator is an important mechanism for removing inhaled particles that stick to the lining of the airways. Material trapped in the mucus is continuously moved toward the pharynx. When mucus reaches the pharynx, it is usually swallowed, expectorated, or removed by blowing one's nose. An important concern is for patients who cannot clear their tracheobronchial secretions (such as an intubated patient, or one unable to cough adequately) because they continue to produce secretions. If the secretions are not removed from the patient by suction or other means, airway obstruction develops.

Stimulating the receptors in the nose, trachea, larynx, or elsewhere in the respiratory tract, either mechanically or chemically, may cause bronchoconstriction, averting deeper penetration of the irritant into the airways, and may also evoke a cough or a sneeze. A *sneeze* results when receptors in the nose or nasopharynx are stimulated; a *cough* results from stimulation of receptors in the trachea. In both the sneeze and the cough, after a deep inhalation, often to almost total lung capacity, a forced expiration occurs against apposed vocal cords and a closed glottis. During this phase of the reflex, intrapleural pressure may rise to more than 100 mmHg. The vocal cords and glottis open suddenly, and pressure in the airways falls rapidly, causing the airways to be compressed and an explosive expiration with linear air flow velocities said to approach the speed of sound. These high air flow rates through the narrowed airways are likely to propel the irritant, along with some mucus, out of the respiratory tract. A sneeze, of course, propels the material through the nose; a cough propels it through the mouth. The cough or sneeze reflex is also useful in helping to move the mucus lining of the airways toward the nose or mouth.

Several mechanisms may be involved in the removal of inhaled material reaching the terminal airways and alveoli, including ingestion by alveolar macrophages, nonspecific enzymatic destruction, entry into the lymphatics, and immunologic reactions.

Alveolar macrophages are large mononuclear ameboid cells found on the alveolar surface. The macrophages may engulf particles and, by lysosomal action, destroy them. Most bacteria are digested in this way. However, some material taken in by the macrophages, such as silica, is not degradable by these cells and may even be toxic to them. If the macrophages bearing such material are not removed from the lung, the material is redeposited in the alveolar surface when the macrophages die. The mean life span of alveolar macrophages is apparently 1 to 5 weeks. Macrophages carrying such nondigestable material are chiefly removed by migration to the mucociliary escalator by way of the pores of Kohn, and eventually through the airways. Particle-containing macrophages may also migrate from the alveolar surface into the interstitium, from which they may enter the lymphatic system or the mucociliary escalator. Cigarette smoke has been shown to inhibit macrophage function. Figure 3–39 summarizes bronchoalveolar pulmonary defense mechanisms.

Nonrespiratory Functions of the Pulmonary Circulation

The normal pulmonary blood volume is about 250 to 300 ml of blood per square meter of body surface area. This would give a typical adult male a pulmonary blood volume of about 500 ml. The pulmonary circulation can therefore act as a *reservoir for the left ventricle*. If left ventricular output is

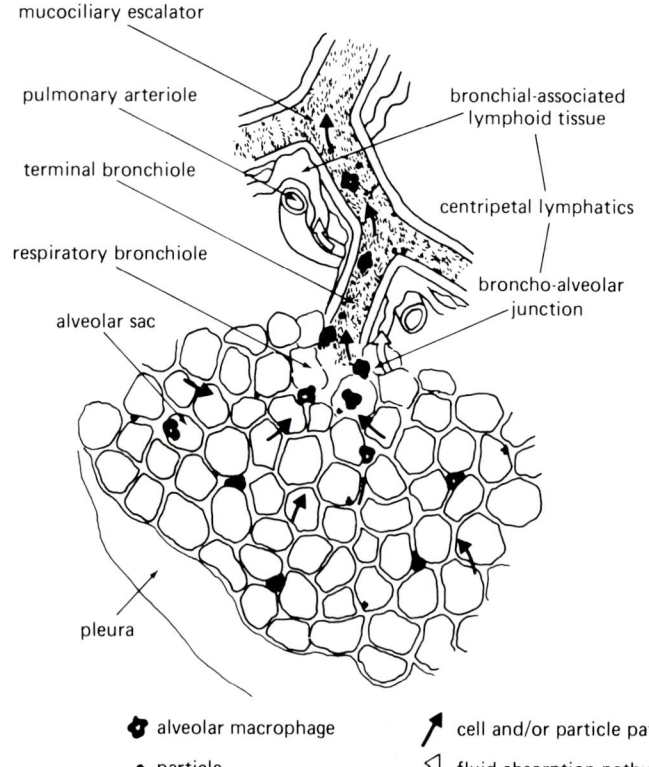

FIGURE 3–39. Diagram of bronchoalveolar defense mechanisms. (Adapted from Green, G.M., Jakab, G.J., Low, R.B., and Davis G.S.: Defense mechanisms of the respiratory membrane. *American Review of Respiratory Disease* 115:479–514, 1977, with permission.)

transiently greater than systemic venous return, that output can be maintained for a few strokes by drawing on blood stored in the pulmonary circulation.

Because all mixed venous blood must pass through the pulmonary capillaries, the pulmonary circulation serves as a *filter,* trapping materials that enter the blood and thus protecting the systemic circulation. The particles filtered may include small fibrin or blood clots, masses of platelets or leukocytes, fat cells, bone marrow, detached cancer cells, gas bubbles, agglutinated erythrocytes (especially in sickle cell anemia), and debris from stored blood or intravenous solutions. If such materials were to enter the arterial side of the systemic circulation, they could occlude vascular beds that have no collateral circulation. Such occlusion would be particularly disastrous if it happened in the vessels supplying blood to the central nervous system or the myocardium.

The lung is able to perform this valuable service because it has many more pulmonary capillaries than are necessary for gas exchange at rest, and because most of the trapped material is removed from the pulmonary circulation within 4 or 5 days. The materials trapped in the pulmonary vascular bed are removed by lytic enzymes in the vascular endothelium, ingestion by macrophages, and penetration to the lymphatic system. Blood administered to patients on cardiopulmonary bypass must be filtered for them because their pulmonary capillary filtration system is circumvented.

The hydrostatic pressure in the pulmonary capillaries, normally far lower than the colloid osmotic pressure of the plasma proteins, tends to draw fluid from the alveoli into the pulmonary capillaries and thus keep the alveolar surface free of liquids other than pulmonary surfactant. Fresh water that is inhaled into the lungs rapidly becomes absorbed into the blood. This quick absorption protects the gas exchange function of the lungs and acts against transudation of fluid from the capillaries to the alveoli.

Drugs or chemical substances that readily diffuse or otherwise pass through the alveolar-capillary barrier rapidly enter the systemic circulation. The lungs are frequently utilized as the route of administration of anesthetic gases, such as halothane and nitrous oxide.

Metabolic Functions of the Lung

Many vasoactive substances are inactivated, changed, or removed from the blood as they pass through the lungs. The endothelium of the vessels of the pulmonary circulation, which has a tremendous surface area in contact with the mixed venous blood, is believed to be the site of this metabolic activity. Prostaglandins E_1, E_2, and $F_{2\alpha}$ are almost completely removed during a single pass through the lungs. On the other hand, prostaglandins A_1 and A_2 and prostacyclin are not affected by the pulmonary circulation. Similarly, about 30% of the norepinephrine and about 80% of the bradykinin in mixed venous blood are removed in one pass through the lungs, but epinephrine and isoproterenol are unaffected. Angiotensin I is converted to angiotensin II in the lung.

Several substances having effects in the lung are known to be synthesized and released by pulmonary cells. The most familiar of these substances, *pulmonary surfactant,* is synthesized in type II alveolar epithelial cells and released onto the alveolar surface. *Histamine* and *serotonin* can be released from mast cells in the lung in response to pulmonary emboli or anaphylaxis, causing bronchoconstriction and possibly initiating other cardiopulmonary reflexes. Alveolar macrophages have also been shown to produce a number of substances. Whatever substance or substances are the *chemical mediators* involved in the hypoxic pulmonary vasoconstriction, they are produced and act in the lung. Many other substances are also produced by the lung cells and released into the alveoli and airways, including mucus and other tracheobronchial secretions, surface enzymes, proteins, immunologically active substances, and other factors. These substances are synthesized in the goblet cells, submucosal gland cells, Clara cells, or macrophages.

Bradykinin, histamine, serotonin, heparin, and prostaglandins E_2 and $F_{2\alpha}$ are all stored in the lung and, under certain circumstances, may be released into the general circulation. For example, heparin, histamine, serotonin, and prostaglandins E_2 and $F_{2\alpha}$ are released during anaphylactic shock.

The lung must be able to respond to injury as well as meet its own cellular energy requirements. Type II alveolar epithelial cells play a major role in the lung's response to injury of type I cells. Investigators have shown that after injury, the type II cells can proliferate and develop into type I cells.

Bibliography

Agostoni, E.: Mechanics of the pleural space. *Physiol. Rev.* 52:57–128, 1972.

Banner, A.S.: Cough: Physiology, evaluation and treatment. *Lung* 164:79–92, 1986.

Barnes, P.J.: Neural control of human airways in health and disease. *Am. Rev. Resp. Dis.* 134:1289–1314, 1986.

Berger, A.J., Mitchell, R.A., and Severinghaus, J.W.: Regulation of respiration. *N. Engl. J. Med.* 297:92–97, 138–143, 194–201, 1977.

Bouhuys, A.: *The Physiology of Breathing.* New York, Grune & Stratton, 1977.

Bruce, E.N., and Cherniack, N.S.: Central chemoreceptors. *J. Appl. Physiol.* 62:389–402, 1987.

Cherniack, N.S., and Widdicombe, J.G. (eds.): Control of breathing, In *Handbook of Physiology*, vol. 2. Bethesda, Md., American Physiological Society, 1986.

Clements, J.A., and Tierney, D.F.: Alveolar instability associated with altered surface tension. In Fenn, W.O., and Rahn, H. (eds.): *Handbook of Physiology*, vol. 2. Washington, D.C., American Physiological Society, 1965, pp 1567–1568.

Comroe, J.H.: *Physiology of Respiration*, 2nd ed. Chicago, Year Book Medical Publishers, 1974.

Comroe, J.H., Forster, R.E., Dubois, A.B., Briscoe, W.A., and Carlsen, E.: *The Lung—Clinical Physiology and Pulmonary Function Tests,* 2nd ed. Chicago, Year Book Medical Publishers, 1962.

Cotes, J.E.: *Lung Function: Assessment and Application in Medicine*, 4th ed. Oxford, Blackwell, 1979.

Davenport, H.W.: *The ABC of Acid-Base Chemistry*, 6th ed. Chicago, The University of Chicago Press, 1974.

Dawson, C.A.: Role of pulmonary vasomotion in physiology of the lung. *Physiol. Rev.* 64:544–616, 1984.

Deffebach, M.E., Charan, N.B., Lakshminarayan, S., and Butler, J.: The bronchial circulation: Small, but a vital attribute of the lung. *Am. Rev. Resp. Dis.* 135:463–481, 1987.

Duffin, J., and Hung, S.: Respiratory rhythm generation. *Can. Anaesth. Soc. J.* 32:124–137, 1985.

Farhi, L.E., and Tenney, S.M. (eds.): Gas exchange. In *Handbook of Physiology*, vol. 4. Bethesda, Md., American Physiological Society, 1987.

Fawcett, D.W.: *Bloom and Fawcett: A Textbook of Histology*, 11th ed. Philadelphia, W.B. Saunders, 1986, pp 731–754.

Fels, A.O.S., and Cohn, Z.A.: The alveolar macrophage. *J. Appl. Physiol.* 60:353–369, 1986.

Fishman, A.P.: Hypoxia on the pulmonary circulation. How and where it acts. *Circ. Res.* 38:221–231, 1976.

Fishman, A.P.: Nonrespiratory functions of the lung. *Chest* 72:84–89, 1977.

Fishman, A.P. (ed.): *Pulmonary Diseases and Disorders.* New York, McGraw-Hill, 1980.

Fishman, A.P. (ed.): *Update: Pulmonary Diseases and Disorders.* New York, McGraw-Hill, 1982.

Fishman, A.P., and Fisher, A.B. (eds.): Circulation and nonrespiratory functions. In *Handbook of Physiology*, vol. 1. Bethesda, Md., American Physiological Society, 1985.

Forster, R.E., II, Dubois, A.B., Briscoe, W.A., and Fisher, A.B.: *The Lung: Physiologic Basis of Pulmonary Function Tests*, 3rd ed. Chicago, Year Book Medical Publishers, 1986.

Fraser, R.G., and Paré, J.A.P.: *Structure and Function of the Lung,* 2nd ed. Philadelphia, W.B. Saunders, 1977.

Gehr, P., Bachofen, M., and Weibel, E.R.: The normal human lung: Ultrastructure and morphometric estimation of diffusion capacity. *Respiration Physiol.* 32:121–140, 1978.

Green, J.F.: *Fundamental Cardiovascular and Pulmonary Physiology*, 2nd ed. Philadelphia, Lea & Febiger, 1987.

Green, G.M., Jakab, G.J., Low, R.B., and Davis, G.S.: Defense mechanisms of the respiratory membrane. *Am. Rev. Resp. Dis.* 115:479–514, 1977.

Grover, R.F., Wagner, W.W., McMurtry, I.F., and Reeves, J.T.: Pulmonary circulation. In Shepherd, J.T., and Abboud, F.M. (eds.): *Handbook of Physiology*, vol. 3. Bethesda, Md., American Physiological Society, 1983, pp 103–136.

Guyton, A.C.: *Textbook of Medical Physiology,* 7th ed. Philadelphia, W.B. Saunders, 1986, pp 465–526.

Harada, R.N., and Repine, J.E.: Pulmonary host defense mechanisms. *Chest* 87:247–252, 1985.

Harris, P., and Heath, D.: *The Human Pulmonary Circulation*, 3rd ed. Edinburgh, Churchill Livingstone, 1986.

Hyatt, R.E.: Dynamic lung volumes. In Fenn, W.O., and Rahn, H. (eds.): *Handbook of Physiology*, vol. 2. Washington, D.C., American Physiological Society, 1965, pp 1381–1398.

Hyatt, R.E.: Expiratory flow limitation. *J. Appl. Physiol.* 55:1–8, 1983.

Hyman, A.L., Lippton, H.L., and Kadowitz, P.J.: Autonomic regulation of the pulmonary circulation. *J. Cardiovasc. Pharm.* 7(Suppl. 3):580–595, 1985.

Kazemi, H., and Johnson, D.C.: Regulation of cerebrospinal fluid acid-base balance. *Physiol. Rev.* 66:953–1037, 1986.

King, R.J.: Pulmonary surfactant. *J. Appl. Physiol.* 53:1–8, 1982.

Kryger, M.H.: Sleep apnea. *Arch. Int. Med.* 143:2301–2303, 1983.

Lambertsen, C.J.: Respiration. In Mountcastle, V.B. (ed.): *Medical Physiology*, 14th ed. St. Louis, C.V. Mosby, 1980, pp 1677–1900.

Levitzky, M.G.: *Pulmonary Physiology,* 2nd ed. New York, McGraw-Hill, 1986.

Macklem, P.T., and Mead, J. (eds.): Mechanics of breathing. In *Handbook of Physiology*, vol. 3. Bethesda, Md., American Physiological Society, 1986.

Milic-Emli, J.: Pulmonary statics. In Widdicombe, J.G. (ed.): *MTP International Review of Sciences: Respiratory Physiology*. London, Butterworths, 1974, pp 105–137.

Murray, J.F.: *The Normal Lung,* 2nd ed. Philadelphia, W.B. Saunders, 1986.

Murray, J.F., Greenspan, R.H., Gold, W.M., and Cohn, A.B.: Early diagnosis of chronic obstructive lung disease. *California Medicine* 116:37–55, 1972.

Nattie, E.E.: Ionic mechanisms of cerebrospinal fluid acid-base regulation. *J. Appl. Physiol.* 54:3–12, 1983.

Netter, F.H.: *The Ciba Collection of Medical Illustration*, vol. 7. Summit, N.J., Ciba, 1979.

Newhouse, M., Sanchis, J., and Bienenstock, J.: Lung defense mechanisms. *N. Engl. J. Med.* 295:990–998, 1045–1052, 1976.

Nunn, J.F.: *Applied Respiratory Physiology,* 2nd ed. London, Butterworths, 1977.

Otis, A.B.: The work of breathing. In Fenn, W.O., and Rahn, H. (eds.): *Handbook of Physiology*, vol. 1. Washington, D.C., American Physiological Society, 1964, pp 463–475.

Pappenheimer, J.R., Comroe, J.H., Jr., Cournand, A., Ferguson, J.K.W., Filley, G.F., Fowler, W.S., Gray, J.S., Helmholtz, H.F., Jr., Otis, A.B., Rahn, H., and Riley, R.L.: Standardization of definitions and symbols in respiratory physiology. *Fed. Proc.* 9:602–605, 1950.

Pitts, R.F.: *Physiology of the Kidney and Body Fluids*, 3rd ed. Chicago, Year Book Medical Publishers, 1974.

Proctor, D.F.: The upper airways. *Am. Rev. Resp. Dis.* 115:97–129, 315–342, 1977.

Proctor, D.F.: Physiology of the upper airway. In Fenn, W.O., and Rahn, H. (eds.): *Handbook of Physiology*, vol. 1. Washington, D.C., American Physiological Society, 1964, pp 309–345.

Proctor, D.F.: The Upper Respiratory Tract. In Fishman, A.P. (ed.): *Assessment of Pulmonary Function.* New York, McGraw-Hill, 1980, pp 3–17.

Proctor, D.F., and Andersen, I. (eds.): *The Nose: Upper Airway Physiology and the Atmospheric Environment.* Amsterdam, Elsevier Biomedical, 1982.

Radford, E.P.: *Tissue Elasticity,* Washington, D.C., American Physiological Society, 1957.

Rodenstein, D.O., and Stanescu, D.C.: The soft palate and breathing. *Am. Rev. Resp. Dis.* 134:311–325, 1986.

Rooney, S.A.: The surfactant system and lung phospholipid biochemistry. *Am. Rev. Resp. Dis.* 131:439–460, 1985.

Roughton, F.J.W.: Transport of oxygen and carbon dioxide. In Fenn, W.O., and Rahn, H. (eds.): *Handbook of Physiology,* vol. 1, Washington, D.C., American Physiological Society, 1964, pp 767–825.

Roussos, C., and Macklem, P.T.: The respiratory muscles. *N. Engl. J. Med.* 307:786–797, 1982.

Roussos, C., and Macklem, P.T. (eds.): *The Thorax.* New York, Marcel Dekker, 1985.

Ryan, U.S.: Metabolic activity of the pulmonary endothelium. *Ann. Rev. Physiol.* 48:268–278, 1986.

Said, S.I.: Metabolic functions of the pulmonary circulation. *Circ. Res.* 50:325–333, 1982.

Sharp, J.T.: Respiratory muscles: A review of old and newer concepts. *Lung* 157:185–199, 1980.

Slonim, N.B., and Hamilton, L.H.: *Respiratory Physiology,* 5th ed. St. Louis, C.V. Mosby, 1987.

Takemura, R., and Werb, Z.: Secretory products of macrophages and their physiological functions. *Am. J. Physiol.* 246:C1–C9, 1984.

Tobin, M.J., Cohn, M.A., and Sackner, M.A.: Breathing abnormalities during sleep. *Arch. Int. Med.* 143:1221–1228, 1983.

Vander, A.J.: *Renal Physiology,* 3rd ed. New York, McGraw-Hill, 1985.

Voelkel, N.F.: Mechanisms of hypoxic pulmonary vasoconstriction. *Am. Rev. Resp. Dis.* 133:1186–1195, 1986.

Wagner, P.D., and West, J.B.: Effects of diffusion impairment on O_2 and CO_2 time courses in pulmonary capillaries. *J. Appl. Physiol.* 33:62–71, 1972.

Weibel, E.R.: Design and structure of the human lung. In Fishman, A.P. (ed.): *Pulmonary Diseases and Disorders,* vol. 1. New York, McGraw-Hill, 1980, pp 224–271.

Weibel, E.R.: *Morphometry of the Human Lung.* Berlin, Springer-Verlag, 1963.

Weibel, E.R.: *The Pathway for Oxygen: Structure and Function in the Mammalian Respiratory System.* Cambridge, Mass., Harvard University Press, 1984.

West, J.B.: Ventilation-perfusion relationships. *Am. Rev. Resp. Dis.* 116:919–943, 1977.

West, J.B.: *Pulmonary Pathophysiology,* 3rd ed. Baltimore, Williams and Wilkins, 1987.

West, J.B.: *Respiratory Physiology—The Essentials,* 3rd ed. Baltimore, Williams and Wilkins, 1985.

West, J.B.: *Ventilation/Blood Flow and Gas Exchange,* 3rd ed. Oxford, Blackwell Scientific Publications, 1977.

Williams, P.L., and Warwick, R.: *Gray's Anatomy,* 36th British ed. New York, Churchill Livingstone, 1980.

Wright, J.R., and Clements, J.A.: Metabolism and turnover of lung surfactant. *Am. Rev. Resp. Dis.* 135:426–444, 1987.

OBJECTIVES

AFTER READING THIS CHAPTER, THE STUDENT WILL BE ABLE TO:

1. Use his or her knowledge of the cardiovascular and pulmonary systems (from material presented in Chapters 2 and 3) to identify the physiologic stresses and cardiopulmonary effects of the following situations and conditions: (a) exercise, (b) hemorrhage, (c) hypoxia, (d) hyperbaric conditions, (e) pregnancy, and (f) surgery.
2. Analyze the integrated responses of the components of the cardiovascular and pulmonary systems to stresses.

4
CARDIOPULMONARY ADJUSTMENTS TO STRESS

CHAPTER OUTLINE

EXERCISE
  Cardiovascular Response to Exercise
    Cardiac Output, Heart Rate, and Stroke Volume
    Blood Pressure and Distribution of Blood Flow
  Pulmonary Response to Exercise

HEMORRHAGE
  Cardiovascular Responses to Hemorrhage
  Renal Responses to Hemorrhage
  Respiratory Responses to Hemorrhage

HYPOXIA
  Causes of Hypoxia
  Effects of Hypoxia
  Response to Hypoxia
  Adaptations to Hypoxia

HYPERBARIC CONDITIONS
  Diving Physiology
    Neck-Deep Immersion
    Breath-Hold Diving
    Scuba Diving

PREGNANCY
  Cardiovascular Effects
  Respiratory Effects
  Eclampsia

SURGERY
  Cardiovascular Effects
  Effects on the Respiratory System

EXERCISE

The main physiologic stress involved in exercise is to supply substrates for the greatly increased metabolic needs of the exercising muscles and to remove the end-products and by-products of metabolism from them. As far as the cardiopulmonary system is concerned, the blood flow and oxygen supply of the skeletal muscles must be increased, and carbon dioxide, hydrogen ions, and heat must be removed from the body.

Cardiovascular Response to Exercise

At the onset of exercise, there is an immediate increase in the heart rate and cardiac output. This response may begin as a result of information sent via collateral fibers from the cortical areas that initiate skeletal muscle movement. It may be a partly learned response, because *anticipation* of exercise also increases the heart rate and cardiac output in some people. It is likely that alterations in cardiovascular and pulmonary control are integrated in the central nervous system, perhaps in the hypothalamus. There may also be receptors within the skeletal muscles themselves that respond to alterations in skeletal muscle metabolism. These "metaboreceptors" are believed to send information indicating the increased skeletal muscle metabolic demand to the cardiovascular and pulmonary controllers.

Cardiac Output, Heart Rate, and Stroke Volume

In normal healthy persons, cardiac output increases nearly linearly with increasing work from about 5 L/min at rest to about 25 L/min at maximal levels. This linear increase is shown in Figure 4–1, in which the work level is represented as *oxygen consumption* (intake) and the cardiac output responses for various arteriovenous oxygen content differences are shown. Oxygen consumption is frequently used as an index of work level because it increases linearly with the amount of work performed, as measured in watts or kilo-pond-meters by using a bicycle ergometer. The normal range of responses is indicated by the shaded area, which crosses over the arteriovenous oxygen content difference lines because the *arteriovenous oxygen content difference* normally increases with increasing work performance.

The increase in cardiac output is brought about by increases in both the heart rate and the stroke volume. *Heart rate* (cardiac frequency) increases linearly with increasing work performed, as shown in Figure 4–2. The mechanism of the increase is an initial withdrawal of vagal parasympathetic tone and a subsequent increase in sympathetic tone to the heart. The increase in heart rate occurs despite a moderate elevation in mean arterial blood pressure, which increases from 90 to 100 mmHg at rest to about 140 mmHg at maximal exercise. The increase in heart rate at a time when blood pressure is increasing indicates that the *baroreceptor reflex* must be reset or attenuated.

The *stroke volume* also increases with increasing work performance in a person in the upright posture. However, the increase is not linear, appearing to plateau at submaximal work levels, as shown in Figure 4–2. The increase in stroke volume results partly from an increase in venous return acting via the Frank-Starling mechanism and partly from increased myocardial contractility caused by increased sympathetic stimulation of the heart. Stroke volume does not increase by much if exercise is done in the supine position, mainly because changing from the upright to the supine position itself causes an increase in stroke volume. This increased stroke volume is a result of decreased pooling of venous blood in the lower extremities and abdomen, causing an increased venous return, with a subsequent increase in central blood volume, central venous pressure, right and left atrial pressures, and pulmonary blood volume.

If cardiac output increases with increasing levels of exercise, *venous return* must also increase. This is accomplished by increased muscular compression of the valved veins of the extremities (the "muscle pumps" in Fig. 2–7); deeper breaths, increasing the pressure gradient for venous return (the "thoracoabdominal pump" in Fig. 2–28); and increased sympathetic tone to the veins causing a decreased capacitance.

Blood Pressure and Distribution of Blood Flow

During exercise, blood flow to the skeletal muscle is greatly increased, rising from about 15% to 20% of the cardiac output at rest to as much as 85% to 90% during severe exercise. During maximal exercise, the four- or fivefold increase in cardiac output over the resting level represents an increase of 15 to 20 times the resting blood flow. This increase in skeletal muscle blood flow is mainly a result of local metabolic autoregulatory factors

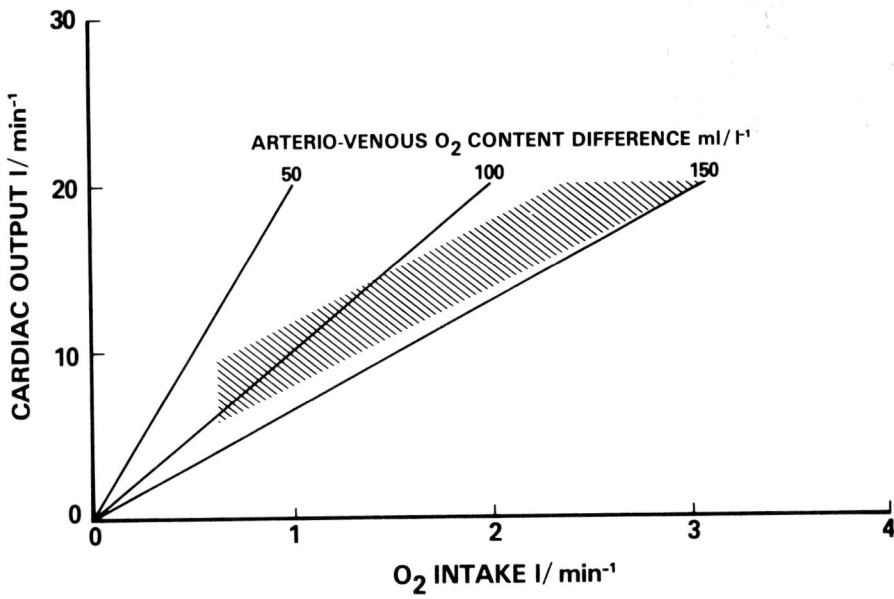

FIGURE 4–1. The normal range of cardiac output during exercise plotted against work load, expressed as $\dot{V}O_2$, for three different arteriovenous O_2 content differences. (From Jones, N.L., and Campbell, E.J.M.: *Clinical Exercise Testing*, 2nd ed. Philadelphia, W.B. Saunders, 1982, with permission.)

causing a vasodilation, thus decreasing the resistance to blood flow. As precapillary sphincters open, capillaries are recruited and the surface area available for exchange between the muscle tissue and the blood increases.

However, the decrease in resistance to blood flow occurs immediately after the onset of exercise (or even in anticipation of exercise), so the response may be initiated by sympathetic cholinergic fibers innervating skeletal muscle arterioles, or by sympathetic adrenergic beta-receptor stimulation of these vessels. Thus, the vasodilation may be initiated via the autonomic nervous system and then maintained by local metabolic autoregulation.

As already noted, during severe muscular exercise, the relative increase in blood flow to the skeletal muscles is greater than the increase in cardiac output. If the great fall in vascular resistance

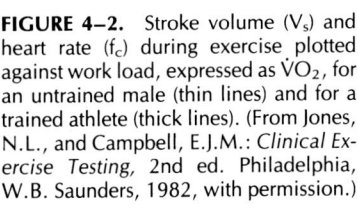

FIGURE 4–2. Stroke volume (V_s) and heart rate (f_c) during exercise plotted against work load, expressed as $\dot{V}O_2$, for an untrained male (thin lines) and for a trained athlete (thick lines). (From Jones, N.L., and Campbell, E.J.M.: *Clinical Exercise Testing*, 2nd ed. Philadelphia, W.B. Saunders, 1982, with permission.)

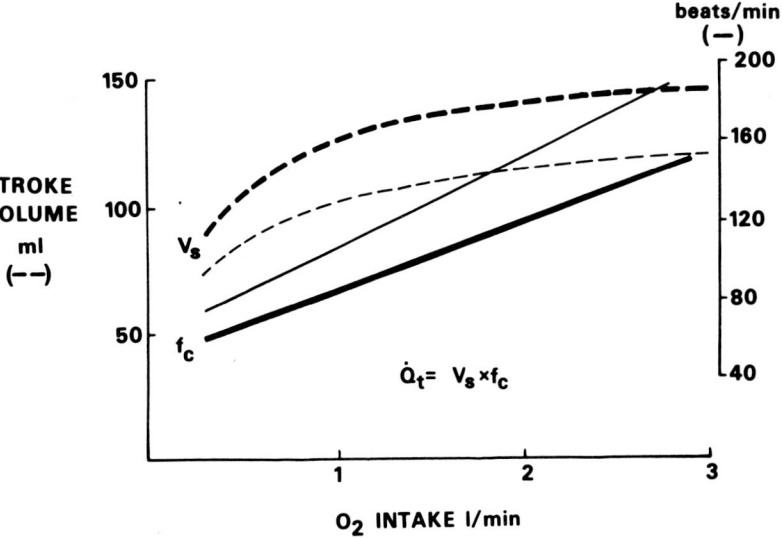

of the skeletal muscle beds exceeds the rise in cardiac output, then the mean arterial blood pressure would be expected to fall. Yet, as mentioned before, mean arterial blood pressure increases during exercise. This increase in mean arterial blood pressure results mainly from an increase in *systolic pressure* (reflecting the increased stroke volume and myocardial contractility), but *diastolic pressure* normally does increase slightly or remains the same. The maintenance of diastolic blood pressure in this situation, in which the resistance to blood flow offered by the skeletal muscle vascular beds is falling more than cardiac output is increasing, indicates that an increase in resistance is occurring in vascular beds other than those of the exercising skeletal muscle. This is accomplished by a sympathetically mediated increase in vascular tone to many other vascular beds, which along with local regulatory factors, *redistributes the cardiac output* during exercise.

Blood flow through nonexercising muscles, kidneys, and splanchnic regions decreases during severe exercise as a result of a sympathetically mediated vasoconstriction. *Coronary* blood flow increases because of a metabolic autoregulatory vasodilation secondary to the increased cardiac work necessary to produce an increased cardiac output. *Cutaneous* blood flow may be greatly increased as the skin acts to promote heat loss from the body. This heat, which is generated during muscle contraction, is removed by the process of sweating, which in turn, releases the vasodilator bradykinin; and by opening the arteriovenous anastomoses and causing dilation of cutaneous resistance and capacitance vessels. These latter responses help to allow direct transfer of heat to the environment. These cutaneous vascular responses are integrated in the hypothalamic thermoregulatory centers. During extremely severe exercise, skin blood vessels may constrict to divert blood flow to the exercising muscle, heart, and brain. As we would expect, total *cerebral* blood flow remains unchanged during exercise as a result of local autoregulatory factors.

Pulmonary Response to Exercise

The acute pulmonary effects of exercise on an untrained person are mainly a function of the increased cardiac output coupled with an increase in alveolar ventilation.

Control of Breathing. *Minute ventilation* increases with exercise. As Figure 4–3 shows, it in-

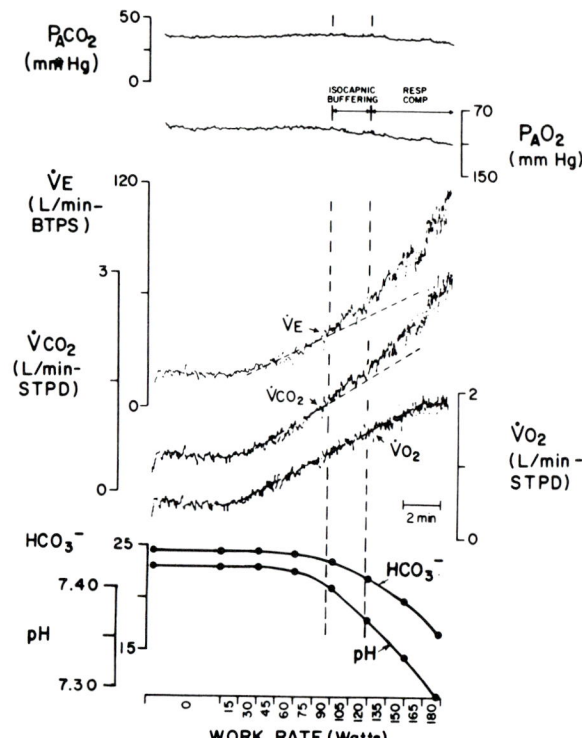

FIGURE 4–3. Continuous measurement of alveolar P_{CO_2} and P_{O_2} (measured as end-tidal), minute ventilation ($\dot{V}_E$), CO_2 production ($\dot{V}_{CO_2}$), oxygen consumption ($\dot{V}_{O_2}$), and the arterial bicarbonate and pH of a normal male subject increasing his work rate on a bicycle ergometer. (From Wasserman, K.: Breathing during exercise. Reprinted by permission of *The New England Journal of Medicine*, 298:780–785, 1978.)

creases linearly with both oxygen consumption and carbon dioxide production up to about 60% of the person's maximal work capacity. Above that level, minute ventilation increases more rapidly than does oxygen consumption, but it continues to rise proportionally with increases in carbon dioxide production. This increase in ventilation above oxygen consumption at high work levels is caused by the increased lactic acid production that results from anaerobic metabolism. The hydrogen ions liberated in this process can stimulate the arterial chemoreceptors directly, and as they are buffered by bicarbonate ions, this also results in production of carbon dioxide in addition to that derived from aerobic metabolism. Thus, there is additional stimulation of the central and peripheral chemoreceptors.

The ventilatory response to a constant level of exercise consists of three phases, as shown in Figure 4–4. At the beginning of exercise, an *immediate* increase in ventilation occurs (Phase I). This phase is followed by one of slowly increasing ven-

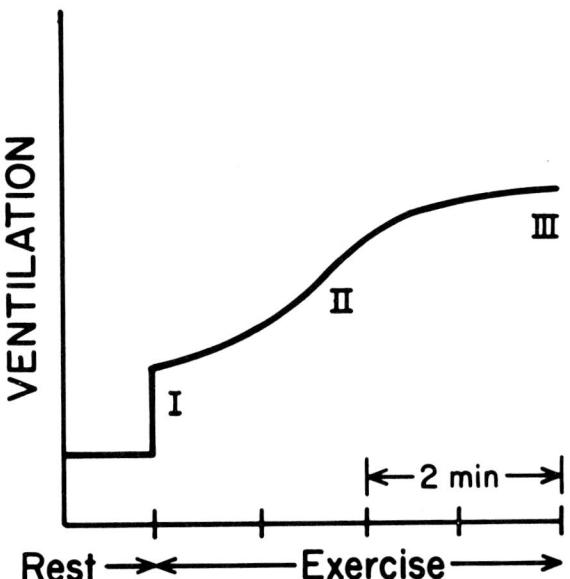

FIGURE 4–4. The pattern of changes in minute ventilation occurring during constant work-rate exercise. (From Wasserman, K.: Breathing during exercise. Reprinted by permission of *The New England Journal of Medicine*, 298:780–785, 1978.)

tilation (Phase II), ultimately rising to a final steady state (Phase III) if the exercise is not too severe. The Phase I increase in ventilation may account for as much as 50% of the total steady state response, although it is usually a smaller fraction of the total.

No single factor can fully account for the ventilatory response to exercise. The immediate increase in ventilation (Phase I) happens too quickly to be a response to changes in metabolism or blood gases. This neural component may be partly a learned response. Experiments have also shown that input to the respiratory centers from proprioceptors in the joints and muscles of the exercising limbs may influence the ventilatory response to exercise. In anesthetized animals, passive movements of the limbs cause an increase in ventilation. As already mentioned, the ventilatory and cardiovascular responses are probably initiated at cortical areas responsible for motor function and may be coordinated (and in part initiated) in an "exercise center" in the hypothalamus.

The *arterial chemoreceptors* do not seem to be implicated in the Phase I response to exercise. In mild or moderate exercise, *mean* arterial P_{CO_2} and P_{O_2} remain relatively constant, even during the increasing ventilation phase (the humoral component), and may actually improve. Note that at moderate exercise levels the P_{AO_2} (and therefore P_{aO_2}) in Figure 4–3 are unchanged. However, patients whose carotid bodies have been surgically removed do show a slower increase in ventilation during Phase II, even in the absence of lactic acidosis. It is possible that the arterial chemoreceptors are responding to greater breath-to-breath fluctuations in blood gases during exercise, despite relatively constant mean P_{aCO_2}'s and P_{aO_2}'s. During exercise levels above the anaerobic threshold, the ventilation of these carotid body–resected patients does not increase further despite metabolic acidosis, demonstrating that the peripheral chemoreceptors are important in this part of the response.

Several investigators have suggested that receptors able to respond to an increased carbon dioxide load in the mixed venous blood may exist in the pulmonary circulation. The metaboreceptors in the exercising muscles may also send information on increased muscle metabolism to the respiratory controllers. The increase in body temperature that results from exercise may also contribute to the ventilatory response.

Alveolar Ventilation. In adults, the normal resting minute ventilation ($\dot{V}_E$) of 5 to 6 L/min can increase to as much as 150 L/min during brief periods of maximal exercise. During exercise, maximal increases in cardiac output are only 4 or 5 times the resting level in healthy adults, compared with a 25-fold potential increase in minute ventilation. Therefore, the cardiovascular system—rather than the respiratory system—is the limiting factor during exercise by normal healthy persons.

As shown in Figure 4–5, at lower work levels, more of the increase in alveolar ventilation is accounted for by an increase in *tidal volume* than by an increase in *breathing frequency*. Breathing frequency increases nearly linearly with work level, whereas the elevation in tidal volume is greater at lower work levels and plateaus at higher work levels. During strenuous exercise, the tidal volume usually increases to a maximum of about 50% to 60% of the vital capacity or, in an average-sized man, about 2.5 to 3.0 liters. This increase in tidal volume apparently occurs more at the expense of the inspiratory reserve volume, with the expiratory reserve volume being somewhat less affected. In healthy adults, strenuous exercise may increase breathing frequency to 30 to 40 breaths/min and in children, as high as 70 breaths/min.

A slight increase in the *anatomic dead space* may occur on inspiration during exercise because the airways distend at high lung volumes; as cardiac output increases, any *alveolar dead space* present at rest normally decreases. As a result, there is either a decrease or no change in *physi-

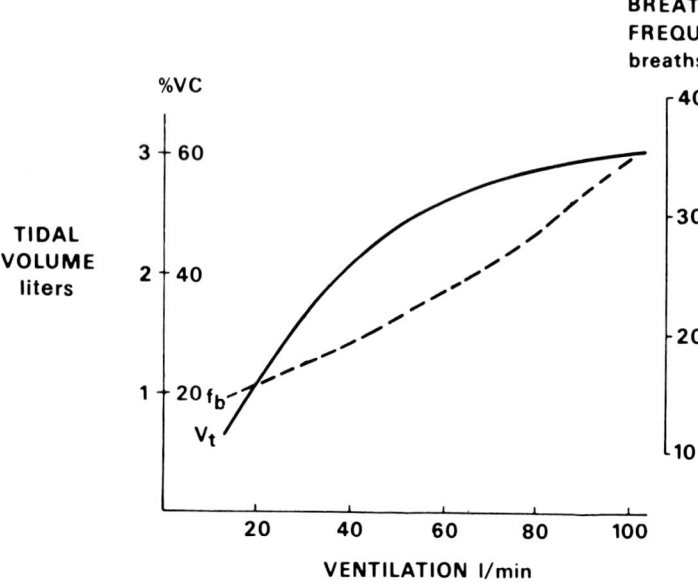

FIGURE 4–5. Changes in tidal volume (V_T) and breathing frequency (f_b) as ventilation increases during increasing work-load exercise. (From Jones, N.L., and Campbell, E.J.M.: *Clinical Exercise Testing*, 2nd ed. Philadelphia, W.B. Saunders, 1982, with permission.)

ologic dead space during exercise. Inasmuch as the tidal volume increases, the ratio of physiologic dead space to tidal volume (V_D/V_T) decreases.

The regional differences in alveolar ventilation that occur in upright lungs are probably diminished during exercise, because during the deeper inspirations, alveoli in more dependent regions of the lung inflate more fully. At higher lung volumes during active expirations, however, these alveoli may also undergo airway collapse. Similarly, alveoli in upper parts of the lungs (with respect to gravity) should deflate more fully during exhalation, resulting in greater ventilation of those upper regions.

Mechanics of Breathing. Because the lungs are less compliant at higher lung volumes, larger tidal volumes result in an increased work of breathing to overcome the *elastic recoil of the lungs* (and the inward recoil of the chest wall at high lung volumes) during inhalation. Of course, the greater elastic recoil of the lungs tends to make exhalation easier, but this is offset by a much greater *airways resistance* component of the work of breathing. Work done to overcome airways resistance is greatly increased by the greater turbulence and dynamic compression of airways during active exhalation. The resistive work of breathing through the nose is particularly increased at high air flow rates: Minute ventilations above about 40 L/min are normally accomplished by breathing through the mouth.

Pulmonary Blood Flow. As mentioned previously, during exercise cardiac output increases linearly with oxygen consumption. *Mean pulmonary artery* and *mean left atrial pressures* increase, but the increase is not as great as that of pulmonary blood flow. Thus *pulmonary vascular resistance* undergoes a *decrease*, which occurs by recruitment and distension of pulmonary vessels. Pulmonary blood vessel recruitment occurs to a greater degree in upper regions of the lung, thus tending to decrease the regional differences in pulmonary blood flow discussed in Chapter 3. We would expect the exercise-induced deeper tidal volumes and active expirations to increase pulmonary vascular resistance. During active expiration, the extra-alveolar vessels should be compressed; during inspiration, the alveolar vessels themselves should be compressed. The decrease in mean pulmonary vascular resistance shows that the effects of recruitment and distension are greater than those of extravascular compression.

Ventilation-Perfusion Relationships. The greater uniformity of regional ventilation and perfusion that occurs during exercise results in a much more uniform distribution of $\dot{V}_A/\dot{Q}$s throughout the lung. Studies of normal persons exercising while upright have shown that the perfusion of upper regions of the lung increases greatly, resulting in nearly uniform $\dot{V}_A/\dot{Q}$s from the bottom to the top of the lung. As Figure 4–6 shows, the ventilation-perfusion ratios are close to 1.0 during exercise, with slightly higher (1.2 to 1.4) ratios in the uppermost and lowermost regions (compare Fig. 3–26).

More detailed investigations of ventilation-per-

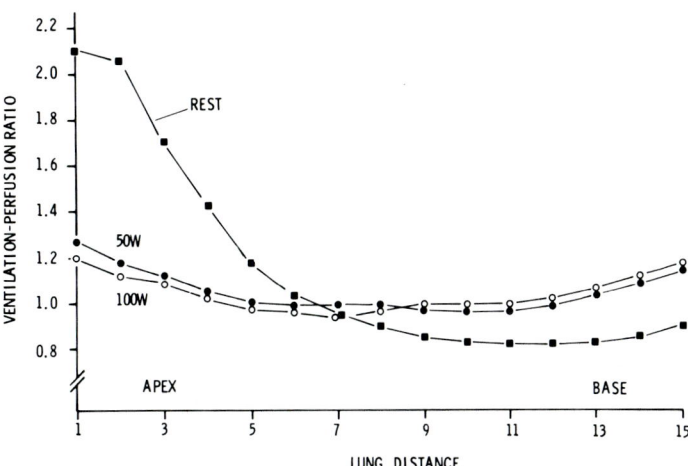

FIGURE 4–6. Normalized mean ventilation-perfusion ratios plotted against distance down the lung for six human subjects at rest and exercising on bicycle ergometers. (From Harf, A., Pratt T., and Hughes, J.M.B.: Regional distribution of $\dot{V}_A/\dot{Q}_C$ in man at rest and with exercise measured with krypton-81. Journal of Applied Physiology 44:115–123, 1978, with permission.)

fusion relationships during severe exercise have revealed that normal subjects have some degree of $\dot{V}/\dot{Q}$ mismatch, perhaps caused by overperfusion of some alveoli. Severe exercise can also cause diffusion limitation of oxygen transfer. Both of these factors may increase the alveolar-arterial oxygen gradient and cause mild arterial hypoxemia.

Diffusion Through the Alveolar-Capillary Barrier. During exercise, the *diffusing capacities* for both oxygen and carbon dioxide normally increase considerably. The increase in diffusing capacity during exercise results largely from the increase in pulmonary blood flow. Recruitment of capillaries in upper regions of the lungs, increases the surface area available for diffusion. As Figure 3–27 shows, the increased linear velocity of blood flow through pulmonary capillaries also reduces the time red blood cells are exposed to the alveolar air, making it less than the 0.75 to 1.2 seconds normally seen at rest. Because the P_{O_2} and P_{CO_2} of the pulmonary capillary blood normally equilibrate with the alveolar P_{O_2} and P_{CO_2} within 0.25 seconds, increasing the velocity of blood flow through the lung increases the diffusing capacity by bringing unequilibrated blood into the lung faster, thus maintaining the partial pressure gradient for diffusion. At very high cardiac outputs, the linear velocity may be so great that diffusion limitation of gas transfer occurs.

Another factor, one depending less on increased cardiac output, that helps to increase diffusion during exercise is the fact that the mixed venous P_{O_2} may be lower and the mixed venous P_{CO_2} may be higher than the levels normally found at rest. These changes in P_{O_2} and P_{CO_2} levels may also help to increase and sustain the partial pressure gradients for diffusion. People with a decreased alveolar surface area or increased alveolar-capillary barrier thickness may become hypoxemic during exercise. As already noted, normal subjects may show diffusion limitation of oxygen transfer during severe exercise.

Oxygen and Carbon Dioxide Transport by Blood. Exercising muscles enhance the loading of carbon dioxide into the blood and the unloading of oxygen from the blood. Oxygen unloading is improved by the decreased P_{O_2} of the exercising muscle and by the rightward shift of the oxyhemoglobin dissociation curve caused by the decreased pH (the Bohr effect), increased P_{CO_2}, and temperature (and possibly 2,3-DPG) found in the exercising muscle. Low capillary P_{O_2}'s should also lead to improved CO_2 loading because lower oxyhemoglobin levels shift the CO_2 dissociation curve leftward (the Haldane effect).

HEMORRHAGE

The initial physiologic stress of hemorrhage is a *loss of blood volume*. Blood loss, whether from the arterial or venous side of the circulation, is likely to result in *decreased venous return, cardiac output,* and *blood pressure*. The cardiovascular, pulmonary, and renal responses to these alterations and their consequences help to return cardiac output and blood pressure toward normal; retain and replace blood volume, body fluids, and electrolytes; and buffer the consequences of anaerobic metabolism resulting from impaired tissue perfusion.

Cardiovascular Responses to Hemorrhage

Decreased blood volume is sensed by the *low-pressure baroreceptors* located in the atria, ventricles, vena cavae, and pulmonary vessels; decreased arterial blood pressure is sensed by the systemic *arterial baroreceptors*. As Figure 4–7 shows, *heart rate* (pulse rate) increases linearly with decreased blood volume. The cardiopulmonary stretch receptors (labelled cardiac receptors) seem to be much more responsive to changes in blood volume than the arterial baroreceptors. It therefore seems likely that the initial increase in heart rate is mainly a result of decreased stretch of cardiopulmonary receptors, especially those known to tonically inhibit the heart rate and blood pressure. This also seems to be the case because the mean arterial blood pressure is usually unchanged after the loss of as much as 10% to 15% of the blood volume of a young healthy adult. With more severe loss of blood volume, the baroreceptors also show decreased activity, as shown in the figure.

Decreased afferent information from the cardiopulmonary receptors and the arterial baroreceptors results in decreased parasympathetic tone to the heart, increased sympathetic tone to the heart and blood vessels, and release of epinephrine and norepinephrine from the adrenal medulla. Heart rate and *myocardial contractility* are increased, thus helping to bring cardiac output toward normal. *Arteriolar tone* is increased, raising the systemic vascular resistance. If we recall that

$$\Delta P = \dot{Q} \times R \quad \text{or}$$
$$MABP - RAP = CO \times SVR$$

we can see that blood pressure maintenance is effected by increasing both output and resistance. Increased sympathetic tone to the veins results in *decreased venous capacitance*, as shown in Figure 4–7. This capacitance decrease helps to bring blood normally pooled in the limbs, gastrointestinal tract, central veins, and pulmonary circulation back to the heart. This effect is occasionally referred to as an autotransfusion. Thus, venous return increases to allow the increase in cardiac output.

The increased sympathetic tone to the arterioles results in a *redistribution of the cardiac output*. Vascular beds mainly under neural control are constricted, allowing a diversion of blood flow to those beds with a better ability to autoregulate.

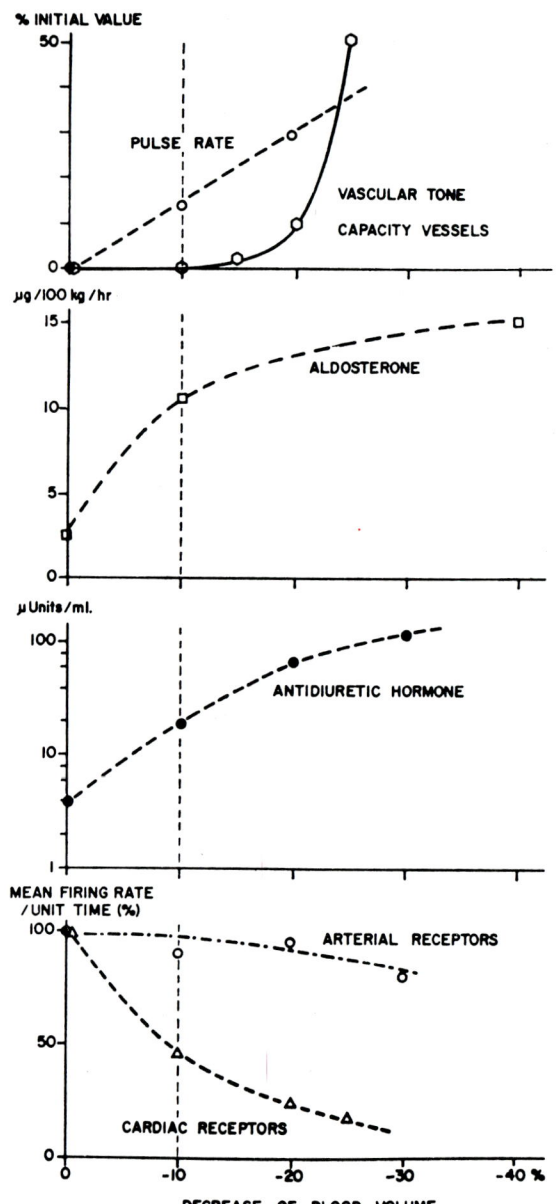

FIGURE 4–7. Changes in heart rate, the tone of compliance vessels of the forearm, level of aldosterone released into the plasma, plasma ADH concentration, and the firing rate arterial and atrial pressure receptors of dogs during a graded hemorrhage experiment. (From Gauer, O.H., Henry, J.P., and Behn, C.: The regulation of extracellular fluid volume. Reproduced with permission, from the *Annual Review of Physiology*, vol. 32. © 1970 by Annual Reviews Inc.)

Blood flow to the skin, gastrointestinal tract, and kidneys—and, to a lesser extent, skeletal muscle—decreases, whereas blood flow to the myocardium and brain is preserved. If arterial blood pressure does fall too low to bring blood to the brain, a loss of consciousness and body posture result. This may almost be thought of as a homeostatic mechanism because the loss of body posture usually puts the brain at the same hydrostatic level as that of the heart. We should also recall that the baroreceptors cease firing at blood pressures below 60 mmHg, so the baroreceptor reflex should be acting maximally at such low pressures.

An indirect effect of the elevated arteriolar (and precapillary) resistance to most vascular beds is an increase in capillary fluid reabsorption. As the arterioles and precapillary sphincters constrict, capillary hydrostatic pressure decreases. This alters the balance between filtration and reabsorption because capillary hydrostatic pressure is the main force driving fluid out of the capillaries. Unfortunately, this so-called autoinfusion becomes limited by the dilution of the plasma proteins. The osmotic effects of the plasma proteins (the capillary oncotic pressure) are normally the main factors retaining fluid in the capillaries and causing its reabsorption from the interstitial space and from the tissue cells themselves. Plasma proteins are lost with the loss of whole blood, and, as interstitial and tissue fluid is drawn back into the circulation because of the decreased capillary hydrostatic pressure, the remaining plasma proteins are diluted and capillary oncotic pressure decreases. The autoinfusion mechanism can bring as much as a liter of fluid back into the circulation within an hour. The hematocrit may also be diluted by this mechanism.

Renal Responses to Hemorrhage

The increase in sympathetic tone to the arterioles and subsequent decrease in capillary hydrostatic pressure have more specific and profound effects in the kidneys than they do in other vascular beds. The simplest of these is that, with renal vasoconstriction, the *glomerular filtration rate* (GFR) is reduced. This results in decreased fluid and electrolytes presented to the kidneys or, looking at it another way, retention of fluid and electrolytes in the circulation with no need for them to be reabsorbed. This mechanism is an effective homeostatic strategy for short periods, but renal hypoperfusion for longer periods may result in renal failure—or even permanent damage to the kidneys.

A second effect of the renal vasoconstriction and subsequent hypoperfusion is activation of the *renin-angiotensin-aldosterone* system. This may be initiated by decreased renal arterial pressure or by decreased sodium load to the macula densa (see Chapter 2). As renin is released, it acts on angiotensinogen to form angiotensin I, which is then converted to angiotensin II in the lungs. Angiotensin II is a potent vasoconstrictor and a mild venoconstrictor, as well as a potentiator of sympathetic activity. Another important effect of angiotensin II is its stimulation of the release of aldosterone into the circulation (see Fig. 4–7). Aldosterone increases sodium reabsorption (and thus water reabsorption) by the kidney. Angiotensin also stimulates the sensation of *thirst*, which may also be increased by decreased stretch of the low-pressure baroreceptors or by changes in osmolarity sensed in the hypothalamus. Thus if a person is conscious after blood loss, he or she will try to replenish body fluids by increasing water intake.

Decreased stretch of the cardiopulmonary volume receptors may also be responsible for the increased blood levels of *antidiuretic hormone* (ADH or *vasopressin*, named after its vasoconstrictor property), which are shown in Figure 4–7. Increased levels of ADH cause water retention by the kidney, resulting in a more concentrated urine. Secretion of atrial natriuretic factor is also likely to be decreased.

Respiratory Responses to Hemorrhage

The decreased venous return and cardiac output resulting from hemorrhage have important pulmonary consequences. Many pulmonary capillaries are likely to be *derecruited* as right ventricular output falls. This should be especially pronounced in upper regions of the lung, leading to an increase in Zone 1 and *alveolar dead space*.

Pulmonary hypoperfusion also results in an increased tendency for the alveoli to collapse. This may be caused by decreased production of pulmonary surfactant. This *atelectasis* results in a decreased pulmonary compliance, an increased work of breathing and development of intrapulmonary *shunts and shunt-like states*. The *mismatching of ventilation and perfusion* may decrease the arterial P_{O_2} and increase the alveolar-arterial oxygen difference. This action may lead to the adult respiratory distress syndrome (see Chapter 5).

As pulmonary blood flow decreases, diffusion through the alveolar-capillary barrier may also be impaired because of both capillary derecruitment and perfusion limitation of gas transfer. This diffusion impairment may contribute to the increased (A-a) P_{O_2}.

Alveolar ventilation increases after hemorrhage. This increase probably results mainly from stimulation of the arterial chemoreceptors by hydrogen ions coming from *lactic acid* formed by anaerobic metabolism in the tissues. The increased lactic acid formation is therefore a result of tissue hypoperfusion secondary to both the decreased cardiac output and the intense reflex vasoconstriction in response to it. Buffering of the hydrogen ions by bicarbonate ions results in the formation of carbonic acid, which dissociates to carbon dioxide and water. The carbon dioxide formed stimulates both the arterial and central chemoreceptors. Ventilation-perfusion imbalance and diffusion problems may depress the arterial P_{O_2} enough to also stimulate the arterial chemoreceptors. It is also possible that decreased arterial baroreceptor afferent input may contribute to the increased ventilation.

The metabolic acidosis and hypoxia secondary to ventilation-perfusion mismatch and diffusion impairment may be sufficient to impair oxygen loading by the blood in the pulmonary capillaries. However, the shape of the oxyhemoglobin dissociation curve is such that oxygen loading is not impaired much until the arterial P_{O_2} falls below 70 mmHg, especially since the rightward shift of the curve caused by elevated hydrogen-ion levels is less affected at higher P_{O_2}'s. The unloading of any oxygen carried to tissues by hemoglobin is enhanced by the low local P_{O_2} and pH.

HYPOXIA

Most of the body relies on aerobic metabolism to provide energy at rest. Although some tissues, like skeletal muscle, are able to switch to anaerobic metabolism for brief periods, others, like the brain, are obligatory aerobes. Hypoxia is a general term meaning decreased oxygen in tissues. It may occur locally or systemically, and it is a stress that can sometimes be life-threatening.

Causes of Hypoxia

Many conditions or situations can lead to tissue hypoxia. They can be classified into four major groups, as shown in Table 4–1.

Hypoxic Hypoxia. Hypoxic hypoxia refers to conditions in which the arterial P_{O_2} is abnormally low. Because the binding of oxygen with the hemoglobin in the arterial blood is mainly determined by the arterial P_{O_2}, such conditions lead to decreased oxygen delivery to the tissues if reflexes or compensatory responses cannot adequately increase the cardiac output or hemoglobin concentration of the blood.

Low Alveolar P_{O_2}. Conditions causing low alveolar P_{O_2}'s lead to low arterial P_{O_2}'s and oxygen contents (unless the hemoglobin concentration is elevated) because the alveolar P_{O_2} determines the upper limit of arterial P_{O_2}. *Hypoventilation* leads to both alveolar hypoxia and hypercapnia (high CO_2). Hypoventilation can be caused by depression or damage of the respiratory centers in the brain by drugs, poisons, or injuries; interference with the nerves supplying the respiratory muscles, as in myasthenia gravis; and altered mechanics of the lung or chest wall caused by restrictive or obstructive conditions.

Ascent to *high altitudes* causes alveolar hypoxia because of the reduced total barometric pressure encountered above sea level. Accidentally reduced $F_{I O_2}$'s during anesthesia or treatment have similar effects. Unlike the case in hypoventilation, alveolar carbon dioxide is *decreased* at high

TABLE 4–1. A Classification of the Causes of Hypoxia

Classification	$P_{A O_2}$	$P_{a O_2}$	$C_{a O_2}$	$P_{\bar{v} O_2}$	$C_{\bar{v} O_2}$	Increased $F_{I O_2}$ Helpful?
Hypoxic hypoxia						
Low alveolar P_{O_2}	Low	Low	Low	Low	Low	Yes
Diffusion impairment	Normal	Low	Low	Low	Low	Yes
Right-to-left shunts	Normal	Low	Low	Low	Low	No
$\dot{V}/\dot{Q}$ mismatch	Normal	Low	Low	Low	Low	Yes
Anemic hypoxia	Normal	Normal	Low	Low	Low	No
CO poisoning	Normal	Normal	Low	Low	Low	Possibly
Hypoperfusion hypoxia	Normal	Normal	Normal	Low	Low	No
Histoxic hypoxia	Normal	Normal	Normal	High	High	No

Reproduced with permission from Levitzky, M.G.: *Pulmonary Physiology.* New York, McGraw-Hill, 1982.

altitudes or with low F_{IO_2}'s because of the reflex increase in ventilation caused by hypoxic stimulation of the arterial chemoreceptors. Hypoventilation and ascent to high altitudes lead to decreased venous P_{O_2} and oxygen content as oxygen is extracted from the already hypoxic arterial blood. Although administration of increased F_{IO_2}'s can alleviate the alveolar and arterial hypoxemia in hypoventilation and ascents to high altitudes, it cannot reverse the hypercapnia resulting from hypoventilation. In fact, giving elevated F_{IO_2}'s to spontaneously breathing patients hypoventilating because of a depressed central response to carbon dioxide may further depress ventilation (see Chapter 3).

Diffusion Impairment. When interstitial fibrosis and intersititial or alveolar edema are present, low arterial P_{O_2}'s and contents with normal or elevated alveolar P_{O_2}'s can result. As already noted, people with a decreased surface area for diffusion, caused for example by emphysema, can be subject to arterial hypoxemia. Diffusion limitation and $\dot{V}/\dot{Q}$ mismatch can also cause hypoxemia in normal people during severe exercise. High F_{IO_2}'s that increase the alveolar P_{O_2} to very high levels may raise the arterial P_{O_2} by increasing the partial pressure gradient for oxygen.

Shunts. True right-to-left shunts, such as anatomic shunts and absolute intrapulmonary shunts, can cause arterial P_{O_2}'s to decrease, whereas alveolar P_{O_2}'s remain normal or even become elevated. Arterial hypoxemia caused by true shunts is not relieved by high F_{IO_2}'s because the shunted blood is not exposed to the high levels of oxygen. At a normal F_{IO_2} of 0.21 the hemoglobin of the *unshunted* blood is nearly saturated with oxygen, and at high F_{IO_2}'s the small additional volume of oxygen *dissolved* in the blood cannot compensate for the low hemoglobin saturation of the shunted blood.

$\dot{V}_A/\dot{Q}c$ Mismatch. Alveolar-capillary units with low ventilation-perfusion ratios contribute to arterial hypoxemia. Units with high $\dot{V}_A/\dot{Q}c$'s do not by themselves lead to arterial hypoxemia, but large lung areas that are underperfused are usually associated with either overperfusion of other units or with low cardiac outputs (see "Hypoperfusion Hypoxia"). Normally, the ventilation-perfusion mismatch is minimized somewhat by the hypoxic pulmonary vasoconstriction and local airway reflexes.

Anemic Hypoxia. Anemic hypoxia is caused by a decrease in the amount of functional hemoglobin. This decrease can result from decreased hemoglobin or erythrocyte production, the production of abnormal hemoglobin or red blood cells, pathologic destruction of erythrocytes or interference with the chemical combination of oxygen and hemoglobin. For example, carbon monoxide poisoning results from the greater affinity of hemoglobin for carbon monoxide than for oxygen. In methemoglobinemia, the iron in hemoglobin has been changed from the Fe^{++} to the Fe^{+++} form, and the latter does not combine with oxygen.

In anemic hypoxia, oxygen content decreases, even when both alveolar and arterial P_{O_2} levels remain normal. Venous P_{O_2} and oxygen content both decrease. Administration of high F_{IO_2}'s does not greatly increase the arterial oxygen content (except perhaps in carbon monoxide poisoning).

Hypoperfusion Hypoxia. Hypoperfusion hypoxia (sometimes called stagnant hypoxia or circulatory hypoxia) is a result of low blood flow. This condition can occur either locally, in a particular vascular bed, or systemically, if cardiac output is low. The alveolar P_{O_2}, arterial P_{O_2}, and oxygen content may be normal, but the reduction in oxygen delivered to the tissues may result in tissue hypoxia. Venous P_{O_2} and oxygen content are low. Raising the F_{IO_2} has little benefit in hypoperfusion hypoxia (unless it directly increases the perfusion) inasmuch as the blood flowing to the tissues is already oxygenated normally.

Histotoxic Hypoxia. Histotoxic hypoxia refers to a poisoning of the cellular machinery that uses oxygen to produce energy. For example, cyanide binds to cytochrome oxidase in the mitochondria and blocks oxidative phosphorylation. Alveolar P_{O_2}, arterial P_{O_2}, and oxygen content may be normal (or even elevated, because low doses of cyanide increase ventilation by stimulating the arterial chemoreceptors). Venous P_{O_2} and oxygen content are elevated because oxygen cannot be utilized normally.

Other Causes of Hypoxia. Tissue edema or fibrosis may result in impaired diffusion of oxygen from the blood to the tissues. If the oxyhemoglobin dissociation curve is shifted very far to the left and hemoglobin releases oxygen only at very low P_{O_2}'s, then the tissues may become hypoxic. This is called affinity hypoxia. Another possibility is a normal tissue oxygen delivery, but the tissue's metabolic demands still exceed the supply. This circumstance is called overutilization hypoxia.

Effects of Hypoxia

With hypoxia, reversible tissue injury or even tissue death can result. The outcome of an hypoxic episode depends on whether the tissue hypoxia is generalized or localized, how severe the hypoxia is, how quickly the hypoxia develops, and how long the hypoxia lasts. Different cell types have different susceptibilities to hypoxia; unfortunately, brain cells and heart cells are the most susceptible.

Cyanosis. A sign of poor transport of oxygen, cyanosis results when more than 5 gm of hemoglobin per 100 ml of arterial blood is in the deoxy state. The skin, nailbeds, and mucous membranes become bluish-purple. Cyanosis indicates that the concentration of deoxyhemoglobin in the arterial blood is abnormally high. Absence of cyanosis, however, does not exclude the presence of hypoxemia because an anemic patient with a low P_{aO_2} may not have sufficient hemoglobin to appear cyanotic. Patients who have abnormally high levels of hemoglobin in their arterial blood, such as those with *polycythemia* (abnormally high levels of erythrocytes), may appear cyanotic without being hypoxemic.

Response to Hypoxia

The response to hypoxia depends on the duration and severity of the hypoxia as well as whether the hypoxia is accompanied by hypocapnia and alkalosis, as seen at high altitudes, or by hypercapnia and acidosis, as seen with hypoventilation and chronic obstructive lung disease. We can look at an ascent to high altitude to consider the responses to acute and chronic hypoxia with hypocapnia and alkalosis. We can then compare them with the responses to the hypoxia with hypercapnia and acidosis of chronic obstructive lung diseases (see Chapter 5).

The total barometric pressure falls with altitude, but not exactly linearly. The barometric pressure is proportional to the weight of the air above it. As the atmospheric air is attracted to the earth's surface by gravity, the compressibility of air causes its density to be greater closer to the earth's surface. This, combined with the fact that gravitational force is inversely proportional to the square of the distance between two objects (here between atmospheric gas and the earth), causes a greater change in barometric pressure per change in altitude closer to the earth's surface than at greater altitudes.

The inspired P_{O_2} falls as the total barometric pressure falls. Oxygen constitutes about 21% of the dry ambient air at any altitude. Assuming that inspired air is heated to body temperature and completely humidified as it is inspired, the partial pressure of water vapor remains at 47 torr.

Thus, $P_{IO_2} = 0.21 \times (P_B - 47\ \text{torr})$, where P_B equals the total barometric pressure.

The alveolar P_{O_2} can be calculated by using the alveolar air equation discussed in Chapter 3:

$$P_{AO_2} = P_{IO_2} - \frac{P_{ACO_2}}{R} + [F]$$

As the alveolar P_{O_2} falls, the arterial P_{O_2} falls. When it decreases enough to stimulate the arterial chemoreceptors, alveolar ventilation is increased. The alveolar P_{CO_2} therefore decreases at high altitudes. For example, at 15,000 feet, the total barometric pressure is about 429 torr. The inspired P_{O_2} is therefore $0.21 \times (429 - 47)$, or 80.2 torr. The alveolar P_{CO_2} is likely to decrease to about 32 torr, resulting in a P_{AO_2} of about 45 torr. At 18,000 feet, the total barometric pressure is about 380 torr; at 20,000 feet, it is 349 torr.

The barometric pressure measured on high mountains may not be exactly that predicted because barometric pressure changes with seasonal weather conditions, and it may also be higher close to the equator.

Commercial airplanes are not usually pressurized to 760 torr but are kept at around 650 torr, corresponding to an altitude of about 5,000 feet. If cabin pressure is lost in an airplane, a person suffers a deterioration of nervous system function, unless he or she inspires supplemental 100% oxygen. The symptoms are mainly due to *hypoxia* and may include sleepiness, laziness, a false sense of well-being, impaired judgment, blunted pain perception, increasing errors on simple tasks, decreased visual acuity, clumsiness, and tremors. Severe hypoxia, of course, may result in a loss of consciousness or even death.

An unacclimatized person who ascends to a moderate altitude may suffer from a group of symptoms known as *acute mountain sickness*. The symptoms of this condition include headache, dizziness, breathlessness at rest, weakness, nausea, sweating, palpitations, dimness of vision, partial deafness, sleeplessness, and dyspnea on exertion. The symptoms are mainly attributed to the secondary hypocapnia and alkalosis caused by hypoxic stimulation of the arterial chemoreceptors, resulting in increased alveolar ventilation. Many of the symptoms of acute mountain sickness can be alleviated by using elevated F_{IO_2}'s to prevent the hypoxic drive of ventilation, or even by elevating the F_{ICO_2} or performing strenuous exercise to prevent the alkalosis. The adaptive response of the body to altitude is mainly dependent on correcting the alkalosis. This response, which is called *acclimatization*, is discussed later.

Source of the Ventilatory Response. The *arterial chemoreceptors* are apparently solely responsible for the increased ventilation; the *central chemoreceptors* are not responsive to hypoxia. Furthermore, as discussed in Chapter 3, arterial hypocapnia results in movement of carbon dioxide out of the cerebrospinal fluid, resulting in an increase in its pH. Thus, not only are central chemoreceptors unresponsive to the hypoxia of altitude, but also their activity is depressed by the hypocapnia and alkalosis of the cerebrospinal fluid.

Effects on the Mechanics of Breathing. The increased alveolar ventilation is mainly effected by an increased *tidal volume*, with an increased *breathing rate* a less constant finding. The work of breathing is therefore increased because of the greater elastic work of generating greater tidal volumes and also because of greater airways resistance. The increased alveolar ventilation is likely to be accompanied by active expiration, resulting in dynamic compression of airways. This airway compression, along with a reflex parasympathetic bronchoconstriction in response to the arterial hypoxemia, results in increased resistance work of breathing. More turbulent airflow, likely to be encountered at elevated rates of alveolar ventilation, may also contribute to the increased airways resistance. Maximum air flow rates may increase because of decreased gas density.

Effects on Distribution of Alveolar Ventilation. There is little change in *anatomic dead space* at high altitudes because of the opposing effects of the reflex bronchoconstriction, which should decrease the dead space, and the increased tidal volumes, which should increase it. Therefore, the ratio of the dead space to the tidal volume decreases as the tidal volume increases. The distribution of the tidal volume should become more uniform as the tidal volume increases.

Effects on Cardiac Output and Pulmonary Blood Flow. *Cardiac output, heart rate,* and *systemic blood pressure* increase at high altitudes. These increases probably result from increased *sympathetic stimulation* of the cardiovascular system secondary to arterial chemoreceptor stimulation, increased lung inflation, and increased circulating catecholamines. The increased sympathetic tone to the systemic vessels should cause a redistribution of the left ventricular output away from nonessential vascular beds, while local hypoxia should dilate the vessels mainly under local control. Venoconstriction helps maintain the increased cardiac output. There may also be a direct stimulatory effect of hypoxia on the myocardium.

In the lungs, alveolar hypoxia stimulates the *hypoxic pulmonary vasoconstriction*. The increase in cardiac output in addition to the hypoxic pulmonary vasoconstriction and sympathetic stimulation of larger pulmonary vessels increases the mean pulmonary artery pressure and tends to eliminate any pre-existing Zone 1 by recruiting previously unperfused capillaries. Adverse consequences of these increases in arterial pressure include vascular distention and engorgement of the lung secondary to the pulmonary hypertension, which may contribute to high-altitude pulmonary edema, and a greatly increased right ventricular work load. With the increase in pulmonary blood flow seen acutely at altitude, along with the more uniform alveolar ventilation, one would expect regional $\dot{V}_A/\dot{Q}$ to become more uniform and closer to 1.0. Surprisingly, studies have not shown striking improvements in ventilation-perfusion relationships at high altitudes.

Effects on Diffusion Through the Alveolar-Capillary Barrier. At high altitudes, the low alveolar P_{O_2} sets the upper limit for the end-capillary blood P_{O_2}. Because this hypoxic hypoxia decreases the oxygen content of the arterial blood, the mixed venous P_{O_2} is also depressed. The even greater decrease in the alveolar partial pressure of oxygen, however, results in a decreased *alveolar-capillary partial pressure gradient*, and the blood P_{O_2} takes longer to equilibrate with the alveolar P_{O_2}. A normal person exerting himself or herself at a high altitude, therefore, might be subjected to diffusion limitation of oxygen transfer. The low alveolar P_{O_2} and the tendency for diffusion limitation of gas transfer to occur at high altitudes are partly offset by the effects of the increased cardiac output and increased pulmonary artery pressure, which in turn, increase the surface area available for diffusion and decrease the time that erythrocytes are within the pulmonary capillaries.

Effects on Oxygen Transport by the Blood. Oxygen loading in the lung is decreased at alveolar P_{O_2}'s low enough to be below the flat part of the oxyhemoglobin dissociation curve, resulting in a low arterial oxygen content. Although hypocapnia may aid slightly in oxygen loading in the lung, it also interferes with oxygen unloading at the tissues. The main immediate compensatory mechanism for maintaining oxygen *delivery* is increased cardiac output. One area of particular difficulty is the cerebral circulation: Hypocapnia causes dramatic cerebral vasoconstriction. This may be partly offset by the cerebral vasodilating effect of the hypoxemia. Thus, the brain may not only receive blood with a low oxygen content, but it also may be subjected to a reduced blood flow.

Adaptations to Hypoxia

As already noted, the adaptations to the chronic hypoxia of high altitudes are called *acclimatization*. Longer-term compensations to high-altitude ascent begin to occur after several hours and continue for days or even weeks.

Renal compensation for respiratory alkalosis begins within a day. Excretion of base increases and hydrogen ions are conserved. Another major compensatory mechanism is *erythropoiesis*, which is initiated in the kidney. Within 3 to 5 days, new red blood cells are produced by the bone marrow, increasing the hematocrit and the oxygen-carrying capacity. Thus, although the arterial P_{O_2} cannot be increased, the arterial oxygen *content* increases by virtue of the increased blood hemoglobin concentration. Increased levels of 2,3-DPG also help to unload oxygen at the tissues.

Hypoxic stimulation of the arterial chemoreceptors persists indefinitely, although it may decrease slightly after prolonged periods at high altitudes. Within a few days, the ventilatory response curve to carbon dioxide shifts to the left. In other words, after several days at high altitude, the ventilatory response is greater for any given alveolar or arterial P_{CO_2}. This increased response probably reflects alterations in central acid-base balance. It is associated with the alleviation of most of the central nervous system symptoms and with a return of the cerebrospinal fluid pH toward normal. This is a result of a reduction of the bicarbonate concentration of the cerebrospinal fluid. The mechanism of this decrease is controversial: Bicarbonate may simply diffuse out of the cerebrospinal fluid, or it may be moved out by active transport, or the reduced CSF levels of bicarbonate may reflect decreased production of bicarbonate as the cerebrospinal fluid is produced.

The increased cardiac output, heart rate, and systemic blood pressure return to normal levels after a month or so at high altitude. This reversal probably reflects a decrease in sympathetic activity or changes in sympathetic receptors. The hypoxic pulmonary vasoconstriction and pulmonary hypertension persist, along with increased blood viscosity resulting from the increased hematocrit, leading to right ventricular hypertrophy and frequently to *chronic cor pulmonale* (right ventricular failure secondary to pulmonary hypertension).

HYPERBARIC CONDITIONS

Elevated ambient pressures have been used for medical purposes for well over 50 years. Although the use of hyperbaric chambers has never been widespread, hyperbaric oxygenation has been successfully employed in the treatment of carbon monoxide poisoning and infection by anaerobic organisms, such as those responsible for gas gangrene, and during open heart surgery and radiation therapy. Currently, hyperbaric chambers are probably used most often to treat decompression sickness, which is described later. They are also used to improve and speed up wound healing. In some hospitals, this is done in large hyperbaric chambers capable of holding 12 or more patients simultaneously.

Among the general public, hyperbaric conditions are most frequently encountered during underwater diving. The stresses and hazards associated with clinically applied hyperbaric pressures are similar to many of those identified with scuba diving. These are mainly a result of the elevated total pressure and the elevated partial pressures of individual gases. The diver has the additional physiologic stresses of decreased effects of gravity, hypothermia, and sensory impairment and the additional risks of interacting with the local marine life.

Diving Physiology

The pressure at the bottom of a column of liquid is directly proportional to the height of the column, the density of the liquid, and gravity. For each 33 feet of seawater (or 34 feet of fresh water), ambient pressure increases by one atmosphere (atm). At a depth of 33 feet of seawater, therefore, total ambient pressure is 1,520 torr.

Body tissues consist mainly of water and are therefore nearly incompressible. However, gases are compressible in accordance with Boyle's law. Thus, in a breath-hold dive, the *volume* of gas in the lungs (and other compressible spaces) is inversely proportional to the depth attained. At a depth of 33 feet (2 atm), lung volume is reduced by half; at 66 feet (3 atm), it is reduced to one third the original volume. As gases are compressed their *densities* increase.

According to Dalton's law, as the total pressure increases, the *partial pressures* of the constituent gases also increase. The biological effects of gases generally depend on their partial pressures rather than their fractional concentrations. According to Henry's law, as the partial pressures of gases increase, the amounts *dissolved* in the tissues of the body also increase.

Neck-Deep Immersion

If a person immerses himself or herself up to the neck in water, major alterations in the cardiovascular and pulmonary systems result by virtue of the increased pressure outside of the thorax, abdomen, and limbs. This positive pressure outside the chest, averaging about 20 cmH$_2$O, opposes the normal outward elastic recoil of the chest wall and decreases the *functional residual capacity* and the *expiratory reserve volume*. The work that is needed to bring air into the lung increases because extra inspiratory effort is necessary to overcome the positive pressure outside the chest. Nonetheless, the *vital capacity* and *total lung capacity* decrease only slightly. Immersion up to the neck in water results in about a 60% increase in the work of breathing.

With increased pressure outside of the limbs and abdomen, less pooling of systemic venous blood occurs in gravity-dependent regions of the body. If the water temperature is less than the body temperature, a sympathetically mediated venoconstriction results, also augmenting *venous return*. As the venous return increases, the central blood volume increases by approximately 500 ml. Right atrial pressure increases from about -2 to $+16$ mmHg, resulting in increases in *cardiac output* and *stroke volume* of about 30%.

The increased central blood volume stimulates stretch receptors in the left atrium and elsewhere in thoracic vessels. This stimulation, in turn, is believed to decrease the secretion of *antidiuretic hormone* (ADH) by the posterior pituitary gland and cause the so-called immersion diuresis. It may also increase the secretion of atrial natriuretic factor (ANF).

Breath-Hold Diving

Many people have a profound bradycardia and intense peripheral vasoconstriction immediately after face immersion, especially into cold water. This transient *diving reflex* is initiated by as yet unknown sensors in the face or nose. A similar, but greater, response is seen in diving mammals, such as whales and seals. The vagally mediated bradycardia decreases the work of the heart, which would otherwise be greatly increased by the sympathetically mediated vasoconstriction. The peripheral vasoconstriction severely limits perfusion to all systemic vascular beds except for the strongest autoregulators, that is, the heart, brain, and lungs. Note that the cardiovascular effects of the diving reflex mimic those produced when the arterial chemoreceptors are stimulated and ventilation cannot increase.

In diving mammals, prolonged dives result in very low tissue P_{O_2}'s in skeletal muscle. This initially releases oxygen from *myoglobin*, a heme protein similar to a single subunit of hemoglobin. Myoglobin is found in human skeletal muscle cells, but it occurs in much greater concentrations in the skeletal muscle of diving mammals. The oxyhemoglobin dissociation curve of myoglobin, each molecule of which can combine with a single molecule of oxygen, is far to the left of that of normal adult hemoglobin. Therefore, at lower P_{O_2}'s considerably more oxygen remains bound to myoglobin so that myoglobin can act to store and transport oxygen in skeletal muscle. As blood courses through the muscle, oxygen is released from hemoglobin and binds to myoglobin. The oxygen then can be released from the myoglobin when conditions such as those encountered in a prolonged dive cause very low P_{O_2}'s.

Breath-hold divers usually hyperventilate before a dive so that typical alveolar P_{O_2}'s and P_{CO_2}'s might be 120 torr and 30 torr, respectively. During a breath-hold dive to a depth of 33 feet, gases are compressed and lung volume decreases. Total gas pressure almost doubles: thus, after the diver has been at 33 feet for 20 seconds, his or her alveolar P_{O_2} is well above 100 torr; at that depth, even after 1 minute the alveolar P_{O_2} is still well above 100 torr. During descent, however, the alveolar P_{CO_2} also increases to well above 40 torr and may increase even more. Thus, the transfer of oxygen from alveolus to blood remains undisturbed until ascent; however, during descent the normal transfer of carbon dioxide from blood to alveolus is reversed, causing the blood to retain a considerable amount of carbon dioxide.

Scuba Diving

Self-contained underwater breathing apparatus, or scuba, consists of a tank full of compressed gas. Also included is a demand regulator that delivers gas at ambient pressure when the diver's mouth pressure decreases (during inhalation) to slightly less than the ambient pressure. Exhaled gas is released into the water as bubbles.

During a dive with scuba gear, gas pressure within the lungs is about equal to the ambient pressure at a given depth. In scuba diving, therefore, the stresses on the respiratory system result mainly from elevated gas densities and partial pressures. The inspiratory work of breathing is not much of a problem at moderate depths because gas is delivered at ambient pressures. Increased gas *density* becomes a problem at very great depths or at high levels of ambient pressure because it increases the airways resistance work of breathing during turbulent flow. During long-term studies on persons simulating dives of more than 2,000 feet inside hyperbaric chambers, for example, all subjects reported that they could breathe only through their mouths; breathing through their noses was too difficult. One reason for replacing nitrogen with helium for deep dives is that the density of helium is only about one seventh that of nitrogen.

Other hazards that may be encountered in diving to great depths or in the practice of hyperbaric medicine include barotrauma, decompression sickness, oxygen toxicity, nitrogen narcosis, and high-pressure nervous syndrome.

Barotrauma. Barotrauma occurs when ambient pressure increases or decreases, but the pressure of a volume of gas trapped in a closed unventilated area of the body cannot equilibrate with it. The barotrauma of descent or compression is called "squeeze." The middle ear can be affected if the eustachian tube is filled with fluid or otherwise clogged so that the person cannot equilibrate it with ambient pressure; the sinuses, lungs (which can result in pulmonary congestion, edema, or hemorrhage), and even cavities in the teeth are subject to this problem. The barotrauma of ascent or decompression can occur if gases are trapped in areas of the body and begin to expand as a diver ascends or as a hyperbaric chamber is decompressed. For example, if during ascent, a diver does not exhale, expanding alveolar gas may overdistend the lung and cause it to rupture (burst lung). This may result in hemorrhage, pneumothorax, or air embolism. Gases that are trapped in the stomach or intestines may cause abdominal discomfort and eructation or flatus as they expand. When a diver rapidly ascends from great depths, barotrauma of the ears, sinuses, and teeth may also occur.

Decompression Sickness. Decompression sickness (also called caisson disease or the bends) occurs when gas bubbles form in the blood and body tissues as the ambient pressure decreases. During a dive, or compression, the increasing ambient pressure causes the partial pressure of gases in the body to increase. The high partial pressure of nitrogen causes this gas, normally poorly soluble, to dissolve in the body fluids and tissues (especially body fat). At great depths, body tissues become supersaturated with nitrogen.

In a rapid ascent, ambient pressure falls quickly, and nitrogen comes out of solution, causing bubbles to form in body tissues and fluids. The effect is like opening a bottle of a carbonated beverage. In production, the soft drink is exposed to hyperbaric pressures of gases, usually carbon dioxide, and then capped. The total pressure in the gas layer above the liquid remains greater than the atmospheric pressure. The gases dissolved in the liquid phase are in equilibrium with the partial pressures in the gas phase, according to Henry's law. When the cap is removed, the gas-phase pressure decreases suddenly and the gas dissolved in the liquid phase comes out of solution, producing bubbles.

In decompression sickness, bubbles may form in the blood, in the joints of the extremities, and in the circulation of the central nervous system. Those bubbles that form in the venous blood usually become trapped in the pulmonary circulation and rarely cause symptoms. If symptoms do occur, they are known as the chokes by divers and include substernal chest pain, dyspnea, and cough, which may be accompanied by pulmonary hypertension, pulmonary edema, and hypoxemia. These symptoms are an extremely dangerous form of decompression sickness. Even more dangerous, of course, are bubbles that form in the circulation of the central nervous system, which may cause brain damage and paralysis. Too rapid decompression may also cause osteonecrosis of joints.

The treatment for decompression sickness is immediate *recompression* in a hyperbaric chamber, to cause the gases to go back into solution, followed by slow decompression. Decompression sickness may be prevented by gradual ascents from great depths (according to decompression tables) and by substituting helium for nitrogen in inspired gas mixtures, because helium is only about one half as soluble as nitrogen in body tissues.

Divers who ascend from submersion with no immediate effects of decompression may later suffer decompression sickness if they travel in an airplane within a few hours of the dive because, as noted previously, cabin pressures in commercial airplanes are normally maintained below 760 torr.

Nitrogen Narcosis. Very high partial pressures of nitrogen directly affect the central nervous system, causing euphoria, loss of memory, clumsiness, and irrational behavior. Occurring at depths of 100 feet or more, this "rapture of the deep" may result in numbness of the arms and legs, disorientation, motor impairment, and ultimately, unconsciousness. The mechanism of nitrogen narcosis is unknown.

Oxygen Toxicity. If 100% oxygen is inhaled at 760 torr, or lower oxygen concentrations are inhaled at higher ambient pressures, both central nervous system and alveolar damage can result, although pulmonary symptoms are rare among divers. The mechanism of oxygen toxicity is unknown but may involve the formation of superoxides or free radicals.

High-Pressure Nervous Syndrome. Tremors

and decreased manual dexterity are associated with exposure to very high ambient pressures, such as those encountered at extreme depths (>250 feet). This high-pressure nervous syndrome (HPNS) usually occurs when nitrogen has been replaced by helium. Adding small amounts of nitrogen to the inspired gas mixture helps to counteract the problem.

PREGNANCY

The course of pregnancy results in significant changes in both the cardiovascular and respiratory systems. These alterations are consequences of hormonal effects, the additional metabolic and nutritional demands of the fetus and its support tissue, and the mechanical effects of the enlarging uterus.

Cardiovascular Effects

Both the *plasma volume* and the *erythrocyte volume* begin to increase between the 6th and 12th week of pregnancy, resulting in about a 40% increase in total blood volume by approximately the 30th week of gestation. After that point, there is little further change in blood volume until the birth of the baby. Although the red blood cell volume increases about 20% to 30% during the same time course, the plasma volume increases 40% to 50%, so the *hemoglobin concentration, erythrocyte count,* and *hematocrit* all fall. The fall in hematocrit from about 42% to about 35%, and the decrease in blood hemoglobin concentration from 14g/100 ml of blood to about 11 to 12 g/100 ml of blood are frequently referred to as the physiological anemia of pregnancy. This "anemia" can be prevented by diet supplementation with iron and folic acid.

The increase in plasma volume results mainly from the effects of elevated levels of estrogen and progesterone, which are secreted in large amounts by the placenta, especially during the last trimester of pregnancy. Estrogen is known to stimulate the hepatic synthesis of angiotensinogen, and estrogen and/or progesterone stimulate renin secretion by the juxtaglomerular cells of the kidney. These two effects result in elevated levels of angiotensin I, which is converted to angiotensin II by converting enzyme in the lung. Increased angiotensin II in the blood acts on the adrenal cortex to stimulate the production and release of aldosterone. The effects of increased aldosterone are to promote sodium and water retention by the kidneys, thus increasing the plasma volume.

Despite the elevated plasma volume, an increase in the resting cardiac output of about 30% to 40%, and increased blood levels of angiotensin II, the *mean arterial blood pressure* decreases slightly during the latter stages of pregnancy. The decrease in diastolic pressure is greater than the decrease in systolic pressure, reflecting a reduction in systemic vascular resistance. This is mainly a result of the development of a large parallel vascular circuit in the blood supply to the uterus, especially the placenta. As discussed in Chapter 2, resistances in parallel add as reciprocals, so the addition of a large parallel circuit decreases the total systemic vascular resistance. Hormonal effects may also be responsible for the decreased vascular resistance.

Cardiac output increases progressively to a maximum of 35% to 50% above normal by about the 30th week of gestation. After this peak is reached, cardiac output decreases rapidly to near nonpregnant levels. The exact mechanism by which the cardiac output increases during pregnancy is not known, but it seems to be related to the increased oxygen demand of the fetus, the decreased systemic vascular resistance, the expanded plasma volume, and reflex and hormonal effects.

The subsequent decrease in cardiac output is most likely a result of compression of the inferior vena cava by the enlarging uterus, causing a decrease in venous return. The effect of vena cava compression on the cardiac output seems to be sensitive to changes in body position. As one would predict, the greatest decrease occurs when cardiac output is measured with the woman in a supine position, compared with measurements made in the sitting or lateral positions. This decrease can result in arterial hypotension in the supine position, with tachycardia, pallor, and a feeling of faintness.

The decrease in cardiac output that occurs during the last 6 to 8 weeks of pregnancy is likely to be the result of a decrease in *stroke volume* because *heart rate* gradually increases during pregnancy, rising by about 12 beats per minute when it peaks around the 32nd week. It then begins to decrease, but it never falls to nonpregnant levels until several days after delivery. The changes in heart rate are likely to be reflex or hormonal effects.

Upward displacement of the diaphragm by the enlarging uterus shifts the position of the heart in the thorax. This shift is seen as a *left axis deviation* in the electrocardiogram.

Respiratory Effects

The effects of pregnancy on the respiratory system result mainly from alterations in the mechanics of the chest wall and vena cava compression caused by the enlarging uterus and from increased oxygen demand and hormone levels.

Compression of the vena cava causes engorgement of the veins and capillaries throughout the respiratory tract, particularly in the nasopharynx and larynx. This engorgement may increase the resistance to airflow in the nasopharynx sufficiently to make breathing through the nose difficult for some women. It may also cause noticeable changes in their voices.

The enlarging uterus alters the conformation of the chest wall. As it pushes upward, the uterus elevates the *resting* level of the diaphragm by a maximum of about 4 cm. However, diaphragmatic movement is not usually affected. The circumference of the thoracic cavity also increases somewhat as the rib cage expands. As would be expected from these changes, the *functional residual capacity* (FRC) begins to decrease at about the 5th month of pregnancy, falling about 20% below the FRC of nonpregnant women at term. Both the *expiratory reserve volume* and the *residual volume* decrease, mainly as a result of the decreased outward elastic recoil of the chest wall but also because of an increased pulmonary blood volume. Because the diaphragm is still able to descend normally when it contracts, the *total lung capacity* decreases little if at all (0 to 5%). Because the functional residual capacity decreases significantly and the total lung capacity does not, the *inspiratory reserve volume* and *inspiratory capacity* increase about 15% to 20%. The *vital capacity* increases slightly or does not change. The *maximal voluntary ventilation* usually remains unchanged.

The *compliance* of the lungs is usually unchanged. Intrapulmonary *airways resistance* decreases mainly due to bronchiolar smooth muscle relaxation resulting from elevated levels of progesterone.

Minute ventilation increases progressively during pregnancy, beginning in the first trimester and reaching levels 50% above normal near term. Because this increase is effected mainly by an increase in *tidal volume*, with only a slight increase in ventilatory rate, and because the anatomic dead space is not altered significantly, the *alveolar ventilation* increases relatively more than the minute ventilation, rising progressively to about 70% above control at term. This increase in tidal volume occurs mainly because of increased diaphragmatic breathing rather than intercostal muscle activity. Although this association of tidal volume with diaphragmatic breathing may seem surprising at first, diaphragmatic motion does not appear to be impeded by the enlarging uterus, as already noted.

The increase in alveolar ventilation is much greater than that in *oxygen consumption*, which only increases to about 20% above nonpregnant levels at term. Much of the increase in ventilation is believed to result from increased levels of progesterone, which is known to stimulate ventilation. This increased alveolar ventilation results in changes in arterial blood gases that begin early in pregnancy. Arterial P_{O_2} increases slightly to a mean of about 106 torr, and arterial P_{CO_2} decreases to a mean of about 32 torr. Arterial pH remains near normal because the buffering capacity of the blood is decreased by renal excretion of bicarbonate and dilution of blood buffers, especially hemoglobin.

Eclampsia

Eclampsia is a severe form of a group of disorders known as the *toxemias of pregnancy*. Preeclampsia or eclampsia generally occurs during the last 16 weeks of gestation and remains only a short time after delivery. It affects 1% to 5% of pregnant women.

Preeclampsia is usually characterized by hypertension, edema, and/or protein in the urine. Mild preeclampsia is usually preceded by a sudden abnormal weight gain. Edema of the lower limbs is a common finding in normal pregnancies because of vena cava compression, but edema of the face or upper extremities often indicates preeclampsia. Treatment with bed rest, salt restriction, diuretics, and antihypertensive drugs at this stage may prevent the disease from progressing. Severe preeclampsia is characterized by more severe proteinuria and higher blood pressure resulting from fluid retention and arterial spasm in many vascular beds. These spasms often cause decreased renal blood flow and glomerular filtration rate, resulting in a low urine output, cerebral or visual disturbances, or even pulmonary edema.

Eclampsia is the most severe form of the disorder. It is characterized by convulsions, which may be severe and also may vary in frequency and duration. The convulsions may be followed by comas. They are frequently accompanied by severe hypertension, renal and hepatic failure, and generalized toxicity. Early labor may be precipitated.

Preeclampsia and eclampsia can be very serious and may result in the death of the mother or child. The incidence of death of the fetus or baby ranges from about 10% in preeclampsia to 35% in eclampsia. Maternal deaths are usually preventable in preeclampsia; they approach 10% in eclampsia.

SURGERY

The cardiopulmonary stresses involved in surgery depend on the kind of operation performed, the duration of the surgery, and whether or not any complications occur. Thoracic surgery, especially if it involves cardiopulmonary bypass, may represent the most severe stress. High abdominal surgery also involves a great stress to the respiratory system because it restricts lung expansion and impedes venous return. Uncontrolled bleeding during surgery represents stresses identical to those of hemorrhage, and steps must be taken to prevent and correct blood loss, hypotension, and decreased cardiac output.

Because so many different factors may be involved in different types of surgery, it is difficult to make general statements concerning surgical stress. However, one group of alterations common to nearly all major operations are those associated with general anesthesia. These include decreased cardiac output, altered lung and chest wall mechanics, and an abnormal distribution of alveolar ventilation resulting in greater ventilation-perfusion mismatch. These problems may be exacerbated by paralysis of the patient and mechanical ventilation involving positive end-expiratory pressure (PEEP), which is discussed in Chapter 20.

Cardiovascular Effects

Almost all general anesthetics are direct *myocardial depressants* to a greater or lesser degree. As discussed in Chapter 2, venous return is aided by muscle contraction (the muscle pump) and by negative-pressure breathing, as intrathoracic pressure becomes more negative and abdominal pressure increases during inspiration (the thoracoabdominal pump). During general anesthesia, these mechanisms may be impaired because of restraint of the patient and muscle relaxants or even paralytic agents used by the anesthetist. If positive-pressure ventilation is used, either by manual compression of the rubber bag on an anesthesia machine or by a mechanical ventilator, alveolar pressure and intrapleural pressure become positive, thus compressing the alveolar vessels and intrathoracic veins. In fact, if PEEP or continuous positive airway pressure (CPAP) are used, intrapleural pressure stays positive throughout the respiratory cycle, as discussed in Chapter 20.

Myocardial depression and impaired venous return combine to decrease *cardiac output*, which may be depressed by as much as 50% by anesthesia and ventilation with PEEP alone. Reduced cardiac output as well as the fact that many general anesthetics and other drugs used during surgery are vasodilators indicates that decreased blood pressure may be a problem during surgery, even without significant blood loss.

Effects on the Respiratory System

Depressed cardiac output by itself tends to compromise tissue oxygen delivery and carbon dioxide elimination. The potential for these problems to occur is enhanced by changes in the respiratory system. Aside from accidentally administering a low FIO_2, having too much dead space, or using improper intubation, the main factors we will consider are changes in respiratory drive in spontaneously breathing anesthetized patients, changes in lung and chest wall mechanics, and changes in the distribution of ventilation and perfusion.

As noted in Chapter 3, nearly all general anesthetics depress the *ventilatory response to carbon dioxide* and may therefore decrease alveolar ventilation and lead to a decreased Pa_{O_2} and an increased Pa_{CO_2}. General anesthesia may also decrease the frequency of the extra deep inspirations referred to as *sighs* in Chapter 3. This may lead to an increased tendency for alveoli to collapse spontaneously, thus elevating the *intrapulmonary shunt* and decreasing the Pa_{O_2}. A paralyzed patient who is being ventilated manually or mechanically must also have sighs administered periodically.

During anesthesia, especially with paralysis, the shape and motion of the chest wall are altered. In a recumbent person, this results in a decreased *functional residual capacity* caused by decreased outward elastic recoil of the chest wall. The diaphragm, especially the more gravity-dependent portion, tends to be positioned farther up in the thorax. There is also an increase in the inward elastic recoil of the lungs and a decreased *lung compliance* that may be partly due to increased atelectasis and partly due to the changes in chest wall mechanics.

The changes in chest wall and lung mechanics appear to cause an alteration in the *distribution of alveolar ventilation.* As noted in Chapter 3, alveolar ventilation is normally not uniformly distributed. When a person is breathing normally from the functional residual capacity, relatively more of the alveolar ventilation occurs in gravity-dependent regions of the lung. In a conscious, spontaneously breathing person in the supine position, therefore, more of the ventilation occurs posteriorly, in lung regions closer to the spine. However, in an anesthetized paralyzed person, alveolar ventilation becomes *more uniform* for two reasons. First, lung expansion seems to occur more by rib cage movement than by diaphragmatic motion. Second, the motion of the diaphragm changes from greater movement posteriorly in the conscious spontaneously breathing person to greater movement anteriorly with anesthesia and paralysis. This change makes sense because, in the conscious spontaneously breathing person, the diaphragm is *contracting*, but in the paralyzed ventilated patient, diaphragmatic motion is *passive*. As the flaccid diaphragm is pushed by the expanding lungs against the contents of the abdominal cavity, it encounters greater resistance posteriorly, where the abdominal contents collect because of hydrostatic forces.

Although at first thought more uniform alveolar ventilation seems desirable during anesthesia and paralysis, it is not. This is because the *distribution of pulmonary blood flow* is not changed to match the altered distribution of alveolar ventilation. The decreased cardiac output may in fact result in greatly decreased perfusion of the now better ventilated regions of the lung as non–gravity-dependent areas are *derecruited* secondary to the decreased perfusion and pulmonary artery pressure. Wellventilated, non–gravity-dependent regions are likely to have high ventilation-perfusion ratios and may even be unperfused, resulting in Zone 1 conditions and contributing to elevated alveolar and physiologic dead space. The distribution of the cardiac output, which is determined primarily by hydrostatic effects, will be mainly to more gravity-dependent regions of the lung, which are relatively less well ventilated. Thus, much of the perfusion of the lung is to units with low ventilation-perfusion ratios or even to intrapulmonary shunts. The fact that this occurs suggests that general anesthetics or other drugs administered during surgery may interfere with the hypoxic pulmonary vasoconstriction.

The combination of increased ventilation of unperfused or poorly perfused alveolar units combined with increased perfusion of unventilated or poorly ventilated units leads to both an elevated arterial-alveolar carbon dioxide gradient and an elevated alveolar-arterial oxygen gradient. Thus, less efficient matching of ventilation and perfusion during general anesthesia and surgery may lead to decreased tissue oxygenation and decreased carbon dioxide elimination.

Bibliography

Asmussen, E.: Muscular Exercise. In Fenn, W.O. and Rahn, H. (eds.): *Handbook of Physiology,* vol. 2. Washington, D.C., American Physiological Society, 1965, pp 939–978.

Begin, R., Epstein, M., Sackner, M.A., Levinson, R., Dougherty, R., and Duncan D.: Effects of water immersion to the neck on pulmonary circulation and tissue volume in man. *J. Appl. Physiol.* 40:273–299, 1976.

Bennett, P.B., and Elliot, D.H. (eds.): *The Physiology and Medicine of Diving,* 3rd ed. London, Baillière Tindall, 1983.

Bisgard, G.E., Will, J.A., Tyson, I.B., Dayton, L.M., Henderson, R.R., and Grover R.F.: Distribution of regional lung function during mild exercise in residents of 3100 m. *Respir. Physiol.* 22:369–379, 1974.

Bonica, J.J.: *Obstetric Analgesia and Anesthesia,* 2nd ed. Amsterdam, World Federation of Anaesthesiologists, 1980, pp 1–22.

Bonica, J.J.: *Principles and Practice of Obstetric Analgesia and Anesthesia.* Philadelphia, F.A. Davis, 1967, pp 13–39, 1127–1147.

Ceretelli, P., and Di Prampero, P.E.: Gas Exchange in Exercise. In Farhi, L.E., and Tenney, S.M. (eds.): *Handbook of Physiology,* vol. 4. Bethesda, Md., American Physiological Society, 1987, pp 297–339.

Collins, V.J.: *Principles of Anesthesiology,* 2nd ed. Philadelphia, Lea & Febiger, 1976, pp 793–804.

Covino, B.G., Fozzard, H.A., Rehder, K., and Strichartz, G. (eds.): *Effects of Anesthesia.* Bethesda, Md., American Physiological Society, 1985.

Dempsey, J.A., Vidruk, E.H., and Mitchell, G.S.: Pulmonary control systems in exercise: Update. *Fed. Proc.* 44:2260–2270, 1985.

Epstein, M.: Water immersion and the kidney: Implications for volume regulation. *Undersea Biomed. Res.* 11:113–121, 1984.

Finley, J.P., Bonet, J.F., and Waxman, M.B.: Autonomic pathways responsible for bradycardia on facial immersion. *J. Appl. Physiol.* 47:1218–1222, 1979.

Gauer, O.H., Henry, J.P., and Behn, C.: The regulation of extracellular fluid volume. *Ann. Rev. Physiol.* 32:547–595, 1970.

Guenter, C.A., Welch, M.H., and Hogg, J.C.: *Clinical Aspects of Respiratory Physiology.* Philadelphia, J.B. Lippincott, 1977, pp 3–37.

Hammond, M.D., Gale, G.E., Kapitan, K.S., Ries, A., and Wagner, P.D.: Pulmonary gas exchange in humans during exercise at sea level. *J. Appl. Physiol.* 60:1590–1598, 1986.

Harf, A., Pratt, T., and Hughes, J.M.B.: Regional distribution of $\dot{V}/\dot{Q}$ in man at rest and with exercise measured with krypton-81 m. *J. Appl. Physiol.* 44:115–123, 1978.

Hills, B.A.: *Decompression Sickness,* vol. 1. Chichester, England, Wiley, 1977.

Hong, S.K., Ceretelli, P., Cruz, J.C., and Rahn, H.: Mechanics of respiration during submersion in water. *J. Appl. Physiol.* 27:535–538, 1969.

Houston, C.S., Sutton, J.R., Cymerman, A., and Reeves, J.T.: Operation Everest II: Man at extreme altitude. *J. Appl. Physiol.* 63:877–882, 1987.

Jones, N.L., and Campbell, E.J.M.: *Clinical Exercise Testing,* 2nd ed. Philadelphia, W.B. Saunders, 1982, pp 10–51.

Lambertsen, C.J.: Hypoxia, altitude and acclimatization. In Mountcastle, V.B. (ed.): *Medical Physiology,* 14th ed. St. Louis, C.V. Mosby, 1980, pp 1843–1872.

Lenfant, C., and Sullivan, K.: Adaptation to high altitude. *N. Engl. J. Med.* 284:1298–1309, 1971.

Levitzky, M.G.: *Pulmonary Physiology,* 2nd ed. New York, McGraw-Hill, 1986. pp 119–122, 210–226.

Little, R.C.: *Physiology of the Heart and Circulation,* 3rd ed. Chicago, Year Book Medical Publishers, 1985, pp 326–341.

Metcalfe, J., and Bissonnette, J.M.: Gas Exchange in Pregnancy. In Farhi, L.E., and Tenney, S.M. (eds.): *Handbook of Physiology,* vol. 4. Bethesda, Md., American Physiological Society, 1987, pp 341–350.

Metcalfe, J., and Ueland, K.: Maternal cardiovascular adjustments to pregnancy. *Progress in Cardiovascular Diseases* 16:363–374, 1974.

Milledge, J.S.: Acute mountain sickness. *Thorax* 38:641–645, 1983.

Mohsenifar, Z., Ross, M.D., Waxman, A., Goldbach, P., and Koerner, S.K.: Changes in distribution of lung perfusion and ventilation at rest and during maximal exercise. *Chest* 87:359–362, 1985.

Murray, J.F.: *The Normal Lung,* 2nd ed. Philadelphia, W.B. Saunders, 1986, pp 261–282.

Nadel, E.R.: Physiological adaptations to aerobic training. *Am. Scientist* 73:334–343, 1985.

Pederson, H., and Finster, M.: Anesthetic risk in the pregnant surgical patient. *Anesthesiology* 51:439–451, 1979.

Rehder, K.: Anaesthesia and the respiratory system. *Can. Anaesth. Soc. J.* 26:451–462, 1979.

Rehder, K., and Marsh, H.M.: Respiratory mechanics during anesthesia and mechanical ventilation. In Macklem, P.T., and Mead, J. (eds.): *Handbook of Physiology,* vol. 3. Bethesda, Md., American Physiological Society, 1986, pp 737–752.

Rehder, K., Sessler, A.D., and Marsh, H.M.: General anesthesia and the lung. *Am. Rev. Resp. Dis.* 112:541–563, 1975.

Rushmer, R.F.: *Cardiovascular Dynamics,* 4th ed. Philadelphia, W.B. Saunders, 1976, pp 246–268.

Schmid, E.R., and Rehder, K.: General anesthesia and the chest wall. *Anesthesiology* 55:668–675, 1981.

Simpson, E.R., and McDonald, P.C.: Endocrinology of pregnancy. In Williams, R.H. (ed.): *Textbook of Endocrinology,* 6th ed. Philadelphia, W.B. Saunders, 1981, pp 420–421.

Smith, J.J., and Kampine, J.P.: *Circulatory Physiology—The Essentials,* 2nd ed. Baltimore, Williams & Wilkins, 1984, pp 219–236, 247–264.

Strauss, R.H. (ed.): *Diving Medicine.* New York, Grune & Stratton, 1976.

Strauss, R.H.: Diving medicine. *Am. Rev. Resp. Dis.* 119:1001–1023, 1979.

Vander, A.J.: *Renal Physiology,* 3rd ed. New York, McGraw-Hill, 1985, pp 70–85, 111–142.

Wagner, P.D., Gale, G.E., Moon, R.E., Torre-Bueno, J.R., Stolp, B.W., and Saltzman, H.A.: Pulmonary gas exchange in humans exercising at sea level and simulated altitude. *J. Appl. Physiol.* 61:260–270, 1986.

Wasserman, K.: Breathing during exercise. *N. Engl. J. Med.* 298:780–785, 1978.

Wasserman, K., and Whipp, B.J.: Exercise physiology in health and disease. *Am. Rev. Resp. Dis.* 112:219–249, 1975.

Wasserman, K., Whipp, B.J., and Casaburi, R.: Respiratory Control During Exercise. In Cherniack, N.S., and Widdicombe, J.G. (eds.): *Handbook of Physiology,* vol. 2. Bethesda, Md., American Physiological Society, 1986, pp 595–610.

Weil, J.V.: Ventilatory Control at High Altitude. In Cherniack, N.S. and Widdicombe, J.G. (eds.): *Handbook of Physiology,* vol. 3: Bethesda, Md., American Physiological Society, 1986, pp 703–727.

West, J.B.: *Everest: The Testing Place.* New York, McGraw-Hill, 1985.

West, J.B., Hackett, P.H., Maret, K.H., Milledge, J.S., Peters, R.M., Jr., Pizzo, C.J., and Winslow, R.M.: Pulmonary gas exchange on the summit of Mount Everest. *J. Appl. Physiol.* 55:678–687, 1983.

West, J.B., and Lahiri, S. (eds.): *High Altitude and Man.* Bethesda, Md., American Physiological Society, 1984.

Whipp, B.J., and Pardy, R.L.: Breathing During Exercise. In Macklem, P.T., and Mead, J. (eds.): *Handbook of Physiology,* vol. 3. Bethesda, Md., American Physiological Society, 1986, pp 605–629.

Williams, J.H., Powers, S.K., and Stuart, M.K.: Hemoglobin desaturation in highly trained athletes during heavy exercise. *Med. Sci. Sports Exerc.* 18:168–173, 1986.

Winslow, R.M., Samaja, M., and West, J.B.: Red cell function at extreme altitude on Mount Everest. *J. Appl. Physiol.* 56:109–116, 1984.

OBJECTIVES

AFTER READING THIS CHAPTER, THE STUDENT WILL BE ABLE TO:

1. Identify the basic problem in each of the following common cardiopulmonary diseases and disorders:
   a. Conditions causing left heart failure, including myocardial infarction, hypertension, and valvular dysfunctions.
   b. Conditions causing right heart failure, including pulmonary vascular disease and valvular dysfunctions.
   c. Obstructive lung disorders, including asthma, chronic bronchitis, emphysema, and upper airway obstructions.
   d. Restrictive lung disorders, including pneumoconiosis, sarcoidosis, diffuse alveolar fibrosis, hypersensitivity pneumonitis, infiltrations, atelectasis, and conditions involving the pleural space.
   e. Restrictive disorders of the chest wall, including musculoskeletal problems, neuromuscular conditions, and obesity.
   f. Other conditions leading to problems in gas exchange, including adult respiratory distress syndrome, infectious diseases of the lung, and lung cancer.
   g. Disorders of the control of breathing.
   h. Respiratory failure.
2. Discuss the causative factor(s) for each of these common cardiovascular and pulmonary disorders
3. Understand the mechanisms that occur in response to these diseases and disorders.
4. Use his or her understanding of normal physiologic responses to predict the consequences of these basic problems.

5
PATHOPHYSIOLOGY OF CARDIOPULMONARY DISEASE

CHAPTER OUTLINE

CARDIOVASCULAR DISEASES
  Left Heart Failure
    Cardiomyopathies
    Ischemic Heart Disease and Myocardial Infarction
    Hypertension
    Valvular Dysfunctions
    Pathophysiology of Left Heart Failure
  Right Heart Failure
    Pulmonary Vascular Diseases
    Valvular Dysfunctions
    Pathophysiology of Right Heart Failure

PULMONARY DISEASES
  Obstructive Disease
    Asthma
    Chronic Bronchitis
    Emphysema
  Obstructions in Upper Airways
  Restrictive Disease
    Pneumoconiosis
    Sarcoidosis
    Diffuse Alveolar Fibrosis
    Hypersensitivity Pneumonitis and Infiltrative Lung Disorders
    Atelectasis
    Chest Wall Restriction
    Skeletal Problems
    Neuromuscular Disorders
    Obesity
    Pathophysiology of Restrictive Diseases
  Adult Respiratory Distress Syndrome
  Infectious Lung Disease
  Lung Cancer
  Disorders of the Control of Breathing
    Central Sleep Apnea
    Obstructive Sleep Apnea
    Other Ventilatory Control Disorders Causing Hypoventilation
    Abnormal Breathing Patterns
    Hyperventilation Syndrome
  Respiratory Failure

CARDIOVASCULAR DISEASES

In this section, our discussion is limited to those conditions that can lead to either left or right ventricular failure. The discussion of congenital cardiovascular defects is deferred to Chapter 6.

Left Heart Failure

We can define left heart failure as any condition in which the left ventricle is unable to produce a cardiac output adequate to meet the demand of the body tissues for blood flow. This definition does not include inadequate cardiac outputs caused by hypovolemia resulting from hemorrhage or dehydration, which might be included under a more general term such as *circulatory failure*. It also omits inadequate cardiac outputs secondary to right ventricular problems, which are discussed in the section on right heart failure. It does include conditions directly affecting the function of the left ventricular muscle, such as *cardiomyopathies* and *myocardial infarction,* and conditions in which left ventricular function is impaired as a result of an elevated pressure or volume work load. Left ventricular failure secondary to *systemic hypertension* or *valvular dysfunctions* is an example of a condition that may cause left heart failure as a result of elevated left ventricular work loads.

Although most of the conditions that can cause left heart failure result in a low cardiac output even under resting conditions (low-output failure), there are some conditions that can cause inadequate tissue perfusion even though cardiac output is elevated above normal (high-output failure). For example, volume overloading of the left ventricle caused by low-resistance connections between the atria or ventricles or by a patent ductus arteriosus or an arteriovenous fistula could cause heart failure even though the output of one or both ventricles is greater than normal.

Low-output cardiac failure can be a result of injury, disease, ionic imbalance, or metabolic disorders of the heart muscle. Infections, endocrine disorders, myocardial ischemia, cardiomyopathies, toxins, drugs, and arrythmias may all directly affect the ability of the heart muscle to depolarize and contract normally.

Diseases affecting the pericardium or conditions causing an accumulation of blood or fluid in the pericardium can interfere with cardiac filling by restricting its expansion in diastole and may therefore cause low cardiac outputs. *Pericarditis,* or inflammation of the pericardium, may be caused by bacterial, viral, or parasitic infection, or by rheumatologic or autoimmune processes. Chronic pericarditis can result in fibrous scarring of the pericardium. This may lead to *pericardial constriction* by the thickened and stiffened pericardium. Tumors also can occur in the pericardium or as secondary or metastatic neoplasms arising from the lungs, breasts, or elsewhere in the body. The space between the outside of the heart and the inside of the pericardium normally contains only about 15 to 20 ml of pericardial fluid, a clear ultrafiltrate of plasma. Accumulation of fluid or blood in the pericardium (*pericardial effusion*) may occur secondary to inflammation, infection, or injury. As Figure 5–1 shows, such an accumulation restricts both venous return and cardiac filling and may severely reduce the cardiac output. If such *cardiac tamponade* (or pericardial tamponade) is not relieved quickly, it can become fatal. Finally, conditions requiring the heart to do more pressure work, such as hypertension or valvular *stenosis* (narrowing), or volume work, such as arteriovenous fistulas or valvular *incompetence,* may lead to heart failure.

Cardiomyopathies

Cardiomyopathy is a nonspecific term indicating diseases or disorders that directly affect the heart muscle itself. Although the cardiomyopathies are probably not a common cause of cardiac failure, it is logical to begin our discussion of cardiac failure with them because they affect the heart muscle directly. Since the symptoms of some cardiomyopathies are sometimes mistakenly attributed to ischemic heart disease (discussed in the next section), the cardiomyopathies may be more common than they are currently believed to be.

Because cardiomyopathy is a nonspecific term denoting all diseases directly affecting the myocardium (as well as those conditions causing cardiac dysfunctions that are not attributable to anything else), there are several different ways of classifying the cardiomyopathies. One way of doing this is to divide them into those conditions that can be attributed to other diseases and those that cannot. *Secondary cardiomyopathies* can occur as a result of myocarditis secondary to bacterial, viral, and parasitic infection, toxins, or severe allergic reactions; infiltrative diseases, such as sarcoidosis and amyloidosis; neuromuscular disorders; connective tissue disorders, such as rheumatoid disease; and metabolic disorders, such as thyroid diseases, glycogen storage diseases, and nutritional deficiencies. *Primary* or *idiopathic* (i.e., of unknown origin) *cardiomyopathies* cannot

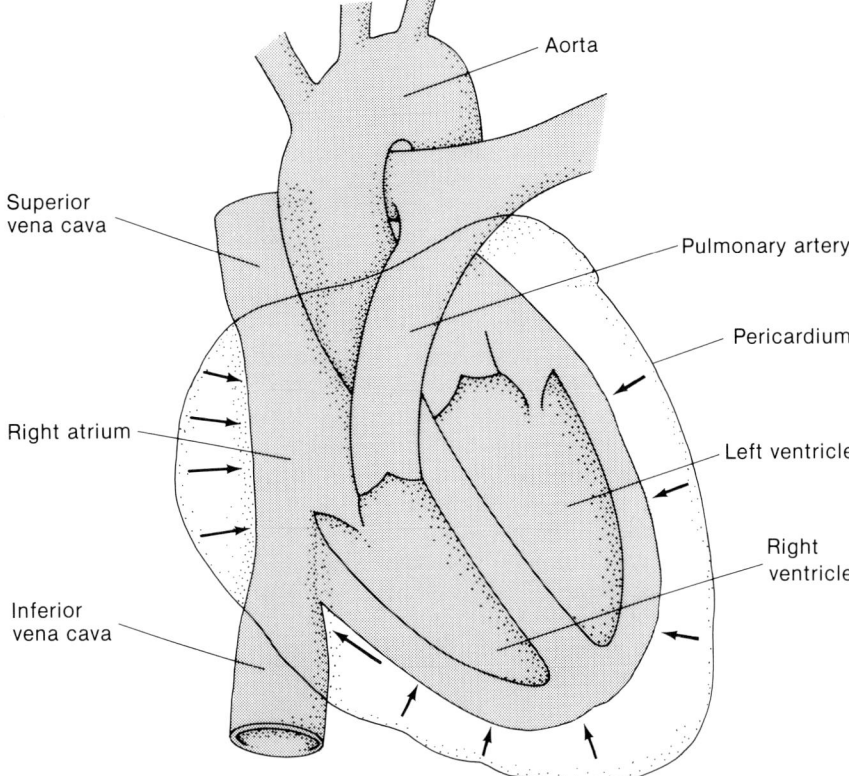

FIGURE 5-1. Cardiac tamponade: Arrows indicate compression of the great veins and restriction of cardiac filling caused by accumulation of blood within the pericardial sac.

be attributed to any other known disease or problem.

Cardiomyopathies may also be classified on the basis of functional and pathologic alterations into *dilated* or *congestive cardiomyopathy*, *hypertrophic cardiomyopathy*, and *restrictive cardiomyopathy*. A patient suffering from a *congestive cardiomyopathy* usually has symptoms of left ventricular dilation, a reduced cardiac output at rest, and other indications of left ventricular failure. Tests usually reveal contractile dysfunction of the other three chambers of the heart as well. To correctly diagnose the condition as congestive cardiomyopathy, one must first exclude volume or pressure overload resulting from hypertension or valvular disease, coronary artery diseases, and pericardial diseases as the cause of the contractile dysfunction.

Hypertrophic Cardiomyopathy, or idiopathic hypertrophic subaortic stenosis, usually results in a marked increase in ventricular wall thickness (especially papillary muscle hypertrophy), a normal or decreased ventricular volume, elevated left ventricular end-diastolic pressure with an *increase* in both the rate of left ventricular pressure development (dP/dt) and ejection fraction (stroke volume/end diastolic volume), and as the alternative term implies, obstruction of the outflow tract of the left ventricle proximal to the aortic valve. Elevated indices of left ventricular contractility with increased left ventricular end-diastolic pressure indicate the hypertrophy that occurs in response to the increased pressure work caused by the outflow tract obstruction results in decreased left ventricular compliance, initially without a depression of ventricular contractile elements.

The exact cause of this obstruction is not known, but in about 30% of such cases, it is seen in several members of the same family. It often affects both ventricles but usually has greater effects on the left side. It appears to develop with hypertrophy and fibrosis of the interventricular septum, occurring first with a marked thickening of the endocardium. A pattern develops so that during systole the anterior leaflet of the mitral valve is pulled into apposition with the interventricular septum and causes both valve and septum to bulge into the outflow tract of the left ventricle. The aortic valve itself is usually normal. Surgical intervention may be necessary to relieve the obstruction in severe cases.

Restrictive Cardiomyopathies occur rarely, usually in association with infiltrative conditions such as amyloidosis, lymphomas, and leukemia. The clinical findings suggest constrictive pericarditis, but the pericardium itself appears normal and has normal compliance characteristics. It is the heart itself, usually the left ventricle, that has become less compliant, resulting in elevated end-diastolic ventricular pressure and atrial pressure, with a decreased cardiac output and perhaps stroke volume.

Ischemic Heart Disease and Myocardial Infarction

The most common pathologic situation leading to cardiac dysfunction is poor perfusion of the heart muscle itself, either as a result of obstruction secondary to clots (*thromboemboli*) or more generalized coronary artery disease, resulting in a progressive narrowing (*stenosis*) of coronary vessels. We can think of the impaired contractility of the myocardium secondary to poor perfusion as an ischemic cardiomyopathy.

Although blood clots (*thrombi*), air bubbles, or fat from bone marrow occasionally may be carried by the blood (such an abnormal blood-borne mass is called an *embolus*) and obstruct or *embolize* coronary blood vessels, by far the most frequent cause of coronary ischemia is an event secondary to coronary heart disease or *atherosclerosis*.

Atherosclerosis is one of the two main disease types that may be referred to by a more generalized term, *arteriosclerosis,* which means hardening of the arteries. It is used to indicate progressive long-standing changes in the structure and mechanical characteristics of the arteries, mainly thickening and stiffening of the vessel walls. The various forms of arteriosclerosis, including atherosclerosis and hypertension, cause almost all heart attacks and strokes. Taken together, heart attack and stroke are the most common causes of death in the United States.

The other major form of arteriosclerosis comprises the alterations that cause *systemic hypertension* (or high blood pressure). Unfortunately, these changes are often referred to as arteriosclerosis, thus leading to confusion because those using the word may not intend to include atherosclerosis in this term. We will use arteriosclerosis to include both atherosclerosis and systemic hypertensive diseases. We can differentiate between the two by the way that the arteries are affected. In systemic hypertension, which is discussed in the next section, small systemic arteries and arterioles are affected. In atherosclerosis, larger arteries, such as the aorta and its major branches, are affected. These include the carotid, cerebral, renal, mesenteric, iliac, femoral, and—most important for our discussion of myocardial ischemic disease—coronary arteries. The second major characteristic distinguishing atherosclerosis from systemic hypertensive disease (besides the hypertension itself) is the characteristic lesion of atherosclerosis, the *atheroma*. Note that a patient may have both hypertensive changes and atherosclerosis.

An atheroma or *atheromatous plaque* is a focal thickening of the innermost layer of an artery (the *intima*—the other two layers are the *media,* or middle layer, and the *adventitia,* or outer layer). It consists of a deposition of cholesterol and cholesteryl ester, fibrous connective tissue, and/or proliferated smooth muscle cells. Atherosclerotic lesions begin to form as isolated atheromas in various larger arteries. As the disease progresses, more and more atheromas develop, and adjacent lesions coalesce to form larger atheromatous plaques. As lipid accumulates, mainly in the form of cholesterol, the intimal layer thickens and begins to narrow the lumen of the artery (Fig. 5–2). Proliferation of fibroblasts (connective tissue cells) occurs, causing the vessels to stiffen. Calcium salts also accumulate in the intimal layer, and collections of dead cells and debris may lead to lighter "hyalinized" areas when viewed with a light microscope.

The effects of the proliferation of atheromatous plaques in the systemic circulation are stenosis, thrombosis, embolism, and aneurysm. As the lesions encroach into the vascular lumens, the resistance to blood flow increases. Irregular, slow blood flow tends to favor the deposition and aggregation of blood platelets and the formation of blood clots. This tendency is greatly increased when the accumulation of lipids and debris ruptures the normally smooth vascular surface, providing both a damaged, irregular surface and the release of thromboxane. Such thrombi may themselves completely occlude arteries, or break off with part of the plaque and be carried by the blood until they lodge in a vessel and occlude it. When this occurs in a coronary vessel, such thrombi and/or emboli may cause a *myocardial infarction;* in the circulation of the brain, they may cause a *cerebrovascular accident* (CVA), or stroke.

An *aneurysm* is a swelling or enlargement of an arterial wall caused by a loss of vascular integrity. The vascular wall may bulge into the lumen, swell outward, or both. Aneurysms bulging into a vessel lumen elevate its resistance to blood flow and may even occlude it. They also form an excellent environment for thrombus formation. The other pos-

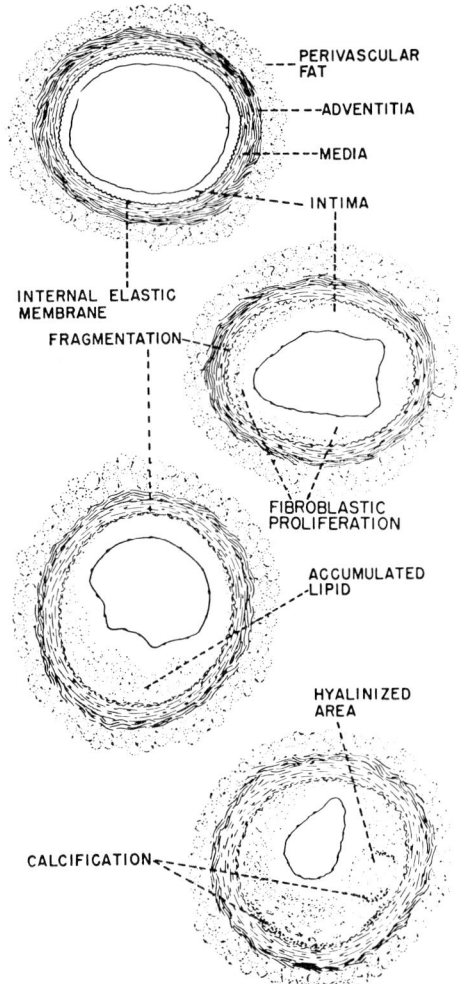

FIGURE 5–2. Progressive alterations in a coronary artery caused by atherosclerosis. The uppermost cross section shows a normal vessel unaffected by atherosclerosis. Early atherosclerosis, shown in the second cross section from the top, is characterized by fragmentation of the internal elastic membrane and a thickening of the intimal layer caused by a proliferation of fibroblasts and an accumulation of mucopolysaccharides. The third cross section shows a progression of encroachment of the vessel lumen caused by lipid accumulation (mainly cholesterol). Finally, the atheroma shows calcifications and hyalinization. (From Rushmer, R.F.: Cardiovascular Dynamics, 4th ed. Philadelphia, W.B. Saunders, 1976, with permission.)

sibility is that the vessel ruptures, allowing blood to leave the vessel. Aneurysms are frequent causative factors in strokes. They may also occur in the aorta itself, with predictably disastrous results.

Ischemic Heart Disease. As atherosclerosis develops, its effects on the coronary vasculature may not produce any symptoms during early stages of the disease. This is because the smaller coronary vessels are still able to dilate in response to increased levels of vasodilator metabolites produced as a result of an increased myocardial metabolic demand. Because normally the coronary arteriovenous oxygen content difference is nearly maximal at rest, the only way the heart can increase its own oxygen supply is to increase coronary blood flow by arteriolar dilation. This is called the *coronary reserve.* In ischemic heart disease, coronary blood flow may be sufficient to meet the metabolic demands of the heart *at rest,* but the vessels can no longer dilate adequately to respond to the increased energy requirements of producing a greater cardiac output, for example, during exercise or even after eating a large meal.

The inability of the coronary circulation to provide blood flow sufficient to meet the increased metabolic demands of the myocardium during exercise is most frequently manifested in the symptom called *angina pectoris* as well as some other symptoms associated with mild heart failure, such as dyspnea (breathlessness), which is discussed shortly. Angina pectoris is a pattern of chest pain that appears to the patient to be localized behind the sternum. This referred pain may also radiate, frequently to the left arm, left shoulder, or even the left side of the face or jaw. The sensation of angina pectoris varies greatly in its severity. During a myocardial infarction, the pain may be intolerable or may be so slight as to be confused with heartburn or indigestion. During ischemic heart disease, it usually takes milder forms, but it is generally sufficient to restrict exercise.

Angina pectoris appears to occur because a limitation of coronary blood flow causes altered metabolism in the affected areas—usually subendocardial, as noted in Chapter 2. The altered metabolism during the ischemia causes release of products that can stimulate what are believed to be free ends of sympathetic afferent nerves in the myocardium. Afferent impulses are carried to the spinal cord at the level of C-7 to T-4 and then relayed to the cerebral cortex via the thalamus. The exact metabolites released during the ischemia that stimulate these receptors are not known but may include kinins, histamine, potassium, and hydrogen ions.

Along with the sensation of angina pectoris, there are both electrocardiographic and mechanical changes associated with myocardial ischemia. The electrocardiographic changes indicate the effects of the myocardial ischemia on the movement of ions within the heart. As we would predict from our discussion of the ionic basis of the electrocardiogram in Chapter 2, transient ischemia first affects the most energy-sensitive aspect of the electrical activity of the heart—repolarization. This is seen in the electrocardiogram as alterations in the T waves, which are often inverted and/or abnormally large during myocardial ischemia (Fig. 5-3B). If the ischemia progresses to cell *injury* during such an episode, as it does frequently, the ST segment is elevated or depressed. As noted in Chapter 2, the ST segment normally falls on the line of zero potential, the isoelectric line. This happens because, at this point in the cardiac cycle, both ventricles are completely depolarized and their repolarization has not yet begun. Thus, there is no net movement of ions into or out of the cell during the ST segment.

During myocardial injury, the cell membrane (the sarcolemma) is not able to maintain its integrity, and ions continue to stream into and out of the myocardial cells. These so-called currents of injury are responsible for depression or elevation of the ST segment (Fig. 5-3C). The characteristic pattern of alterations in the T wave and ST segment of the electrocardiogram seen during myocardial ischemia and injury is one of the major diagnostic aspects of cardiopulmonary stress testing. These tests, which are discussed in Chapter 11, usually involve having the patient exercise by jogging or walking on a treadmill or climbing a small series of steps while the ECG and other cardiopulmonary variables are monitored.

As already noted, ischemia and injury cause alterations in myocardial mechanical function in addition to producing angina pectoris and electrocardiographic alterations. Those areas of the myocardium that receive inadequate perfusion suffer depressed contractile function because local hypoxia prevents normal aerobic metabolism and normal energy production. Affected areas become less compliant during diastole, the stroke volume and ejection fraction decrease, and cardiac output and blood pressure may fall unless the Frank-Starling relationship and/or compensatory reflex mechanisms can maintain them. Left ventricular end-diastolic volume and pressure are likely to increase.

Transient episodes of angina pectoris and the other alterations mentioned before are usually self-limiting in a person with long-standing coronary artery disease. As the person begins to exercise, he or she experiences angina pectoris and stops the increased activity. However, sudden death frequently occurs as a result of ischemic heart disease, most often because of the rapid development of lethal arrhythmias such as ventricular fibrillation. These arrhythmias can develop during such episodes because of the ionic alterations produced by the ischemia and because of the increased excitability of the myocardium caused by high local levels of catecholamines. Norepinephrine and epinephrine are released either as part of cardiovascular reflexes (e.g., the baroreceptor reflex) or in response to the sensation of chest pain and the anxiety associated with it.

More precise characterization of portions of the coronary vasculature affected by atherosclerosis can be obtained by *radionuclide imaging techniques* and by *coronary angiography*. Perfusion scans after injection of radiolabeled cations, such as thallium, rubidium, cesium, or potassium, can reveal unperfused areas of the myocardium. Similarly, during coronary angiography, a radiopaque solution is injected into the ostia of the coronary arteries. Nonperfused or poorly perfused coronary vessels do not show up as the radiopaque material visibly flows through the perfused vessels.

Treatment of coronary artery disease may entail *vasodilating* drugs, such as nitroglycerin and calcium channel blockers; *beta-adrenergic blockers* to decrease cardiac metabolic demands and prevent arrhythmias; and *anticoagulants*. Severe angina pectoris may require relief by *percutaneous transluminal coronary angioplasty,* a technique in which the balloon tip of a special catheter is worked into the stenotic region and inflated during fluoroscopy; or by *coronary bypass surgery,* during which a graft constructed from a normal blood vessel from elsewhere in the body is surgically implanted to bypass the coronary obstruction.

There are a few people with coronary atherosclerosis who do not experience angina pectoris and may therefore be unaware that they have ischemic heart disease. They may die suddenly and unexpectedly, probably as a result of arrhythmias. Another small group of patients experience angina pectoris and other related symptoms at times not associated with exercise or other stresses on the cardiovascular system. This effect is probably a result of abnormally muscular and reactive coronary arteries that go into spasm. These patients therefore suffer from myocardial ischemia related to coronary *vasospasm* rather than atherosclerosis.

Myocardial Infarction. Another potentially lethal consequence of ischemic heart disease is myocardial infarction. An *infarct* is a region of necrotic (i.e., dead) tissue caused by ischemia. Thus, when myocardial *injury* was discussed in the previous section, we used the term *injury* to denote potentially *reversible* damage to the myocardium. If the ischemia is not too long in duration, the myocardial cells may recover and regain their contractility. On

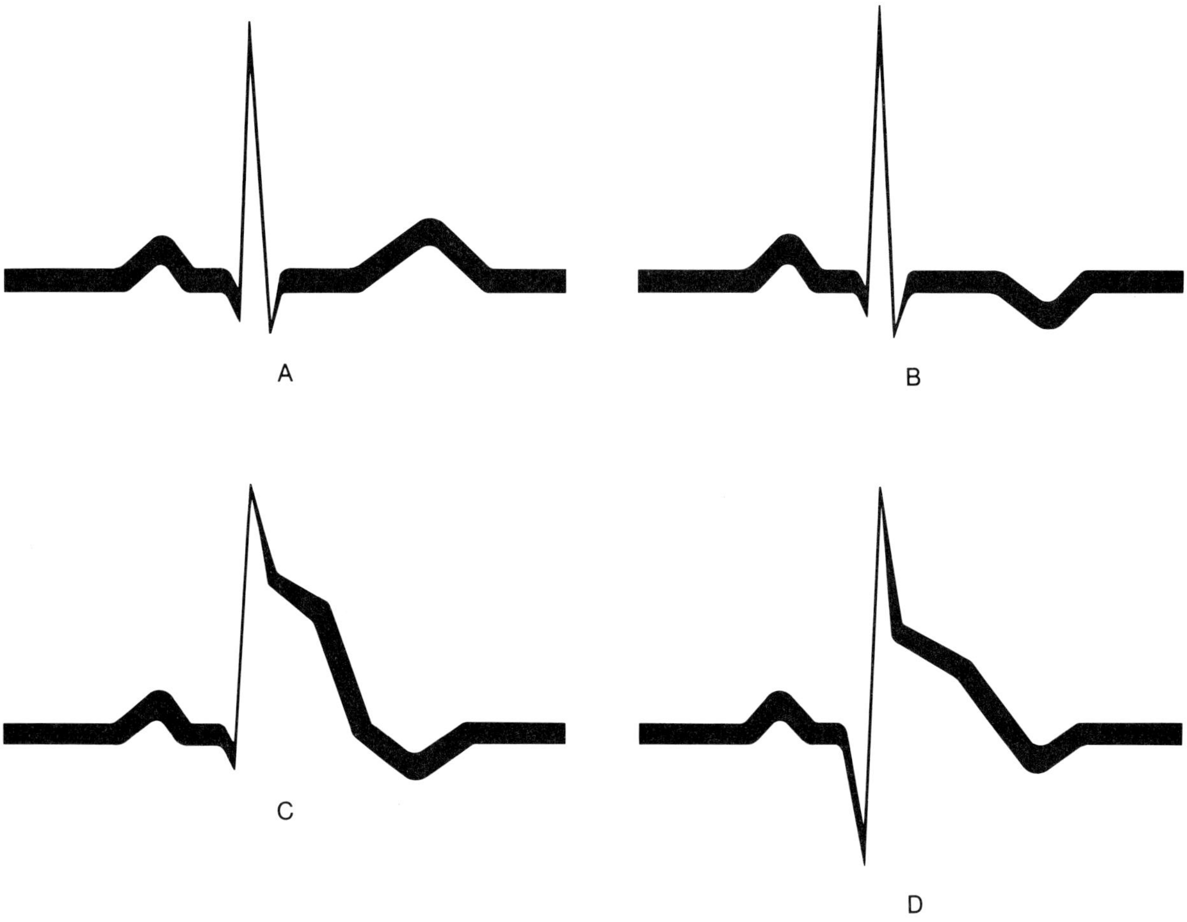

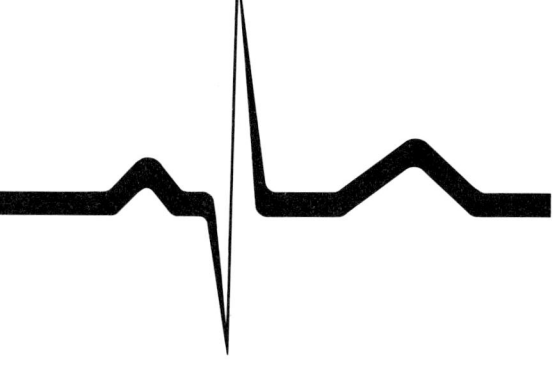

FIGURE 5–3. Progressive alterations in the electrocardiogram following myocardial ischemia, injury and infarction. *A,* Normal. *B,* Ischemia (note the inverted T wave). *C,* Ischemia with injury (note the ST elevation resulting from currents of injury). *D,* Ischemia with injury and infarction (note the prominent S waves, representing tissue no longer electrically excitable). *E,* Old infarct (note the prominent *S* wave without ST segment or T-wave abnormalities).

the other hand, if the ischemia is not relieved, the injury progresses to infarction.

In atherosclerosis, myocardial infarction usually occurs as a result of atheromatous plaques and/or thrombi associated with them, either occluding the coronary artery branch where they have formed, or breaking off and traveling downstream as emboli to occlude vessels. As already mentioned, blood clots, detached fat cells, and air bubbles sometimes cause myocardial infarction, and coronary vasospasms may also play a role.

If a sizable thrombus that had formed on an atheromatous plaque were to break loose in the coronary circulation, it would likely be carried by the blood until it completely occluded a branch of a coronary artery. As it blocked blood flow to the region of the myocardium normally supplied by that branch of the vessel (in humans, the coronary circulation does not have many *collateral vessels* connecting downstream branches of adjacent arteries), the resulting ischemia and hypoxia would interfere with the metabolism of that region. As the metabolic machinery became impaired, the affected myocardium would no longer be able to function.

If a portion of left ventricular muscle were affected, it would bulge out, while unaffected areas of the ventricle continue to contract during systole. At the same time, the electrocardiogram would show signs of ischemia and injury (see Figs. 5–3B and C). The area of the ventricle unable to contract would contribute nothing to the stroke volume (in fact, it would subtract from it), and stroke volume, cardiac output, and blood pressure would decrease unless cardiovascular reflexes (mainly the baroreceptor reflex) could compensate. The ejection fraction would decrease, and left ventricular end-diastolic volume and pressure and pulmonary venous pressure would increase. The patient would probably experience severe angina pectoris.

As the injury proceeded irreversibly to infarction, the electrocardiographic pattern would change to one like that seen in Figure 5–3D. Prominent Q waves are electrocardiographic evidence of an infarct. They represent an area of the myocardium that is no longer electrically excitable. Vectors that normally cancel out those in the opposite direction are no longer present, and the mean electrical axis is momentarily "pulled" away from the infarcted area.

Figure 5–3D shows a prominent Q wave, ST elevation, and T wave inversion, indicating the coexistence of ischemia, injury, and infarct. This pattern is typical during myocardial infarction, with a central area of necrotic tissue surrounded by a ring of injured tissue (the *border zone*) that may be possible to save and an outermost region that is merely ischemic (Fig. 5–4). Figure 5–3E shows an electrocardiographic pattern associated with an old healed infarct, as would be seen in a person who had survived a myocardial infarction. Signs of ischemia and injury are gone, with only prominent Q waves remaining. Such a pattern would be seen days after the infarction and would persist indefinitely until the patient had another infarction and/or died.

The diagnosis of myocardial infarction is based on one or more of the following symptoms: chest pain, which can range from mild discomfort to excruciating pain, dyspnea or breathlessness, palpitations, syncope, nausea, and anxiety. The characteristic electrocardiographic changes already described are often accompanied by arrhythmias with either tachycardia or bradycardia, hypotension, heart murmurs, abnormal lung sounds, and evidence of abnormal ventricular wall motion (*dyskinesis*). Chest radiographs may show signs of pulmonary vascular congestion or edema.

During infarction of the left ventricle, right heart catheterization with a Swan-Ganz catheter would reveal elevated pulmonary artery and pulmonary capillary wedge pressures, the latter reflecting the increased left ventricular end-diastolic pressure (LVEDP). Left heart catheterization would show decreased left ventricular dP/dt in addition to the increased LVEDP.

Echocardiography may show dyskinesis and abnormalities of wall thickness. Various radionuclide imaging techniques can show poor or absent perfusion of the infarcted area (perfusion scans using intravenous radiolabeled thallium, rubidium, cesium, potassium, or red blood cells) or preferential uptake of some radiolabeled tracers by acutely infarcted tissue.

Also associated with myocardial infarction are other signs of tissue damage, including elevated plasma potassium ion levels and the appearance of intracellular myocardial enzymes such as the

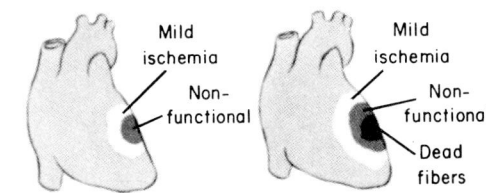

FIGURE 5–4. Concentric zones of myocardial ischemia, injury, and infarction. (From Guyton, A.C.: *Textbook of Medical Physiology*, 7th ed. Philadelphia, W.B. Saunders, 1986, with permission.)

cardiac forms of creatine phosphokinase (CPK), serum glutamic-oxaloacetic transaminase (SGOT), and lactate dehydrogenase (LDH) in the blood.

The outcome of a myocardial infarction depends on the size and location of the region affected. Areas of the right ventricle and atria can be infarcted as well as the left ventricular infarction discussed here. These are usually less serious because the atria and right ventricle do not have to perform as much pressure work as does the left ventricle. Infarctions involving pacemaker or high-speed conducting tissue of the heart may lead to all sorts of arrhythmias, many of which are described in Chapter 8. As already noted, arrhythmias may occur without involvement of the pacemaker high-speed conduction pathway, and ventricular fibrillation may be a lethal outcome of a myocardial infarction. Other potential sequelae of myocardial infarction include heart failure with either peripheral or pulmonary congestion and edema, which are discussed later in this chapter, and cardiac tamponade, which may occur following the weakening of the infarcted area and its subsequent rupture, allowing blood to fill the pericardial sac.

Hypertension

Hypertension means high blood pressure. In common usage, the term hypertension by itself, without any modifiers, means *systemic arterial hypertension* and does not refer to high blood pressure in the pulmonary artery (*pulmonary hypertension*) or the portal vein of the liver (*portal hypertension*). Systemic arterial hypertension can be caused by a number of diseases and disorders and should not be considered as a single disease.

Definition of Hypertension. The clinical definition of systemic arterial hypertension is somewhat controversial because the *range* of normal blood pressure is not clearly defined. Furthermore, the mean "normal" arterial blood pressure increases with age in nearly every society that has been studied. Mean *diastolic* arterial blood pressure increases from 75 to about 85 mmHg between approximately 21 to 45 years of age and increases very slightly thereafter. Mean *systolic* arterial blood pressure increases more rapidly and continues to increase at about the same rate through the later decades of life, rising from about 120 mmHg at 21 years of age to about 150 mmHg at 75 years of age. These age-related changes are mainly a result of structural alterations in the aorta and large arteries, which become less distensible, primarily because of changes in the mechanical properties of the collagen and elastin fibers of these vessels. Thus, clinical decisions on whether a particular patient's blood pressure constitutes hypertension and should be treated depend on what is considered to be the normal range for a person in that age group.

Causes of Hypertension. Hypertension is a condition that can be caused by many diseases and factors. Blood pressure is a function of the cardiac output and systemic vascular resistance, and anything that can interfere with the normal *regulation* of these components may produce hypertension. Additionally, long-standing hypertension can perpetuate hypertension itself because high blood pressure appears to cause changes in the structure of blood vessels, especially a thickening of the arterial wall, and it may also cause an adaptive "resetting" of the baroreceptor reflex to a higher blood pressure level.

Generally, systemic arterial hypertension can be classified by the etiologic factors involved in its production. Cases of hypertension for which no clear cause can be determined are termed *essential hypertension* (or *primary* or *idiopathic hypertension*). Cases that can be attributed to other diseases or conditions are called *secondary hypertension*.

Many renal diseases can cause a secondary systemic arterial hypertension (*renal hypertension*), because the kidney is both directly involved in blood pressure regulation and it indirectly affects blood pressure as it regulates body fluids, electrolytes, and especially blood volume. Any disease that inactivates or destroys a sufficient amount of renal tissue to impair its ability to eliminate an elevated plasma volume may lead to hypertension caused by hypervolemia. Acute glomerulonephritis is an example of a renal parenchymal disease that can cause systemic arterial hypertension.

The kidney's participation in the regulation of systemic arterial blood pressure is mediated through the renin-angiotensin-aldosterone system (see Chapter 2). Any disease or condition that impairs renal arterial blood flow leads to increased release of renin by the juxtaglomerular cells of the kidney. The elevated plasma renin activity converts angiotensinogen to angiotensin I, which is subsequently converted to angiotensin II. Angiotensin is a potent arteriolar constrictor, it potentiates sympathetic effects, and it stimulates aldosterone release, leading to sodium retention and plasma volume expansion. Renal atherosclerosis, fibrotic proliferation of the vessel wall, embolic obstruction, compression or obstruction by tumors, and the results of trauma are all possible causes of hypertension secondary to decreased renal blood flow (*renovascular hypertension*). The kidney may also normally produce a substance (or substances) that tonically decreases systemic arterial blood pressure.

Several endocrine disorders can cause systemic arterial hypertension. One of the rarest of these is also the easiest to understand. *Pheochromocytoma* denotes tumors of the medullary portion of the adrenal gland (or other tissue) that can produce and secrete epinephrine and norepinephrine. Patients with these tumors may have persistent hypertension and/or episodes of severe hypertension, tachycardia, headache, nausea, perspiration, chest pain, and anxiety. Adrenergic blocking drugs can temporarily reduce the blood pressure. The tumors must be surgically excised.

The adrenal cortex is also susceptible to tumors (or occasionally simply hyperplasia) that can result in an overproduction and secretion of aldosterone. This is called *primary aldosteronism* (Conn's disease). Patients with this disorder often have hypertension caused by both hypervolemia (resulting in an elevated cardiac output) and elevated systemic vascular resistance. The hypervolemia is a result of increased sodium and water retention. These patients also suffer from hypokalemia. Other endocrine disorders associated with hypertension include Cushing's syndrome (glucocorticoid excess resulting from various causes), excess mineralocorticoids (for reasons other than those noted above), thyroid hormone disorders, and acromegaly (excess growth hormone in adults). Oral contraceptives may also be associated with hypertension in some cases. We have already discussed the hypertension associated with toxemia of pregnancy in Chapter 4.

Hypertension caused by abnormalities in the central nervous system is referred to as *neurogenic hypertension*. Although *anxiety* has often been linked to elevated blood pressure, no clear-cut relationship has been demonstrated. *Elevated intracranial pressure* reflexly causes systemic arterial hypertension (see Chapter 2). This response (the *Cushing response*) maintains cerebral perfusion if intracranial pressure is elevated by the growth of a tumor, overproduction or decreased removal of CSF, or extravasated blood. Other diseases or disturbances of the central nervous system can also lead to hypertension.

Coarctation of the Aorta is a congenital narrowing of the aorta in the region of the ductus arteriosus. The hypertension associated with aortic coarctation is thought to be mainly a result of the mechanical obstruction and decreased capacitance of the aorta. However, it is also possible that part of the hypertension is a result of other mechanisms, including autoregulatory dilation of arterioles distal to the coarctation, and the renal pressor mechanisms previously discussed. Thus, it appears that pressure proximal to the narrowed region may be increased in order to maintain the perfusion of the vessels distal to it.

Essential or Primary Hypertension is systemic arterial hypertension not directly attributable to the causative factors discussed above. However, it is possible that any of them (or any combination of them) may ultimately be demonstrated to be important in its etiology. Similarly, it is also possible that essential hypertension is not a single disease entity. For one thing, some people with essential hypertension have high blood pressure all of the time. They are said to have *fixed* or *established hypertension*. Others have intermittent episodes of high blood pressure. They are said to have *labile hypertension*. The term *malignant hypertension* is used to describe patients with very rapidly developing increases (over 1 to 2 years) in blood pressure. As is apparent from the name, this condition is associated with very high mortality, especially that resulting from strokes.

Finally, there are some conditions that lead to systolic hypertension without much of an increase in diastolic pressure. These are results of either elevated left ventricular stroke volumes or decreased distensibility of the aorta. For example, complete heart block results in very low heart rates. Because of increased time for ventricular filling, left ventricular end-diastolic volume and pressure are elevated. Stroke volume is increased by the Frank-Starling mechanism. However, diastolic pressure is likely to be normal or low because of greater time for blood to flow out of the arterial tree before the next stroke volume is ejected into it. Similarly, aortic valve incompetence (discussed in the next section), a patent ductus arteriosus (discussed in the next chapter), and arteriovenous fistulas all result in elevated stroke volumes with increased diastolic runoff. Thyrotoxicosis (excess thyroid hormone) usually affects systolic blood pressure more than it does diastolic pressure. Arteriosclerosis or coarctation of the aorta should also affect systolic blood pressure more than diastolic blood pressure by decreasing the distensibility of the aorta.

The treatment of a particular patient's hypertension depends on whether its source can be identified. If the hypertension is secondary to another disease state, treatment is likely to focus on the underlying cause of the hypertension. If an underlying cause cannot be determined, or if the hypertension persists despite treatment of the causative factor, then a number of treatment modalities are available. These mainly include the use of beta-adrenergic blocking drugs, calcium channel blockers, angiotensin-converting enzyme (ACE) inhibitors, thiazide and other types of diuretics, and other vasodilating drugs (see Chapter 15).

Valvular Dysfunctions

Diseases and disorders of the aortic valve and mitral valve may lead to left ventricular hypertrophy or failure or both. *Aortic stenosis* and *aortic insufficiency* can overburden the left ventricle, as can *mitral insufficiency*. *Mitral stenosis* puts an increased pressure load on the right ventricle; it is discussed in the section on right heart failure. Note that valves may suffer from a combination of stenosis and insufficiency and that some diseases often affect several of the valves in both the right and left ventricle simultaneously. Echocardiography, which allows a graphic interpretation of cardiac valve function, is useful in the diagnosis of valvular dysfunctions.

Aortic Stenosis is seen most frequently as a result of rheumatic fever, and it usually occurs with mitral valve dysfunction following this disease. Rheumatic fever is an occasional sequela to upper respiratory tract bacterial infections that results in inflammation of the heart, often including the cardiac valves and pericardium. When aortic stenosis occurs as an isolated uncomplicated lesion (as discussed here), it is usually either a congenitally obstructed valve (especially when seen in patients under 15 years old), a congenitally abnormal valve that degenerates later in life (patients 15 to 65), or a normal valve that degenerates later in life from atherosclerosis or other problems (patients over 65).

The initial physiologic consequence of aortic stenosis is that the left ventricle must do more work to deliver the same stroke volume through a higher resistance to blood flow. Because the stenosis usually develops slowly, the ventricle can adapt to the increased resistance to blood flow by developing greater pressure. Remember that local autoregulatory mechanisms work to maintain blood flow to the various organs of the body, whereas the systemic arterial baroreceptor reflex attempts to maintain systemic arterial pressure by increasing sympathetic tone to the heart and some vascular beds.

Cardiac catheterization reveals the important features of the pathophysiology of aortic stenosis. Figure 5–5 shows two traces obtained simultaneously from catheters in a patient with aortic stenosis. The narrowed stenotic valve has greatly increased the pressure gradient between the left ventricle and the aorta during systole. Compare this figure with the aortic and ventricular pressure traces in Figure 2–19. In order to maintain aortic pressure at a reasonable level, left ventricular pressure must be increased substantially. Also note how slowly the aortic pressure rises during ventricular systole in the patient with aortic stenosis shown in Figure 5–5, whereas aortic pressure normally rises almost simultaneously with ventricular pressure.

As aortic stenosis progresses from mild obstruction to nearly complete obstruction (the patient from whom Figure 5–5 was obtained had severe obstruction), a predictable sequence of physiologic alterations and their associated symptoms occurs. The response of the left ventricle to a chronic pressure load is *hypertrophy,* and increase in muscle mass and wall thickness. Although the left ventricular end-diastolic volume and end-systolic volume do not increase initially, as the stenosis progresses they will increase, and the ejection fraction will decrease.

The increased energy demand of the elevated pressure development, combined with increased blood flow required by the increased mass of muscle tissue, place a great stress on the coronary circulation and may result in myocardial ischemia. Coronary blood flow may be further compromised if aortic pressure falls (especially diastolic), because aortic pressure provides the energy for coronary perfusion. Thus, the presenting symptoms of aortic stenosis are usually fatigue, dyspnea, and/or syncope (fainting or feeling faint), especially during exercise. Because resistance takes *time* to overcome, the increased heart rate of exercise does not increase cardiac output efficiently. Angina pectoris and symptoms of left ventricular failure are common in later stages in older patients.

Aortic stenosis is almost always associated with a systolic heart murmur that begins with the opening of the aortic valve (after S_1) and ends before it closes (before S_2). It is loudest over the aortic area (see Chapters 7 and 8) and is usually diamond-shaped on a phonocardiogram. A *thrill* (vibrations felt over the skin) may also be present over the aortic area. The electrocardiogram should show signs of hypertrophy (e.g., increased amplitudes of the QRS complex) and may also indicate ischemia (e.g., altered T waves and ST depression or elevation). Chest radiographs should show an enlarged ventricle in later stages, due to both hy-

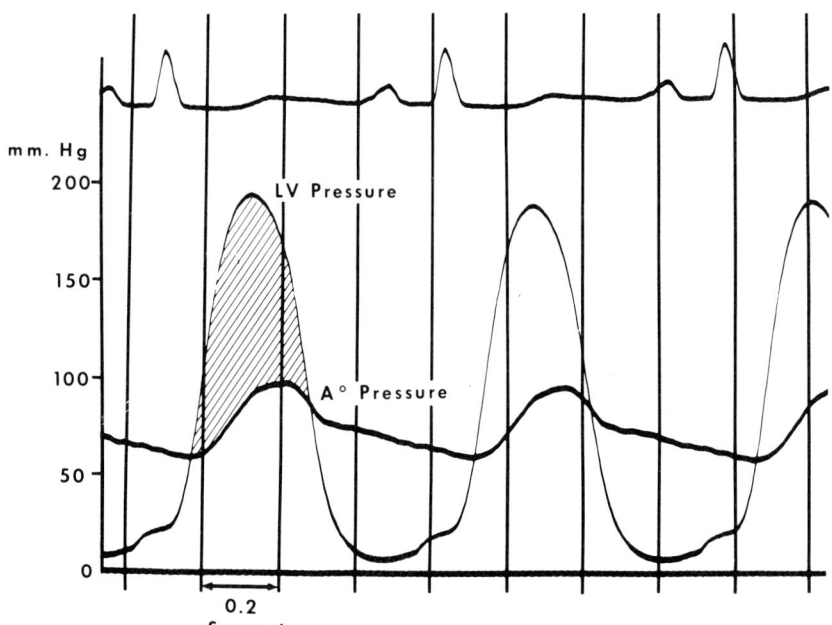

FIGURE 5-5. Cardiac catheterization data from a patient with severe aortic stenosis. Top trace represents ECG. (A° pressure = aortic pressure; LV pressure = left ventricular pressure.) Note the large systolic pressure gradient between the left ventricle and the aorta (shaded area). (From Sodeman, W.A., Jr., and Sodeman, T.M. (eds.): *Sodeman's Pathologic Physiology: Mechanisms of Disease*, 6th ed. Philadelphia, W.B. Saunders, 1979, with permission.)

pertrophy and dilation of the ventricle. The treatment for aortic stenosis is to surgically replace the valve with a prosthetic valve or xenograft or allograft. Note that idiopathic hypertrophic subaortic stenosis has many symptoms in common with aortic stenosis.

Aortic Insufficiency or *aortic regurgitation*, is a condition in which the aortic valve is no longer competent. That is, it no longer closes completely during diastole. Although rheumatic heart disease remains the major etiologic factor of aortic insufficiency, many other disorders can cause it. These include congenital abnormalities, aortitis secondary to syphilis, aneurysms, Marfan's syndrome, bacterial endocarditis, severe hypertension, and chest wall trauma.

The physiologic problem in aortic insufficiency is evident if we consider the cardiac cycle (see Fig. 2–19). As the left ventricle relaxes, left ventricular pressure normally falls far below aortic pressure. This pressure drop can occur because the aortic valve normally closes as soon as ventricular pressure falls just below that in the aorta. The blood in the arterial tree cannot flow backward into the ventricle; instead, it flows through the resistance vessels into the peripheral tissues.

If the aortic valve does not close properly, as the left ventricle relaxes, blood flows backward into the left ventricle. The volume of these *retrograde* blood flows varies according to the severity of the incompetency of the valve, but values between 20 and 80 ml/beat are not uncommon, and much higher values have been observed. Consider that a 70 kg man normally has a stroke volume of about 70 ml. To maintain a normal cardiac output, the left ventricle must generate a very large *total* stroke volume to produce an adequate *net* stroke volume (the stroke volume after regurgitated volume has been subtracted). Thus, aortic incompetence puts a volume load on the left ventricle. The left ventricle is able to meet this demand early in the disease because of the Frank-Starling mechanism. The volume of blood regurgitated into the left ventricle during diastole results in a very large left ventricular end-diastolic volume and elevated left ventricular end-diastolic pressure. Additional demand for cardiac output (e.g., during exercise) can initially be met with sympathetically mediated increases in contractility and heart rate.

The hemodynamic effects of aortic insufficiency are shown in the cardiac catheterization traces in Figure 5-6. As we would predict from our knowledge of the cardiac cycle, reflux of blood from the aorta into the left ventricle during diastole and very large stroke volumes result in very large aortic pulse pressures. During systole, the increased stroke volumes ejected into the aorta result in high systolic pressures, even if the distensibility of the aorta is normal. During diastole, rapid regurgitation of blood back into the ventricle results in low aortic diastolic pressure. The pulse pressure (systolic minus diastolic), therefore, is elevated. Left ventricular systolic pressure is also elevated because of the increased stroke volume; further-

conditions that put an abnormal pressure load on the heart, such as systemic arterial hypertension or aortic stenosis; and conditions that put a volume load on the heart, such as aortic or mitral insufficiency and arteriovenous shunts. Note that some people may have heart disease without symptoms of failure. They are said to be *compensated*. Patients showing symptoms of failure are said to be *decompensated*.

In this section, the pathophysiologic aspects of left ventricular failure are discussed. We have already noted most of these in the preceding sections; nearly all of them are easy to predict if we consider how the problem affects the physiologic mechanisms already covered in Chapters 2 and 3.

As the left ventricle fails, it is no longer able to perform work (stroke work = stroke volume × aortic pressure). Patients are weak and feel fatigued. As Figure 5–9 shows, this results in a downward shift in the Frank-Starling curve (see also Fig. 2–21), so for a given left ventricular end-diastolic pressure (labeled LV filling pressure), less left ventricular stroke work is performed. As the failure progresses, the stroke volume decreases. If pulmonary venous return exceeds the output of the left ventricle, left ventricular end-diastolic pressure increases (Figs. 5–9 and 5–10). At high left ventricular end-diastolic volumes, the function of the already impaired ventricle can be exacerbated because, according to Laplace's Law,

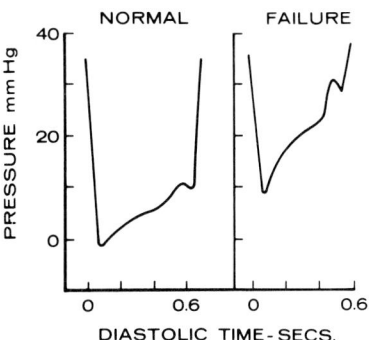

FIGURE 5–10. Left ventricular diastolic pressure traces of normal and failing left ventricles. Note the elevated left ventricular diastolic pressure and more rapid diastolic pressure increase with filling during failure. (From Sodeman, W.A., Jr., and Sodeman, T.M., (eds.): *Sodeman's Pathologic Physiology: Mechanisms of Disease*, 6th ed. Philadelphia, W.B. Saunders, 1979, with permission.)

$T = P \times r$. As the radius of the dilated ventricle increases, it must generate more wall tension to generate the same pressure. During diastole, left atrial pressure is dependent on (and slightly higher than) left ventricular pressure, so it increases also.

Because there are no valves between the left atrium and pulmonary veins or in the pulmonary veins themselves, both pulmonary venous pressure and pulmonary capillary hydrostatic pressure increase. This leads to pulmonary vascular congestion, which decreases pulmonary compliance. As pulmonary capillary hydrostatic pressure continues to increase, pulmonary interstitial edema may develop. The decreased pulmonary compliance and stimulation of pulmonary "J" receptors by pulmonary vascular congestion and interstitial edema may cause dyspnea (a feeling of shortness of breath), especially on exertion or episodically at night (paroxysmal nocturnal dyspnea). Patients may also experience orthopnea (less dyspnea if they sit up or stand, than if they lie down). The pulmonary interstitial edema may interfere with gas exchange in the lungs and may even progress to life-threatening alveolar flooding. Such cases of pulmonary edema must be relieved rapidly.

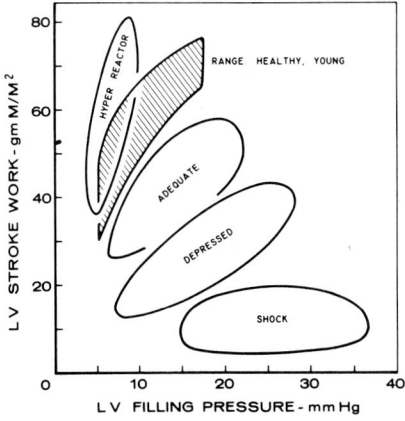

FIGURE 5–9. Ranges of left ventricular work curves ("Starling curves") for normal young healthy adults; those with enhanced responses (for example, during sympathetic stimulation); and those with varying degrees of left ventricular depression. Note that sympathetic stimulation shifts the curve to the left and makes it steeper, and depression shifts the curve to the right and decreases its slope. (From Sodeman, W.A., Jr., and Sodeman, T.M., (eds.): *Sodeman's Pathologic Physiology: Mechanisms of Disease*, 6th ed. Philadelphia, W.B. Saunders, 1979, with permission.)

The effects of an inadequate left ventricular output on the systemic circulation are mainly a result of the reduced perfusion of the peripheral tissues, either as a direct consequence of the decreased perfusion *pressure* or as a consequence of compensatory reflexes like the baroreceptor reflex. Patients may appear confused or forgetful as a result of insufficient cerebral blood flow. Baroreceptor reflex–mediated increases in sympathetic tone (parasympathetic tone is decreased) usually result in tachycardia, cutaneous vasoconstriction, perspiration, and decreased gastrointestinal and renal blood flow. Decreased perfusion of metabolically active tissues may lead to a reduced mixed venous oxygen content. (Recall that oxygen consumption = blood flow × arteriovenous oxygen content difference.) The reduced mixed venous oxygen content, along with mismatched ventilation and perfusion in the lung and impaired diffusion because of pulmonary vascular congestion and edema, decrease the arterial oxygen content and PaO_2. The decreased arterial oxygen content and reduced cutaneous perfusion may cause the patient to appear cyanotic.

Reduced renal perfusion decreases the ability of the kidneys to eliminate fluid volume. As renal perfusion pressure is decreased, the glomerular filtration rate is decreased, renin is released, and the angiotensin-aldosterone system is activated. Elevated levels of aldosterone cause sodium and water retention and exacerbate the buildup of fluid in the lungs and peripheral tissues, thus tending to increase the blood volume. It is also possible for left ventricular failure to cause right ventricular failure by increasing pressures in the pulmonary circulation. This is sometimes called *backward failure*. We will discuss right ventricular failure shortly, but at this point, we can predict that it will lead to systemic venous congestion and hypertension, and possibly peripheral edema.

The retention of fluid secondary to impaired renal perfusion, along with pulmonary vascular congestion and edema and the possibility of venous congestion and peripheral edema, have resulted in the use of the term *congestive heart failure* for patients with these symptoms. If congestive heart failure is not treated, it can progress to a state called *shock*. In this case, because the shock is secondary to cardiac failure, it would be called *cardiogenic shock*. We can define shock as a state in which the heart and/or peripheral vasculature are unable to maintain adequate perfusion of the vital organs. Shock may also be a result of trauma, hemorrhage, infection, and burns. It is characterized by hypotension, tachycardia, sweating, pallor, decreased urine production, cyanosis, acidosis, hyperventilation, and altered mental status, especially loss of consciousness. Note that these correspond to the alterations from hemorrhage (see Chapter 4). The decreased perfusion of peripheral tissues in shock can lead to changes in metabolism that can cause irreversible damage in some tissues, especially the brain and heart.

Treatment of congestive heart failure involves an immediate attempt to reduce the preload and/or afterload on the heart, increase cardiac performance, restore the perfusion of peripheral tissues, and relieve the pulmonary and systemic vascular congestion. The preload and much of the congestion are usually relieved by using strong diuretic drugs to decrease body fluids. Peripheral vasodilators like nitroglycerin or adrenergic blocking drugs are used to decrease the afterload of the left ventricle and restore peripheral perfusion. Positive inotropic agents like digitalis are used to improve cardiac performance and increase the stroke volume. Of course, over the long term, the underlying cause of the failure should be alleviated or removed, if possible. This may include valve replacement, treatment of hypertension, coronary bypass, angioplasty operations or even heart transplants.

Right Heart Failure

Right heart failure can be defined as any condition in which the right ventricle is unable to produce an output adequate to keep pace with venous return. The major feature of right heart failure is therefore *venous congestion,* with an elevated central venous pressure. The right ventricle can better adapt to an increased volume load than it can to an increased pressure load, so right ventricular failure is much more likely to result from such conditions as pulmonary vascular diseases, primary pulmonary diseases with secondary pulmonary hypertension, valvular dysfunctions (pulmonary and mitral valve stenosis), and left ventricular failure causing pulmonary vascular congestion and hypertension. These are in addition to conditions that may directly affect the right ventricular muscle, such as myocardial ischemia, infarction, and cardiomyopathies, which have already been discussed.

Pulmonary Vascular Diseases

Although pulmonary hypertension is said to exist when pulmonary artery pressure is increased by 5 to 10 mmHg above the normal average pressure of 25/10 (with a mean of 15 to 18), a pressure of 35/15 with a mean of 25 has little clinical significance. Mean pulmonary artery pressures above 30 to 35 mmHg, however, may compromise the right ventricle.

Table 5–1 lists some of the main conditions that can cause pulmonary hypertension. These can be divided into diseases and disorders that occlude or obliterate pulmonary blood vessels and those that

TABLE 5–1. Classification of the Causes of Pulmonary Hypertension

Occlusion of Blood Vessels
Pulmonary emboli
Pulmonary vasculitis
Primary pulmonary hypertension
Pulmonary veno-occlusive disease

Obliteration of Blood Vessels
Emphysema
Interstitial infiltration
Surgical resection

Hypoxia with Normal Lungs
Obesity
Neuromuscular diseases
Upper airway obstruction
Chronic mountain sickness

Hypoxia with Abnormal Lungs
Chronic bronchitis
Alveolar infiltrations
Bronchial asthma
Kyphoscoliosis

From Hinshaw, H.C., and Murray, J.F.: *Diseases of the Chest*, 4th ed. Philadelphia, W.B. Saunders, 1980, with permission.

cause hypoxia and hypercapnia, either as a result of primary diseases of the lung or secondary to other respiratory problems or disorders.

Occlusion of Pulmonary Blood Vessels. Portions of the pulmonary vasculature can be occluded by emboli, vasculitis, smooth muscle hypertrophy, and fibrous tissue proliferation. *Pulmonary emboli* usually occur as a result of blood or fibrin clot formation elsewhere in the body. As noted previously, such emboli are carried by the venous blood to the lungs, where they lodge in small vessels. Most pulmonary emboli are caused by acute injuries or the immobility of limbs (usually the legs) following injury or surgery. Immobility leads to venous *stasis* (poor blood flow with blood collecting and stagnating in the veins), thus predisposing a person to the formation of blood clots. Obesity and pregnancy may also cause venous stasis. Pulmonary emboli usually are an acute problem because the fibrinolytic capabilities of the pulmonary vascular endothelium (see Chapter 3) can break such clots down within 4 or 5 days. Under most circumstances, the fact that all pulmonary capillaries are not normally perfused at resting cardiac outputs allows recruitment of unaffected vessels and prevents pulmonary hypertension, except in the most severe cases. Although rare, some patients have chronic recurrent pulmonary embolisms that may occlude a sufficient portion of the pulmonary vasculature to cause chronic pulmonary hypertension. The emboli may be of various sizes, or more rarely small and fairly uniform clots, originating in the leg veins.

The symptoms of pulmonary embolism are dependent on the size and number of the emboli. Small emboli may be asymptomatic. Accumulation of many small emboli does decrease the ability to recruit pulmonary capillaries, so exercise may provoke dyspnea and syncope. Pulmonary hypertension may be present, even at rest. Larger pulmonary emboli are usually associated with dyspnea, pleuritic pain, and *hemoptysis* (coughing up blood). Massive pulmonary embolism can produce circulatory collapse, shock, severe dyspnea, chest pain, tachypnea with shallow breaths, tachycardia, fever, and occasionally, cyanosis.

Diagnosis of pulmonary embolism is based on chest radiographs; electrocardiograms, which may show right ventricular strain or hypertrophy; arterial blood gases, which may indicate an arterial-alveolar CO_2 gradient and hypoxemia; lung scans for the distribution of ventilation and perfusion; pulmonary angiography; and fibrinogen scanning.

Treatment of patients with pulmonary embolism usually involves maintenance of the patient's blood pressure and blood gases, prevention of more emboli, attempts to dissolve the emboli present, and if necessary, surgical removal of large emboli. Patients are treated with anticoagulants, such as *heparin* or *warfarin,* to prevent further thrombus formation. Fibrinolytic drugs, such as *urokinase* and *streptokinase,* may be used to break down existing thrombi. Surgical procedures in the past aimed at preventing the movement of venous thrombi to the lungs have included ligating or clipping large veins, but these procedures are no longer widely employed. A more commonly used procedure is the intravenous insertion of a *vena cava "umbrella" filter* under fluoroscopy. The filter is maneuvered into the vena cava with the umbrella closed. It is then opened so that it can trap emboli, which can be removed. In cases of massive pulmonary embolism, *pulmonary embolectomy* may be attempted to surgically remove the clots from the pulmonary vasculature.

Although the enzymatic machinery of the pulmonary vasculature is able to break down many substances presented to it, many other foreign substances provoke granulomatous inflammatory reactions. Such substances may include living parasites, their products, or their eggs, as in schistosomiasis; or insoluble organic or inorganic material, such as the impurities in preparations taken by chronic intravenous drug abusers. These inflammatory reactions may cause irreversible occlusion of pulmonary vessels widespread enough to remove a sufficient number of parallel pathways for blood flow to result in intractable pulmonary hypertension.

Several systemic diseases can cause *pulmonary vasculitis* (inflammation of pulmonary blood vessels) severe enough to cause pulmonary hypertension. These include scleroderma, rheumatoid arthritis, and systemic lupus erythematosis—all diseases associated with collagen proliferation.

Primary Pulmonary Hypertension is the term for pulmonary hypertension that cannot be attributed to any known cause. This small group of patients does seem to be suffering from a specific disease because the symptoms and course of the disease as well as the pathologic picture are similar in all patients. Although primary (or idiopathic) pulmonary hypertension is seen in both sexes and all age groups, it appears to occur most frequently in young to middle-aged women. The presenting symptoms usually include fatigue and dyspnea on exertion. These are caused by lesions in the pulmonary arteries, including greatly thickened arterial walls with narrowing of the arterial lumen by hypertrophied medial smooth muscle and proliferating intima. Later stages of the disease are characterized by the so-called *plexiform lesions,* in which dilated aneurysmic small muscular pulmonary arteries display a proliferation of intimal cells into the vessel lumen with smaller capillary-like channels permitting some blood flow through them. Other indications of advanced disease include necrosis, thrombosis, and aneurysms.

Primary pulmonary hypertension is a rapidly progressing irreversible disease for which there is no effective therapy. As the disease progresses, pulmonary hypertension becomes more and more severe, with pulmonary artery pressures of 90 mmHg or more a frequent finding. Vascular occlusion and elevated pulmonary artery pressure cause right ventricular hypertrophy, restriction of cardiac output, and ultimately, failure. Death usually occurs within 2 to 8 years of the diagnosis.

Another rare disorder, called *pulmonary veno-occlusive disease,* causes proliferative fibrous occlusion of small- and medium-sized pulmonary veins throughout the lungs. Patients with this disease, usually children or young adults, may suffer from severe dyspnea and pulmonary edema on exertion. Pulmonary venous thrombosis, possibly caused by viral infections, may be etiologic factors in this disease. Pulmonary hypertension, congestion, edema, and right ventricular hypertrophy are usually found in patients with pulmonary veno-occlusive disease. Typically they die within one year of the onset of its symptoms.

Obliteration of Blood Vessels. Any disease, condition, or surgical procedure that causes the loss or obliteration of a significant portion of the pulmonary vascular bed can cause an increase in pulmonary vascular resistance. If cardiac output is maintained or elevated, pulmonary hypertension may result.

Emphysema (discussed in greater detail later) destroys alveolar septa and thus obliterates large numbers of pulmonary capillaries. However, since only about half of the pulmonary capillaries are normally perfused at resting cardiac outputs, others can be recruited as emphysema progresses. "Pure" emphysema does not usually involve significant alveolar hypoxia, so pulmonary hypertension with consequent right ventricular failure is not seen until the very late stages of pure emphysema.

Many lung diseases of differing origins result in diffuse granulomatous reactions or fibrous tissue infiltrations of the pulmonary parenchyma. Pulmonary capillaries and other small vessels may be obliterated by these processes. Because of the vast number of pulmonary vascular pathways, pulmonary hypertension and right ventricular hypertrophy and failure do not usually occur until the advanced stages of such diseases as sarcoidosis, diffuse alveolar interstitial fibrosis, pneumoconiosis, and related conditions. Similarly, a considerable amount of lung tissue can be surgically resected without causing pulmonary hypertension. As much as 60% to 70% of the total pulmonary vascular bed may be removed without the development of pulmonary hypertension at resting cardiac outputs. It is reasonable to assume that a similar amount can be obliterated without the development of pulmonary hypertension.

Hypoxia with Normal or Abnormal Lungs. As noted in the section on control of pulmonary vascular resistance, alveolar hypoxia (and/or hypercapnia) causes an active constriction of the pulmonary vasculature. *Hypoxic pulmonary vasoconstriction* can be an important mechanism for diverting blood flow away from poorly ventilated alveoli, thereby reducing the pulmonary venous admixture and helping to maintain arterial P_{O_2}. However, many diseases of the respiratory system may directly or indirectly cause chronic hypoxia of large regions of the lungs, or even all of the alveoli. Such diseases, some of which are listed in Table 5–1, can cause chronic pulmonary hypertension and right ventricular hypertrophy and may even lead to right ventricular failure. Hypoxia may place the additional stresses of an increased cardiac output and increased blood viscosity (secondary to erythropoiesis) on the right ventricle.

Cor Pulmonale can be defined as right ventric-

PATHOPHYSIOLOGY OF CARDIOPULMONARY DISEASE

ular hypertrophy, dilation, and/or even failure secondary to diseases of the lungs or respiratory system. Thus, cor pulmonale is a result of pulmonary hypertension caused by pulmonary vascular occlusion, obliteration, or chronic vasoconstriction.

Valvular Dysfunctions

Pulmonary stenosis and insufficiency, mitral stenosis, and tricuspid insufficiency all have the potential to lead to right ventricular failure. Because of the ability of the right ventricle to accommodate a volume load, pulmonary and tricuspid insufficiency do not often cause right ventricular failure. Tricuspid stenosis may cause systemic venous congestion and symptoms similar to those of right ventricular failure, even though the right ventricle is unaffected.

Pulmonary Stenosis may be a congenital condition or may be acquired by disease processes. It is analogous to aortic stenosis in the systemic circulation. Constriction of the pulmonary valve increases the resistance to blood flowing from the right ventricle during systole, and therefore, the right ventricle must generate higher systolic pressures to maintain an adequate output. The magnitude of the increase in systolic pressure is dependent on the extent of the stenosis—pressures up to 200 mmHg have been recorded. If such pressure loads develop gradually, the right ventricle hypertrophies to meet the increased work demand. The right ventricular wall may increase in mass until it is as thick as that of the left ventricle. The lumen of the chamber becomes more rounded instead of the normal right ventricular crescent-shaped chamber.

Many patients with pulmonary stenosis and no other problems have no symptoms at all until the condition has progressed to severe constriction. When present, the main symptoms are related to the restriction of cardiac output—fatigue and dyspnea on exertion. The diagnostic signs include a loud murmur (rising in intensity to peak in the first half of systole); large R waves and right axis deviation (indicating right ventricular hypertrophy); large peaked P waves (indicating right atrial enlargement) in the ECG; and high right ventricular systolic pressures with a large pressure drop across the stenotic valve. Surgical correction is usually required. Cardiac catheterization findings in pulmonary stenosis are shown in Figure 5–11.

Mitral Stenosis is most frequently caused by rheumatic fever. The basic pathophysiologic problem is increased resistance to blood flow through the mitral valve. Left atrial diastolic pressure rises if the left atrium cannot pump the whole volume of blood returning from the lungs via the pulmonary veins through the elevated resistance to blood flow. Left atrial systolic pressure must be increased to produce a larger pressure gradient in order to maintain blood flow, and the left atrium hypertrophies. Because there are no valves between the left atrium, the pulmonary veins, capillaries, and arteries, these increased pressures are transmitted backward, causing pulmonary hypertension. This leads to right ventricular hypertrophy and may cause right ventricular failure.

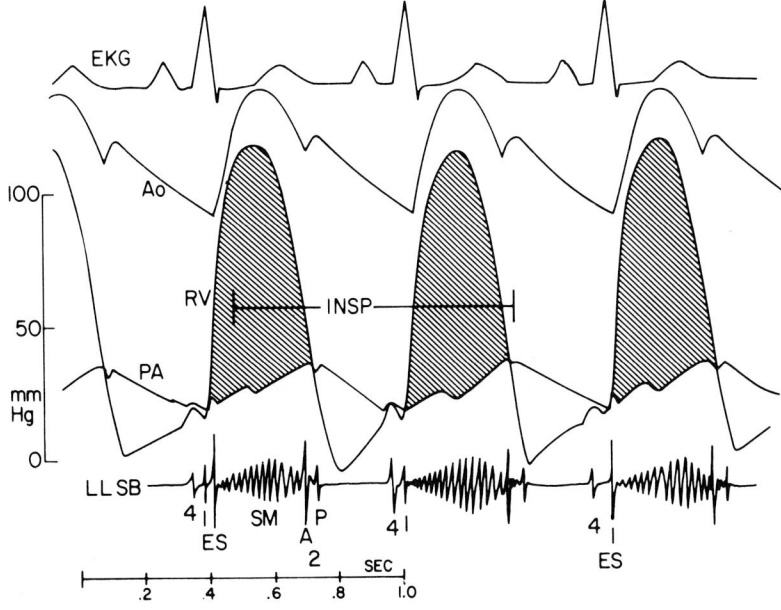

FIGURE 5–11. Cardiac catheterization data from a patient with stenosis of the pulmonary valve. (Ao = aortic pressure; RV = right ventricular pressure; PA = pulmonary artery pressure; INSP = inspiration; SM = systolic murmur; ES = ejection sound.) Note the large systolic pressure gradient between the right ventricle and the pulmonary artery (shaded area), the greatly elevated right ventricular systolic pressure, the slow rise of pulmonary artery pressure, and the murmur during systole. (From Ross, G., Jr., (ed.): *Pathophysiology of the Heart.* New York, Masson, 1982, with permission.)

The main symptoms of mitral stenosis are dyspnea (especially *orthopnea*), resulting from pulmonary vascular congestion, and fatigue and poor exercise tolerance because of restricted cardiac output. Left atrial hypertrophy often leads to atrial flutter or fibrillation, which may be episodic or chronic. This, in turn, may lead to irregular ventricular beats and bradycardia, giving the patient *palpitations* because of large aortic pulse pressures. Atrial fibrillation may also precipitate episodes of pulmonary edema and dangerous systemic arterial thromboemboli because of blood stasis in the left atrium. High pulmonary vascular pressures may also cause small vessels to rupture, resulting in hemoptysis.

Auscultation of patients with mitral stenosis usually reveals a first heart sound and a second pulmonary (P_2) sound of increased intensities and a low-amplitude, low-frequency diastolic murmur (diastolic rumble) as turbulent flow occurs as blood passes through the stenotic mitral valve during ventricular filling. There may also be a sound as the valve opens (the opening snap). The ECG usually shows a prolonged and sometimes double-peaked P wave ("P-mitrale") and large R waves and right-axis deviation because of left atrial and right ventricular hypertrophy, respectively. As already noted, atrial fibrillation may be present. As Figure 5–12 shows, the most important finding on cardiac catheterization is a diastolic gradient between the left atrium and left ventricle, with elevated left atrial pressures during both systole and diastole. Surgical treatment of mitral stenosis is usually required, either to open the stenosis (*commissurotomy*) or replace the valve with a prosthesis.

Pathophysiology of Right Heart Failure

The main causes of right ventricular failure all involve acute or chronic pressure overload of the right ventricle. Conditions capable of producing chronic pulmonary hypertension include diseases of the pulmonary vasculature itself, diseases of the lungs or respiratory system causing alveolar hypoxia and provoking chronic hypoxic pulmonary vasoconstriction (including residence at high altitudes), mitral stenosis, pulmonary valve stenosis, and left ventricular failure.

The main signs of right ventricular failure are those of *venous congestion*. Elevated systemic venous pressure results in prominent distention of the jugular and peripheral veins and engorgement of the organs with a large capacity to store venous blood, such as the liver, spleen, and kidneys, which may be evident on palpation. The splanchnic vascular bed may also be engorged. Chronic venous congestion of the liver may lead to liver dysfunction and cirrhosis.

The other main result of elevated systemic venous pressure is the extravasation of fluid in sys-

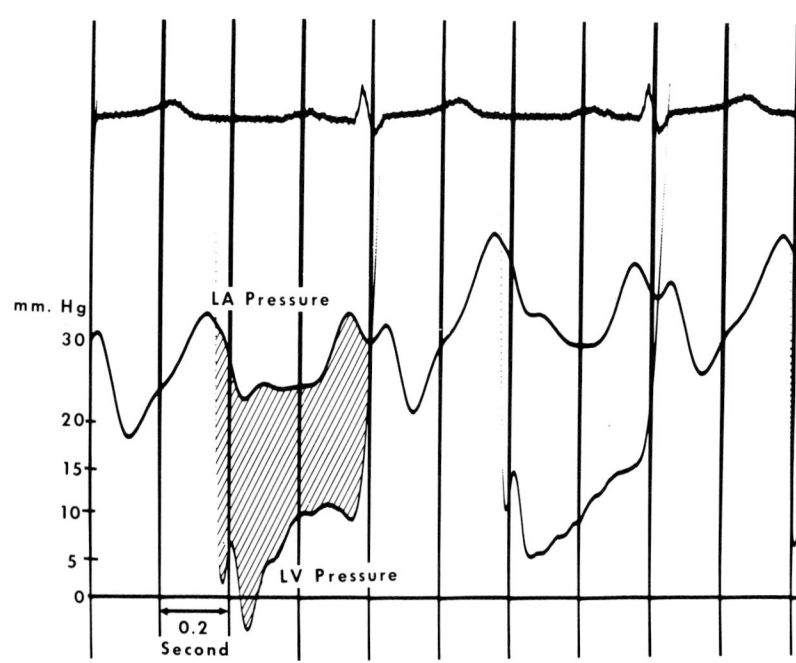

FIGURE 5–12. Cardiac catheterization data from a patient with mitral stenosis. Top trace represents ECG. (LA pressure = left atrial pressure; LV pressure = left ventricular pressure [scale expanded to show diastolic pressure in greater detail]). Note the diastolic pressure gradient between the left atrium and the left ventricle (shaded area) and the greatly elevated left atrial pressure. (From Sodeman, W.A., Jr., and Sodeman, T. M., (eds.): *Sodeman's Pathologic Physiology: Mechanisms of Disease*, 6th ed. Philadelphia, W.B. Saunders, 1979, with permission.)

temic capillaries. As noted in Chapter 2, increased venous pressure increases capillary hydrostatic pressure. As capillary hydrostatic pressure increases, the balance of "Starling forces" in the systemic capillaries is altered to favor filtration of fluid out of systemic capillaries. As edema fluid is produced, it tends to collect in gravity-dependent regions, so swelling of the ankles and feet during the day is a common finding in decompensated patients. In later stages, it may advance up the legs to the genitalia. Pressing the swollen areas with one's fingers squeezes the edema fluid out and temporarily leaves depressions that last a few minutes (pitting edema). Fluid may also be extravasated into serous cavities (effusion), especially the peritoneal cavity. The collection of fluid in the peritoneal cavity is called *ascites*. Pleural effusion may also occur, causing hydrothorax. Cyanosis may also be present in right heart failure.

PULMONARY DISEASES

In this section, the pathophysiology of pulmonary diseases is considered. Perhaps it would be more accurate to say the pathophysiology of the *respiratory system* because some of the problems discussed do not directly affect the lungs but cause dysfunction of other components of the respiratory system, such as the chest wall or respiratory control centers in the brain. Respiratory disorders are often grouped into those that interfere with air flow, which are called *obstructive diseases,* those that restrict lung or chest-wall expansion, which are called *restrictive diseases,* and those that obliterate the gas exchange surface. (Most diseases in this last group are included in the restrictive disease group because they give a similar pattern of pulmonary function test results.) Disorders of the control of breathing are also discussed in this section.

Obstructive Disease

The most common obstructive diseases are those that decrease air flow through the tracheobronchial tree and small airways. These include *asthma, emphysema,* and *chronic bronchitis.* The last two diseases are frequently considered together as *chronic obstructive pulmonary disease* (COPD). The upper airways and larger branches of the tracheobronchial tree may be obstructed by other factors, including accidental inhalation of foreign objects (especially common in young children), the growth of neoplasms or tumors, or trauma.

Asthma

Asthma is usually a disease of *episodic* dyspnea caused by airway obstruction, that is, the patient experiences distinct periods of difficulty in breathing, between which he or she may have no obvious respiratory dysfunction. The episodes of airway obstruction are associated with *constriction* of hypertrophied bronchiolar smooth muscle, *inflammation* and edema of the mucosa and submucosa of the airways, and excessive viscous *secretions* of the tracheobronchial tree. Each of these three features contributes to the obstruction of the airways.

It does not appear that asthma can be attributed to any single etiologic factor, and it must therefore be defined in rather general terms, especially because the episodes of obstructive dyspnea may be precipitated by many different factors. Thus, asthma is conventionally defined as a disorder characterized by *hyperreactivity* of the trachea and bronchi to many stimuli, resulting in a generalized bronchoconstriction or bronchospasm that may become less severe either spontaneously or as a result of therapeutic intervention. Thus, asthma is also referred to as *reactive airway disease*.

Cases of asthma can be attributed to allergic, infectious, environmental, psychological, and physical factors. Perhaps the easiest to understand are those of patients who respond to specific precipitating factors, such as inspired pollens, mold spores, animal fur or dander, or specific types of dusts. Such patients are said to suffer from *allergic* or *extrinsic asthma*. Extrinsic asthma is usually seen in children and young adults. Patients with no identifiable specific stimulus that provokes asthma attacks are said to suffer from *idiosyncratic* or *intrinsic asthma*. Intrinsic asthma usually develops in middle age.

Allergic asthmatics have elevated blood levels of an immunoglobulin E (IgE) antibody specific to the precipitating allergen. They often have a family history of allergies or asthma. They may demonstrate seasonal variations in the frequency of their symptoms, and they have positive skin test reactions to the allergen that precipitates the asthma attacks.

Intrinsic asthmatics either have no known specific allergen that precipitates their attacks or else do not have elevated levels of IgE antibodies to the initiating factor even if it has been identified. Their attacks may be initiated by drugs, such as aspirin or indomethacin (both are nonsteroid anti-inflammatory drugs that block reactions in the prostaglandin pathway), psychological or emotional states, or even exercise, especially in cold environments.

Although people of all ages may suffer from asthma, it is mainly seen as a childhood disease. Many children who develop asthma before 16 years of age have decreasing frequency and severity of symptoms as they get older; more than half have no further symptoms as adults. On the other hand, patients who develop asthma during their adult years tend to have more chronic problems; less than a third of these patients have a spontaneous complete loss of their symptoms.

At least two different pathways appear to be involved in the production of the bronchoconstriction, inflammation, and mucous plugging of airways in asthma. The first is the series of immunological pathways involved in allergic or extrinsic asthma; the second is the parasympathetic cholinergic innervation of the airways, which is probably involved in idiosyncratic or intrinsic asthma.

Immediate Hypersensitivity—Type I Immune Reaction

Initial exposure to the antigenic portion of allergens causes plasma cells in the lymphoid tissue of the respiratory mucosa to release IgE molecules specific for the antigen. These IgE molecules bind to receptors in the cell membranes of mast cells (and basophils), *sensitizing* them. The sensitized mast cells, which are found throughout the mucosa and submucosa of the nasal passages, upper airways, and tracheobronchial tree, can then react with the antigen on subsequent exposure to the allergen (Fig. 5–13). On re-exposure, each antigen molecule reacts with two membrane-bound IgE molecules on the surface of the sensitized mast cells and *activates* the mast cell. The mast cells are biochemically activated to release several types of stored mediators and to produce and release others. These mediators and their effects are summarized in Table 5–2.

Preformed Histamine is released from basophilic storage granules in the mast cells. Histamine can cause constriction of both large and small airways. Small-airway constriction appears to be a direct consequence of histamine; large-airway constriction occurs both because of direct effects of histamine on bronchial smooth muscle and via a vagal reflex in response to its stimulation of airway irritant receptors. Histamine can increase capillary permeability and cause venoconstriction, both of which may lead to edema formation in the mucosa and submucosa and contribute to airway obstruction. Histamine also may stimulate mucous gland secretions and contribute to mucous plugging of airways in asthma. However, because antihistamines have little influence on the symptoms of asthma, it is likely that histamine is only a contributing factor, not the main mediator in asthma.

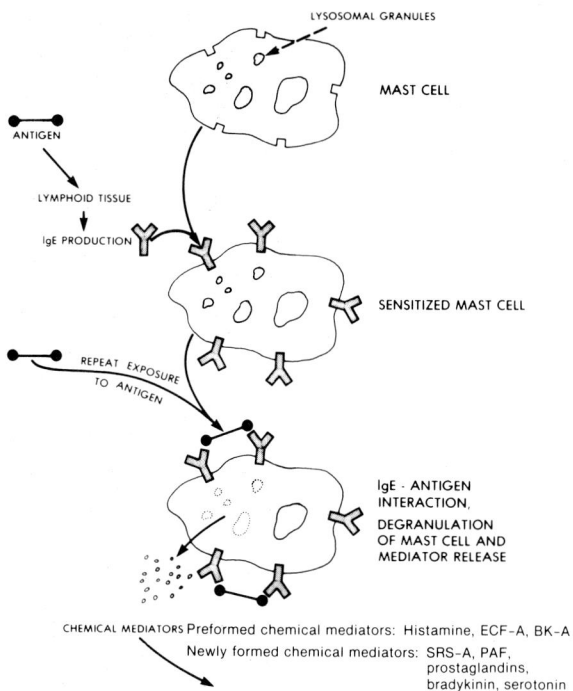

FIGURE 5–13. Reactions in Type I hypersensitivity. Antigens stimulate lymphoid tissue to produce specific IgE antibodies. The IgE antibodies attach to the surfaces of mast cells, sensitizing them. Upon re-exposure to the antigen, the antigen attaches to two IgE molecules on the sensitized mast cell surfaces, stimulating the release of chemical mediators. (From Costello, J.F.: Asthma. In Hinshaw, H.C., and Murray, J.F.: *Diseases of the Chest*, 4th ed. Philadelphia, W.B. Saunders, 1980, with permission.)

The Slow-Reacting Substance of Anaphylaxis (SRS-A) also appears to be involved in asthma. SRS-A is not found preformed in mast cells, so it is probably formed and released when mast cells are activated, although it may be released by other lung cells. Recently, SRS-A has been shown to be a group of several different compounds called *leukotrienes*, which are produced by one of the arachidonic acid metabolic pathways. As Figure 5–14 shows, alternative pathways of arachidonic acid metabolism produce various prostaglandins, prostacyclin, and thromboxanes. The leukotrienes of

TABLE 5–2. Chemical Mediators of Immediate Hypersensitivity

Mediator	Form in Tissues	Actions	Importance in Asthma
Histamine	Formed	Contracts smooth muscles. Increases vascular permeability. Stimulates pain and irritant receptors. Stimulates exocrine secretions.	Major, but probably little effect without other factors.
Slow-reacting substance of anaphylaxis (SRS-A) (leukotrienes C_4, D_4, and E_4)	Precursor	Contracts smooth muscle. Increases vascular permeability. Dilates microvasculature. Stimulates airway secretions.	Probably important. May prolong immediate hypersensitivity response.
Serotonin (5-hydroxytryptamine)	Precursor	Mediator of inflammatory response in animals. Dubious significance in man.	Negligible.
Eosinophilic chemotactic factor of anaphylaxis (ECF-A)	Formed	Chemotaxis and inactivation of eosinophils	Unknown. May inactivate SRS-A.
Bradykinin	Precursor	Constricts bronchial smooth muscle. Increases venular permeability. Vasodilation.	Uncertain. The vasodilator and permeability effects may contribute to mucosal edema.
Platelet-activating factor (PAF)	Precursor	Aggregation of platelets and release of serotonin and prostaglandins. Contracts smooth muscle.	Unknown.
Prostaglandins	Precursor	Regulation of bronchomotor tone and pulmonary vascular resistance.	Major, in both bronchoconstrictor and bronchodilator effects.

From Hinshaw, H.C., and Murray, J.F.: *Diseases of the Chest*, 4th ed. Philadelphia, W.B. Saunders, 1980, with permission.

SRS-A may produce sustained contraction of bronchiolar smooth muscle and may also increase vascular permeability.

Platelet-Activating Factor (PAF) and several other mediators may be released by activated mast cells (see Table 5–2). PAF causes platelets to aggregate and release serotonin and prostaglandins. PAF may be related to thromboxane. *Bradykinin* may also cause bronchoconstriction and lead to bronchial mucosal edema. Increased eosinophils are usually seen in the sputum and in the peripheral blood in people with allergic asthma. *Eosinophil chemotactic factor of anaphylaxis (ECF-A)*, *basophil kallikrein of anaphylaxis (BK-A)*, *serotonin*, and several *prostaglandins* may also be involved in the immunologically mediated mechanism of extrinsic asthma.

Innervation of Bronchial Smooth Muscle. Because idiosyncratic or intrinsic asthmatics do not appear to owe their symptoms to specific allergens with IgE-mediated responses, another mechanism in the production of their obstruction, inflammation, and mucous plugging must be sought. As noted in Chapter 3, the airways are innervated both by parasympathetic cholinergic fibers and sympathetic adrenergic fibers. Stimulation of parasympathetic fibers causes airway constriction and bronchial mucous gland secretion. Stimulation of the sympathetic fibers produces relaxation of bronchial smooth muscle and inhibits glandular secretions. Thus, the patency of muscular airways

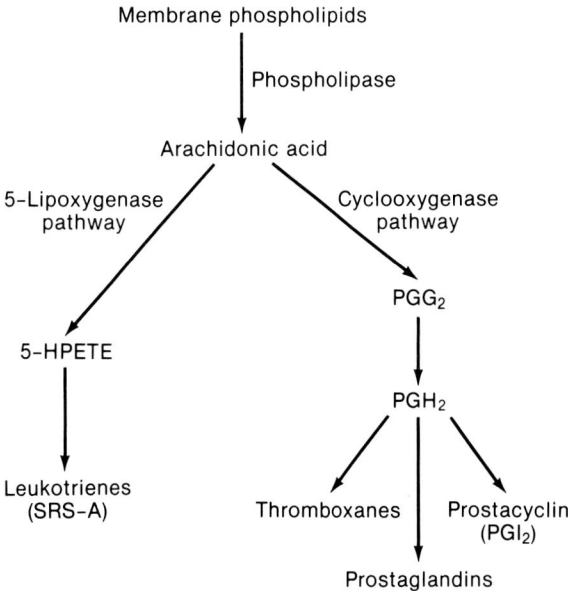

FIGURE 5–14. Diagram of the arachidonic acid pathways.

is maintained by a balance of parasympathetically initiated contraction of bronchial smooth muscle, which is believed to be mediated via cyclic guanosine monophosphate (cyclic GMP) and sympathetically β_2-receptor–mediated relaxation of bronchial smooth muscle, which is believed to act via cyclic adenosine monophosphate (cyclic AMP).

The airways respond to stimulation of irritant receptors with a parasympathetically mediated reflex constriction (see Chapter 3). The afferent pathway for this reflex is via the vagus (and trigeminal nerves for those receptors in the nasal mucosa). Thus, hyperirritability of these irritant receptors, or exaggerated efferent responses to their stimulation may explain the hyperreactive airways response of intrinsic asthmatics to such irritant stimuli as cigarette smoke, noxious chemicals, dusts, cold, and/or exercise. It is also likely that emotional asthma attacks work through this pathway. Histamine and other mediators released in immunologically mediated extrinsic asthma may also stimulate these irritant receptors and activate the vagal pathway. A partial blockade or dysfunction of the sympathetic β_2-receptors of the airway smooth muscle may also be involved in the pathogenesis of asthma in some intrinsic asthmatics.

Pathophysiology of Asthma

Asthma is a disease of *episodic* airway obstruction, so pulmonary function tests are often within normal limits between asthma attacks. During episodes of asthma, pulmonary function tests demonstrate *airway obstruction* and *hyperinflation*. Note that some patients with asthma do show evidence of obstruction on pulmonary function testing during asymptomatic periods, and some asthmatics do suffer some symptoms between attacks.

Pulmonary function tests were introduced in Chapter 3 and are discussed in greater detail in Chapter 9. The main problem during an asthma attack is airway obstruction resulting from severe constriction of hypertrophied bronchial smooth muscle, inflammation of the mucosa and submucosa of the airways, and viscous mucus in the airways. This obstruction is reflected in increased airways resistance and decreases in all measurements of all time-dependent lung volumes (the dynamic lung volumes). As noted before, resistance takes *time* to overcome.

During an asthma attack, airways resistance may increase as much as fivefold. The forced vital capacity (FVC), forced expiratory volume in one second (FEV_1), the FEV_1/FVC, the midmaximal expiratory flow rate (MMEFR), and the peak expiratory flow rate (PEFR) are all decreased. A key diagnostic feature of asthma is that the decrease in dynamic lung volumes that occurs during an attack should be partly alleviated with bronchodilator therapy.

The lung volumes and capacities show a pattern of *hyperinflation* during asthma. The elevated airways resistance leads to a greatly increased work of breathing, both directly and indirectly because of the hyperinflation. Asthma patients breathe at high lung volumes for two reasons. The first is that the bronchospasm, inflammation, and mucous plugs lead to airway closure, gas trapping, and elevated residual volume and functional residual capacity. Thus, the end-expiratory volume increases. Second, breathing at high lung volumes helps to decrease the elevated airways resistance by taking advantage of increased alveolar elastic recoil at the higher lung volumes. The increased alveolar elastic recoil helps hold small airways open by *traction* or tethering (see Chapter 3). Of course, this leads to greatly increased work of breathing on *inspiration* because, at high volumes, the lungs are less compliant.

The high alveolar elastic recoil does help provide the driving force for air flow during expiration, which may be either passive or may be active in more severe cases of asthma. Thus, the work of breathing is increased during asthma attacks because of increased airways resistance on inspiration and expiration, especially if it is active, and because of decreased lung compliance (and inward chest wall recoil) during inspiration at high lung volumes.

Obstructive diseases, such as asthma and COPD, that lead to hyperinflation are frequently associated with inspiratory muscle fatigue. The increased inspiratory work of breathing caused by the great inward elastic recoil of the lungs and chest wall at high lung volumes is exacerbated by less efficient inspiratory muscle function in hyperinflated states. The contracted inspiratory muscles, especially the flattened diaphragm, develop less tension because they are at a shorter length (see Chapter 2). Furthermore, as the diaphragm flattens, it becomes less efficient at generating negative intrapleural pressure because of Laplace's law: At a greater radius of curvature, the diaphragm must develop more tension to generate the same transdiaphragmatic pressure gradient. Indeed, contraction of a very flattened diaphragm pulls the lower ribs inward and converts it to an expiratory muscle. This is called *Hoover's sign*.

Inspiratory muscle fatigue may be relieved with

temporary mechanically assisted ventilation. Inspiratory muscle performance may be improved with drugs such as theophylline.

It is also possible to improve diaphragmatic function by altering the body posture and contracting the abdominal muscles to raise abdominal pressure and therefore decrease the radius of curvature of the diaphragm.

Briefly summarized, the alterations in static lung volumes and capacities during an asthma attack are as follows. The residual volume (RV), functional residual capacity (FRC), and total lung capacity (TLC) are all likely to be increased—the RV and FRC because of airway closure, gas trapping, and the tendency to breathe at high lung volumes, and the TLC because of increased inspiratory muscle strength. The shift to higher lung volumes to make use of increased alveolar elastic recoil may be partly the result of reflex effects. Because the residual volume and functional residual capacity increase much more than the total lung capacity, the expiratory reserve volume (ERV), inspiratory reserve volume (IRV), inspiratory capacity (IC), and vital capacity (VC) are all likely to be decreased.

Arterial blood gases during an acute asthmatic episode show a pattern of hypoxemia with hypocapnia and alkalosis (e.g., a PaO_2 of 55, a $PaCO_2$ of 30, and a pH of 7.48). These can be explained by ventilation-perfusion mismatching with a secondary hyperventilation that is not capable of correcting the hypoxemia. The $\dot{V}_A/\dot{Q}_c$ mismatching is a result of a poor distribution of alveolar ventilation caused by local areas of greatly elevated airways resistance. Diffuse areas of constricted and inflamed airways and mucous plugs lead to many collapsed, unventilated, or poorly ventilated alveoli distributed unevenly throughout the lungs. Any mixed venous blood not diverted away from these poorly ventilated or unventilated regions by the hypoxic pulmonary vasoconstriction, therefore, constitutes a shunt or shunt-like state and contributes to the low arterial P_{O_2}. As already noted, hypoxic pulmonary vasoconstriction is not a very strong response (especially during alkalosis), and studies have shown that such poorly ventilated and unventilated areas continue to be perfused with significant amounts of mixed venous blood. As the hypoxemia and anxiety associated with the attack develop, ventilation is increased. Increased ventilation of already well-ventilated and perfused units does little to increase the arterial oxygen content (the hemoglobin in the pulmonary venous blood draining such regions is already nearly saturated with oxygen), but it does increase carbon dioxide elimination, thus accounting for the respiratory alkalosis.

In many cases, an asthma attack may progress to more severe obstructive limitation of ventilation. In severe cases, hyperventilation may convert to hypoventilation with accompanying hypercapnia and acidosis as well as more severe hypoxia. This may progress further to *status asthmaticus*, a severe, prolonged asthma attack that cannot be relieved by conventional therapy for acute attacks.

The symptoms of an acute asthma attack, which may develop suddenly or gradually, are mainly *dyspnea*, (especially on inspiration), and *wheezing*. Coughing and sputum production are often present. Therapy for asthma is primarily pharmacologic (see Chapter 15).

Chronic Bronchitis

Although chronic bronchitis and emphysema are two separate entities, many patients with COPD have elements of both diseases, and their symptoms reflect either a combination of both or the predominate one. Thus, "pure" chronic bronchitis and "pure" emphysema represent two ends of a continuum of various types of chronic airflow obstruction. Patients with findings indicative mainly of emphysema are frequently called *pink puffers*, for reasons discussed shortly, and are said to suffer from type A chronic obstructive pulmonary disease. Patients with findings indicative mainly of chronic bronchitis are frequently called *blue bloaters* and are said to suffer from type B disease. In many cases, however, either the patient suffers from both emphysema and chronic bronchitis or their symptoms and clinical findings do not clearly fall into either the type A or type B category.

Chronic bronchitis is defined clinically as *excessive mucus production*, usually with *cough* and *expectoration*. The conventional clinical definition further specifies that the symptoms of excessive mucus production, cough, and expectoration must be present on most days of at least 3 months of the year for at least 2 successive years and that other possible causes of these symptoms, such as bronchiectasis or tuberculosis, must be excluded.

Chronic bronchitis thus defined covers patients with disease varying in severity from those suffering from a mild morning cough with some sputum production and no other symptoms to those with severe airway obstruction resulting in dyspnea, hypoxia, and hypercapnia. These may be referred to as *simple chronic bronchitis* and *chronic obstructive bronchitis*, respectively.

Pathologic Alterations in Chronic Bronchitis. In "pure" chronic bronchitis, the pathologic changes are seen in the conducting airways. The excessive secretion of mucus results from an increase in the number and size of mucus glands and frequently the goblet cells in the conducting airways. Airflow obstruction is a result of both increased amounts of mucus in the airways and a narrowing of the airways, probably secondary to inflammation. The viscosity of the mucus may also be increased, which could affect air flow as well as reduce the efficiency of the mucociliary escalator. This may contribute to the recurring pulmonary infections suffered by these patients. Although hypertrophy and hyperreactivity of bronchial smooth muscle is not usually thought to occur in "pure" chronic bronchitis, many patients diagnosed as having chronic bronchitis do respond to bronchodilators and may actually suffer from a mixture of both asthma and chronic bronchitis.

Etiology of Chronic Bronchitis, like that of emphysema, is poorly understood. Cigarette smoking and environmental factors, such as air pollution, occupational hazards, recurrent infections, and genetic factors, may all play a role in causing chronic bronchitis or predisposing a person to get this disease. Cigarette smoke may irritate the airways chronically, causing release of mucus and hypertrophy of the glands. It also decreases the activity of the cilia of the airways.

Pathophysiology and Clinical Findings in Chronic Bronchitis. Table 5–3 summarizes the clinical and physiologic findings in the emphysematous (type A) and bronchitic (type B) extremes of chronic obstructive pulmonary disease. It is possible that many of the differences seen between patients with these two syndromes reflect differences in the patient's control of breathing rather than in the underlying pathology. Patients with chronic bronchitis are characterized by sputum

TABLE 5–3. Clinical, Roentgenographic, and Physiologic Findings in Patients with Type A (Emphysematous) and Type B (Bronchial) Varieties of COPD

Findings	Type A	Type B
Clinical		
Dyspnea	Early onset, steadily progressive	Intermittent during intercurrent infection
Sputum	Scant and mucoid	Early onset, copious
Weight loss	Often marked	Slight or absent
Percussion of chest	Hyperresonant	Normal
Auscultation of chest	Breath sounds remote, rales unusual	Rales and rhonchi frequent
Cor pulmonale	Late manifestation	Common
Polycythemia	Absent	Present
Cyanosis	Absent	Present
Roentgenographic		
Anterior-posterior diameter	Increased	Normal
Diaphragm	Low, flat, moves poorly	Nearly normal position
Peripheral markings	Attenuated	Increased
Cardiac shadows	Small and vertical	Normal or enlarged
Physiologic		
Lung volumes		
Vital capacity	Normal or decreased	Markedly decreased
Total lung capacity	Increased	Normal
Functional residual capacity	Increased	Increased
Residual volume	Increased	Markedly increased
Mechanics of ventilation		
FEV_1/FVC	Markedly decreased	Markedly decreased
Maximal expiratory flow	Markedly decreased	Markedly decreased
Specific airways conductance	Decreased	Decreased
Distribution of ventilation	Markedly abnormal	Markedly abnormal
Diffusing capacity	Markedly decreased	Normal
Gas exchange		
P_{O_2}	Slightly decreased	Markedly decreased
P_{CO_2}	Normal	Increased
pH	Normal	Decreased
(Alveolar-arterial) P_{O_2}	Slightly increased	Markedly increased
Right-to-left shunt	Absent	Absent
Wasted ventilation	Markedly increased	Slightly increased

From Hinshaw, H.C., and Murray, J.F.: *Diseases of the Chest*, 4th ed. Philadephia, W.B. Saunders, 1980, with permission.

production and coughing, with a pattern of hypoxia and hypercapnia secondary to the obstruction of air flow as the disease progresses.

Airway obstruction, mainly from mucus occlusion of small airways, causes gas trapping and increases the functional residual capacity and residual volume. The vital capacity is reduced because the residual volume increases with no change in the total lung capacity. Airflow obstruction results in profound decreases in all of the dynamic lung volumes, such as the FEV_1 and FEV_1/FVC, flow-volume curves, and the peak expiratory flow rate. The specific airways conductance is decreased (conductance is the inverse of resistance, which is increased) because of the airway obstruction.

Obstruction of small airways with subsequent gas trapping leads to a maldistribution of alveolar ventilation. Any blood flow to such poorly or nonventilated alveoli results in ventilation-perfusion mismatch. As already discussed, the hypoxic pulmonary vasoconstriction is a weak response, so many obstructed alveoli contribute to this shunt-like state. This lowers the arterial Po_2 and thus contributes to the increased alveolar-arterial oxygen gradient. The profound chronic hypoxia leads to erythropoiesis, thus causing polycythemia. The low PaO_2 and high hematocrit contribute to cyanosis. Carbon dioxide retention may lead to incredibly high $PaCO_2$'s in patients with chronic bronchitis. The arterial and CSF pH may be only slightly decreased, however, because of renal and CSF bicarbonate retention. Cor pulmonale is a frequent finding in chronic bronchitis because of the pulmonary hypertension resulting from alveolar hypoxia and hypercapnia and because of the increased blood viscosity resulting from polycythemia.

Therapeutic Management of Chronic Bronchitis includes attempts to remove possible causative factors and to reduce airways resistance, as well as physiotherapy and supplemental oxygen. Cessation of smoking may reverse or at least slow down the pathologic alterations of chronic bronchitis, especially if it is done early in the course of the disease. Changes in the home or work environment may also be helpful. As already noted, some patients with chronic bronchitis do respond to bronchodilators, so such drugs should be considered. Steroids may be used to reduce inflammation, and antibiotics are used to control the recurrent infections. Physiotherapy including postural drainage and other measures aimed at clearing the airways of mucus may help patients with chronic bronchitis. Increasing the FIO_2 is necessary to bring the arterial Po_2 nearer to normal and may also help to relieve pulmonary hypertension. However, it does not alleviate the hypercapnia of chronic bronchitis.

Emphysema

Pulmonary emphysema is best defined anatomically rather than clinically. It is a disease of the terminal exchange units, characterized by *destruction of alveolar septa*. This destruction has consequences in both the mechanics of breathing and the gas exchange function of the lungs.

Pathologic Alterations. Pulmonary emphysema is classified by pathologists as being centrilobular, panlobular, paraseptal, or irregular, depending on the sites of pathology within the lungs. (Note that emphysema refers to any pathologic accumulation of air in body tissues, so subcutaneous, mediastinal, and interstitial emphysema are not usually related to pulmonary emphysema; in common usage, emphysema is used to discuss pulmonary emphysema.) No matter what the pathologic classification (which is usually too late to be of interest to the therapist anyway), destruction of alveolar septal tissue represents a loss of potential gas exchange surface area, a potential decrease in pulmonary capillary blood volume, and a loss of alveolar elastic support of small airways and blood vessels in the lungs.

Etiology. As was the case with chronic bronchitis, the etiology of pulmonary emphysema is poorly understood. Cigarette smoking, environmental and occupational hazards, and genetic factors may all play a role. Because emphysema appears to be a disease in which alveolar septa are destroyed by the lung's own enzyme systems, these etiologic factors must act on the lung indirectly by affecting the lung's enzymatic control mechanisms.

In normal people, proteolytic enzymes, such as trypsin, elastases, and collagenases, are found in the lysosomes of circulating leukocytes and in alveolar macrophages. These enzymes are used to destroy engulfed bacteria and other particulate matter (see Chapter 3). Under normal circumstances, these enzymes remain bound within the membranes of the lysosomes inside phagocytic cells until they die. When the proteolytic enzymes are released from the lysosomes upon the death of the cells, they are usually neutralized by enzymes from another system (the antiprotease system) and are thus prevented from digesting pulmonary parenchymal tissue. Of these antiproteolytic enzymes, the best known is *alpha₁-antitrypsin,* which not only inhibits trypsin, but also inhibits elastase and collagenase.

One subgroup of emphysema patients suffers

from a genetically mediated deficiency of alpha$_1$-antitrypsin. They tend to have a relatively pure form of panlobular emphysema that appears to cause damage especially in the lower lung regions. Cigarette smoking may contribute to emphysema by causing release of proteolytic enzymes from phagocytic cells or by killing the cells and causing a passive release of the enzymes as their lysosomes degenerate.

Pathophysiology and Clinical Findings in patients with "pure" emphysema (type A) are shown in Table 5–3. These patients, although dyspneic, tend to maintain their arterial P$_{O_2}$'s reasonably well and are not usually cyanotic. As already noted, destruction of alveolar septa results in a loss of alveolar elastic recoil. This elastic recoil in the alveolar septa helps to oppose airway closure during forced expiration (see Fig. 3–17).

The loss of alveolar elastic recoil in emphysema therefore manifests itself as increased static pulmonary compliance, total lung capacity, functional residual capacity, and residual volume. The total lung capacity is determined by the opposition of alveolar elastic recoil and the inward elastic recoil of the chest wall to the force of the inspiratory muscles. With fewer alveolar septa to confer inward elastic recoil on the lungs, the total lung capacity increases. Similarly, the functional residual capacity represents the balance point between the inward recoil of the lungs and the outward recoil of the chest wall. Therefore, the FRC increases in emphysema. The residual volume is increased in emphysema because of the greater tendency for airway closure to occur during forced expiration. This is a result of both the loss of alveolar septal traction on the small airways and loss of connective tissue in the airways themselves. Airway closure therefore occurs at higher lung volumes in patients with emphysema. Because the residual volume may increase more than the total lung capacity does, the vital capacity is either normal or decreased.

The greater effects of dynamic compression of airways during forced expiration result in decreases in all measurements of airflow, including the FEV$_1$, the FEV$_1$/FVC, and peak expiratory flow. Flow-volume curves also show evidence of airway obstruction in emphysema. The distribution of ventilation, as determined with nitrogen washout curves or other techniques, is abnormal.

As one might predict, indices of gas exchange show many abnormalities. The diffusing capacity is reduced (especially during exercise) because of a loss of surface area for gas exchange. Although there may be a small increase in the perfusion of poorly ventilated alveoli in the patient with emphysema, their main problem is more likely to be overventilation of poorly perfused alveoli. This may be a consequence of the loss of capillaries and of the ease of inflation of highly compliant large alveoli formed by destruction of alveolar septae. These alterations are reflected in the patients' blood gases, which may show only a slightly decreased arterial P$_{O_2}$ at rest. On the other hand, they may become hypoxemic during exercise because of either diffusion limitation of gas exchange secondary to loss of alveolar-capillary surface area or, more likely, decreased mixed venous P$_{O_2}$ caused by an inability to increase the cardiac output sufficiently.

As already noted, chronic bronchitis and emphysema are rarely seen in the pure forms. The two patterns or syndromes described in Table 5–3 may therefore partly reflect differences in the ability of patients with varying combinations of the two underlying pathologic mechanisms of chronic obstructive pulmonary disease to meet the increased demands of the work of breathing. This may be a function of differences in their central respiratory control mechanisms or differences in the work of breathing itself. Some may be more sensitive to carbon dioxide than others, or some may be unable to perform the work of breathing even though ventilatory drive is increased.

Therapy and Management of emphysema are similar to that for chronic bronchitis, including cessation of smoking, removal of environmental factors, and reduction of airways resistance by physiotherapy, such as instruction in *pursed-lip breathing*. This adds downstream resistance during expiration and therefore helps hold small airways open. Many patients with emphysema initiate pursed-lip breathing or make grunting vocalizations to add downstream resistance without being instructed to do so.

Obstructions in Upper Airways

Obstructions in the upper airways can be either acute or chronic in nature. Obviously, *acute upper airway obstruction* is an imminently dangerous situation, with the immediate threat of asphyxiation. Acute upper airway obstruction is caused most frequently by aspiration of vomit or foreign bodies, such as foodstuffs or pieces of plastic toys by children under 2 years old. Removal of the obstructing material can be effected using suction, manually (by using a laryngoscope or bronchoscope), surgically, or by the *Heimlich maneuver*. The Heimlich maneuver consists of grasping the person with an acutely obstructed upper airway from behind by pressing the fist of one hand with the palm of the other hand, into the person's upper abdomen between the navel and the breastbone. If this is done with a strong, rapid upward motion, it usually generates sufficient upstream pressure to dislodge the foreign body.

Chronic Upper Airway Obstructions present different pathophysiologic pictures, depending on whether they are located extrathoracically or intrathoracically and whether they are *fixed* or *variable*. If the obstruction is variable, its effects on the airway are dependent on the transmural pressure gradient at the obstruction. As the inside pressure minus the outside pressure *increases*, the diameter of the obstructed lumen increases and resistance through the obstruction decreases. As the inside pressure minus the outside pressure *decreases*, the diameter of the obstructed lumen decreases, and the resistance through the obstructed lumen increases. A *fixed obstruction* is not affected by the transmural pressure gradient at the site of the obstruction. Fixed obstructions are most commonly caused by scarring that makes the region too stiff to be affected by the transmural pressure gradient. The obstruction is therefore similar on both inspiration and expiration, no matter whether it is extrathoracic or intrathoracic. This is shown in the inspiratory and expiratory flow-volume curves in the top panel of Figure 5–15.

Variable Extrathoracic Obstructions may be caused by tumors, fat deposits, weakened or flabby pharyngeal muscles (as in obstructive sleep apnea), enlarged lymph nodes, inflammation, or paralyzed vocal cords. As shown in the middle panel of Figure 5–15, the variable extrathoracic occlusion during a forced expiration is distended because the pressure inside increases. Thus, the expiratory flow-volume curve appears normal. During inspiration, the walls of the occlusion are narrowed, so the inspiratory flow-volume curve is truncated.

Variable Intrathoracic Obstructions of the upper airways are most commonly caused by tumors. During inspiration, the intrapleural pressure becomes more negative, so the transmural pressure gradient increases and resistance falls. During a forced expiration, the positive intrapleural pressure compresses the walls of the obstruction, and resistance increases. Thus, the expiratory flow-volume curve is affected more than the inspiratory curve, as shown in the bottom panel of Figure 5–15. This pattern is similar to what might be seen in a flow-volume curve obtained from someone with chronic obstructive pulmonary disease. Chronic variable upper airway obstructions are sometimes misdiagnosed as chronic bronchitis or emphysema because of their many similarities.

Restrictive Disease

Any condition that interferes with normal lung expansion during inspiration can be considered a restrictive disease. Thus, disorders that increase the inward elastic recoil of the lungs and/or chest wall are typical restrictive diseases. Conditions such as pneumothorax and hydrothorax, which diminish the mechanical interdependence of the lung and chest wall or interfere with the movement of the lungs, and musculoskeletal and neuromuscular disorders that impair the motion of the chest wall or contraction of the inspiratory muscles are also included in this category.

Pneumoconiosis

The term *pneumoconiosis* does not refer to a specific disease. It is a general term used to represent a number of conditions characterized by chronic or permanent *deposition of inhaled dusts* in the lungs and the tissue reaction that occurs in response to the presence of these particles. Most of these dusts are composed of particles too small to be filtered from the inspired air (see Chapter 3) but too large to remain suspended in it. Thus, the particles that can cause pneumoconiosis are usually between 1 and 5 μm in diameter and cannot be degraded by the alveolar macrophages. Because the source of these dusts is from the patient's own environment, most of the pneumoconioses are related to a specific harmful dust, usually produced or encountered in the patient's occupation. Thus, the pneumoconioses are also called *occupational lung diseases*. The tissue reactions to the agent causing the pneumoconiosis differ, depending on the nature of the offending dust itself. All involve *inflammation* and *fibrosis* in response to the retained particles. Some may also involve *direct injury* caused by the offending particles, immunologic reactions to the particles, and/or even malignant neoplasms if a carcinogenic agent is involved.

The pneumoconioses include such diseases as silicosis, asbestosis, coal worker's pneumoconiosis, and diseases caused by inhalation of talc, iron oxide, aluminum ores, fiberglass, and cement. *Silicosis* is caused by chronic inhalation of *silica* (silicon dioxide), the main constituent of sand. Ex-

208 PATHOPHYSIOLOGY OF CARDIOPULMONARY DISEASE

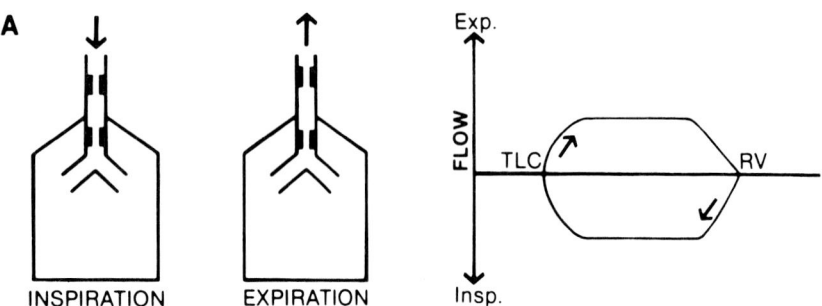

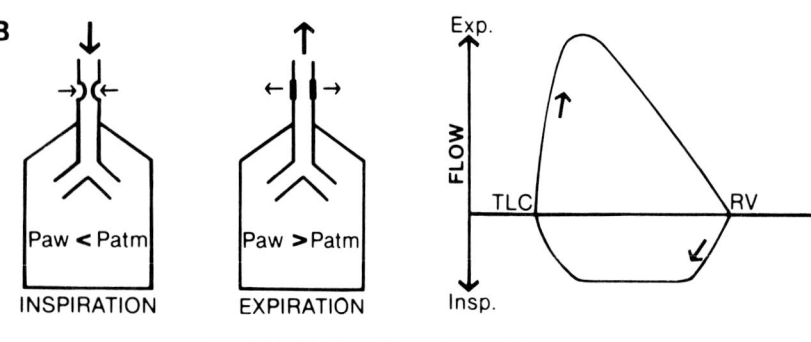

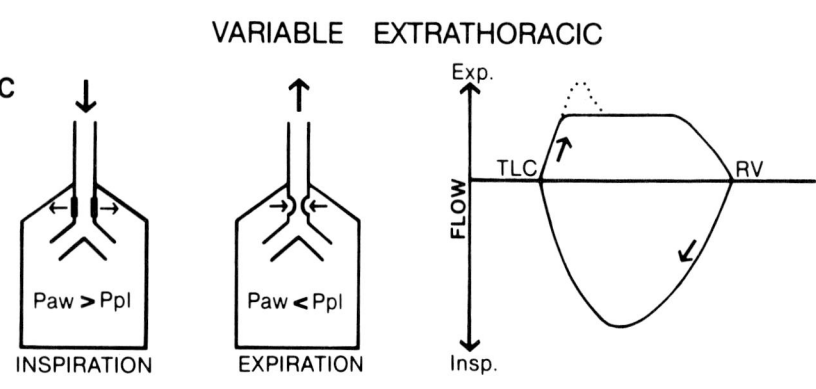

FIGURE 5–15. Inspiratory and expiratory flow-volume curves representing the patterns in: *A*, Fixed intra- or extrathoracic obstruction. *B*, Variable extrathoracic obstruction. *C*, Variable intrathoracic obstruction. (Reproduced with permission from Burrows, B., Knudson, R.J., Quan, S.F., and Kettel, L.J.: *Respiratory Disorders: A Pathophysiologic Approach*, 2nd ed. Copyright © 1983 by Year Book Medical Publishers, Inc., Chicago.)

posure to air-borne silica often occurs in mining or tunneling, because many rocks are composed mostly of silica. Silicosis is also a hazard in sandblasting and in industries in which finely ground sand is used.

Asbestosis is caused by chronic inhalation of asbestos, a term used to denote a number of different kinds of silicates (compounds containing silicon, usually oxygen and one or more metallic bases, such as calcium, magnesium, or aluminum). Asbestos is mainly used for thermal insulation because of its apparently unique resistance to heat. Asbestosis is seen in patients who have worked in the mining, milling, cutting, and installation of asbestos as well as in the demolition or renovation of buildings or ships that have asbestos insulation.

Chronic exposure to air-borne asbestos entails not only the risk of parenchymal asbestos fiber deposition, inflammation, and fibrosis but also predisposes the affected person to neoplasms, such as mesotheliomas (usually malignant), bronchogenic carcinoma, and other malignancies.

Coal miners are at risk of developing both *coal worker's pneumoconiosis* (black lung disease) and chronic bronchitis. Many may get both diseases, but some get only one.

Sarcoidosis

Sarcoidosis is a disease that can affect several organs of the body. It often involves the lungs. About a third of patients with sarcoidosis experience dyspnea. Pulmonary dysfunction is often the initial complaint that brings the patient with sarcoidosis to the physician, and it is the most frequent cause of disability and death in these people.

Sarcoidosis is characterized by granulomatous lesions that may be present in many other organs, including the skin, lymph nodes, liver, and less frequently, the central nervous system, heart, and skeletal muscle. The pulmonary involvement usually consists of a general fibrotic thickening of the interstitium of the alveolar walls with granulomas scattered throughout them. This generalized fibrotic infiltration of the lungs usually results in a pattern of symptoms associated with pulmonary restriction. Obstruction of the airways, especially upper airways such as the nasal mucosa, by granulomas also occurs occasionally.

Sarcoidosis is usually first seen in young adults. It is much more common in blacks than other groups and is seen slightly more frequently in females than males. It is associated with many different immunologic abnormalities, but at present, its cause is unknown. The prognosis is usually good. The main treatment is aimed at reducing the granulomas and fibrosis with corticosteroids.

Diffuse Alveolar Fibrosis

Diffuse alveolar fibrosis (or idiopathic fibrosing alveolitis, interstitial pneumonitis, or pulmonary fibrosis) is a nonspecific term referring to inflammation of the alveolar walls with interstitial fibrosis when no specific etiologic agent can be determined. There is often a cellular infiltrate that includes lymphocytes, plasma cells, and granulocytes; immunologic factors and complexes may also be found. This condition probably represents the end result of the lung's response to many kinds of injuries and infections. It affects males and females with equal frequency. The fibrosis usually results in a restrictive disease pattern with a progressive development of dyspnea. The prognosis is usually poor. Treatment is mainly corticosteroids to suppress the inflammation.

Hypersensitivity Pneumonitis and Infiltrative Lung Disorders

Inhalation of many kinds of organic dusts can cause pulmonary diseases resulting in pulmonary fibrosis. Many of the cases labelled idiopathic pulmonary fibrosis or diffuse alveolar fibrosis are probably hypersensitivity pneumonitis for which no specific organic dust has been identified.

Chronic inhalation of specific organic dusts is usually related to a person's occupation. Thus, the different types of hypersensitivity pneumonitis have names like farmer's lung (exposure to moldy hay), sugar cane worker's lung or bagassosis (exposure to mold on sugar cane), bird-breeder's lung (exposure to bird feathers, droppings, and serum), and mushroom-worker's lung. The most commonly implicated agents are fungi and bacteria. The pathogenesis of the diseases usually involves immunologic reactions leading to inflammation and alveolar interstitial fibrosis. Treatment usually involves corticosteroids as well as avoidance of the dust. The prognosis is usually good.

Systemic diseases that frequently cause infiltrative fibrosis in the lungs include systemic lupus erythematosus (pleural effusions are much more common than fibrosis in this disease, however), scleroderma, and rheumatoid arthritis.

Atelectasis

Atelectasis means incomplete expansion of the lung either at birth (primary atelectasis) or later in life, when it is often simply referred to as a collapsed lobe or lung if a discrete area is involved. *Miliary atelectasis* is used to denote widespread collapse of very small areas of the lung, usually on the level of the gas exchange units themselves. Atelectasis may be caused by loss of the integrity of the visceral pleura, for example, by spontaneous rupture of a *bleb* or *bulla*; or by loss of integrity of the thoracic wall, for example, by a stab wound or other injury resulting in a *pneumothorax*, as well as by *pleural effusions* or other conditions resulting in blood or fluid in the thorax (hemothorax or hydrothorax); *neoplasms*; and *bullae* or *blebs*. Atelectasis may also result from the absorption of alveolar air distal to obstructed airways (*absorption atelectasis*). Absorption atelectasis is a particular hazard in patients unable to clear their airway secretions.

Although atelectasis represents a form of restrictive pulmonary disease, it is more obviously a potential ventilation-perfusion balance problem. Any pulmonary blood flow to such unventilated areas represents a right-to-left shunt that lowers the arterial P_{O_2}. The hypoxic pulmonary vasoconstriction should divert some blood flow away from these unventilated areas, but this response is rarely completely effective. Stimulation of the Hering-Breuer deflation reflex plus possible hypoxemic stimulation of the arterial chemoreceptors may lead to rapid shallow breathing and dyspnea. Hypoxemia may be sufficient to cause cyanosis. Treatment consists of re-expansion of the collapsed area, removal of the space-occupying fluid, lesion, or tumor encroaching on the lung's expansion, and prevention of subsequent incidents of atelectasis.

Chest Wall Restriction

Any condition that interferes with the expansion of the chest wall during inspiration acts as a restrictive disease. These include conditions that restrict the movement or flexibility of the components of the chest wall, such as obesity, chest trauma, spinal cord injury, musculoskeletal disorders, and conditions that affect the control and strength of the inspiratory muscles.

Skeletal Problems

Kyphoscoliosis commonly leads to a restrictive pattern of lung disease. *Kyphosis* is an anterior-posterior curvature of the spine that usually causes little restriction of inspiration. *Scoliosis* is a lateral curvature of the spine that may cause significant restriction because it distorts the thoracic cavity. Kyphoscoliosis is a combination of both, and it almost always results in severe restriction. The altered chest wall mechanics lead to decreased lung volumes, ventilation-perfusion mismatch, hypoxemia, and sometimes even cor pulmonale. Most cases of kyphoscoliosis appear during adolescence and are of unknown origin.

Ankylosing Spondylitis causes fusion of the spinal vertebrae and the costovertebral joints. Although the movement of the diaphragm is usually well-maintained, thoracic wall compliance is decreased. Nonetheless, this disease does not usually have profound effects on ventilation or on arterial blood gases.

Neuromuscular Disorders

Any condition that partially impairs the strength or control of the respiratory muscles can result in a pattern of symptoms representative of restrictive pulmonary disease. Neuromuscular diseases, such as myasthenia gravis, Guillain-Barré syndrome, or poliomyelitis, can in mild cases lead to inspiratory restriction. Severe cases causing paralysis of the respiratory muscles lead to respiratory failure.

Myasthenia Gravis is a fairly rare disease in which an autoimmune reaction (an immune response to a patient's own body protein as if it were a foreign antigen) causes a decreased number of acetylcholine receptors in the neuromuscular junctions of skeletal muscle. This results in weak, easily fatigued skeletal muscles, usually beginning with the extraocular, facial, pharyngeal, neck, and upper limb muscles. Involvement of the diaphragm and intercostal muscles is rarely seen early in the course of the disease but is quite common in its later stages (50% to 60% of all cases). This can be very serious and may lead to ventilatory failure. Diagnosis of myasthenia gravis is based on improved muscle performance in response to anticholinesterase drugs, such as edrophonium chloride (Tensilon), nerve conduction tests, and electromyograms. The treatment of myasthenia gravis usually involves anticholinesterases and immune system suppression with cortisone-like drugs. Some cases of myasthenia gravis are associated with tumors of the thymus gland (thymomas), so patients with myasthenia gravis are screened for such tumors, which can be surgically removed. These patients are usually permanently cured following thymectomy.

Guillain-Barré Syndrome or acute idiopathic polyneuritis is a paralytic disease of unknown cause that is frequently, but not always, associated with influenza-like infections. The onset of the disease is usually manifested by skeletal muscle weakness, often beginning with the legs. The disease rapidly progresses to maximum weakness and/or varying degrees of paralysis within 2 to 4 weeks. About 20% to 50% of these patients require intubation and mechanical ventilation. Diagnosis is based on the history and symptoms of muscle weakness with evidence of slowed nerve conduction. Peripheral nerves show evidence of demyelination. Treatment is mainly supportive. About 85% of the patients make a complete or nearly complete recovery, after an average of about 8 weeks on a ventilator (approximate range is 2 weeks to 30 months).

Poliomyelitis, once a very common disease, is an acute viral infection that can destroy spinal and bulbar (medullary) motoneurons, often leading to skeletal muscle paralysis. It frequently causes respiratory failure sufficient to require mechanical ventilation, usually with a *Drinker respirator* (a negative-pressure respirator, referred to as the iron lung; see Chapter 19). The use of preventive vaccines has nearly eliminated this disease from North America.

Amyotrophic Lateral Sclerosis is another motoneuron disease that can cause respiratory failure in its later stages.

Diseases that directly affect skeletal muscle can also cause respiratory insufficiency requiring mechanical ventilation. These include myotonic dystrophy, Duchenne's muscular dystrophy, and some metabolic diseases.

Paralysis of one side of the diaphragm severely

decreases ventilation on that side. The affected side of the diaphragm moves *upward* into the thorax during inspiration (paradoxical movement) because of the negative pressure generated by displacement of the mediastinum toward the other side of the thorax as the other leaflet of the diaphragm contracts, and by contraction of the other muscles of inspiration. Bilateral paralysis of the diaphragm can cause significant decreases in the functional residual capacity and total lung capacity, especially when the patient is in the supine position, because the flaccid diaphragm is pushed into the thorax by the contents of the abdomen.

Paralysis of the intercostal muscles without paralysis of the diaphragm does not usually have much of an effect on resting ventilation. This is because the intercostals are normally only responsible for about one third of the resting tidal volume.

Obesity

Severely obese patients usually show a restrictive pattern of symptoms and pulmonary function test results, including decreased thoracic cage compliance and decreased functional residual capacity. Their residual volumes and total lung capacities are usually within normal limits, indicating that they have sufficient strength to overcome the decrease in chest-wall compliance. Ventilation of lower lung regions is usually impaired, without an effective redistribution of pulmonary blood flow to better-ventilated lung regions. This ventilation-perfusion imbalance may lead to hypoxemia. All of these alterations are usually attributed to impaired movement of the chest wall and an increased work of breathing caused by the accumulation of excess adipose tissue in the abdomen and around the rib cage.

A small number of very obese patients develop a pattern of symptoms referred to as the *pickwickian syndrome* (named after a character in Charles Dickens' *Pickwick Papers*). The syndrome is characterized by hypoventilation with hypoxemia, hypercapnia, and carbon dioxide insensitivity as well as pulmonary hypertension and polycythemia. This pattern often leads to right ventricular failure (cor pulmonale) and peripheral edema. One of the most important features of this syndrome is uncontrollable sleepiness (*somnolence*) during the daytime. Although these alterations have usually been attributed to the greatly increased work of breathing caused by the decreased chest-wall compliance previously discussed, it is now clear that the progression to pickwickian syndrome is associated with *obstructive sleep apnea*. Obstruction of the upper airways by pharyngeal muscle relaxation during sleep is exacerbated by accumulation of adipose tissue in the neck region. Periods of obstructive sleep apnea may occur many times during the night and usually result in the patient waking up gasping for air (obviously, the consequences of not waking up are far worse). This sleep disturbance leads to chronic somnolence during the daytime. It is not known why some obese patients progress to carbon dioxide insensitivity, cor pulmonale, and respiratory failure and others do not.

Pathophysiology of Restrictive Diseases

In previous sections, many conditions that can be called restrictive lung diseases are discussed. Because these conditions are the products of numerous etiologies and pathologic processes, it is not possible to completely generalize the pathophysiology of the restrictive diseases. Nonetheless, all show alterations in the lung volumes and capacities, and in compliance of the lungs or chest wall. Some lead to ventilation abnormalities and ventilation-perfusion mismatching; others may lead to diffusion impairment.

Lung Volumes and Capacities. Alterations in lung and chest-wall compliance (or elastic recoil) can have profound influences on the lung volumes and capacities. Decreased lung compliance (or increased inward elastic recoil of the lungs) is seen in many restrictive diseases, including diffuse alveolar fibrosis, sarcoidosis, and atelectasis. Decreased chest-wall compliance (especially decreased outward elastic recoil near the functional residual capacity) is seen in kyphoscoliosis, arthritis, and obesity. One might predict that these should lead to a decreased functional residual capacity. Total lung capacity and residual volume are usually reduced; inspiratory and expiratory reserve volumes should be decreased accordingly.

The vital capacity is generally decreased in restrictive diseases because the decrease in total lung capacity is usually greater than the decrease in residual volume. This is because the residual volume is largely determined by small airway closure, which is opposed by the increased alveolar septal traction in restrictive disease caused by alveolar fibrosis. The forced vital capacity (FVC) and forced expiratory volume in the first second (FEV_1) are both usually decreased because of the decrease in total lung capacity and/or decreased chest-wall compliance or muscle strength. The FEV_1/FVC, however, may be normal or elevated in conditions that lead to increased inward elastic recoil of the alveoli.

Ventilation and Ventilation-Perfusion Matching. Some of the restrictive disorders, such as those causing decreased lung compliance, lead patients to hyperventilate, despite the increased work of breathing on inspiration and the lack of hypoxemia. The source of the hyperventilation is believed to be a reflex from the lungs or chest wall. Other restrictive diseases, such as those affecting chest-wall compliance or motion, may lead to hypoventilation and hypoxemia. These include kyphoscoliosis, obesity, and neuromuscular disorders. Many restrictive diseases lead to ventilation-perfusion mismatch and consequent hypoxemia.

Diffusion Impairment. Restrictive diseases caused by alveolar fibrosis represent a thickening of the alveolar-capillary barrier and are therefore expected to lead to a decreased diffusing capacity. Although a reduction in the diffusing capacity sufficient to cause hypoxemia at rest is rarely seen in these patients, they may show significant diffusion impairment when they exercise.

Adult Respiratory Distress Syndrome

The adult respiratory distress syndrome (ARDS) is not really a single disease. It is a term used to describe the end stages of a variety of diseases and conditions that directly or indirectly injure the gas exchange units of the lung. Thus, clinical terms that have been used to describe this syndrome include shock lung, congestive atelectasis (a good description of the lung in ARDS), post-traumatic respiratory distress syndrome, post-perfusion lung, pump lung, post-cardiopulmonary bypass lung, blast lung, Da Nang lung, acute respiratory failure (ARF), respirator lung, adult hyaline membrane disease, and many others. Conditions associated with ARDS are shown in Table 5–4.

Adult respiratory distress syndrome is characterized by acute severe hypoxemia, dyspnea, decreased lung compliance and functional residual capacity, diffuse atelectasis, infiltrations, and edema of noncardiac origin occurring in previously healthy persons.

Pathologic Alterations. The main pathologic changes in ARDS include diffuse alveolar atelectasis and fluid and erythrocytes in the interstitium of the lung and, in later stages, in the alveoli. Hyaline membranes consisting of proteins (mainly fibrinogen) may be seen upon histologic examination of the alveoli of patients with ARDS in its later stages. This protein was carried into the alveoli in the edema fluid.

Etiology. ARDS appears to be caused by diffuse damage to the gas-exchange surface of the lung. There does not seem to be a single etiologic factor. Injury to either the alveolar epithelium or capillary endothelium or both may cause ARDS, although capillary endothelial injury is probably more common. The loss of capillary integrity may be caused by toxins; humoral vasoactive sub-

TABLE 5–4. Conditions Associated with Adult Respiratory Distress Syndrome

Hemodynamic Disturbances
  Shock of any etiology
  Increased intracranial pressure (including seizures)

Infectious Causes
  Gram-negative sepsis
  Viral pneumonia
  Bacterial pneumonia
  Fungal pneumonia (rare)
  Pneumocystis carinii

Trauma
  Fat emboli
  Lung contusion
  Nonthoracic trauma (including head injury)

Liquid Aspiration
  Gastric juice
  Fresh or salt water (drowning)
  Hydrocarbon fluids

Drug Overdose
  Heroin
  Methadone
  Propoxyphene
  Barbiturates
  Colchicine
  Salicylates
  Ethchlorvynol

Inhaled Toxins
  Oxygen (high concentrations)
  Smoke
  Corrosive chemicals (NO_2, Cl_2, NH_3, phosgene, cadmium)

Hematologic Disorders
  Intravascular coagulation
  Massive blood transfusion
  Postcardiopulmonary bypass

Metabolic Disorders
  Pancreatitis
  Uremia
  Paraquat ingestion

Miscellaneous
  Lymphangitic carcinomatosis
  Eclampsia
  Postcardioversion
  Radiation pneumonitis (rare)

From Hinshaw, H.C., and Murray, J.F.: *Diseases of the Chest*, 4th ed. Philadephia, W.B. Saunders, 1980, with permission.

stances, such as prostaglandins, histamine, or catecholamines; excessive sympathetic tone to the pulmonary vasculature; components of the blood-clotting system, especially platelets; or immunologic reactions. A second major etiologic feature may involve the production, inactivation, or utilization of pulmonary surfactant because diffuse alveolar atelectasis and decreased pulmonary compliance are seen in ARDS.

Pathophysiology. Abnormalities in pulmonary surfactant production or interference with its function by edema fluid lead to decreased pulmonary compliance and a low functional residual capacity. Miliary atelectasis occurs as unstable alveoli throughout the lungs collapse. Loss of more and more functioning alveoli add to the loss of pulmonary compliance.

Continued perfusion of unventilated or poorly ventilated alveoli constitutes shunts and shunt-like states. These low (or zero) ventilation-perfusion ratios are the primary cause of the low arterial Po_2 with diffusion impairment the other contributing factor. Hypoxemia may lead to increased respiratory drive, dyspnea, and cyanosis.

Management. The management of ARDS mainly involves establishment of a patent airway, mechanical ventilation, increasing the FiO_2, and positive end-expiratory pressure (PEEP). Increasing the FiO_2 without PEEP does not usually relieve the hypoxemia, indicating that pulmonary blood flow to collapsed alveoli is the primary source of the low arterial Po_2. An occasional large positive-pressure tidal volume (a sigh or deep breath) helps to expand collapsed alveoli. PEEP prevents more spontaneous atelectasis from occurring.

Infectious Lung Disease

Because there are many different infectious pulmonary diseases that may primarily affect the upper airways, lower airways, gas-exchange surface of the lung, pleural surface, chest wall, or control of breathing, there are really no unifying pathophysiologic features of the infectious pulmonary diseases. Therefore, we will not discuss all the infectious diseases in this chapter. Two infectious pulmonary diseases that deserve mention are pneumonia and tuberculosis.

Pneumonia (also referred to as pneumonitis) is a term describing inflammation of the lung parenchyma with the alveoli filling with an exudate of cells, especially polymorphonuclear leukocytes. The clinical features depend on which type of organism causes the pneumonia (pneumonia can be caused by many viruses and bacteria and occasionally by noninfectious material as well) and the general condition of the patient, but ventilation-perfusion mismatch and hypoxemia are often seen. If the patient is debilitated by age or other diseases, pneumonia can be fatal.

Pneumonia may primarily affect the air spaces, especially of an entire lung lobe (lobar pneumonia); the small airways, often causing distal atelectasis (bronchial pneumonia); or the interstitium (interstitial pneumonia). Some of the bacteria that commonly cause pneumonia include *Streptococcus pneumoniae, Staphylococcus aureus, Haemophilus influenzae, Pseudomonas aeruginosa, Escherichia coli, Klebsiella pneumoniae,* and *Legionella pneumophila* and *micdadei*. Some common viral causes of pneumonia include influenza A and B viruses, adenoviruses, respiratory syncytial virus, and parainfluenza viruses. Fungal causes of pneumonia include species of *Aspergillus* and *Candida, Histoplasma capsulatum*, and *Coccidioides immitis*. An organism called *Pneumocystis carinii*, which is likely a protozoan, frequently causes pneumocystis pneumonia in patients with suppressed immune systems. It is common in patients with acquired immunodeficiency syndrome (AIDS) which is discussed in Chapter 12.

Patients occasionally become infected with pathogens during a stay in a hospital. Such hospital-acquired infections are referred to as *nosocomial infections*. Nosocomial pneumonias are frequently caused by pathogens that would be unusual causative agents of pneumonia in patients infected outside of the hospital (community-acquired pneumonia). Enteric gram-negative bacilli, such as *Klebsiella pneumoniae* and *Escherichia coli*, and *Staphylococcus aureus* are common causes of hospital-acquired pneumonias but not community-acquired pneumonias.

Examination of a patient with pneumonia usually reveals fever, chills, tachypnea, tachycardia, and dullness on percussion of the chest, but all may be absent. Similarly, there may or may not be abnormal breath sounds, cough, expectoration, chest pain, and evidence of pneumonia on chest radiographs. The most definitive and useful diagnostic procedures involve the collection, gross and histologic examination, and culture of expectorated sputum. Sputum culturing is also important in order to determine the most effective antibiotic to use to treat the patient (see Chapter 12). If appropriate expectorated sputum cannot be obtained, *transtracheal aspiration* with a needle inserted percutaneously via the cricothyroid space may be necessary.

Tuberculosis is caused by a *Mycobacterium* bacillus. The primary infection usually results from the inhalation of *Mycobacteria* into the respiratory tract. The extent of the infection depends on the dose of the bacteria and the patient's general condition. The bacteria are ingested by alveolar macrophages but are not destroyed by them. Instead the bacteria multiply inside the macrophages. The bacteria also are carried to regional lymph nodes, where they sensitize T lymphocytes, thus generating a delayed hypersensitivity reaction to the bacilli. The primary lesion, the *tubercle* composed mainly of macrophages and T cells, forms within about 6 weeks of the initial infection. Beginning at this time, the patient shows a positive skin reaction to the antigen. Most patients have only a mild, short illness on initial exposure to the bacillus. After the hypersensitivity reaction, the lesion heals and the affected lymph nodes calcify. However, some bacteria may get into the blood and be carried to other organs, where they may remain in an inactive state for years. Later, they may *reactivate* and begin to reproduce, causing active disease in the lungs, kidneys, or bones. The site of this reactivation is often the apex of the lung because the relatively high ventilation-perfusion ratio there results in high P_{O_2}'s favorable to these bacteria.

Cough and sputum production are the most common early symptoms of pulmonary tuberculosis. The cough is not usually severe, and the symptoms are often mistaken for a lingering cold. If blood vessels in the lungs are damaged, there may be blood in the sputum. In advanced stages of the disease, the patient may cough up large quantities of blood. Other symptoms of advanced tuberculosis include chest pain, fever, sweating at night, fatigue, weight loss, and loss of appetite. Although tuberculosis may lead to rapid death, it occurs more commonly as a long-term, progressively worsening disease.

The diagnosis of tuberculosis is mainly based on skin tests, chest radiographs, and laboratory tests. *Skin tests* can determine if a person has been infected with tubercle bacilli in the past. However, such tests do not tell the physician whether the active disease is present. All types of skin tests are based on specific allergic reactions to the tubercle bacilli. The body develops the allergy to the bacilli within a few weeks after the primary infection. *Chest radiographs* may reveal tubercles or other signs of tuberculosis in the lungs. They are usually done after a skin test has indicated a previous infection. However, chest radiographs done for other reasons sometimes reveal the presence of tubercles. *Laboratory tests* of the patient's sputum can determine if bacilli are present. Sputum samples are treated with histochemical stains to make the bacilli visible under the microscope. If bacilli are present, they are *cultured*—that is, grown in laboratory dishes or test tubes. Culturing determines whether they are *Mycobacterium tuberculosis* or other bacilli. It also helps find out which drugs will be most effective against the bacteria.

Tuberculosis can usually be treated successfully with drugs. Isoniazid (INH) is one of the most effective antituberculosis drugs. Other effective drugs include rifampin, ethambutol, para-aminosalicylic acid (PAS), streptomycin, and pyrazinamide. These drugs stop the bacteria from multiplying and allow the body's natural defenses to work against the disease. Two or more drugs are usually prescribed at one time because tubercle bacilli may become resistant to only one medication.

Lung Cancer

Lung cancer is one of the most common kinds of malignancy and a frequent cause of death. Malignancies in the lung can be either *primary* or *metastatic*. Metastatic lung cancer is common (as is metastatic liver cancer) because cancer cells carried in the venous blood may settle in the lungs (or liver) and proliferate. The lung is a common site of metastasis because the entire venous drainage of the body passes through the lungs.

The pathophysiology of lung cancer depends on the site and cell type of the cancer. Cell types include *squamous-cell carcinomas,* which most often arise from large airways and produce symptoms of obstruction; *adenocarcinomas,* which usually begin more peripherally and may not produce any symptoms until the cancer is far advanced; *undifferentiated carcinomas,* both large-cell and small-cell (or oat-cell) types; and *alveolar cell* carcinomas. Oat-cell carcinomas often produce ectopic hormones, such as ACTH, serotonin, or parathyroid hormone, and may mimic endocrine diseases.

The most common cause of lung cancer is cigarette smoking. Other causes include exposure to substances such as asbestos and beryllium and to radiation. Treatment includes surgical removal, when possible, chemotherapy, and radiation therapy.

Disorders of the Control of Breathing

We have already discussed many disorders in the control of breathing in this chapter and in Chapter 3. These include carbon dioxide insensitivity secondary to chronic airway obstruction, lung or chest wall restriction, obesity, and drug overdoses. We have also noted several neuromuscular diseases as well as obstructive sleep apnea.

Central Sleep Apnea

In obstructive sleep apnea, the controllers of breathing are issuing the command to breathe, but upper airway obstruction prevents airfow. In *central* sleep apnea, there is an absence of medullary respiratory center output sufficient to drive the respiratory muscles. Thus, central sleep apnea can be distinguished from obstructive sleep apnea (in the setting of a sleep laboratory) by the cessation of the electrical activity of the diaphragm and intercostal muscles and the lack of alterations in intrathoracic pressure during periods of no airflow at the nose and mouth. In contrast, periods of obstructive sleep apnea are accompanied by diaphragmatic and intercostal muscle activity and large fluctuations in intrathoracic pressure.

Studies carried out in a sleep laboratory are called *polysomnography* and usually include a collection of electroencephalograms (EEGs), electromyograms (EMGs), electrocardiograms (ECGs), electro-oculograms (EOGs), airflow data, and arterial oxygen saturations (as determined noninvasively with a transcutaneous ear oximeter, which is also called pulse oximetry). Many other physiologic variables may also be determined.

The cause of central sleep apnea is not known. It may be related to the apnea seen in neonates and infants with *sudden infant death syndrome* (SIDS), which is discussed in the next chapter. We have already seen in Chapter 3 that normal healthy people have a reduced sensitivity to carbon dioxide during sleep, so that $PaCO_2$ increases 5 to 6 torr. Obstructive sleep apnea is far more common than central sleep apnea. Some patients have *mixed sleep apnea,* which is usually seen as episodes of central sleep apnea followed by obstructive sleep apnea.

Central sleep apnea may be treatable with respiratory stimulant drugs, such as medroxyprogesterone. Electrical pacemakers for the phrenic nerves may be effective for some patients.

Obstructive Sleep Apnea

Obstructive sleep apnea is the most common form of sleep apnea. It occurs primarily in men between the ages of 40 and 60. As already noted, its clinical features include repetitive episodes of obstructive apnea followed by arousal into the awake state. Because the respiratory controller *does* function during obstructive sleep apnea, it is probably more accurate to classify this as an obstructive disease of the upper airway. Occlusion of the upper airway usually occurs in the oropharynx as the tongue and soft palate come into apposition with the posterior wall of the pharynx. During inspiration, the muscles of the oropharynx normally contract to help hold the airway open in opposition to the negative airway pressure generated by the muscles of inspiration. In obstructive sleep apnea, the airway is not held open because (1) the pharyngeal muscles are too weak, (2) there is too much fat around the pharynx, (3) the tongue is enlarged or displaced, or (4) other components of the upper airways are constricted or congested.

Patients with sleep apnea are likely to experience very loud snoring between apneic periods and to make grunting and gurgling sounds as they reach arousal. During the apneic periods, they may show pronounced breathing efforts. Indeed, the loud snoring and apneic periods frequently make the patient's bed partner as important as the patient during the history-taking.

The most important daytime symptom of obstructive sleep apnea is excessive sleepiness (*hypersomnolence*). As the severity of the disease increases, this progresses from daytime drowsiness and inattentiveness to episodes of involuntary sleep, which may even occur while the patient is driving a car. Affected persons may also complain of morning headaches and undergo personality changes.

Prolonged recurrent apneic periods resulting in hypoxia and hypercapnia (which are probably the source of the headaches) can cause numerous cardiopulmonary alterations, including arrhythmias, pulmonary hypertension, and even cor pulmonale, systemic hypertension, polycythemia, and sudden nocturnal death.

Treatment of obstructive sleep apnea is dependent on the patient and the severity of the problem. Correction of the upper airway problem by surgery may be possible in many patients. Avoidance of drugs (especially alcohol) that depress ventilation is very important. Respiratory stimulant drugs, such as protriptyline, progesterone, and aminophylline, may also be helpful. If all other forms of therapy are ineffective and the patient's problem is severe, a chronic tracheostomy may be necessary—despite the consequent problems in speaking and airway clearance. The tracheostomy need only be open during sleep, so normal speech is possible during the daytime.

Other Ventilatory Control Disorders Causing Hypoventilation

Medullary infections, trauma, hypotension, and ischemia all can interfere with normal automatic respiratory control and cause hypoventilation. In some congenital medullary disorders (such as the Arnold-Chiari malformation) or medullary infections or inflammations (such as bulbar poliomyelitis or encephalitis), the medullary pacemaker (probably the dorsal respiratory group, as noted in Chapter 3) or the medullary chemoreceptor may not function properly. Such patients usually breathe irregularly (see the section on ataxic breathing discussed later) and hypoventilate in both the sleeping and waking states, even though they can hyperventilate *voluntarily*. This is called *idiopathic hypoventilation,* or primary alveolar hypoventilation, if it cannot be attributed to any other neurologic cause. It is most frequently referred to as *Ondine's curse,* after a mythologic character. Such patients are candidates for electric phrenic nerve pacemakers.

Abnormal Breathing Patterns

Abnormal breathing patterns include tachypnea, Kussmaul's respiration, Cheyne-Stokes respiration, Biot's respiration, and ataxic respiration.

Tachypnea is rapid breathing such as that after a pulmonary embolus develops. *Kussmaul's respiration* is very deep tidal volumes with little or no increase in breathing frequency. This condition is often seen in response to metabolic acidosis. *Cheyne-Stokes respiration* is a complex breathing pattern consisting of periods of breath-by-breath increases in tidal volume until a peak tidal volume is reached. Tidal volume then decreases with each successive breath until a period of apnea occurs. Ventilatory rate may also be affected. Then this crescendo-decrescendo cycle is repeated. Cheyne-Stokes breathing is often associated with lesions in the cerebral hemispheres, cerebral vascular accidents, and is also seen in persons unacclimatized to high altitudes. It may be a result of cycles of hyperventilation until there is no carbon dioxide drive to breathe followed by a buildup of carbon dioxide until ventilation is stimulated. It is as though the sensors for carbon dioxide and oxygen and the central ventilatory control mechanisms are out of phase with each other. This seems reasonable because Cheyne-Stokes breathing is also seen in patients with slow blood circulation, such as those in heart failure or near death.

Biot's respiration, or cluster breathing, consists of clusters of about four or five deep, gasping breaths (but not with regular increases and then decreases in tidal volume) alternating with periods of apnea. It is seen most commonly in diseases of or trauma to the medulla or pons. *Ataxic respiration* consists of totally irregular tidal volumes and breathing frequency.

Hyperventilation Syndrome

Although hyperventilation can be caused by some types of encephalitis or meningitis as well as by lesions of the pons, some otherwise healthy patients display a syndrome caused by chronic hyperventilation secondary to anxiety or similar emotional states. Most of the symptoms are attributable to respiratory alkalosis secondary to chronic hyperventilation, including dyspnea, shortness of breath, and chest pain or tightness; faintness or dizziness, clouded mentation, and feelings of being distanced from reality; numb, tingling, and cold extremities; muscle tremors and spasms; palpitations, tachycardia, and arrhythmias; and fatigue and weakness.

Respiratory Failure

Respiratory failure is a nonspecific term used to describe the consequences of many of the respiratory diseases and disorders described in this chapter. Respiratory failure can be defined most easily on the basis of arterial blood gases. Respiratory failure is therefore a state in which the dysfunction(s) in a patient's respiratory system are so great that he or she can no longer compensate to maintain his or her arterial blood gases within "normal" limits. Thus, respiratory failure is defined in terms of hypoxemia and/or hypercapnia. By normal, we mean what is normal for a person of that age and condition and excluding the effects of intracardiac shunts or respiratory compensations for other problems.

Respiratory failure can be either acute, chronic, or both. That is, a person in chronic respiratory failure that is not life-threatening (for example, mild hypoxemia and hypercapnia with metabolic compensation for the acidosis, such as that seen in someone with chronic bronchitis) may have acute respiratory failure *superimposed* on the chronic respiratory failure by a pulmonary infection.

The symptoms and signs of respiratory failure involve the central nervous system as well as the respiratory and cardiovascular systems, and they depend on the cause of the failure, including restlessness, personality changes, confusion, irritability, headaches, somnolence, seizures, and coma; tachycardia (or bradycardia), hypertension (or hypotension), and bounding pulses; dyspnea and tachypnea (or apnea); and cyanosis.

Part III of this book is largely devoted to the treatment of respiratory failure. Treatment may include establishment of an artificial airway, mechanical ventilation with positive end-expiratory pressure, and increasing the F_IO_2.

Bibliography

Bates, D.V., Macklem, P.T., and Christie, R.V.: *Respiratory Function in Disease*, 2nd ed. Philadelphia, W.B. Saunders, 1971.

Berte, J.B.: *Pulmonary Emergencies*. Philadelphia, J.B. Lippincott, 1977.

Burrows, B., Knudson, R.J., Quan, S.F., and Kettle, L.J.: *Respiratory Disorders: A Pathophysiologic Approach*, 2nd ed. Chicago, Year Book Medical Publishers, 1983.

Cherniack, R.M., and Cherniack, L.: *Respiration in Health and Disease*, 3rd ed. Philadelphia, W.B. Saunders, 1983.

Cohn, P.F.: *Clinical Cardiovascular Physiology*. Philadelphia, W.B. Saunders, 1985.

Emes, J.H., and Nowak, T.J.: *Introduction to Pathophysiology: Basic Principles of Disease Processes*. Baltimore, University Park Press, 1983.

Fishman, A.P. (ed.): *Pulmonary Disease and Disorders*. New York, McGraw-Hill, 1980.

Fishman, A. P. (ed.): *Update: Pulmonary Diseases and Disorders*. New York, McGraw-Hill, 1982.

Fraser, R.G., and Paré, J.A.: *Diagnosis of Diseases of the Chest*, 2nd ed. Philadelphia, W.B. Saunders, 1977.

Frohlich, E.D. (ed.): *Pathophysiology: Altered Regulatory Mechanisms in Disease*, 3rd ed. Philadelphia, J.B. Lippincott, 1984.

Guyton, A.C.: *Textbook of Medical Physiology*, 7th ed. Philadelphia, W.B. Saunders, 1986.

Harris, P.D., and Heath, D.: *The Human Pulmonary Circulation*, 3rd ed. Edinburgh, Churchill Livingstone, 1986.

Hinshaw, H.C., and Murray, J.F.: *Diseases of the Chest*, 4th ed. Philadelphia, W.B. Saunders, 1980.

Kaminski, M.J., and Young, R.R.: Neuromuscular and neurological disorders affecting respiration. In Roussos, C., and Macklem, P.T. (eds.): *The Thorax*. New York, Marcel Dekker, 1985, pp 1023–1087.

Kryger, M.H. (ed.): *Pathophysiology of Respiration*. New York, John Wiley and Sons, 1981.

Leitch, A.G.: Asthma-mechanisms and management. *Clinical Notes on Respiratory Diseases* 21(1):3–9, 1982.

Moser, K.M. (ed.): *Pulmonary Vascular Diseases*. New York, Marcel Dekker, 1979.

Netter, F.H.: *The Ciba Collection of Medical Illustrations*, vol. 5. Summit, N.J., Ciba, 1969.

Netter, F.H.: *The Ciba Collection of Medical Illustrations*, vol. 7. Summit, N.J., Ciba, 1979.

Paré, J.A., and Fraser, R.G.: *Synopsis of Diseases of the Chest*. Philadelphia, W.B. Saunders, 1983.

Ross, G., Jr. (ed.): *Pathophysiology of the Heart*. New York, Masson, 1982.

Rushmer, R. F.: *Cardiovascular Dynamics*, 4th ed. Philadelphia, W.B. Saunders, 1976.

Sharp, J. T.: The respiratory muscles in emphysema. *Clin. Chest Med.* 4:421–432, 1983.

Smith, L.H., Jr., and Thier, S.O. (eds.): *Pathophysiology: The Biological Principles of Disease*, 2nd ed. Philadelphia, W.B. Saunders, 1985.

Sodeman, W.A., Jr., and Sodeman, T.M. (eds.): *Sodeman's Pathologic Physiology: Mechanisms of Diseases*, 7th ed. Philadelphia, W.B. Saunders, 1985.

Tisi, G.M.: *Pulmonary Physiology in Clinical Medicine*, 2nd ed. Baltimore, Williams & Wilkins, 1983.

Weir, E.K., and Reeves, J.T. (eds.): *Pulmonary Hypertension*. Mount Kisco, N.Y., Futura, 1984.

Weiss, E.B.: Bronchial asthma. *Ciba Clinical Symposia* 27(1–2):1–72, 1975.

West, J.B.: *Pulmonary Pathophysiology: The Essentials*, 3rd ed. Baltimore, Williams & Wilkins, 1987.

OBJECTIVES

AFTER READING THIS CHAPTER, THE STUDENT WILL BE ABLE TO:

1. Understand the cardiopulmonary alterations that occur with fetal and neonatal development, childhood growth, and aging.
2. Describe the embryologic development of the cardiovascular and pulmonary systems and relate that development to perinatal cardiopulmonary pathophysiologic states.
3. Describe the anatomy and physiology of the fetal circulation.
4. Discuss the physiologic and potential pathophysiologic cardiopulmonary alterations that occur at birth.
5. Predict the physiologic consequences of the major perinatal cardiopulmonary pathologic states.
6. Describe the cardiopulmonary developmental changes that occur during childhood.
7. Discuss the pathophysiology of the major pulmonary diseases of childhood.
8. Predict the physiologic effects of aging on the cardiopulmonary system.

6
CARDIOPULMONARY CHANGES THROUGH LIFE

CHAPTER OUTLINE

EMBRYOLOGIC DEVELOPMENT OF THE CARDIOVASCULAR AND PULMONARY SYSTEMS
  Development of the Heart
  Development of the Systemic Arteries
  Development of the Lungs
FETAL CIRCULATION
  The Placenta
  Anatomy and Physiology of Fetal Circulation
CARDIOPULMONARY ALTERATIONS AT BIRTH
  Alterations in the Respiratory System
  Alterations in the Circulation
PERINATAL PATHOPHYSIOLOGY
  Cardiovascular Disorders
    Atrial Septal Defects
    Ventricular Septal Defects
    Patent Ductus Arteriosus
    Coarctation of the Aorta
    Tetralogy of Fallot
    Transposition of the Great Vessels
    Persistent Truncus Arteriosus
    Persistent Fetal Circulation

  Pulmonary Disorders
    Choanal Atresia
    Infant Respiratory Distress Syndrome
    Bronchopulmonary Dysplasia
    Meconium Aspiration
    Tracheoesophageal Fistulas
    Diaphragmatic Hernia
    Apnea of Infancy and Sudden Infant Death Syndrome
    Transient Tachypnea of the Newborn
  Retrolental Fibroplasia
DEVELOPMENTAL CHANGES IN THE CARDIOPULMONARY SYSTEM DURING CHILDHOOD
  Postnatal Cardiovascular Development
  Postnatal Pulmonary Development
PEDIATRIC PATHOPHYSIOLOGY
  Croup and Epiglottitis
  Bronchiolitis
  Cystic Fibrosis
PHYSIOLOGIC CONSEQUENCES OF AGING
  Changes in the Cardiovascular System
  Changes in the Respiratory System

EMBRYOLOGIC DEVELOPMENT OF THE CARDIOVASCULAR AND PULMONARY SYSTEMS

The embryologic development of the cardiovascular and respiratory systems is briefly summarized in this section to provide the background of the morphology, physiology, and pathophysiology of prematurely born infants and many congenital and perinatal problems.

Development of the Heart

The cardiovascular system is probably the first system to assume its normal adult function in the embryo, with blood flow beginning after only the 3rd week of development. The heart starts to form 18 to 19 days after fertilization. Two endocardial *heart tubes* develop and then start to fuse at about day 21 (Fig. 6–1A and B). During the next 2 days, the heart tube, which is growing much faster than the developing blood vessels to which it is attached, dilates and begins to form constrictions that start to separate it into chambers and vessels—the *atrium, ventricle, truncus arteriosus, sinus venosus*, and the *bulbus cordis* (Fig. 6–1C). Note that at this stage blood flows upward from the sinus venosus to the atrium and then to the ventricle, which is located above the atrium. The continued rapid development of the heart tube causes it to double over on itself, forming the U-shaped bulboventricular loop by about the 24th day (Fig. 6–1D). As heart growth continues, the atrium is pushed upward and the ventricle is pushed downward, resulting in the more familiar configuration of the atrium above the ventricle.

The single atrium and the single ventricle of the developing heart are each divided into left and right chambers during the period between the middle of the 4th week and the end of the 5th week after fertilization. The communication between the atrium and the ventricle, which is called the *atrioventricular canal* at this stage, is divided into left and right atrioventricular canals by the development of *endocardial cushions* that then fuse (Fig. 6–2).

The atrial septum begins to form as a membrane

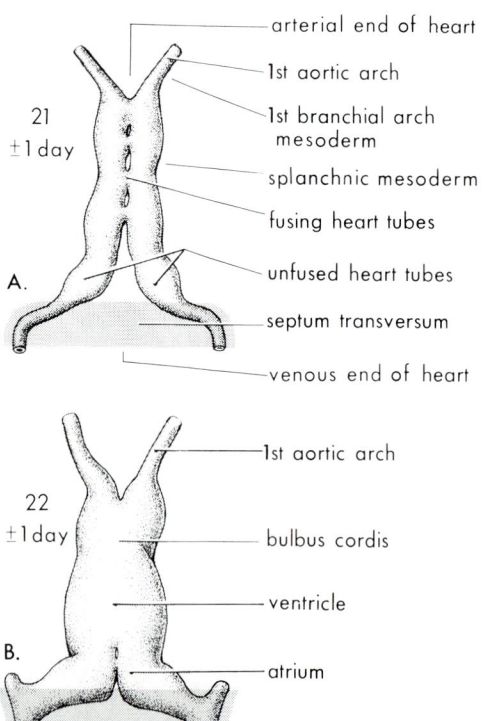
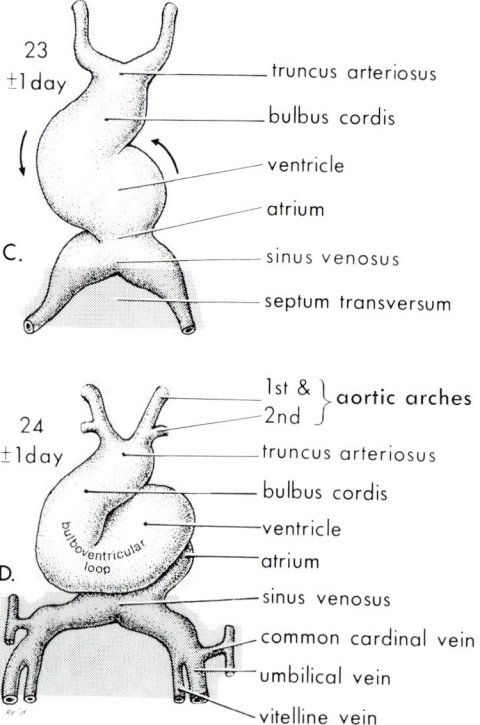

FIGURE 6–1. Development of the fetal heart during the 4th week of life. The approximate day after conception is indicated to the left of each of the figures. (From Moore, K.L.: *Before We Are Born: Basic Embryology and Birth Defects*, 2nd ed. Philadelphia, W.B. Saunders, 1983, with permission.)

called the *septum primum* grows from the upper part of the atrium toward the fused endocardial cushions (Figs. 6–2D and 6–3B). The opening remaining between the septum primum and endocardial cushions is called the *foramen primum*. The septum primum eventually fuses with the endocardial cushions, thus closing the foramen primum. However, during this time, perforations appear in the upper part of the septum primum, forming a new opening called the *foramen secundum* (Figs. 6–3C and D). Another membrane, the *septum secundum*, then begins to grow from the upper part of the atrium, eventually covering the foramen secundum. An orifice remaining in the septum secundum is called the *foramen ovale*. Although it is covered by the septum secundum, the thin lower part of the septum primum is not fused to the septum secundum. Thus, the septum primum acts as the valve of the foramen ovale until after birth. During this period, the left part of the sinus venosus starts to form the coronary sinus, while the right part becomes part of the wall of the right atrium.

The ventricular septum begins to form as a ridge of muscle that projects from the lower part of the single ventricle (Figs. 6–2D and 6–3B). This *interventricular septum* grows toward the fused endocardial cushions (Figs. 6–3C and D). The resulting *interventricular foramen* exists until complete fusion of the septum and the endocardial cushions at about the end of the 7th week of gestation. During this period, spirally arranged ridges appear in the truncus arteriosus. These truncal ridges (Figs. 6–4B and C) fuse to form the aorticopulmonary septum that separates the pulmonary trunk from the aorta (Fig. 6–4E). After the interventricular foramen closes, the right ventricle is connected with the pulmonary artery and is therefore separate from the left ventricle, which is connected with the aorta. The bulbus cordis is ultimately incorporated into the ventricular walls. Figures 6–4G and H demonstrate how the spiral arrangement of the aorticopulmonary septum results in the aorta and pulmonary trunk twisting about each other as they leave the heart.

Development of the Systemic Arteries

Six pairs of *aortic arch arteries* (also called branchial arch arteries) arise from the truncus arteriosus and terminate in the dorsal aorta of the same side. As shown in Figure 6–5, these aortic arch arteries do not all exist at the same time. During

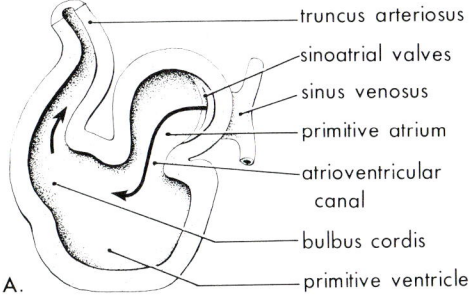
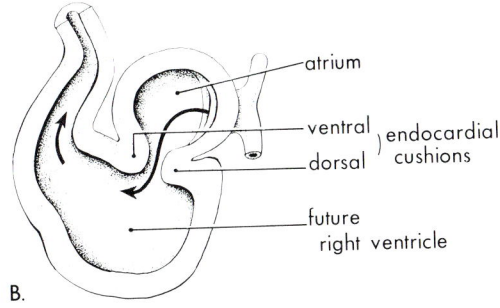
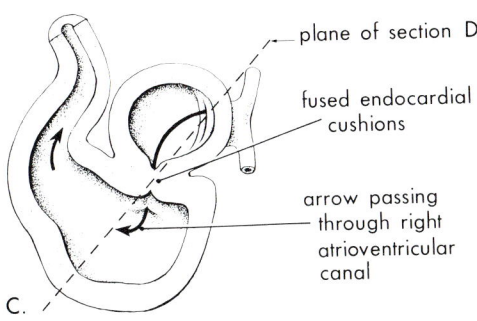
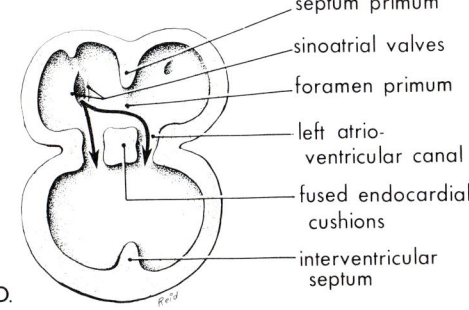

FIGURE 6–2. Development of the chambers of the fetal heart during the 4th and 5th weeks of gestation. *A* to *C*, Sagittal sections showing the fusion of the endocardial cushions to separate the atria from the ventricles. *D*, Frontal section showing fusion of the endocardial cushions. (From Moore, K.L.: *Before We Are Born: Basic Embryology and Birth Defects*, 2nd ed. Philadelphia, W.B. Saunders, 1983, with permission.)

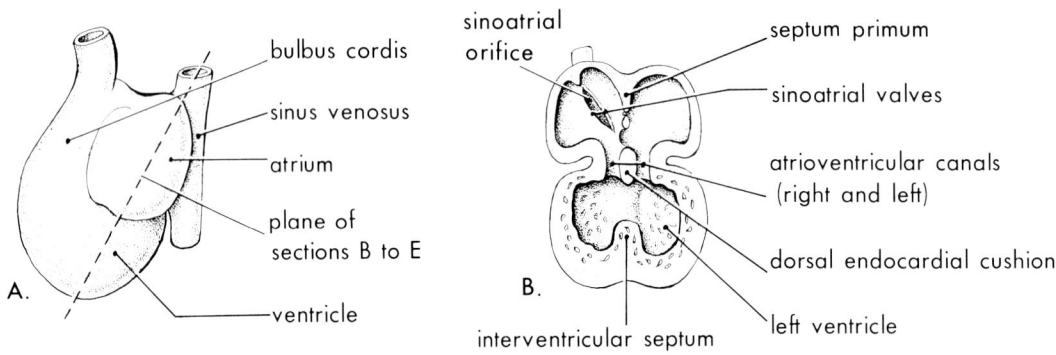
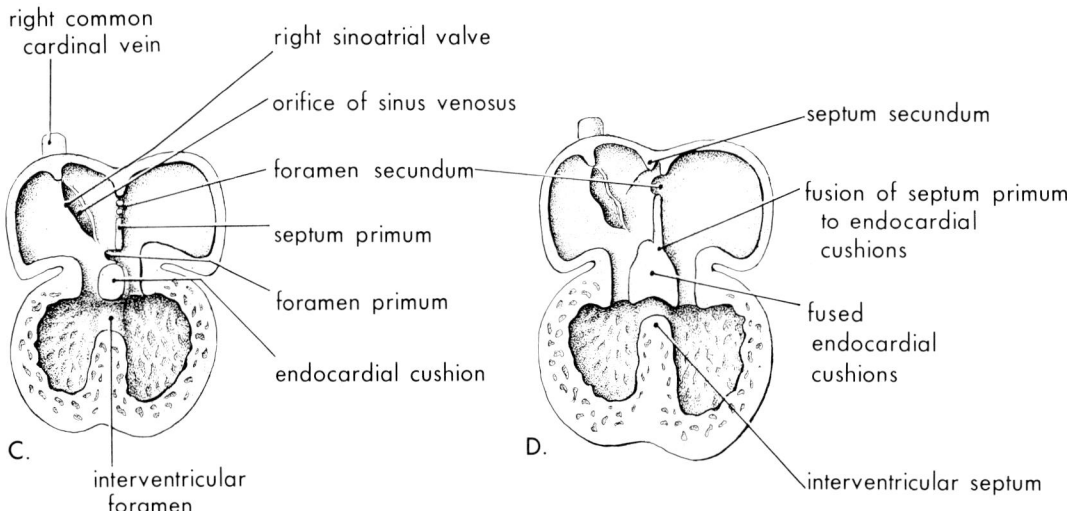
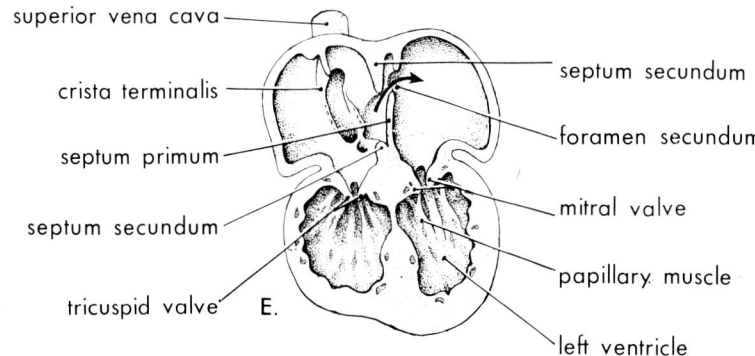

FIGURE 6–3. Development of the fetal heart during the 4th to 8th weeks of gestation, showing the fusion of the endocardial cushions to separate the atria from the ventricles and the development of the interatrial and interventricular septas to separate the left and right hearts. A, Dotted line shows the plane of the section in B to E. B, Heart at about 28 days of gestation. C, Heart at about 30 days. D, Heart at about 35 days. E, Heart at about 8 weeks. (From Moore, K.L.: *Before We Are Born: Basic Embryology and Birth Defects,* 2nd ed. Philadelphia, W.B. Saunders, 1983, with permission.)

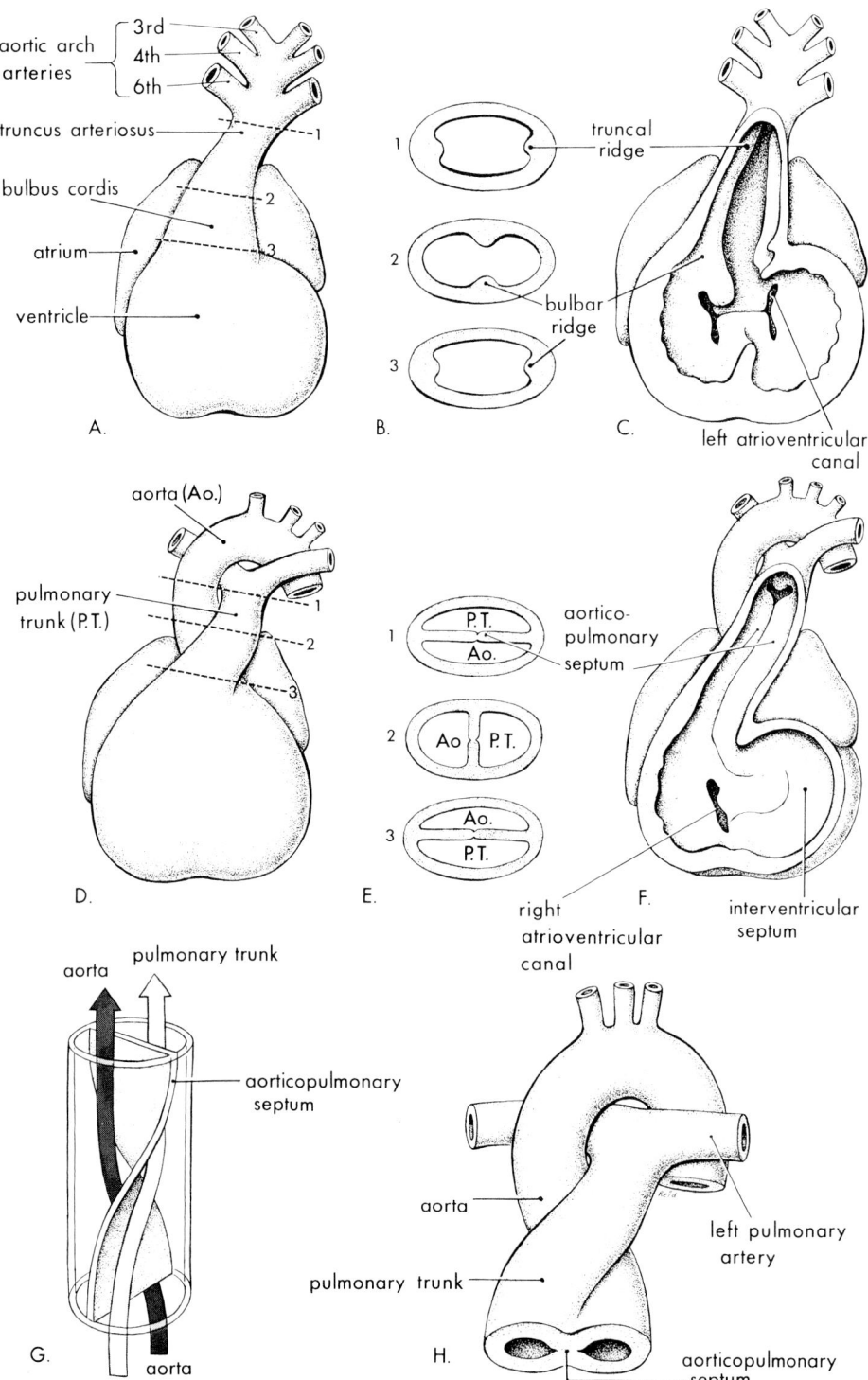

FIGURE 6–4. Development of the aorta and pulmonary trunk from the truncus arteriosus and bulbus cordis. The fetal heart at 5 weeks of gestation: *A*, ventral view of the heart; *B*, Transverse sections through the truncus arteriosus and bulbus cordis at sites indicated in *A*; *C*, the heart at 5 weeks of development, shown with the ventral wall removed. The fetal heart at 6 weeks of development: *D*, ventral view of the heart; *E*, transverse sections through the aorta and pulmonary trunk showing the aorticopulmonary septum at sites indicated in *D*; *F*, the heart at 6 weeks of development, shown with the ventral wall removed. *G*, Illustration of the spiral development of the aorticopulmonary septum. *H*, Final form of the aorta and pulmonary artery. (From Moore, K.L.: *Before We Are Born: Basic Embryology and Birth Defects*, 2nd ed. Philadelphia, W.B. Saunders, 1983, with permission.)

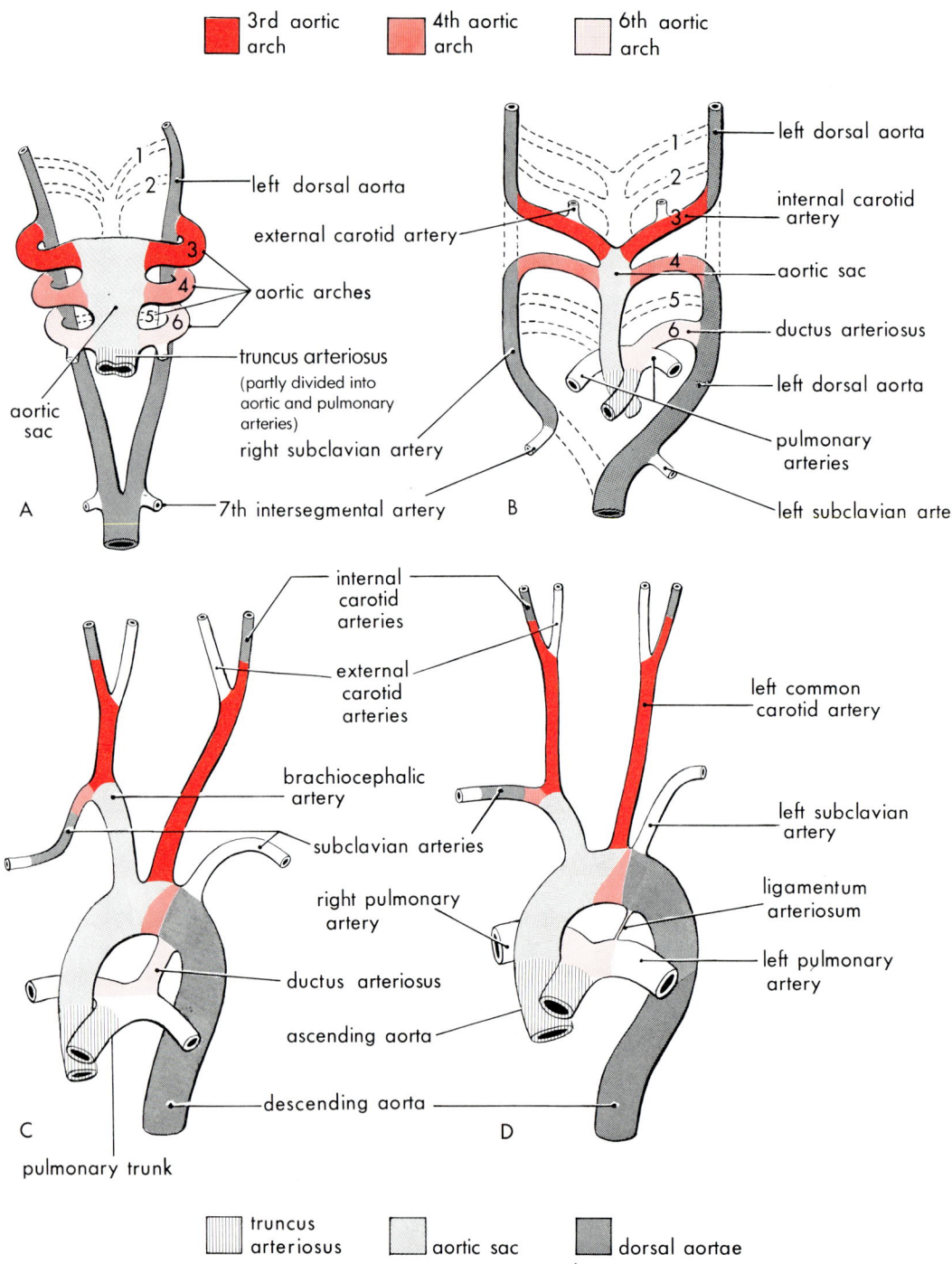

FIGURE 6–5. Development of the pulmonary trunk and the aortic arch and its main branches from the aortic sac, dorsal aorta, truncus arteriosus, and aortic arch arteries of the fetus. *A*, At 6 weeks of gestation. *B*, At 7 weeks. *C*, At 8 weeks of gestation. *D*, At 6 months after birth. (From Moore, K.L.: *Before We Are Born: Basic Embryology and Birth Defects*, 2nd ed. Philadelphia, W.B. Saunders, 1983, with permission.)

the 6th to 8th weeks of development, the first and second pairs of aortic arch arteries (shown at day 24 in Fig. 6–1D) disappear, and the proximal parts of the third pair become the common carotid arteries. These join the dorsal aorta to form the internal carotid arteries (Figs. 6–5B and C). The left fourth aortic arch artery becomes part of the arch of the aorta; the right becomes the initial portion of the right subclavian artery. The fifth aortic arch artery disappears. The left part of the sixth aortic arch artery develops into part of the left pulmonary artery, and part remains as a connection between the aorta and the pulmonary artery called the *ductus arteriosus*. Part of the right sixth aortic arch artery develops into the right pulmonary artery.

Development of the Lungs

The embryologic development of the lungs is simple compared with that of the heart and major arteries. Unlike the heart, however, the lungs are not ready to assume their main adult function until late in fetal development. Lung development is usually divided into three stages: the *glandular stage*, *canalicular stage*, and *alveolar stage*.

Glandular Stage (5 to 16 weeks). The airways of the respiratory system are derived from the *laryngotracheal groove* of the embryo. This groove begins to form as an outpouching of the primitive pharynx during the 4th week after gestation. This outpouching, or *diverticulum*, grows away from the pharynx, forming a separate *lung bud* (Fig. 6–6A). The folds in the tracheoesophageal structure grow toward each other, ultimately fusing to form the *tracheoesophageal septum* (Fig. 6–6B). The septum thus separates the developing larynx and tracheobronchial tree from the esophagus (Fig. 6–6C).

The lung bud splits into two *bronchopulmonary buds* during the end of the 4th week of development (Figs. 6–6B and C). These buds push out into the pleural cavities and become the two mainstem bronchi. During the 5th week after conception, the right bronchopulmonary bud gives rise to three secondary buds, and the left bronchopulmonary bud gives rise to two secondary buds (Figs. 6–6D and E). The secondary buds ultimately develop into the right upper, right middle, and right lower lobes; and the left upper and lower lobes. Figure 6–6F shows the developing lungs at 6 weeks after conception; Figure 6–6G shows the developing lungs at 8 weeks after conception. The tertiary buds shown in these figures develop into the bronchopulmonary segments (see Fig. 3–4). As the lungs continue to grow, they are covered by the visceral pleura; at the same time, the thoracic cavity is lined with the parietal pleura.

The structure of the tracheobronchial tree develops and matures during this same period. Mesenchymal cells surround the endodermal lining of the laryngotracheal tube and give rise to the connective tissue, cartilage, and smooth muscle of the larynx and trachea. The epithelium and glands of the tracheobronchial tree are derived from the endoderm. The C-shaped tracheal cartilages begin to appear during the 8th week after conception, and cilia begin to form in the tracheal lining by about the 10th week. Mucous glands begin to appear in the upper part of the tracheobronchial tree in the 12th week of development and are seen farther down the tree shortly thereafter. Thus, cartilage is present in the mainstem bronchi by the 10th week of development and in segmental bronchi by the 12th week; cilia appear in the mainstem bronchi at the 12th week and in segmental bronchi at the 13th week; and mucous glands appear in the bronchi at the 13th week and begin to produce mucus only a week later.

The pulmonary arteries begin to develop from the sixth aortic arch artery during the 5th and 6th weeks after conception (Fig. 6–5B). The pulmonary arteries grow and branch parallel to the growth of the branches of the two mainstem bronchi. Pulmonary veins develop from the wall of the left atrium, starting at about 4 weeks after conception. Bronchial arteries develop from the dorsal aorta, starting in the 7th to 8th week, and form many connections with the pulmonary circulation.

Development of the lower portions of the tracheobronchial tree and the alveolar-capillary gas exchange units occurs during the second and third stages of fetal lung development, the *canalicular stage* and *alveolar stage*. All three stages are indicated in the lowermost portion of Figure 6–7, which summarizes the time course of the important aspects of lung development.

Canalicular Stage (16 to 26 weeks). The glandular stage of lung development is usually said to end during the 15th to 16th week of fetal development. Up to this point the lungs resemble glands upon microscopic inspection because they consist of small branching airways lined with a large number of mucous glands. During the canalicular stage the lumens of the airways enlarge, and the terminal bronchioles give rise to respiratory bronchioles. The respiratory bronchioles then divide into alveolar ducts and *terminal air sacs*, which later develop into alveolar cells. Pulmonary capillaries and lymphatics begin to form during this period.

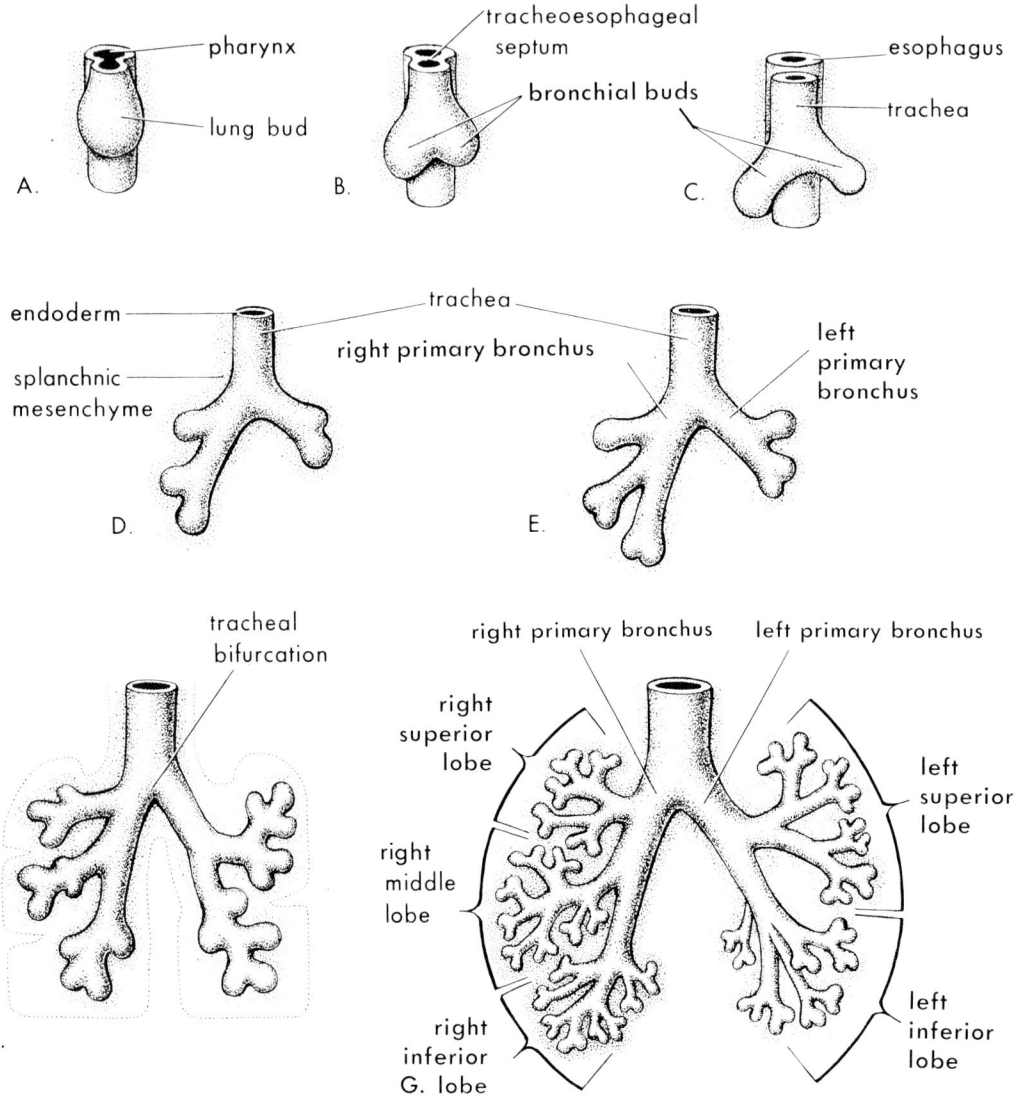

FIGURE 6–6. Ventral views of the development of the fetal tracheobronchial tree. *A* to *D*, At 4 weeks of development. *E* to *F*, At 5 weeks, *G*, At 6 weeks. (From Moore, K.L.: *Before We Are Born: Basic Embryology and Birth Defects,* 2nd ed. Philadelphia, W.B. Saunders, 1983, with permission.)

A diagrammatic sketch of the microscopic appearance of the lung at the end of the canalicular period is shown in Figure 6–8A.

Alveolar Stage (26 weeks to birth). During the final stage, the capillary network proliferates around the developing alveoli, and the immature cuboidal epithelial alveolar cells shown in Figure 6–8A begin to differentiate into flattened (squamous) type I alveolar epithelial cells or the cuboidal type II alveolar epithelial cells, as shown in Figure 6–8B. These begin to produce functional pulmonary surfactant after about the 7th month of gestation.

Thus, by the time a normal fetus has developed for 7 to 8 months, the lungs are capable of their main adult function of gas exchange between the blood and the external environment. At the end of the normal gestation period of 40 weeks, almost all of 23 branchings (or generations) of the airways have occurred, resulting in a number of alveolar ducts approximately one tenth that of the adult and a number of alveoli approximately one fifteenth that of the adult. The pulmonary circulation has developed, and pulmonary capillaries have proliferated around the alveoli, forming a surface area for gas exchange approximately one twentieth that

CARDIOPULMONARY CHANGES THROUGH LIFE 227

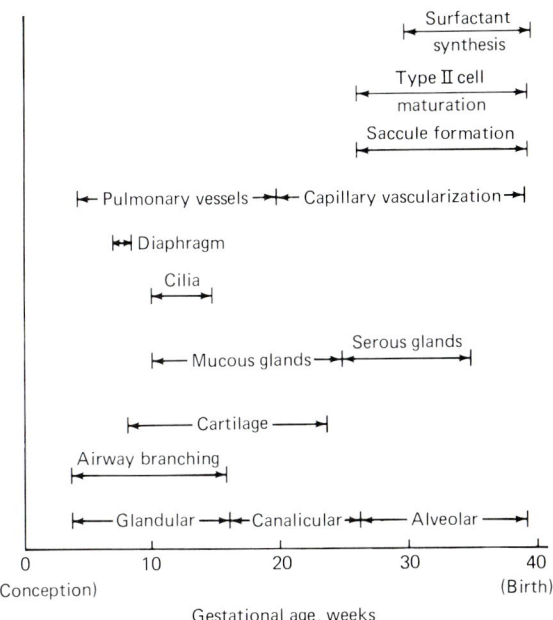

FIGURE 6–7. The time course of different aspects of fetal lung development. (From Brody, J.S.: Lung development, growth and repair. In Fishman, A.P. (ed.): *Pulmonary Diseases and Disorders.* New York, Mc-Graw-Hill, 1980, with permission.)

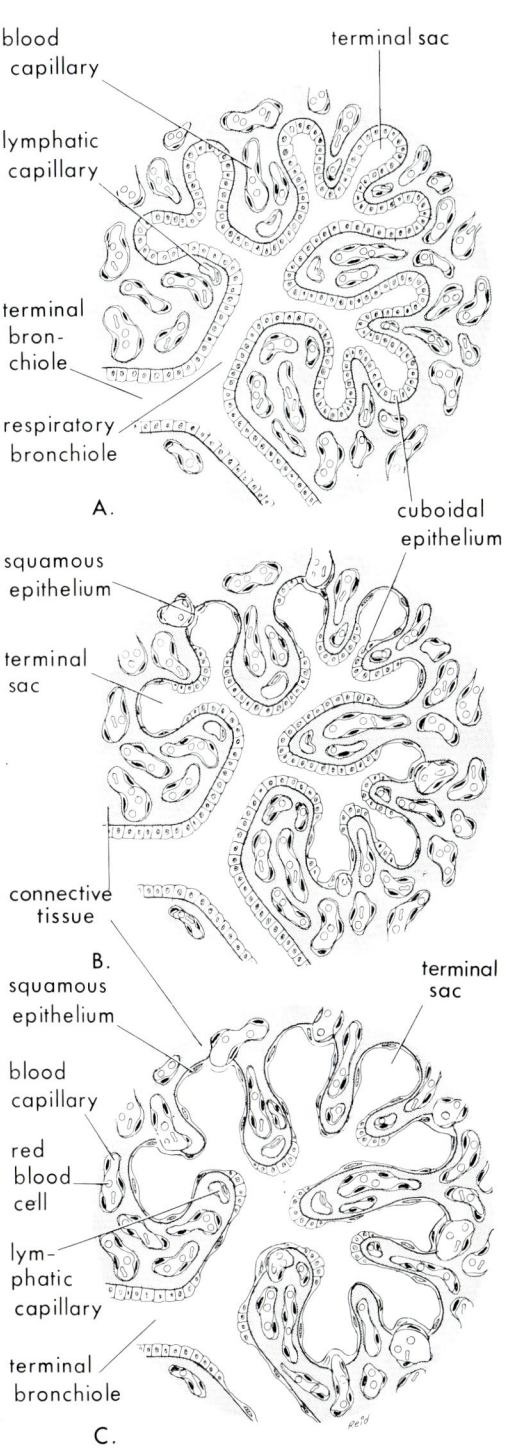

FIGURE 6–8. Diagrams of the microscopic appearance of the fetal lung: *A,* At 24 weeks of gestation. *B,* At 26 weeks of gestation. *C,* At birth. (From Moore, K.L.: *Before We Are Born: Basic Embryology and Birth Defects,* 2nd ed. Philadelphia, W.B. Saunders, 1983, with permission.)

of the adult. Furthermore, pulmonary surfactant is being produced by the type II alveolar epithelial cells.

At birth, the lungs are partly inflated with a mixture of amniotic fluid and secretions from the glands of the tracheobronchial tree. The lungs must be inflated with the neonate's first breath and the fluid must also be removed. But before the events associated with the neonate's first breath are discussed, we must first consider the anatomy and physiology of the fetal circulation.

FETAL CIRCULATION

There are several important differences between the circulation of the fetus and that of the adult. These include the presence of the placenta, the ductus venosus, the foramen ovale, and the ductus arteriosus. The two ventricles of the fetus pump in parallel; in the adult, the two ventricles pump in series.

The Placenta

Gas exchange between the fetus and mother occurs in the placenta, so the placenta acts as the lung of the fetus. The fetus absorbs nutrients from the mother's blood in the placenta and delivers waste products to the mother's blood there as well, so the placenta also acts as the gastrointestinal tract and kidney of the fetus.

The placenta weighs about a half kilogram at birth and thus constitutes about 14% of the weight of the fetus. After the fertilized ovum is implanted in the wall of the uterus, blood-filled sinuses developed between the endometrium of the uterus and the surface of the embryo. These sinuses are supplied with arterial blood from the *uterine artery* of the mother and are drained by her *uterine veins*. As the embryo grows, fetal capillaries form projections into the sinuses. These projections develop into the *chorionic villi*, which interdigitate with the maternal blood sinuses and increase the area of contact between the fetal and maternal circulations. The increased surface area for diffusion is necessary because the thickness of the diffusion barrier is much greater in the placenta than in the adult lung.

The placenta receives blood low in oxygen (the P_{O_2} is about 25 mmHg) and high in carbon dioxide (the P_{CO_2} is about 50 mmHg) from the fetus via the umbilical arteries (Fig. 6–9). As this blood travels through the placental capillaries of the fetus, it is exposed to the maternal blood with a P_{O_2} of about 100 mmHg and P_{CO_2} of about 36 mmHg (recall from Chapter 4 that pregnant women hyperventilate because of elevated progesterone levels). Blood returning from the placenta to the fetus has a P_{O_2} of only about 35 mmHg and a P_{CO_2} of about 45 mmHg. This is partly a result of the inefficient diffusion between the maternal and fetal portions of the placenta resulting from the thickness of the diffusion barrier and partly a result of the high oxygen consumption of the placenta itself.

Two factors assist in gas transfer between the fetus and the mother. Fetal hemoglobin concentration is higher than that of the adult, so the oxygen carrying capacity of fetal blood may be greater than that of the adult. The oxyhemoglobin dissociation curve of fetal blood is also shifted to the left (Fig. 6–10). Thus, fetal hemoglobin (HbF) has a greater affinity for oxygen than adult hemoglobin (HbA) at the same P_{O_2}. HbF consists of two alpha subunit chains and two gamma chains, whereas HbA has two alpha chains and two beta chains. Part of the reason that HbF has a greater affinity for oxygen than does HbA is that 2,3-DPG has little effect on the affinity of HbF for oxygen. Fetal hemoglobin concentration may be as high as 18 to 20 grams Hb/100 ml blood, and its P_{50}, as low as 19 mmHg. Synthesis of beta chains normally begins about 6 weeks before birth, and nearly all of the HbF is usually replaced by HbA by the time an infant is 4 months old. Fetal oxygen consumption is about 7 ml/min/kg or about 20 to 25 ml/min near term.

Anatomy and Physiology of Fetal Circulation

The *umbilical vein* carries "arterial" blood from the placenta to the fetus (Fig. 6–9). As already noted, its P_{O_2} ranges from 30 to 35 mmHg. After giving rise to branches that supply the left two thirds of the liver, the umbilical vein joins the *portal sinus* (a branch of the *portal vein*) to form the *ductus venosus*. Flow in the portal sinus is from the umbilical vein to the portal vein. Therefore, the right third of the liver, which is supplied by branches of the portal vein, receives a mixture of umbilical vein blood and portal venous blood with a lower P_{O_2}.

The ductus venosus runs along the underside of the liver and joins the *inferior vena cava*. The blood in the inferior vena cava drains the abdominal viscera and lower extremities, so its P_{O_2} is very low (about 14 mmHg) *below* its connection with the ductus venosus. Inferior vena cava blood *above* the ductus venosus has a higher P_{O_2} because of the blood in the ductus venosus that came from the umbilical vein.

The blood entering the heart via the inferior vena cava is divided into two streams by a projection of the atrial septum called the *crista dividens*. Most of the blood passes through the open *foramen ovale* and enters the left atrium, thus bypassing the lungs. (In the fetus, the left atrium extends dorsally beneath the rest of the heart to join the inferior vena cava at the foramen ovale.) The rest of the blood from the inferior vena cava joins blood draining the head and upper extremities via the *superior vena cava* and blood draining the myocardium via the *coronary sinus* in the right atrium. This blood passes into the right ventricle and is pumped to the lungs via the pulmonary artery. The P_{O_2} of the blood in the pulmonary artery is approximately only 20 mmHg because it is a mixture of the relatively well-oxygenated inferior vena cava blood and blood low in oxygen from the head, upper extremities, and myocardium. The P_{O_2} of the blood in the aorta, on the other hand, is 25 to 30 mmHg because it is mainly inferior vena cava blood, with only a small contribution from the pulmonary veins.

As already noted, the two fetal ventricles pump in parallel, rather than in series. In contrast to the

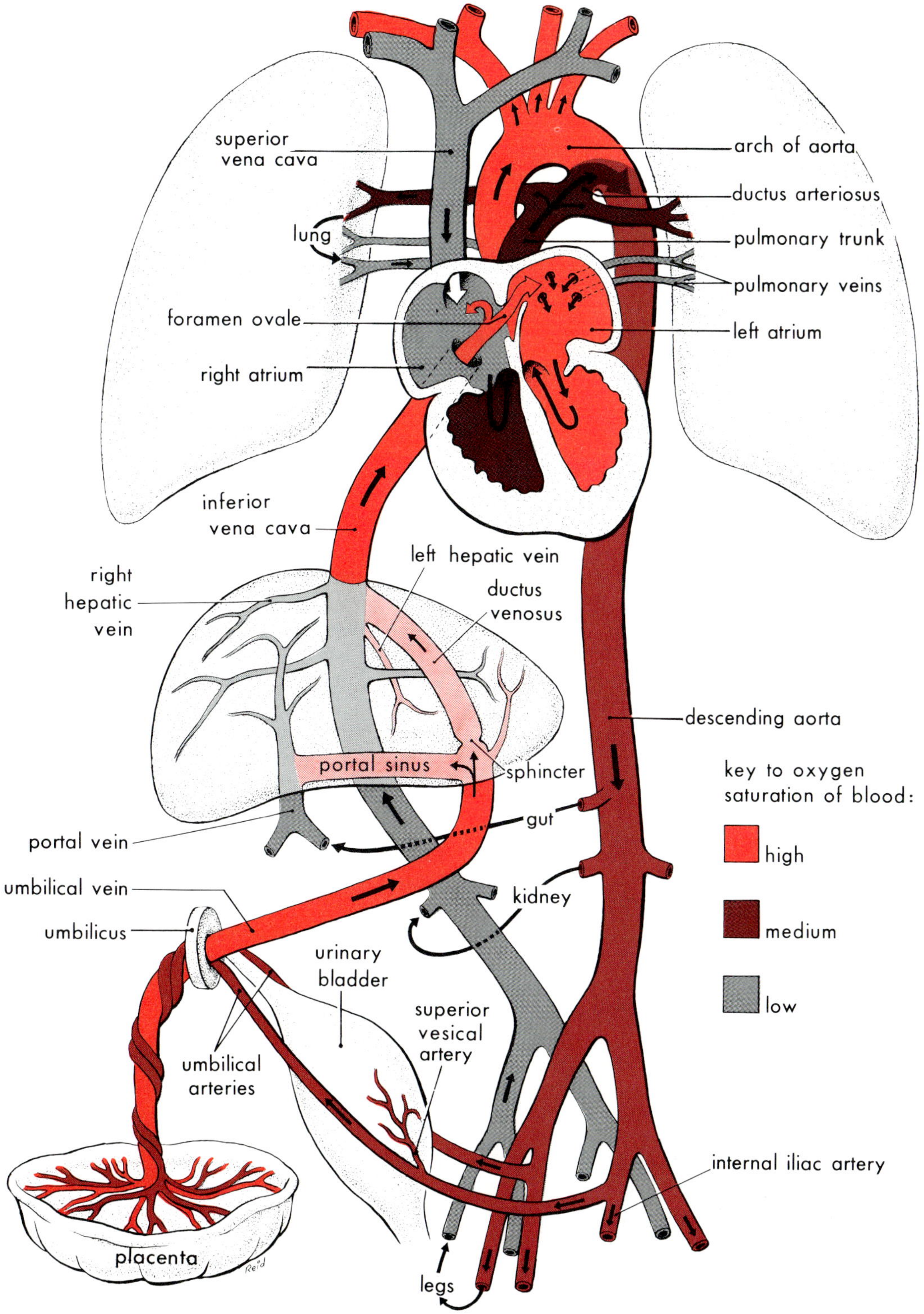

FIGURE 6–9. Diagram of the fetal circulation just before birth. (From Moore, K.L.: *Before We Are Born: Basic Embryology and Birth Defects,* 2nd ed. Philadelphia, W.B. Saunders, 1983, with permission.)

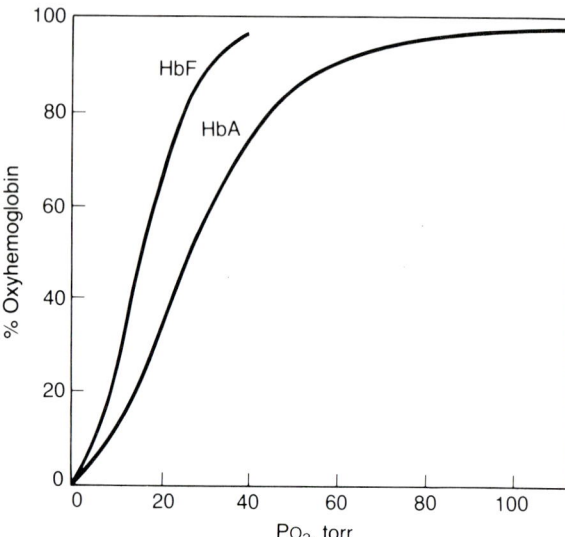

FIGURE 6–10. Oxyhemoglobin dissociation curves of blood from a fetus (HbF) and blood from an adult (HbA).

situation in the adult, they are similar in size and muscular development. Pulmonary artery pressure is several mmHg greater than aortic pressure. Only 5% to 15% of the right ventricular output passes through the lungs because they are collapsed and offer much greater resistance to blood flow. Instead, most of the right ventricular output passes through the open *ductus arteriosus* into the aorta.

Blood is pumped by the left ventricle to the heart, brain, and upper extremities before the connection of the pulmonary artery with the aorta at the ductus arteriosus. The brain and heart are therefore supplied with blood that has a relatively high P_{O_2} of 25 to 30 mmHg. Blood in the descending (or abdominal) aorta, on the other hand, is a mixture from both ventricles, and it has a lower P_{O_2} (20 to 23 mmHg). More than half of the combined output of the two ventricles perfuses the placenta via the umbilical arteries. The rest supplies the abdominal viscera and lower extremities.

Fetal mean arterial blood pressure increases during the last third of normal pregnancies to about 55 mmHg. During that time, the heart rate decreases. These changes are associated with the development of the autonomic nervous system of the fetus, especially the arterial baroreceptor and chemoreceptor reflexes.

CARDIOPULMONARY ALTERATIONS AT BIRTH

At birth, the neonate's lungs must take over the gas exchange function from the placenta. This is accomplished by initiation of the first breath, aeration of the lungs, resorption of fluid from the air spaces, and a series of changes in the neonate's cardiovascular system.

Alterations in the Respiratory System

Intrapleural pressures estimated to be from -30 to -70 cmH$_2$O are necessary to overcome the surface tension of the alveoli, the tissue resistance of the lungs and chest wall, and the viscosity of the liquid in the airways to expand the lungs and generate the first breath. The fetus begins to make respiratory movements in utero during the later stages of gestation. These movements are believed to be important in the development of the strength of the respiratory muscles.

Several chemical and physical stimuli may combine to initiate the neonate's first breath. These include drive from both the arterial chemoreceptors and the central chemoreceptors caused by hypoxia and/or hypercapnia, the sensation of the reduction in ambient temperature, and tactile sensations, including pain.

Alveoli open serially, that is, one after the other, because of both Laplace's law and the structural interdependence of the alveolar septa. Inflation of the alveoli is probably nearly complete within a few breaths, especially if the baby cries.

Prenatal liquids appear to be removed from the lungs by several mechanisms, including osmosis into the capillaries, lymphatic drainage after diffusion into the interstitium, and even pinocytosis. During labor, prenatal fluid from the upper airways is expelled into the pharynx by mechanical compression of the thoracic cage. At delivery, this process may be assisted by the physician aspirating the fluid.

Alterations in the Circulation

Cessation of umbilical blood flow occurs even if the umbilical cord is not clamped and tied. Umbilical blood flow continues after delivery but decreases rapidly. The mechanism of the decrease in umbilical blood flow is not known, but it may involve compression of the umbilical cord in the uterus during delivery, catecholamines from the neonate's adrenal medulla, or exposure to the cold ambient air.

Closure of the foramen ovale occurs within a few minutes after delivery. This is partly because of the cessation of umbilical vein blood flow following clamping of the umbilical cord, which decreases venous return and lowers right atrial pressure; and partly because inflating the lungs increases pulmonary blood flow and therefore increases left atrial pressure. These two factors tend to reverse the pressure gradient across the foramen ovale, and the valve closes. The valve usually becomes adherent to the edge of the foramen ovale within a few days of birth.

Elimination of the low resistance pathway for blood flow through the placenta increases systemic vascular resistance and ends blood flow through the ductus venosus. Fibrosis and closure of the ductus venosus occurs within about 7 days after birth, but the mechanism is not well understood.

Expansion of the neonate's previously collapsed lungs by its first breath results in a rapid decrease in pulmonary vascular resistance, a decrease in pulmonary artery pressure, and a sixfold to tenfold increase in pulmonary blood flow. Pulmonary vascular resistance may fall as a result of mechanical effects by the expanding alveoli, which should lengthen vessels and pull some open by traction; the establishment of an air-liquid interface; relief of pulmonary vasoconstriction caused by hypoxia and possibly hypercapnia; and release of pulmonary vasodilators, such as prostacyclin.

Aortic pressure increases after birth because of increased sympathetic stimulation and because of cessation of perfusion of the placenta, which removes a large parallel pathway for blood flow. The increased aortic blood pressure, coupled with decreased pulmonary artery pressure, reverses the pressure gradient for blood flow through the ductus arteriosus, and blood begins to flow from the aorta to the pulmonary artery within about an hour after birth. The ductus arteriosus begins to constrict within a few hours after birth but does not close completely for 1 to 8 days.

The stimulus that initiates constriction of the ductus arteriosus is believed to be the elevation in systemic arterial P_{O_2} that occurs after birth. The mechanism causing the constriction may involve decreased release of vasodilators (such as prostacyclin, prostaglandin E_2, or acetylcholine) or increased release of catecholamines, constrictor prostaglandins, or bradykinin. After final occlusion of the ductus arteriosus by contraction of its vascular smooth muscle, its wall is replaced by fibrous tissue. This usually occurs within 2 or 3 weeks after birth.

PERINATAL PATHOPHYSIOLOGY

After discussing the embryology, growth, and development of the fetal pulmonary and cardiovascular systems, we can now consider the pathophysiology of the major cardiopulmonary disorders of the neonate.

Cardiovascular Disorders

The most common cardiovascular disorders of the neonate include atrial and ventricular septal defects, patent ductus arteriosus, coarctation of the aorta, tetralogy of Fallot, transposition of the great vessels, and persistent fetal circulation.

Atrial Septal Defects

There are two main types of atrial septal defects (ASDs). One type occurs in the area of the foramen ovale (see Fig. 6–3) and may involve perforations in the valve of the foramen, abnormal or excessive resorption of the septum primum, or defective development of the septum secundum. Each of these can result in a *patent foramen ovale*. The second type occurs when the septum primum doesn't fuse with the endocardial cushions, which causes a *patent foramen primum*. This is often seen with mitral valve malformations.

Expansion of the lung and changes in the cardiovascular system that occur at birth normally increase left atrial pressure and decrease right atrial pressure. Thus, left atrial pressure normally exceeds right atrial pressure. In a person with an atrial septal defect, blood therefore flows from the left atrium back into the right atrium through the defect. Because the right atrium is still receiving all of the systemic venous return, this additional quantity of oxygenated blood from the left atrium imposes a large volume load on the right atrium and right ventricle and may greatly increase pulmonary blood flow. The increase in pulmonary blood flow does not usually lead to an increase in systemic blood flow because of the baroreceptor reflex, autoregulation, and other mechanisms discussed in Chapter 2. Most of the excess pulmonary venous return goes back through the atrial septal defect into the right atrium. Thus, right ventricular output may be two or three times the left ventricular output in a resting patient who has an atrial septal defect. During exercise, however, left ventricular output may increase without any further increase in right ventricular output as systemic vascular resistance falls.

As noted in Chapter 5, the right ventricle responds much better to a volume load than to a pressure load. Indeed, most cases of congenital atrial septal defects are asymptomatic until the person is a young adult. Then, the symptoms are usually an increased susceptibility to fatigue and dyspnea on exertion.

The heart is usually only slightly enlarged. Pulmonary hypertension, right ventricular hypertrophy, and signs of right ventricular failure are all rarely encountered in patients with atrial septal defects. A systolic murmur of mild intensity and medium pitch is often present, usually in the pulmonary area of the precordium. Cardiac catheterization should demonstrate an elevated right atrial Po_2 and may also show the left atrial to right atrial pressure gradient. Electrocardiographic features usually include signs of right axis deviation, and large peaked P-waves may be seen. First-degree A–V block and right bundle branch block are also frequent findings. Surgical repair of the atrial septal defect is usually recommended.

Ventricular Septal Defects

Ventricular septal defects (VSDs) are a very common congenital cardiac disorder. They may be caused by incomplete closure of the interventricular foramen and by failure of the muscular part of the interventricular septum to fuse with the endocardial cushions and the aorticopulmonary septum (see Figs. 6–3 and 6–4).

Large ventricular septal defects result in blood flow from the left ventricle through the defect and into the right ventricle during systole. Large ventricular septal defects also result in transmission of left ventricular *pressure* through the defect and may elevate right ventricular systolic pressure to levels nearly equal to left ventricular systolic pressure. The increased blood flow into the right ventricle, along with the increased right ventricular systolic pressure, leads to increased pulmonary blood flow, pulmonary vascular congestion, and pulmonary hypertension. These, in turn, decrease the compliance of the lungs and increase the patient's inspiratory work of breathing and susceptibility to interstitial pulmonary edema and pneumonia. The left ventricle must do increased volume work to perfuse the systemic circulation.

Infants with small ventricular septal defects may be asymptomatic. Symptoms of infants with large ventricular septal defects include slow weight gain and a pale, delicate appearance. Respiratory infections, feeding difficulties and heart failure are often seen.

Patients with small ventricular septal defects usually have louder systolic murmurs than those with larger ones. Radiography may show enlargement of either or both ventricles, depending on the size of the defect. The main pulmonary arteries are usually enlarged, and the aorta may appear smaller than normal. The electrocardiogram usually shows right axis deviation and hypertrophy of both ventricles. Cardiac catheterization reveals an increased right ventricular Po_2 and pulmonary hypertension.

Small ventricular septal defects are not usually treated surgically. Larger defects may be treated in two stages. First, a band may be placed around the pulmonary artery to decrease the pulmonary vascular congestion and hypertension. When the infant grows large enough to permit the more severe open-heart surgery, the band is removed and the defect is closed.

Patent Ductus Arteriosus

The pathophysiologic effects of a patent ductus arteriosus depend on the diameter of the connection between the aorta and pulmonary artery. A large patent ductus arteriosus results in large volumes of blood taking this low-resistance pathway from the left ventricle into the pulmonary artery during systole and a continued movement of blood from the aorta into the pulmonary artery during diastole. This results in low aortic diastolic pressures, large pulse pressures, increased left ventricular volume work, and elevated pulmonary artery pressure and blood flow. The last two may lead to a greater risk of interstitial pulmonary edema and congestive heart failure. A small patent ductus arteriosus may not lead to any symptoms during early childhood, with a characteristic continuous murmur and the possibility of left ventricular enlargement later in life.

A large patent ductus arteriosus often results in a radiograph showing an enlarged left atrium, left ventricle, and aorta. The ECG may show evidence of left ventricular hypertrophy or biventricular hypertrophy. Cardiac catheterization should demonstrate a high pulmonary artery Po_2 in the blood *distal* to the patent ductus and may also show pulmonary hypertension.

Treatment of patent ductus arteriosus is usually with pharmacologic prostaglandin synthetase inhibitors like indomethacin or by surgical closure.

Coarctation of the Aorta

Coarctation, or narrowing, of the aorta usually occurs as a result of an abnormal development of the fourth and sixth aortic arch arteries. The narrowing of the aorta usually takes place just above or just below the ductus arteriosus. *Preductal* coarctations (those above the ductus arteriosus) are usually seen in infants and usually involve other cardiac abnormalities, especially patent ductus arteriosus. *Postductal* coarctation (those occurring below the ductus arteriosus) are not usually associated with other cardiac abnormalities and are not usually discovered until adulthood. Patients with severe narrowing of the aorta often develop large networks of collateral vessels, usually branches of the subclavian and intercostal arteries.

The main pathophysiologic effects of coarctation of the aorta usually reflect systemic hypertension above the coarctation rather than hypoperfusion below the coarctation, although some adult patients do complain of cold feet. Patients may have numerous headaches but may have no symptoms at all during childhood. Long-standing hypertension above the coarctation may cause left ventricular hypertrophy and congestive heart failure. Aortic rupture and cerebrovascular accidents are also seen occasionally, usually in young adults.

Clinical findings usually include weaker femoral pulses than brachial pulses, hypertension above the coarctation and lower arterial pressure below the coarctation, and sometimes a systolic murmur. Cardiac catheterization and angiography should give evidence for the coarctation. Left ventricular hypertrophy may be apparent on chest radiography and on electrocardiograms.

Surgical correction of coarctation of the aorta usually involves resection and end-to-end anastomosis of the aorta.

Tetralogy of Fallot

The tetralogy of Fallot is a congenital combination of four cardiac defects: a *ventricular septal defect*, an *"overriding" aorta* (the opening of the aortic valve is directly over the interventricular septal defect), *pulmonary stenosis*, and *right ventricular hypertrophy*. These four abnormalities are probably the result of a single embryologic problem because they occur together so often.

The pathophysiologic effects of the tetralogy of Fallot include decreased pulmonary blood flow, resulting from pulmonary stenosis; elevated right ventricular systolic pressure, because of the ventricular septal defect and pulmonary stenosis; mixture of systemic venous blood from the right ventricle into the left ventricle (especially if the pulmonary stenosis is severe) via the ventricular septal defect; and, therefore, *cyanosis*. Thus, the patient suffering from the tetralogy of Fallot may become increasingly cyanotic and have a progressively lower systemic arterial Po_2 if the pulmonary stenosis worsens because of less blood passing through the lung to be oxygenated and more shunting of venous blood into the aorta. At first, cyanosis may only occur when the infant eats, cries or defecates (sometimes it leads to unconsciousness and even convulsions); later, it may be a constant finding. The children are usually underdeveloped and dyspneic and may have clubbing of the fingers and toes.

Children with tetralogy of Fallot usually have loud systolic heart murmurs and a "boot-shaped" appearance of the heart in radiographs (because right ventricular hypertrophy elevates the apex and the small pulmonary artery leaves a concavity in the upper left border of the cardiac silhouette) and show evidence of right ventricular and right atrial hypertrophy, including right axis deviation and peaked P waves. Cardiac catheterization usually reveals equal pressures in the two ventricles. The treatment of tetralogy of Fallot is usually by one of a number of complicated surgical procedures.

Transposition of the Great Vessels

Complete simple transposition of the great vessels occurs as a result of a failure of the aorticopulmonary septum to follow a spiral course during the partitioning of the truncus arteriosus (see Fig. 6–4). The right ventricle therefore pumps systemic venous blood into the aorta and the left ventricle pumps oxygenated blood back into the lungs. If no other cardiac defects are present, none of the oxygenated blood coming from the lungs can be distributed to the systemic circulation and the neonate dies almost immediately. If other defects, such as atrial or ventricular septal defects or a patent ductus arteriosus, are present, the infant may survive long enough for surgical measures to be attempted. There are other congenital forms of transposition of the great vessels and also transposition of the pulmonary veins.

Persistent Truncus Arteriosus

In persistent truncus arteriosus, the spiral-shaped aorticopulmonary septum, shown in Figure 6–4G and H, does not form completely, resulting in a single arterial trunk supplying the systemic and pulmonary arteries. There is usually a large ventricular septal defect located directly beneath the orifice of the common arterial trunk so that both ventricles empty into it. This often results in markedly increased pulmonary blood flow that can produce congestive heart failure within the first few weeks of life, even though the baby may appear normal at birth. The congestive heart failure is usually treated with digitalis and diuretics until a surgical correction can be performed.

Persistent Fetal Circulation

Persistent fetal circulation is a syndrome in which the neonate suffers from *pulmonary artery hypertension*, caused by a continuation of high pulmonary vascular resistance, and/or *systemic arterial hypoxemia*, caused by *right to left shunts* through a patent ductus arteriosus or foramen ovale. The condition is associated with infants born of normal-length pregnancies, but with sustained periods of intrauterine hypoxemia. Severe hypoxemia and acidosis may occur at birth. The syndrome is often associated with *transient myocardial ischemia* and tricuspid valve insufficiency.

High pulmonary artery pressures caused by persistent pulmonary vasoconstriction can force systemic venous blood through the patent ductus arteriosus if pulmonary artery pressure exceeds aortic pressure. Similarly, elevated right atrial pressure forces systemic venous blood through the foramen ovale if right atrial pressure exceeds left atrial pressure. Each of these situations can lead to systemic arterial hypoxemia and cyanosis. Systemic arterial perfusion is normally maintained unless the hypoxemia causes decreased left ventricular contractility. If the ductus arteriosus does close before the elevated pulmonary vascular resistance is relieved, possible consequences include right ventricular failure secondary to its increased workload and a restriction of pulmonary venous return to the left ventricle, thus limiting or decreasing the systemic cardiac output.

Treatment of persistent fetal circulation syndrome includes attempts to decrease pulmonary vascular resistance by increasing alveolar P_{O_2} (to inhibit hypoxic pulmonary vasoconstriction), relieving acidosis, and using pulmonary vasodilators as well as attempts to maintain left ventricular output. Hyperventilation may be used to increase alveolar P_{O_2} and increase the arterial pH.

Pulmonary Disorders

The most common pulmonary disorders of the neonate include choanal atresia, infant respiratory distress syndrome, meconium aspiration, tracheoesophageal fistula, and diaphragmatic hernia.

Choanal Atresia

Neonates are usually considered to breathe through the nose preferentially, but some are believed to be *unable* to breathe through the mouth during sleep. This may be a result of either upper airway obstruction, resulting from apposition of the tongue and soft palate, or because the respiratory control mechanisms have not yet developed sufficiently to switch from nasal to oral breathing when the nasal air passages are obstructed. Such an obligate nasal breather would only ventilate his or her alveoli during crying in periods of nasal airway obstruction. Obligatory nose breathing is believed to contribute to sudden infant death syndrome, but the evidence is unclear.

The *choana* or *internal nares* were discussed in Chapter 3. The choana are the openings of the nasal passages into the nasopharynx. Complete bilateral obstruction of the opening into the nasopharynx, called bilateral *choanal atresia*, may be either membranous or bony. A neonate with bilateral choanal atresia may be in severe respiratory distress at birth, although most start to breathe through their mouths after their first episode of crying. However, these infants usually show symptoms of severe breathing problems, including cyanosis and chest *retractions* (that is, the soft tissues of the chest are pulled inward during inspiration, clearly delineating the ribs and sternum), during feeding. The diagnosis is usually made on observation of ineffective respiratory efforts with the mouth held closed. Failure of a flexible probe or dye to pass into the pharynx confirms the diagnosis of choanal atresia. Choanal atresia may be seen in several members of the same family and is often associated with other congenital disorders.

Although some infants with choanal atresia adapt to mouth breathing and do reasonably well, others may die from a failure to breathe orally, an inability to tolerate feeding, or aspiration. Treatment involves surgical opening of the choana; until this can be done, the patency of the infant's oral airway must be maintained.

Infant Respiratory Distress Syndrome

Infant respiratory distress syndrome (IRDS), also called *hyaline membrane disease*, is a disorder commonly seen in prematurely born neonates, especially those with low birth weights. This syndrome was associated with very high neonatal mortality until about 25 years ago when great advances in understanding the disorder and its treatment began to occur. Deaths caused by IRDS are now rare in infants born after 7 months of gestation and weighing more than 1.5 kg.

Symptoms of IRDS usually occur within 6 to 8 hours after birth and include cyanosis, an elevated respiratory rate, chest retractions, abdominal protrusion on inspiration, and dilation of the nares. These are signs of *hypoxemia* and *acidosis* resulting from hypoventilation, right-to-left shunts, and *labored breathing on inspiration*. Severely affected neonates may whimper, cry, or grunt on each expiratory effort. Systemic hypotension and hypothermia are also common in neonates with IRDS, as is persistent patency of the ductus arteriosus.

At autopsy, the lungs from infants who died from IRDS are airless, purple, and resemble the liver in gross appearance. Upon microscopic inspection, the lungs show such complete *atelectasis* that individual alveoli are difficult to see. The other characteristic histopathologic feature of IRDS is the presence of the so-called *hyaline membranes,* which give the disorder its other common name. These membranes, which are usually seen in cases in which the neonate lived more than a few hours with the disease, line whatever portions of the lung that show air spaces. Because most or all of the alveoli are collapsed, the hyaline membranes are usually present only in the terminal bronchioles and alveolar ducts. Pulmonary vascular congestion and even hemorrhage may also be seen. The hyaline membrane, which consists mainly of proteins, appears to be entirely derived from substances from the blood and the injured alveolar epithelium, although it was once thought to represent aspirated amniotic fluid or gastric contents.

The main cause of IRDS is that functional pulmonary surfactant is not usually produced by the fetal lung until the 7th month of gestation. As discussed in Chapter 3 (see Fig. 3–14), pulmonary surfactant normally lines the alveolar surface, and it has two main functions.

The first function of pulmonary surfactant is that it *lowers the overall surface tension* of the alveoli. This decreases the inward elastic recoil of the lungs, making them more compliant and decreasing the work of breathing during inspiration. Therefore, a prematurely born infant whose lungs are not yet producing pulmonary surfactant has to work much harder to inspire its tidal volume, which is about 14 to 16 ml in a normal infant. This can be seen in Figure 6–11, which compares a pulmonary pressure-volume curve from a neonate with normal lungs with one from a neonate with IRDS. Normal lungs excised from a neonate who died from nonpulmonary causes are much more compliant than those excised from a neonate who died from IRDS. Thus, the slopes of both the inspiratory and expiratory curves of the normal lungs are much steeper than those from the lungs of a neonate who died from IRDS. A baby with IRDS has to develop much greater transpulmonary

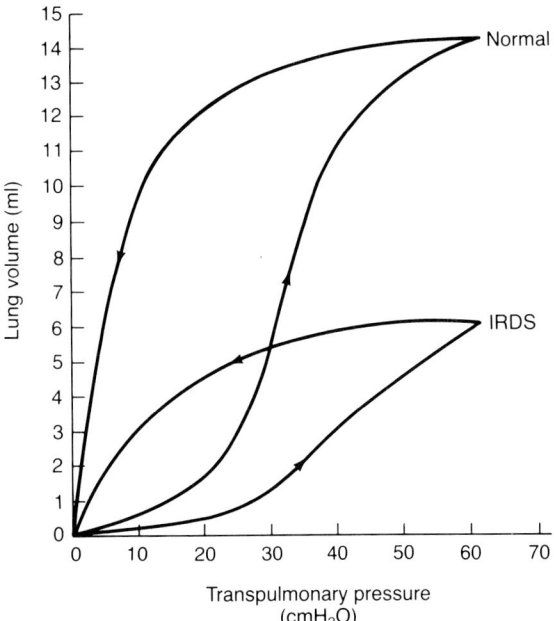

FIGURE 6–11. Pressure-volume curves of lungs from a normal infant and from a premature infant with infant respiratory distress syndrome (IRDS).

pressures to generate a normal tidal volume, so it must breathe at a lower tidal volume and faster respiratory rate. Because a neonate's chest wall is normally very compliant (that is, it has much less outward elastic recoil than an adult's), the increased inward elastic recoil of the lungs of a baby with IRDS also results in a low functional residual capacity.

The second function of pulmonary surfactant is that it *stabilizes alveoli and helps to prevent atelectasis* by equalizing the pressures inside alveoli of different sizes. As discussed in Chapter 3, pulmonary surfactant decreases the surface tension of smaller alveoli and increases the surface tension of larger alveoli (see Figure 3–14). This prevents the pressure in smaller alveoli from exceeding that in larger alveoli, as would be predicted by Laplace's law (see Figure 3–13). Thus, the neonate with IRDS is at much greater risk of alveolar atelectasis throughout the lungs. If many alveoli do collapse, any mixed venous blood that continues to perfuse these atelectatic alveoli constitutes an intrapulmonary shunt and therefore decreases the arterial P_{O_2}.

The treatment of IRDS primarily involves increasing the F_{IO_2} to increase the P_{aO_2}, the use of mechanical ventilators to relieve the infant from the great work of breathing on inspiration, and positive end-expiratory pressure to prevent atelectasis and maintain the functional residual capacity. Positive end-expiratory pressure means that airway and alveolar pressures are kept greater than atmospheric pressure at the end of expiration. The complications caused by these treatments may include pulmonary oxygen toxicity, pneumothorax, pneumomediastinum, and possibly cerebrovascular hemorrhage. (It is not clear whether the intracranial hemorrhage is caused by the disorder itself or the high airway pressures used in its treatment.)

Other aspects of the treatment of IRDS include surgical or pharmacologic closure of the ductus arteriosus if it is patent, maintenance of body temperature, correction of acid-base disturbances, and surfactant replacement. In many cases, administration of pharmacologic blockers of dilator prostaglandin synthesis (such as indomethacin) or constrictor prostaglandins may cause closure of the ductus arteriosus. Replacement of pulmonary surfactant with synthetic or animal-derived surfactant is currently being done experimentally and in clinical trials and may prove to be a very useful treatment.

The administration of *glucocorticoids* is known to stimulate and accelerate fetal lung maturation. Administration of glucocorticoids at least 24 hours before birth has been shown to greatly reduce the incidence of IRDS in prematurely born infants. Sometimes, it is also possible to inhibit labor with drugs (tocolytics) to give the glucocorticoids time to work. Because the ratio of lecithin to another phospholipid called sphingomyelin in the amniotic fluid (the L:S ratio) increases dramatically when the fetus begins to produce pulmonary surfactant (remember that pulmonary surfactant is primarily dipalmitoyl lecithin), *amniocentesis* may indicate whether glucocorticoids will be beneficial. During amniocentesis, a long catheter is inserted (following a local anesthetic) through the pregnant woman's skin and abdominal wall into the uterus. A sample of the amniotic fluid can then be withdrawn so that the L:S ratio can be determined. An L:S ratio greater than or equal to 2:1 usually indicates adequately mature lungs to maintain ventilation. Amniocentesis is also used to sample fluid and obtain shed fetal cells for chromosome analysis. The presence of neural tube defects (such as spina bifida), Down syndrome, Tay-Sachs disease and other disorders in the developing fetus, can thus be determined.

Bronchopulmonary Dysplasia

Bronchopulmonary dysplasia is a nonspecific term used to describe *chronic* pulmonary insufficiency in babies born prematurely and subsequently treated for IRDS. Problems may be intermittent, with episodes of atelectasis, hyperaeration, and sometimes pneumothorax and interstitial air. The infant often appears to be doing well but may have a sudden onset of severe respiratory distress or apnea. A left-to-right shunt via a patent ductus arteriosus is a common finding at 1 to 2 weeks of age, which may be accompanied by pulmonary edema.

Pathologic findings in bronchopulmonary dysplasia seem to indicate a pattern of continuous injury and repair of lung tissue. The pathogenesis of the disease is not completely understood, but it appears to result from the use of high levels of oxygen (oxygen toxicity), and high airway pressures (barotrauma), or both. It is possible that the immature, surfactant-deficient lung may be especially sensitive to these stresses. On autopsy, the lungs show regions of inflammation and scarring mixed with regions with destruction of alveoli and capillaries that resemble emphysema. Some areas appear underdeveloped with alveoli that do not appear to have divided and smaller, thicker pulmonary arteries than are normal for the infant's age. There is usually a loss of the ciliated epithelium of the airways, with mucous plugs and debris in the airways and alveoli.

Therapy for bronchopulmonary dysplasia is mainly supportive with care taken to avoid worsening the oxygen toxicity and barotrauma. The disease usually proves fatal within a few weeks, or it may continue for months with either death or recovery the outcome.

Meconium Aspiration

Meconium is the first stool of the newborn, and it appears in utero in about 10% to 20% of all pregnancies. Its presence in utero is often, but not always, associated with fetal distress. Fetal *aspiration* of amniotic meconium into the respiratory tract is likely to lead to neonatal respiratory distress.

At birth, an infant who aspirated meconium usually has depressed breathing, which may be irregular and gasping. Labored breathing, tachypnea, retractions, and cyanosis may be present. The symptoms and course of the infant's disease are dependent on the volume of meconium aspirated, how deeply it penetrated the airways, and whether it can be easily removed by laryngoscopy and suction.

Treatment of meconium aspiration includes attempting to remove the obstruction with suction, aspiration of the stomach to prevent vomiting and further aspiration, chest physiotherapy (CPT), oxygen therapy, and antibiotics. Mechanical ventilation with positive end-expiratory pressure may also be used, if necessary.

Tracheoesophageal Fistulas

Tracheoesophageal fistulas are fairly common congenital anomalies resulting from incomplete fusion of the tracheoesophageal folds (Figs. 6–6A and B). Such an incomplete fusion results in a communication between the trachea and esophagus. A number of different types of tracheoesophageal fistulas have been seen in infants; four types are shown in Figure 6–12. The one labeled *A* is by far the most common form. Tracheoesophageal fistulas are often seen in infants with other congenital abnormalities.

The clinical manifestations of tracheoesophageal fistula are partly dependent on the type of malformation but are usually seen at the time of the infant's first feeding. The infant characteristically regurgitates immediately and sometimes then aspirates, causing choking and gagging. As soon as the diagnosis is confirmed by radiologic and other means, the tracheoesophageal fistula should be corrected immediately by surgery.

Diaphragmatic Hernia

Congenital defects of the diaphragm frequently cause movement of the abdominal viscera into the thoracic cavity. This usually occurs on the left side of the diaphragm. The extent of the problem to the neonate and the symptoms seen are dependent on the volume of the thoracic cavity occupied by abdominal viscera and on how early in the development of the fetus the hernia occurred. Large herniations of the diaphragm that occur fairly early during fetal development can cause *pulmonary hypoplasia,* especially on the herniated side of the thorax. This hypoplasia (that is, retarded development of the lung), usually involves a decreased number of bronchial branchings and airways, although the number of alveoli per branch may be normal. The alveoli may be smaller than normal, and the pulmonary circulation may also be underdeveloped. Large volumes of abdominal viscera in the thoracic cavity interferes with lung expansion and may also shift the heart's position and impede blood flow. Infants with very small diaphragmatic hernias may be asymptomatic; those with large ones may suffer severe respiratory distress; some are even unable to initiate their first breaths.

Treatment of infants with diaphragmatic hernias involves oxygenation (without overexpansion of the underdeveloped lungs), minimizing intestinal distention with gastrointestinal suction, and im-

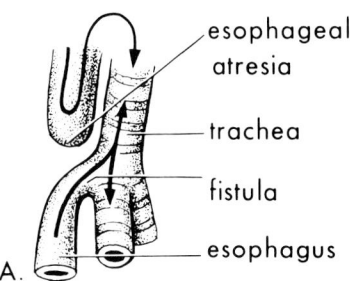
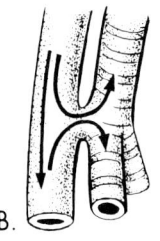
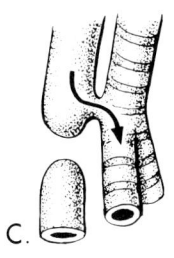
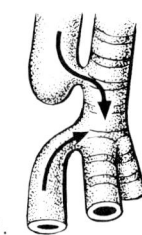

FIGURE 6–12. Four common forms of tracheoesophageal fistulas. Esophageal atresia (*A*) occurs in about 90% of the cases of tracheoesophageal fistulas. (From Moore, K.L. *Before We Are Born: Basic Embryology and Birth Defects,* 2nd ed. Philadelphia, W.B. Saunders, 1983, with permission.)

mediate surgery to correct the herniated diaphragm.

Apnea of Infancy and Sudden Infant Death Syndrome

Apnea of infancy (or neonatal apnea) is a nonspecific syndrome that can be arbitrarily defined as an unexplained and frightening episode of the cessation of breathing for 20 seconds or more or a shorter cessation of breathing associated with bradycardia, cyanosis or pallor, and usually limpness. In many (but not all) cases, it is associated with *sudden infant death syndrome* (SIDS), in which case it may be referred to as a "near-miss" incident. SIDS is also a nonspecific syndrome that refers to the sudden unexpected death of an infant that *cannot* be explained by any autopsy findings, such as meningitis, intracranial hemorrhage, myocarditis or child abuse. Babies with apnea of infancy have 10 to 30 times as great a risk of SIDS as other infants.

There are many potential causes of the apnea of infancy, including reflex apnea and bradycardia caused by stimulation of receptors around the larynx by food or small amounts of refluxed gastric contents (laryngeal chemoreceptor apnea), seizure disorders, infections, upper airway obstruction, incompletely developed peripheral or central chemoreceptors or respiratory controller, especially in premature babies (apnea of prematurity), a failure of automatic respiratory rhythmicity (Ondine's curse), cardiac arrhythmias and congenital heart disease, tumors, anemia, and ionic or metabolic disturbances.

Therapeutic measures include respiratory and cardiac monitoring, and support of the cardiopulmonary system. If a treatable cause can be identified, then appropriate medical or surgical care should be administered.

Transient Tachypea of the Newborn

Transient tachypnea of the newborn is a syndrome found in neonates, usually born at term, in which they demonstrate abnormally high ventilatory rates (as high as 120 breaths/min) during their first hours of life. These high respiratory rates are not associated with significant retractions, cyanosis, abnormal arterial pH and $P{CO_2}$, or cardiovascular abnormalities. Chest radiographs usually suggest interstitial and even alveolar edema and congestion of the lymphatics (thus the syndrome's other name, wet-lung disease), providing evidence that the syndrome is caused by delayed reabsorption of fetal lung liquid. The lungs usually begin to clear spontaneously within 1 day, although it may take 13 to 17 days to be completed.

Retrolental Fibroplasia

Treatment of prematurely born infants in respiratory distress with very high fractional concentrations of oxygen can lead to a very serious condition called *retrolental fibroplasia*. Retrolental fibroplasia, which is also known as retinopathy of the premature, is a proliferation of fibrotic tissue behind the lens of the eye that can cause permanent blindness. This fibrosis is believed to be a consequence of alterations in the blood vessels of the eye, caused either by the high $P{O_2}$ of the arterial blood perfusing the eye or by periods of hypoxia *followed* by hyperoxia.

The threat of retrolental fibroplasia often represents a difficult dilemma in the treatment of prematurely born neonates with IRDS. Although $F{I O_2}$'s of 0.40 or less are considered safe for short periods of time, even lower $F{I O_2}$'s may cause retrolental fibroplasia if they are administered for greater durations. However, such elevated $F{I O_2}$'s may be necessary to prevent hypoxemia and thus allow for the infant's survival. Therefore, the prematurely born infant's arterial blood gases, especially the arterial $P{O_2}$, must be carefully monitored, especially during elevated $F{I O_2}$'s.

DEVELOPMENTAL CHANGES IN THE CARDIOPULMONARY SYSTEM DURING CHILDHOOD

Because fetal cardiovascular growth and development are far more complete at term than those of the respiratory system, the childhood developmental changes seen in the respiratory system are more striking than those of the cardiovascular system.

Postnatal Cardiovascular Development

Once the dramatic cardiovascular alterations normally associated with birth (cessation of blood flow to the placenta; increased pulmonary blood flow; and closure of the foramen ovale, ductus venosus, and ductus arteriosus) have occurred, most of the developmental changes seen in the cardiovascular system are related to changes in body mass and configuration and organ function.

The myocardium, especially the left ventricle, matures and increases its ability to generate pressure and pump greater volumes. This is important because the neonate has little ability to increase the stroke volume and therefore must increase cardiac output by increasing the heart rate. Bradycardic neonates may have difficulty maintaining their cardiac outputs.

Resting cardiac output increases with age from about 750 ml/min at birth to about 5L/min at 16 to 18 years old. This increase is, however, only seen when cardiac output is expressed in *absolute terms* (L/min). If it is expressed per kilogram of *body weight,* it actually falls from about 200 ml/kg/min at birth to about 100 ml/kg/min in teenagers. This decrease is especially rapid during the first couple of years. If cardiac output is expressed per square meter of *body surface area,* it stays fairly constant during postnatal growth and development. Thus, it appears that resting cardiac output is most closely related to body surface area and that changes in body configuration result in a decrease in the ratio of body weight to body surface area. Another explanation is that growth results in greater increases in limb size and muscle mass than it does in the weight of the visceral organs. Blood flow to resting muscles and long bones is very low compared with that of other organs.

Heart rate decreases from about 150 beats/min at birth to approximately 70 beats/min in the young adult. Stroke volume therefore increases with age and does so somewhat faster than cardiac output. Mean systemic blood pressure increases from about 60 mmHg at birth to the normal adult mean pressure of approximately 95 mmHg. Systemic vascular resistance decreases with growth and development, if it is expressed per square meter of body surface area.

Pulmonary artery pressure and pulmonary vascular resistance both decrease during the first year of life as the smooth muscle of the medial layer of the pulmonary vessels decreases in thickness. Mean pulmonary artery pressure falls from about 50 mmHg at birth to nearly the adult mean pressure of approximately 15 mmHg within about a year after birth. Pulmonary blood flow, of course, stays relatively constant, if it is expressed per square meter of body surface area. As the pressure work done by the right ventricle decreases, the relative thickness of the right ventricular wall also decreases.

Postnatal Pulmonary Development

Many important, if not completely understood, changes occur in the physiology of the upper airways during infancy and the first 4 or 5 years of life. These may result from the growth of tissue or the development of better neural mechanisms and reflex controls, or both. One of the most important changes that take place concerns the relative positions of the larynx and the epiglottis. The larynx and epiglottis are located higher with respect to the cervical vertebrae in the child than in the adult. Most of the time, especially during nursing, the neonate's epiglottis and uvula make contact with the soft palate, thus allowing the neonate to swallow and breathe through the nose at the same time. This is also the reason that some infants under 3 to 5 months of age appear to be able to breathe through their mouths only when they are crying. As the infant grows, the larynx and epiglottis gradually move downward, so by age 5, the epiglottis can hardly make contact with the uvula. In the adult, the larynx opens into the lower part of the pharynx, so the lower pharnyx is the pathway for both food and air.

The relatively large epiglottis, tonsils, and adenoids of the infant and small child appear to be particularly sensitive to certain kinds of bacterial infections and may seriously impede airflow when they are inflamed. This problem may be made worse by the relatively soft laryngeal cartilages of the infant because they may tend to collapse on inspiration. Dilation of the nares and much of the pharyngeal muscle contraction associated with inspiration also gradually decrease during the first few months of life. Reflexes and complex coordinated activities, such as the cough reflex and speech, develop during the first years of life.

The tracheobronchial tree continues to grow and develop after birth, and there is an exponentially increasing number of alveoli for at least the first 8 years. Unlike adults in whom the large airways are the site of the greatest airways resistance, in small children smaller more peripheral airways are the major site of airways resistance. The diameter, length and cross-sectional areas of the airways all increase from infancy to adulthood, with greater increases in the diameter and cross-sectional area than in the length of the individual larger airways. By 3 months of age, 21 of the 23 generations of airways have already developed. The total number of respiratory airways (including alveolar ducts) increases from about 1.5 million at birth to the adult figure of 14 million by age 8. The *total* cross-sectional area of the smaller airways increases much more than that of the larger airways because of their much greater number.

The total number of alveoli increases from about 24 million at birth to about 280 million at age 8. In other words, about 90% of the adult alveoli have developed. Alveoli increase in size as well as number during this period. The average alveolus increases from about 50 μ in diameter to 150 to 250 μ in diameter by the early teenage years, with little further increase thereafter. This increase in alveolar size may represent changes in the distribution of alveolar elastin and collagen and increased outward elastic recoil of the chest wall in addition to growth of alveolar septal tissue.

Pulmonary capillaries proliferate along with the increased number and size of the alveoli and continue to increase in number after the alveoli stop. The alveolar-capillary interface is believed to be about 2.8 m^2 in the newborn, about 6.5 m^2 at 3 months, and about 32 m^2 by age 8. Because the adult alveolar-capillary surface area is about 70 m^2, the continued increase in the number of pulmonary capillaries doubles the surface area available for gas exchange after age 8. The lungs of a newborn infant weigh about 50 gm; those of a 12- to 14-year-old, 400 gm; and those of an adult, 800 gm.

The functional residual capacity increases with the growth and development of the lungs. The increase is directly and linearly related to the height of the child (or the length of the infant). The tidal volume stays fairly constant (expressed per weight) at 7 to 10 ml/kg from birth to adulthood, as does the anatomic dead space, which is about 2 ml/kg throughout the same period. Thus, the ratio of dead space to tidal volume also stays constant. Oxygen consumption decreases from 6 to 8 ml/kg/min in the infant to about 3.9 ml/kg/min in the adult. The infant's alveolar ventilation is 100 to 150 ml/kg/min; this is about twice that of the adult. Since infants and adults have about the same tidal volume per weight, it is not surprising that they have a higher respiratory rate: about 40 breaths/min compared with 13 breaths/min for the adult.

The standard lung volumes and capacities, which cannot be determined by conventional (voluntary) means in infants and young children, all increase linearly with height between ages 6 and 18. Total lung capacity and vital capacity increase slightly more rapidly than does residual volume.

PEDIATRIC PATHOPHYSIOLOGY

Upper respiratory infections, croup and epiglottitis, bronchiolitis, and cystic fibrosis are among the most commonly occurring respiratory disorders of the child. Another common problem involving the respiratory system in children is foreign object aspiration (see Chapter 5). Most of the cardiovascular problems seen in children have already been discussed in this chapter or in Chapter 5.

Croup and Epiglottitis

Croup is a nonspecific term applied to a syndrome that can be caused by a number of upper respiratory tract infections. The symptoms are caused by rhinitis, laryngitis, and tracheobronchitis. It is characterized by difficulty in breathing accompanied by inspiratory *stridor* (abnormal breathing sounds usually caused by laryngeal obstruction); chest retractions; and often hoarseness, harsh "barking" coughing, and fever. The stridor seems to be related to laryngeal edema in addition to inflammation. Most cases of croup are not serious, but those involving severe *epiglottitis* can be fatal.

Viruses are probably responsible for most cases of croup, although 15% or so are caused by bacterial infections, especially *Haemophilus influenzae*, type B. This bacterial infection is associated with an extremely rapid enlargement of the epiglottis and fever; the epiglottitis it produces can cause life-threatening obstruction of the upper airways of infants, requiring immediate use of an artificial airway.

Treatment of croup includes maintaining the patency of the upper airways with intubation, if necessary, and the use of a humidifying mist and supplemental oxygen. Aerosolized racemic epinephrine is sometimes administered to help dilate the bronchioles and constrict the blood vessels of the airways. Steroids may be given to decrease the inflammation, and antibiotics are used to combat the infection causing the problem.

Bronchiolitis

Acute bronchiolitis frequently leads to serious problems in infants and children. Bronchiolitis refers to inflammation of the bronchioles, which may affect both the larger and smaller generations of airways. *Chronic bronchiolitis* is usually seen as part of the picture in cases of chronic bronchitis and is implied by the use of that term. Acute bronchiolitis in the adult is usually caused by either infections or by inhalation of noxious gases or substances suspended in the inspired air. In the child, acute bronchiolitis is almost always caused by infections.

Acute bronchiolitis can cause serious problems in the child because it usually affects both the large and small airways; the obstruction of the small airways may be sufficient to cause significant impairment of gas exchange. The obstruction is caused by the inflammation, cell exudates, edema, and increased mucus secretion by the affected airways. It may be severe enough to cause severe arterial hypoxemia and carbon dioxide retention. The airway obstruction may be made worse by reflex constriction of the smooth muscles of the small airways caused by stimulation of irritant receptors in the upper airways. Treatment of bronchiolitis is aimed at removing the source of the inflammation and maintaining the blood gases.

Cystic Fibrosis

Cystic fibrosis, which is also called mucoviscidosis or fibrocystic disease, is a common genetic disease that affects the exocrine glands. It involves many organs besides the lungs, especially the pancreas. Cystic fibrosis appears to cause increased secretion of an abnormally viscous mucus, leading to obstruction of exocrine gland ducts and the vessels into which the mucus is discharged. Thus, the airways, paranasal sinuses, mucus-secreting salivary glands, pancreatic duct, gastrointestinal tract, bile duct, cervix, and other organs may be involved in this multisystem disease. Although the disease is known to have a genetic basis, the precise defect is unknown. Cystic fibrosis is inherited as an autosomal recessive trait, and it is therefore assumed that both parents must be heterozygous carriers for their child to get the disease.

The symptoms of cystic fibrosis are usually first seen during infancy or early childhood, but in some cases, they are not seen until adolescence or even early adulthood. Virtually all patients who survive early infancy develop respiratory problems, and pulmonary dysfunctions are the cause of death in most cases. Neonates who die of cystic fibrosis often die of acute intestinal obstruction.

The first changes that can be seen in the airways of children with cystic fibrosis are hypertrophy of bronchial glands and alterations in the appearance of goblet cells. The increased secretion of viscous mucus may overwhelm the mucociliary escalator, or the *ciliary function may be impaired* either directly or indirectly by the disease. Accumulation of mucus in the airways causes obstruction. This problem is made worse by repeated bronchial infections. These infections result from the apparent excellence of the abnormal bronchial secretions to serve as a growth medium for bacteria and fungi, and the decreased effectiveness of the mucociliary escalator. Cystic fibrosis may also impair the function of alveolar macrophages.

Recurrent bronchial infections usually cause permanent structural damage of the airways, especially *bronchiectasis*. Bronchiectasis is defined as a permanent dilation of one or more bronchi caused by the destruction of the structural components of the bronchial wall.

The diagnosis of cystic fibrosis is usually based on the presence of two or more of the following: chronic obstructive airways disease, exocrine pancreatic disease (as established on the basis of abdominal or digestive disturbances and abnormal pancreatic exocrine function), a family history of cystic fibrosis, and abnormally high chloride levels in the sweat. The sweat test is described in Chapter 14.

The main respiratory symptoms associated with cystic fibrosis include chronic cough, wheezing, and as the obstruction worsens, the symptoms associated with chronic obstructive diseases, such as hyperinflation. As the obstruction worsens it leads to hypoventilation, progressive hypoxemia, cyanosis, clubbing of the digits, pulmonary hypertension, and ultimately, cor pulmonale.

Treatment of cystic fibrosis involves mist and aerosol therapy, segmental postural drainage, chest therapy, and physical activity, all of which are aimed at assisting mucociliary clearance and increasing the removal of sputum to relieve and prevent further airway obstruction. Other therapy includes bronchodilators to remove any bronchoconstrictive component of the obstruction, antibiotics to treat respiratory tract infections, oxygen, and pulmonary vasodilators to relieve hypoxia, decrease pulmonary hypertension, and decrease right ventricular work. Disorders of the other organ systems can also be treated.

PHYSIOLOGIC CONSEQUENCES OF AGING

Aging causes major changes in the function of many of the organ systems of the body. We will concentrate on the changes that occur in the cardiovascular and respiratory systems.

Changes in the Cardiovascular System

As normal healthy adults age, they encounter little decrease in cardiovascular function at rest. However, the ability of adults to increase their cardiovascular performance during stresses such as exercise decreases progressively with age. The progressive decrease in maximal cardiovascular function that occurs with aging is a result of structural alterations in the cardiovascular system. These structural alterations are in many ways similar to those that occur in the respiratory system with aging.

Structural Alterations. There is a progressive increase in the ratio of collagen to elastin in the walls of arteries and veins as people get older. Because collagen is much less distensible than elastin, this results in *decreased compliance* (or increased stiffness) of the aorta and the large arteries and veins, both radially and longitudinally. The walls of the ventricles probably also become less compliant.

Functional Alterations at Rest. The decrease in vascular distensibility, along with some degree of atherosclerotic alteration of the arterial tree, tends to increase systemic vascular resistance and therefore increase systemic diastolic blood pressure with age. The decreased distensibility (or compliance) of the aorta means that for the same stroke volume, aortic systolic pressure causes a greater increase above diastolic pressure. Thus, the pulse pressure increases with age. Because pulse pressure and diastolic pressure both increase with age, the systolic pressure increases more with age than diastolic. The valves of the heart may also stiffen with age.

The elevated afterload on the left ventricle represented by these increases in pressure increases the stroke work of the left ventricle. As the pressure work increases, the left ventricle is less able to generate stroke volume (especially *increases* in stroke volume), so the resting cardiac output, cardiac index, and stroke index all decrease with age. The increased afterload also usually results in some degree of cardiac enlargement, resulting both from dilation during diastole and from muscular hypertrophy. The hypertrophy of the left ventricle slows contraction and relaxation.

Functional Alterations During Exercise. The structural changes in the cardiovascular system that occur with aging have a much greater effect on the response to exercise than at rest. The maximum work capacity, as determined by the maximal oxygen uptake, decreases linearly with age after about 20 years of age. This is mainly a result of a decreased ability to increase the cardiac output (or index), both by increasing stroke volume and by increasing heart rate. This decreased ability to increase the cardiac output may be a consequence of the increased stiffness of the aorta, arterial tree, and cardiac valves; the increased systemic vascular resistance; a decreased contractility of the ventricles; or a decreased effectiveness of the Frank-Starling mechanism. Several of these changes may be the result of a decreased effectiveness of or responsiveness to the sympathetic nervous system.

Changes in the Respiratory System

The growth and development of the respiratory system ends at about 20 years of age. As a result, most people with normal healthy cardiopulmonary systems reach their maximum performance levels on pulmonary function tests between 20 and 25 years of age and experience a progressive decline as they get older.

The alterations of the respiratory system that occur with aging are summarized in Table 6–1. The

TABLE 6–1. Summary of the Effects of Aging on the Respiratory System: Relationship of Changes in Structure to Changes in Function

Loss of alveolar elastic recoil:
    Increased static pulmonary compliance
    Decreased pulmonary elastic recoil pressure
    Increased functional residual capacity
    Decreased support of small airways
    Greater effect of dynamic compression
    Decreased dynamic lung volumes
    Increased residual volume
    Increased closing volume, gas trapping
    Decreased dynamic pulmonary compliance
    Less uniform alveolar ventilation
    Ventilation-perfusion mismatch
    Decreased response to hypoxia and hypercapnia

Alterations in chest wall structure and decreased respiratory muscle strength:
    Decreased chest wall compliance
    Increased residual volume
    Decreased vital capacity, dynamic lung volumes
    Decreased maximum voluntary ventilation
    Decreased response to hypoxia and hypercapnia

Loss of alveolar surface area and changes in the pulmonary circulation:
    Ventilation-perfusion mismatch
    Increased alveolar dead space
    Decreased diffusing capacity
    Decreased arterial P_{O_2}
    Increased (A-a) P_{O_2}

Reproduced with permission from Levitzky, M.G.: Effects of aging on the respiratory system. *The Physiologist* 27:102–107, 1984. American Physiological Society, Bethesda, Maryland.

functional alterations are listed according to the structural changes thought to be responsible for them.

Structural Alterations. The structural changes that occur in the respiratory system with age primarily affect the alveoli and alveolar ducts, the rib cage and respiratory muscles, and the pulmonary vasculature.

Alveoli and Alveolar Ducts. After about age 40, alveolar ducts and respiratory bronchioles begin to enlarge. This results in a larger fraction of the lung volume consisting of alveolar ducts and a smaller volume of the lung consisting of alveoli. The *alveolar surface area* decreases with age, although it is not known whether this reflects a decrease in the number of alveolar septa or changes in their configuration. At the same time, there is a degeneration of the elastic fibers in the walls of the alveoli and alveolar ducts that provide much of the structural support of the alveoli. There are also changes in the cross-linking between collagen fibers, elastin fibers, and each other. Although the exact nature of these alterations in structure is not well known, they appear to be the source of *increased lung compliance* and *decreased pulmonary elastic recoil*. There may also be age-related changes in the composition and turnover of pulmonary surfactant.

Chest Wall. The *costal cartilages* calcify with age, resulting in decreased compliance and mobility of the rib cage. At the same time, the spaces between *spinal vertebrae* decrease, and the degree of kyphotic spinal curvature increases, leading to a shorter thorax with an increased anterior-posterior diameter. A greater deposition of abdominal and thoracic adipose tissue may also contribute to the decreased chest wall compliance of many elderly people. Finally, the strength of the muscles of breathing decreases with age.

Pulmonary Vasculature. There is an increase in the thickness of larger pulmonary arteries with age, especially of the intimal and medial layers. Although resting mean pulmonary artery pressure and pulmonary vascular resistance do not usually increase with age, the pulmonary vasculature becomes less distensible, and there may be fewer unopened capillaries to recruit. The result of these changes is that, during exercise, mean pulmonary artery pressure may increase more and pulmonary vascular resistance may decrease less than they do in younger individuals. Pulmonary capillary blood volume decreases with age as a consequence of either loss of or changes in the configuration of alveoli and alveolar septa as well as a decrease in the cardiac index of the elderly.

Larger Airways. Bronchial cartilage shows a tendency to calcify in the aged. This is probably the main cause of the slight increase in dead space seen in older people.

Functional Alterations. Aging causes changes in the lung volumes and capacities, the mechanics of breathing, gas exchange (diffusing capacity and arterial P_{O_2}), the control of breathing, exercise capacity, and pulmonary defense mechanisms.

Lung Volumes and Capacities. The changes that occur in the standard lung volumes and capacities with aging are shown in Figure 6–13. Although the *total lung capacity* (TLC) has been demonstrated in several studies to decrease with age, if the TLC data are normalized for the decrease in height that is seen in the elderly, then there is no change in the total lung capacity with age, as shown in the figure. The decreased height of the elderly is a result of the decrease in the size of the intervertebral spaces as well as the fact that in *cross-sectional studies* (studies in which people of different age groups are studied simultaneously) subjects from younger generations are taller than those from

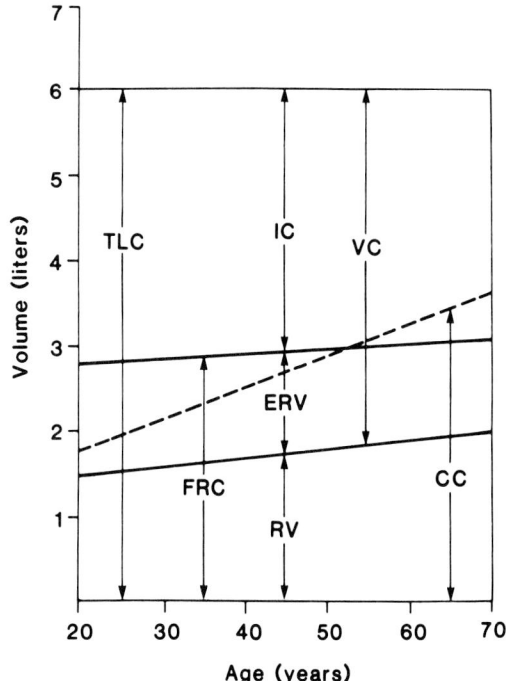

FIGURE 6–13. Diagram of the alterations in the standard lung volumes and capacities occurring with age. (TLC, = total lung capacity; FRC = functional residual capacity; ERV = expiratory reserve volume; RV = residual volume; IC = inspiratory capacity; VC = vital capacity; CC = closing capacity.) (From Levitzky, M.G.: Effects of aging on the respiratory system. *The Physiologist* 27:102, 1984, with permission by the American Physiological Society.)

older generations at the same age, probably as a result of better nutrition. Numerous studies have shown that the *residual volume* (RV) increases with age, as does the ratio of the RV to the TLC. Because the TLC is unchanged by aging (if normalized for height changes) and the RV increases, the *vital capacity* (VC) decreases with age. Studies on the effects of aging on the *functional residual capacity* (FRC) have yielded variable results: Some have shown no change in the FRC; others have demonstrated that the FRC and FRC/TLC increase, but not as much as the RV and RV/TLC, respectively. These different findings may reflect differences in the way the FRC was determined in different studies because the helium dilution and nitrogen washout techniques do not include gas trapped behind closed airways, whereas the body plethysmograph technique does. As discussed later, there may be appreciable gas trapping at this lung volume in elderly people. Most recent studies have shown that the FRC increases with age. Because even those studies that have shown an increasing FRC with age have shown greater increases in RV, the *expiratory reserve volume* (ERV) decreases with age. The *inspiratory capacity* (IC) decreases with age in those studies showing an increasing FRC.

Mechanics of Breathing. As already noted, the *elastic recoil* of the *lungs* decreases with age, especially at higher lung volumes. This is seen as a a leftward shift of the lung recoil pressure curve. *Static pulmonary compliance,* which is the inverse of the elastic recoil, increases with age. *Dynamic pulmonary compliance* decreases and becomes more frequency dependent with age. This probably reflects increased resistance to airflow in small airways more than it does decreased compliance of alveolar units, especially since static lung compliance increases. The increased resistance to airflow in small airways is probably mainly a result of decreased alveolar elastic recoil leading to decreased support of small airways.

The *compliance of the chest wall* decreases with age. The chest wall recoil pressure curve is shifted to the right and is less steep, indicating a greater inward recoil pressure and less compliance of the chest wall. Chest wall elastic recoil also shifts from outward to inward at a much lower lung volume.

The *closing volume* or *closing capacity* (CC) increases from about 30% of the total lung capacity at age 20 to about 55% at age 70 (see Fig. 6–13). The closing volume may exceed the functional residual capacity in elderly people, which suggests that they may have airway closure and poorly ventilated or unventilated alveoli at resting lung volumes.

As discussed in Chapter 3, airway closure usually begins to occur in the lower regions of the lung of a normal young person who is standing or sitting in an upright posture. Small airways in lower regions of the lung are more likely to collapse than those in upper lung regions because alveoli there are at lower volumes and therefore have less elastic recoil helping to hold small airways open, and because intrapleural pressure is higher (less negative at the FRC and more positive during a forced expiration) than in upper regions. Thus, the pattern of greater ventilation in lower lung regions seen in normal young subjects cannot occur in the elderly, and more ventilation is distributed to upper lung regions. This may result in less efficient matching of ventilation and perfusion in the lung and may contribute to the decreasing arterial P_{O_2} seen with aging.

The *dynamic measurements of lung volume* decrease with age. The maximal expiratory flow rate, the maximal midexpiratory flow rate, the forced expiratory volume in one second (FEV_1), and the ratio of FEV_1 to forced vital capacity (FVC) all decrease with age. This is probably a result of decreasing strength of the expiratory muscles, decreasing chest wall compliance, and an increasing tendency for airways to close during forced expiratory efforts, causing gas trapping in the lungs. These factors also explain the increase in the residual volume. The maximum voluntary ventilation (MVV), which is the maximum volume of air that can be breathed in and out in 12 or 15 seconds (expressed in liters/minute), also decreases with age. However, this is a rather nonspecific test.

Pulmonary Gas Exchange. The arterial P_{O_2} decreases progressively and linearly with age, falling from approximately 95 torr at age 20 to about 75 torr at age 70. The P_{O_2} of well-ventilated alveoli does not change, so the *alveolar-arterial oxygen gradient,* or (A-a) P_{O_2}, increases progressively with age by the same amount. The factors that determine the (A-a) P_{O_2} include the physiologic shunt, which increases slightly from less than 5% at age 20 to approximately 15% at age 70, the matching of ventilation and perfusion, and the diffusing capacity.

Ventilation and perfusion are not matched as well in the lungs of the elderly as in younger subjects. Alveolar ventilation becomes less uniform with age, which is probably attributable to airway closure in lower lung regions causing more ventilation of upper lung regions, as discussed before.

Normally, there is greater perfusion of lower lung regions in young healthy adults. Preferential ventilation of upper lung regions of the elderly without decreasing blood flow to lower regions and increasing blood flow to upper regions results in disturbed ventilation-perfusion relationships. Ventilation-perfusion studies have shown only slightly increased blood flow to upper lung regions in the elderly. The alveolar dead space increases in the elderly, probably because of a decreased cardiac index, leading to unrecruited pulmonary capillaries. Age-related structural alterations of pulmonary vessels may occur that attenuate the strength of the hypoxic pulmonary vasoconstriction.

The *pulmonary diffusing capacity* ($D_L CO$) decreases progressively and linearly with age, falling approximately 20% over the course of adult life. This decrease is probably a result of decreased alveolar surface area as well as a decrease in the pulmonary capillary blood volume. The decrease in diffusing capacity may not have as great an effect on the (A-a) P_{O_2} as the $\dot{V}/\dot{Q}$ mismatch. There are no consistent age-related alterations in *arterial P_{CO_2}*. This may be a result of the greater diffusivity of carbon dioxide through the alveolar-capillary barrier and the differences in the oxygen and carbon dioxide dissociation curves.

Control of Breathing. The *ventilatory responses to both hypoxia and hypercapnia* have been shown to decrease with age. These decreased responses could be a result of any combination of several alterations in the respiratory system that occur with age, including decreased sensitivity of the central and arterial chemoreceptors or alterations in the central respiratory controller. However, it is much more likely that the attenuated responses to hypoxia and hypercapnia reflect decreased strength of the respiratory muscles and alterations in the mechanics of the lung and chest wall. The occurrence of snoring and obstructive sleep apnea also increase with aging (see Chapter 5).

Exercise Capacity. The ability to perform exercise, as indicated by the *maximal oxygen uptake* ($\dot{V}_{O_2}$max), decreases progressively and linearly with age, falling about 35 percent between the ages of 20 and 70. The main cause of the decreased ability to exercise is probably a decreased ability to increase the cardiac output, although many of the alterations discussed above may also contribute.

Pulmonary Defense Mechanisms. The elderly have fewer cilia lining their airways than do younger individuals, which probably leads to a decreased efficiency of the *mucociliary escalator*. Elderly people also show decreased *reflex responses* to mechanical or chemical stimulation of the upper airways or tracheobronchial tree.

Bibliography

Avery, M.E., Fletcher, B.D., and Williams, R.G.: *The Lung and its Disorders in the Newborn Infant*, 4th ed. Philadelphia, W.B. Saunders, 1981.

Brody, J.S.: Lung Development, Growth, and Repair. In Fishman, A.P. (ed.): *Pulmonary Diseases and Disorders*. New York, McGraw-Hill, 1980, pp 298–314.

Comroe, J.H., Jr.: Premature science and immature lungs, Parts, I, II, and III. *Am. Rev. Resp. Dis.* 116:127–135, 311–323, 497–518, 1977.

Gerhardt, T., Hehre, D., Feller, R., Reifenberg, L., and Bancalari, E.: Pulmonary mechanics in normal infants during first 5 years of life. *Pediatr. Pulmonol.* 3:309–319, 1987.

Hinshaw, H.C., and Murray, J.F.: *Diseases of the Chest*, 4th ed. Philadelphia, W.B. Saunders, 1980, pp 591–605.

Keele, C.A., Neil, E., and Joels, N.L.: *Samson Wright's Applied Physiology*, 13th ed. Oxford, Oxford University Press, 1982, pp 585–597.

Leape, L.L.: *Patient Care in Pediatric Surgery*. Boston, Little, Brown, 1987.

Levin, D.L., Morriss, F.C., and Moore, G.C. (eds): *A Practical Guide to Pediatric Intensive Care*, 2nd ed. St. Louis, C.V. Mosby, 1984.

Levitzky, M.G.: The effect of aging on the respiratory system, *The Physiologist* 27:102–107, 1984.

Matthews, L.W., Dearborn, D.G., and Tucker, A.S.: Cystic fibrosis. In Fishman, A.P. (ed.): *Pulmonary Diseases and Disorders*, New York, McGraw-Hill, 1980, pp 600–613.

Miller, R.D.: Obstructing lesions of the larynx and trachea: Clinical and pathophysiologic aspects. In Fishman, A.P. (ed.): *Pulmonary Diseases and Disorders*. New York, McGraw-Hill, 1980, pp 490–502.

Moore, K.L.: *Before We Are Born: Basic Embryology and Birth Defects*, 2nd ed. Philadelphia, W.B. Saunders, 1983.

Moore, K.L.: *The Developing Human: Clinically Oriented Embryology*, 3rd ed. Philadelphia, W.B. Saunders, 1982.

Murray, J.F.: *The Normal Lung*, 2nd ed. Philadelphia, W.B. Saunders, 1986.

Netter, F.H.: *The Ciba Collection of Medical Illustrations*, vol. 5. Summit, N.J., Ciba, 1969, pp 112–164.

Netter, F.H.: *The Ciba Collection of Medical Illustrations*, vol. 7. Summit, N.J., Ciba, 1979, pp 34–43, 107–115.

Polgar, G., and Weng, T.R.: The functional development of the respiratory system: From the period of gestation to adulthood. *Am. Rev. Resp. Dis.* 120:625–695, 1979.

Reid, L.: Chronic Obstructive Lung Diseases. In Fishman, A.P. (ed.): *Pulmonary Diseases and Disorders*. New York, McGraw-Hill, 1980, pp 507–508.

Rodenstein, D.O., Kahn, A., Blum, D., and Stănescu, D.C.: Nasal occlusion during sleep in normal and near-miss for sudden death syndrome infants. *Clin. Resp. Physiol.* 23:223–226, 1987.

Ross, G.: *Pathophysiology of the Heart*. New York, Masson, 1982, pp 257–291.

Rudolph, A.M.: *Congenital Diseases of the Heart*, Chicago, Year Book Medical Publishing, 1974.

Rushmer, R.F.: *Cardiovascular Dynamics*, 4th ed. Philadelphia, W.B. Saunders, 1976, pp 446–496.

Scarpelli, E. M. (ed.): *Pulmonary Physiology of the Fetus and Newborn Child.* Philadelphia, Lea and Febiger, 1975.

Shepherd, J.T., and Vanhoutte, P.M.: *The Human Cardiovascular System: Facts and Concepts,* New York, Raven, 1979, pp 269–279.

Smith, J.J., and Kampine, J.P.: *Circulatory Physiology—The Essentials,* 2nd ed. Baltimore, Williams & Wilkins, 1984, pp 237–243.

Stalcup, S.A., and Mellins, R.B.: Acute respiratory distress in the newborn infant. In Fishman, A.P. (ed.): *Pulmonary Diseases and Disorders.* New York, McGraw-Hill, 1980, pp 1653–1666.

Weibel, E.R.: *The Pathway for Oxygen: Structure and Function in the Mammalian Respiratory System.* Cambridge, Mass., Harvard University Press, 1984, pp 211–230.

Williams, P.L., and Warwick, R. (eds.): *Gray's Anatomy,* 36th ed. Philadelphia, W.B. Saunders, 1980, pp 180–196, 207–210.

II
ASSESSMENT OF CARDIOPULMONARY DISEASE

OBJECTIVES

AFTER READING THIS CHAPTER, THE STUDENT WILL BE ABLE TO:

1. Describe the organization of the general medical history.
2. Describe the technique of obtaining a cardiopulmonary history.
3. Discuss the significance of historical findings associated with dyspnea, chest pain, cough, and expectoration.
4. Discuss the importance of obtaining information about allergic disorders and personal and occupational history.
5. Describe the procedures of inspection, palpation, percussion, and auscultation of the cardiovascular and pulmonary systems.
6. Discuss abnormal findings observed during the assessment of cardiopulmonary function.

7
HISTORY AND PHYSICAL EXAMINATION

CHAPTER OUTLINE

THE MEDICAL HISTORY
  General Medical History and Physical
  Obtaining the Cardiopulmonary History
    Dyspnea
    Chest Pain
    Cough and Expectoration
    Hemoptysis
    Allergic Disorders and Personal-
      Occupational History
PHYSICAL EXAMINATION OF
CARDIOPULMONARY FUNCTION
  Inspection
    Thoracic Contours
    Respiratory Patterns
    Cyanosis
    Clubbing of Digits
    Nutritional Status
  Palpation
    Heart Rate and Rhythm
    Movement of the Chest
    Tracheal Position
    Lymph Nodes and Tumors
    Tactile Fremitus
  Percussion
  Auscultation
    Use of the Stethoscope
    Heart Sounds
    Lung Sounds

The medical record is a document containing a patient's medical and social history, along with information on the diagnostic and therapeutic interventions initiated for his or her present illness. The record is useful to the respiratory care practitioner because (1) it contains information that can guide therapy and (2) it can serve as legal evidence for insurance claims or litigation associated with suspected malpractice. Because of its legal importance, the medical record should be prepared carefully and written clearly and succinctly, with dates, times, and authorships recorded for each entry.

Typically, the medical record remains in the custody of the admitting institution. The contents of this record are considered by law to be *privileged* and must be protected from access by unauthorized persons.

THE MEDICAL HISTORY

To obtain a useful medical history, the examiner must have a thorough knowledge of cardiopulmonary disease states and their associated pathophysiologic findings. The reliability and validity of the medical history are affected considerably by the skill with which the interview is conducted. Failure to establish rapport with the patient can result in misinformation, either because the patient failed to understand the questions or felt a lack of confidence in the person performing the interview. When obtaining a medical history, therefore, one should be especially careful to choose the simplest and most direct phrases possible in order not to confuse the patient.

General Medical History and Physical

The organization of the history and physical examination performed by the admitting physician follows a standardized sequence that varies only slightly among physicians (Table 7–1). Although the respiratory therapist is primarily interested in the patient's cardiopulmonary status, valuable information regarding extrathoracic manifestations of cardiovascular and/or pulmonary diseases can be obtained from the general medical history and physical.

Obtaining the Cardiopulmonary History

Once an impairment of cardiopulmonary function has been noted by the attending physician, it is useful for the therapist to obtain a detailed history of the patient's cardiovascular and pulmonary function. This analysis should focus on the following symptoms: dyspnea, chest pain, cough and expectoration, and hemoptysis. Additional information should be obtained on allergies and personal and occupational history.

Dyspnea

Most patients seek medical attention for diseases of cardiovascular or pulmonary origin after experiencing an abnormal amount of breathlessness. The sensation of *dyspnea*, or shortness of breath, is a subjective complaint that is extremely variable among individuals. For this reason, various rating scales have been proposed to facilitate the assessment of dyspnea. These rating scales provide a reference that allows the patient to describe his or her shortness of breath in terms of physical activity.

Dyspnea may result from a variety of causes, including decreased oxygen in the air (as occurs when one ascends to a high altitude), airway obstruction, respiratory muscle weakness and fatigue, pneumonia, pulmonary embolism, pulmonary vascular congestion, arteriovenous shunts in the heart or lungs, cardiac valvular disorders, anemia, and emotional disorders. Of particular importance is dyspnea that is influenced by postural changes.

Orthopnea is a type of dyspnea that occurs when a patient assumes a recumbent position. It is most often associated with left heart failure but it can also occur with severe pulmonary diseases. *Paroxysmal nocturnal dyspnea* is a form of orthopnea that is perceived by the patient while sleeping. Typically, the paroxysmal nocturnal dyspnea occurs 1 to 2 hours after the patient has fallen asleep. To relieve the dyspnea, the patient awakens and assumes a sitting position. Paroxysmal nocturnal dyspnea differs from simple orthopnea because it usually requires 20 or 30 minutes of sitting upright to relieve the shortness of breath, whereas simple orthopnea can be relieved with only 5 minutes of sitting upright. Since orthopnea is relieved when the patient assumes a more upright position, inquiry as to the patient's postural sleeping habits (e.g., the number of pillows he or she requires to relieve the sensation of breathlessness) is often used a rough indication of the degree of pulmonary congestion.

Chest Pain

Thoracic pain is associated with a variety of cardiovascular and pulmonary disorders. Angina pec-

TABLE 7–1A. Patient History

HOSPITAL REGULATION:
ALL POSITIVE AND IMPORTANT NEGATIVE FINDINGS SHALL BE RECORDED.

Date _____ Time _____ A.M. / P.M.

ORDER OF RECORDING

1. Chief Complaint
2. History of Present Illness
3. History of Past Illness
    a) childhood
    b) adult
    c) operations
    d) injuries
    e) drugs
4. Family History
5. Social History
6. Systemic Review
    a) General
    b) Head–Eyes–Ears–Nose–Throat
    d) Neck
    e) Respiratory
    f) Cardiovascular
    g) Gastrointestinal
    h) Genitourinary
    i) Gynecological
    j) Locomotor
    k) Neuropsychiatric
7. Signature

_____ M.D.
SIGNATURE

TABLE 7–1B. Physical Examination

HOSPITAL REGULATION:
ALL POSITIVE AND IMPORTANT NEGATIVE FINDINGS SHALL BE RECORDED.

Date _____ Time _____ A.M./P.M.

Temp. _____ Pulse _____ Resp. _____ Blood Pressure _____

ORDER OF RECORDING

1. General
2. Skin
3. Eyes
4. Ears
5. Nose
6. Mouth
7. Throat
8. Neck
9. Chest
10. Heart
11. Abdomen
12. Genitalia
13. Lymphatic
14. Blood Vessels
15. Locomotor
16. Extremities
17. Neurological
18. Rectal
19. Vaginal
20. Diagnosis
21. Signature

_____ M.D.
SIGNATURE

Courtesy of East Jefferson General Hospital, Metairie, La.

toris, myocardial infarction, pericarditis, myocarditis, pulmonary embolism, pneumonia, rib fracture, and pneumothorax are just a few examples. When questioning the patient about his or her chest pain, the examiner should inquire about precipitating factors, the pain's anatomic location, and its quality and duration.

Chest pain of cardiac origin is commonly precipitated by exertion, intense emotion, or ingestion of a large meal. The pain is typically described as either constricting or pressing (as occurs with angina pectoris and myocardial infarction) or sharp (as occurs with pericarditis and pulmonary embolism). In cases of angina pectoris and myocardial infarction, the maximum intensity of pain occurs in the precordial and retrosternal regions and extends with less intensity into the neck and to the left and right hemithoraces. It may radiate into one or both of the arms, usually the left. The duration of pain associated with angina pectoris varies from 1 to 30 minutes, whereas the pain of myocardial infarction may last several days.

Chest pain of pulmonary origin involves the chest wall, the parietal pleura, the major airways, the diaphragm, or the mediastinum; the lung parenchyma and visceral pleura covering it are insensitive to pain stimuli. *Chest wall pain* resulting from trauma (e.g., rib fracture) is well localized and very sharp. The pain is increased by deep breathing and coughing and is referred to as *pleuritic pain* because of the similarity to the pain associated with pleurisy (i.e., inflammation of the pleura). Patients afflicted with a pneumothorax or extensive atelectasis may experience occasional pain. This pain is thought to be due to traction on the parietal pleura by adhesions that are attached to the moving visceral pleura. *Visceral pain,* such as that which occurs with neoplasms of the major bronchi or contusions of the lung, is less localized and dull. *Diaphragmatic pain* is usually felt along the superior ridge of the trapezius muscle and along the costal margins of the affected side. Intercostal neuritis (shingles, or herpes zoster), acute myositis, esophageal spasm, spinal cord compression, hyperventilation, and psychogenic factors may also contribute to the perception of chest pain.

Cough and Expectoration

Afferent excitatory stimuli arising from irritation of pulmonary structures (i.e., the pharynx, larynx, trachea, bronchi, and pleura) and extrapulmonary structures (e.g., auricular branch of the vagus nerve) result in the generation of a cough. The efferent arc of the cough reflex, which is mediated through innervation of the respiratory, laryngeal, and abdominal muscles, when activated, results in a short inspiratory phase followed by closure of the glottis and contraction of the abdominal muscles. With opening of the glottis, a forceful expiration occurs to expel the material that acted as the irritant.

Sputum production often accompanies cough when pulmonary irritation leads to transudation or exudation of fluid within the lung. Normally, less than 100 ml of sputum is produced daily and is usually swallowed. Excessive volumes of sputum should be noted and the sputum's color, odor, turbidity, and consistency recorded. Laboratory analysis of sputum samples may also be indicated to determine if any abnormal bacterial growth exists. As discussed in Chapter 12, culture and sensitivity tests are important in the successful treatment of persons experiencing respiratory infections. Note that sputum can be examined only when a sufficient amount is collected. Typically, the patient is instructed to collect expectorant in a clear container (Fig. 7–1).

Sputum may be described as *serous, mucoid, purulent, seropurulent,* or *mucopurulent.* The presence of *bronchial casts* and *pneumoliths* are also notable findings.

Stringy mucoid sputum is characteristically produced by patients during asthma paroxysms. Purulent sputum indicates the presence of an infectious disease process. Patients with pneumonia or who are in the resolving phases of pulmonary tuberculosis typically produce small amounts of purulent sputum, whereas those with lung abscesses, chronic bronchitis, bronchiectasis, and bronchopulmonary fistula produce large amounts of purulent sputum. Sudden expectoration of a large volume of sputum after a short illness, usually indicates the presence of a lung abscess. Patients with chronic bronchitis and bronchiectasis usually produce increasing amounts of sputum, up to as much as 200 to 500 ml/day. Chronic bronchitics produce purulent sputum that is mucoid, sticky, and gray or white in color. When the sputum from a patient with bronciectasis is allowed to settle, it characteristically divides into three layers: the top layer has a mucoid consistency, the middle layer is composed of clear fluid, and the bottom layer has a purulent appearance.

Hemoptysis

When examining a sputum sample, it is also important to note any blood that may be present.

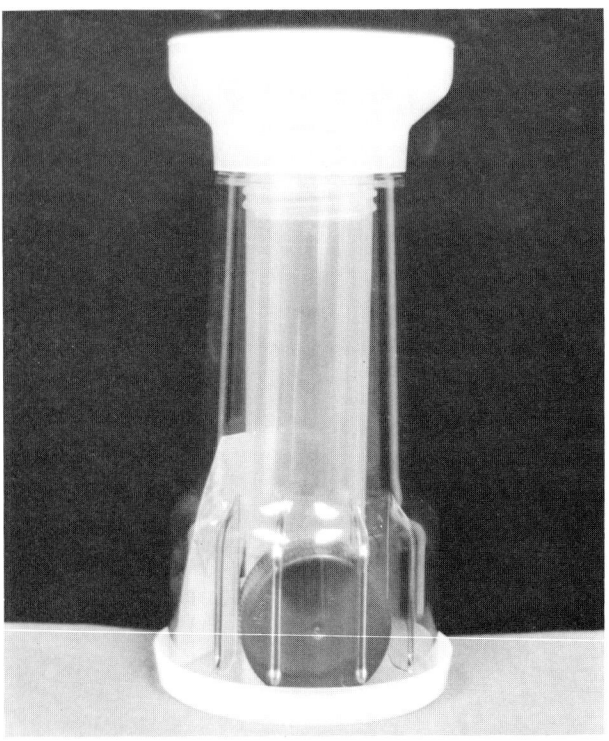

FIGURE 7-1. Sputum collection container.

Hemoptysis is the coughing up of blood or blood-stained sputum. The source of blood may be the mouth, nasopharynx, trachea, intrapulmonary bronchi, or the lung parenchyma. Massive bleeding can occur with pulmonary tuberculosis, lung abscesses, pulmonary embolism and infarction, bronchiectasis, mitral stenosis, and bronchiogenic carcinoma. Copius amounts of tenacious blood in the sputum occurs with klebsiella pneumonia. The presence of pink frothy sputum is associated with pulmonary edema, as occurs during left heart failure.

Hematemesis, or the vomiting of blood, may contribute to the amount of blood expectorated and is often confused with the diagnosis of hemoptysis. Hematemesis can result from ulceration of the esophagus, esophageal neoplasms, esophageal varices from the portal circulation, peptic ulcers, gastric carcinoma, hiatal hernia, gastritis, severe retching, or abdominal surgery. Table 7-2 shows the differential diagnosis of hemoptysis and hematemesis. Both conditions can be treated with drugs or surgery or both, depending on the severity of the bleeding.

Allergic Disorders and Personal-Occupational History

Defense of the body against foreign antigens (e.g., microorganisms, toxins, neoplasms, drugs, or pollen) involves the activation of cellular and humoral immunologic defense mechanisms. Alterations in immune activity may result in allergic reactions that can lead to problems in about 10% of the U.S.

TABLE 7-2 Differential Diagnosis of Hemoptysis and Hematemesis

Feature	Hemoptysis	Hematemesis
Prodrome	Tingling in throat, desire to cough	Nausea, stomach distress
Onset	Blood is coughed up; retching may accompany	Blood is vomited; coughing may accompany
Appearance	Some portions frothy	Never frothy
Color	Portions may be bright red	Uniformly dark red
pH reaction	Alkaline	Acid
Content	Leukocytes, microorganisms, hemosiderin-laden macrophages	Food particles
Past history	Lung disease	Alcoholism, peptic ulcer, liver disease
Anemia	Occasionally present	Common
Stools (at onset)	Guaiac negative	Guaiac positive

From Hinshaw, H.C., and Murray, J.F.: *Diseases of the Chest*, 4th ed. Philadelphia, W.B. Saunders, 1980, p 11, with permission.

population. Thus, a history of allergy should be noted because it may become important when one tries to differentiate the causative factors contributing to cardiopulmonary impairment. A history of recurrent upper respiratory infections and/or atopy (e.g., bronchial asthma) usually signals the presence of altered immunologic defense of the respiratory system, which may be the source of a pathophysiologic process.

Information concerning environmental factors (e.g., seasonal variations or contact with toxic chemicals or pets) that elicit allergic responses also may aid in the cardiopulmonary diagnosis and therapeutic regimen. Smoking habits, including the quantity of tobacco consumed (e.g., for cigarette smokers, this can be expressed in pack years—2 pack of cigarettes per day for 5 years equals a 10 pack-year history of smoking) and the manner in which it is consumed, are useful correlates with the frequency and severity of cardiopulmonary dysfunctions (e.g., bronchitis, emphysema, angina pectoris, myocardial infarction).

Details about the patient's occupational history, including places and types of employment, and the duration of each job may provide important information about the patient's disease. For example, exposure to silica-bearing rocks, asbestos, nitrogen dioxide fumes, or moldy hay may predispose the patient to the development of one of the pneumoconioses discussed in Chapter 4.

Acquisition of a complete cardiopulmonary history, coupled with the recognition of extrathoracic alterations that affect circulatory and/or respiratory function, facilitates the second aspect of assessment, *physical examination*.

PHYSICAL EXAMINATION OF CARDIOPULMONARY FUNCTION

The medical history furnishes information on the chronology and symptoms associated with the patient's present illness. The physical examination reveals physical signs of disease. Symptoms are subjective information that are perceived by the patient; signs are objective manifestations of disease perceived by the examiner.

We stated earlier in this chapter that acquisition of a meaningful medical history requires a knowledge of pathophysiologic states and their associated symptoms. For the successful completion of a cardiopulmonary assessment, the cardiopulmonary specialist should have a working knowledge of the procedures involved in the physical assessment of the heart and lungs: *inspection, palpation, percussion,* and *auscultation*. The ability of a practitioner to associate abnormal physical findings with historical data can only be accomplished through repeated examination of normal subjects and patients afflicted with cardiopulmonary impairments.

Inspection

Inspection of cardiopulmonary function should focus on the following signs: thoracic contours; respiratory rate, depth, and rhythm; symmetry of chest wall movements during the respiratory cycle; the presence of central and/or peripheral cyanosis; clubbing of the digits; and overall nutritional status.

Thoracic Contours

Figure 7–2 shows several of the more common chest wall contours that should be noted in the cardiopulmonary assessment. Recognition of thoracic deformities may help to delineate the source of impairment (e.g., barrel chest is an obvious sign of air-trapping associated with obstructive pulmonary disease).

Respiratory Patterns

While the patient is seated upright, observe the length and depth of successive respiratory cycles. Compare these data for several breathing cycles to determine whether any abnormal breathing patterns are discernible. Variations in the character of breathing affect the amount of work required to sustain efficient gas exchange.

Figure 7–3 shows how varying the respiratory rate could affect the mechanical work of breathing in a normal subject, a patient with obstructive pulmonary disease (e.g., emphysema), and a patient with restrictive pulmonary disease (e.g., pulmonary fibrosis). As this figure shows, for any given alveolar ventilation, there is an optimum respiratory frequency at which the work of breathing is minimal. Normal subjects breathe at respiratory rates of 10 to 15 breaths/minute. At rates less than 10 breaths/minute, the flow resistance decreases but the elastic resistance of the respiratory system increases. Conversely, at respiratory rates greater than about 15 breaths/minute, frictional resistance increases and elastic work decreases. Patients with obstructive pulmonary diseases typically choose to breathe at slow respiratory rates and large tidal volumes. By using this breathing pattern, they minimize air trapping and, therefore, reduce the

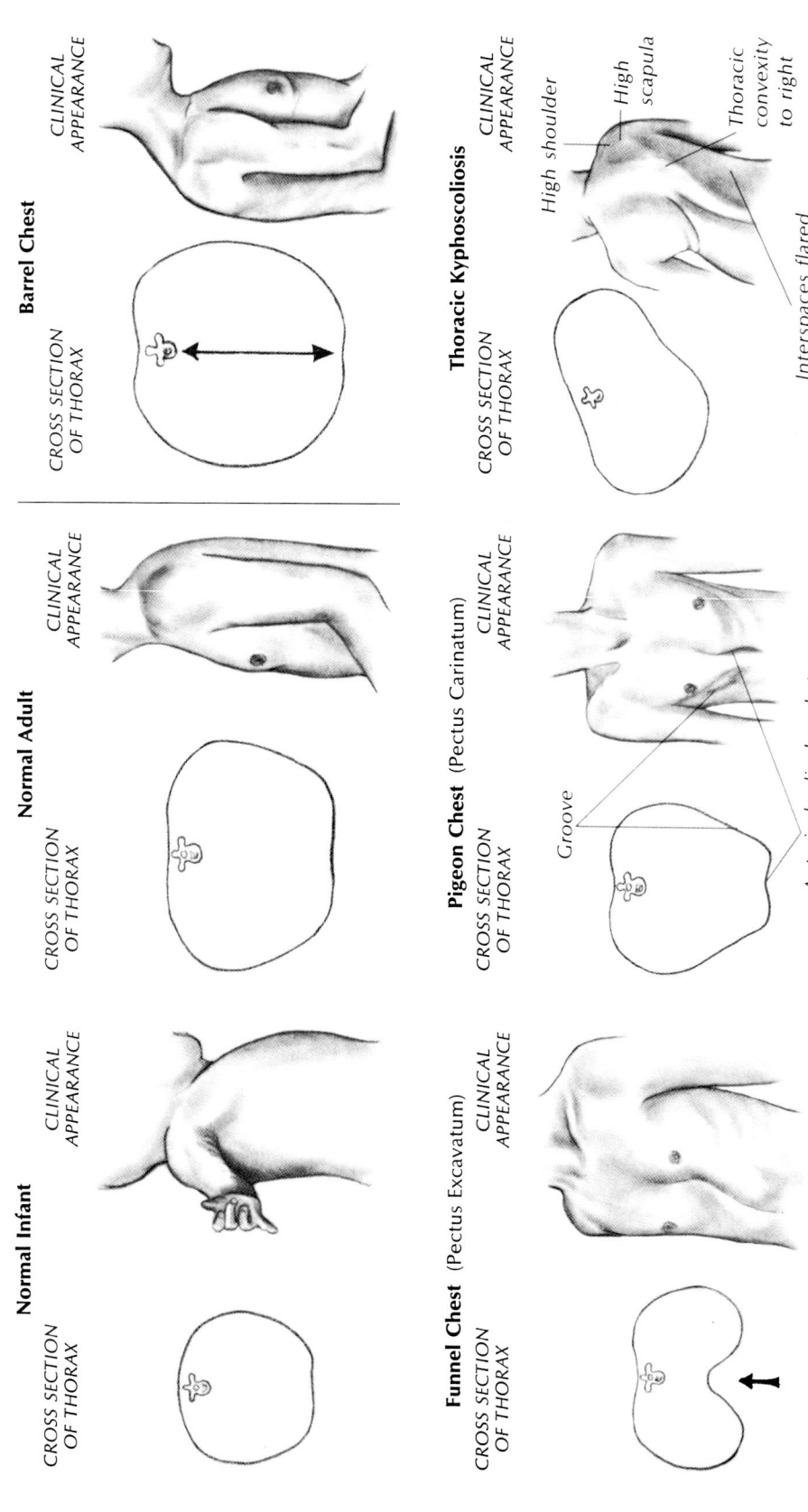

FIGURE 7–2. Chest wall contours. (From Bates, B.: *A Guide to Physical Examination*, 4th ed. Philadelphia, J.B. Lippincott, 1987, with permission.)

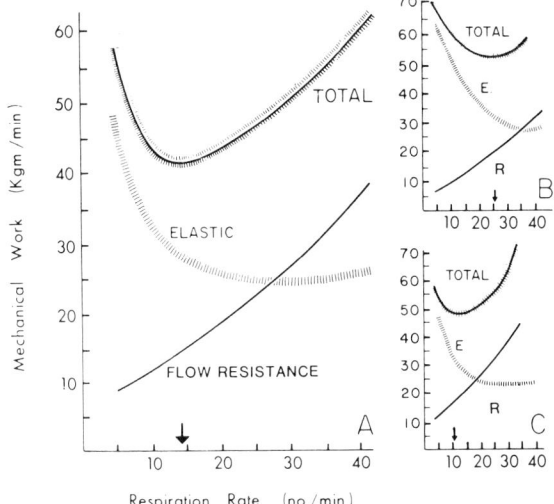

FIGURE 7–3. Relationship between respiratory rate and the mechanical work of breathing at a given alveolar ventilation. (From Cherniack, R.M., and Cherniack, L.: *Respiration in Health and Disease,* 3rd ed. Philadelphia, W.B. Saunders, 1983, with permission.)

work of breathing. In patients with restrictive pulmonary diseases, such as pulmonary fibrosis or kyphoscoliosis, elastic resistance is increased. These patients choose to breathe at high respiratory rates and shallow tidal volumes because a considerable amount of work is required to overcome the increased elastic resistance.

Very high respiratory rates with shallow tidal volumes may also result from dyspnea of cardiac or respiratory origin, anxiety, or simply from environmental factors (e.g., climatic conditions). Continued use of the accessory muscles of respiration (e.g., parasternal, substernal, and intercostal retractions) is a sign of respiratory distress and should be dealt with promptly.

Chest trauma that causes multiple rib fracture can result in a *flail chest*, which is a paradoxical movement of the chest wall at the site of the fractures (i.e., the chest wall moves inward during inspiration and outward during expiration). This paradoxical movement occurs because the chest wall in the affected area is drawn inward during inspiration by the increasing negative intrathoracic pressure; the outward movement of the chest wall during expiration occurs when the intrathoracic pressure rises above atmospheric pressure.

Cyanosis

Cyanosis is a bluish coloration of the skin or mucous membranes that results from the presence of excess unsaturated hemoglobin. Classically, cyanosis is said to occur when more than 5 gm of deoxygenated hemoglobin are present per 100 ml of blood. Note that this definition is generally accepted for persons having normal hemoglobin levels (i.e., 12 to 18 gm/100 ml of whole blood); however, in cases of anemia (decreased hemoglobin) or polycythemia (increased hemoglobin), the above definition is not accurate. Anemic patients do not appear cyanotic unless they are severely hypoxemic, whereas polycythemic patients require considerably lower percentages of deoxygenated hemoglobin to produce the bluish discoloration of cyanosis.

Central cyanosis is detected by observing mucous membranes (e.g., tongue, gums, or lining of the cheeks). *Peripheral cyanosis* is detected by noting discoloration of the extremities (e.g., nailbeds). Central cyanosis is a primary manifestation of cardiac and/or ventilatory impairment, whereas peripheral cyanosis occurs in peripheral vascular obstruction or occlusion.

Clubbing of Digits

Clubbing of the digits can be associated with both intra- and extrathoracic abnormalities. Congenital cardiac disease (e.g., right-to-left intracardiac shunts), subacute bacterial endocarditis, and cor pulmonale represent intrathoracic examples; osteoarthropathy and cirrhosis of the liver represent extrathoracic diseases associated with clubbing of the digits. Although the exact cause of this phenomenon is unknown, its presence, particularly when associated with cyanosis, can be used as an indication of the severity of a cardiopulmonary disease. Figure 7–4 illustrates the anatomic changes that occur with clubbing of the digits.

Nutritional Status

Assessment of the nutritional status of an individual can provide important information about the person's general health and his or her capacity to endure physiologic stress. Table 7–3 outlines some

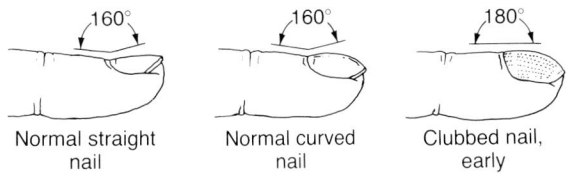

FIGURE 7–4. Clubbing of the digits. (From Cherniack, R.M., and Cherniack, L.: *Respiration in Health and Disease,* 3rd ed. Philadelphia, W.B. Saunders, 1983, with permission.)

TABLE 7–3. Features of the Clinical History Suggesting Malnutrition

1. Recent weight loss (>10% of usual body weight).
2. Restricted oral intake of nutrients (e.g., clear liquid diet or the administration of intravenous infusions of simple solutions only for the preceding 10 days or more.)
3. Protracted nutrient loss as a result of vomiting diarrhea, or surgical resection of portions of the gastrointestinal tract.
4. Increased metabolic needs due to recent surgery or trauma, infections, fever, extensive burns, recent pregnancy, or lactation.
5. Chronic disease or impaired function of any major organ system.
6. Fad diets, eccentric behavior, or social or family disruption.
7. Use of drugs with antinutrient or catabolic properties, such as corticosteroids, immunosuppressants, and anticonvulsants.

of the prominent features of a clinical history that can aid in identifying patients who either have or are at high risk for developing malnutrition. Table 7–4 is a partial list the clinical manifestations of malnutrition.

During the initial physical assessment, the patient's overall physical and mental condition should be noted. As discussed in Chapter 12, more

TABLE 7–4. Partial Listing of Physical Manifestations of Malnutrition

Cutaneous
    Thin, shiny skin
    Drying or scaling of skin
    Easily pluckable hair
    Lackluster nails
    Decubitus ulcer
    Jaundice, hyperpigmentation, xanthomas, seborrhea
    Nonhealing surgical wounds
Mouth and Mucus Membranes
    Absent teeth or ill-fitting dentures
    Angular fissures of the mouth
    Pallor
Musculoskeletal
    Growth retardation
    Weakness and atrophy of the muscles
    Epiphyseal swelling
Neurologic
    Opthalmoplegia
    Ataxia
    Coma, convulsions, and paralysis
Abdominal and Gastrointestinal
    Hepatomegaly
    Ascites
    Small bowel distension
    Lymphadenopathy or tumors
General appearance
    Edema
    Obesity
    Cachectic appearance
    Pregnancy

detailed analysis of a patient's nutritional status involves *anthropometric measurements,* including the patient's age, weight, and height; *biochemical measurements,* such as nitrogen excretion, serum albumin levels, serum transferrin levels, and serum lipid levels; *immunologic assessment* through skin testing; and *indirect calorimetry,* or the quantitation of energy expenditure through measurements of inspired and expired gases (i.e., oxygen consumption and carbon dioxide production).

Palpation

The act of feeling with the hand, or palpation, enables the clinician to assess: (1) heart rate and rhythm, (2) symmetry of chest wall motion and diaphragmatic excursions, (3) position of the trachea, (4) presence of enlarged lymph nodes, (5) tactile fremitus, defined shortly, and (6) turgor, warmth or coldness, and moistness of the skin. Human touch also helps to establish a closer patient-practitioner relationship, which is sometimes thwarted in an environment overshadowed by mechanical and electronic monitoring devices. Palpation, therefore, not only provides information about anatomic and physiologic function but also helps to strengthen the rapport required to successfully treat patients.

Heart Rate and Rhythm

Effective left ventricular rate may be counted by lightly pressing one's finger against one of the peripheral arteries. The radial, carotid, brachial, and femoral arteries are generally used for this measurement (Fig. 7–5).

The resting heart rate of a healthy adult usually ranges from 60 to 100 beats/minute, depending on the person's physical condition. The pulse rate increases with exertion, with excitement, and after a large meal is ingested.

Changes in resting rhythm of the pulse usually signals the presence of some process that is interfering with the normal conduction of electrical impulses throughout the heart. Figure 7–6 illustrates several different types of arterial pulse waves that can be determined with palpation of the peripheral arteries. In the normal pulse wave, the primary wave begins with a swift upstroke to the peak of systolic pressure, followed by a more gradual decline in amplitude. At the end of ventricular ejection, a secondary and normally smaller upstroke occurs, the dichrotic notch, caused by the rebounding of blood against the closed aortic valve.

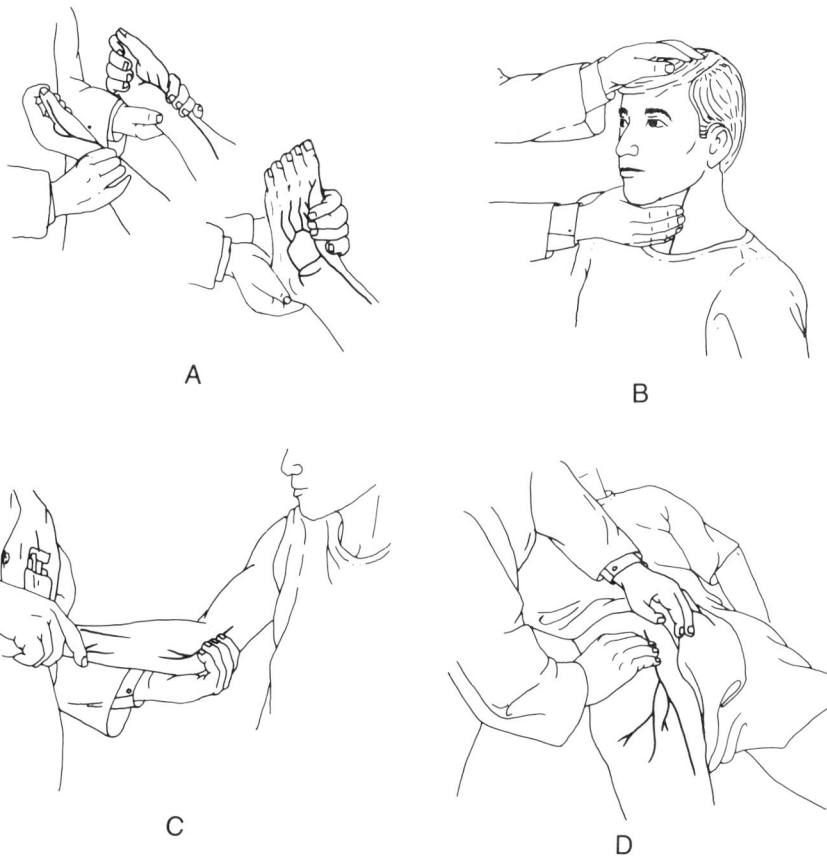

FIGURE 7–5. Examination of the pulses: *A*, Radial and dorsalis pedis. *B*, Carotid. *C*, Brachial (epitrochlear). *D*, Femoral. (From Judge, R.D., Zuidema, G.D., and Fitzgerald, F.T.: *Clinical Diagnosis: A Physiological Approach*, 4th ed. Boston, Little Brown 1982.)

(Note that the dichrotic notch is not normally palpable.) A *bounding pulse,* caused by a fast upstroke and downstroke, is typically encountered in aortic regurgitation, essential hypertension, and thyrotoxicosis. *Pulsus alternans* is characterized by a normal rhythm; however, the amplitude of the pulse wave alternates between high and low volumes, indicating the presence of severe myocardial weakness. *Pulsus paradoxus,* or inspiratory weakening of the pulse is thought to result from the traction of the diaphragm on a distended pericardium. It is associated with pericardial effusion, constrictive pericarditis, or cardiac tamponade.

Movement of the Chest

Palpation is an excellent way to evaluate the extent of chest wall movement during a respiratory cycle. As Figure 7–7 shows, both hands are simultaneously placed over the shoulders of the patient, then over the subclavicular spaces, and finally over the abdomen. While performing these maneuvers, the degree of thoracic and abdominal movement that occur with each breath should be noted. Diaphragmatic excursions are observed by placing the hands over the lower anterior chest wall with the thumbs over the right and left costal margins. As the patient inspires, the thumbs should move apart equally. Factors that cause the diaphragm to lose its normal dome-shaped contour (e.g., hyperinflation or pleural effusion) causes the costal margins to move inward on inspiration.

Tracheal Position

The position of the trachea can be determined by placing the tip of an extended index finger into the suprasternal notch (Fig. 7–8). Tracheal deviation toward the affected lung occurs in atelectasis and localized pulmonary fibrosis, whereas tracheal shifting away from the affected side can occur with pneumothorax and contralateral pleural effusion.

Lymph Nodes and Tumors

The presence of enlarged lymph nodes in the neck and head region can be ascertained by palpation of the areas shown in Figure 7–9. Lymphadenopathy (i.e., enlargement of the lymph nodes) can be

260 HISTORY AND PHYSICAL EXAMINATION

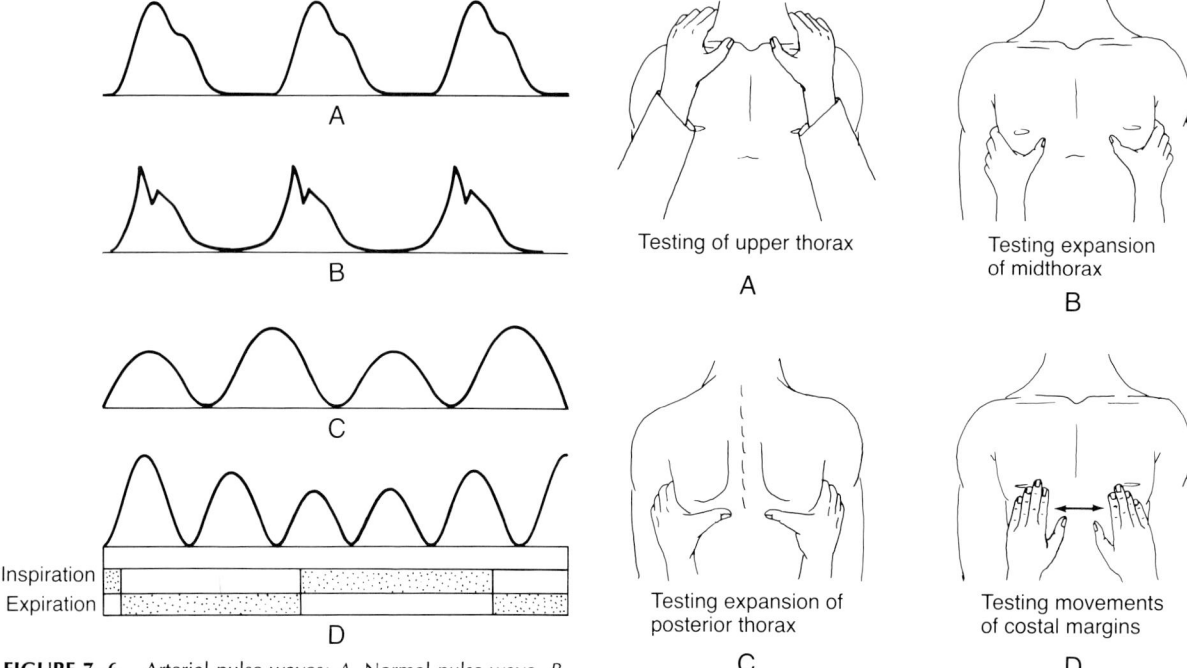

FIGURE 7–6. Arterial pulse waves: *A*, Normal pulse wave. *B*, Bounding pulse. *C*, Pulsus alternans. *D*, Pulsus paradoxus. (Adapted from DeGowin, E.L., and DeGowin, R.L.: *Bedside Diagnostic Examination*, 3rd ed. New York, Macmillan, 1976.)

FIGURE 7–7. Palpation for chest wall movements. (Adapted from DeGowin, E.L., and DeGowin, R.L.: *Bedside Diagnostic Examination*, 3rd ed. New York, Macmillan, 1976.)

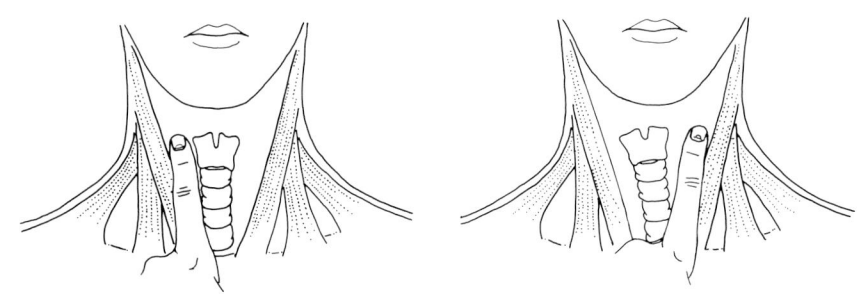

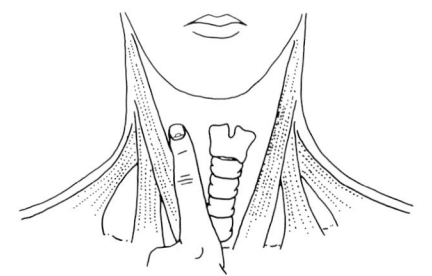

FIGURE 7–8. Determining tracheal position. (From Lehrer, S.: *Understanding Lung Sounds*. Philadelphia, W.B. Saunders, 1984.)

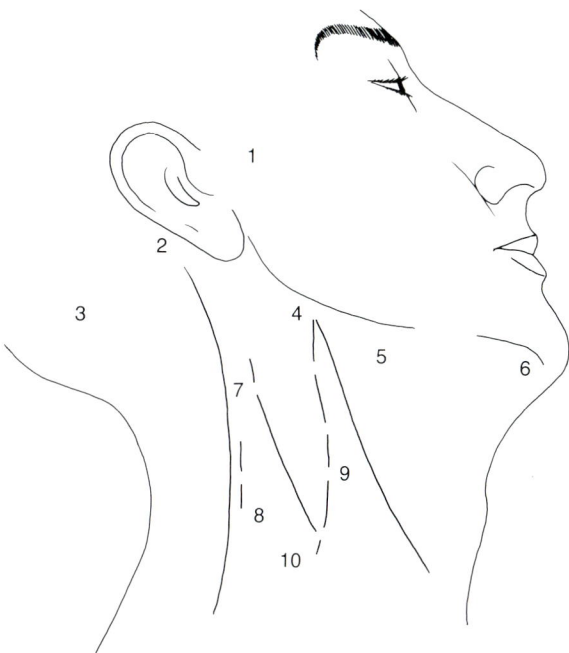

FIGURE 7-9. Lymph node regions in the neck: Preauricular (1), posterior auricular (2), occipital (3), tonsillar (4), submaxillary (5), submental (6), superficial cervical (7), posterior cervical chain (8), deep cervical chain (9) and supraclavicular (10). (Adapted from Bates, B.: *A Guide to Physical Examination*, 4th ed. Philadelphia, J.B. Lippincott, 1987.)

localized or generalized. Regional lymphadenopathy results from local infections, whereas generalized lymphadenopathy occurs in systemic disorders, such as leukemia, tuberculosis, sarcoidosis, and rheumatic arthritis.

The presence of thoracic and extrathoracic tumors should also be noted because these lesions may restrict lung movement and thus lead to atelectasis and possibly respiratory failure.

Tactile Fremitus

Tactile fremitus is a voice-generated vibration (also called a thrill) transmitted to the chest wall. These vibrations may be perceived by placing the palms against the chest wall bilaterally over areas that correspond to the various lung subdivisions. (Figure 7-10 illustrates the surface anatomy of various bronchopulmonary segments.) The intensity of the vibration is less when passing through a gaseous medium than a liquid, semisolid, or solid material. Therefore, increased fremitus on one side indicates that the lung is less aerated than the contralateral segments. Depending on the location, this difference in fremitus may represent a normal anatomic finding or indicate the presence of a pathophysiologic process. Pathology can usually be differentiated by having the patient say "ninety-nine" or "one, two, three."

Decreased fremitus is associated with pneumothorax, pleural thickening, or when there is fluid in the pleural space. Increased fremitus is associated with atelectasis and tissue consolidation, as occurs in lobar pneumonia.

Percussion

Percussion is performed by tapping body structures to produce sound. *Immediate percussion* is performed by striking the chest wall with either the palmar aspect of the middle finger or the tip of the index and middle fingers held tightly together. *Mediate percussion* involves the use of one hand placed firmly against the chest wall with one finger acting as a *pleximeter*. Using the tip of the middle finger of the opposite hand as the *plexor*, the clinician strikes the *pleximeter* and notes the resonance of the sound produced.

Percussion should begin with location of the cardiac and hepatic borders. Note the gastric tympany. Continue the percussing procedure by moving symmetrically from the thorax to the lower abdomen, tapping each side with equal intensity.

A number of terms are used by clinicians to denote the quality of sounds produced during percussion. *Flatness* is the sound produced by percussing a mass, similar to that produced when percussing the thigh muscle. *Resonance* describes the sound produced when a normal lung is percussed. *Dullness* describes a decrease in resonance, and *hyperresonance* indicates an increase in the perception of sound. Figure 7-11 illustrates the regions over the normal thorax where each of these sounds can be elicited during percussion.

Although newer techniques, such as computed tomography, magnetic resonance imaging, and ultrasound, have virtually replaced percussion as a primary diagnostic tool, it should be remembered that percussion still remains a very useful method for confirming suspected abnormalities of anatomic or physiologic function.

Auscultation

Auscultation is the act of listening for sounds generated within the body. The first detailed description of heart and lung sounds was made by René Théophile Hyacinthe Laënnec, who between 1816 and 1819, used auscultation to characterize varia-

262 HISTORY AND PHYSICAL EXAMINATION

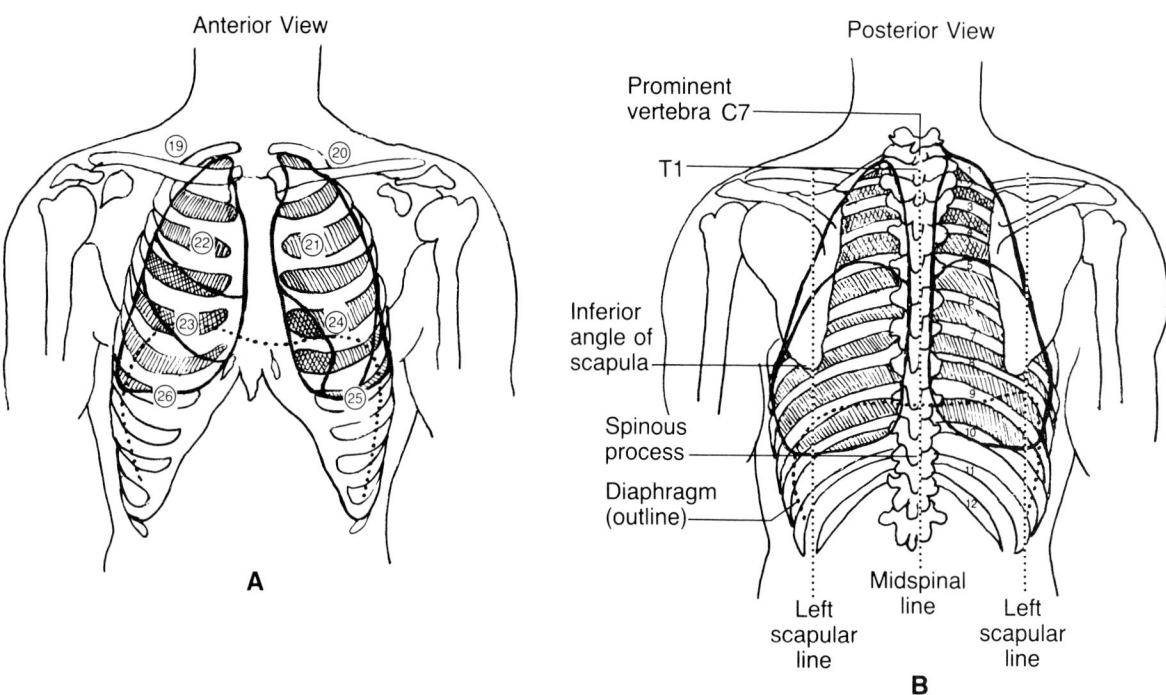

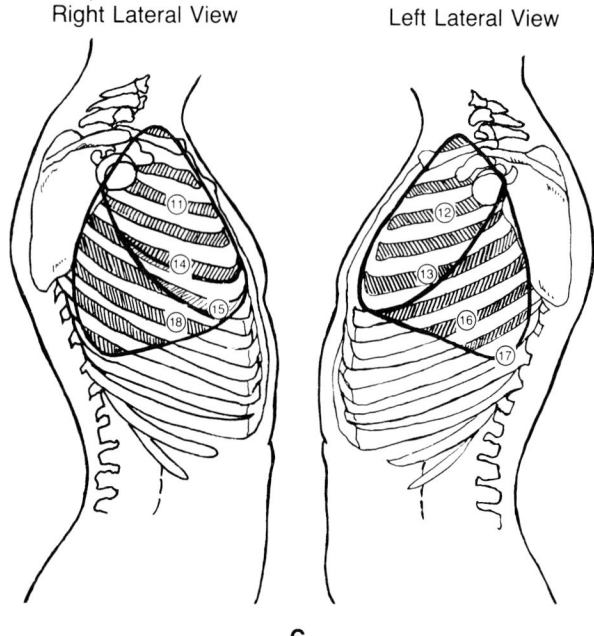

FIGURE 7–10. Surface anatomy of the thorax showing the approximate location of the various bronchopulmonary segments. (From Tilkian, A.G., and Conover, M.B.: *Understanding Heart Sounds and Murmurs,* 2nd ed. Philadelphia, W.B. Saunders, 1984, with permission.)

tions in the sounds produced during contraction of the heart and the movement of air into and out of the lungs. Since these initial studies, many physicians and scientists have contributed to our understanding of both normal and abnormal sounds heard during auscultation. Although a complete review of these studies is not given here, the reader can find several excellent reviews of the history and development of this technique in this chapter's bibliography.

Use of the Stethoscope

The stethoscope is an instrument that conveys a vibrating column of air from the body wall to the ear. The sounds transmitted through the stetho-

HISTORY AND PHYSICAL EXAMINATION   263

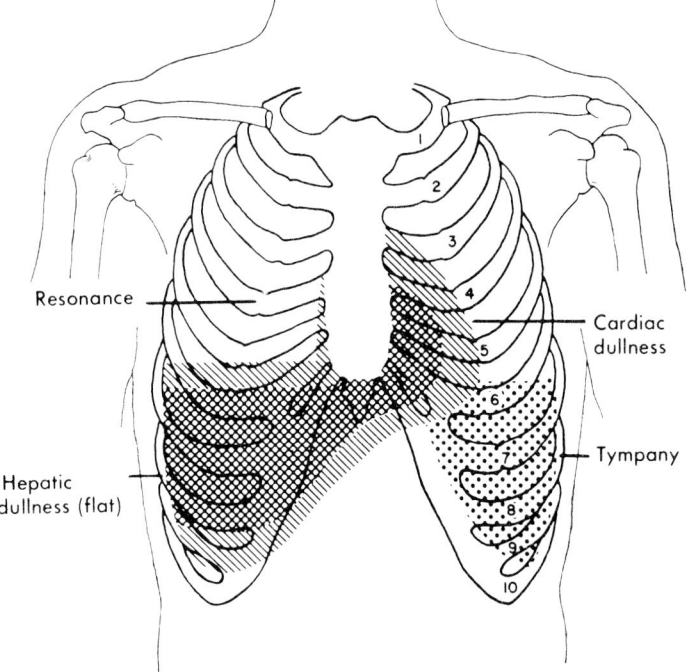

FIGURE 7–11. Regions over the normal thorax where resonance, dullness, and tympany can be elicited during percussion. (Reproduced by permission from: Prior, J.A., Silberstein, J.S., and Stang, J.M.: *Physical Diagnosis,* 6th ed. St. Louis, 1981, The C.V. Mosby Co.)

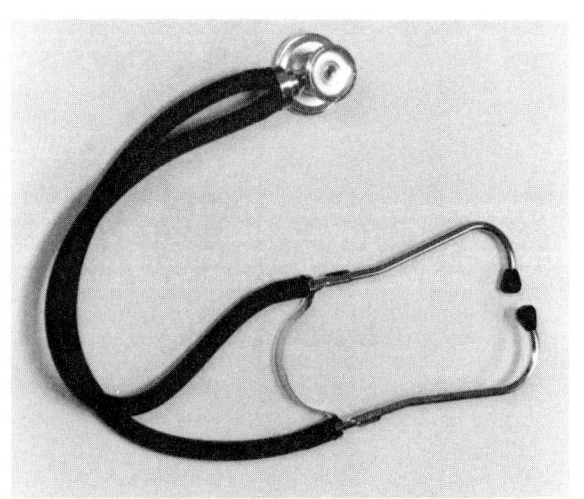

FIGURE 7–12. Stethoscope. (Courtesy of Hewlett-Packard, Palo Alto, CA.)

scope vary in frequency (the number of sound vibrations per second, measured in *hertz*), intensity (amplitude, measured in *decibels*), and duration (measured in *seconds*). The stethoscope is used by the cardiopulmonary specialist because heart and lungs sounds occur in a frequency range to which the human ear is relatively insensitive.

Modern stethoscopes consist of a combination of two chest pieces, tubing, a binaural headset, and eartips (Fig. 7–12). The bell chest piece is used for listening to low-pitched sounds (e.g., the first heart sound), whereas the closed diaphragm chest piece is used for listening to high-pitched sounds (e.g., the second heart sound or lung sounds). The tubing connecting the chest pieces to the binaurals is about 30 cm long. The binaurals and eartips should fit snugly, yet comfortably.

For optimal results, the patient should be auscultated in a quiet, well-ventilated room. For auscultation of the heart, the patient should be listened to first while he or she is seated upright and then in the left lateral decubitus position (i.e., patient is lying on the left side). Auscultation should proceed from the apex of the heart to the mitral area, up the left border of the heart to the pulmonic area, and finally to the aortic area (Fig. 7–13). The procedure should be done slowly, and the quality of sounds heard over each area noted carefully. Be aware that the sounds heard at the apex of the heart have a greater intensity when the patient is in the left lateral decubitus position. This occurs because the heart is located closer to the chest wall in this body position. (The point of maximum intensity (PMI) is the site where heart sounds are heard with the greatest intensity.)

Lung sounds are best heard while the patient is in an upright seated position. Auscultation of the lungs should proceed by the sequence shown in Figure 7–14. Extraneous noises, such as muscle, joint, or tendon movements, hair movements against the chest piece, or inadvertent touching of the stethoscope tubing should be taken into account to avoid confusion with abnormal sounds that result from altered physiology. Note that auscultation should not be performed over clothing because the clothing can act as a sound filter and alter the perception of sound.

The technique of auscultation offers the clinician an easy way to assess the condition of the heart,

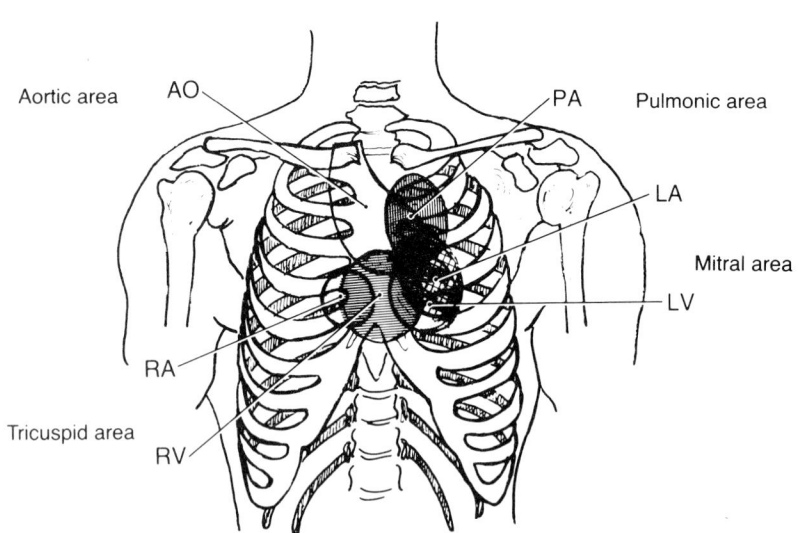

FIGURE 7–13. Auscultation of the heart. (From Tilkian, A.G., and Conover, M.B.: *Understanding Heart Sounds and Murmurs*, 2nd ed. Philadelphia, W.B. Saunders, 1984, with permission.)

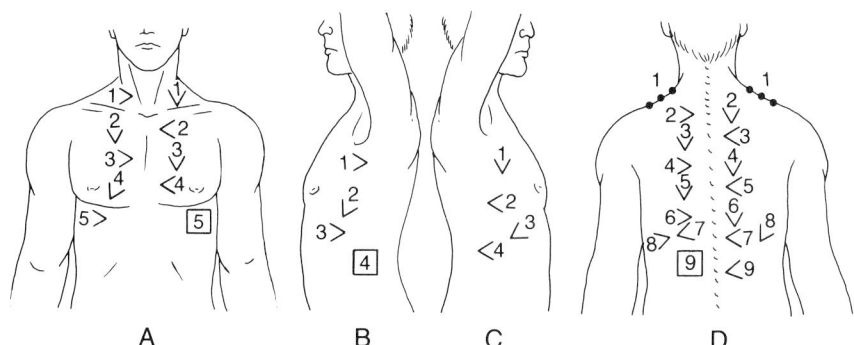

FIGURE 7–14. Auscultation of the lungs. (From Lehrer, S.: *Understanding Lung Sounds*. Philadelphia, W.B. Saunders, 1984, with permission.)

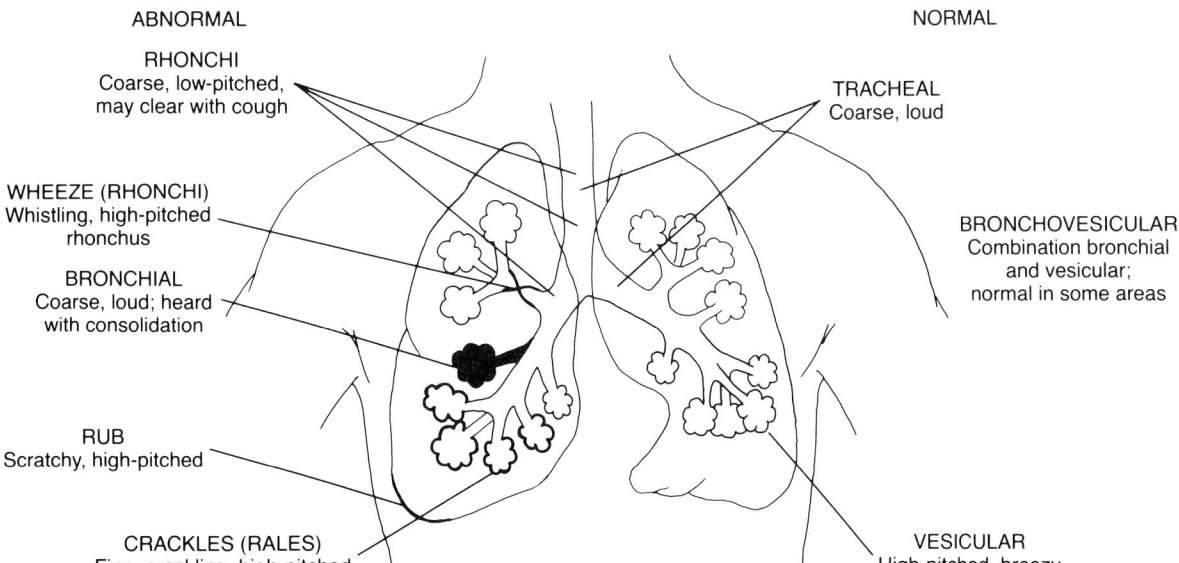

FIGURE 7–15. Representation of normal breath sounds and abnormal sounds in the chest. (From Judge, R.D., Zuidema, G.D. and Fitzgerald, F.T.: *Clinical Diagnosis: A Physiological Approach*, 4th ed. Boston, Little, Brown 1982.)

lungs, pleura, and abdomen. Remember, however, that the stethoscope should be used only after sufficient information has been obtained from the history and physical examination.

Heart Sounds

Although cardiac sounds were initially thought to be created by the opening and closing of the heart valves, the exact origin of these sounds remains to be determined. Currently, experts believe that they result from the generation of turbulent blood flow (see Chapter 2). When one or more of the valves close, vibrations occur as blood is dammed within the heart and great vessels. These vibrations are transmitted to the chest wall, creating the characteristic lubb-dubb sound of the normal heart. Classically, only two sounds are usually described, S1 and S2. S1 (or lubb) is associated with closure of the atrioventricular valves (i.e., tricuspid and mitral valves), and S2 (or dubb) results from closure of the semilunar valves (i.e., pulmonic and aortic valves). Note that the length of ventricular systole can be approximated by determining the time interval between the S1 and S2 sounds. Conversely, ventricular diastole occurs during the interval between S2 and the next S1 sound. A third (S3) and fourth (S4) sound may also be heard by the experienced listener. S3 is thought to occur as blood rushes into the ventricles during early ventricular diastole, and S4 results from atrial systole that occurs in late ventricular diastole. S3 and S4 sounds are difficult to hear in an adult, but may be more easily heard in children because a child's chest wall is less thick and does not filter the sound as in an adult's.

The presence of abnormal heart sounds or *murmurs* generally occurs when blood is forced through a structure having a reduced cross-sectional area, and a greater amount of turbulent flow is generated. Murmurs are usually described according to their timing (at what part of the cardiac cycle the murmur occurs), location (the anatomic position where the murmur exhibits the maximum sound intensity), its pattern (whether it is uniform in intensity or whether its intensity rises, also called *crescendo,* or diminishes, also called *decrescendo*), and its pitch (low-pitched or high-pitched).

Phonocardiography, the recording and analysis of heart sounds, is an ideal way to illustrate various types of murmurs. As discussed in Chapter 8, the presence of a cardiac murmur may indicate some pathophysiologic process and usually warrants the use of more sophisticated testing procedures to define the abnormality (e.g., electrocardiography or echocardiography).

Lung Sounds

Since Laënnec first described the auscultatory findings associated with the movement of air into and out of the lung, a considerable amount of discussion has arisen as to the most appropriate terms to use when describing normal and abnormal lung sounds. The following is a summary of the criteria for describing lung sounds based on the suggested nomenclature adopted by the American Thoracic Society (ATS) and the American College of Chest Physicians (ACCP). Figure 7-15 summarizes the various types of lung sounds and their appropriate anatomic locations.

Normal Breath Sounds. Four types of breath sounds are heard over the normal chest: vesicular, bronchial, bronchovesicular, and tracheal sounds. *Vesicular Sounds* are low-pitched sounds heard over most of the periphery of the lung. These sounds have a characteristic rustling quality, which is more prolonged in inspiration than expiration. (The term *vesicular* was derived from the initial belief that these sounds were generated by the movement of air into and out of the alveoli, which were originally called vesicles.)
Bronchial Sounds are high-pitched vibrations that are normally heard directly over the lower part of the sternum. A distinct pause occurs between inspiration and expiration, with the expiratory phase lasting longer than the inspiratory phase. Bronchial sounds heard over the periphery of the lung are considered to be abnormal and may indicate lobar consolidation or atelectasis.
Bronchovesicular Sounds are, as the name implies, a mixture of bronchial and vesicular sounds. They are normally heard over the first and second intercostal spaces (anteriorly) and between the scapulae (posteriorly). The duration of inspiration is normally equal to that of expiration.
Tracheal Sounds are heard over the extrathoracic portions of the trachea. These high-pitched "tubular" sounds have a harsh quality. Expiration is heard for a longer period than inspiration.

Abnormal Breath Sounds. Abnormal breath sounds are generally classified as (1) adventitious sounds, (2) irregularly transmitted sounds, and (3) diminished breath sounds.

Adventitious Sounds. There are four basic types of adventitious sounds: crackles, wheezes, stridor, and pleural friction rubs.

Crackles (or *rales*) are usually described as short, explosive, discontinuous sounds. They are characterized according to quantity, pitch, amplitude, and timing. Quantitatively, they are referred to as scanty or profuse; qualitatively, they are described as high-pitched or low-pitched, loud or faint, inspiratory, expiratory or both, and regular or random. Current theory suggests that crackles result from an explosive equalization of pressure that occurs when air rushes into previously closed alveoli. This theory seems reasonable since the timing of crackles relates closely to changes in transpulmonary pressure.

In general, early inspiratory crackles are associated with obstructive pulmonary dysfunctions, whereas late inspiratory crackles are associated with restrictive disorders. Expiratory crackles are most often associated with bronchiectasis.

Wheezes (or *rhonchi*) are continuous musical sounds that are believed to result when air flows through a constricted bronchus. Wheezes are also described according to pitch, amplitude, and timing. Additionally, they may be characterized as monophonic or polyphonic.

Monophonic wheezes consist of a single musical tone. These sounds may be heard singly or in synchrony. They are typically heard during inspiration. Polyphonic wheezes are composed of several musical notes that are heard during expiration. Polyphonic wheezes are generally heard in patients with obstructive pulmonary diseases; however, they may also be produced by a healthy person during a forced expiration. (The wheeze produced by healthy subjects during a forced expiration is thought to result from the generation of high air flow rates rather than from pathologic changes.)

Stridor is often confused with monophonic wheezing because it possesses a musically constant pitch. It differs from monophonic wheezing in intensity (stridor is much louder than wheezing) and in that it is produced by air flowing through a constricted larynx or trachea. Stridor usually begins as a purely inspiratory sound but may progress to both the inspiratory and expiratory phases of breathing as the degree of obstruction increases. Viral croup, epiglottitis, diphtheria, laryngomalacia, vocal cord paralysis, and inhalation of foreign bodies can produce stridor.

Pleural friction rubs are nonmusical sounds that are similar to crackles in quality. Friction rubs are produced by the movement of inflamed parietal and visceral pleura over each other. These sounds differ from crackles, being usually more prolonged and lower in pitch. Friction rubs are typically described as the sound produced when two pieces of leather are rubbed together, whereas the crackles elicited from pathologic changes in the lung sound similar to the sounds of hairs rubbed together next to the ear.

Irregularly Transmitted Sounds. Egophony, whispered pectoriloquy, and bronchophony are used to describe the transmission of abnormal breath sounds. It is generally thought that consolidation of lung tissue is chiefly responsible for the generation of these sounds.

To determine whether abnormally transmitted sounds are present, the examiner listens to the patient's chest with a stethoscope as the patient enunciates certain letters or phrases.

Egophony may be elicited by having the patient say the letter *E*. Because of the filtering characteristics produced when voiced sounds travel through consolidated tissue, the *E* sound will be perceived as an *A*, which is referred to as *E to A egophony*. This transition occurs because the lower frequency characteristics of the *E* sound are filtered resulting in the transmission of primarily high-frequency sounds, like those associated with saying *A*. Figure 7–16 is a sound spectrograph illustrating this phenomenon.

Under normal circumstances, whispered sounds are not heard at the chest wall. However, in atelectasis or consolidation, high-pitched components of a whisper can be heard through the chest wall. This is referred to as *whispered pectoriloquy*. *Bronchophony* is similar to whispered pectoriloquy in that, when a portion of the lung becomes airless, high-pitched sounds are transmitted with greater clarity.

Each of the abnormally transmitted sounds results when the filtering characteristics of the lung are altered. Having the subject say "one, two, three" or "ninety-nine" is a convention and by no means the only way to elicit the signs of altered sound transmission during auscultation.

Diminished Breath Sounds. The intensity of breath sounds is diminished if, for some reason, the bronchi are completely occluded so there is no airflow or if the patient's lungs are abnormally hyperinflated. Patients with pneumothorax, atelectasis, pleural effusion, localized pulmonary fibrosis, or emphysema typically demonstrate diminished breath sounds. Inadvertent intubation of the right mainstem bronchus during the placement of an endotracheal tube also causes a reduction in breath sounds over the left lung.

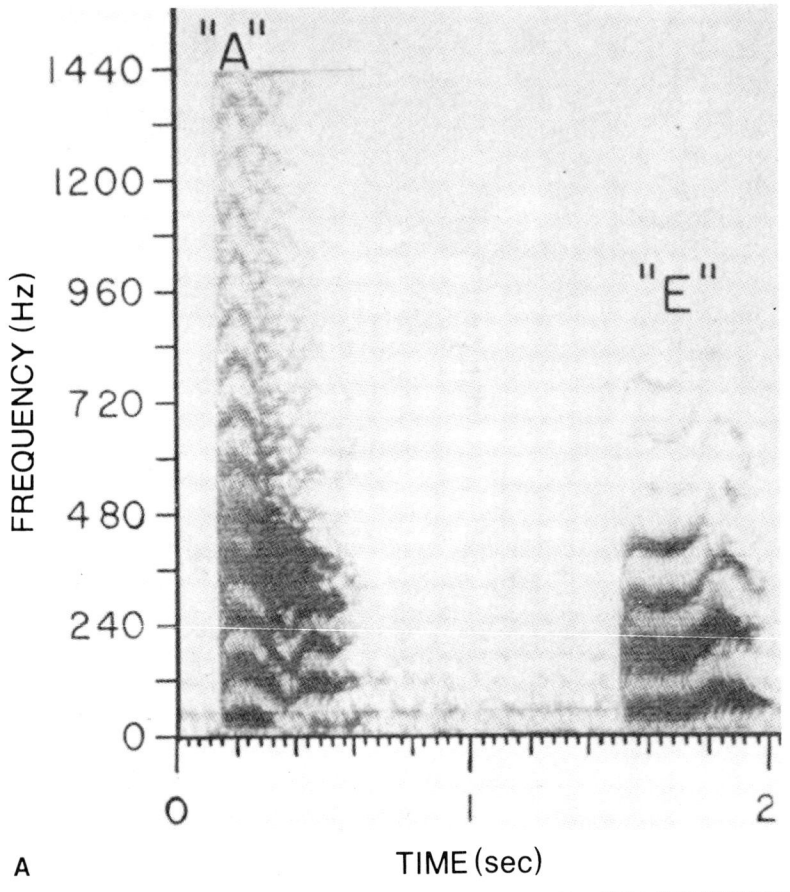
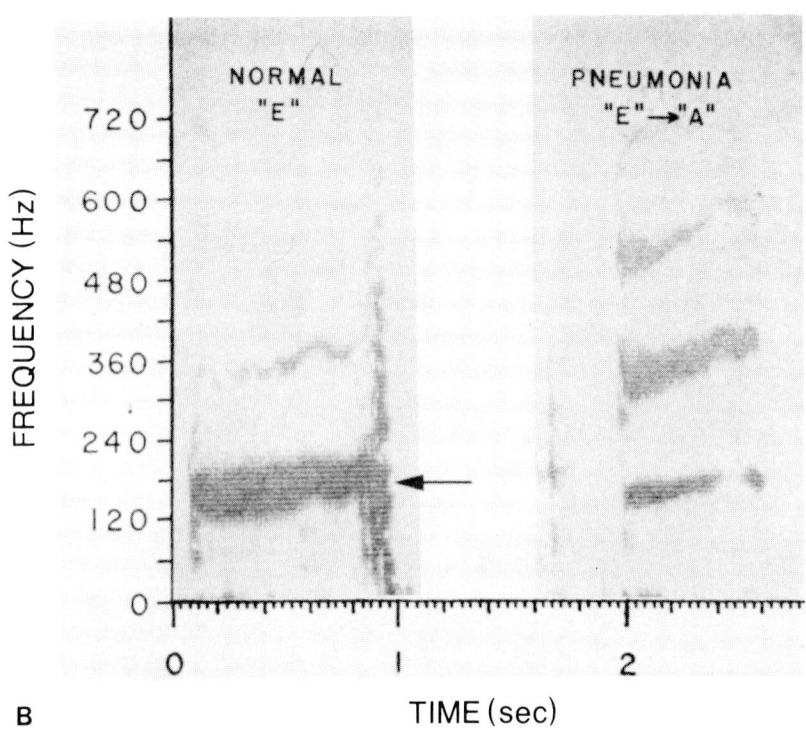

FIGURE 7–16. Sound spectrograph illustrating "E" to "A" egophony. (From Lehrer, S.: *Understanding Lung Sounds*. Philadelphia, W.B. Saunders, 1984, with permission.)

Bibliography

ACCP-ATS Joint Committee on Pulmonary Nomenclature: Pulmonary Terms and Symbols. *Chest* 67:583, 1975.

Andrews, J.L., and Badger, T.L.: Lung sounds through the ages. From Hippocrates to Laënnec to Osler. *JAMA* 241:2,625, 1979.

Bedford, D.E.: The ancient art of feeling the pulse. *Br. Heart J.* 13:423, 1951.

Bishop, P.J.: Evolution of the stethoscope. *J. Royal Soc. Med.* 73:448, 1980.

Bouhuys, A.: *The Physiology of Breathing*. New York, Grune and Stratton, 1977.

Chang, E.K.: *A Clinical Manual of Cardiovascular Medicine*. Norwalk, Conn., Appleton-Century-Croft, 1984.

Cherniack, R.M., and Cherniack, L.: *Respiration in Health and Disease*, 3rd ed. Philadelphia, W.B. Saunders, 1983.

Daniloff, R., Schuckers, G., and Feth, L.: *The Physiology of Speech and Hearing*. Englewood Cliffs, N.J., Prentice-Hall, 1980.

DeGowin, E.L., and DeGowin, R.L.: *Bedside Diagnostic Examination*, 3rd ed. New York, Macmillan, 1976.

Forgacs, P.: Crackles and wheezes. *Lancet* 2:203, 1967.

Forgacs, P.: Lung sounds. *Br. J. Dis. Chest.* 63:1, 1969.

Forgacs, P.: The functional basis of pulmonary sounds. *Chest* 73:399–405, 1978.

George, R.B., Light, R.W., and Matthay, R.A.: *Chest Medicine*. New York, Churchill Livingstone, 1983.

Hinshaw, H.C., and Murray, J.F.: *Diseases of the Chest*, 4th ed. Philadelphia, W.B. Saunders, 1980.

Judge, R.D., Zuidema, G.D., and Fitzgerald, F.T.: *Clinical Diagnosis: A Physiological Approach*, 4th ed. Boston, Little, Brown, 1982.

Leathan, A.: Auscultation of the heart since Laënnec. *Thorax* 36:95, 1981.

Lehrer, S.: *Understanding Lung Sounds*. Philadelphia, W.B. Saunders, 1984.

Luisada, A.A.: Sounds and pulses as aids to cardiac diagnosis. *Med. Clin. North Am.* 64:3, 1980.

Nath, A.R., and Capel, L.H.: Inspiratory crackle, early and late. *Thorax* 29:223, 1974.

Nath, A.R., and Capel, L.H.: Inspiratory crackles and mechanical events of breathing. *Thorax* 29:685, 1974.

Nunn, J.F.: *Applied Respiratory Physiology*, 2nd ed. Boston, Butterworth, 1977.

Perloff, J.K.: *Physical Examination of the Heart and Circulation*. Philadelphia, W.B. Saunders, 1982.

Prior, J.A., Silberstein, J.S., and Stang, J.M.: *Physical Diagnosis*, 6th ed. St. Louis, C.V. Mosby, 1981.

Ozawa, Y., Smith, D., and Craig, E.: Origin of the third heart sound. I. Studies in dogs. *Circulation* 67:393, 1983.

Ozawa, Y., Smith, D., and Craig, E.: Origin of the third heart sound. II. Studies in human subjects. *Circulation* 67:399, 1983.

Sakamoto, T., Kusukawa, R., MacCanon, D.M., and Luisada, A.A.: Hemodynamic determinants of the amplitude of the first heart sound. *Circ. Res.* 16:45, 1965.

Tilkian, A.G., and Conover, M.B.: *Understanding Heart Sounds and Murmurs*. Philadelphia, W.B. Saunders, 1984.

OBJECTIVES

AFTER READING THIS CHAPTER, THE STUDENT WILL BE ABLE TO:

1. Describe the components of a typical electrocardiograph.
2. Describe electrode placement for a standard 12-lead ECG.
3. Determine the heart rate and the mean electrical axis of the heart from an electrocardiogram.
4. Describe cardiac arrhythmias encountered in patients with cardiovascular disease.
5. Discuss artificial pacing of the heart.
6. Describe noninvasive and invasive methods for determining arterial blood pressure.
7. Describe the components of an electronic pressure monitoring system.
8. Discuss right heart catheterization using the Swan-Ganz catheter.
9. Discuss the use of left heart catheterization in the diagnosis of various cardiac diseases, such as intracardiac shunts and coronary artery disease.
10. Understand the use of hemodynamic data in diagnosing and treating critically ill patients.
11. Discuss how noninvasive techniques like echocardiography and phonocardiography are used in the assessment of cardiovascular diseases.

8
CARDIOVASCULAR ASSESSMENT

CHAPTER OUTLINE

ELECTROCARDIOGRAPHY
  The Electrocardiograph
    Electrodes
    Lead Configurations
    ECG Recorders
  The Normal Electrocardiogram
    Determination of Heart Rate
    Electrical Axis
  Interpretation of Electrocardiograms
    Heart Rate
    Abnormal Sinus Rhythms
    Heart Blocks
    Premature Contractions
    Tachyarrythmias
    Myocardial Ischemia and Infarction
    Pacemakers
HEMODYNAMIC MONITORING
  Determination of Arterial Blood Pressure
    Noninvasive Methods
    Invasive Methods
  Right Heart Catheterization
    Basic Features of the Swan-Ganz Catheter
    Placement of the Swan-Ganz Catheter
  Left Heart Catheterization
  Determination of Cardiac Output
    Direct Fick Method
    Indicator Dilution Methods
  Interpretation of Cardiac Profiles
    Stroke Volume
    Cardiac Work
    Vascular Resistance
NONINVASIVE CARDIOVASCULAR TECHNIQUES
  Echocardiography
  Phonocardiography

CARDIOVASCULAR ASSESSMENT

In addition to the history and physical examination, a complete assessment of the heart and circulation requires that the physician use specialized tests, such as electrocardiography and hemodynamic monitoring. It is important that the respiratory therapist have an understanding of the technical and physiologic principles involved in these tests in order to effectively treat patients with various types of cardiovascular disease. In this chapter, several noninvasive and invasive techniques that are routinely used in the diagnosis and treatment of patients with heart disease are reviewed.

ELECTROCARDIOGRAPHY

The electrocardiogram (ECG) is a graphic representation of the voltage changes that occur in the heart during a cardiac cycle. Because the heart can be considered as an electrical generator enclosed within a volume conductor (the body contains an aqueous electrolyte solution that can conduct electrical impulses throughout the body), electrical potentials measured between various points on the body surface can be related to electrical impulses traveling throughout the heart.

In healthy subjects, the appearance of the electrocardiogram remains relatively constant, even though the heart rate may change considerably. For patients with heart disease, pathologic alterations in the excitability, rhythmicity, and conductivity of the heart can result in significant changes in the magnitude and duration of the ECG waveform. In Chapter 2, the electrophysiologic basis of the ECG waveform was discussed; here we will review the equipment and techniques that are commonly used to record ECGs as well as how various pathologic conditions can affect a patient's electrocardiogram.

The Electrocardiograph

The major components of an electrocardiograph are illustrated in Figure 8–1. *Electrodes*, which are in contact with the skin of the patient, act as transducers to convert ionic potentials into electrical impulses. These electrical impulses are transferred by wires, called *leads*, to the inputs of an amplifier before being registered on an output display. In many of the newer systems, microprocessors are included for on-line analysis of ECG tracings. These computer systems produce preliminary interpretations of a patient's ECGs, which can be used to guide the physician in treating the patient.

Electrodes

Three types of electrodes are routinely used in clinical electrocardiography: (1) plate, (2) suction-cup, and (3) floating electrodes.

The plate and suction-cup types of electrodes are made of silver, nickel, or a similar alloy with high conductivity (Fig. 8–2). A thin coat of conduction jelly or electrolyte paste, which reduces the impedance of the skin-electrode interface, is applied evenly to the electrode before it is attached to the patient's body surface. (For plate electrodes, rubber straps are used to hold the electrode in place while the ECG is recorded.) Because these electrodes adhere loosely to the patient's skin, the major difficulty encountered when using these electrodes usually involves electrode movement artifacts.

Floating electrodes typically contain a silver-silver chloride electrode that is encased in a plastic housing and covered with electrolyte paste or conductive jelly (Fig. 8–3). The entire electrode assembly can be attached to the patient with a double-sided adhesive ring, which adheres to both the plastic surface of the electrode and the patient's skin. These electrodes are referred to as floating electrodes because the only conductive path between the electrode and the patient's skin is the electrolyte paste or jelly. Disposable electrodes, which are pre-gelled and ready for use, are also available, thus eliminating the need for cleaning and care of electrodes after each use. As Figure 8–4 shows, disposable electrodes have snap connectors, which are used to attach them to the ECG lead wires.

Lead Configurations

As discussed in Chapter 2, the standard electrocardiogram includes 12 leads: 6 extremity (limb) leads and 6 precordial (chest) leads. The limb leads, which define the frontal plane of the heart, are divided into three bipolar leads (i.e., leads I, II, and III) and three augmented unipolar leads (i.e., leads aVR, aVL, and aVF). The chest leads (i.e., leads V1 to V6) define the transverse plane of the heart and are all unipolar. Remember that a bipolar lead records the voltage difference between a positive and a negative electrode; a unipolar lead measures the electrical potential at the site of the positive or active (sensing) electrode relative to an indifferent electrode, which for practical purposes, is considered to be zero.

Figure 8–5 shows electrode placement and lead configurations that are routinely used to record a

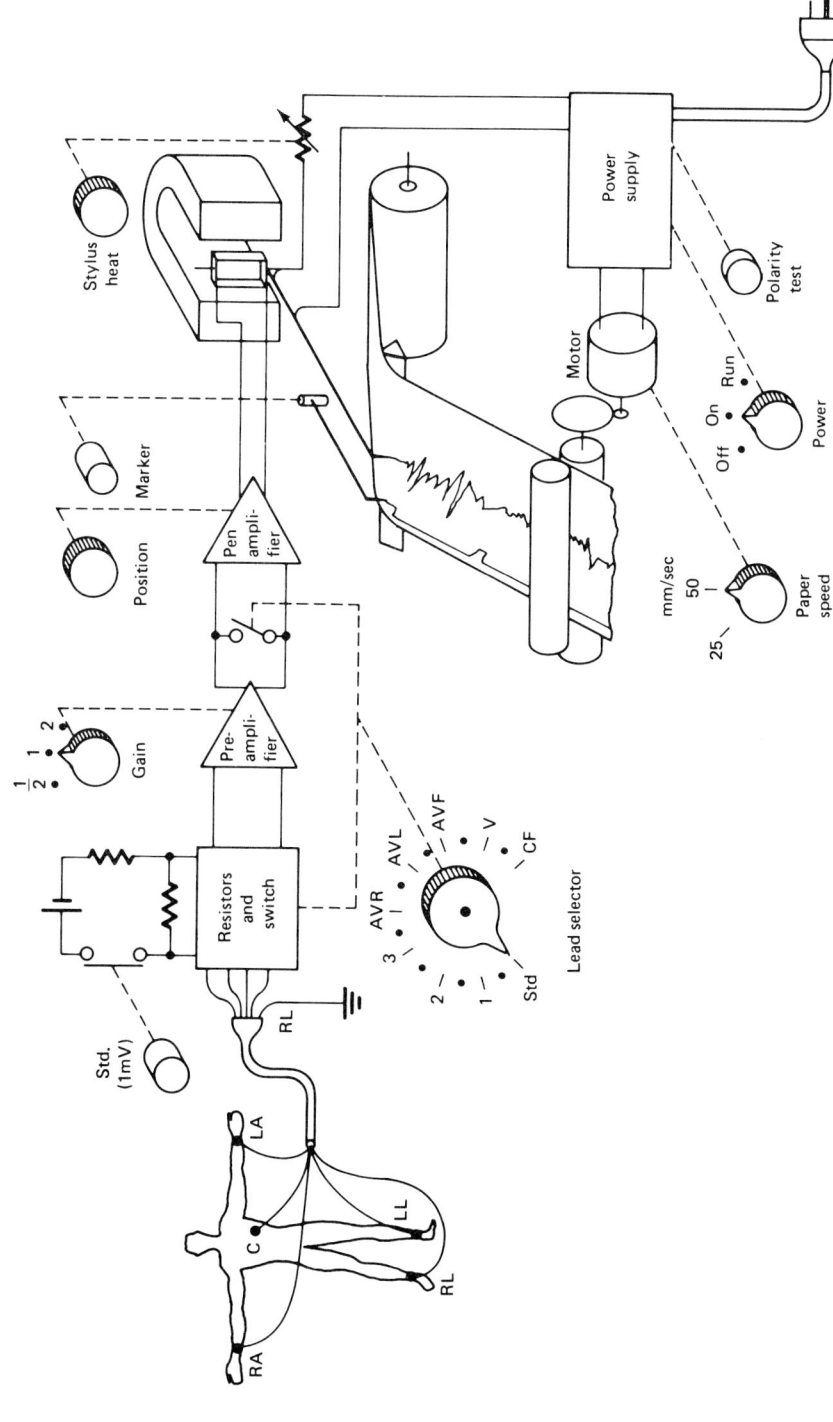

FIGURE 8-1. Major components of an electrocardiograph (ECG). (From Cromwell, L., Weibell, F.J., and Pfeiffer, E.A.: *Biomedical Instrumentation and Measurements*. Englewood Cliffs, N.J., Prentice-Hall, 1980, with permission.)

274 CARDIOVASCULAR ASSESSMENT

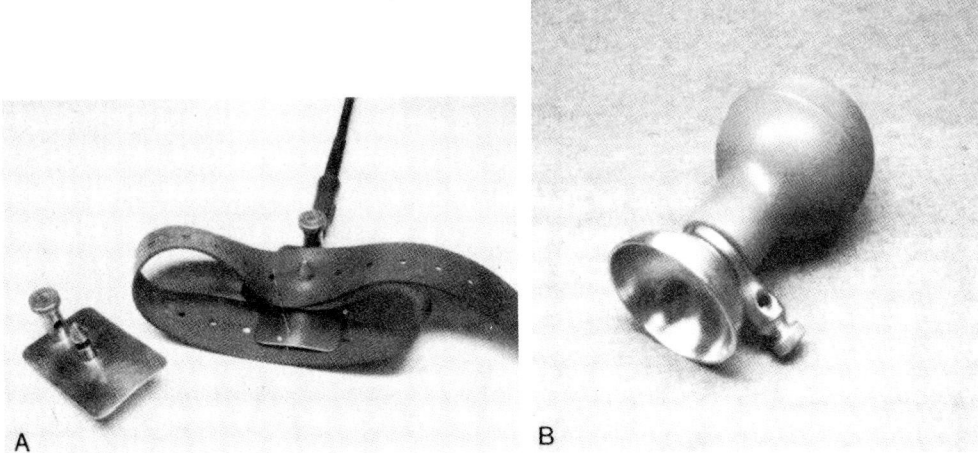

FIGURE 8–2. Plate (*A*) and suction cup (*B*) electrodes used in electrocardiography. (From Cromwell, L., Weibell, F.J., and Pfeiffer, E.A.: *Biomedical Instrumentation and Measurements,* 2nd ed. Englewood Cliffs, N.J., Prentice-Hall, 1980, with permission.

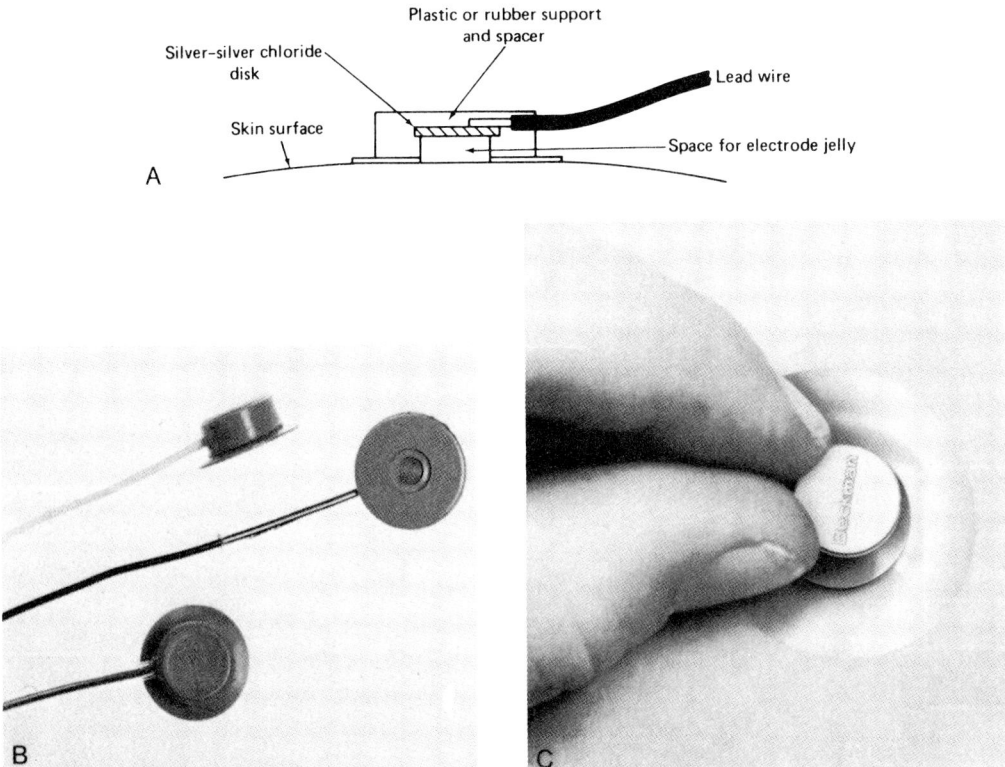

FIGURE 8–3. *A,* Diagram of floating skin surface electrode. *B,* Floating skin surface electrode. *C,* Application of floating skin surface electrode. (Courtesy of Beckman Instruments, Inc., Fullerton, CA.)

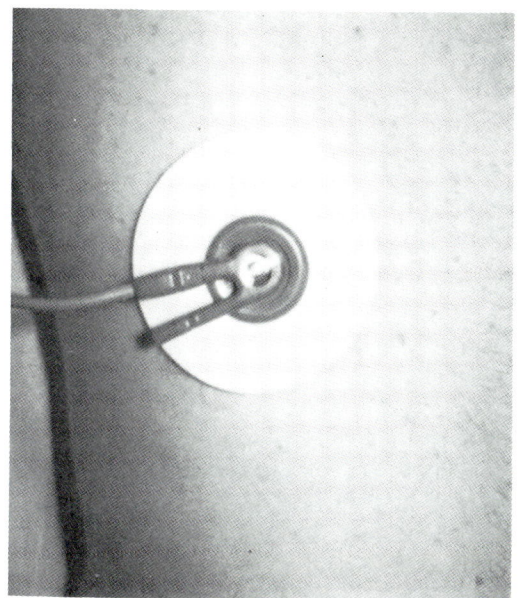

FIGURE 8–4. Disposable floating electrode. (Courtesy of Beckman Instruments, Inc., Fullerton, CA.)

standard 12-lead ECG. Note that for patients with *congenital cardiac anomalies* or *dextrocardia*, additional right precordial leads (i.e., leads V3R, V4R, V5R, V6R) may be used. Special lead configurations are also available for recording ECGs of patients in the critical care setting and during exercise. The modified chest lead, MCL_1 (also referred to as the *Marriott* lead—named for the physician who invented it), involves a placement of the positive electrode in the standard V1 position (fourth intercostal space to the right of the sternum), while the negative electrode is placed just below the outer part of the left clavicle. The ground electrode can be positioned anywhere on the body surface, but it is usually placed just under the outer part of the right clavicle. We will discuss ECG lead configurations used during exercise testing in more detail in Chapter 11.

ECG Recorders

The typical ECG recorder includes a differential amplifier with filtering circuits and an output display, such as a strip chart recorder or cathode ray tube (CRT). The differential amplifier and filtering circuits serve to increase the power output of the electrical signal detected by the surface electrodes and to remove extraneous electrical interference. Electrical interference, or "noise," can be caused by action potentials generated by skeletal muscle (electromyographic interference), fluorescent lights, and television and radio signals as well as by other electrical monitoring devices. A special circuit that allows for a 1 millivolt (mV) standardization signal to be introduced into the system is also included in the central processing unit so that the output display can be calibrated. In the older ECG systems, a lead selector switch is used to access information from each of the 12 standard leads. Newer systems contain microprocessors that automatically access each of the standard 12 leads in sequence.

Commercial instruments that use strip chart recorders as the output display are commonly referred to as *electrocardiographs;* whereas those systems that use cathode ray tubes (CRTs) are called *ECG monitors*. In most direct-writing strip chart recorders, the ECG is inscribed on a moving sheet of heat-sensitive paper with an electrically-heated stylus. The paper upon which the ECG is recorded is ruled in lines 1 mm apart, both vertically and horizontally. When properly standardized, a 1 mV input should cause a 10 mm deflection on the vertical axis. The horizontal axis is used to measure the passage of time. When the ECG is recorded at a paper speed of 25 mm per second (the standard ECG paper speed), a 1-mm space corresponds to 0.04 seconds.

CRTs are most commonly used to monitor the electrocardiograms of patients in intensive care units (Fig. 8–6). They are also used for continuous monitoring of patients during cardiac catheterization and exercise testing. It is a common practice to calibrate the CRTs to read 20 mm/mV on the vertical axis and a sweep speed of 50 mm per second. Most ECG monitors are equipped with alarm systems to alert the clinician of significant changes in heart rate. A single-channel pen recorder is usually incorporated into the monitor to register abnormal ECG waveforms. Coronary care units (CCU) may have CRTs that can simultaneously display ECGs from several patients. This allows the nursing staff to view a number of patient's ECGs at one central location.

The Normal Electrocardiogram

Waveforms and Intervals. Figure 8–7 shows a normal 12-lead ECG. The *P wave,* which represents atrial depolarization, is normally 0.1 to 0.3 mV in amplitude and 0.06 to 0.10 seconds in duration. It is upright in all leads except aVR. The *P-R segment,* which corresponds to the atrioventricular conduction time, falls on the isoelectric line and ranges from 0.12 to 0.20 seconds. Septal

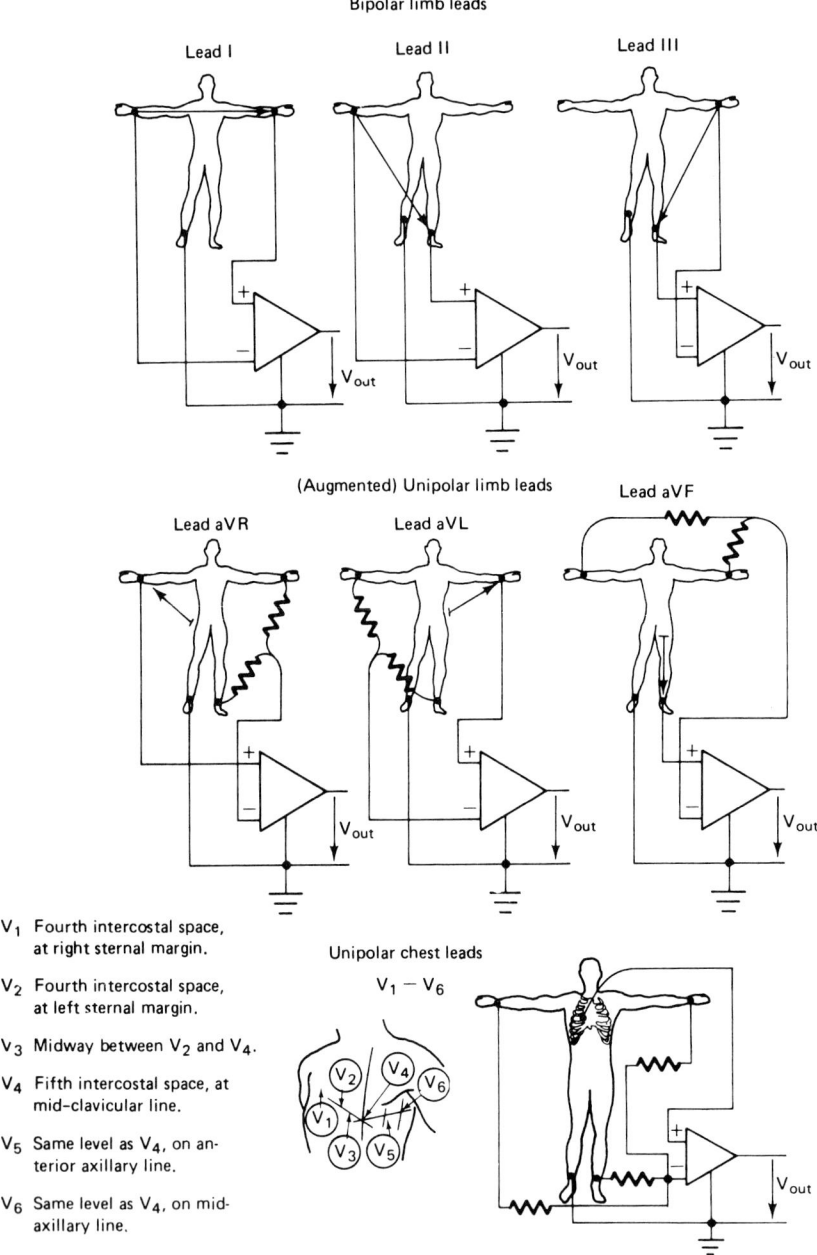

FIGURE 8–5. Electrode placement and lead configurations for a standard 12-lead ECG. (From Cromwell, L., Weibell, F.J., and Pfeiffer, E.A.: *Biomedical Instrumentation and Measurements*. Englewood Cliffs, N.J., Prentice-Hall, 1980, with permission.)

and ventricular depolarizations are associated with the *QRS complex* and typically last from 0.06 to 0.12 seconds. The amplitudes of the Q, R, and S waves vary with the anatomic position of the heart, the direction and rapidity of the ventricular depolarization, the lead being examined, and the amount of electrically excitable tissue present. In normal subjects, the largest QRS complexes appear in those leads that face the left side of the heart (i.e., leads I, II, aVL, V5, and V6).

The *S-T segment* occurs between the end of ventricular depolarization and the beginning of ventricular repolarization and therefore is normally isoelectric. It typically lasts from 0.10 to 0.16 seconds. The junction between the QRS complex and the S-T segment is called the *J-point*; it is sometimes used to identify shifts in the S-T segment, such as those that occur during cardiac ischemia and infarction. The *T wave* represents ventricular repolarization, and it normally has an

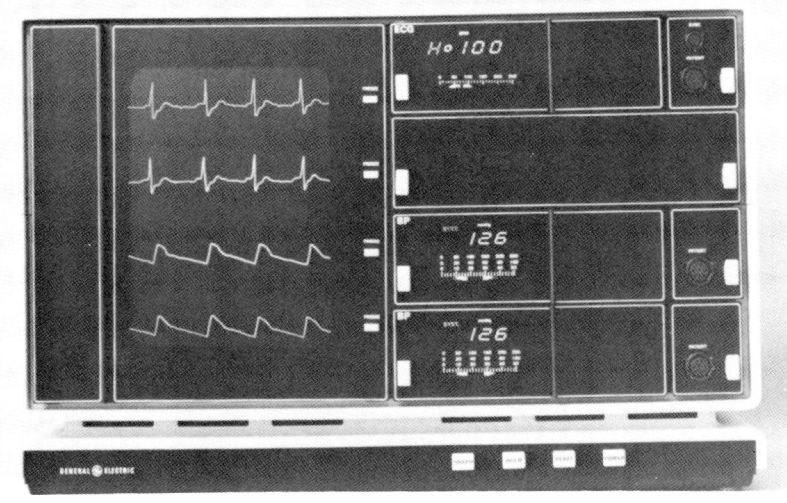
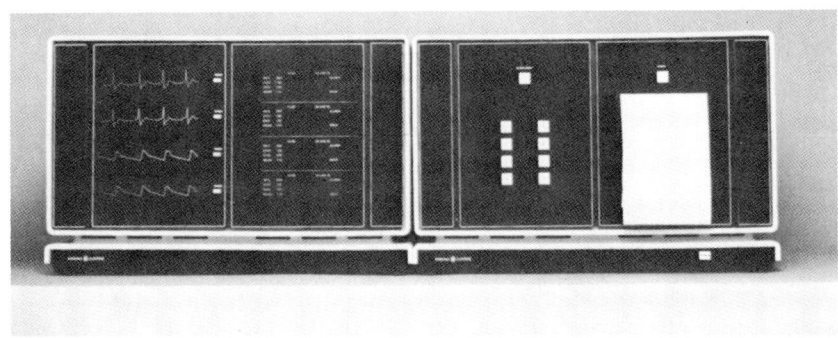

FIGURE 8–6. Typical ECG monitor used in a critical care unit. (Courtesy of General Electric Company, Medical Systems Division, Milwaukee, WI.)

amplitude of 1 to 3 mV and is 0.10 to 0.20 seconds in duration (the T wave is usually in the same direction as the QRS complex). The *Q-T segment*, which corresponds to the time required for contraction of the ventricles, is measured from the beginning of the Q wave to the end of the T wave. The duration of the Q-T segment depends on the heart rate; it is generally about 0.40 seconds for heart rates between 60 and 100 beats per minute. In children and young adults, a *U wave,* which is thought to represent remnants of ventricular repolarization and/or afterpotentials from the papillary muscles may also be present. The amplitude and duration of the U wave are considerably less than those of the T wave.

Determination of the Heart Rate

The most practical method to determine the heart rate from an electrocardiogram is to count the number of cardiac cycles during a 6-second interval and multiply this number by 10. This can be easily accomplished because most ECG paper has vertical markings on the top of the paper corresponding to 3-second intervals when the paper speed is 25 mm per second (Fig. 8–8). If the vertical markings are absent, the rate can be calculated by counting the number of millimeters between two successive P waves (or R waves) and dividing 1,500 by this number (25 mm per second equals 1,500 mm per minute). Although these methods are quite accurate for subjects with normal rhythms, they are less reliable in patients with arrhythmias.

Electrical Axis

As discussed in Chapter 2, the heart's mean electrical axis is a term commonly used to describe the direction and magnitude of the electrical activity of the heart. Ordinarily, the frontal plane electrical axis is determined from the standard limb leads.

278 CARDIOVASCULAR ASSESSMENT

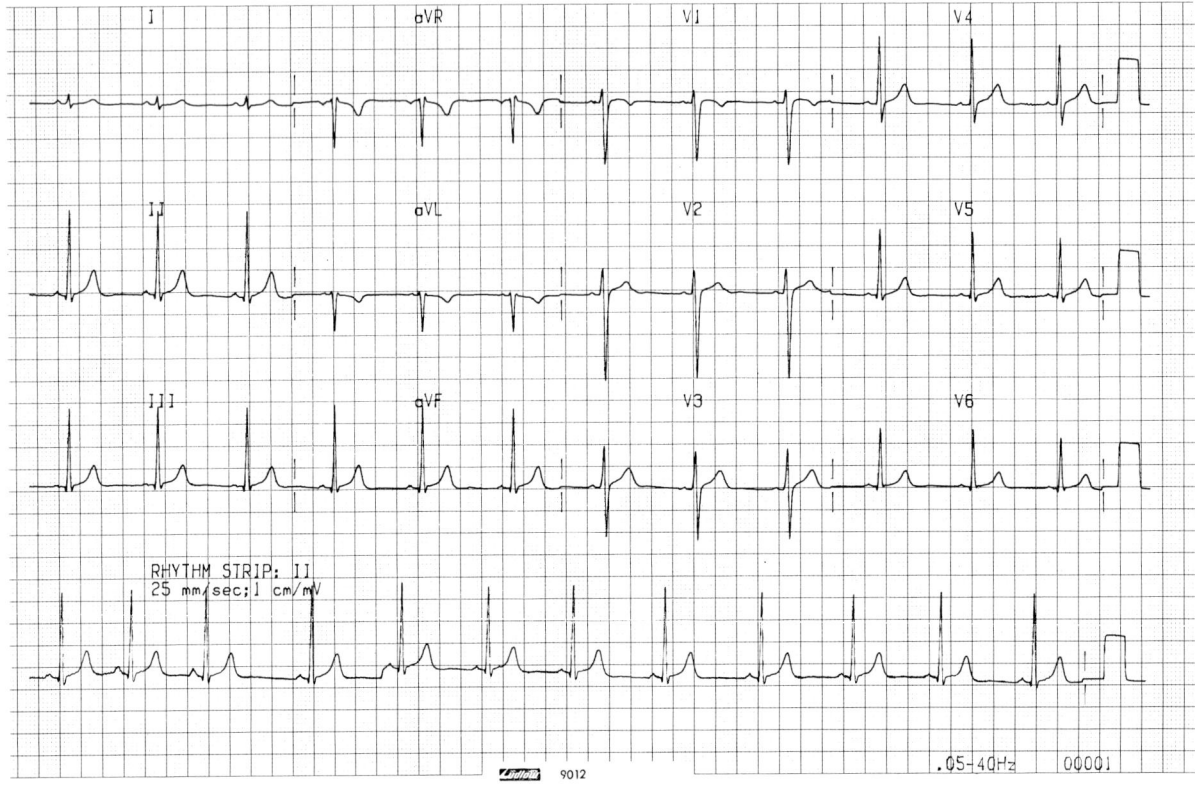

FIGURE 8–7. Standard 12-lead ECG. Note that the waveform in lead aVL is negative in this subject.

Figure 8–9 illustrates an easy method to do this. In healthy subjects, the mean electrical axis is between 0 and 90 degrees because of the anatomic position of the heart in the chest and because the muscle mass of the left ventricle is approximately three times greater than that of the right ventricle. The axis rotates to the left in normal hearts during the expiration and when a subject lies down because the diaphragm rises. Rotation to the right occurs during inspiration and when a person assumes a standing position. As the following sections explain, chronic changes in the mean electrical axis of the heart occur in pathologic conditions, such as left or right ventricular hyper-

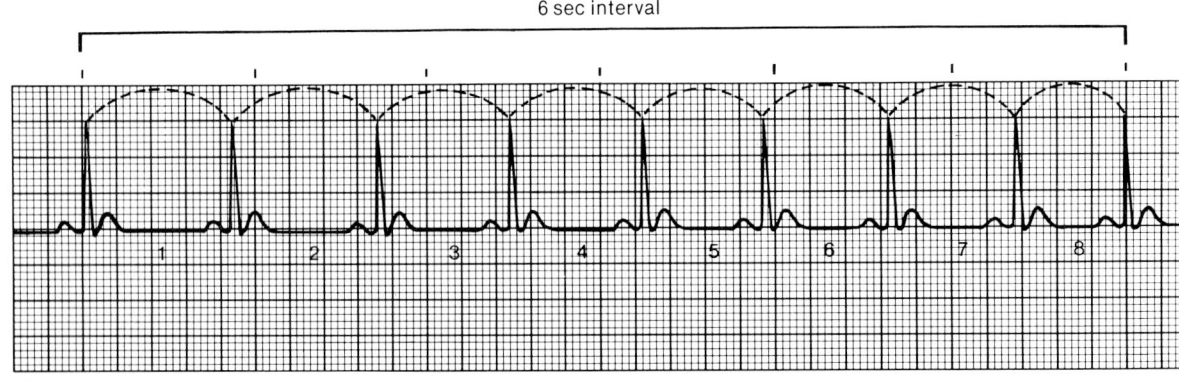

FIGURE 8–8. Calculating the heart rate from a standard ECG tracing: First, count the number of QRS in a 6-second period (note the 3-second time marks at the top of the ECG paper). Then, multiply this number by 10 to get the rate per minute. (From Brown, K.R., and Jacobson, S.J.: *Mastering Dysrhythmias: A Problem Solving Guide*. Philadelphia, F.A. Davis, 1988, with permission.)

CARDIOVASCULAR ASSESSMENT

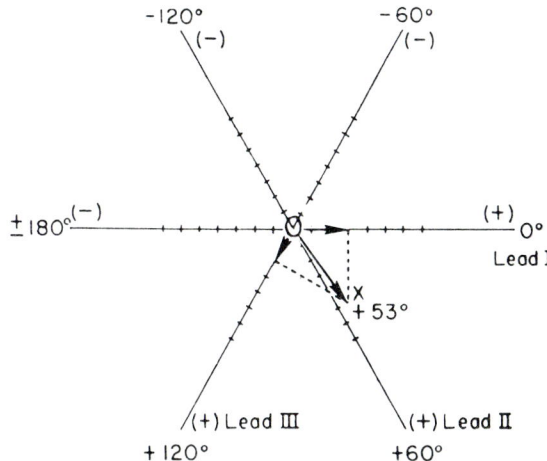

FIGURE 8–9. Determining the mean electrical axis of the heart. (From Little, R.C., and Little, W.C.: *Physiology of the Heart and Circulation*, 4th ed. Chicago, Year Book, 1989, with permission.)

trophy, myocardial infarction, and right and left bundle branch blocks.

Interpretation of Electrocardiograms

Abnormal cardiac rhythms or *arrhythmias* (also called *dysrhythmias*) can be caused by abnormalities in the rhythmicity of the heart's pacemaker, by altered conductivity of electrical impulses through the heart, and by the spontaneous generation of abnormal impulses in the atria, ventricles, and the Purkinje fibers (i.e., *ectopic* or *premature beats*). The following is a brief description of some of the major cardiac arrhythmias.

Heart Rate

Normally, the heart rate is determined by the number of times that the SA node depolarizes per minute. In a healthy sedentary adult, the average resting heart rate is between 60 and 100 beats per minute. Athletes typically show slower resting heart rates than sedentary subjects due to greater stroke volumes.

Tachycardia, which literally means a rapid heart rate, is usually defined as a resting heart rate greater than 100 beats per minute. Stimulation of the autonomic nervous system, as occurs with the administration of sympathomimetic drugs (e.g., isoproterenol or epinephrine) or drugs that block parasympathetic impulses to the heart (e.g., atropine) cause considerable increases in heart rate. Tachycardia can also result from exertion, ingestions of large quantities of caffeine or nicotine, fever, hypotension, anemia, pulmonary emboli, myocardial ischemia, congestive heart failure, and thyrotoxicosis.

Bradycardia refers to heart rates less than 60 beats per minute. It can be caused by increased vagal tone, as occurs with carotid sinus stimulation or following the administration of β-adrenergic blocking agents (e.g., propranolol). Bradycardia is also associated with hypothermia, eye surgery, increased intracranial pressure, cervical and mediastinal tumors, myxedema, vomiting, and vasovagal syncope.

Abnormal Sinus Rhythms

Respiratory Sinus Arrhythmia refers to a regular acceleration of the heart rate during inspiration followed by a slowing of the heart rate during expiration. Although this variation in heart rate can be quite significant, the QRS complexes are all preceded by P waves and the P-R interval has a normal duration. Respiratory sinus arrhythmias are a common finding in children and young adults.

Electrocardiograms showing sinus tachycardia, sinus bradycardia, and respiratory sinus arrhythmia are illustrated in Figure 8–10.

Heart Blocks

Conduction disturbances or *heart blocks* may occur anywhere in the heart when the refractory period at a certain point in the conduction path is abnormally prolonged. In general, they are divided into three categories: (1) sinoatrial (SA), (2) atrioventricular (AV), and (3) intraventricular blocks.

Sinoatrial (SA) Blocks occur when the impulse generated at the SA node is blocked before it can enter the atrial muscle. As Figure 8–11 shows, the electrocardiogram is characterized by a sudden cessation of P waves due to the absence of atrial depolarizations. The contour of QRS complex is normal but the R-R intervals are prolonged. Transient sinoatrial blocks usually do not produce symptoms. Prolonged sinoatrial blocks can cause dizziness and syncope, particularly if the ventricular "escape" rhythm is slow (i.e., when the SA node impulse is not conducted to the ventricles, slower pacemakers in the AV node or ventricles will initiate a heart cycle).

Atrioventricular Blocks occur when impulses generated by the SA node are slowed or blocked in or near the AV node. Clinically, AV blocks are

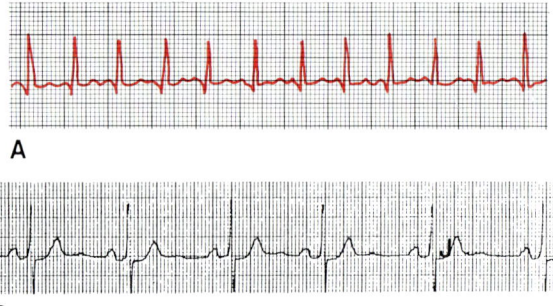

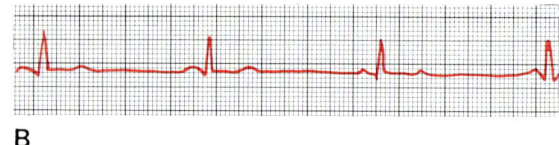

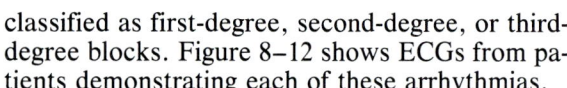

FIGURE 8–10. *A*, Sinus tachycardia. *B*, Sinus bradycardia. *C*, Respiratory sinus arrhythmia with U waves.

classified as first-degree, second-degree, or third-degree blocks. Figure 8–12 shows ECGs from patients demonstrating each of these arrhythmias.

First-degree AV blocks are characterized by a prolongation of the P-R interval (longer than 0.20 seconds), although every atrial impulse does elicit ventricular excitation. Patients with first-degree AV blocks are generally asymptomatic if they do not have any other cardiovascular problems.

Second-degree AV blocks occur when some of the impulses originating at the SA node fail to pass through the AV node into the ventricles. The electrocardiogram shows "dropped" beats (that is, P waves not followed by QRS complexes) as a result of a failure to conduct every impulse from the atria to the ventricles. In many cases, electrocardiographers differentiate two types of second-degree AV blocks: the *Mobitz Type I* (or Wenckebach) AV block and the *Mobitz Type II* AV block. In the Mobitz Type I block, there is a progressive prolongation of the P-R interval until a P wave is not followed by a QRS complex. In the Mobitz Type II block, not every impulse generated in the atria is conducted into the ventricles, and thus the atrial rate is a multiple of the ventricular rate. (Atrioventricular ratios are often used to describe the number of impulses conducted from the atria to the ventricles, e.g., a 2:1 second-degree block means that for every two impulses generated in the atria, only one is conducted into the ventricles.) Mobitz Type I blocks usually do not require treatment; permanent artificial pacemakers are usually required for the treatment of sustained Mobitz Type II blocks.

Third-degree blocks result from a complete blocking of impulses from the SA node through the AV node. The SA node and the atria continue to depolarize at a normal or elevated rate, but the ventricles "escape" to a slower rate. The electrocardiogram therefore shows an atrial rate (P-P intervals) that is completely dissociated from the ventricular rate (R-R intervals). Treatment of third-degree blocks may necessitate the insertion of a permanent artificial pacemaker if the ventricular rate is too low to permit normal activity.

Intraventricular Blocks. The most common forms of intraventricular conduction disturbances are the *bundle branch blocks,* which occur when cardiac impulses are delayed or blocked in either the right or left branches of the Purkinje fiber system. The hallmark of this type of arrhythmia is the prolongation of the QRS complex because, distal to the block, ventricular excitation must spread by cell-to-cell conduction.

Figure 8–13A shows an electrocardiogram from a patient with a *right bundle branch (RBB) block.* Note the presence of P waves and that the QRS complex is prolonged (greater than 0.12 seconds). There is usually a characteristic rSR' pattern in the right precordial leads (i.e., leads V1, V2, and V3) and a prolonged deep S wave in the left precordial leads (i.e., leads V4, V5, and V6) caused by presence of cell-to-cell conduction through the right ventricle (not shown in the figure). Vectorial analysis demonstrates that the mean electrical axis in RBB blocks is shifted to the right (more than 90 degrees). Right bundle branch blocks are associated with hypertensive cardiac disease, cardiac tumors, rheumatic heart disease, myocarditis, pulmonary emboli, and congenital cardiac defects.

Left bundle branch (LBB) blocks (Fig. 8–13B) are characterized by the absence of Q waves in the left limb leads (i.e., leads I and aVL) and in the left precordial leads (i.e., leads V4, V5, and V6). The QRS complexes in the left precordial leads show an rsR' pattern. The mean electrical axis in

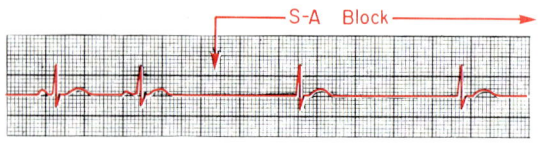

FIGURE 8–11. Sinoatrial (SA) block.

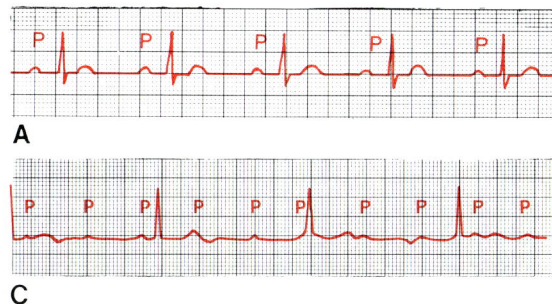

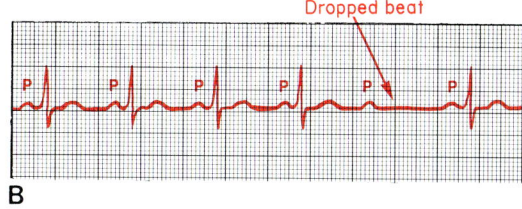

FIGURE 8–12. Atrioventricular (AV) block: *A,* Prolonged P-R interval (first degree). *B,* Partial AV block (second degree, Mobitz Type II). *C,* Complete AV block (third degree).

LBB blocks is shifted to the left (less than 0 degrees). Although LBB blocks are less common than RBB blocks, they are almost always indicative of coronary artery disease or systemic hypertension. Other possible etiologies of LBB blocks include aortic stenosis, myocarditis, and congenital cardiac diseases.

Premature Contractions

Premature contractions are caused by action potentials that originate and propagate from ectopic foci in the atria, the AV node, the Purkinje fibers, and ventricles. Figure 8–14 shows ECGs from patients with various types of premature beats.

Premature atrial contractions (PACs) results when an atrial ectopic focus produces an abnormal P wave earlier than expected. Because the impulse does not originate in the SA node, the P wave does not appear like the other P waves in the same lead. In *nodal premature beats,* the AV node fires before the SA node initiates a normal cardiac cycle. Because the impulse is transmitted into the ventricles and causes ventricular depolarization, the ECG shows a normally occurring QRS complex that appears early and is not preceded by a P wave.

In *premature ventricular contractions* (PVCs), the duration of QRS complex is prolonged, and its amplitude is increased. The T wave following the PVC (if it can be distinguished) has an electrical

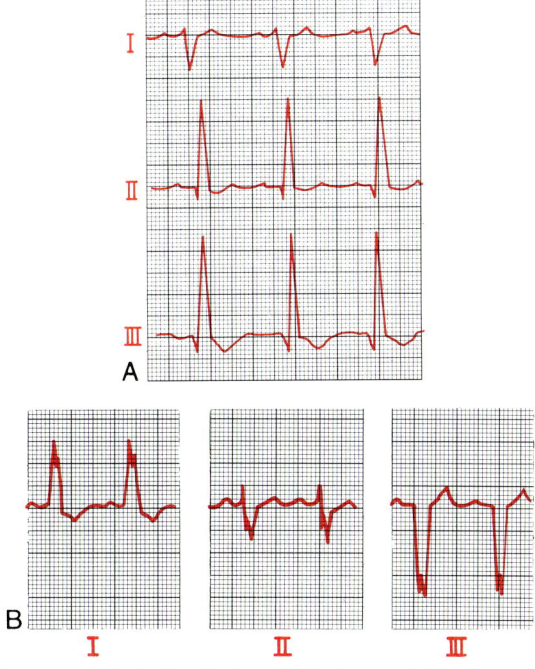

FIGURE 8–13. *A,* Right bundle branch block. *B,* Left bundle branch block.

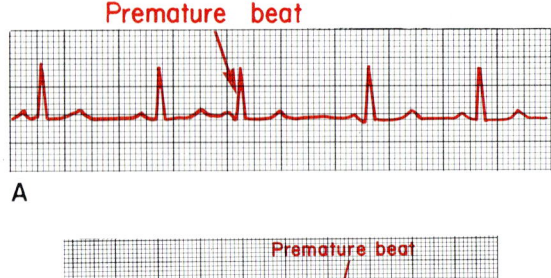

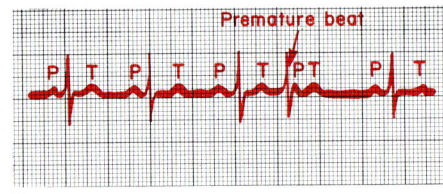

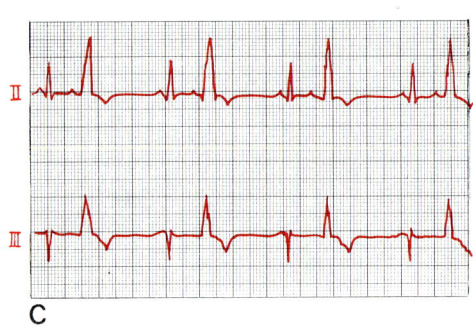

FIGURE 8–14. *A*, Premature atrial contraction. *B*, Nodal premature contraction. *C*, Premature ventricular contraction.

potential that is opposite to the QRS complex. Note that following a PVC, the ventricles are refractory to the next impulse conducted from the atria, which should occur at its normal interval. Consequently, an interval referred to as a *compensatory pause* continues until the ventricle is stimulated by the following atrial impulse. PVCs may occur alone or coupled with a normal beat—when this occurs, the patient is said to be in *bigeminy*. Repetitive premature ventricular contractions can be extremely dangerous and should be treated aggressively if tachycardia is present. The treatment of PVCs usually involves the administration of oxygen and antiarrhythmic drugs, such as lidocaine (see Chapter 15).

Spontaneous ectopic beats can be caused by hypoxia, localized ischemia, heart failure, digitalis toxicity, and following the administration of sympathomimetric amines, such as isoproterenol. Premature contractions can occur in normal individuals who consume excessive amounts of caffeine, alcohol, and nicotine. PVCs can be induced during cardiac catheterization if the catheter irritates the ventricular endocardium.

Tachyarrhythmias

Figure 8–15 illustrates four types of tachyarrhythmias: *atrial flutter, atrial fibrillation, ventricular tachycardia,* and *ventricular fibrillation*. The exact mechanisms responsible for these arrhythmias are not fully understood, but it is believed that they are caused by reverberating impulses that are generated at ectopic foci in the atria and ventricles.

In *atrial flutter*, aberrant atrial foci depolarize at rates of 250 to 300 beats per minute while the ventricular rate is about 150 beats per minute caused by a slowed conduction of impulses in the AV node. As Figure 8–15A shows, P waves are replaced by sawtooth flutter waves (sometimes referred to as F waves). Atrial flutter is most often associated with underlying valvular and coronary artery disease.

As with atrial flutter, *atrial fibrillation* is characterized by gross irregularities in both atrial and ventricular depolarization. On the ECG, P waves are replaced by atrial fibrillatory waves, which are small irregular waves of variable amplitude and morphology (Fig. 8–15B). Because the ventricles usually appear to respond randomly to the rapid

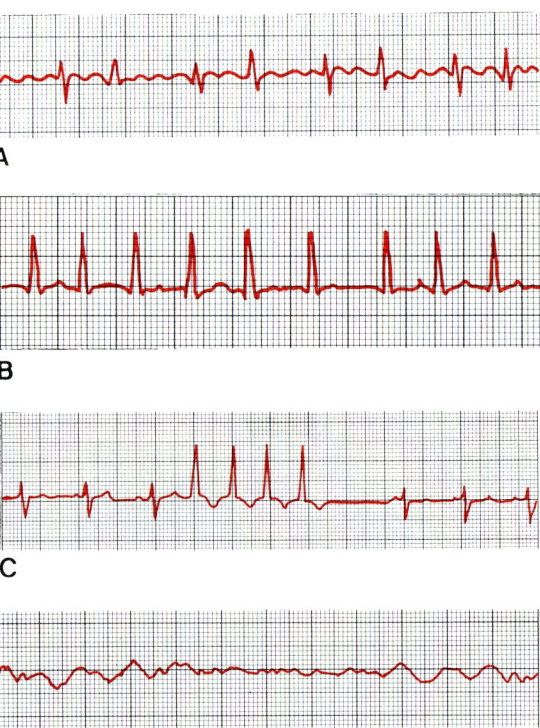

FIGURE 8–15. *A*, Atrial flutter. *B*, Atrial fibrillation. *C*, Ventricular tachycardia. *D*, Ventricular fibrillation.

atrial depolarization, the ventricular rate may be between 150 and 175 beats per minute. The QRS complexes can appear at regular intervals but they are usually irregularly spaced. Atrial fibrillation can occur as a sequel to atrial flutter, or it may occur alone in such diseases as mitral stenosis, ischemic heart disease, thyrotoxicosis, or chronic pericarditis. It is also a common finding during exercise in patients who have previously experienced a myocardial infarction.

Both atrial flutter and atrial fibrillation can be treated with drugs like procainamide and quinidine, which decrease the excitability of atrial tissue. Additionally, ventricular rates may be slowed by administering digitalis or propranolol, both of which delay the conduction of impulses from the atria through the AV node.

Ventricular tachycardia is commonly defined as six or more consecutive premature ventricular contractions. The ventricular rate may vary from 120 to 300 beats per minute. At the higher rate (i.e., about 300 beats per minute), the rhythm is called ventricular flutter. The QRS complexes are prolonged (greater than 0.12 seconds) because of the cell-to-cell conduction that occurs as impulses emanating from the ectopic foci in the ventricles spread through the ventricular muscle. Ventricular tachycardia and flutter may be complications of myocardial ischemia and infarction, excessive adrenergic stimulation, or toxicity to digitalis.

Ventricular tachycardia can be treated by cardioversion (i.e., restoration of normal rhythm by using electrial shock). If ventricular tachycardia or ventricular flutter is sustained in a patient, *ventricular fibrillation* (totally disorganized ventricular depolarization) can occur. The ECG of a patient with ventricular fibrillation shows a loss of the typical PQRST waves (Fig. 8–15D). The physiologic consequences of this type of arrhythmia include the absence of any effective ventricular contractions and, thus, the loss of arterial blood pressure. Unlike atrial fibrillation, ventricular fibrillation is a life-threatening arrhythmia that must be treated immediately with cardiopulmonary resuscitation (CPR). CPR involves the establishment of a patent airway so that the patient can be ventilated either by mouth-to-mouth breathing or with a manually operated resuscitator. External chest wall compressions, pharmacologic agents to maintain the circulation, and the employment of electrical defibrillation may also be needed.

Myocardial Ischemia and Infarction

When coronary blood flow is severely limited, as occurs with atherosclerosis, the heart's oxygen demand exceeds its oxygen delivery and myocardial ischemia results. In Chapter 4, the pathophysiologic changes that occur in myocardial ischemia and infarction were discussed. Table 8–1 sum-

TABLE 8–1. Localization of Myocardial Infarcts

Anterior Infarcts	
Anterolateral (Occlusion of the anterior interventricular branch of the left coronary artery)	Deep Q waves in precordial Leads V3 to V5. Loss of R waves in the left precordial leads (V4 and V5). ST segment elevation in lead I; ST segment depression in lead III.
Anteroseptal (Occlusion of the right division of the interventricular branch of the coronary artery)	Deep Q wave in precordial leads V2 and V3. Normal QRS complexes in limb leads I, II, and III. S-T segment depression in limb lead II.
Apical (Occlusion of the terminal portions of the anterior interventricular branch of the left coronary artery)	Loss of R waves with deep Q waves in limb lead I and in precordial leads V3 and V4. ST segment elevation in lead I; S-T segment depression in lead III.
Anterobasal (Occlusion of a branch of the circumflex artery)	Small Q wave in limb lead I; large Q waves in precordial lead V6. S-T segment elevation in leads I and V6. T wave inversion in leads I and V6.
Posterior Infarcts	
Posteroseptal (Occlusion of the right coronary artery)	S-T segment depression in precordial leads V3 and V4.
Posteroinferior (Occlusion of the posterior interventricular branch of the right coronary artery)	Large Q waves in limb leads II and III and aVF. S-T segment depression in leads I, V3, and V4; S-T segment elevation in lead aVF.
Posterolateral (Occlusion of the circumflex artery)	Q waves in leads aVL and V6. S-T segment elevation and T wave inversion in limb leads II, III, and aVL.

marizes the ECG changes associated with myocardial infarction at various locations within the heart. Note that the most characteristic findings involve S-T segment changes, T wave inversion, and Q waves. S-T depression occurs generally when "currents of injury" originate in the subendocardium (remember that a current of injury relates to current flow between pathologically depolarized tissue and normally polarized tissue). S-T elevation is associated with decreased blood flow in the subepicardial tissue. If tissue necrosis does not extend throughout the wall of the heart, T wave inversion is all that is typically present. Q waves usually result when the myocardial infarction involves the entire heart wall.

Pacemakers

As mentioned earlier, artificial electrical pacing of the heart is sometimes used to treat patients with second-degree (Mobitz Type II) and third-degree (complete) heart blocks.

The essential elements of an artificial pacemaker are shown in Figure 8–16. These include: (1) a power supply, which is usually a small mercury or lithium-iodide battery; (2) an electronic circuit to regulate the timing and intensity of the impulses; and (3) a lead, which contains electrodes to deliver the impulses to the heart.

In general, pacemakers are classified as either external or internal systems. External systems consist of an externally-worn generator connected to electrodes that are positioned either within or on the myocardium. Temporary transvenous catheters containing electrodes attached to the tip of the catheter can be inserted through a peripheral vein and positioned in the heart with the aid of fluoroscopic and electrocardiographic monitoring. Internal systems are entirely surgically implanted inside the patient's body. Usually, the pulse generator is secured in a subcutaneous pocket below the clavicle or in the subcostal area, and the electrodes are positioned within the heart.

Two types of pacing modes are available for both the external and internal systems. The simplest type is the fixed-rate mode, which delivers electrical impulses independent of any natural cardiac activity. The more sophisticated *demand* systems can be programmed so that the output of the pulse generator is either inhibited or triggered by naturally occurring impulses. In the inhibited type, no output impulses are produced as long as naturally occurring ventricular depolarizations (R waves) are present. In the triggered type devices, the impulse generator delivers an output impulse after a naturally occurring atrial impulse is sensed by the pacemaker.

The major problems encountered by patients with artificial pacemakers involve battery failure and electrical interference. Implanted devices typically must be replaced every 5 to 10 years. Various sources of electromagnetic energy can emit impulses that can interfere with signal reception in demand-type pacemakers. Patients with artificial pacemakers should therefore avoid devices such as microwave ovens, diathermy units, and automobile ignition systems.

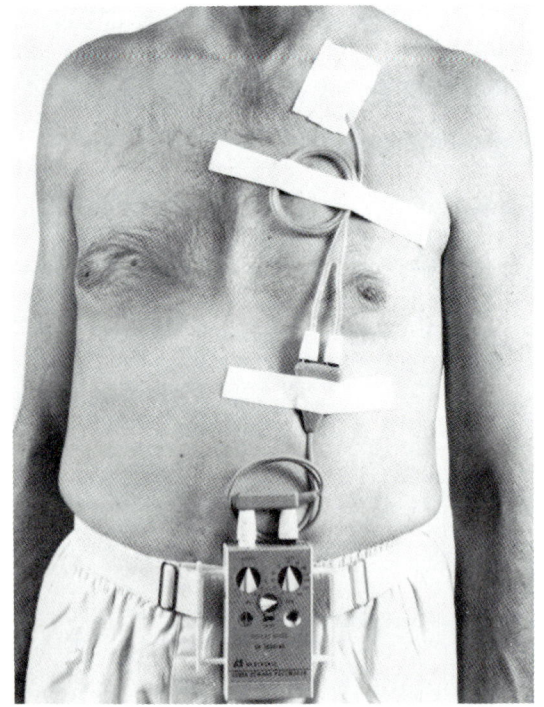

FIGURE 8–16. Artificial pacemaker. (Courtesy of Medtronics, Minneapolis, MN.)

HEMODYNAMIC MONITORING

Hemodynamic monitoring provides valuable information on the pressure, flow, and resistance characteristics of the cardiovascular system. Generally, hemodynamic monitoring techniques are classified as being either noninvasive or invasive.

CARDIOVASCULAR ASSESSMENT

Determination of the Arterial Blood Pressure

Noninvasive Methods.

The most widely used technique for determining systemic arterial blood pressure involves a *sphygmomanometer,* which is a device that consists of a mercury or aneroid manometer, an inflatable compression cuff, and a pressure source, which is usually a hand bulb and a pressure control valve (Fig. 8–17). The blood pressure is usually determined from the brachial artery with the patient in a sitting or recumbent position. It is important that the patient be relaxed when you are determining blood pressure.

The following list summarizes the method used for determining blood pressure with a sphygmomanometer:

1. The deflated compression cuff is applied evenly and snugly to the patient's arm. When using the brachial artery, the cuff should be placed so that the bottom edge of the cuff is 2 to 3 centimeters above the antecubital fossa. Note that the width of the cuff should be approximately 40% of the circumference of the patient's arm. (The standard adult cuff is 5 inches wide; pediatric sizes range from 1½ inches for infants to 3 inches for children under 5 years old.)

2. The radial artery (in the arm being used for the measurement) is palpated, and the heart rate and rhythm are noted.

3. The cuff is inflated to about 30 mm above the pressure at which the radial pulse disappears.

4. The cuff is then deflated at a rate of about 3 to 5 mmHg per heartbeat. The pressure at which the radial pulse returns should be used as the systolic pressure.

5. The cuff is then completely deflated.

6. The cuff is reinflated to about 30 millimeters above the systolic pressure determined by palpation.

7. A stethoscope is placed over the brachial artery and the cuff is gradually deflated at a rate of 3 to 5 mmHg per heartbeat. The pressure at which a tapping sound first appears is recorded as the systolic pressure and the pressure at which these sounds disappear during the cuff deflation is the diastolic pressure. The tapping sounds (referred to as the *Korotkoff* sounds) are caused by turbulent blood flow that occurs when blood is forced through the partially occluded artery. As the diameter of the vessel becomes larger with deflation of the compression cuff, blood flow becomes more laminar and the tapping sound ceases.

8. The cuff is then completely deflated.

Automated systems that use a self-contained cuff inflation device can be programmed to inflate and deflate at various time intervals. Contact microphones, which are located in the cuff are positioned over the artery and used to detect the Korotkoff sounds as the cuff is deflated. As with the manual technique, the pressure recorded when the first sound occurs is the systolic pressure and the pressure measured at the last Korotkoff sound is the diastolic pressure.

The most common errors encountered when determining the arterial blood pressure with a sphyg-

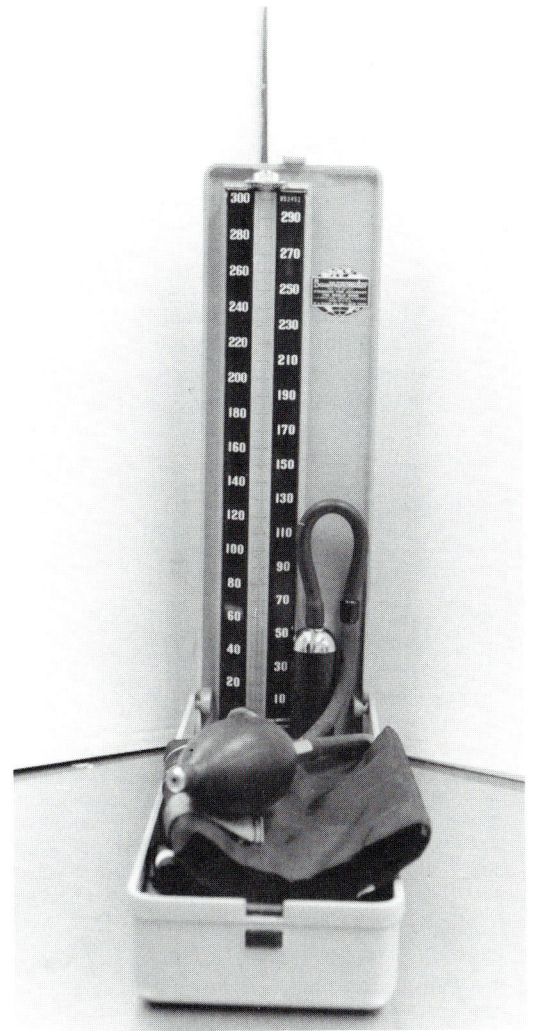

FIGURE 8–17. Sphygmomanometer. (Courtesy of W.A. Baum, New York.)

momanometer include failure to use the proper cuff size, improper positioning of the cuff on the arm, improper deflation of the compression cuff, and mechanical problems, which can result from a defective pressure control valve or from old porous connecting tubing.

Invasive Methods

Direct measurements of systemic arterial pressure require the insertion of a catheter into a peripheral artery either by a percutaneous technique or by a surgical cutdown technique. Pressure changes are sensed by a physiologic pressure transducer and converted into an electrical signal that can be displayed on a meter, a strip chart recorder, or an oscilloscope.

Peripheral Artery Catheterization. The most common sites for insertion of a peripheral artery catheter are the radial, brachial, and femoral arteries. Although accessibility of the artery as well as institutional preference usually dictate the site of catheter insertion, percutaneous insertion of the catheter into the radial artery is the most widely used technique. Table 8–2 summarizes the recommended technique for inserting and maintaining an arterial line. Our discussion is limited to arterial lines here because this topic is discussed in more detail in the analysis of arterial blood gases (see Chapter 10).

Physiologic Pressure Transducers are electronic devices that convert mechanical motion into electronic signals. In general, they are classified according to the physical principle used to sense pressure changes. Figure 8–18 shows several different types of physiologic pressure transducers.

TABLE 8–2. Recommended Technique for Inserting and Maintaining Systemic Artery Lines

1. Do Allen test prior to radial artery cannulation. Ischemic complications will be lowest if ulnar artery refill time is <5 seconds.
2. Use sterile technique for insertion (antiseptic preparation, gloves, drapes).
3. Choose percutaneous insertion over surgical cutdown when possible.
4. Use 20-gauge catheter if patient's wrist circumference is small.
5. Use continuous flush system with a nondextrose solution (normal saline) containing heparin.
6. Use transducer with disposable dome.
7. Assess daily:
   a. Catheter site for evidence of inflammation
   b. Distal extremity for evidence of ischemia.
8. Limit cannulation to 4 to 5 days at one site.
9. Remove catheter for:
   a. Distal ischemia
   b. Local infection
   c. Persistently damped pressure tracing
   d. Difficulty with blood withdrawal.

From Matthay, R.A., Wiedemann, H.P., and Matthay, M.A.: Cardiovascular function in the intensive care unit: Invasive and noninvasive monitoring. *Respiratory Care* 30:432–449, 1985, with permission.

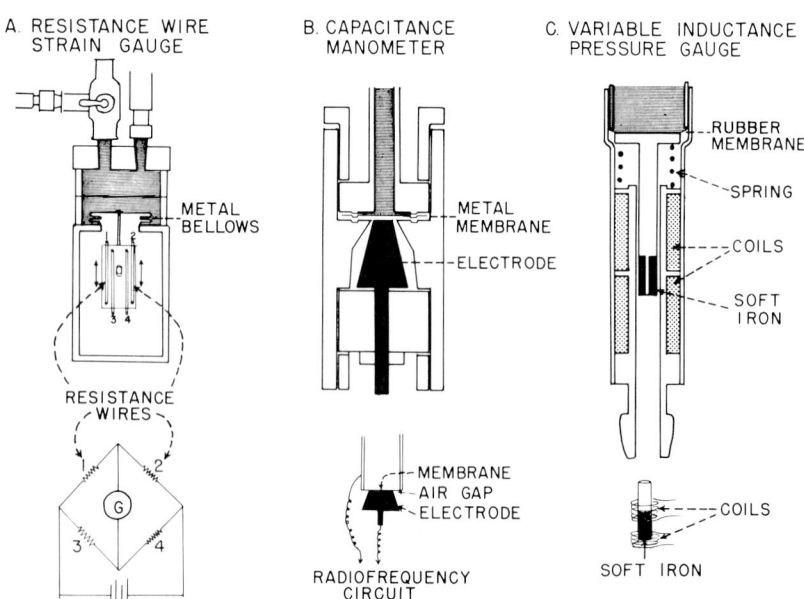

FIGURE 8–18. Physiologic pressure transducers: *A*, Resistance wire strain gauge. *B*, Capacitance manometer. *C*, Variable inductance pressure gauge. (From Rushmer, R.F.: *Organ Physiology: Structure and Function of the Cardiovascular System*, 2nd ed. Philadelphia, W.B. Saunders, 1976, with permission.) (*A* and *B* from Lilly, J.C.: Electrical capacitance diaphram manometer. *Review of Scientific Instruments* 13:34–37, 1942. *C* from Gauer, O.H., and Gienapp, E.: Miniature pressure recording device. *Science* 112:404, 1950.)

Because the *strain gauge* transducer is the most widely used, our discussion is limited to this type of transducer.

In the strain gauge transducer, a thin metal diaphragm is attached to four resistance wires. The wires function as a *Wheatstone bridge,* which is an electronic device that contains two sets of resistors in parallel. One branch of the circuit has a fixed resistance (R1 + R2) while the second is a variable resistor (R3 + R4)—that is, the resistance varies as the physical dimensions of the resistive wire change. As pressure is applied to the diaphragm, the wires change in length and diameter, thus changing the resistance of the Wheatstone bridge. This change in electrical resistance causes a current change that can be amplified and displayed on an oscilloscope or a direct writing pen recorder.

Amplifiers-Output Displays. Electrical signals acquired from the transducer are typically small and must be amplified into a form that is visible to the user. In pressure monitoring, these electrical signals are usually converted into standard units of millimeters of mercury (mmHg), before they are displayed on a meter located on the front panel of the monitor. In most intensive care units, oscilloscopes are routinely used to continuously monitor pressure changes generated within the systemic circulation (e.g., a peripheral artery, such as the radial artery) and the pulmonary circulation (e.g., the pulmonary artery). These oscilloscopes, or CRTs, can simultaneously display the patient's pressure waveform and his or her ECG.

System Calibration. When monitoring critically ill patients, all components of the system should be calibrated at regular intervals in order to establish a relationship between the magnitude of the patient's arterial pressure and the corresponding deflection on the output display. To accomplish this, a known stepwise increase in pressure is applied to the transducer's diaphragm using a sphygmomanometer placed at the level of the patient's heart. For measurements of arterial blood pressure, increments of 25 to 50 mmHg of mercury pressure up to a maximum deflection of 200 mmHg are routinely used. (Remember that atmospheric pressure is considered to be 0 mmHg.)

Right Heart Catheterization

Since the introduction of the balloon-tipped, flow-directed catheter by Swan and his colleagues in 1970, catheterization of the right heart chambers and the pulmonary artery has become a routine procedure in most intensive care units. Proper placement of the *Swan-Ganz catheter* enables the clinician to continuously monitor a patient's pulmonary artery pressure as well as indirectly assess fluid balance by using the pulmonary artery wedge pressure (PAWP), also referred to as the pulmonary capillary wedge pressure or PCWP, as an indication of the left ventricular pressures and volumes. Additionally, these catheters can be used to obtain mixed venous blood samples, which reflect oxygen utilization by the peripheral tissues. As discussed in Chapter 9, mixed venous sampling is used to calculate pulmonary venous admixture or shunts.

The electronic pressure monitoring systems that are used for measuring systemic artery pressures can also be used to monitor right heart and pulmonary artery pressures (Fig. 8-19). Note, however, that when calibrating the system for right

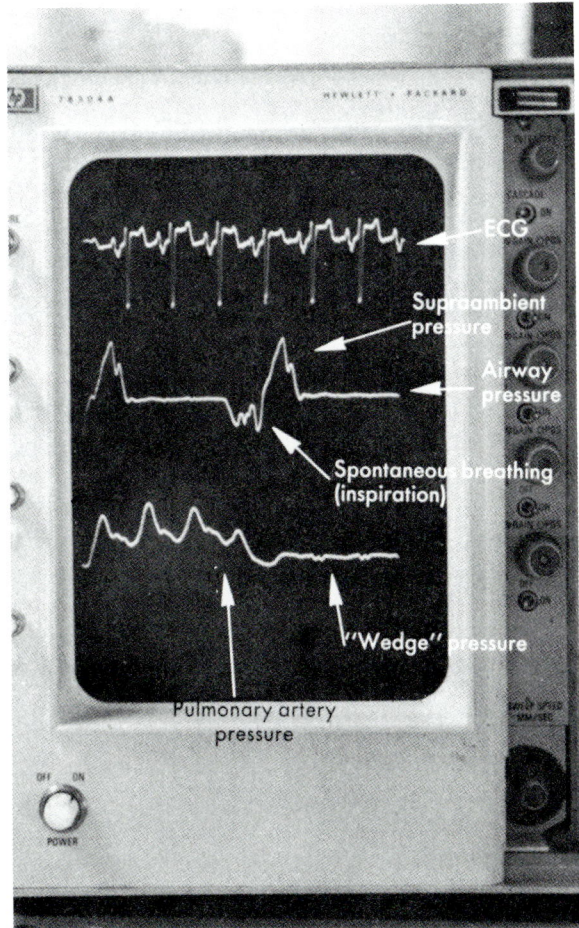

FIGURE 8–19. Electronic monitoring system. (Courtesy of Hewlett-Packard, Palo Alto, CA.)

288 CARDIOVASCULAR ASSESSMENT

heart catheterization, the output display should be set to read in increments of 5 to 10 mmHg up to a maximum deflection of 50 mmHg.

Basic Features of the Swan-Ganz Catheter

The Swan-Ganz catheter is a multiple lumen catheter constructed of polyvinylchloride that is available in both adult and pediatric sizes (Fig. 8–20). The standard adult catheter is 110 cm in length and is either 5 or 7 French in external diameter (the French number divided by π equals the diameter in mm). The pediatric catheter is 60 cm in length and is either 4 or 5 French in external diameter. All catheters are marked at 10 cm increments.

Dual lumen catheters have one lumen that connects to a balloon located at the tip of the catheter and a second lumen that runs the length of the catheter, terminating at a port at the distal end of the catheter. In most cases, air can be used to inflate the balloon. However, in situations where the catheter may be introduced into the left side of the circulation (e.g., right to left shunt), the balloon is inflated with carbon dioxide so that, in case the balloon ruptures, the carbon dioxide is absorbed rather than released into the circulation as an air bubble (the 4 and 5 French sizes have a balloon capacity of 0.8 ml and the 7 and 8 French sizes have balloon capacities of 1.5 ml). The second lumen can be used to monitor blood pressure and to obtain mixed venous blood samples. Usually, a heparinized flush solution is continuously run through the catheter at a rate of 1 to 5 ml per hour (except when making pressure measurements) to prevent clot formation, because the lumen is so small.

Triple lumen catheters have an additional lumen, which is connected to a proximal port located 30 cm from the tip of the catheter. When the catheter is placed properly, the proximal port is located in the area of the right atrium, so the third lumen can be used to monitor the central venous pressure (CVP).

Thermodilution catheters have a fourth lumen, which contains electrical wires that connect a thermistor (located approximately 2 cm from the tip of the catheter) to a cardiac output computer like the one shown in Figure 8–21. In the thermodilution cardiac output determination, cold physiologic saline (0.9% NaCl) or 5% dextrose in water (D_5W) is injected into a proximal port while the thermistor at the distal end of the catheter measures changes in blood temperature that occur as the cold saline or dextrose is diluted by the blood. This technique is discussed in greater detail later in this chapter.

Placement of the Swan-Ganz Catheter

Swan-Ganz catheters may be inserted percutaneously or by venous cutdown with only the aid of continuous pressure monitoring and the ECG,

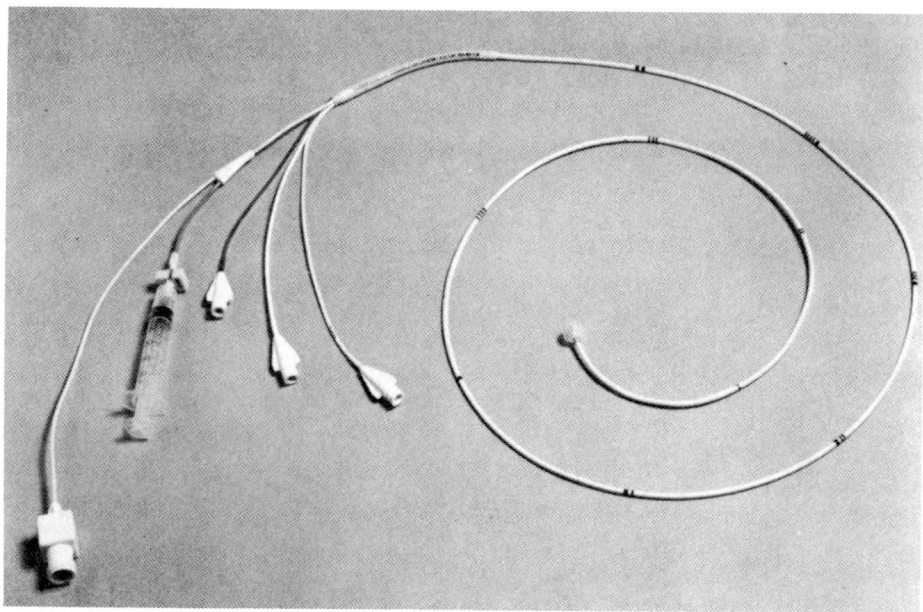

FIGURE 8–20. Swan-Ganz catheter. (Courtesy of Edwards-American Hospital Supply, Santa Ana, CA.)

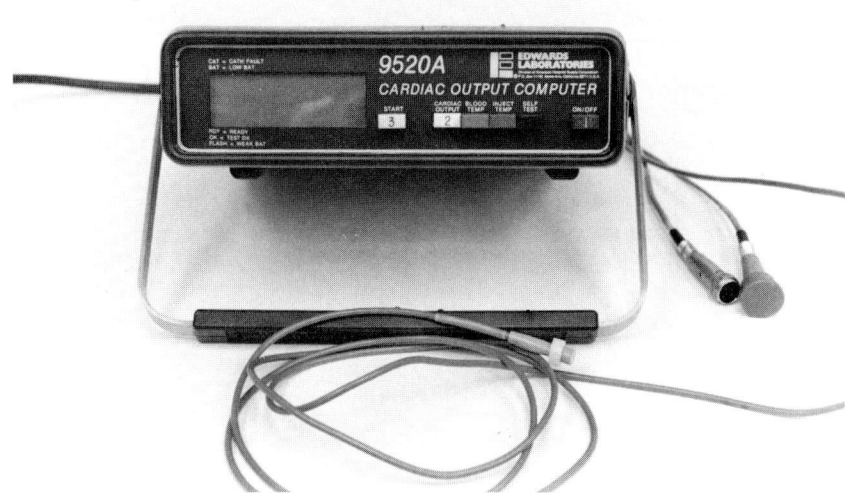

FIGURE 8–21. Thermodilution cardiac output computer. (Courtesy of Edwards-American Hospital Supply, Santa Ana, CA.)

thus eliminating the need for fluoroscopy. Percutaneous insertion may be performed via the subclavian, internal jugular, external jugular, femoral, or antecubital veins; surgical cutdown is sometimes necessary if the antecubital vein route is used. Although the physician's prior experience usually determines the access route chosen, the advantages and disadvantages of using each site should be reviewed prior to insertion. Table 8–3 lists some of the complications encountered during right heart catheterization with the Swan-Ganz catheter. Several articles that discuss the potential complications of Swan-Ganz catheterization are listed in the bibliography.

Once the venous access route has been achieved, the catheter is advanced slowly until it enters the intrathoracic vessels. One method of determining the distance required to enter the intrathoracic veins is to note the 10 cm markers on the catheter as it is inserted. When this method is used, this distance is approximately 40 to 50 cm if the antecubital vein is used; 30 to 40 cm if the femoral vein is used; and 10 to 15 cm if the internal or external jugular route is used. Another method to determine if the catheter is in the intrathoracic vessels is to observe the venous pulse tracings during catheter insertion. These tracings show a sudden increase in respiratory fluctuations as the tip enters the intrathoracic veins.

The balloon is then inflated so that the catheter can be flow-directed by the blood as it passes through the right atrium and right ventricle into the pulmonary artery. Once in the pulmonary artery, the catheter is advanced until it wedges in a distal pulmonary artery. The pulmonary artery wedge position can be identified easily because the pulmonary artery wedge pressure is characteristically lower than the pulmonary artery pressure (see Fig. 8–19). Also, when the catheter occludes a distal pulmonary artery, a continuous column of blood equilibrates between the left atrium and the distal port located at the tip of the catheter. The wedge pressure tracings will therefore show a left atrial waveform (i.e., a, c, and v waves). Once the PAWP has been measured, the balloon is deflated. (Note that the balloon should be inflated only for a few seconds when measuring the wedge pressure.) Figure 8–22 shows the pressure tracings obtained as a Swan-Ganz catheter was passed from

TABLE 8–3. Complications of Balloon-Flotation Right Heart Catheterization

1. Arrhythmias
   a. Transient premature ventricular contractions (PVCs)
   b. Sustained ventricular tachycardia
   c. Ventricular fibrillation
   d. Atrial fibrillation
   e. Atrial flutter
2. Right bundle-branch block
3. Pulmonary infarction
4. Pulmonary artery rupture
5. Catheter-related infections
6. Balloon rupture
7. Catheter knotting
8. Endocardial damage to:
   a. Valve cusps
   b. Chordae tendineae
   c. Papillary muscles
9. Complications at insertion site
   a. Pneumothorax
   b. Arterial puncture
   c. Venous thrombosis or phlebitis
   d. Air embolism

From Wiedemann, H.P., Matthay M.A., and Matthay, R.A.: Cardiovascular-pulmonary monitoring in the intensive care unit. Chest 85:537–549, 656–658, 1984, with permission.)

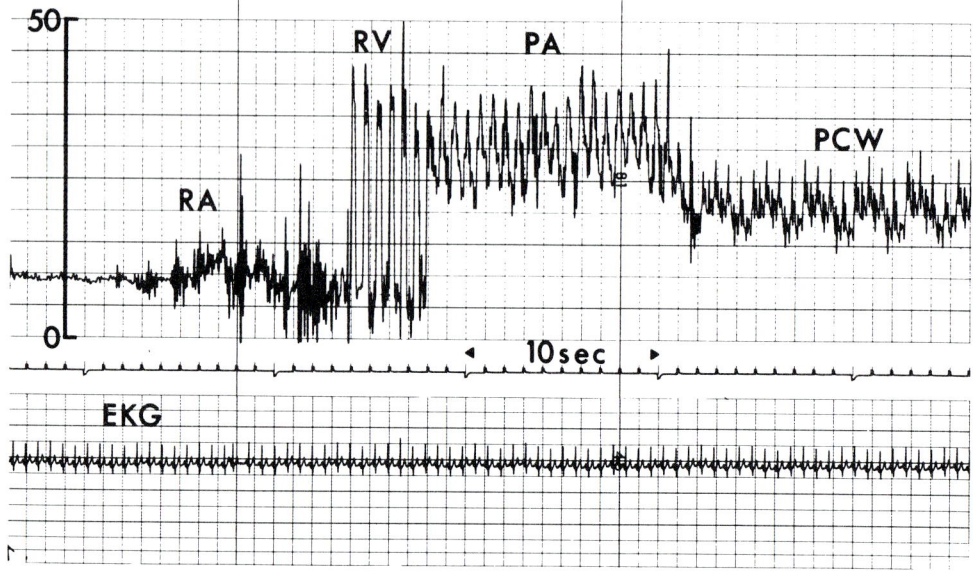

FIGURE 8–22. Pressure tracings during passage of a Swan-Ganz catheter. (RA = right atrial pressure; RV = right ventricular pressure; PA = pulmonary arterial pressure; PCW = pulmonary capillary wedge pressure.) (From Grossman, W.: *Cardiac Catheterization and Angiography*, 3rd ed. Philadelphia, Lea & Febiger, 1986, with permission.)

a peripheral vein through the vena cava, right atrium, right ventricle, and pulmonary artery and into the pulmonary artery wedge position.

Left Heart Catheterization

Catheterization of the left heart is routinely used to measure left atrial, left ventricular, and aortic blood pressures; to assess the mechanical function of the mitral and aortic valves; to establish the presence of an intra-atrial or intraventricular shunt; and to assess the integrity of the blood vessels supplying the heart. The procedure is usually performed in a specially designed laboratory that is equipped with a fluoroscopic unit, which contains a source of x-rays, an image intensifier, and an image recording system. The recording system is usually a video camera and monitor. These recording techniques are referred to as *cine* methods because the camera can record up to 100 pictures per minute and thus provide a "motion picture" of the heart. These cine recordings are used almost exclusively in cardiac angiography (thus, *cine angiography*).

The catheter can be inserted, either percutaneously or by surgical cutdown, through a peripheral artery and then advanced into the aorta, across the aortic valve into the left ventricle, and finally into the left atrium. By connecting the catheter to a pressure monitoring system, blood pressures in the aorta and left heart chambers can be recorded as the catheter is inserted. This is particularly important in the diagnosis of conditions involving valvular stenosis or incompetency, as discussed in Chapter 5. Intracardiac shunt can be identified by determining the left atrial and left ventricular oxygen saturations. Normally, the left atrium and left ventricle contains blood that is almost completely saturated with oxygen (the oxygen saturation is greater than 95%). In patients with right to left intracardiac shunts, blood samples obtained from the left heart have oxygen saturations that are significantly reduced. Left to right intracardiac shunts can be identified by simultaneously catheterizing the right and left heart. Mixed venous blood samples obtained with right heart catheterization from the right ventricle or the pulmonary artery have oxygen saturations that may approximate the left heart or arterial blood oxygen saturations.

Imaging of the coronary vessels can be accomplished by selectively injecting a radiopaque dye into either the right or left coronary arteries. This is usually done with one of the specially designed catheters shown in Figure 8–23. By recording the flow of dye through the coronary vessels, the physician can identify areas of reduced blood flow and actually quantitate the level of obstruction. The information obtained from coronary angiography can be used by the cardiologist and the cardiovascular surgeon to guide therapeutic intervention, such as coronary angioplasty or coronary artery bypass surgery.

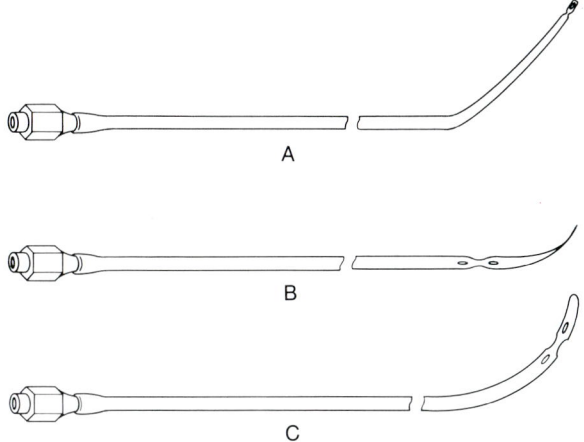

FIGURE 8–23. Left heart catheters: *A*, Sones catheter. *B*, Lehman-ventriculography catheter. *C*, Eppendorf catheter.

Determination of Cardiac Output

Direct Fick Method

According to the Fick principle, the total uptake of a substance by an organ ($\dot{V}_x$) is determined by the blood flow through the organ per time ($\dot{Q}$) and the arteriovenous difference of the substance across the organ ($Ca_x - C\bar{v}_x$):

$$\dot{V}_x = \dot{Q} \times (Ca_x - C\bar{v}_x)$$

If we assume that the output of the right ventricle is equal to the output of the left ventricle, then cardiac output can be determined by simultaneously measuring the total uptake of oxygen by the lungs ($\dot{V}O_2$, also known as oxygen consumption) and the arteriovenous oxygen difference across the lung ($CaO_2 - C\bar{v}O_2$). (This method therefore determines *pulmonary blood flow,* or *PBF.*) The oxygen consumption is derived from measurements of the volumes and oxygen concentrations in a subject's inspired and expired gases while the arteriovenous oxygen difference is determined by measuring the oxygen contents of blood samples drawn from a systemic artery and the pulmonary artery. Table 8–4 is a summary of the calculations involved in a direct Fick cardiac output determination.

Indicator Dilution Methods

In the *Stewart-Hamilton dye dilution technique,* a known amount of dye, like Evan's blue or indocyanine green (cardiogreen) is injected intravenously as a bolus. The passage of the dye through

TABLE 8–4. A Direct Fick Cardiac Output Determination

If	$\dot{V}O_2 = \dot{Q} \times (CaO_2 - C\bar{v}O_2)$
Then	$\dot{Q} = \dot{V}O_2 \div (CaO_2 - C\bar{v}O_2)$
	$\dot{V}O_2 = \dot{V}_I F_I O_2 - \dot{V}_E F_E O_2$
	$CaO_2 = (Hb \times 1.34)SaO_2 + PaO_2 \times 0.003$
	$C\bar{v}O_2 = (Hb \times 1.34)S\bar{v}O_2 + P\bar{v}O_2 \times 0.003$
	$\dot{Q} = 250$ ml/min $\div 50$ ml/L whole blood
	$\dot{Q} = 5$ L/min

the pulmonary artery and its appearance and changing concentration in the arterial blood are recorded by continuously withdrawing blood samples from a peripheral artery (e.g., radial, brachial, or femoral). The samples are passed through a detector, such as a densitometer, which determines their concentration in the blood. As shown in Figure 8–24, the resultant time-concentration curve shows an initial rapid rise followed by a gradual decline in concentration that is interrupted by a secondary rise due to recirculation and thus reappearance of the dye.

The cardiac output can be calculated using the following relationship:

$$\dot{Q} = I \div Co$$

where $\dot{Q}$ is the cardiac output measured (in liters per minute), *I* is the total amount of dye injected (in milligrams per minute), and *Co* is the average concentration of dye in the first pass (in milligrams per liter). The first-pass curve is therefore extrapolated with time to eliminate the effects of recirculation, as shown in the figure. Thus, *Co* can be determined as the area under the first-pass curve by planimetry or through computer methods in which the area computation is accomplished electronically.

The dye dilution cardiac output technique is used in many cardiac catheterization laboratories because of its accuracy and simplicity. However, note that the cardiac output is inaccurate in the presence of intracardiac shunts and in patients with low cardiac outputs. The downslope of the curve may be prolonged, and it is difficult to differentiate recirculated dye from that of the first-pass dye.

For the *thermodilution cardiac output technique,* sterile cold physiologic saline or 5% dextrose in water (D_5W) is injected through the proximal port of an indwelling Swan-Ganz catheter, and a small thermistor located at the tip of the catheter senses changes in the temperature of the

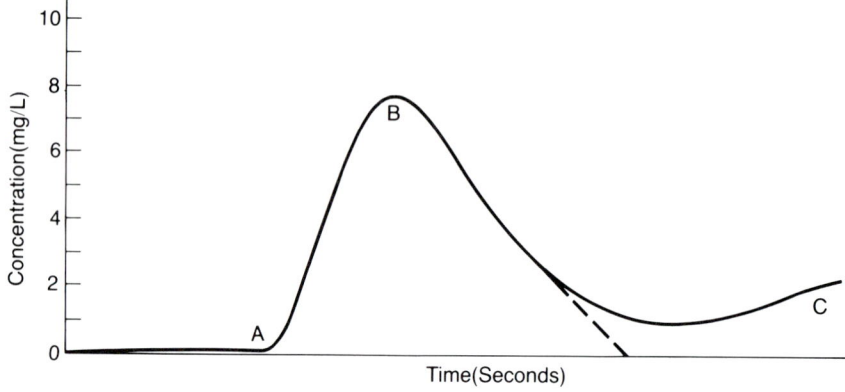

FIGURE 8–24. Time-concentration curve from a dye dilution cardiac output determination.

blood. In general, syringes with 10 ml of normal saline or D_5W are used as the indicator. The syringes are cooled to 0°C by immersion in an ice water bath. It is important that the injectate syringe is equilibrated at the temperature of the water bath because the computer's temperature probe (which is used to determine the temperature of the injectate) is usually submerged in the water bath. (Many of the newer systems do not require cold injectate but require only room temperature solutions for measuring cardiac output by the thermodilution technique.)

The thermodilution technique is the most widely used method for determining the cardiac output because it has distinct advantages over the dye dilution technique—namely, an arterial puncture is not required; measurements require only injection of small volumes so multiple measurements can be made, and there is essentially no problem with recirculation. Inaccuracies in thermodilution cardiac output can occur in patients with tricuspid valve insufficiency, intracardiac shunts, and low cardiac outputs. For patients on mechanical ventilation, timing of the injections to a particular phase of the respiratory cycle, usually the end-expiratory level, produces consistent measurements.

Interpretation of Cardiac Profiles

Stroke Volume (SV)

The stroke volume is defined as the volume of blood pumped by either the right or left ventricle with each cardiac contraction. It is calculated by dividing the cardiac output by the heart rate. In many cases, the stroke volume is expressed relative to the individual's body surface area—as the *stroke index* (SI), which is calculated by dividing the stroke volume by the body surface area (SI = SV ÷ BSA) (Appendix C contains a nomogram for calculating body surface area). In normal subjects, the average resting SV is between 60 and 70 ml per heartbeat (SI = 40 to 50 ml/m²). A good estimate of the normal resting SV is 1 ml per kilogram of body weight.

As discussed in Chapter 2, the main factors that influence the stroke volume include the preload, the afterload, and the contractility of the ventricles. The *preload* is the volume of blood in the ventricle just before contraction (e.g., *left ventricular end-diastolic volume,* or LVEDV; in normal subjects, the LVEDV can be estimated with the PAWP). The *afterload* is the pressure that the ventricle has to pump against with each contraction (i.e., mean pulmonary artery pressure for the right ventricle and mean aortic blood pressure for the left ventricle—thus the afterload is proportional to the *pulmonary vascular resistance* (PVR) and the *systemic vascular resistance* (SVR), respectively). The *contractility* of the ventricular muscle, may be defined as the property of ventricular muscle to generate tension in response to an appropriate stimulus without an increase in muscle fiber length or LVEDV (remember that contractility is not the same as the Frank-Starling relationship).

The SV may be reduced because of:
1. Decreases in preload or venous return, such as during tachycardia, cardiac tamponade, and extreme vasodilation (high intrathoracic pressures caused by excessive amounts of *positive end-expiratory pressure (PEEP) therapy* may also cause a reduction in venous return by compressing intrathoracic vessels).
2. Increases in afterload, such as occurs in pulmonary and systemic hypertension, or pulmonary or aortic valvular stenosis.
3. Decreases in contractility that are related to heart failure, hypoxemia, myocardial infarction, acidosis, or hypercapnea.

Increases in stroke volume are associated with

increases in preload, increases in contractility, and decreases in afterload. Bradycardia results in an increase in SV by causing an increase in LVEDV. Stimulation of the sympathetic nervous system, as occurs during exercise, causes an increase in SV through augmentation of heart's contractility. Administration of positive inotropic agents (e.g., epinephrine, isoproterenol, dopamine) increases the stroke volume by increasing the contracility of the heart.

Cardiac Work

The work performed by the heart during each contraction is considered to be equal to the product of the pressure generated by the heart and the volume of the blood pumped. *Left cardiac work* (LCW) is the work performed by the left ventricle as it ejects blood each minute. The *right cardiac work* (RCW) is the work of the right ventricle each minute as it ejects blood. Note that atrial work is usually not included in the calculation of the LCW or the RCW because of the relatively small pressures generated in these chambers during a cardiac contraction.

In hemodynamic monitoring, left and right cardiac work are usually expressed as stroke work, which is the amount of work done by the heart per beat. Thus, *left ventricular stroke work* is calculated as:

$$LSW = MAP \times SV \times 0.00136$$

where *MAP* is the mean arterial blood pressure, *SV* is the stroke volume, and 0.00136 is a conversion factor to convert milliliters-mmHg to gram-meters. Similarly, *right ventricular stroke work* is calculated as:

$$RSW = MPAP \times SV \times 0.00136$$

where *MPAP* is the mean pulmonary artery pressure. *LSW* and *RSW* are usually indexed to body surface area (LSW/BSA and RSW/BSA, respectively). Normal values for LSWI are between 0.50 and 0.60 kg-m/m^2. RSWI is normally between 0.07 and 0.10 kg-m/m^2.

Any condition that increases stroke volume or the mean pressure generated by the ventricle results in increased cardiac work.

Vascular Resistance

Remember from Chapter 2 that $\Delta P = \dot{Q} \times R$, so that $R = \Delta P \div \dot{Q}$. The resistance or opposition to blood flow offered by the systemic and pulmonary vascular beds (SVR and PVR, respectively) is therefore usually calculated as:

$$SVR = \frac{MAP - RAP}{SBF} \times 80$$

and

$$PVR = \frac{MPAP - MLAP}{PBF} \times 80$$

where *MAP, RAP, MPAP,* and *MLAP,* are the mean pressures in the aorta, right atrium, pulmonary artery, and left atrium in mmHg and *SBF* and *PBF* are the systemic and pulmonary blood flows (normally equal to the cardiac output) in L/min. The constant 80 is a conversion factor used to covert mmHg/L/min to dyne sec cm^{-5}.

The normal range of SVR is 900 to 1,500 dyne sec cm^{-5} while that of PVR is between 100 and 250 dyne sec cm^{-5}. Vascular resistance may be indexed to body surface area by multiplying the SVR and PVR by the body surface area. The normal systemic vascular resistance when indexed to the body surface area (the *systemic vascular resistance index,* or SVRI) is about 2,000 dyne sec cm^{-5}/m^2 and that of the pulmonary vascular resistance (the *pulmonary vascular resistance index,* or PVRI) is approximately 300 dyne sec cm^{-5}/m^2.

SVR may be increased directly by systemic vasoconstriction. It may be increased in left ventricular failure and hypovolemia as a result of a baroreceptor response. Polycythemia causes an increase in SVR by increasing the viscosity of the blood (remember that $R = 8\eta l \div \pi r^4$, where η is the viscosity of blood). SVR may be decreased by systemic vasodilation, such as occurs with moderate hypoxemia or following the administration of pharmacologic agents like nitroglycerin, hydralazine, or verapamil.

Increases in PVR are associated with increases in the pressure gradient between the pulmonary artery and the left atrium; it is also associated with conditions that cause a decrease in the cardiac output. Alveolar hypoxia causes an increase in PVR by causing constriction of the pulmonary arterioles and thus raising the MPAP. When cardiac output decreases, derecruitment of the pulmonary vessels causes an increase in PVR. Administration of pulmonary vasodilator agents, such as acetylcholine, prostaglandin E, and prostacyclin result in a decreased PVR.

NONINVASIVE CARDIOVASCULAR TECHNIQUES

The use of noninvasive cardiovascular techniques, particularly echocardiography and phonocardiography, have increased significantly during the past decade. These techniques provide both qualitative and quantitative data about the anatomy and function of the cardiovascular system, while causing only a minimum risk to the patient.

Echocardiography

Echocardiography is the general term used to describe procedures that utilize ultrasound to examine the heart and blood vessels. The movement of structures within and around the heart are recorded as reflected sound waves or echoes. Figure 8–25 shows a typical echocardiograph. A piezoelectric crystal functions as a transmitter and receiver of high-frequency vibrations. Short repetitive pulses of sound waves with a frequency between 1 and 7 megahertz are emitted from the transducer at a rate of 200 to 2,000 pulses per second. Echoes returning from an acoustically reflective interface are detected by the crystal during the intervals between pulse transmission and displayed on an oscilloscope or a video monitor.

The two echocardiographic scanning techniques most commonly used in cardiac ultrasound are *M-mode* and *real time* (2-D) scanning. In M-mode scanning, cardiac structures are displayed relative to time and the distance of the structure from the transducer. In 2-D scanning, cardiac structures are displayed as a two-dimensional picture (i.e., the picture shows that length and width of the structure being examined).

Echocardiography has been shown to be quite useful in the diagnosis of mitral and aortic stenosis and regurgitation, pericardial effusions, intracardiac tumors, and congenital cardiac defects, such as interatrial and interventricular septal defects.

Phonocardiography

A phonocardiogram is a graphic recording of sounds and pulses that originate in the heart and great vessels. These sound waves are detected by placing a microphone designed to detect low-frequency sound waves on the chest.

As Figure 8–26 shows, the normal phonocardiogram includes 2 to 4 waves. The first wave is associated with the opening of the aortic and pul-

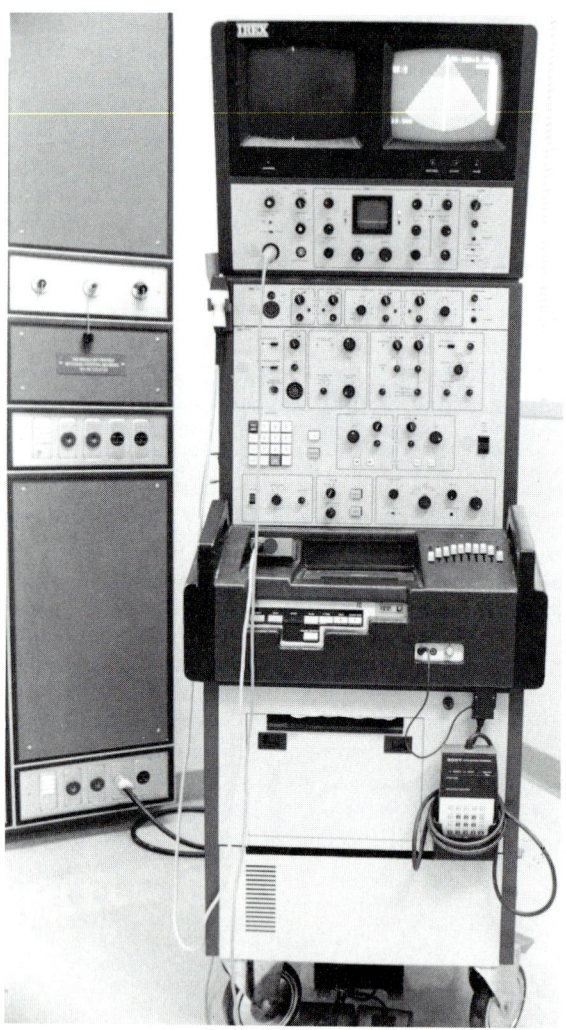

FIGURE 8–25. A typical echocardiograph unit. (Courtesy of Hewlett-Packard, Palo Alto, CA.)

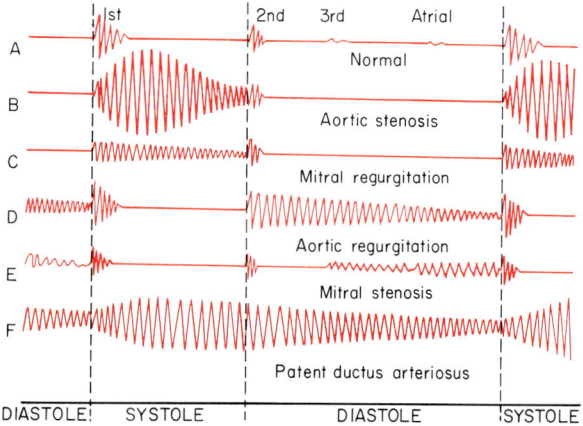

FIGURE 8–26. Phonocardiograms: *A*, Normal. *B*, Aortic stenosis. *C*, Mitral regurgitation. *D*, Aortic regurgitation. *E*, Mitral stenosis. *F*, Patent ductus arteriosus. (From Guyton, A.C.: *Textbook of Medical Physiology*, 7th ed. Philadelphia, W.B. Saunders, 1986, with permission.)

monary valves and the closure of the mitral and tricuspid valves (beginning of ventricular systole). The second sound corresponds to the opening of the mitral and tricuspid valves and the closure of the aortic and pulmonary valves (beginning of ventricular diastole). The third and fourth heart sounds are related to the rapid inflow of blood into the ventricles during diastole and atrial contraction, respectively. The third and fourth heart sounds are not normally audible in most subjects.

Figure 8–26 also shows several examples of phonocardiograms for patients with *murmurs*. Phonocardiography is useful in detecting valvular abnormalities as well as certain congenital cardiac defects, like a *patent ductus arteriosus*. Aortic stenosis is an example of a systolic murmur because when blood is ejected from the left ventricle through a narrowed (stenotic) aortic valve, a "nozzle" effect is created resulting in severe turbulence at the aortic root. Mitral regurgitation is also considered to be an example of a systolic murmur, however, with this type of abnormality, blood is pushed through an incompetent mitral valve during ventricular systole causing a swishing sound that is transmitted to the left atrium. Aortic regurgitation and mitral stenosis are representative of diastolic murmurs. In aortic regurgitation, blood flows back into the left ventricle during ventricular diastole due to an incompetent aortic valve. For mitral stenosis, as blood flows from the left atrium to the left ventricle, it must overcome an increased resistance offered by a stiff mitral valve. Because the pressure in the left atrium rarely rises above 30 mmHg, a large pressure for forcing blood from the left atrium to the left ventricle never develops. Thus, the abnormally generated sounds of mitral stenosis are relatively weak and may not be heard.

BIBLIOGRAPHY

Berne, R.M., and Levy, M.N.: *Cardiovascular Physiology,* 4th ed. St. Louis, C.V. Mosby Company, 1981.
Braunwald, E.: *Heart Disease: A Textbook of Cardiovascular Medicine,* 3rd ed. Philadelphia, W.B. Saunders, 1988.
Burch, G.E., and Winsor, T.: *A Primer of Electrocardiography,* 6th ed. Philadelphia, Lea and Febiger, 1972.
Chung, E.K.: *Electrocardiography: Practical Applications With Vectorial Principles,* 2nd ed. Hagerstown, Md., Harper & Row, 1980.
Chung, E.K.: *Non-Invasive Cardiac Diagnosis.* Philadelphia, Lea & Febiger, 1976.
Civetta, J.M., and Gabel, J.C.: Flow-directed pulmonary artery catheterization in surgical patients: Indications and modifications of technic. *Ann. Surg.* 176:753, 1972.
Cranefield, P.F., and Wit, A.L.: Cardiac arrhythmias. *Annu. Rev. Physiol.* 41:459, 1979.
Criley, J.M., and Ross, R.S.: *Cardiovascular Physiology.* Tampa, Fla., Tampa Tracings, 1971.
Cromwell, L., Weibell, F.J., and Pfeiffer, E.A.: *Biomedical Instrumentation and Measurements.* Englewood Cliffs, N.J., Prentice-Hall, 1980.
Daily, E.K., and Schroeder, J.S.: *Techniques in Bedside Hemodynamic Monitoring.* St. Louis, C.V. Mosby, 1985.
Ganz, W., Donoso, R., Marcus, H.S., Forrester, J.S., and Swan, H.J.C.: A new technique for measurement of cardiac output by thermodilution in man. *Am. J. Cardiol.* 27:392, 1971.
Grossman, W.: *Cardiac Catheterization and Angiography,* 3rd ed. Philadelphia, Lea & Febiger, 1986.
Guyton, A.C.: *Textbook of Medical Physiology,* 7th ed. Philadelphia, W.B. Saunders, 1986.
Houser, S.R.: Cardiac electrophysiology: Cellular events that underlie the ECG. *Journal of Cardiovascular and Pulmonary Technique* 8(3):44–50, 1980.
Littmann, D.: *The Electrocardiogram: Part Five.* Dallas, American Heart Association, 1973.
Mohrman, D.E., and Heller, L.J.: *Cardiovascular Physiology,* 2nd ed. New York, McGraw-Hill, 1986.
Pollard, D., and Seliger, E.: *An Implementation of Bedside Physiological Calculations.* Palo Alto, Hewlett-Packard Company, 1985.
Rushmer, R.F.: *Organ Physiology: Structure and Function of the Cardiovascular System,* 2nd ed. Philadelphia, W.B. Saunders, 1976.
Swan, H.J.C., Ganz, W., Forrester, J. et al.: Catheterization of the heart in man with use of a flow-directed balloon-tipped catheter. *N. Engl. J. Med.* 283:447, 1970.
Swan, H.J.C., and Ganz, W.: The use of balloon-tipped, flow-directed catheters in monitoring patients with acute myocardial infarction. In Corday, E., and Swan, H.J.C. (eds.): *Myocardial Infarction.* Baltimore, Williams & Wilkins, 1973.
Wiedemann, H.P., Matthay, M.A., and Matthay, R.A.: Cardiovascular-pulmonary monitoring in the intensive care unit (Part 1). *Chest* 85(4):537–549, 1984.
Winsor, T.: *The Electrocardiogram in Myocardial Infarction.* Summit, N.J. Ciba-Geigy Corporation, 1973.
Yang, S.S., Bentivoglio, L.G., Maranhao, V., and Goldberg, H.: *From Cardiac Catheterization Data to Hemodynamic Parameters,* 2nd ed. Philadelphia, F. A. Davis, 1978.

OBJECTIVES

AFTER READING THIS CHAPTER, THE STUDENT WILL BE ABLE TO:

1. Understand the physiologic basis of pulmonary function tests.
2. Discuss how these tests are used in the diagnosis and treatment of pulmonary diseases.
3. Describe the procedures and instrumentation used in the measurement of the vital capacity and its subdivisions.
4. Discuss the use of inert gas dilution and plethysmographic techniques for the measurement of residual volume.
5. Describe compliance measurements and their use in the evaluation of the elastic properties of the lungs and chest wall.
6. Describe airway resistance measurements and the use of these measurements in the diagnosis and treatment of obstructive pulmonary diseases.
7. Discuss bronchoprovocation in the diagnosis of hypersensitive airway disease.
8. Discuss the measurements of maximum inspiratory and expiratory pressures.
9. Discuss the use of the single-breath oxygen test and the multibreath nitrogen washout technique to assess the distribution of ventilation.
10. Discuss the determination of lung diffusing capacity and the effect of disease on gas transport between the alveoli and the blood.
11. Discuss several methods that are used to assess ventilation-perfusion relationships in the lung.
12. Discuss the pulmonary function tests used to assess the control of breathing.

PULMONARY ASSESSMENT

CHAPTER OUTLINE

DETERMINATION OF LUNG SUBDIVISIONS
  Spirometry
    Volume-Collecting Devices
    Flow-Sensing Devices
  Determination of Vital Capacity
  Determination of Residual Volume, Functional Residual Capacity, and Total Lung Capacity
    Helium Dilution Technique
    Nitrogen Washout Technique
    Body Plethysmography
  Interpretation of Static Lung Volume Measurements
ASSESSMENT OF THE LUNG'S ELASTIC PROPERTIES
  Static Lung Compliance
  Dynamic Lung Compliance
  Interpretation of Lung Compliance Measurements
DYNAMIC LUNG FUNCTION
  Maximum Voluntary Ventilation
  Forced Vital Capacity
  Flow-Volume Analysis
  Airway Resistance
  Maximum Inspiratory and Expiratory Pressures
  Bronchoprovocation
DETERMINATION OF THE DISTRIBUTION OF VENTILATION
  Single-Breath Oxygen Test
  Multibreath Nitrogen Washout Test
DETERMINATION OF LUNG DIFFUSING CAPACITY
  Single-Breath Carbon Monoxide Test
ASSESSMENT OF VENTILATION-PERFUSION
  Calculation of Physiologic Deadspace
  Calculation of Physiologic Shunt
  Alveolar-Arterial Oxygen Differences
ASSESSMENT OF THE CONTROL OF BREATHING
  Ventilatory Response to Inhaled Hypercapnic Gas Mixtures
  Ventilatory Response to Inhaled Hypoxic Gas Mixtures
  Respiration and Sleep

PULMONARY ASSESSMENT

During the past 25 years, pulmonary function tests have become essential for the diagnosis and treatment of pulmonary diseases (Table 9–1). Until recently, clinical pulmonary function tests have primarily been used to study pulmonary mechanics; however, recent technologic advances have made it relatively easy for the cardiopulmonary specialist to evaluate the distribution of ventilation, ventilation-perfusion relationships, lung diffusing capacity, the control of breathing, and metabolic rate.

The physiologic basis of pulmonary function testing has been discussed in Chapter 3, and the pathophysiologic findings associated with various pulmonary disorders have been presented in Chapter 5. In this chapter, the procedures and instruments commonly used in pulmonary diagnostic tests as well as the clinical application of these tests in the management of pulmonary diseases are discussed.

DETERMINATION OF LUNG SUBDIVISIONS

The lung is conventionally divided into four standard volumes and four standard capacities (see Figs. 3–20 and 9–1). As stated previously, the resting size of the lungs depends on the physical characteristics of an individual (age, sex, height, weight, and body surface area), but the volume of gas present in the lungs at any instant is determined by the mechanical properties of the lungs and chest wall and the activity of the respiratory muscles (see Chapter 3). Lung volume determinations can therefore be used to identify abnormalities of respiratory system mechanics. These measurements are also used in calculations of lung and chest wall compliance, airway resistance, lung diffusing capacity, and the ratio of forced expiratory volumes to the vital capacity.

TABLE 9–1. Indications for Pulmonary Function Testing

1. To establish baseline respiratory system function (e.g., preoperative evaluation of patients about to undergo thoracic or abdominal surgery).
2. To identify individuals at risk for developing pulmonary dysfunctions (e.g., occupational screening).
3. To establish the presence of obstructive or restrictive pulmonary disease.
4. To follow the progress of a pulmonary disease once a diagnosis has been made.
5. To monitor the effectiveness of therapeutic interventions.

The vital capacity and its subdivisions (tidal volume and inspiratory and expiratory reserve volumes) are measured directly with a *spirometer,* but the residual volume, which is the volume of gas remaining in the lungs after a complete exhalation, must be measured with indirect techniques, such as *nitrogen washout, helium dilution, and body plethysmography*. The determination of the vital capacity and its subdivisions is often used as a screening test in subjects suspected of having respiratory system dysfunctions. Measurement of the residual volume is usually reserved for those subjects demonstrating an abnormality during simple spirometry.

Spirometry

A *spirometer* is used to measure the volume of gas exchanged at the airway opening. There are two basic types of spirometers: volume-collecting and flow-sensing devices. The water-seal spirometer, the dry-rolling seal spirometer, and the bellows spirometer are examples of volume-collecting devices; the differential pressure pneumotachograph, the hot-wire anemometer, and the turbine flowmeter are flow-sensing devices.

Volume-Collecting Devices

The *water-seal spirometer* consists of a mouthpiece and tubing connected to a lightweight bell that is inverted over a water bath (Fig. 9–2A). As the subject breathes into the mouthpiece, the bell moves up and down with each expiration and inspiration, respectively. The volume of gas exchanged is registered on a rotating drum of graph paper (the kymograph) by a pen connected to the bell. These spirometers are available in a variety of sizes, with bell capacities ranging from 7 to 14 L. Removable flutter valves and a carbon dioxide absorber (containing calcium carbonate) can be added to the system for rebreathing studies. Because the kymograph can be rotated at both slow and fast speeds (typically, 32, 160, 300, and 1,920 mm per second), these instruments can be used to measure both static and dynamic lung volume changes.

In the *dry-rolling seal spirometer,* the bell and water reservoir are replaced by a movable piston that is attached to a flexible Silastic rubber seal (Fig. 9–2B). Displacement of the piston is recorded by a potentiometer that creates a voltage proportional to the volume of gas contained in the spirometer.

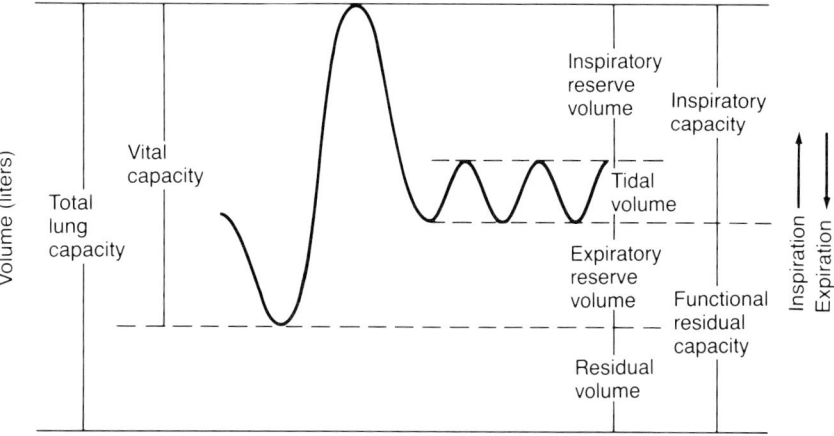

FIGURE 9–1. Standard lung volumes and capacities. The y axis = liters; the x axis = seconds.

Bellows spirometers are expandable devices that resemble the schematic in Figure 9–2C. As the subject exhales into the system, the bellows moves a distance that is proportional to the volume of gas exchanged. A direct writing pen or a potentiometer attached to the free wall of the bellows is used to register volume changes in the system.

Flow-Sensing Devices

Differential pressure pneumotachographs (or pneumotachometers) are flow-sensing devices based on the principle that air flowing through a fixed resistance creates a pressure difference that is primarily a function of its volume flow. According to Poiseuille's law, the pressure difference is equal to flow times resistance (for laminar flow). The *Fleisch* pneumotachograph, the most common of this type, uses a set of parallel capillary tubes to create a fixed resistance and cause laminar airflow (Fig. 9–3A). These capillary tubes are encased within a heating element, which serves to remove any condensation that accumulates while a subject is breathing through the device. Such an accumulation would increase the resistance to airflow. An electronic transducer, attached to pressure taps upstream and downstream of the fixed resistance, is used to determine the pressure difference that occurs as air flows through the device. As already noted, the pressure gradient across the resistance determined by this differential air pressure transducer is directly proportional to the airflow for *laminar* flow, but it is proportional to the square of the airflow for *turbulent* flow (see Chapter 3). Obstructions to airflow caused by bends in the tubing, uneven connections, or the physical properties of the gas being analyzed therefore influence the airflow and may affect the accuracy of these measurements. Newer differential pressure pneumotachographs, which use wire mesh rather than capillary tubes as the fixed resistance, are also used in many pulmonary function testing systems. Although they differ in construction, they follow the same principles used in the Fleisch pneumotachograph.

The *hot-wire anemometer* contains a platinum element that is heated to a temperature of 50°C by an electric current (Fig. 9–3B). As the subject exhales into the spirometer, air flows around the element, which causes the element to become cooled. Because the amount of heat lost is directly related to the specific heat of the gas being breathed, the airflow rate can be determined by measuring the current needed to keep the platinum element at a temperature of 50°C.

The *turbine flowmeter* uses a rotating vane to measure airflow (Fig. 9–3C). In a photosensitive flowmeter, every time the turbine rotates, one of its blades interrupts a beam of light that is focused on a photocell and produces an electronic pulse that is counted by a digital circuit. The greater the airflow, the faster the turbine spins, resulting in a greater number of pulses.

Spirometric Standards. In 1978, the American Thoracic Society (ATS) approved a series of recommendations for instruments and techniques used in clinical spirometry. Table 9–2 summarizes the instrument specifications that have been set forth by this ATS statement on spirometry. (For a complete review of these standards, the reader is encouraged to read the complete ATS statement in the article by Gardner and colleagues listed in the Bibliography.) It should be noted that these are minimal standards, and an instrument used in clinical or occupational screening programs should therefore at least meet these standards.

300 PULMONARY ASSESSMENT

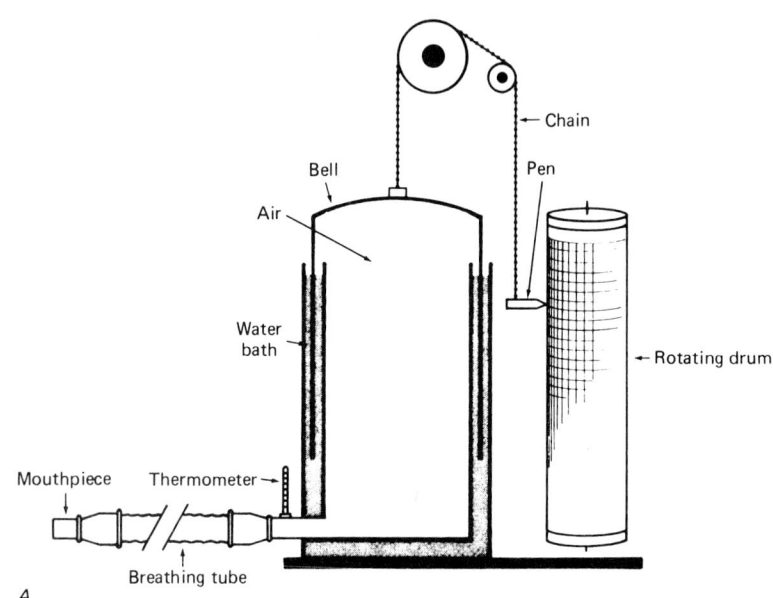

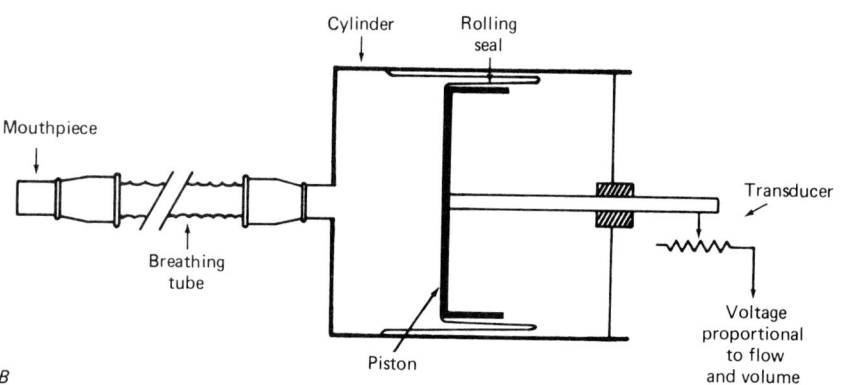

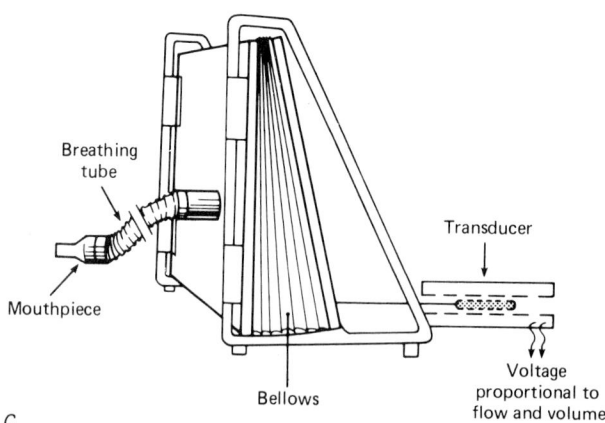

FIGURE 9–2. Examples of volume-collecting spirometers: A, Water-seal spirometer. B, Dry-rolling seal spirometer. C, Bellows spirometer. (From Fishman, A.P. (ed.): *Pulmonary Diseases and Disorders*. New York, McGraw-Hill, 1980, with permission.)

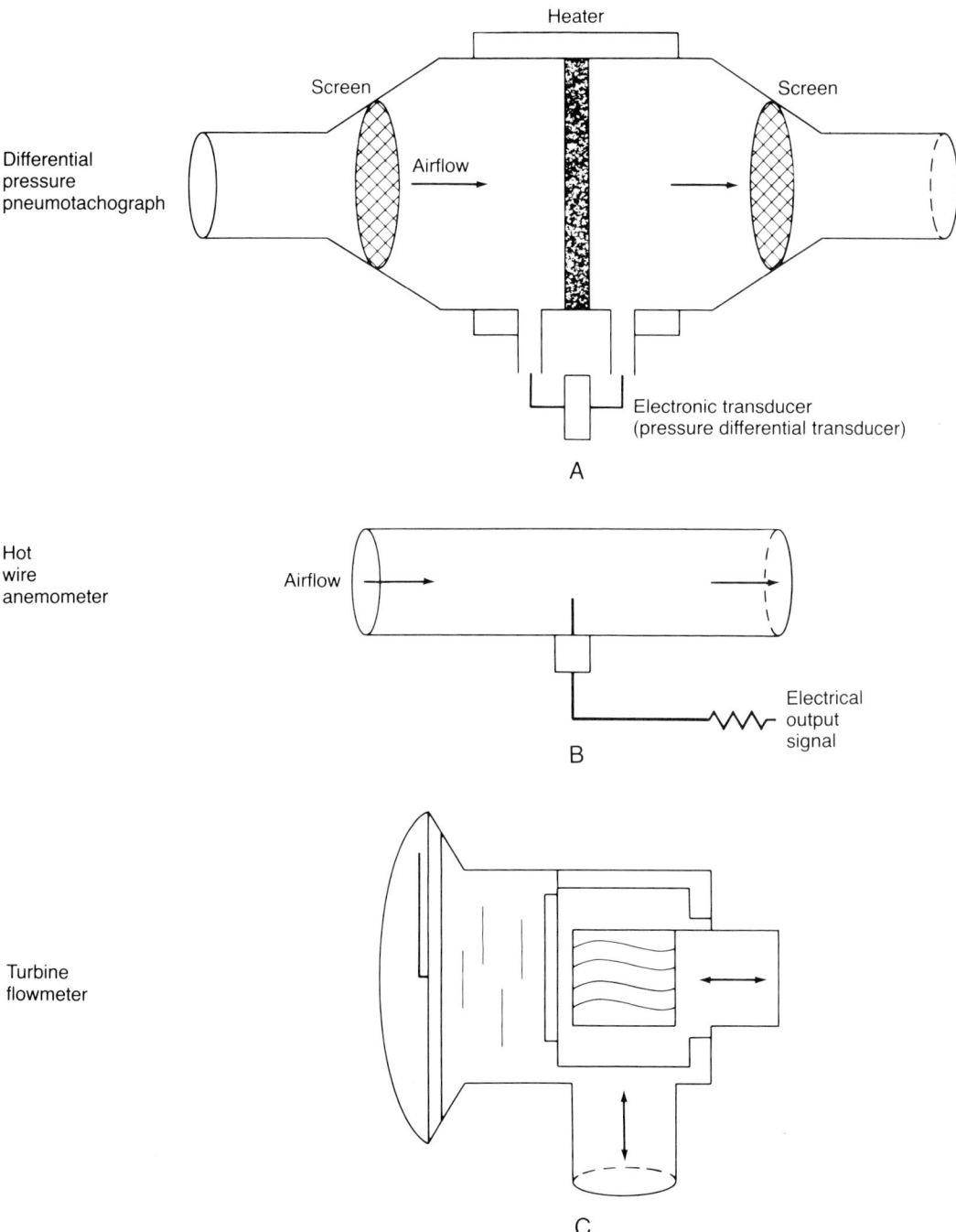

FIGURE 9–3. Examples of flow-sensing spirometers: *A*, Differential pressure pneumotachograph. *B*, Hot-wire anemometer. *C*, Turbine flowmeter.

TABLE 9-2. Minimal Spirometry Standards by the American Thoracic Society

Test	Range/Accuracy BTPS (liter)	Flow Range (liter/sec)	Time (sec)	Start Point	Resistance and Back Pressure	Test Signals
VC	7 liter ± 3% of reading or 50 ml, whichever is greater	0 → 12	30	—		Calibrated syringe
FVC	7 liter ± 3% of reading or 50 ml, whichever is greater	0 → 12	10.0	—		Two simulated FVC signals in range (1) FVC = 5 liter; τ = 0.4 sec (2) FVC = liter; τ = 2.4 sec
FEV_t	7 liter ± 3% of reading	0 → 12	t	Back extrapolate or equivalent	Less than 1.5 cm H_2O liter/sec at 12.0 liter/sec flow	Same as FVC
FEV_1			1.0			
FEF 25–75%	7 liter ± 5% of reading or 0.1 liter/sec, whichever is greater	0 → 12	10.0	—	Same as FEV_t	Same as FVC
$\dot{V}$	12 liter/sec ± 5% of reading or 0.2 liter/sec, whichever is greater	0 → 12	10.0	—	Same as FEV_t	Manufacturer proof
MVV	Sine wave 250 liter/min at 2 liter to ± 5% of reading	0 → 12 ± 5%	12 to 15 ± 3%	—	Pressure less than ± 10 cm H_2O at 2 liter TV 2.0 Hz	Sine wave pump 0 → 4 Hz ± 10% at ± 12 liter/sec

(From Gardner, R.M., Baker, C.D., Boennle, A.M. Jr., et al.: ATS statement—Snowbird workshop on standardization of spirometry. Am. Rev. Resp. Dis. 119:831–838, 1979, with permission. Courtesy of the American Lung Association)

Determination of Vital Capacity

Before beginning the test, anthropometric data should be obtained from the patient. These data, which include sex and age (in years) along with height (in centimeters) and weight (in pounds), are used to calculate *predicted values* for the patient. A number of regression equations have been determined for calculating the predicted values. These equations can be found in some of the references listed at the end of this chapter. Note that for patients with kyphoscoliosis, the height can be estimated from measurements of arm span. Figure 9-4 shows how arm span measurements are made as well as the correction factors used to estimate height.

Once the preliminary data mentioned above have been obtained, the technician should take a few minutes to explain the procedure to the patient. It is important that the patient understand the instructions for performing the test because a lack of understanding may result in a poor effort during testing and thus in erroneous data.

To begin the test, the patient is seated comfortably in front of the spirometer and instructed to loosen any restrictive clothing, such as a necktie, brassiere, or belt (for children, spirometry is best performed with the child standing). The patient's body position is important because it affects lung volumes. With noseclips in place, the patient is instructed to breathe quietly through the mouthpiece into and out of the spirometer until a stable end-tidal expiratory level (i.e., functional residual capacity [FRC]) is achieved. The patient is then instructed to perform a maximum inspiration followed by a slow and complete expiration to the residual volume. Alternatively, the vital capacity and its subdivisions can be determined by measuring the expiratory reserve volume and the inspiratory capacity in separate maneuvers. This latter technique may yield larger volumes in the elderly and in patients with obstructive pulmonary disease for reasons that are not entirely clear at this time.

The volumes measured by the spirometer are recorded at ambient temperature and pressure, saturated (ATPS), which are the conditions inside the spirometer. By convention, these measurements are converted to body temperature and ambient pressure, saturated (BTPS), that is, the conditions in the patient's lungs. This conversion is done so that lung volume determinations can be

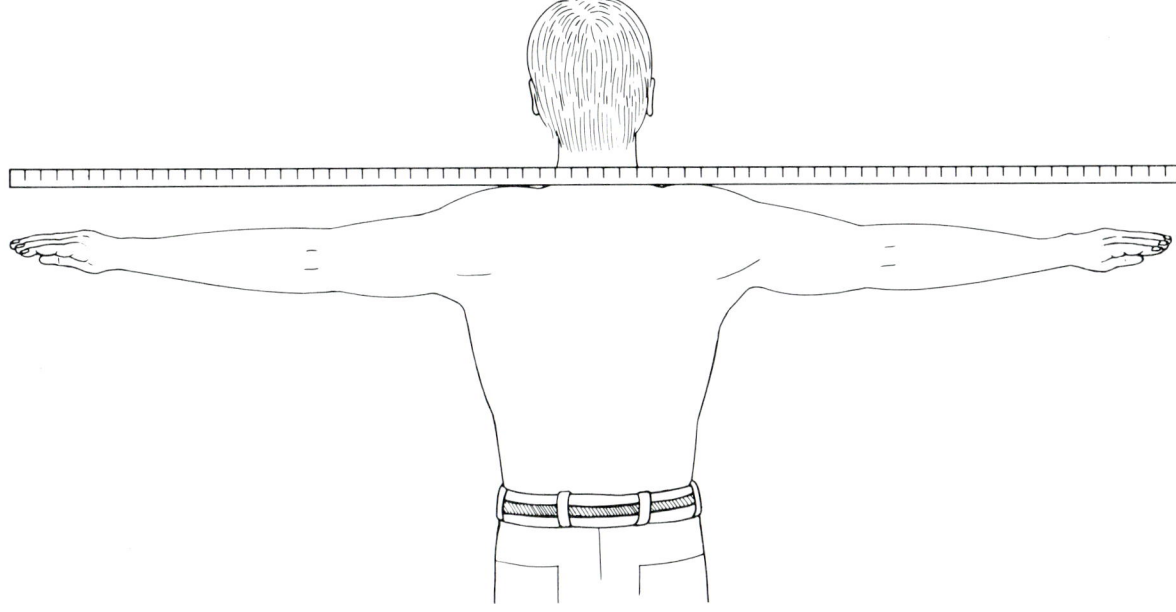

FIGURE 9–4. Arm span measurements used for the estimation of height.

Patient's arms are fully extended from the sides. A measurement in centimeters is taken from the tip of the middle finger of the right hand to the tip of the middle finger of the left hand. The *span* measured is then applied to the following formula:

Height (in cm) = span (in cm) − correction factor*

Correction Factors

Age (yrs)	Boys	Girls	Age (yrs)	Boys	Girls
1	−2.5	−3.0	9	0.0	1.2
2	−2.8	−3.6	10	0.0	1.0
3	−3.0	−4.1	11	0.0	0.0
4	−3.0	−3.8	12	2.0	0.0
5	−3.3	−3.6	13	3.3	0.0
6	−2.5	−3.3	14	3.3	0.0
7	−2.5	−2.0	15	4.3	1.3
8	−1.2	−1.8	16	4.6	1.3

EXAMPLE: What is the predicted height of a 5 year old male patient with severe scoliosis?

span = 125 cm; correction factor = −3.3

Thus, 125 − (−3) = 128.3 cm

compared between laboratories with different environmental conditions (ambient temperature and barometric pressures). A list of conversion factors commonly used in clinical laboratories is presented in Table 9–3.

Determination of Residual Volume, Functional Residual Capacity, and Total Lung Capacity

As stated previously, the residual volume is the volume of gas remaining in the lungs at the end of a maximum expiration. In the pulmonary function laboratory, the residual volume is usually determined by measuring the functional residual capacity and subtracting the expiratory reserve volume, which is measured separately during simple spirometry. The FRC or end-tidal expiratory level is determined because it is a very reproducible lung volume for a subject to attain and, therefore, increases the accuracy as well as the precision of the residual volume measurement. Two types of tests are routinely used to determine the residual volume, the functional residual capacity, and the total lung capacity. These include inert gas dilution tests and body plethysmography.

Inert gas dilution tests, which include the open-circuit nitrogen washout technique and closed-circuit helium dilution technique, can determine the

TABLE 9–3. Correction Factors Used in Pulmonary Function Testing to Convert Gas Volumes from ATPS to BTPS*

When Ambient Temperature (°C) Is	Factor to Convert Volume to BTPS Is
20	1.102
21	1.096
22	1.091
23	1.085
24	1.080
25	1.075
26	1.068
27	1.063
28	1.057
29	1.051
30	1.045
31	1.039
32	1.032
33	1.026
34	1.020
35	1.014

* Note that these correction factors have been calculated for a barometric pressure of 760 torr.

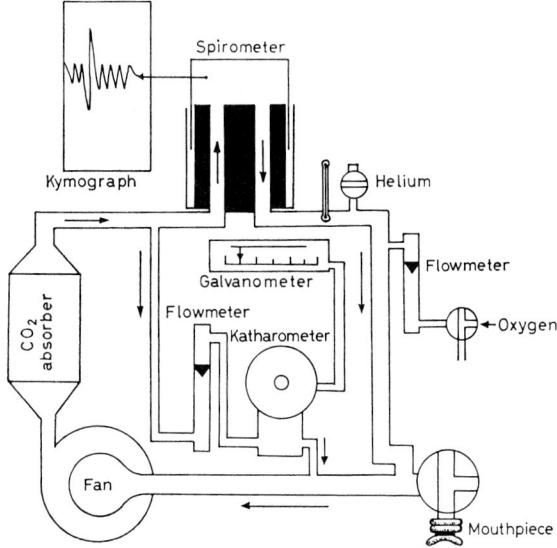

FIGURE 9–5. Instrument used to determine functional residual capacity by helium dilution. (From Cotes, J.L.: *Lung Function*. Oxford, Blackwell Scientific Publications, 1979, with permission.)

volume of gas that is in communication with the major airways. Body plethysmography measures the compressible volume of gas within the thorax. In normal, healthy subjects, all three techniques give similar values for each of the three volumes. However, in patients with pulmonary disease, the inert gas dilution tests may underestimate lung volumes because of airway closure and air trapping.

Helium Dilution Technique

The helium dilution test is based on the principle that if the total amount of a substance dissolved in a volume is known and its concentration can be measured, then the volume in which the substance is dissolved can be determined because amount equals volume times concentration. To perform the helium dilution test, the subject breathes into and out of a closed system containing a known concentration of helium (approximately 10% to 15%). Helium is used because it is not absorbed (or produced) by the pulmonary capillary blood. As Figure 9–5 shows, the system consists of a spirometer, a source of oxygen to replace what is used by the subject, a carbon dioxide absorber, and a fan that ensures that the gas within the circuit is adequately circulated. A helium analyzer, which works on the principle of thermal conductivity, is used to determine the concentration of helium present in the system. (In Figure 9–5, the flowmeter, katharometer, and galvanometer constitute the helium analyzer.)

The patient begins and ends the test at end-tidal expiration and continues to rebreathe into the system until there is no difference between the helium concentration in the spirometer and that in his or her lungs. The FRC can then be determined using the following relationship:

$$F_{He\ (initial)} \times V_{spiro\ (initial)} = F_{He\ (final)} (V_{spiro} + V_{lung})_{[final]}$$

If the total amount of helium present in the spirometer initially equals the total amount of helium in the spirometer plus that in the patient's lungs at the end of the test, determination of the decrease in the concentration of helium present in the system allows the volume of gas added to the system (or the FRC) to be calculated.

Nitrogen Washout Technique

The open-circuit nitrogen washout test is based on the knowledge that air contains a fixed percentage of nitrogen and that the concentration of nitrogen in the lungs of a patient breathing room air is approximately equal to this percentage (about 80%). Thus, by determining the amount of nitrogen present in the patient's lungs at the end of a tidal expiration, the functional residual capacity can be calculated.

The system used to perform this test is shown in Figure 9–6. The patient breathes 100% oxygen through a one-way (non-rebreathing) valve until virtually all of the nitrogen in the lungs is washed out. The volume of expired gas is determined by having the subject exhale into a large spirometer (i.e., Tissot spirometer) while the concentration of expired nitrogen is monitored with an analyzer, such as a mass spectrometer, a gas chromatograph, or an ionization chamber. The test is begun after the subject achieves a stable end-tidal expiratory level and is continued until the concentration of nitrogen during expiration is less than 1.2%. Because all of the nitrogen in the system was contained in the patient's lungs at the beginning of the test and is in the spirometer at the end of the test, the volume of gas in the patient's lungs at the start of the test can be calculated. By noting the volume of gas collected in the spirometer and the average nitrogen concentration of the total volume of expired gas, the FRC can be calculated with the following equations:

1. Vol lung (FRC) × Conc lung N_2 (FRC)

    = Vol spirometer × Conc spirometer N_2

2. FRC (uncorrected)

$$= \frac{\text{Total expired volume in spirometer} \times \text{Percent nitrogen in spirometer}}{\text{Percent nitrogen in lung (FRC)}}$$

3. FRC (corrected)

    = FRC (uncorrected) × BTPS factor

Normal subjects usually complete the test in 2 to 3 minutes, whereas patients with pulmonary diseases such as emphysema, bronchitis, asthma, and space-occupying lesions in the major airways require considerably longer periods of time to wash the nitrogen out. As we will discuss later in this chapter, breath-by-breath analysis of expired nitrogen concentrations during the test, and measurement of the time required for washout, are also useful indicators of the distribution of ventilation.

Body Plethysmography

The plethysmographic, or pneumatometric, technique is the most accurate of the indirect methods for measuring functional residual capacity. By applying Boyle's law, the body plethysmograph (or body box) can be used to measure the compressible gas volume within a subject's thorax. For clinical pulmonary function testing, three types of body boxes are available: the constant volume, variable pressure type (pressure box), the constant pressure, variable volume (volume box) and pressure corrected, variable volume (flow box) plethysmographs. In this chapter, our discussion is limited to the pressure box because it is the one most commonly used.

As Figure 9–7 shows, the body box consists of an airtight chamber that contains a pneumotachometer, pressure transducers, and a mouthpiece-shutter assembly. The pneumotach and transducers allow for the measurement of airflow at the mouth as well as the pressure at the mouth and the box pressure while a patient is seated within the plethysmograph and breathing through the mouthpiece. For measurement of FRC, the patient first breathes tidally through the mouthpiece-shutter assembly. At the end of a tidal expiration, the shutter at the mouth is closed, and the patient is instructed to make a gentle panting maneuver, which causes a rhythmic compression and decompression of the thorax. By occluding the airway, airflow becomes zero and thus, the mouth pressure approximates the alveolar pressure. Measurements of the box pressure changes, which are assumed to be proportional to the alveolar pressure and, thus the alveolar volume, are used to reflect thoracic gas volume changes. The pressure-volume changes that occur at the end of the tidal breath are then used to calculate the FRC with the following formulas:

$$P_1V_1 = P_2V_2 \text{ (Boyle's law)}$$

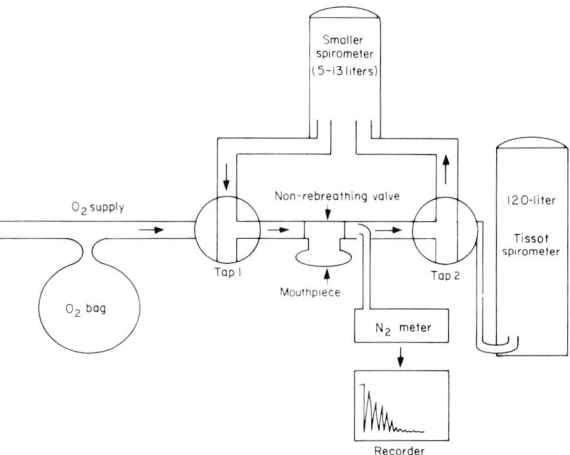

FIGURE 9–6. Instrument used to determine functional residual capacity by nitrogen washout. (From Jalowayski, A.A., and Dawson, A.: Measurement of lung volume. The multiple breath nitrogen method. In Clausen, J.L., (ed.): *Pulmonary Function Testing. Guidelines and Controversies. Equipment, Methods, and Normal Values.* New York, Academic Press, 1982, with permission.)

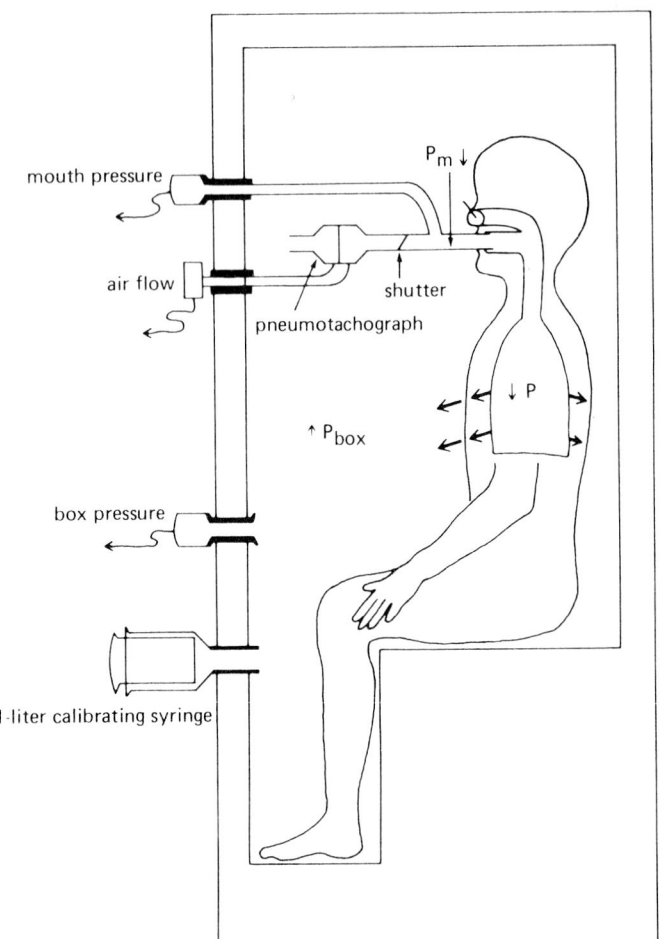

FIGURE 9-7. The body plethysmograph for determining functional residual capacity. The subject is seated in the small, airtight chamber and breathes through the apparatus shown. By monitoring the subject's airflow with a pneumotachograph, the operator can briefly occlude the subject's airway at end-expiration. As the subject makes an inspiratory effort against the closed airway, the pressure in the chamber (P_{box}) increases, and the pressure at the subject's mouth (P_M) decreases. The subject's functional residual capacity can then be calculated. (From Levitzky, M.G.: *Pulmonary Physiology*, 2nd ed. New York, McGraw-Hill, 1986, with permission.)

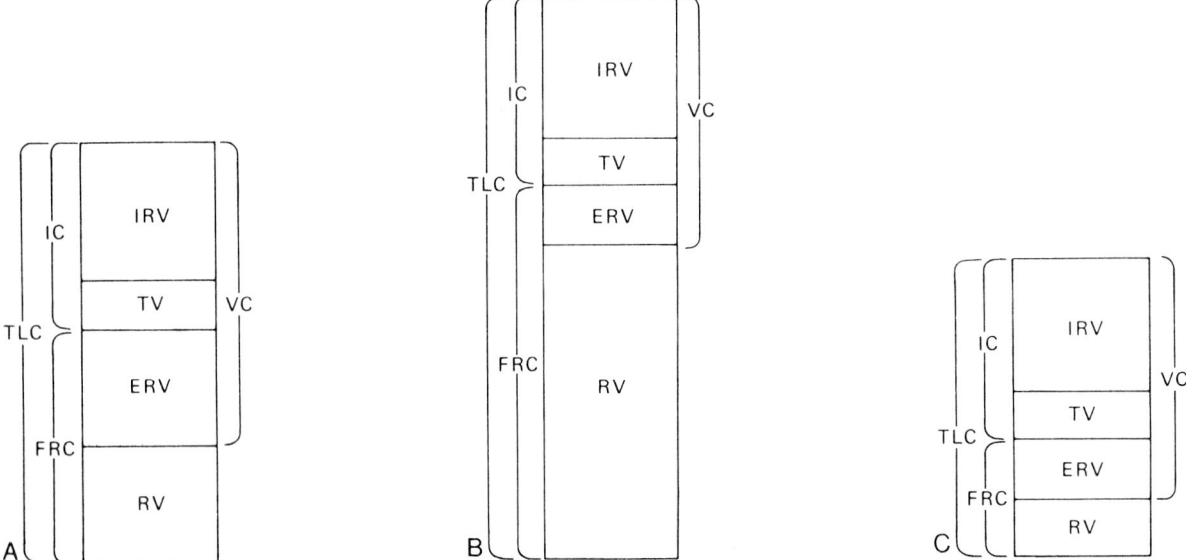

FIGURE 9-8. Static lung volume determinations from: *A*, Normal subject. *B*, Patient with obstructive lung disease. *C*, Patient with restrictive lung disease. (From Levitzky, M.G.: *Pulmonary Physiology*, 2nd ed. New York, McGraw-Hill, 1986, with permission.)

where P_1 is the mouth pressure at FRC (or barometric pressure), V_1 is the volume of gas in the thorax at end-tidal expiration, P_2 is the pressure change that occurs with an inspiratory effort, and V_2 is the volume change that occurs with an inspiratory effort. Rearranging this equation to obtain the volume at FRC, the equation now becomes:

$$V_1 = P_2 V_2 \div P_1$$

or

$$V_{FRC} = \frac{(P_{FRC} - \Delta P)(V_{FRC} + \Delta V)}{P_{FRC}}$$

Interpretation of Static Lung Volume Measurements

Measurements of vital capacity, residual volume, functional residual capacity, and total lung capacity are useful in the differential diagnosis of *obstructive* and *restrictive* pulmonary diseases. In obstructive lung diseases, such as emphysema or bronchitis, the vital capacity may be normal or reduced, while the residual volume, functional residual capacity, and total lung capacity are elevated. The vital capacity becomes reduced as the ratio of residual volume to total lung capacity (RV/TLC) increases. Patients with restrictive disorders, such as pulmonary interstitial fibrosis, chest wall abnormalities, or obesity show reductions in their vital capacities primarily due to reduced total lung capacities. The functional residual capacity, the residual volume, and the inspiratory capacity may also be reduced in these patients. Figure 9–8 shows lung volume measurements for three persons who possess similar anthropometric data: a normal subject, a patient with obstructive lung disease, and a patient with restrictive lung disease.

ASSESSMENT OF THE LUNG'S ELASTIC PROPERTIES

The elastic properties of the lung can be evaluated by determining lung compliance, which is defined as the change in lung volume that occurs with a given change in transpulmonary pressure (remember that under static conditions the transpulmonary pressure equals the alveolar pressure minus the intrapleural pressure). Static lung compliance is determined when no air is flowing. Lung volume changes are recorded with a spirometer or body plethysmograph, while changes in transpulmonary pressure are reflected by changes in the intrapleural pressure. The intrapleural pressure can be estimated with an esophageal balloon, which is swallowed by the subject being tested and then positioned in the lower third of the esophagus.

To perform the test with a body plethysmograph, the patient is seated in the body box and instructed to breathe into a mouthpiece-shutter assembly similar to the one used in the thoracic gas volume measurements. He or she is then told to inspire to total lung capacity and exhale slowly. As the patient exhales, the airway is intermittently occluded with the shutter, and the esophageal pressures for several lung volumes from total lung capacity to functional residual capacity are recorded. Because the mouth pressure reflects alveolar pressure when there is no airflow, transpulmonary pressure can therefore be calculated with the esophageal estimates of intrapleural pressure. Note that the lung volume measurements are derived from the body box volume changes rather than the mouth pressures because exhalation against an occluded airway causes some compression of the lung volume, and lung volume measurements made at the mouth are not accurate. Lung volume changes for compliance determinations may be obtained with a spirometer, if a body plethysmograph is unavailable.

Dynamic Lung Compliance

These measurements are obtained by monitoring the esophageal pressure while lung volume changes during tidal breathing are determined using a body plethysmograph. The patient breathes at a rate of approximately 12 to 15 times per minute, and the inspiratory tidal volume is determined. This volume is then divided by the transmural or intrapleural pressure difference between points of zero airflow (i.e., end-expiration and end-inspiration).

To determine the frequency dependence of compliance, the patient is asked to vary his or her breathing frequency while attempting to keep the tidal volume constant (this can be accomplished by having the patient observe his or her tidal volumes, which can be displayed on an oscillocope). Note that for each dynamic compliance measurement, the average inspiratory tidal volume should be calculated for a minimum of 10 breaths.

Interpretation of Lung Compliance Measurements

Static lung compliance is used to assess the elastic recoil properties of the lungs and chest wall. It is usually determined only for lung volumes between total lung capacity and functional residual capacity, because esophageal estimates of intrapleural pressure for lung volumes below FRC would include expiratory muscular forces, which affect the intrapleural pressure. The slope of the compliance curve during the tidal volume is most often used as a clinical expression of the static lung compliance because of the nonlinearity of the compliance curve near TLC and RV (see Chapter 3). Other methods of reporting data obtained during compliance measurements include the *maximum static recoil pressure*, which is the transpulmonary pressure measured at total lung capacity, and the *coefficient of retraction*. The maximum static recoil pressure is sometimes used as an index of the elasticity of the lungs. The coefficient of retraction is the static recoil pressure relative to the corresponding lung volume. It is calculated by dividing the elastic recoil pressure by the lung volume at which it is determined.

Static lung compliance decreases and elastic recoil pressures increase in fibrotic lung diseases,

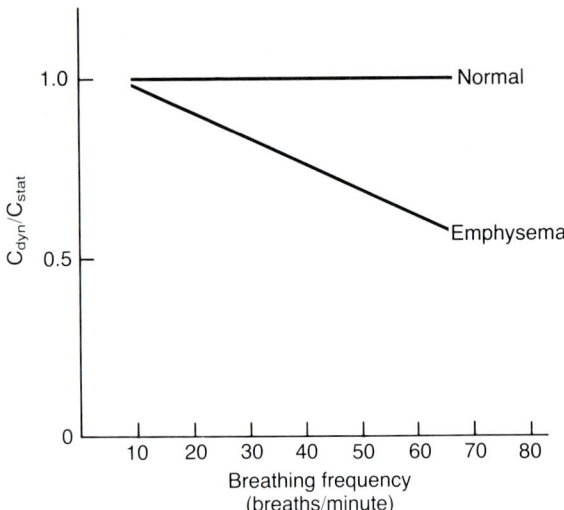

FIGURE 9–10. Ratio of C_{dyn} to C_{stat} for a normal subject and a patient with emphysema.

such as pulmonary interstitial fibrosis, sarcoidosis, or any of the pneumoconioses (see Chapter 5). Static lung compliance is increased and elastic recoil pressures are reduced in pulmonary emphysema patients because of the destruction of lung parenchyma. Lung compliance is also increased in normal subjects over 50 years old as a result of alterations in the elastin and collagen fibers within the lung (Fig. 9–9). Dynamic (frequency-dependent) compliance changes occur in diseases in which there is an asynchronous filling and emptying of lung units caused by increases in airway resistance and/or altered lung compliance. This is most obvious in patients with pulmonary emphysema. In these patients, the ratio of dynamic compliance to static lung compliance decreases as the breathing frequency increases (Fig. 9–10).

DYNAMIC LUNG FUNCTION

Besides the elastic properties of the lungs and chest wall, the mechanical efficiency of ventilation is also influenced by the resistance of the airways and the strength of the respiratory muscles. Some of the tests used to monitor the dynamic properties of the respiratory system include maximum voluntary ventilation, forced expiratory and inspiratory vital capacities, flow volume analysis, airway resistance, and maximum inspiratory and expiratory pressures.

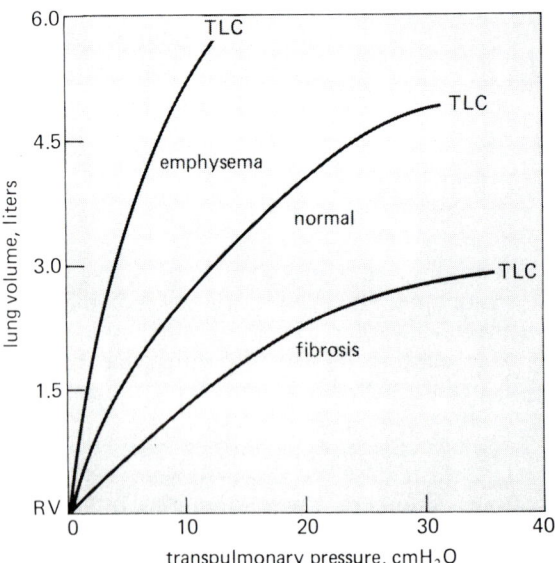

FIGURE 9–9. Expiratory flow-volume traces from a normal subject, a patient with obstructive lung disease, and a patient with restrictive lung disease. (From Levitzky, M.G.: *Pulmonary Physiology*, 2nd ed. New York, McGraw-Hill, 1986, with permission.)

Maximum Voluntary Ventilation

The maximum voluntary ventilation (MVV) is defined as the total volume of air that a patient can move into and out of his or her lungs per minute. It is determined by measuring the total ventilation of the patient while he or she performs a maximum breathing effort (breathing as fast and deep as possible) over a 12-second period. The MVV is then calculated by multiplying the total volume of air exchanged in 12 seconds by 5.

The difference between the MVV and the resting minute ventilation is called the *breathing reserve*. A decreased breathing reserve is associated with dyspnea and a reduction in exercise tolerance. The use of MVV measurements in exercise testing is discussed in Chapter 11.

Forced Vital Capacity

The maximum airflow rates during forced expiratory and inspiratory maneuvers and the volume of air expired in specific time intervals provide valuable information about the flow-resistive properties of the respiratory system. The test is performed by having the patient make a maximum inspiration to TLC, followed by a maximum (forced) expiration to RV. When the residual volume is reached, the patient is then asked to make a maximum (forced) inspiration back to TLC (Fig. 9–11). Several measurements can be obtained from this type of two-stage vital capacity maneuver, including:

1. The forced expiratory vital capacity (FEVC) and the forced inspiratory vital capacity (FIVC). The lung volume changes equal the difference between TLC and RV.
2. The forced expiratory volumes in 1 ($FEV_{1.0}$) and 3 ($FEV_{3.0}$) seconds, which are determined by measuring the volumes of gas exhaled by the patient at 1 and 3 seconds, respectively.
3. The $FEV_{1.0\%}$ and the $FEV_{3.0\%}$, which are calculated by dividing the $FEV_{1.0}$ and $FEV_{3.0}$, respectively, by the vital capacity.
4. The forced expiratory flow between 25% and 75% of the vital capacity (FEF_{25-75}, also known as the maximum midexpiratory flow rate, or MMEFR). It is calculated by dividing the lung volume change that occurs between 25% and 75% of the forced vital capacity by the time interval between these two points. The FEF_{25-75} represents the average airflow during the "effort-independent" portion of the forced vital capacity and thus may be used to assess small airway function.
5. The peak expiratory and inspiratory flow rates (PEF and PIF). The peak flows are determined by calculating the airflows (volume/time) that occur at the beginning of expiration and inspiration, respectively.

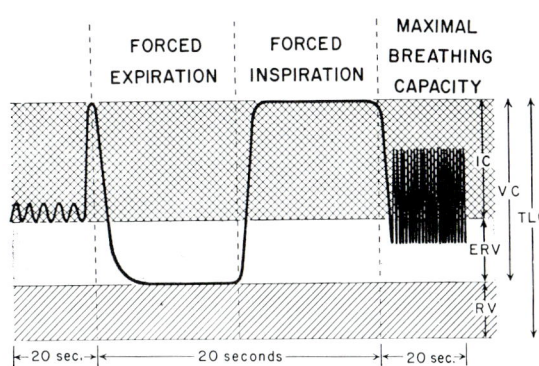

FIGURE 9–11. Volume time tracing of the forced vital capacity from a normal subject. (Reproduced with permission from Forster, R.E., Dubois, A.B., Briscoe, W.A., and Fisher, A.B.: *The Lung, Physiologic Basis of Pulmonary Function Tests*, 3rd ed. Copyright © 1986 by Year Book Medical Publishers, Inc., Chicago.)

Flow-Volume Analysis

Maximum flow-volume loops provide valuable information about the relationship between instantaneous airflow and the volume of air in the lungs. As Figure 9–12 shows, characteristic flow-volume contours can be demonstrated for normal subjects as well as for patients with obstructive and restrictive disorders.

In normal subjects, the peak expiratory airflow occurs near TLC, and then declines as the subject continues to exhale to RV. On inspiration, airflow increases greatly as the airways are pulled open by the large negative pressures generated by the inspiratory muscles. At approximately 25% to 50% of TLC, the airflow reaches a plateau and remains fairly constant until the subject reaches about 75% of his or her total lung capacity, at which point it begins to decrease.

For a patient with an obstructive pulmonary disease, such as emphysema or bronchitis, the expiratory portion of the flow-volume loop is concave, indicating that the airflow decreases precipitously as the patient exhales. As discussed in Chapter 3, this reduction in airflow results from dynamic compression of the airways, which oc-

AIRWAYS RESISTANCE

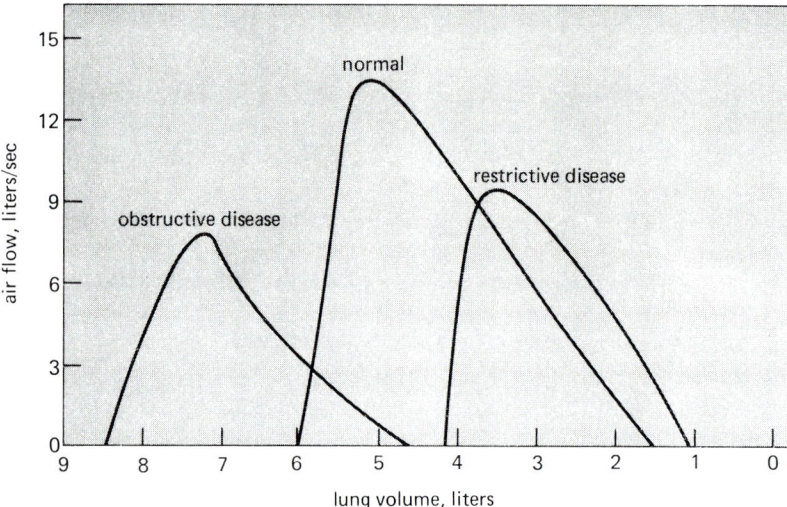

FIGURE 9–12. Expiratory flow-volume curves for a normal subject, a patient with obstructive disease, and a patient with a restrictive disease. (From Levitzky, M.G.: *Pulmonary Physiology*, 2nd ed. New York, McGraw-Hill, 1986, with permission.)

curs as the patient exerts greater expiratory effort and from decreased alveolar elastic recoil. The inspiratory portion of the curve from the patient with obstructive disease shows decreases in maximum airflow rates throughout the inspiration, probably from the effects of hyperinflation on the inspiratory muscular force that can be achieved (i.e., alterations in the length-tension relationships of the inspiratory muscles). (As discussed in Chapter 5, more extensive analysis of flow-volume loops can be used to differentiate intrathoracic and extrathoracic airway obstructions [see Fig. 5–15].)

Flow-volume loops from patients with restrictive pulmonary disease are similar in contour to the normal subject's loop during both expiration and inspiration. Restrictive pulmonary disease can be distinguished from a normal tracing by noting that the flow-volume curve is shifted to the right and that the maximum volume of air expired or inspired during the maneuver is reduced. Inspiratory airflow rates may be low in patients with restrictive disease because of reduced respiratory system compliance; however, this usually does not occur until the disease has progressed to a severe level.

Airway Resistance

In the pulmonary function laboratory, airway resistance is usually determined with the aid of a body plethysmograph. In this test, airway resistance is measured as a ratio of changes in alveolar pressure to airflow at the mouth. To make this determination, the patient is seated within a body box and instructed to breathe tidally into the mouthpiece-shutter assembly, similar to the one used in the thoracic gas volume determinations. At the end of a tidal inspiration, the airway is occluded with the shutter, and the patient is told to pant at a rate of approximately two to three times per second. While the patient continues to pant, the shutter is opened, allowing him or her to pant into and out of a pneumotachograph attached to the mouthpiece-shutter assembly. As the patient pants against the closed shutter, changes in mouth pressure and box pressure are recorded and displayed on the body box's oscilloscope (as Figure 9–13A shows, changes in mouth pressure are plotted on the y-axis while changes in box pressure are plotted on the x-axis). During the open-shutter pant, airflow and changes in box pressure are recorded and displayed on an oscilloscope (as Figure 9–13B shows, airflow is plotted on the y-axis and changes in box pressure are plotted on the x-axis). By calculating the slope of each curve and assuming that the pressure measured at the mouth when no air is flowing is equivalent to the alveolar pressure, airway resistance can be determined:

$$Raw = \frac{\Delta P_{Mouth} \div \Delta P_{Box}}{\dot{V}_{Mouth} \div \Delta P_{Box}}$$

$$Raw = \frac{\Delta P_{Mouth}}{\dot{V}}$$

Note that measurements of airway resistance involve both inspiratory and expiratory airflow. The loops generated can therefore be used to calculate

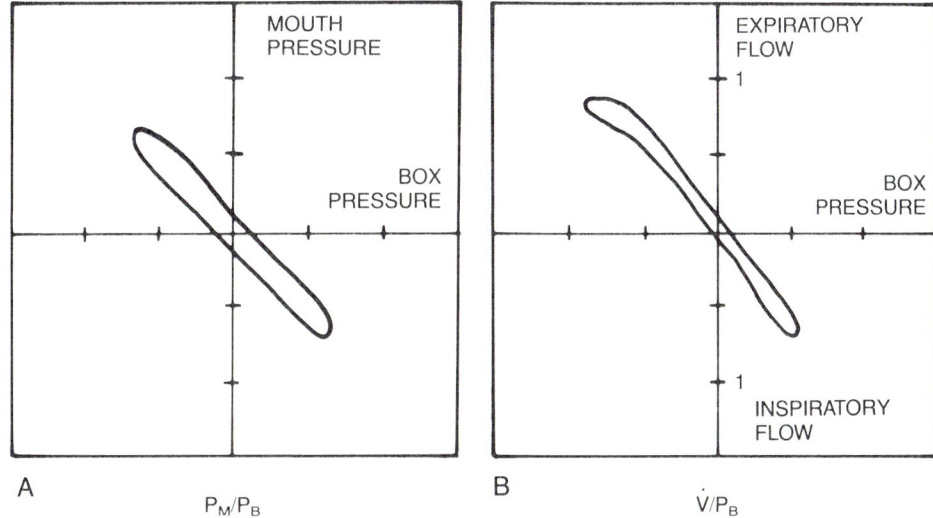

FIGURE 9-13. Plethysmographic pressure-flow loops illustrating how airway resistance measurements are made: *A*, Mouth pressure versus box pressure. *B*, Airflow versus box pressure. (Reproduced with permission from Conrad, S.A., Kinasewitz, G.T., and George, R.B.: *Pulmonary Function Testing. Principles and Practice.* New York, Churchill Livingstone, 1984, p. 146.)

both inspiratory and expiratory resistances. In normal subjects, these two are equal; however, in patients with obstructive pulmonary disease, expiratory airway resistance may be greater than inspiratory airway resistance. It is generally agreed that the inspiratory resistance measurement should be reported. Additionally, in normal subjects, airway resistance is constant at all flow rates encountered during a panting maneuver, while in patients with airway obstruction, airway resistance measurements may increase at high rates of airflow because of decreases in dynamic compliance. Decreased dynamic compliance results in curvilinear pressure-flow plethysmographic recordings. To alleviate this problem, airway resistance measurements are often standardized to flow rates of 0.5 L per second.

An alternate method of expressing airway resistance is *airway conductance* (Gaw), which is the inverse of the airway resistance. Specific conductance is an expression of the airway conductance relative to the lung volume at which Gaw is determined.

Maximum Inspiratory and Expiratory Pressures

The simplest approach to assessing respiratory muscle strength is to measure the maximum inspiratory and expiratory pressures that a patient can attain. (Remember, however, that the maximum respiratory pressures measured also include elastic recoil forces that result from the lungs and chest wall.) This can be easily accomplished with a mouthpiece and a three-way valve connected to a direct-reading pressure gauge. The pressure gauge should be linear from 0 to +100 mmHg and from -10 to -100 mmHg. Figure 9-14 shows the equipment required to perform these measurements. To ensure accuracy, the pressure gauge should be checked periodically using a blood pressure manometer or by measuring the maximum respiratory pressures of a normal individual who works in the laboratory.

The techniques used to determine maximum respiratory forces are relatively easy. The patient is

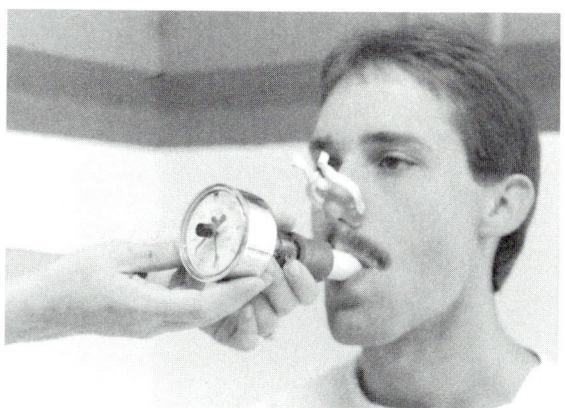

FIGURE 9-14. Equipment used to measure maximal respiratory pressures.

seated upright, with noseclip in place, and instructed to breathe into and out of the mouthpiece. With the three-way valve open to room air, the patient is asked to exhale to residual volume. The valve is turned to the closed position, and the patient is told to make a maximum inspiratory effort for at least 3 seconds. The maximum negative pressure attained after the first second is then recorded. To determine the maximum expiratory force, the three-way valve is returned to the open position, and the patient is instructed to inhale to total lung capacity. When he or she reaches this volume, the valve is closed and the patient is told to make a forceful expiration for 3 seconds. The maximum positive pressure is then recorded. Both maximum inspiratory and expiratory pressures should be recorded a minimum of three times because a lack of patient effort or leakage of air caused by an incomplete seal around the mouthpiece can cause erroneous data. Note that maximum inspiratory and expiratory pressures are measured starting at RV and TLC, respectively, for several reasons; elastic recoil forces of the lungs and chest wall are maximum at these lung volumes, and the inspiratory and expiratory muscle length-tension relationships are at their optimal levels.

In general, the maximum inspiratory pressures in a normal subject are at least -60 mmHg while the maximum expiratory pressures are in the range of $+90$ to $+100$ mmHg. Note that maximum respiratory pressures are useful in monitoring patients with neuromuscular diseases, such as myasthenia gravis and poliomyelitis. Maximum expiratory pressures are useful in assessing the maximum force that a patient can generate during a cough, while maximum inspiratory pressures are often used when weaning patients from mechanical ventilation.

Bronchoprovocation

These tests are usually performed in patients with respiratory symptoms to determine whether *reversible* airway obstruction is the underlying cause. The most commonly used provocation methods include: (1) sympathomimetic and parasympathomimetic drugs and (2) exercise. Our discussion here is limited to pharmacologic bronchoprovocation. The diagnosis of exercise-induced bronchospasm is presented in Chapter 11. The information gained from bronchoprovocation tests can be used to determine whether a patient will benefit from bronchodilator therapy.

Sympathomimetics (Bronchodilators). When airway obstruction is detected in routine pulmonary function tests, an aerosolized bronchodilator is usually administered to determine whether reversible airway obstruction is present. Usually, after a baseline forced vital capacity maneuver is performed by the patient, the drug is administered, and after 15 minutes, the pulmonary function tests are repeated. The bronchodilators used most often include: isoproterenol, metaproterenol, albuterol, and isoetharine. Improvement in the forced expiratory volume in 1 second ($FEV_{1.0}$) of at least 10%, or a 15% to 20% decrease in residual volume, is considered to be a positive response to the bronchodilator. Note that patients should not receive medications, such as cromolyn sodium, or antihistamines for 24 hours prior to the bronchoprovocation tests. Additionally, patients should be instructed not to smoke or consume coffee, tea, or chocolate for 4 to 6 hours before performing the test because ingestion of these substances may alter airway reactivity.

Parasympathomimetics (Bronchoconstrictors). Analogs of acetylcholine, such as methacholine and histamine, are used to diagnose patients with suggestive histories of asthma but with normal physical examinations and normal pulmonary function tests. During the test, the patient performs a series of inhalations of increasing concentrations of the bronchoconstricting drug (e.g., 1, 5, 10, and 25 mg/ml), and maximum expiratory vital capacity is measured after each inhalation. Patients demonstrating a positive response to the drug have a 20% decrease in the $FEV_{1.0}$ (note that the bronchoconstricting effect of these drugs can be reversed with bronchodilators, such as metaproterenol). It should be pointed out that patients with severe obstructive pulmonary diseases, such as chronic bronchitis, may also show a positive response to bronchoprovocation with methacholine and histamine.

DETERMINATION OF THE DISTRIBUTION OF VENTILATION

We have already discussed how normal physiologic factors can influence the distribution of ventilation (see Chapter 3). Pathologic alterations in the resistance and/or compliance characteristics of the lungs can result in a maldistribution of ventilation and lead to significant alterations in gas exchange. The pulmonary function tests routinely used to assess the distribution of ventilation include the single-breath oxygen test and the multibreath nitrogen washout test.

Single-Breath Oxygen Test

The SBO_2 (Fowler's test) is performed by having a patient first inspire 100% oxygen, starting at the residual volume, going up to the total lung capacity, and then exhaling back to the RV into a spirometer equipped with a nitrogen analyzer. Plotting the percent nitrogen measured at the mouth as a function of the expired lung volume as the patient exhales results in a tracing like the one in Figure 9–15.

To understand how the curve is generated, consider what happens during this maneuver. First, the patient exhales to the residual volume. Because of the gradient of intrapleural pressure from the top of the lung to the bottom, alveoli at the top are more distended than those at the bottom. The upper alveoli contain a larger portion of the gas volume left in the lungs at the end of expiration (and therefore a greater amount of nitrogen) than those in the more dependent portions of the lungs (i.e., lower lobes).

The patient then inspires 100% oxygen to total lung capacity. Although the initial portions of the inspiration enter the upper lobes of the lungs, most of the 100% oxygen enters alveoli in the lower lobes of the lungs (note that the first part of the breath that enters the alveoli is from the conducting airways, which contain 80% nitrogen at the end of the maximum expiration). Thus, at the end of the maximum inspiration of 100% oxygen from RV, a higher concentration of nitrogen can be found in the alveoli in the upper lobes of the lung compared with the more dependent alveoli in the lower lobes. The conducting airways contain 100% oxygen.

The patient then exhales to the residual volume, and the percent nitrogen and expired gas volume are measured. The initial expired gas (phase I) is composed of 100% oxygen from the conducting airways. The next portion of gas exhaled (phase II) is a mixture of deadspace gas and alveolar gas. The third portion of gas exhaled by the patient (phase III) is composed of mixed alveolar gas (from alveoli in the upper and lower lung lobes)

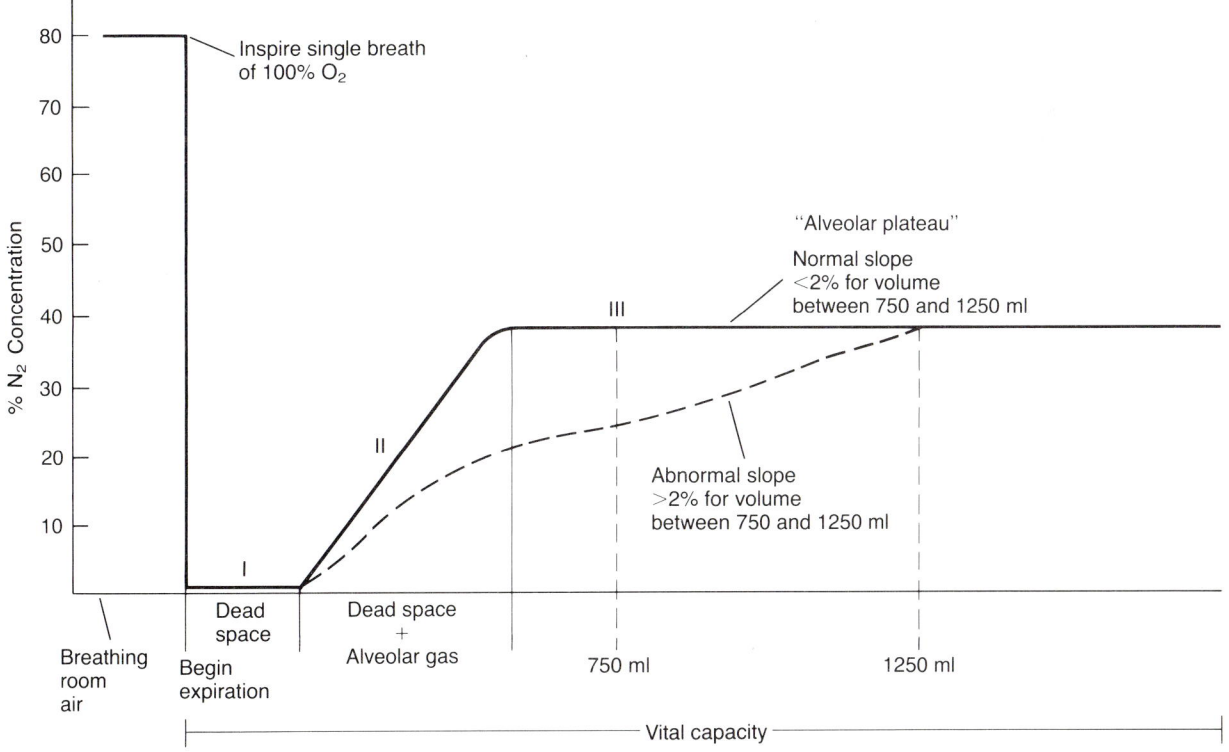

FIGURE 9–15. Graph of a single-breath oxygen test from a normal subject (solid line) and a patient with emphysema (dashed line). Note that the emphysema patient shows a large increase in expired nitrogen concentration between 750 and 1,250 ml of the expired volume.

and is sometimes referred to as the *alveolar plateau*. In normal subjects, a phase IV can also be determined. It has been shown that this phase occurs as nitrogen-rich alveoli at the lung apices continue to empty following closure of the small airways in the bases of the lungs (which are exposed to greater intrapleural pressures and have less alveolar elastic recoil traction). This *closing volume* measurement has been proposed as a test to determine early small airway disease in the asymptomatic population. The closing volume is calculated by subtracting the residual volume from the lung volume at which phase IV begins. The *closing capacity* is calculated by adding the closing volume to the residual volume. Although the closing volume test is not widely used in pulmonary diagnostics, it can be used to show a number of physiologic mechanisms that occur during a respiratory cycle.

In normal adult subjects, the anatomic deadspace, which is approximately 150 ml (or 1 ml per pound of body weight), can be measured by determining the volume of expired air at 50% of phase II. Normal healthy subjects show a fairly constant expired nitrogen concentration during the beginning of phase III (between 750 and 1,250 ml of the expired volume). However, those with many alveoli supplied by small airways with abnormally high resistance to airflow show a rising nitrogen concentration during phase III (a 2% or greater increase). This is because these alveoli receive little of the 100% oxygen and also because they empty more slowly than those supplied by normal airways. Thus, because they contribute increasing expired nitrogen toward the end of the expiration, it may be difficult to distinguish phase II from phase III and determine a closing volume in the single-breath oxygen tracing from a person with maldistribution of ventilation.

Multibreath Nitrogen Washout Test

Distribution of ventilation can be assessed by measuring the concentration of nitrogen in the lungs of a patient at the conclusion of a 7-minute nitrogen washout test. Normal subjects can wash out 98% of the nitrogen in their lungs within 7 minutes. The nitrogen concentration in the lungs of a patient with a maldistribution of ventilation, such as from obstructive pulmonary disease, is higher than 2% at the end of 7 minutes. With the introduction of spirometers equipped with rapid responding nitrogen analyzers, breath-by-breath measurements of percent nitrogen and expired lung volumes can be recorded and used to distinguish fast and slow alveoli. By plotting the expired lung volume versus the logarithm of the percent nitrogen, distribution of ventilation can be assessed by noting the slope of the resultant curve. As Figure 9–16 shows, normal subjects show a rapid decrease in the slope of this curve compared with patients with emphysema. The decreased slope for the patient with emphysema results from the presence of alveoli that have increased resistance and/or decreased compliance.

DETERMINATION OF LUNG DIFFUSING CAPACITY

As discussed in Chapters 1 and 3, the factors that influence the diffusion rate of a gas through a semipermeable membrane are described by Fick's law of diffusion, which is:

$$\dot{V}gas = A \times D \times (P_1 - P_2) \div T$$

where $\dot{V}gas$ is the volume of gas diffusing through the membrane per unit time, A is the surface area available for diffusion, D is the diffusion coefficient or diffusivity of the gas crossing the membrane (this is related to the solubility and molecular weight of the gas), $P_1 - P_2$ is the partial pressure gradient of the gas across the membrane, and T is the thickness of the membrane.

In the pulmonary function laboratory, the diffusion characteristics of the alveolar-capillary barrier can be assessed by measuring the rate of uptake of gases, such as oxygen or carbon monoxide, for a given partial pressure gradient of the gas between the alveoli and pulmonary capillaries. The units of this measurement, which is called the *diffusing capacity* (D_{LX}), are ml/min/mmHg because it is derived from the following relationship:

$$D_{LX} = \frac{\dot{V}x}{P_{AX} - P_{CX}} = ml/min/mmHg$$

This equation is really just a rearrangement of Fick's law of diffusion because the area, diffusivity, and thickness factors contribute to the D_{LX} term as shown below:

$$D_{LX} = \frac{\dot{V}x}{P_{AX} - P_{CX}} = \frac{A \times D}{T}$$

Clinically, three kinds of methods are used to determine lung diffusing capacity. These include steady state, rebreathing, and single-breath methods for oxygen and carbon monoxide. The steady

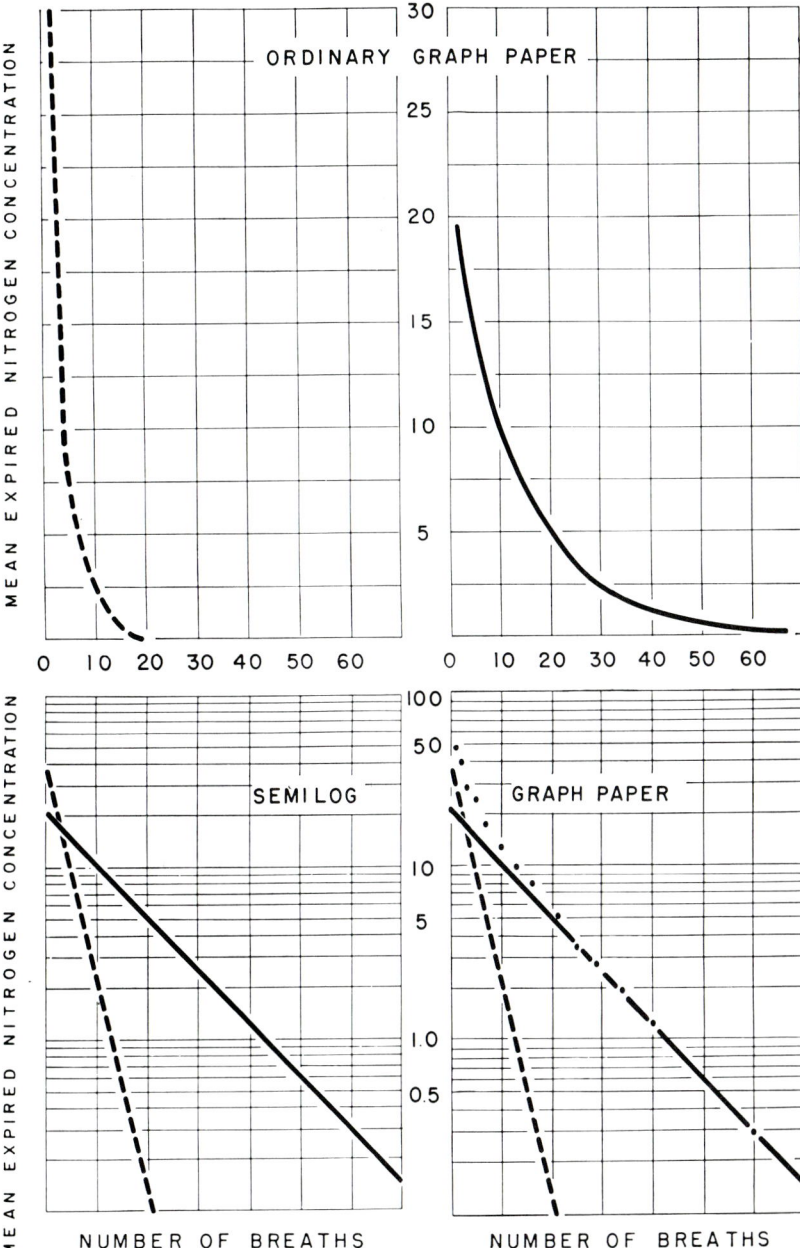

FIGURE 9–16. Expired lung volume versus the number of breaths plotted on ordinary graph paper (top) and on semi-log paper (bottom) for a normal subject (*A*) and a patient with emphysema (*B*). (Reproduced with permission from Forster, R.E., Dubois, A.B., Briscoe, W.A., and Fisher, A.B.: *The Lung, Physiologic Basis of Pulmonary Function Tests,* 3rd ed. Copyright © 1986 by Year Book Medical Publishers, Inc., Chicago.)

state and rebreathing methods are most often used to determine diffusing capacity in exercising patients, while the single-breath method is commonly used to assess diffusing capacity in resting patients. Our discussion is limited to the single-breath (carbon monoxide) technique because it is used most often in clinical pulmonary function laboratories.

Single-Breath Carbon Monoxide Test

In the single-breath carbon monoxide test (or $D_{L_{CO}}$), the patient is seated upright and allowed to breathe through a three-way valve that can be opened either to room air or to a reservoir containing a gas mixture of 0.3% carbon monoxide, 21% oxygen, 10% helium, and the balance of nitrogen. With the valve turned to room air, the patient is instructed to expire to residual volume. At the end of the maximum expiration, the three-way valve is turned to the reservoir, and the patient is asked to inspire maximally and then hold his or her breath for 10 seconds. The end-expiratory gas, which is free of deadspace gas, is then collected and analyzed. Carbon monoxide is used as a tracer gas in this test because it is not normally found in high concentrations within the pulmonary capillary blood and it has such a high affinity for hemoglobin (approximately 210 times greater than oxygen) that essentially none of it remains dissolved in the plasma. Thus, carbon monoxide uptake is not limited by a decrease in its pressure gradient across the membrane (as occurs in *perfusion-limited* transfer of gases, such as nitrous oxide) but rather by the diffusion characteristics of the alveolar-capillary membrane and hemoglobin content of the red blood cells in contact with alveolar air (its transfer is *diffusion-limited*).

The calculation of single-breath carbon monoxide diffusing capacity is therefore performed using the following equation:

$$D_{L_{CO}} = \frac{\dot{V}_{CO}}{P_{A_{CO}} - P_{c_{CO}}}$$

where $\dot{V}_{CO}$ equals the uptake of carbon monoxide by the pulmonary capillaries per minute, $P_{A_{CO}}$ equals the partial pressure for carbon monoxide in the alveoli, and $P_{c_{CO}}$ is the mean partial pressure of carbon monoxide in the pulmonary capillaries. If we assume that the amount of carbon monoxide normally present in the pulmonary capillaries is negligible, then the $D_{L_{CO}}$ can be determined from the uptake of carbon monoxide per minute and the mean alveolar partial pressure of carbon monoxide, or

$$D_{L_{CO}} = \frac{\dot{V}_{CO}}{P_{A_{CO}}}$$

Note that diffusing capacity is influenced by lung volume. Helium is included in the gas mixture so that the alveolar volume at which the lung diffusing capacity is measured can be determined by a simple dilution calculation (alternatively, the lung volume at which the diffusing capacity measurement is made can be determined by measuring the volume of air inspired and adding this to the residual volume, which had been determined using indirect techniques or body plethysmography). The $D_{L_{CO}}$ should be reported with the alveolar volume at which the measurement was made (this is usually reported as the $D_{L_{CO}}/V_A$).

Lung diffusing capacity is decreased in diseases associated with:
1. A decreased surface area available for diffusion, such as emphysema or the removal of a lung (lobectomy).
2. An increase in the thickness of the alveolar-capillary barrier, such as interstitial or alveolar fibrosis and interstitial or alveolar edema.
3. A decreased hemoglobin concentration, such as anemia.
4. A ventilation-perfusion mismatch, such as that caused by pulmonary emboli.

Conversely, lung diffusing capacity is increased by conditions that are associated with:
1. An increase in the alveolar-capillary surface area available for diffusion, such as during exercise or elevations in pulmonary artery pressure.
2. An increase in red blood cell volume, such as occurs in polycythemia.

Table 9–4 summarizes various conditions that can alter the lung diffusing capacity.

ASSESSMENT OF VENTILATION-PERFUSION

A number of methods are available to assess the presence or location of areas of the lung with mismatched ventilation and perfusion. These methods include calculations of the physiologic deadspace, and the physiologic shunt, determination of differences between the alveolar and arterial P_{O_2}s and P_{CO_2}s, and findings on lung scans after inhaled and intravenously administered ^{133}Xe.

Calculation of Physiologic Deadspace

The amount of wasted ventilation (i.e., the amount of ventilation that does not participate in gas exchange) can be calculated using the Bohr equation. This equation is based on the concept that any measurable volume of carbon dioxide found in the mixed expired gas must come from alveoli that are both ventilated and perfused. This is because inspired air contains negligible amounts of carbon dioxide; therefore, the CO_2 in the expired gas must be from the mixed venous blood. Furthermore, inspired air remaining in the anatomic deadspace or

TABLE 9–4. Evaluation of D_{LCO}

Abnormality	Pathophysiology	Examples
Increased D_{LCO}	1. Increase in pulmonary capillary blood volume.	Left heart failure, left-to-right shunts (atrial septal defect, anomalous pulmonary venous return), exercise, altitude, supine position.
	2. Increase in red blood cells.	Early in polycythemia.
Decreased D_{LCO}	1. Deficiency in red blood cells.	Anemia.
	2. Loss of pulmonary capillary bed with relatively normal lung volume.	Multiple pulmonary emboli, early collagen-vascular disease, early in sarcoidosis and miliary tuberculosis.
	3. Loss of functioning alveolar-capillary bed with increased lung volume.	Emphysema.
	4. Loss of functioning alveolar-capillary bed with decreased lung volume.	Pulmonary resection, idiopathic interstitial fibrosis, asbestosis, scleroderma lung disease, histiocytosis-X, sarcoidosis, pneumonia.
	5. Failure of inspired air to reach alveoli (i.e., poor distribution of ventilation), with low, normal, or increased lung volume.	Severe bronchospasm. Frequently with emphysema.

(From Ayers, L.N., Whipp, B.J., and Ziment, I.: *A Guide to the Interpretation of Pulmonary Function Tests,* 2nd ed. New York, Pfizer Pharmaceuticals, 1978, with permission.)

entering unperfused alveoli will leave the body as it entered, i.e., no P_{CO_2}.

The physiologic deadspace ratio is calculated using the following equation:

$$\frac{V_{D_{CO_2}}}{V_T} = \frac{PaCO_2 - PeCO_2}{PaCO_2}$$

where the $PaCO_2$ is determined from arterial blood gas analysis and the P_{CO_2} of mixed expired gas is determined using a CO_2 meter (e.g., a nondispersive infrared CO_2 analyzer). The physiologic deadspace, as calculated by the Bohr equation, includes *both* the anatomic and the alveolar deadspace, as noted in Chapter 3. If the $PaCO_2$ is greater than the P_{CO_2} determined by sampling end-tidal CO_2, then the physiologic deadspace is probably greater than the anatomic deadspace. Thus, a significant arterial-alveolar difference in carbon dioxide means that there is significant alveolar deadspace.

Once the V_D/V_T is measured, the deadspace volume can be calculated by determining the tidal volume with a spirometer and multiplying this value by V_D/V_T.

Anatomic deadspace decreases with bronchoconstriction or compression on the airways. It increases with bronchodilation or increased traction of the airways.

Alveolar deadspace normally decreases during exercise and in situations in which the cardiac output is increased. It is increased in situations in which portions of the pulmonary vasculature are occluded by blood clots or other material in the venous blood (pulmonary embolism); in situations in which venous return is reduced, leading to low right ventricular output (hemorrhage); or in situations in which alveolar pressure is high (positive pressure ventilation).

Calculation of Physiologic Shunt

In Chapter 3, we defined right-to-left shunts as the mixing of venous blood that has not been oxygenated (or fully oxygenated) into the arterial blood. Physiologic shunts are divided into anatomic and intrapulmonary shunts, with intrapulmonary shunts being subdivided into absolute shunts ($\dot{V}/\dot{Q}=0$) and "shunt-like states" (areas of low $\dot{V}/\dot{Q}$).

Clinically, we can estimate the physiologic shunt by using the shunt equation, or

$$\frac{\dot{Q}s}{\dot{Q}t} = \frac{Cc'_{O_2} - Ca_{O_2}}{Cc'_{O_2} - C\bar{v}_{O_2}}$$

where $\dot{Q}s/\dot{Q}t$ equals the physiologic shunt, Cc'_{O_2} equals end-capillary oxygen content, Ca_{O_2} equals arterial oxygen content, and $C\bar{v}_{O_2}$ equals mixed venous oxygen content. Arterial and mixed venous oxygen contents can be determined if blood samples are obtained from a systemic artery and from the pulmonary artery (for mixed venous blood). The oxygen content of blood at the end of pulmonary capillaries with well-matched ventilation and perfusion cannot be measured directly and therefore must be calculated from the *alveolar air equation* (see Chapter 3).

The *shunt equation* divides all alveolar-capillary units into two groups: those with well-matched ventilation and perfusion and those with ventilation-perfusion ratios of zero. Thus, the shunt equation combines absolute shunts (including anatomic shunts) and shunt-like areas into a single conceptual group. The resultant ratio of shunt flow to cardiac output, often referred to as *venous admixture*, is the part of the cardiac output that would have to be perfusing absolutely unventilated alveoli to cause the systemic arterial oxygen content obtained from a particular patient. A much larger portion of the cardiac output could be overperfusing poorly ventilated alveoli and yield the same ratio.

The relative contributions of absolute intrapulmonary shunts and shunt-like states to the calculated shunt flow can be estimated by repeating the measurements and calculations while the patient is breathing a normal or slightly elevated inspired concentration of oxygen, and then while he or she is breathing a very high concentration of inspired oxygen, e.g., F_{IO_2}'s of 0.95 to 1.00. At low F_{IO_2}'s the calculated shunt flow will include both the true shunts and the alveolar-capillary units with low ventilation-perfusion ratios. After the patient has breathed 100% oxygen for 20 to 30 minutes, even alveoli with low $\dot{V}/\dot{Q}$'s have high enough alveolar P_{O_2}'s to completely saturate the hemoglobin in the blood perfusing them. These latter units therefore no longer contribute to calculated $\dot{Q}s/\dot{Q}t$, and the new calculated shunt should include only areas of absolute shunt. (Note: prolonged breathing of very high F_{IO_2}'s may lead to absorption atelectasis of poorly ventilated alveoli that remain perfused, and so this test may alter what it is trying to measure when high F_{IO_2}'s are used.)

Alveolar-Arterial Oxygen Differences

From our discussion so far, you should understand that CO_2 normally shows complete equilibration across the alveolar-capillary membrane, so that the end-capillary P_{CO_2}'s equal the alveolar P_{CO_2}'s. Additionally, you've learned that approximately 3 to 5% of the cardiac output normally bypasses the pulmonary circulation (by flowing through anatomic shunts) and mixes with blood returning via the pulmonary veins to the left atrium, resulting in what is referred to as the normal *physiologic shunt*.

In normal healthy individuals, this normal venous admixture, plus a normal degree of regional $\dot{V}/\dot{Q}$ mismatch and some diffusion gradient, results in an alveolar-arterial oxygen difference of 5 to 15 torr. Larger than normal differences between alveolar and arterial P_{O_2} may be caused by larger right-to-left shunts, abnormal mismatching of ventilation and perfusion, and diffusion impairments. (Note that the $P(A-a)O_2$ may not be elevated in cases of hypoventilation, in which both alveolar and arterial P_{O_2}'s are reduced.)

To determine the $P(A-a)O_2$, the P_{AO_2} is calculated using the alveolar air equation, and the P_{aO_2} is measured using standard arterial blood gas analysis.

ASSESSMENT OF THE CONTROL OF BREATHING

The classic tests used to evaluate the control of breathing involve the inhalation of hypercapnic and hypoxic gas mixtures. During the past two decades, investigators have extended the analyses of respiratory control by studying the ventilatory responses to various stimuli, such as elastic and resistive loads, exercise, and sleep. Although these tests can be used to document alterations in the control of breathing, they provide limited information about the location of the dysfunction. Furthermore, conditions that impair the mechanics of breathing may result in decreased responses to hypercapnia and hypoxia even if the respiratory control mechanisms themselves are not impaired. Thus, control of breathing studies must be interpreted along with other pulmonary function data. In the following sections, only those tests commonly performed in clinical pulmonary function laboratories are discussed. Further information on specialized techniques used to assess the control of breathing can be found in the references listed at the end of this chapter.

Ventilatory Response to Inhaled Hypercapnic Gas Mixtures

The physiologic response to increasing levels of carbon dioxide in the inspired air is mediated through the central controller in the brain stem, the central chemoreceptors in the medulla, and peripheral chemoreceptors in the carotid bodies and the aortic bodies. The most common technique used to estimate the ventilatory response to inhaled carbon dioxide (typically a 7% carbon dioxide, 93% oxygen mixture) is to relate the minute ventilation and the arterial $P{CO_2}$ attained while the subject breathes the gas mixture. As Figure 9–17 shows, this relationship is linear for healthy subjects. The slope of this line, which is used as a measure of the responsiveness to carbon dioxide, averages 1.5 to 2.0 L/min/m²/mmHg. Patients with chronic obstructive pulmonary diseases, such as emphysema and chronic bronchitis, have a depressed response to inhaled carbon dioxide. Metabolic alkalosis, opiate alkaloids and their derivatives, barbiturates, and most anesthetics also depress the response to carbon dioxide. Metabolic acidosis and hypoxia enhance the response to inhaled carbon dioxide.

Ventilatory Response to Inhaled Hypoxic Gas Mixtures

The ventilatory response to hypoxia arises solely from the peripheral chemoreceptors. As Figure 9–18 shows, during isocapnic breathing, normal healthy subjects demonstrate a curvilinear ventilatory response for PaO_2 between 20 and 100 torr.

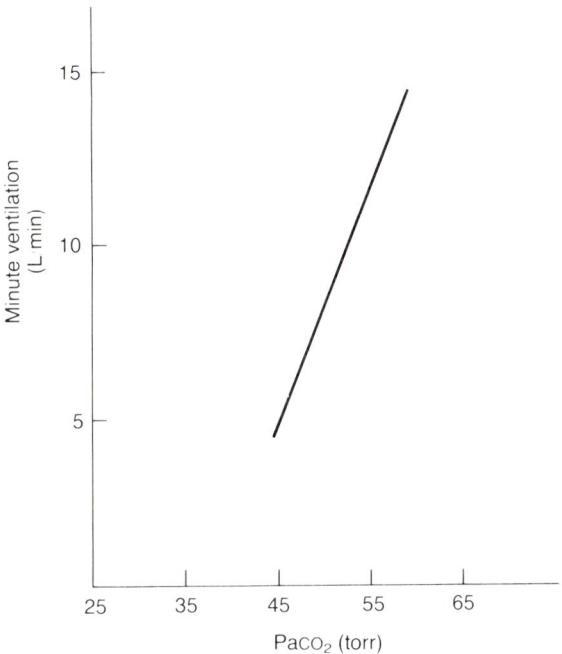

FIGURE 9–17. Ventilatory response to breathing CO_2.

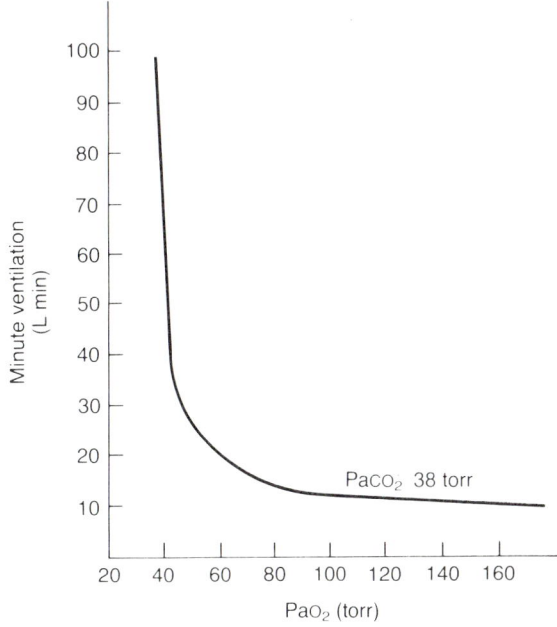

FIGURE 9–18. Ventilatory response to breathing hypoxic gas mixtures.

Note that in the absence of the peripheral chemoreceptors, the effect of increasing degrees of hypoxia is direct depression of the central respiratory controller. These studies are usually performed with gas mixtures containing 15% to 21% oxygen and the rest nitrogen.

Respiration and Sleep

As discussed in Chapter 5, sleep-related disorders associated with respiratory control dysfunctions are classified as: (1) *obstructive sleep apnea,* (2) *central sleep apnea,* and (3) *mixed apnea.*

Obstructive sleep disorders result from upper airway occlusion and are identified by a cessation of airflow in the presence of a continued respiratory effort. Central sleep apnea is characterized by a lack of all respiratory effort for periods exceeding 10 seconds or the equivalent of three respiratory cycles. Mixed apnea is characterized by a cessation of both airflow and respiratory effort.

Although information obtained from a patient and his or her family and a physical assessment may provide useful information about sleep-related disorders, *polysomnography,* which usually includes all-night monitoring of airflow, respiratory inductive plethysmography, and oximetry, is required to diagnose the presence of sleep apnea. Figure 9–19 shows polysomnograms from two patients with obstructive and central sleep apnea.

320 PULMONARY ASSESSMENT

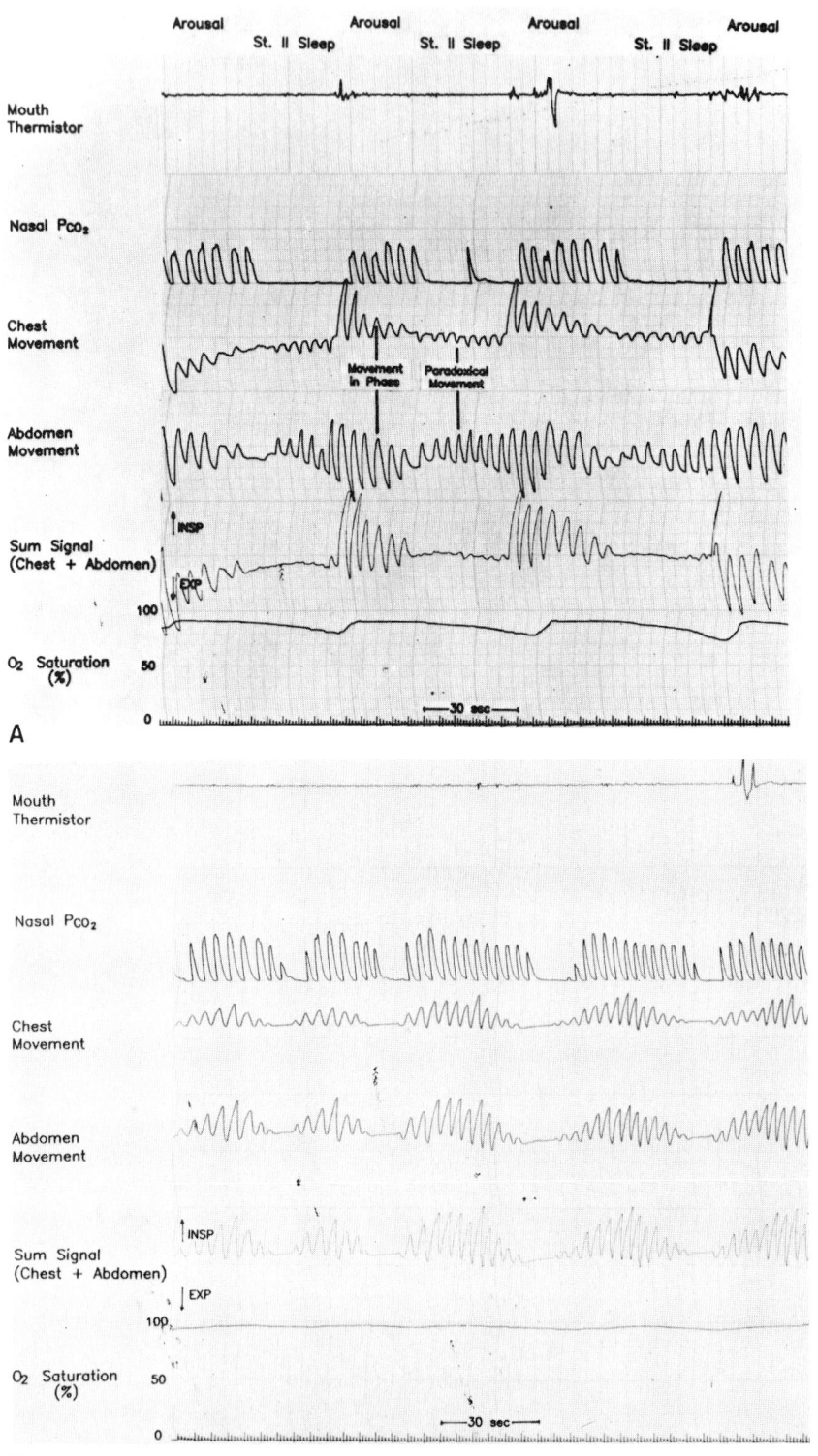

FIGURE 9–19. Polysomnogram from patients with: *A,* Obstructive sleep apnea. *B,* Central sleep apnea. Note that in the patient with obstructive sleep apnea, there is persistent movement of the abdomen and chest sensors (inductance plethysmography), with the absence of airflow at the mouth (thermistor tracing nasal P_{CO_2}). For the patient with central sleep apnea, there is a complete cessation of abdominal and chest wall movements as well as an absence of airflow at the mouth. (From Miller, A. (ed.): *Pulmonary Function Tests. A Guide for the Student and House Officer.* Orlando, Grune & Stratton, 1987, with permission.)

Note that polysomnography may also include electroencephalography (EEG), electro-oculography (EOG), electromyography (EMG), and electrocardiography (ECG).

Bibliography

Anthonisen, N.R.: Tests of mechanical function. In Macklem, P.T., and Mead, J. (eds.): *Handbook of Physiology,* vol. 3. Bethesda, MD, American Physiological Society, 1986.

Askanazi, J., Nordenstrom, J., Rosenbaum, S.H., et al.: Nutrition for the patient with respiratory failure: Glucose versus fat. *Anesthesiology* 54:373–377, 1981.

Bass, H.: The flow-volume loop: Normal standards and abnormalities in chronic obstructive pulmonary disease. *Chest* 63:171–176, 1973.

Black, L.F., and Hyatt, R.E.: Maximal respiratory pressures: Normal values and relationship to age and sex. *Am. Rev. Resp. Dis.* 99:696–702, 1969.

Black, L.F., and Hyatt, R.E.: Maximal static respiratory pressures in generalized neuromuscular disease. *Am. Rev. Resp. Dis.* 103:641–650, 1971.

Black, L.F., Offord, K., and Hyatt, R.E.: Variability in the maximal expiratory flow volume curve in asymptomatic smokers and nonsmokers. *Am. Rev. Resp. Dis.* 110:282–292, 1974.

Blackburn, G.L., Bistrian, B.R., Maini, B.S., et al.: Nutritional assessment of the hospitalized patient. *JPEN* 1:11–22, 1977.

Clausen, J.L., (ed.) *Pulmonary Function Testing. Guidelines and Controversies. Equipment, Methods, and Normal Values.* New York, Academic Press, 1982.

Conrad, S.A., Kinasewitz, G.T., and George, R.B.: *Pulmonary Function Testing, Principles and Practice.* New York, Churchill Livingstone, 1984.

Cormier, Y., and Belanger, J.: Contribution of gas exchange to slope of phase III of the single breath nitrogen test. *J. Appl. Physiol.* 50:1,156–1,160, 1981.

Cotes, J.L.: *Lung Function.* Oxford, Blackwell Scientific Publications, 1979.

Crapo, R.O., and Morris, A.H.: Standardized single breath normal values for carbon monoxide diffusing capacity. *Am. Rev. Resp. Dis.* 123:185–189, 1981.

Crapo, R.O., Morris, A.H., and Gardner, R.M.: Reference spirometric values using techniques and equipment that meet ATS recommendations. *Am. Rev. Resp. Dis.* 123:659–664, 1981.

Cropp, G.J.A.: Guidelines for bronchial inhalation challenges with pharmocologic and antigenic agents. *Am. Thorac. Soc. News* Spring, 1980, pp. 11–19.

Ferris, B.G., Anderson, D.O., and Zickmantel, R.: Prediction values for screening tests of pulmonary function. *Am. Rev. Resp. Dis.* 91:252–261, 1965.

Forster, R.E., Dubois, A.B., Briscoe, W.A., and Fisher, A.B.: *The Lung, Physiologic Basis of Pulmonary Function Tests,* 3rd ed. Chicago, Year Book, 1986.

Gaensler, E.A.: Analysis of the ventilatory defect by timed vital capacity measurement. *Am. Rev. Tuberc.* 64:256–278, 1951.

Gardner, R.M., Baker C.D., Boennle, A.M. Jr., et al.: ATS statement—Snowbird workshop on standardization of spirometry. *Am. Rev. Resp. Dis.* 119:831–838, 1979.

Gilbert, R., Auchincloss, J.H., and Bleb, S.: Measurement of maximal inspiratory pressure during routine spirometry. *Lung* 155:23–32, 1978.

Holley, H.S., Milic-Emili, J., Becklake, M.R., et al.: Regional distribution of pulmonary ventilation and perfusion in obesity. *J. Clin. Invest.* 46:475–481, 1967.

Hutchinson, J.: On the capacity of the lungs and on respiratory functions. *Med. Chir. Soc. (London) Trans.* 29:137, 1846.

Jalowayski, A.A., and Dawson, A.: Measurement of lung volume. The multiple breath nitrogen method. In Clausen, J.L., (ed.): *Pulmonary Function Testing. Guidelines and Controversies. Equipment, Methods, and Normal Values.* New York, Academic Press, 1982.

Knudson, R.J., Burrows, B., and Lebowitz, M.D.: The maximal expiratory flow-volume curve: Its use in the detection of ventilatory abnormalities in a population study. *Am. Rev. Resp. Dis.* 114:871–879, 1979.

Knudson, R.J., Slatin, R.C., Lebowitz, M.D., et al.: The maximal expiratory flow-volume curve. Normal standards, variability and effects of age. *Am. Rev. Resp. Dis.* 113:587–600, 1976.

Milic-Emili, J., Henderson, J.A.M., Dolovich, M.B., et al.: Regional distribution of inspired gas in the lung. *J. Appl. Physiol.* 21:749–759, 1966.

Miller, A.: *Pulmonary Function Tests in Clinical and Occupational Lung Disease.* New York, Grune and Stratton, 1985.

Miller, A.: *Pulmonary Function Tests. A Guide for the Student and the House Officer.* Orlando, Grune and Stratton, 1987.

Morris, A.H., Kanner, R.E., Crapo, R.O., et al.: *Clinical Pulmonary Function Testing: A Manual for Uniform Laboratory Procedures,* 2nd ed. Salt Lake City, Utah, Intermountain Thoracic Society, 1984.

Morris, J.F., Koski, A., and Johnson, L.C.: Spirometric standards for healthy nonsmoking adults. *Am. Rev. Resp. Dis.* 103:57–67, 1971.

Ogilvie, C.M., Forster, R.E., Blackmore, W.S., et al.: A standardized breath holding technique for the clinical measurement of the diffusing capacity of the lung for carbon monoxide. *J. Clin. Invest.* 36:1–17, 1957.

Polgar, G., and Promadhat, V.: *Pulmonary Function Testing in Children: Techniques and Standards.* Philadelphia, W.B. Saunders Co., 1971.

Rahn, H., Otis, A.B., Chadwick, L.E., et al.: The pressure-volume diagram of thorax and lung. *Am. J. Physiol.* 146:161–178, 1946.

Rodarte, J.R., Hyatt, R.E., and Westbrook, P.R.: Determination of lung volume by single and multiple breath nitrogen washout. *Am. Rev. Resp. Dis.* 126:515–520, 1982.

Ruppel, G.: *Manual of Pulmonary Function Testing.* St. Louis, C.V. Mosby, 1982.

Sharp, J.G., Danon, J., Druz, W.S., et al.: Respiratory muscle function in patients with chronic obstructive pulmonary disease. *Am. Rev. Resp. Dis.* 110:154–167, 1974.

Shoenburg, J.B., Beck, G.H., and Bouhuys, A.: Growth and decay of pulmonary function in healthy blacks and whites. *Resp. Physiol.* 33:367–393, 1978.

Smith, A.A., and Gaensler, E.A.: Timing of forced expiratory volume in one second. *Am. Rev. Resp. Dis.* 112:882–885, 1971.

Spriggs, E.A.: The history of spirometry. *Br. J. Dis. Chest* 72:165–180, 1978.

Westenkow, D.R., Cutler, C.A., and Wallace, W.D.: Instrumentation for monitoring gas exchange and metabolic rate in critically ill patients. *Crit. Care Med.* 12(3):183–187, 1984.

Woolcock, A.J., Vincent, N.J., and Macklem, P.T.: Frequency dependence of compliance as a test for obstruction in the small airways. *J. Clin. Invest.* 48:1,097–1,106, 1969.

Wynn, J.W., Block, A.J., Hemenway, J., et al.: Disordered breathing and oxygen saturation during sleep in chronic obstructive lung disease. *Am. J. Med.* 66:573–579, 1979.

OBJECTIVES

AFTER READING THIS CHAPTER, THE STUDENT WILL BE ABLE TO:

1. Differentiate values actually measured by electrodes in a blood gas analyzer from values that are calculated.
2. Describe the proper technique for obtaining a sample of arterial blood for blood gas analysis from an arterial line and by arterial puncture.
3. List common complications associated with obtaining a sample of arterial blood. Describe and explain the purpose of an Allen's test.
4. Explain the proper technique for obtaining a sample of mixed venous blood for blood gas analysis and state some problems associated with improper technique.
5. Summarize the steps for appropriate interpretation of arterial blood gas values.
6. Discuss the clinical interventions for hypoxia. Describe pathologic conditions that may be induced by hyperoxia.
7. Relate the influence of P_{CO_2} and bicarbonate levels on the pH of blood.
8. List the eleven acid-base states and give examples of clinical conditions that may induce these states.
9. Compare invasive versus noninvasive methods of monitoring cardiopulmonary status. List commonly used noninvasive monitors and their most frequent clinical applications.

10
ANALYSIS OF BLOOD GASES AND ACID-BASE BALANCE

CHAPTER OUTLINE

BLOOD GAS ANALYSIS
  The pH Electrode
  The P_{CO_2} Electrode
  The P_{O_2} Electrode
  Blood Gas Analyzer Calculations
OBTAINING SPECIMENS FOR BLOOD GAS ANALYSIS
  Arterial Blood Gas Analysis
  Arterial Puncture
  Arterial Catheterization
  Mixed Venous Blood Gas Analysis
  Other Sites for Blood Gas Samples
INTERPRETING BLOOD GASES
  Interpretation of Arterial Blood Gases
    Evaluation of Oxygenation
    Evaluation of Acid-Base Status
    Compensated Acid-Base States
    Uncompensated Acid-Base States
    Mixed Respiratory and Metabolic Acid-Base States
  Interpretation of Venous Blood Gases
  Interpretation of Capillary Blood Gases
  Interpretation of Umbilical Blood Gases
TRANSCUTANEOUS P_{O_2} AND P_{CO_2}
OXIMETRY
  Co-Oximetry
  Venous Oximetry
  Pulse Oximetry
CAPNOGRAPHY
  Infrared Absorption Analysis
  Mass Spectrometry

324 ANALYSIS OF BLOOD GASES AND ACID-BASE BALANCE

The physical principles that govern the way gases are carried in the blood and other fluids are discussed in Chapter 1. Oxygen must be delivered to the body cells for use in aerobic metabolism to produce adenosine triphosphate (ATP). When one glucose molecule is broken down (catabolized) aerobically in the mitochondrion, 36 ATP molecules are produced in addition to water and carbon dioxide. This mitochondrial process is called oxidative phosphorylation because oxygen is consumed when low-energy adenosine diphosphate (ADP) is converted to high-energy ATP by the addition of phosphate (phosphorylation).

Anaerobic (without oxygen present) metabolism produces only two ATP molecules for each glucose molecule catabolized. Lactic acid is produced as a waste product from this inefficient form of metabolism. Obviously, much more ATP is produced by aerobic breakdown of a glucose molecule than by anaerobic breakdown.

ATP is a vital molecule inside the cell because it produces energy for different types of cellular work:

1. ATP is necessary to supply energy for the enzymes responsible for transporting material across cell membranes. Thus, Na^+/K^+ ATPase requires energy from the breakdown of ATP to move sodium and potassium through the cellular membrane.

2. Mechanical work, such as the sliding of actin and myosin filaments upon each other inside of muscle cells to produce muscular contraction, requires energy from ATP.

3. ATP is utilized to provide energy for synthetic biochemical processes in the cell that produce large or complex molecules (anabolism). For example, the energy of ATP is used to form the bonds between amino acids (peptide bonds) when proteins are formed.

In order to be consumed during aerobic metabolism, oxygen enters the cell as the final step of a transport pathway beginning in the air outside of the body. First, air is inhaled into the lungs, then the oxygen diffuses across the alveolar-capillary membrane, enters the blood cells, and combines with hemoglobin. The circulatory system carries the blood from the lung capillaries to the capillaries of all the other tissues of the body. The oxygen diffuses out of the slow-moving capillary blood and into the cells of the tissues. Finally, it arrives at the mitochondria, where oxygen concentration is lowest because of its constant consumption.

Almost all cells are within 70 μ from a capillary, so the distance that oxygen must diffuse to reach the cell is relatively small. (Remember that a red blood cell is 7 to 10 μ in diameter.) The pathway for carbon dioxide removal from the cells is the same as that for oxygen entry, but in the opposite direction; carbon dioxide is carried in the venous blood to the lungs, where it diffuses into the alveoli.

A sample of blood from any systemic artery should have the same oxygen tension as the blood in the aorta. This is because the blood is completely mixed as it passes through the left ventricle, and little diffusion of the oxygen through arterial walls occurs because of their thickness and because the flow is so rapid through the arteries. An uncommon exception is a perinatal condition called preductal coarctation (narrowing) of the aorta in which the arteries of the lower extremities have a lower oxygen tension than those in the head and upper extremities.

If the arterial blood has low oxygen tension (hypoxemia), the diffusion of oxygen into the tissues may be inadequate for their metabolic demands (hypoxia), resulting in anaerobic metabolism. If hypoxia persists, cell damage and death can result. The rapidity at which cell death occurs depends upon the degree of hypoxia and the metabolic rate of the tissues, as well as their ability to produce energy by anaerobic metabolism. The muscle cells and connective tissues of a severed limb survive even if the circulation is re-established after several hours of total hypoxia. On the other hand, the cells of the brain, heart, and kidney can be destroyed after only a few minutes of hypoxia.

This chapter deals with several instruments that are used to monitor the status of the respiratory system. The machines used to perform blood gas analysis are among the most clinically useful and therefore most commonly used monitors. The blood gas analyzer is a machine that actually determines three things: (1) pH, (2) partial pressure of oxygen dissolved in the plasma (P_{O_2}), and (3) partial pressure of carbon dioxide (P_{CO_2}) dissolved in the plasma of the blood that has been instilled into the blood gas machine. The bicarbonate concentration of the plasma can also be calculated from the pH and P_{CO_2}. Usually, the blood gas analyzer is used to measure these three things in arterial blood to obtain information on oxygen uptake and carbon dioxide removal in the lung, as well as the patient's acid-base status.

Although they do not usually provide the diagnosis of a specific disease state, arterial blood gases are good indicators of the overall status of the cardiopulmonary system. Normal arterial blood gases suggest adequate functioning of the respiratory system. Abnormal blood gases indicate a problem somewhere in the cardiopulmonary system and, even more importantly, can indicate the severity of the problem.

Blood gas analysis of venous blood gives information on the uptake of oxygen by the tissues and, when compared with the measurements from arterial blood, gives information on the adequacy of oxygen delivery to the tissues. Venous blood gases are also used in the calculation of the shunt equation.

Measurement of arterial and venous blood gases is considered invasive monitoring because it requires a puncture through the skin and blood vessel walls to obtain the samples. Because they produce fewer complications, less invasive or noninvasive techniques are becoming more popular, although they may have the drawbacks of being less accurate and providing less information. Transcutaneous oxygen and carbon dioxide analyzers are fairly noninvasive instruments for measuring arterial P_{O_2} and P_{CO_2} through the skin without perforating it. Capnography and mass spectrometry give information on respiratory status noninvasively by evaluation of exhaled gases.

BLOOD GAS ANALYSIS

Chemical analysis of a blood sample for its oxygen and carbon dioxide concentration was described by Van Slyke and Neil in 1924. The cumbersome but very accurate device called the Van Slyke apparatus is still used as a reference device for standardization purposes. The sample for analysis is placed into a chamber in this device where the carbon dioxide and oxygen from the sample is liberated. Next, a chemical that absorbs carbon dioxide is added to the chamber and the loss in volume represents the carbon dioxide in the sample. Then an oxygen absorber is added, and the change in volume represents the oxygen that was in the sample.

Instruments in common use for blood gas analysis are much simpler to use, although their development has been rather recent (Fig. 10–1). Modern blood gas analyzers are fully automated, requiring only injection of collected samples into the machine and occasional calibration with standard solutions. Usually, calibration of the blood gas machine is performed at the beginning of each day's shift and whenever a question arises regarding the accuracy of a measurement. Commercially prepared reference solutions are available to check the reliability of the blood gas measurement and for quality control. Routine maintenance is fairly

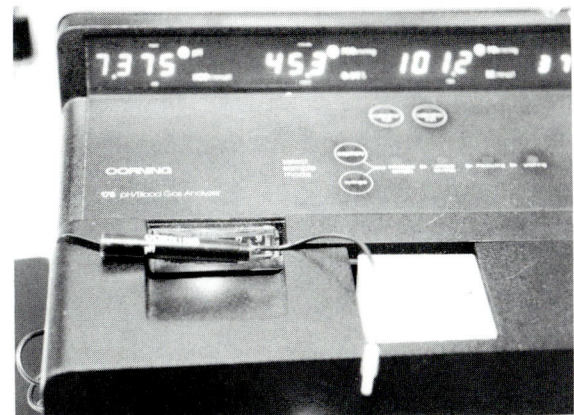

FIGURE 10–1. A blood gas analyzer and electrode.

infrequent but requires the changing of membranes and fluids according to the specific manufacturer's recommendations.

A blood gas analyzer determines the pH, P_{CO_2}, and P_{O_2} of the sample by electrochemical analysis using three different types of electrodes. The electrodes and sample in a blood gas analyzer are maintained at a constant temperature (usually body temperature) and anaerobic conditions. More recently developed blood gas analyzers require a very small sample for analysis (less than 1 ml). The use of a microprocessor in the blood gas analyzer allows values of other parameters, such as bicarbonate, oxygen saturation, and base excess, to be displayed, but these values are calculated from the information obtained by the electrodes.

The pH Electrode

The electrode in the blood gas analyzer that determines pH is called the Sanz electrode. This type of electrode contains a buffer solution of known pH (6.840) that is separated from the blood specimen being analyzed by a special type of glass membrane. Although ordinary glass is an insulator to the conduction of electricity, this special glass contains metals that allow the conduction of electrons. If the pH of the solution being analyzed is the same as the pH of the buffer solution, there is no electrical gradient across the glass membrane because the concentration of positively charged hydrogen ions is the same on both sides of the membrane. The pH of the blood solution being analyzed is almost always higher than the pH of the reference solution so that an electrical gradient exists across this special glass membrane.

As noted in Chapters 1 and 2, the chemical gradient across a cell membrane (high potassium inside the cell and low potassium outside the cell, high sodium outside the cell and low sodium inside the cell) produces the resting membrane potential. Therefore, a difference in ion concentrations on the two sides of a membrane can produce an electrical gradient. The electrical output of the measuring electrode is balanced against the electrical output of a reference electrode. The electrical potential of the reference electrode is constant. Calomel (chemical name, mercurous chloride) is contained in this reference electrode and produces the constant potential. The electrical output of the measuring cell is converted to pH units by using precise buffer solutions recommended by the National Bureau of Standards. Because the electrical potential difference is a linear function of the pH, calibration with two separate solutions of known pH (usually 6.840 and 7.384) is sufficient for accurate blood pH measurement.

The P_{CO_2} Electrode

The P_{CO_2} electrode is a Sanz pH electrode with a slight modification. The pH electrode is bathed in a bicarbonate solution enclosed in an elastic silicone membrane. This membrane separates the blood sample from the bicarbonate solution but is permeable to carbon dioxide. The carbon dioxide diffuses out of the blood and into the bicarbonate solution where it reacts to form carbonic acid and hydrogen ions. The hydrogen ions produce a potential that the pH electrode can measure. The pH change of the bicarbonate solution surrounding the pH electrode is directly proportional to the P_{CO_2} of the sample in contact with the membrane. This type of P_{CO_2} electrode, developed in the late 1950s, is called the Severinghaus electrode. The P_{CO_2} electrode is calibrated by sequentially exposing the membrane to two gas mixtures with a precise concentration of carbon dioxide (5% and 10%), so that a specific pH generated corresponds to a specific P_{CO_2}. As with the pH electrode, the pH gradient across the glass membrane inside the P_{CO_2} electrode produces an electrical gradient that is balanced against the electrical output of a calomel reference electrode.

The P_{O_2} Electrode

The third electrode component of a blood gas analyzer is used to determine the P_{O_2} of the blood sample. The P_{O_2} electrode is based on a different principle than that of the pH and P_{CO_2} electrodes.

The P_{O_2} electrode commonly used in blood gas analyzers consists of a silver and a platinum wire immersed in a KCl solution. The silver wire tends to release electrons, and the platinum wire tends to accept electrons. The rate of electron flow through the KCl solution is accelerated proportionally by the concentration of oxygen present in the solution. The KCl solution is separated from the blood sample being tested by a membrane that is oxygen-permeable. This type of electrode is called a Clark electrode and was developed in the late 1950s.

The more oxygen present in the blood sample, the more oxygen diffuses into the KCl solution, and the greater the rate of electron flow. The resulting current is directly proportional to the number of oxygen molecules and thus the P_{O_2}'s. The electrode is calibrated by exposing it to gases with specific P_{O_2}'s.

The KCl solution in a P_{O_2} electrode can conduct electricity from the silver wire to the platinum wire much better in the presence of oxygen. Normally, the KCl solution of the P_{O_2} electrode is enclosed anaerobically within the blood gas analyzer. The only oxygen that can enter this KCl solution comes from the blood samples undergoing analysis that are placed against the membranes surrounding the KCl solution. The increase in conductivity in the electrode is proportional to the amount of oxygen contained in the blood sample.

Blood Gas Analyzer Calculations

Based on the measurements obtained by the pH, P_{CO_2}, and P_{O_2} electrodes, the microcomputer inside the blood gas analyzer can calculate certain values such as oxygen saturation, bicarbonate level, and base excess. It is important to realize that these additional values are only calculated and not determined directly. Certain assumptions are made to facilitate these calculations that may produce significant error in these derived values.

The oxygen saturation is obtained from the P_{O_2} determined by the analyzer and the oxygen-hemoglobin dissociation curve. The effects of the measured pH, P_{CO_2}, and temperature on the curve are also taken into account. However, the effects of 2,3-DPG and other forms of hemoglobin, such as fetal hemoglobin, carboxyhemoglobin, or methemoglobin, are *not* taken into account. A more precise determination of oxygen saturation can be made by oximetry, which is discussed later in this chapter. Determination of P_{50} (the P_{O_2} at which the hemoglobin is 50% saturated) can also be performed.

The bicarbonate level is determined by microcomputer analysis of measured pH and P_{CO_2}. The pH of the blood sample results from the net effects of the volatile, respiratory acid (carbon dioxide) and the nonvolatile, metabolic acids on the hydrogen ion concentration of the blood.

With certain reservations, it is generally accepted that a proportional change in pH results from alteration of the ratio between the concentration of bicarbonate ions (HCO_3^-) and of dissolved carbon dioxide molecules plus carbonic acid (H_2CO_3). The interrelationship that the blood gas machine microcomputer uses for calculating the amount of bicarbonate is given in a form of the Henderson-Hasselbalch equation:

$$pH = pK' + \log \frac{[HCO_3^-]}{(\text{Diss. } CO_2 + H_2CO_3)}$$

In this equation, the pK' is assumed by the blood gas analyzer to have a constant value of 6.1. However, changes in temperature, pH, and variations in plasma ionic strength can cause pK' to vary widely, which is not accounted for.

Carbonic acid exists in trace amounts and may be ignored clinically. The P_{CO_2} of the plasma in mmHg can be converted to the concentration of dissolved carbon dioxide in millimols per liter by use of the proportionality constant 0.03.

Thus, the above equation may be represented in the more clinically useful form:

$$pH = 6.1 + \log \frac{[HCO_3^-]}{(0.03 \times P_{CO_2})}$$

This is the formula used by the blood gas machine for bicarbonate calculation following measurement of pH and P_{CO_2}. When pH is 7.40 and P_{CO_2} is 40 mmHg, the calculated bicarbonate is 24 mM/L. The usual ratio of bicarbonate to dissolved carbon dioxide is 20.

Measurement of total carbon dioxide and bicarbonate is not performed by present blood gas machines. Remember that calculations of bicarbonate and total carbon dioxide are sometimes based on faulty assumptions, so the resulting values are rough approximations. Actual measurement of total carbon dioxide and bicarbonate may be necessary for appropriate treatment of the critically ill.

The base excess is also calculated by the microprocessor in the blood gas analyzer by determining the difference between the calculated bicarbonate level and the bicarbonate level that is normal for the measured P_{CO_2} (see Fig. 3–32). Normal values for all blood gas parameters are discussed later.

OBTAINING SPECIMENS FOR BLOOD GAS ANALYSIS

It is important to use the proper technique in obtaining samples for blood gas analysis for two reasons:

1. If a poor sample is obtained, it is difficult (if not impossible) to evaluate the patient's respiratory status accurately.
2. If an improper technique is used to obtain the sample, the patient may sustain severe injuries, such as the loss of a limb or a stroke.

Arterial Blood Gas Analysis

Arterial blood gases are among the most useful indicators of respiratory status. Obtaining arterial blood is technically difficult but becomes easier with experience. Arterial blood can be obtained by puncturing an artery with a needle, withdrawing blood into a syringe, and then removing the needle from the artery. However, if the patient requires frequent samples for blood gases and other laboratory tests, a catheter is usually placed into the artery and secured so that repeated puncture of the artery is not necessary. This is called establishing an arterial line. Arterial lines are used for continuous blood pressure monitoring as well as blood sampling.

Originally, only glass syringes were used for obtaining samples for blood gas analysis because gases (especially carbon dioxide) can diffuse easily through plastic syringes, rendering the results less accurate than those obtained when glass syringes are used. However, it was later found that if the plastic syringes were immediately placed in ice, and the samples are promptly injected into the blood gas machine, the results are comparable to those obtained using glass syringes. Icing blood gas samples also slows the metabolism of the blood cells which would alter blood gas values as the blood cells use oxygen. The blood gas syringe should be heparinized to prevent clotting of the blood sample in the syringe. Blood clots not only produce erroneous values for the blood gases, but also clog the analyzer tubing. Such clots are difficult and time-consuming to remove. The barrel of the syringe should be wet with heparin and excess heparin removed from the syringe because it can produce acidification of the sample. The blood gas analyzer would incorrectly interpret this as low bicarbonate and metabolic acidosis. Heparin dilution also affects the Po_2 and Pco_2 of the sample. Care must also be taken to avoid air bubbles in the blood gas syringe because these equilibrate with the gases in the blood sample, causing erroneous results.

Arterial Puncture

If an arterial catheter is not present, arterial blood must be obtained by an arterial puncture. This is usually obtained at the radial artery but is occasionally performed at other sites where pulses are palpable.

Before performing a radial arterial puncture, an Allen's test, watching the return of skin blood flow after separate release of compression of the radial and ulnar arteries, is performed to insure adequacy of collateral perfusion to the hand. This test helps assure that adequate blood flow to the fingers is maintained by the ulnar artery following catheterization of the radial artery. Arterial blood can be obtained from other sites including the brachial, femoral, ulnar, dorsalis pedis, or tibialis arteries.

In adults, a 22- or 23-gauge needle is usually used because it provides sufficient flow without producing too much damage to the artery. The wrist is placed in a hyperextended position and the needle is inserted with its bevel facing up and at a 45-degree angle to the skin of the wrist where the radial artery is most superficial (Fig. 10–2). With glass syringes or commercially available plastic blood gas syringes, the force of the arterial pressure is usually sufficient to push the plunger backward and fill the syringe chamber without requiring aspiration. The syringe must be held very steady as it fills. Only a milliliter or less is required for most types of modern analyzers. After the specimen is obtained, the needle is withdrawn, any air bubbles are removed by holding the syringe with the needle pointing up, allowing the bubbles to float to the top, and pushing them out of the syringe and needle with the plunger. The syringe is capped after it is removed to maintain an anaerobic sample. At the same time, pressure is immediately applied over the puncture site for 5 minutes, using a dry gauze to stop bleeding and prevent hematoma formation. Pressure should be held longer if the patient is receiving anticoagulants.

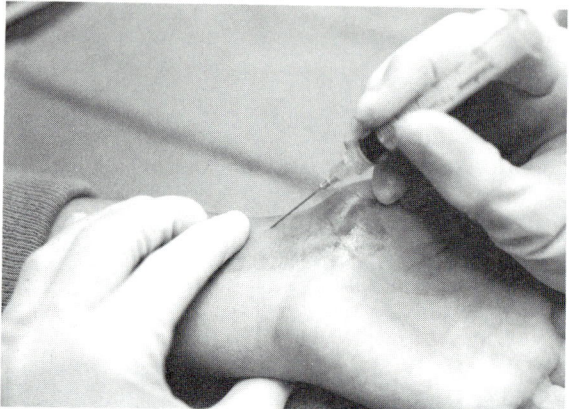

FIGURE 10–2. Proper angle for inserting needle for arterial puncture.

There are many complications associated with arterial puncture, including hematoma formation, nerve damage, and pain. A hematoma can compress the artery, obstructing perfusion distally and also make subsequent arterial puncture difficult. Intra-arterial clot formation and occlusion also occur fairly frequently and may result in tissue necrosis and even the loss of the limb. To help prevent this, avoid using large needles and perform the arterial puncture where collateral circulation is adequate. For example, the brachial artery should be avoided in infants because it is fairly small and is the only blood supply to the arm and hand. Arteriovenous fistulas are occasionally produced by puncturing through the wall of an artery into a vein, and these may require surgical repair. Infection, embolization, and hemorrhage have already been mentioned as complications of arterial puncture.

Arterial Catheterization

The insertion of an arterial catheter is similar to performing an arterial puncture. The most common site is the radial artery, but other large arteries can also be catheterized. As with arterial puncture, an Allen's test is performed before catheterizing the radial artery. The wrist is placed in the hyperextended position and usually fixed to an arm board. Local anesthetic (without epinephrine) is infiltrated into the skin and periarterial area. This is for patient comfort and also to reduce arterial spasm. After threading the catheter into the artery, a sterile dressing is applied, and the catheter is secured with tape. Arterial cutdown (surgical exposure and catheterization of the artery) is sometimes required when attempts at percutaneous catheterization are unsuccessful. Figure 10–3 shows two types of arterial catheterization sets.

If an arterial catheter is in place, obtaining blood for arterial blood gas analysis is fairly simple. In some hospitals, insertion of arterial catheters is performed only by physicians, while others allow arterial catheterization by properly trained non-physicians. It is important to know hospital policy before attempting this procedure.

Obtaining a blood sample from an arterial line is a relatively simple procedure. A stopcock, which also acts as a connector in the arterial line tubing, serves as a port for obtaining arterial blood samples. The steps for obtaining a blood sample from an arterial line are listed in Table 10–1.

Arterial puncture and sampling from an arterial line require careful adherence to aseptic techniques to prevent infection. Additionally, clinicians must follow blood and body fluid precautions when handling blood gas samples to reduce the risk to the clinician for contracting disease from the patients (see Chapter 12).

Prolonged arterial catheterization necessitates the use of a continuous flush mechanism to irrigate the catheter with a heparinized solution at a low flow rate (about 3 ml/hour). Commercially available arterial line sets also have a rapid flush mechanism for quickly clearing the tubing. The irrigating solution comes from a bag of normal saline containing one to two units of heparin per milliliter pressurized to 300 mmHg. Prolonged or frequent rapid flushing of the catheter should be avoided because large amounts of fluid in unknown volumes can be rapidly introduced into the patient. This is especially important in neonates. Neonatal arterial lines are connected to infusion pumps that provide a continuous flush rate of 1 ml or less per hour. Also, cases have been reported of *retrograde embolization* of clots and bubbles (that is, forcing them backwards through the catheter into the aorta) during prolonged flushing of an arterial catheter. This can result in cerebral vascular embolization and stroke if they are carried to the central circulation.

TABLE 10–1. Obtaining a Blood Sample from an Arterial Line

1. Attach syringe to stopcock port.
2. Turn stopcock to close irrigation port while opening the tubing from the patient to the syringe.
3. Aspirate the flush solution from the tubing as well as 1–2 ml of blood.
4. Turn stopcock halfway between flush port and syringe port so that neither are in continuity with the patient or each other.
5. Remove the flush aspirating syringe, replace with a heparinized syringe and turn the stopcock to allow aspiration of blood from the patient into the syringe.
6. Turn the stopcock to re-establish continuity between the flush and the patient. Remove the sample syringe, debubble, cap; the syringe should be placed in ice or in refrigerator, if there will be a delay before the sample can run.
7. Flush arterial line until clear.

In addition to providing access for arterial blood gas sampling and blood sampling for other laboratory tests, arterial lines are often also used for continuous monitoring of arterial blood pressure. Many different types of tubing and transducers are commercially available, and the instructions for a particular brand should be followed carefully. Tightness of connections must be assured because a disconnected arterial line can result in a rapid loss of blood.

Mixed Venous Blood Gas Analysis

Mixed venous blood samples are occasionally analyzed to determine the adequacy of oxygen delivery to body tissues as well as to calculate the shunt or pulmonary venous admixture. These calculations are discussed in the next section. True mixed venous blood can only be obtained from a catheter in the pulmonary artery. Blood samples from a central (CVP) line are not true mixed venous blood samples. The oxygen content of the blood in the superior vena cava is low because it drains from the upper extremities and brain where the oxygen extraction is high. The oxygen content of inferior vena cava blood, on the other hand, is relatively higher because much of it is blood drained from the kidneys, which extract relatively small

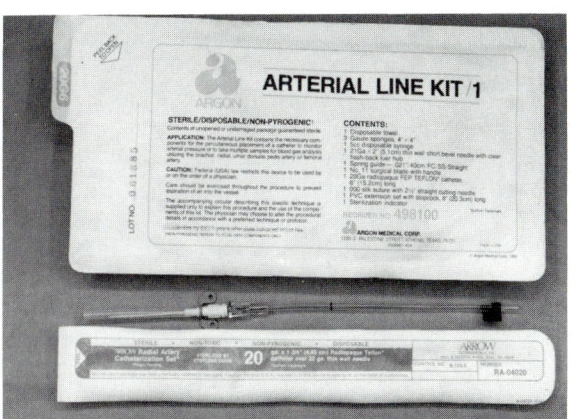

FIGURE 10–3. Arterial catheterization sets.

amounts of the oxygen delivered by their abundant blood flow (about 25% of the cardiac output). Furthermore, true mixed venous blood cannot be obtained from the right atrium or ventricle because of channeling of the blood returning from the inferior or superior vena cava. Thus, true mixed venous blood can only be obtained from the pulmonary artery. When arterial and venous blood samples are drawn for blood gas analysis and hemodynamic profile, it is unnecessary that they be drawn simultaneously. The time between drawing the two should be kept to a minimum, however, so that changes in the patient's status do not add new variables to interpreting the results. They should be drawn simultaneously if they are to be used for calculating the shunt.

Pulmonary artery catheters are fairly long, so an adequate volume (8 to 10 ml) must be withdrawn before aspiration of the venous blood specimen begins. Avoid excess heparin in the syringe, and aspirate slowly, taking about one minute to obtain the specimen. If the pulmonary artery catheter is aspirated too rapidly, arterialization of the venous sample may occur as blood that has passed through the pulmonary capillaries and gone into the pulmonary veins may be forcibly aspirated back past the pulmonary capillaries again into the pulmonary artery and into the syringe. This is avoided by slow aspiration.

Other Sites For Blood Gas Samples

Neonates requiring intensive care are commonly catheterized via the umbilical artery in order to obtain specimens for arterial blood gas analysis and other laboratory tests. There are two arteries in the umbilical cord that may be catheterized relatively more easily and with fewer complications than the smaller arteries elsewhere in the neonate's body. If umbilical artery catheterization is unsuccessful, arterial catheterization elsewhere in the neonate is quite difficult and frequently results in complications. This has fostered the development of noninvasive instruments for this age group such as *transcutaneous Po_2 and Pco_2 monitors* as well as *pulse oximetry*, discussed later.

In neonates, when an arterial sample cannot be obtained, a capillary blood gas (CBG) is occasionally performed to obtain an approximation of the infant's oxygenation, ventilation, and acid-base status. This is done by pricking the infant's finger or heel with a lancet (finger stick or heel stick) and collecting the blood in a heparinized capillary tube for blood gas analysis.

Blood gas analyzers can also be used to analyze fluids other than blood. For example, cerebrospinal fluid, pleural fluid, and even exhaled or inhaled gases can be analyzed for pH, Po_2 and/or Pco_2 with a blood gas analyzer. Typical values from the different sites are discussed in their respective sections of this chapter.

INTERPRETING BLOOD GASES

Use of proper methods for obtaining and analyzing samples for blood gas determinations is essential to obtain valid data upon which to base clinical decisions. However, valid data are only the preliminary step in interpretation and correlation with the patient's clinical status. If indicated, the next step might then be some form of oxygen therapy, mechanical ventilation, or treatment of metabolic acidosis or metabolic alkalosis. Re-evaluation by repeated blood gases follows the treatment to determine if it is appropriate and successful in achieving therapeutic goals.

Interpretation of Arterial Blood Gases

Arterial blood is the most common type of sample submitted for blood gas analysis. Interpretation of the blood gas measurements obtained is based on the knowledge of the normal range for these values. The following blood gas values are for healthy, young adults at sea level breathing atmospheric gas composed of 21% oxygen and 79% nitrogen. The normal pH range for arterial blood (pHa) is 7.35 to 7.45. The range for Pco_2 in arterial blood ($Paco_2$) is normally 35 to 45 mmHg. The Po_2 of arterial blood is normally 80 to 100 mmHg, with a hemoglobin oxygen saturation greater than 95%. Normal Po_2 decreases with age, starting at about 20 to 30 years (see Chapter 6). The calculated plasma bicarbonate concentration is normally 22 to 26 mEq/L. For meaningful blood gas analysis (Table 10–2), knowledge of the patient's clinical condition is essential. Casual blood gas interpretation by evaluating the difference between the actually measured blood gas values and some predetermined normal values may not be appropriate for the patient under evaluation. Care must be taken to differentiate the "normal" values previously mentioned from appropriate values, which may be normal for an individual in a different clin-

TABLE 10–2. Interpretation of Arterial Blood Gas Values

For appropriate interpretation of arterial blood gas values, follow these steps:
1. Determine patient's clinical condition.
2. Estimate blood gas values that would be appropriate for that condition.
3. Examine P_{O_2} and percent hemoglobin saturation to evaluate oxygenation and decide if they are different from expected values.
4. Examine pH, P_{CO_2}, bicarbonate and base excess values to evaluate acid/base status and determine if they are different from expected values.

ical situation. For example, if an arterial blood gas analysis reveals a P_{O_2} of 100 mmHg, your first impression may be that this individual is normal. However, if he is breathing 100% oxygen, then there is a significant abnormality in his cardiopulmonary system's ability to oxygenate his blood.

Evaluation of Oxygenation

Many situations can result in an arterial P_{O_2} that is different from the previously mentioned normal values for young adults, which would still be appropriate for a particular patient. In contrast to young adults, extremely young or old patients normally have a decreased oxygenating ability, as discussed in Chapter 6. The effects of scuba diving or high altitudes on atmospheric pressure can produce arterial P_{O_2} values that seem abnormal. Breathing gas mixtures with a different oxygen concentration than that of the atmosphere can likewise produce changes in arterial P_{O_2}. A fetus would normally be expected to have quite a low Pa_{O_2}.

By now, you should be getting the impression that normal Pa_{O_2} is more correctly based on what is appropriate for the patient under consideration. Arterial P_{O_2} is expected to be slightly less than alveolar P_{O_2}. This results from the normally occurring anatomic shunt (see Chapter 3), which allows unoxygenated blood to mix with blood that has already flowed past the pulmonary alveolar capillaries and become oxygenated as well as some normal degree of V̇/Q̇ mismatch and, possibly, diffusion impairment. The $P_{A_{O_2}}$ is determined by the alveolar air equation, which takes into account the percentage of oxygen in the inspired gas ($F_{I_{O_2}}$), the atmospheric pressure and effects of carbon dioxide in the alveoli (see Chapter 3). Normally, we would expect the Pa_{O_2} to be about 5 to 10 mmHg less than the room air $P_{A_{O_2}}$. This is sometimes called the A-a oxygen gradient. A rapid but inexact approximation of Pa_{O_2} for different inspired oxygen concentrations is calculated by multiplying the percentage of inspired oxygen by 5. For example, a patient breathing 100% oxygen would be expected to have a Pa_{O_2} of about 500 mmHg. Arterial blood gases are considered abnormal if the Pa_{O_2} is inappropriately low compared with the predicted $P_{A_{O_2}}$. The usual causes of this are right-to-left shunts, diffusion impairment, or ventilation/perfusion mismatch. If both $P_{A_{O_2}}$ and Pa_{O_2} are low, the blood gases are also considered abnormal, but they are appropriate in the presence of a low $P_{A_{O_2}}$. Causes of low $P_{A_{O_2}}$ include hypoventilation (increased Pa_{CO_2}), low inspired oxygen concentration and high altitude (low atmospheric pressure).

A Pa_{O_2} less than 40 mmHg should be considered a life-threatening condition. Occasionally, a patient with, for example, chronic obstructive pulmonary disease (COPD) or cardiac defects (right-to-left cardiac shunt) will survive with a Pa_{O_2} in this low range. Long-term hypoxemia produces certain compensatory changes, such as an elevated hemoglobin concentration, which increases oxygen delivery. Vascular and cellular changes (2,3-DPG) also permit an individual to tolerate chronic hypoxemia. However, these individuals have poor tolerance to increased activity levels and generally have shortened life spans. Patients who previously have had normal arterial Pa_{O_2}'s and suddenly become severely hypoxic lack these compensatory mechanisms. Acute, severe hypoxemia can be rapidly fatal but fortunately is usually more easily and more successfully treatable than chronic hypoxemia (Table 10–3).

When the arterial P_{O_2} is less than 60 mmHg but greater than 40 mmHg, the therapeutic modalities are the same as for severe hypoxemia but are not quite as urgent. Hemoglobin saturation is still fairly high in this range of P_{O_2} (75% to 90%) so that oxygen content of the blood is maintained. However, timely intervention is still necessary because, from this range of values, a further decrease in P_{O_2} will produce a precipitous drop in hemoglobin saturation.

When the arterial P_{O_2} is above 60 mmHg, hemoglobin saturation is above 90%, so the oxygen content of the blood is near maximal. Suppose again that the arterial P_{O_2} is 100 mmHg, but the patient is breathing 100% oxygen. There is something seriously wrong with the patient's ability to oxygenate the blood, or there is an abnormally large venous admixture (shunt). In itself, an arterial P_{O_2} of 100 mmHg is not a cause for concern,

TABLE 10–3.   Interventions for Acute, Severe Hypoxemia

1. Initiation of mechanical ventilation if patient is apneic or hypoventilating.
2. Increase inspired oxygen concentration to 100%.
3. Auscultation of both lung fields to determine adequacy of ventilation.
   a. Unable to ventilate—consider intubation, cricothyrotomy, or tracheostomy.
   b. If still unable to ventilate, consider aspirated object in airway—Heimlich maneuver.
   c. Unilateral inability to ventilate—consider tension pneumothorax (must be relieved), inadvertent bronchial intubation, or bronchial foreign body.
4. If appropriate, administration of expiratory positive airway pressure—to help prevent atelectasis and improve ventilation/perfusion matching.
5. Other measures to reduce airway obstruction and atelectasis—bronchodilators, mucolytics, postural drainage, chest physical therapy, IPPB, incentive spirometry, coughing, and suctioning.

but the fact that it should be much higher is. If the inspired oxygen concentration is reduced to atmospheric, the patient may become seriously hypoxic, so further investigation is warranted. An additional area of concern is the risk of oxygen toxicity, which occurs when the inspired oxygen concentration is above 50% for several hours (see Chapter 16).

If the PaO$_2$ is higher than the PAO$_2$ calculated from the alveolar air equation, then some sort of error is the most likely explanation. A bubble of air in the blood gas sample, an inspired oxygen concentration higher than expected, or even confusing blood from different patients can produce this disparity. While it is appropriate to consider hypoxemia a hazardous and possibly lethal condition, hyperoxia also presents certain hazards. We have already mentioned the dangers of lung damage from oxygen toxicity caused by prolonged inspiration of high oxygen concentrations. Additionally, breathing high oxygen concentrations tends to remove the nitrogen from the alveoli. Alveoli that are poorly ventilated from such conditions as airway obstruction from retained secretions are more likely to collapse as the oxygen is removed by the pulmonary capillary blood flow. The loss of this so-called nitrogen splint hastens such *absorption atelectasis.*

A special problem in neonates is the risk of the damaging effect of elevated arterial PO$_2$ on the development of the blood vessels inside the eyes. Infants weighing less than 1,500 gm at birth who receive oxygen supplementation are at an increased risk for retinopathy of prematurity (ROP), such as retrolental fibroplasia. Current theories of the pathogenesis of ROP indicate a disruption of the normal sequence of retinal blood vessel growth by premature birth and by vasoactive substances such as oxygen, carbon dioxide, hydrogen ions, free radicals, and other agents.

Regardless of the mechanism, progressive vascular damage can eventually produce edema, hemorrhage, scarring and detachment of the retina. This can lead to complete loss of vision, but usually varying degrees of glaucoma, myopia, and strabismus occur.

Infants delivered before 35 weeks of gestation or who weigh less than 1,800 gm who required supplemental oxygen should have an ophthalmologic examination. Active disease can frequently be successfully treated by cryotherapy (application of cold to the external surface of the sclera).

Evaluation of Acid-Base Status

Although pH is the blood gas measurement usually listed first, it is sometimes useful to think of it last when considering acid-base status because the interaction of the carbon dioxide and bicarbonate levels determines the pH of the blood. For example, if the Pco$_2$ is high and the bicarbonate level low, then the pH must be quite low.

As previously discussed, the blood gas machine actually measures the pH and Pco$_2$ of the sample and then calculates the bicarbonate concentration. Predicting how the interaction of the Pco$_2$ and bicarbonate levels affects the blood pH is fairly simple under most circumstances:

1. For every 10 mmHg increase in blood Pco$_2$ above 40, the pH tends to decrease 0.05 pH units. For example, if the Pco$_2$ were 70, the pH would tend to decrease from the normal 7.40 by 0.15 units to a pH of 7.25.
2. For every 10 mmHg decrease in Pco$_2$ below 40 mmHg, the pH tends to increase approximately 0.1 pH units. For example, a Pco$_2$ of 20 mmHg would tend to increase the pH to 7.60.
3. Any 5 mEq/L change in bicarbonate level from normal would tend to produce a 0.08 pH change. For instance, if the bicarbonate level is 35 mEq/L (10 mEq/L above normal), this would tend to raise the pH 0.16 to 7.56.
4. The influences of the Pco$_2$ and bicarbonate can be combined to determine the corresponding pH of the blood. For example, if Pco$_2$ is 50 and bicarbonate is 30, then the Pco$_2$ would tend to lower the pH 0.05 units while the bicarbonate would tend to raise the pH 0.08 units. The net result is 0.08 − 0.05 = 0.03 elevation in pH (7.43).

After evaluating the interactions of the blood carbon dioxide and bicarbonate levels on the blood pH, the acid-base status is described. There are only 11 possible acid-base states, which are listed in Table 10–4.

Compensated Acid-Base States

Although the pH is not quite returned to normal, compensated acid-base states show normal functioning of compensatory mechanisms. Compensation takes time to occur. It also can be described in degrees such as slightly, partially, or nearly fully compensated states, depending on how successful the compensatory mechanism is in returning the pH toward 7.40. It is essential to note that overcompensation does not occur. Compensatory mechanisms are effective at returning pH to near normal values but do not overshoot a normal pH. For example, an acidosis is not compensated for so much that an alkalosis results.

Compensated Respiratory Acidosis. Compensated respiratory acidosis usually results from conditions producing chronic hypoventilation, such as airways obstruction caused by COPD, tracheal stenosis, laryngeal web, or airway tumors; pickwickian syndromes; or neuromuscular disease, such as muscular dystrophy or Guillain-Barré syndrome. With time, the acidosis produced by excess carbon dioxide is compensated for by the kidney's excretion of metabolic acid and reabsorption of bicarbonate.

Compensated Respiratory Alkalosis. Hyperventilation (chronic or at least of several days duration) results in compensated respiratory alkalosis. For example, mechanical hyperventilation is used to clinically control intracranial pressure in head trauma or neurosurgical patients. Hyperventilation lowers P_{CO_2} and initially causes alkalemia, which produces constriction of the normal brain blood vessels. Cerebrovasoconstriction reduces intracranial volume, which tends to lower intracranial pressure. With time, compensatory mechanisms, such as decreased acid excretion and increased bicarbonate excretion by the kidneys, produce a lowered bicarbonate level which returns the blood pH toward normal. The respiratory alkalosis is compensated for by metabolic acidosis, and the cerebrovasoconstricting effect is lost. This important effect on intracranial pressure is discussed further in Chapter 20.

Compensated Metabolic Acidosis. Accumulation of excess nonvolatile acid from either increased production or decreased excretion results in metabolic acidosis. Causes of metabolic acidosis include lactic acidosis (from anaerobic metabolism when oxygen demand is greater than oxygen supply), ketoacidosis (from uncontrolled diabetes mellitus), or certain types of poisoning (salicylate overdose). Renal failure results in decreased urinary excretion of metabolic acid, which causes metabolic acidosis. Usually, metabolic acid accumulates at such a rate that respiratory compensation (hyperventilation) occurs almost simultaneously.

In the differential diagnosis of metabolic acidosis, a clinically useful tool is the *anion gap*. The sum of Cl^- and HCO_3^- is subtracted from Na^+, all in mEq/L:

$$\text{anion gap} = Na^+ - (Cl^- + HCO_3^-).$$

The normal range of the anion gap is 8 to 16 mEq/L. An increased anion gap is seen in forms of metabolic acidosis that are due to increased levels of organic acids (such as diabetic ketoacidosis, lactic acidosis, renal failure, or toxicity from salicylates, methyl alcohol, ethylene glycol, or certain other chemicals). Metabolic acidosis with a normal anion gap is most commonly caused by diarrhea, renal tubular acidosis, ureterosigmoidostomy, or administration of NH_4Cl or carbonic anhydrase inhibitors such as acetazolamide (Diamox). The or-

TABLE 10–4. Acid-Base States

pH	P_{CO_2}	HCO_3^-	Description of Acid-Base Status
Normal	Normal	Normal	Normal
↓	↑↑	↑↑	Compensated respiratory acidosis
↑	↓↓	↓↓	Compensated respiratory alkalosis
↓	↓↓	↓↓	Compensated metabolic acidosis
↑	↑↑	↑↑	Compensated metabolic alkalosis
↓↓	↑↑	↑	Uncompensated respiratory acidosis
↑↑	↓↓	↓	Uncompensated respiratory alkalosis
↓↓	—	↓↓	Uncompensated metabolic acidosis
↑↑	—	↑↑	Uncompensated metabolic alkalosis
↓↓↓	↑↑	↓	Mixed (respiratory and metabolic) acidosis
↑↑↑	↓↓	↑	Mixed (respiratory and metabolic) alkalosis

Adapted from Levitzky, M. G.; *Pulmonary Physiology*, 2nd ed. New York, McGraw-Hill, 1986, with permission.

ganic acids act as anions increasing the difference between the routinely measured electrolytes.

Compensated Metabolic Alkalosis. Excessive excretion of metabolic acid or administration of alkalinizing drugs produces metabolic alkalosis. In the presence of metabolic alkalosis, respiratory compensation (hypoventilation) usually occurs rapidly, resulting in the maintenance of blood pH near normal. However, if the metabolic alkalosis is severe, extreme hypoventilation may ensue, resulting in hypoxia, atelectasis, and sputum retention. Mechanical ventilatory support may be mandated in especially severe cases. Causes of metabolic alkalosis include prolonged nasogastric suctioning (removal of gastric secretions which removes hydrochloric acid from the stomach), many diuretic drugs (which promote urinary excretion of potassium, hydrogen and chloride ions), and fluid and electrolyte imbalances which result in hypochloremia (low chloride levels) and hypokalemia (low blood potassium levels).

Uncompensated Acid-Base States

These states occur either when there hasn't been enough time for compensation to occur or when something else prevents compensation from occurring.

Uncompensated Respiratory Acidosis. If a patient stops breathing, carbon dioxide rapidly accumulates, increasing about 5 mmHg per minute of apnea. Obviously, pH decreases rapidly. Renal compensatory mechanisms occur gradually over several hours to increase metabolic acid excretion. Therefore, acute hypoventilation results in uncompensated respiratory acidosis until compensatory mechanisms have time to return the blood pH toward normal. A compensated respiratory acidosis suggests that the hypoventilation is long-standing—at least of several hours' duration. Uncompensated respiratory acidosis is therefore a more alarming finding because it suggests a recent deterioration in the patient's ability to ventilate. Uncompensated respiratory acidosis can also herald further worsening of the patient's ability to ventilate spontaneously, possibly progressing to the point of complete ventilatory failure.

Uncompensated Respiratory Alkalosis. Acute hyperventilation results in uncompensated respiratory alkalosis until renal compensatory mechanisms have time to excrete bicarbonate, retain metabolic acid and return blood pH toward normal. Head trauma, certain nervous disorders (such as anxiety) and controlled mechanical hyperventilation are the most common causes. Normally, a person cannot spontaneously hyperventilate to severe respiratory alkalosis because the respiratory center reduces ventilatory drive.

Uncompensated Metabolic Acidosis and Alkalosis. These are quite uncommon states because the presence of too much or too little metabolic acid almost immediately triggers respiratory compensation via the peripheral and central chemoreceptors and respiratory centers. Only if the chemoreceptors or respiratory centers are impaired or the patient is on controlled mechanical ventilation or unable to alter ventilation does uncompensated metabolic acidosis or uncompensated metabolic alkalosis occur. Severe metabolic acidosis that is uncompensated or poorly compensated is sometimes treated by administration of sodium bicarbonate (see Chapter 15).

Mixed Respiratory and Metabolic Acid-Base States

When both the respiratory and metabolic mechanisms act to shift pH in the same direction, the cumulative effect is a profound pH change that can be life-threatening.

Mixed Acidosis. The combination of both respiratory and metabolic acidosis (simply called mixed acidosis) produces an extremely low blood pH. Accumulation of carbon dioxide and metabolic (lactic) acid is commonly encountered in an unresuscitated patient suffering cardiopulmonary arrest. The cessation of the circulatory system causes lactic acid accumulation while the coexisting apnea results in a rapidly increasing blood P_{CO_2}.

Mixed Alkalosis. Combined respiratory and metabolic alkalosis produces an elevated blood pH that can also be life-threatening. These conditions increase the affinity of hemoglobin for oxygen so that less oxygen is released to the tissues. This can result in dangerous tissue hypoxia. Unfortunately, mixed alkalosis is seen frequently in patients suffering cardiopulmonary arrest who are over-resuscitated. Overzealous mechanical ventilation and sodium bicarbonate administration can rapidly convert a patient with mixed acidosis into one with mixed alkalosis.

Occasionally, a patient has two pathologic processes simultaneously that produce complex acid-base disorders, such as mixed respiratory acidosis and metabolic alkalosis (as in a patient with COPD and hypokalemia). These complex disorders are often difficult to differentiate from compensated states unless both diagnoses, as well as their severity, are appreciated when attempting to interpret the blood gases. Clinical correlation is necessary for accurate blood gas interpretation.

Interpretation of Venous Blood Gases

Mixed venous blood gas (VBG) analysis is quite valuable for indicating therapy for the critically ill or high-risk patient. This technique is not routinely used because it requires the placement of a catheter into the pulmonary artery, which carries a substantial risk of complications. For the severely ill patient, however, the risks of pulmonary artery catheterization are outweighed by the benefits resulting from the more appropriate management based on the data obtained. We have already discussed the importance of proper technique for obtaining mixed venous blood for analysis earlier in this chapter. Venous blood gases can be used to obtain an approximation of the patient's acid-base status. Venous P_{CO_2} is approximately 5 mmHg higher than arterial P_{CO_2}; venous pH is about 0.04 units lower than arterial pH. The degree of oxygenation of the mixed venous blood is usually the most clinically useful measurement obtained from mixed venous blood gas analysis. Venous oxyhemoglobin saturation, $P\bar{v}_{O_2}$, and hemoglobin concentration are used to determine mixed venous oxygen content ($C\bar{v}_{O_2} = P\bar{v}_{O_2} \times 0.003$ + venous saturation × hemoglobin content × 1.34). In normal young adults, the $P\bar{v}_{O_2}$ is approximately 40 mmHg, venous saturation is about 75% and hemoglobin concentration is normally 15 gm/dl. Mixed venous oxygen content is thus about 15 ml of oxygen per deciliter of blood. Continuous monitoring of mixed venous hemoglobin saturation can also be performed with venous oximetry, discussed later in this chapter.

When the mixed venous oxygen content is compared with the arterial oxygen content in a calculation called the *the arterial-venous (A-V) oxygen content difference*, information on the adequacy of the blood flow to the tissues can be obtained. Normally, the Ca_{O_2} is 20 ml of oxygen per deciliter of blood while the $C\bar{v}_{O_2}$ is 15 ml of oxygen per deciliter of blood, which makes the A-V oxygen content difference about 5 ml of oxygen per deciliter of blood. This means that, normally, when 100 ml of blood (1 dl) passes through the capillary from a systemic artery into a systemic vein, about 5 ml of oxygen is given up by the blood and taken up by the tissues. When the A-V oxygen content difference is greater than 5 ml of oxygen per deciliter of blood, this usually implies inadequate cardiac output (the blood stays in the capillaries for a longer time so that more oxygen is extracted). On the other hand, when the A-V oxygen difference is less than 5 ml of oxygen per deciliter of blood, then this suggests excessive cardiac output (the blood is in the capillaries for a short period or may even bypass a capillary so that not much oxygen is extracted before the blood enters the veins). At certain stages of sepsis, particularly with gram-negative organisms, the A-V oxygen difference becomes less than 5 ml of oxygen per deciliter of blood. This is because the toxins from the infection cause arterial-venous anastomoses to open, which allows the blood to bypass the capillaries, so oxygen extraction is diminished. This causes the venous oxygen content to rise while the tissues develop lactic acidosis from relative anoxia from the decreased perfusion of the tissue capillaries.

The basis of the A-V oxygen content difference calculation is the Fick equation ($Ca_{O_2} - C\bar{v}_{O_2}$ = total body oxygen consumption per minute divided by cardiac output). Total body oxygen consumption per minute is the body's oxygen demand while the cardiac output times Ca_{O_2} is oxygen supply. The relationship between supply and demand is the amount of oxygen extracted from the blood as it passes through the systemic capillaries. If cardiac output is known, then oxygen consumption per minute can be determined. Mixed venous blood gases are very important in determining the adequacy of cardiac output to deliver oxygen to meet the tissues' metabolic demands.

The determination of mixed venous oxygen content ($C\bar{v}_{O_2}$) is also necessary for use in the shunt equation:

Percent of shunt

$$= (Cc'_{O_2} - Ca_{O_2}) \div (Cc'_{O_2} - C\tilde{v}_{O_2})$$

$$Cc'_{O_2} = (1.34 \times Hb) + (0.003 \times P_{A O_2}).$$

A clinically useful form of the alveolar air equation from Chapter 3 is:

$$P_{AO_2} = F_{IO_2}(P_{atm} - P_{H_2O}) - (Pa_{CO_2} \div RQ).$$

The venous oxygen content is necessary for the shunt formula because it helps determine how much the shunted (venous) blood will tend to lower the oxygen content of the arterial blood. For example, if the venous blood has a relatively high oxygen content, then an intrapulmonary shunt would produce less reduction in the arterial oxygen content than would occur if the venous blood had very little oxygen. Calculation of the shunt is very useful for the clinical management of a critically ill patient. Shunt calculations are useful to indicate improvement or worsening of pulmonary functions. Measuring the percent of the shunt has also been used to determine the optimal level of positive end-expiratory pressure (PEEP) in patients with severe lung pathology. Several estimated or modified shunt equations have been suggested but are not recommended because they make assumptions that are unreasonable for critically ill patients.

Interpretation of Capillary Blood Gases

In patients who are very young, uncooperative, or have received numerous arterial punctures, arterial blood may be difficult or impossible to obtain. Technically easier, less traumatic, but slightly less meaningful evaluation of the patient's respiratory status can be obtained by using capillary blood gases. An area of skin, usually on the heel, is heated with warm compresses to increase the blood flow. A skin prick in the area provides blood that should be collected as anaerobically as possible. The P_{O_2} of such a sample is relatively meaningless unless severe hypoxia is present (P_{O_2} less than 35 mmHg). The pH and P_{CO_2} of such a sample is much more meaningful because arterial, capillary and venous measurements of these values are usually fairly close, as described previously. A high P_{CO_2} in a capillary blood gas is a fairly good indicator of hypoventilation.

Interpretation of Umbilical Blood Gases

Sampling the blood from a vein in the umbilical cord at the time of delivery is most valuable for determining the presence of acidemia, which would strongly suggest fetal distress from such things as decreased placental blood flow or a kinked umbilical cord. The level of oxygenation of the umbilical blood is less meaningful because it can change rapidly. The pH of the blood from a baby's scalp is occasionally determined while it is still in the uterus. A low scalp blood pH suggests fetal distress.

TRANSCUTANEOUS P_{O_2} AND P_{CO_2}

The transcutaneous P_{O_2} ($P_{tc}O_2$) can be determined with a noninvasive monitor consisting of a miniaturized Clark electrode (similar to those used in blood gas analyzers to measure P_{O_2}) combined with a heating coil. Adhesive and gel are used to anaerobically attach the electrode to the patient. The skin under the electrode is usually heated to 44°C, which produces localized vasodilation and increased diffusion of oxygen through the skin into the electrode. These devices are most useful in infants because their $P_{tc}O_2$ closely correlates with Pa_{O_2}. In adults, the correlation is very unreliable because of thickening of the skin, and so this type of monitor is used almost exclusively on infants.

The $P_{tc}O_2$ is also an indicator of tissue oxygenation. Some clinicians calculate the $P_{tc}O_2/PaO_2$ ratio as an index of oxygen delivery. $P_{tc}O_2$ is not useful as a replacement for PaO_2 but rather as a continuous noninvasive indicator of tissue oxygenation.

The location of the electrode on the patient's body also affects the accuracy of its measurement. For best results the electrode should be on the anterior chest or head where the skin is well perfused, flat, and not excessively hairy. Hypothermia or hypotension also decreases the accuracy of this type of monitor because they cause reflex vasoconstriction.

The transcutaneous P_{CO_2} ($P_{tc}CO_2$) monitor is basically a pH electrode that is modified to read out P_{CO_2}. This electrode must also be heated to cause vasodilation. These monitors usually give $P_{tc}CO_2$'s that are closely correlated to $PaCO_2$'s (probably because carbon dioxide diffuses so well). Some monitors are available that perform both transcutaneous measurements.

Drawbacks to the use of transcutaneous monitors include burns on the skin and unreliability from poor or changing skin perfusion. These monitors require several minutes for sufficient heating of the skin and equilibrium to occur when they are being set up. In addition, the $P_{tc}CO_2$ monitor electrode must be calibrated using a tank of compressed gas.

Although P_{O_2}'s and P_{CO_2}'s obtained by the use of these monitors are not the same as those obtained from arterial blood samples, they can be used in conjunction with blood gases to wean pediatric patients from mechanical ventilation and high inspired oxygen concentrations, thus greatly decreasing the number of blood gases that must be obtained and reducing the risk of complications from arterial punctures.

Conjunctival P_{O_2} and P_{CO_2} electrodes are similar to transcutaneous electrodes and provide similar measurements. Complications associated with their use include conjunctivitis.

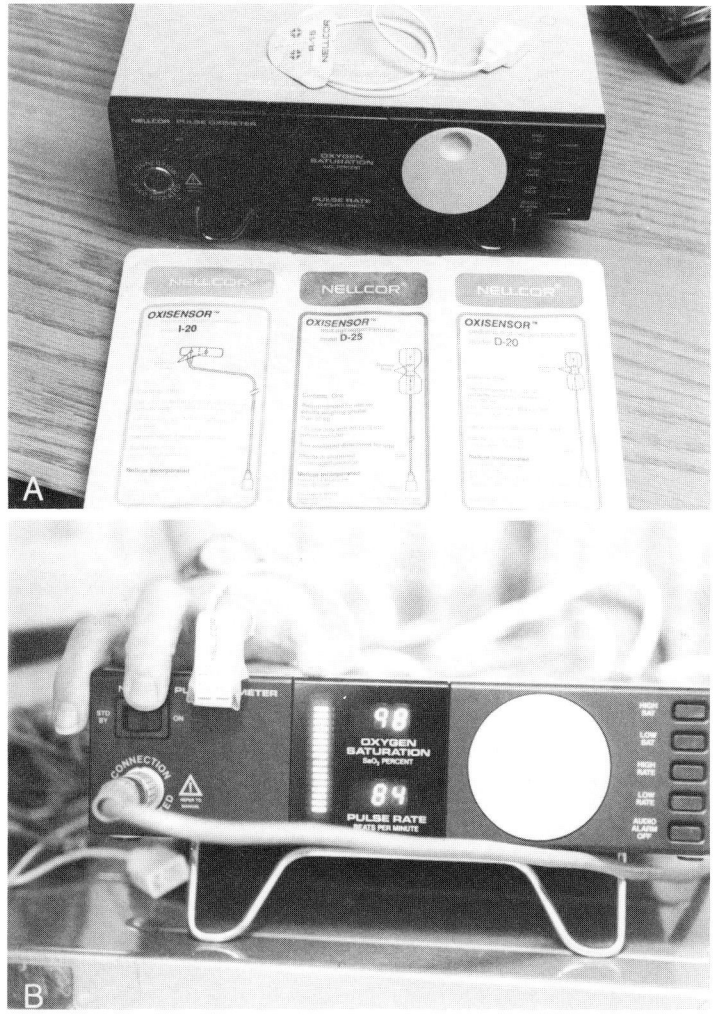

FIGURE 10–4. *A*, Pulse oximeter and cuvettes. Note the three disposable finger cuvettes in front of the machine and a nasal cuvette on top. *B*, Finger cuvette in place with the machine operating.

OXIMETRY

Oxygen saturation of hemoglobin can be determined indirectly by analysis of the color of reflected light. Cardiopulmonary clinicians use the blood's color as a rough index of the patient's respiratory status. Well-oxygenated blood usually appears bright red, while hypoxemia is associated with dark blood (cyanosis) easily observable in the nail beds, conjunctiva, and oral mucosa. Oximetry quantitates this relationship between the oxygenation of the blood and its color.

Co-Oximetry

A co-oximeter is an instrument that measures percent oxyhemoglobin, percent carboxyhemoglobin, and percent methemoglobin in an anticoagulated blood sample. It also calculates total hemoglobin and oxygen content. The blood sample is aspirated into the machine, mixed with a diluent, hemolyzed, and brought to a constant temperature (usually 37°C) in the absorption chamber. Light of four specific wavelengths is passed through the chamber to a photodetector for determination of the absorption characteristics of the sample. Because each of the previously mentioned species of hemoglobin absorbs a different wavelength, a microprocessor can determine the concentrations based on the absorbancies observed. Samples for use in this instrument are collected in the same manner as for blood gas analysis and are frequently performed on the remainder of a sample following blood gas analysis.

Venous Oximetry

By using fiber-optic bundles contained inside a pulmonary artery catheter, the color (wavelength reflected) of the mixed venous blood in the pulmonary artery can be determined. The oxygen saturation of the hemoglobin that corresponds to the reflected wavelength is determined by using a microprocessor. Obviously, venous oximetry is an invasive method and is not usually used by itself but rather as an additional facet of a multilumen pulmonary artery catheter whose other functions include a sampling port for mixed venous blood, thermodilution cardiac output measurements, measurement of pulmonary artery pressures, and access for infusions (see Chapter 8). Determination of mixed venous oxygen saturation ($S\bar{v}O_2$) provides continuous monitoring of the adequacy of oxygen delivery. The primary factors affecting $S\bar{v}O_2$ are the arterial oxygen content, the cardiac output, and the oxygen consumption. The relationship of these factors is given in the Fick equation (see Chapter 5):

$$CO = \dot{V}O_2 \div (CaO_2 - C\bar{v}O_2)$$

Invasive arterial oximetry catheters are also available and have been used in the umbilical arteries of newborns.

Pulse Oximetry

Noninvasive oximetry determines oxygen saturation using the same principle of light absorption that invasive oximetry uses. This type of noninvasive monitor determines both the pulse rate and the arterial saturation. Pulse oximetry is commonly used clinically and is the standard of care for patients undergoing anesthesia and surgery. The most common site of application of the sensor is upon the patient's finger. The sensor (cuvette) consists of a light-emitting portion which is placed on one side of the finger while the photo sensor is on the other side of the finger.

There are many types of pulse oximetry cuvettes especially modified for application at different sites. Figure 10–4 shows a pulse oximeter and cuvettes for application to the finger, earlobe, or bridge of the nose with different sizes available for adults, children, and neonates. Very few complications are associated with the use of this monitor, such as electrical hazards, burns from malfunctioning equipment, or digital necrosis from restricted blood flow. Pulse oximetry has problems with interference from electrocautery or patient movement. New types of pulse oximeters with electrical filters and a means to detect the patient's ECG are commercially available and more reliably monitor the hemoglobin saturation. Research into factors influencing the accuracy of pulse oximetry (the effects of atypical hemoglobin or fingernail polish) continue to define the usefulness of this monitor.

The wavelengths of light transmitted between pulsations is electronically subtracted from the wavelengths of light transmitted through the tissues during a pulsation. The pulse represents the addition of arterial blood to the tissues so the subtraction of nonpulse background wavelengths leaves only those wavelengths provided by the arterial blood.

CAPNOGRAPHY

Capnography is a noninvasive determination of the carbon dioxide concentration in respiratory gases to monitor ventilatory function. Instruments that perform these measurements use either infrared absorption analysis or mass spectrometry.

Infrared Absorption Analysis

The elements that form a molecule and the arrangement of these elements (configuration) as they are bonded together to form a molecule result in individual light absorption characteristics for specific molecules. Carbon dioxide absorbs infrared light, and the degree of absorption depends on the number of molecules and thus the concentration of carbon dioxide present. Water vapor has a similar absorption pattern to carbon dioxide, but fortunately, there is a wavelength of infrared light that is absorbed by carbon dioxide and not by water vapor molecules. High concentrations of nitrous oxide molecules, which also absorb infrared light, may cause erroneous determinations of carbon dioxide concentrations in the gas mixture. Modern carbon dioxide analyzers, especially those designed for use in the operating room, provide electronic compensators for this effect of nitrous oxide.

Respiratory gases are sampled from the patient's airway through a small-diameter tube. The gas passes through a filter or separation chamber to keep water and solid particles out of the analyzing chamber. The carbon dioxide concentration of the aspirated gas varies with the phases of ventilation (Fig. 10–5). The carbon dioxide waveforms should be relatively square with minimal carbon dioxide in the inspired gas, or in gas from the beginning of expiration, when the anatomic deadspace gas is being exhaled. If the alveolar plateau is nearly flat, the exhaled carbon dioxide concentration should correspond well with the arterial P_{CO_2} (unless there is significant alveolar deadspace). The height, frequency, shape and base line of the carbon dioxide waveform reflect characteristics of the patient's ventilatory pattern.

An elevated base line suggests rebreathing of respiratory gases, which may be caused by such things as a valve failure in a ventilatory circuit or saturation of the carbon dioxide absorber in the anesthesia circuit. Absence of a carbon dioxide waveform following attempted endotracheal intubation suggests that the endotracheal tube may actually be in the esophagus. Sudden disappearance of the carbon dioxide waveform from an endotracheal tube that had been previously normal suggests ventilator failure, disconnection from the ventilator, occluded endotracheal tube, inadvertent extubation, or an occluded sampling tube. A sudden decrease in the carbon dioxide waveform may suggest sudden pulmonary hypotension (causing increased alveolar deadspace) or embolism, or cardiac arrest. On the other hand, an increase in the carbon dioxide waveform suggests either increased carbon dioxide production, (such as occurs with malignant hyperthermia) or hypoventilation. The status of the cardiopulmonary system may be determined by monitoring the waveform of the carbon dioxide concentration and life-threatening problems can be rapidly ascertained.

Using a collecting chamber, such as a Douglas bag, mixed expired P_{CO_2} ($P\bar{e}_{CO_2}$) can be measured in the exhaled gases. Using this value, as well as the Pa_{CO_2} from an arterial blood gas sample, phys-

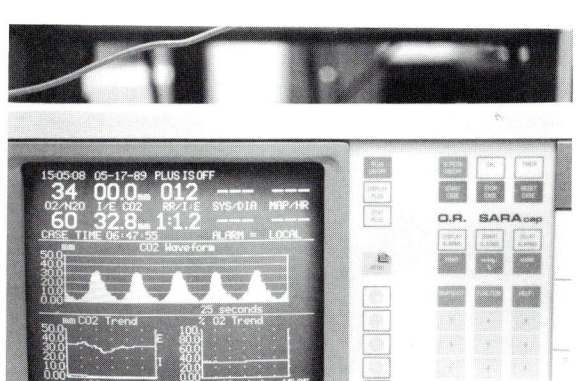

FIGURE 10–5. Normal capnographic waveform.

iologic deadspace can be determined from the Bohr equation:

$$\frac{V_D}{V_T} = (P_{aCO_2} - P\bar{e}_{CO_2}) \div P_{aCO_2}$$

V_D represents physiologic deadspace while V_T is tidal volume. By using a spirometer with the Douglas bag, carbon dioxide production ($\dot{V}_{CO_2}$) can also be determined.

Deadspace and carbon dioxide production studies are commonly performed on patients in intensive care units to determine the adequacy of their ventilation, cardiovascular status, and metabolic state. The steady state ratio of $\dot{V}_{CO_2}$ to oxygen consumption ($\dot{V}_{O_2}$) is the respiratory quotient (RQ = $\dot{V}_{CO_2} \div \dot{V}_{O_2}$), and an RQ greater than one suggests the patient is getting excess carbohydrate in his or her diet. This frequently occurs in critically ill patients receiving parenteral hyperalimentation. This excessive dietary carbohydrate could be deleterious to the critically ill patient in two ways: The conversion of the excess carbohydrate to fat utilizes a metabolic pathway that releases a lot of carbon dioxide at a time when the patient's ventilatory abilities may be marginal. Also, as the excess carbohydrate is converted to fat, it is stored in the liver. This could elevate the diaphragm, interfering with the mechanics of ventilation at a time when the patient needs to eliminate the excess carbon dioxide produced. When excess carbon dioxide production and elevated RQ are found, reduction in carbohydrate alimentation may allow successful weaning from mechanical ventilation (see Chapter 12).

Mass Spectrometry

Mass spectrometers are being increasingly used to monitor respiratory gases during surgery as well as in the intensive care unit. A mass spectrometer ionizes gas molecules, then collects and counts these ions according to their mass-charge ratio.

Two main types of mass spectrometers are currently in use. The magnetic sector type accelerates the ions through a magnetic field that forces them into circular paths with radii proportional to the mass of the ion. Ions of the same mass follow the same path, ending with them striking a specific collector. The more strikes that a collector registers, the greater the current it generates. This is then translated into a greater concentration of that type of molecule. The quadrupole mass spectrometer operates in a similar manner, but instead of having a constant magnetic field and several collectors, it has a single collector and shifting magnetic field. By varying the intensity of the magnetic field, the entire mass spectrum can be scanned in a few milliseconds. Because of its rapid measurements, one mass spectrometer can be used to monitor several patients sequentially. In addition to the respiratory gases, the concentrations of anesthetic agents can be monitored. These noninvasive instruments are quite expensive and require considerable routine maintenance.

Adams, A.P., Morgan-Hughes, J.O., and Sykes, M.K.: pH and blood gas analysis. *Anaesthesia* 23:47, 1968.

Avery, G.B., and Glass, P.: Retinopathy of prematurity: What causes it? In Kliegman, R.M., and Behrman, R.E. (eds.): *Current Controversies in Perinatal Care*. Philadelphia, W.B. Saunders, 1988, pp 917–928.

Bates, R.G.: *Electrometric pH Determination*. New York, John Wiley & Sons, 1954.

DeVoe, W.M.: Prevention of retinopathy of prematurity. *Seminars in Perinatology* 12:373–380, 1988.

Flear, C.T.G., Covington, A.K., and Stoddart, J.D.: Bicarbonate or CO_2? (Editor's correspondence). *Arch. Intern. Med.* 144:2285-2287, 1984.

Hahn, C.E.W., and Foex, P.: Intravascular in vivo P_{O_2} and P_{CO_2} measurements. In Spence, A.A. (ed.): *Respiratory Monitoring in Intensive Care*. Edinburgh, Churchill Livingstone, 1982, pp 56–66.

Jones, N.L.: *Blood Gases and Acid/Base Physiology*. New York, Thieme-Stratton, 1980.

Levitzky, M.G.: *Pulmonary Physiology*, 2nd ed. New York, McGraw-Hill, 1986.

Mohler, J.G.: The basics for clinical blood gas evaluation. In Wilson, A.F. (ed): *Pulmonary Function Testing: Indications and Interpretations*. New York, Grune and Stratton, 1985.

Noback, C.R.: Intraoperative monitoring. In Kaplan, J.A. (ed.): *Thoracic Anesthesia*. New York, Churchill Livingstone, 1983, p 222.

Operators Manual, 282, *Co-oximetrics*. Instrumentation Laboratory, Inc. Catalogue #79282, 1980.

Operators Manual, 813, *pH Blood Gas Analyzer*. Instrumentation Laboratory Inc., Catalogue #79813, 1976.

Rosan, R.C., Enlander, D., and Ellis, J.: Unpredictable error in calculated bicarbonate homeostasis during pediatric intensive care: The delusion of fixed pK'. *Clin. Chem.* 29(1):69–79, 1983.

Sarnquist, F.H., Todd, C., and Whitcher, C.: Accuracy of a new noninvasive oxygen saturation monitor. *Anesthesiology* 53(Suppl.):163, 1980.

Severinghaus, J.W.: Transcutaneous monitoring of arterial P_{CO_2}. In Spence A.A. (ed.): *Respiratory Monitoring in Intensive Care*. Edinburgh, Churchill Livingstone, 1982, p 90.

Shapiro, B.A., Harrison, R.A., and Wilton, J.R.: *Clinical Application of Blood Gases*. 3rd ed. Chicago, Year Book, 1982.

Siggaard-Andersen, O., Norgaard-Pedersen, B., and Rem, J.: Hemoglobin pigments. Spectrophotometric determination of oxy-, carboxy-, met-, and sulfhemoglobin in capillary blood. *Clin. Chim. Acta* 42:85, 1972.

Smallout, B.: *A Quick Guide to Capnography and Its Use in Differential Diagnosis*. Palo Alto, CA, Hewlett-Packard, 1983, pp 3–7.

Sodal, F.E., and Swanson, G.D.: Mass spectrometry: Current technology and implications for anesthesia. In Aldrete, J.A., Lowe, H.J., and Virtue, R.W. (eds.): *Low Flow and Closed System Anesthesia*. New York, Grune and Stratton, 1979, pp 167–182.

Valtin, H., and Gennari, F.J.: *Acid-Base Disorders: Basic Concepts and Clinical Management*. Boston, Little, Brown and Company, 1987.

Waller, J.L., Kaplan, J.A., Bauman, D.I., and Carver, J.M.: Clinical evaluation of a new fiberoptic catheter oximeter during cardiac surgery. *Anesth. Analg.* 61:676, 1982.

Whitesell, R.C., Dhamee, M.S., and Munchi, C.: Transcutaneous P_{O_2} monitoring in adults. *Anesthesiology* 53(Suppl.):372, 1980.

OBJECTIVES

AFTER READING THIS CHAPTER, THE STUDENT WILL BE ABLE TO:

1. Understand the physiologic response to exercise.
2. Summarize the normal cardiopulmonary response during a maximum exercise effort.
3. Name the types of work tests that are routinely used in clinical exercise laboratories to assess physiologic reserve capacity.
4. Describe the instruments used to monitor cardiopulmonary changes during exercise.
5. Discuss multistage exercise tests.
6. Describe several laboratory approaches used to evaluate patients with defects in cardiorespiratory gas transport.
7. Describe the components of an exercise prescription.

11
CLINICAL EXERCISE TESTING

CHAPTER OUTLINE

REVIEW OF NORMAL CARDIOPULMONARY RESPONSE DURING EXERCISE
MODES OF EXERCISE TESTING
   Step Tests
   Cycle Ergometers
   Treadmills
TESTING PROCEDURES
   The Cardiac Stress Test
   The Cardiopulmonary Stress Test
   Test for Exercise-Induced Bronchospasm
   Emergency Procedures
DATA COLLECTION
   Heart Rate and Electrocardiography
   Arterial Blood Pressure
   Cardiac Output
   Respiratory Volumes and Flows
   Metabolic Measurements
DATA ANALYSIS
   Maximum Oxygen Consumption
   Electrocardiography
   Oxygen Pulse
   Breathing Reserve (Dyspneic Index)
   Wasted Ventilation ($\dot{V}_D/\dot{V}_T$)
   Anaerobic Threshold
EXERCISE PRESCRIPTIONS

During exercise, oxygen consumption increases linearly with the amount of work performed up to a maximum volume, or maximum oxygen consumption (V_{O_2} max). This increase in the total body oxygen consumption is made possible by (1) increased cardiac output by increased heart rate and cardiac stroke volume, (2) increased alveolar ventilation, (3) increased diffusion rate of oxygen between the lungs and pulmonary capillaries, and (4) increased amount of oxygen extracted by the muscles. Chapter 5 discussed the physiologic factors that influence these changes. In this chapter, the various methods used in clinical exercise testing and how this type of testing is used to assess cardiopulmonary reserve capacity are discussed.

REVIEW OF NORMAL CARDIOPULMONARY RESPONSE DURING EXERCISE

Figure 11–1 summarizes the cardiopulmonary changes that occur in a typical adult performing a maximum exercise effort by pedaling a bicycle ergometer. Note that the heart rate, blood pressure, cardiac output, minute ventilation, tidal volume, breathing frequency, and fractional concentrations of expired oxygen and carbon dioxide are measured directly during the test, whereas the oxygen consumption, carbon dioxide production, respiratory quotient, stroke volume, oxygen pulse and deadspace–to–tidal volume ratio are derived from the measured variables.

MODES OF EXERCISE TESTING

The most important factors to consider when choosing an exercise mode for clinical testing are (1) the types of muscle groups that the patient will use to perform the test (i.e., the size and number of the muscles used and whether or not they are weight-bearing), (2) the types of measurements that will be recorded during the test, and (3) whether the patient can perform the test. In clinical exercise testing, three modalities are routinely used to assess physical work capacity: *step tests, cycle ergometers,* and *treadmills.*

Step Tests

The simplest and least expensive method of exercise testing is the step test. This test, which was introduced by Selig in 1905 and later standardized by Master and his colleagues in the 1940s (e.g., Master's two-step test), involves electrocardiographic monitoring of a patient while he or she performs a certain number of continuous ascents and descents of a two-stair step (Fig. 11–2). The height of the stair step is kept constant while the number of ascents that the patient is instructed to make is determined using his or her age, sex, and weight. Because of its simplicity, Master's two-step test is still considered to be a useful test that can be conducted in a physician's office or as a screening device for those participating in a sports program or who are attempting to qualify for certain occupations.

Cycle Ergometers

Cycle ergometers are considered to be the most versatile of all of the exercise modes. Both foot-pedal ergometers and arm-crank ergometers are available so that patients can perform exercise in either an upright or a supine position. The handlebars and the saddles of cycle ergometers should be adjustable to accommodate patients of different sizes.

Two types of cycle ergometers are commonly used in physiologic testing: *mechanical* and *electromechanical* cycles (Fig. 11–3). In the mechanical type, a patient performs work against a resistance, created by braking one of the wheels of a modified bicycle or by tightening a strap on a flywheel. Because the power output of this device is influenced by the pedaling frequency, the power output can be controlled by having the patient pedal the cycle at a constant rate (e.g., the pedaling frequency can be set by using a metronome).

In the electromechanical type, the patient pedals against an electrically produced resistance. In general, variations in the pedaling frequency between 50 and 70 revolutions per minute do not affect the power output of electromechanical cycles significantly. For clinical work tests, the electromechanical cycle ergometers and arm crank ergometers that provide a constant and known power output, which is independent of the pedaling frequency, have been found to be the most useful.

Treadmills

Motor-driven treadmills have been widely used by cardiologists in North America for the diagnosis of coronary artery disease. Many clinicians choose treadmill exercise over other forms of exercise be-

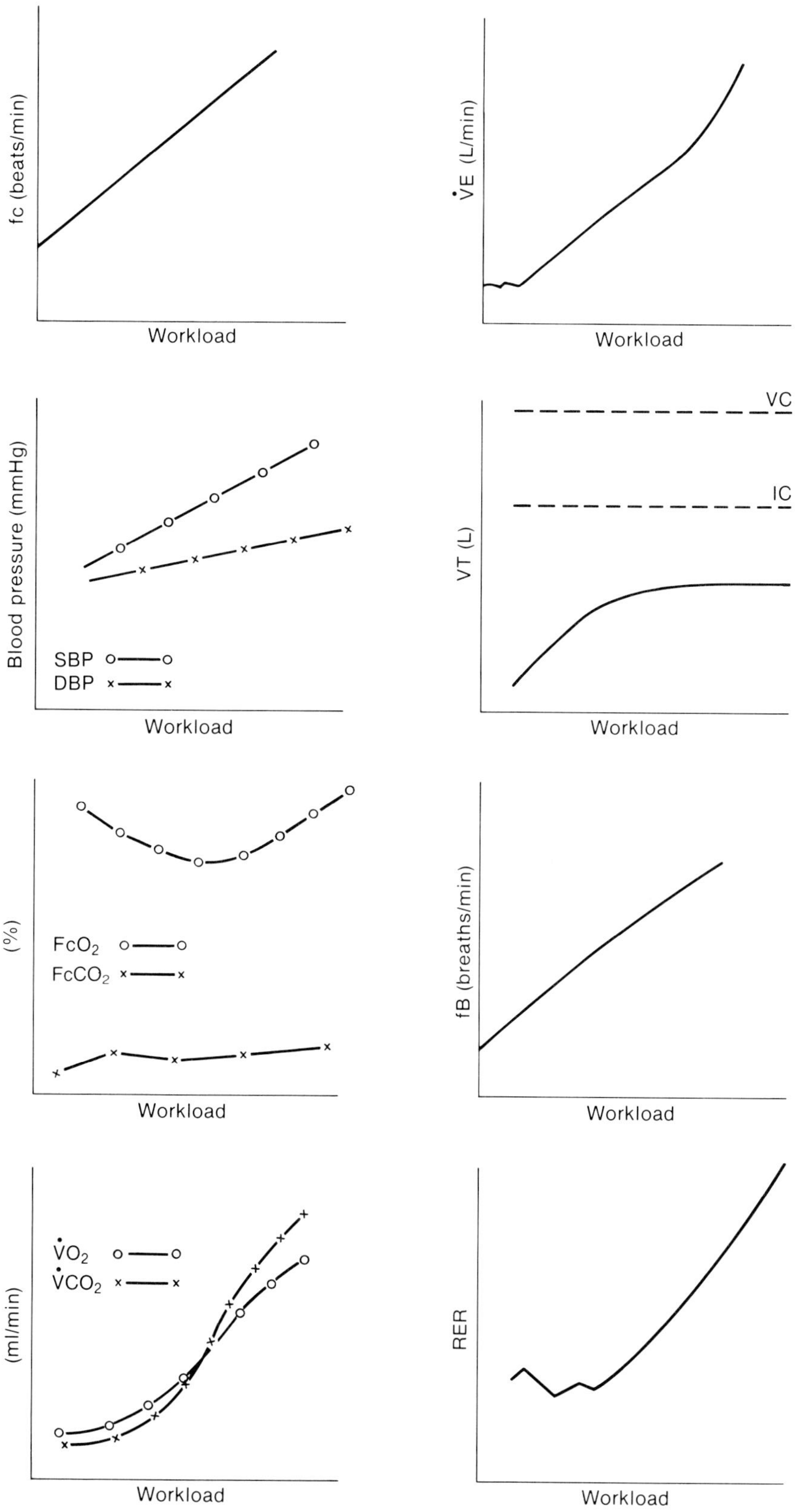

FIGURE 11–1. Cardiopulmonary changes during an incremental exercise test by an adult male on a bicycle ergometer.

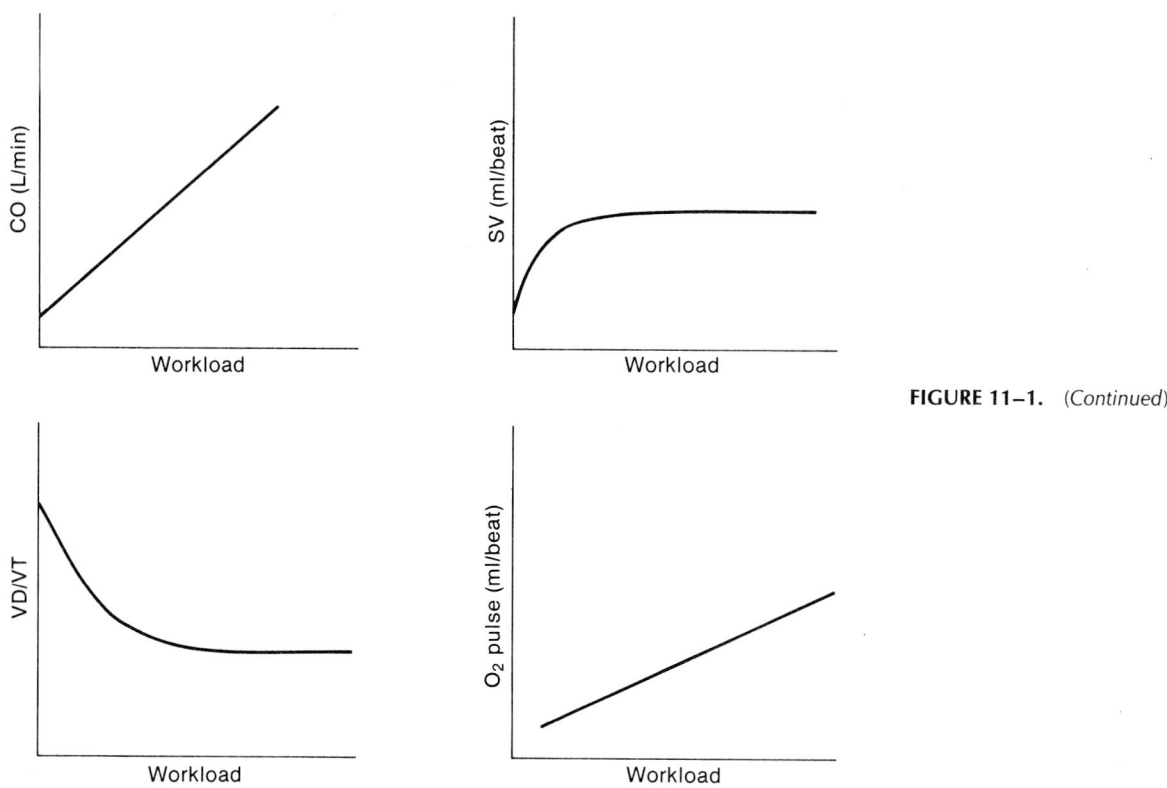

FIGURE 11–1. (Continued)

cause they feel that walking is a universal activity that can be accomplished by almost everyone. In treadmill exercise, the amount of work that a patient performs is determined by his or her weight as well as by the incline and speed of the treadmill. Note that when patients are performing exercise on a treadmill, they *should not hold onto the siderails* since this affects the workload. In clinical exercise testing, treadmills that can be adjusted from 0% to 14% grade and from 1 to 10 miles per hour have been shown to be acceptable (Fig. 11–4).

TESTING PROCEDURES

Before a patient performs an exercise test, a full history and physical examination should be obtained. When a patient is suspected of having cardiac or pulmonary dysfunction, the pretesting evaluation should also include pulmonary function tests (particularly static and dynamic lung volumes), carbon monoxide diffusing capacity ($D_{L_{CO}}$), maximum voluntary ventilation (MVV), airflow response to bronchodilators (if the patient has evidence of airflow obstruction), arterial blood gases, as well as a resting ECG, and the determination of systemic blood pressure. These resting data can then be used by the attending physician to determine whether the patient demonstrates any of the contraindications to exercise testing (Table 11–1).

If the patient does not demonstrate any of the contraindications to exercise testing, the physician

TABLE 11–1. Contraindications to Exercise Testing

1. Recent acute myocardial infarction
2. Unstable angina
3. Uncontrolled ventricular dysrhythmia
4. Uncontrolled atrial dysrhythmia which compromises cardiac function
5. Congestive heart failure
6. Severe aortic stenosis
7. Suspected or known dissecting aneurysm
8. Active or suspected myocarditis
9. Thrombophlebitis or intracardiac thrombi
10. Recent systemic or pulmonary embolus
11. Acute infection
12. Third-degree heart block
13. Significant emotional distress (psychosis)
14. A recent significant change in the resting ECG
15. Acute pericarditis

From American College of Sports Medicine: *Guidelines for Exercise Testing and Prescription,* 3rd ed. Philadelphia, Lea and Febiger, 1986, with permission.

CLINICAL EXERCISE TESTING 347

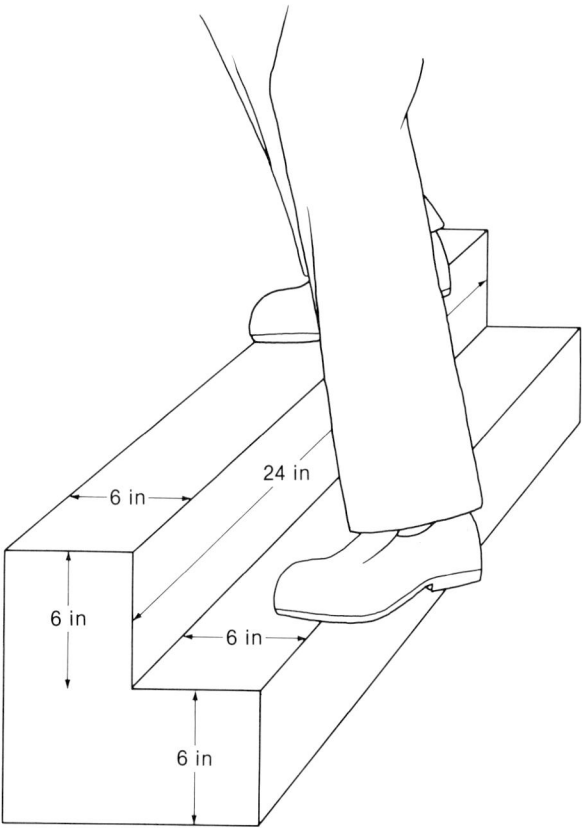

FIGURE 11–2. Step tests.

can then choose an exercise strategy that is suited to the patient's physical ability. Table 11–2 lists four exercise strategies that can be used to evaluate exercise performance. Note that these strate-

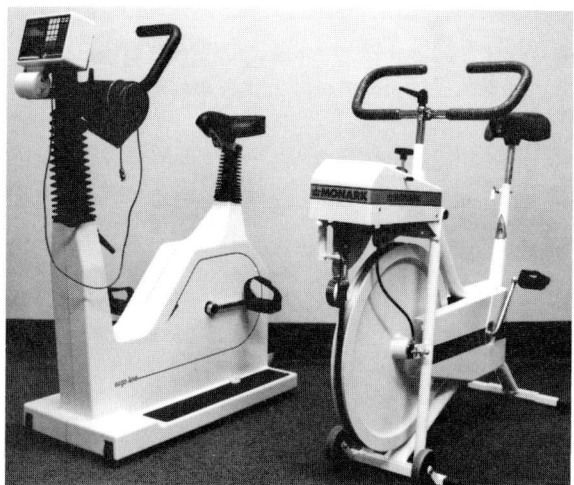

FIGURE 11–3. Mechanical and electromechanical cycle ergometers.

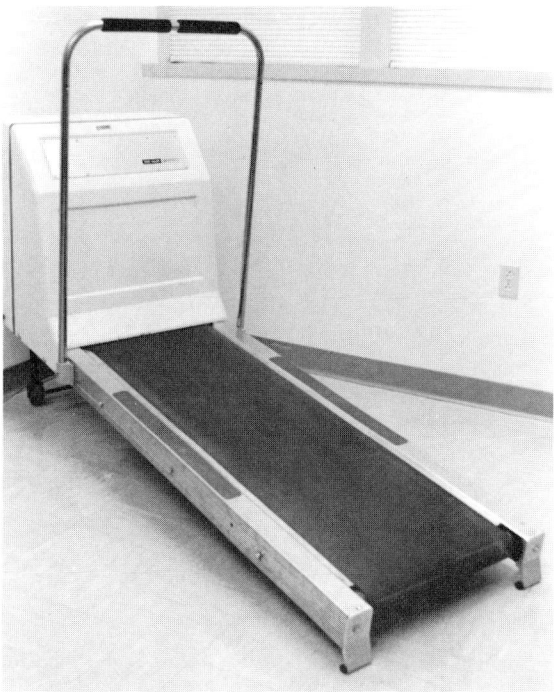

FIGURE 11–4. Treadmill. (Courtesy of Cambridge Instruments, Cambridge, MA.)

gies can involve submaximal or maximal tests, achieved with a single work load, a discontinuous series of increasing work loads, or a continuous series of increasing work loads. The measurements made during these tests can range from simple noninvasive measurements of heart rate, blood pressure, and electrocardiograms to fairly complex measurements of inspired and/or expired airflows,

TABLE 11–2. Summary of Measurements Made in Stage 1 to Stage 4 Exercise Tests

Stage 1:	Always recorded—heart rate, blood pressure, electrocardiogram, ventilation, tidal volume, symptoms. Optional measurements made when indicated—mixed expired O_2 and CO_2 concentrations, O_2 saturation by ear oximetry, and postexercise plasma lactate concentration.
Stage 2:	Always recorded—heart rate, blood pressure, electrocardiogram, ventilation, tidal volume, mixed expired O_2 and CO_2 concentrations, end-tidal P_{CO_2}, mixed venous P_{CO_2}.
Stage 3:	As for Stage 2 with arterial or capillary P_{O_2}, P_{CO_2}, pH, and lactate concentration.
Stage 4:	Pulmonary float catheter with pressure measurements.

From Jones, N.L., and Campbell, E.J.M.: *Clinical Exercise Testing,* 2nd ed. Philadelphia, W.B. Saunders, 1982, with permission.

respiratory frequency, expired gas concentrations, arterial blood gases, and intravascular pressures. In the following sections, several exercise protocols routinely used in clinical exercise testing are described.

The Cardiac Stress Test

This is a noninvasive procedure in which the patient's heart rate, blood pressure, and electrocardiogram are monitored continuously as he or she performs an incremental work test. The test can be conducted with a treadmill (Table 11–3) or a cycle ergometer. Measurements are made before the test begins (while the subject is at rest), at the end of each stage, and for at least 15 minutes after the test is completed or until any evidence of cardiac or respiratory problems has subsided. Most healthy subjects have no problem in completing all of the stages, whereas patients with coronary artery disease are usually limited either by their symptoms (e.g., angina or dyspnea) or because one of the safety limits listed in Table 11–4 has been reached.

TABLE 11–3. Treadmill Exercise Test Protocols

Stage	Duration (min)	Speed (mph)	Grade %	Approx. $\dot{V}O_2$ (ml/kg/min)	Mets
Bruce Protocol*					
0*	3	1.7	0	8	2.0
½*	3	1.7	5	12	3.1
1	3	1.7	10	18	4.8
2	3	2.5	12	25	6.8
3	3	3.4	14	34	9.6
4	3	4.2	16	46	13.2
5	3	5.0	18	55	16.1
6	3	5.5	20		
7	3	6.0	22		
Naughton Protocol					
1	2	3	0	10	2.5
2	2	3	2.5	14	3.5
3	2	3	5	18	4.7
4	2	3	7.5	21	5.6
5	2	3	10	24	6.4
6	2	3	12.5	28	7.5
7	2	3	15	32	8.7
8	2	3	17.5	35	9.5
9	2	3	20	38	10.7
10	2	3	22.5	42	11.9

* Sheffield modification: begin at stage 0. Original Bruce: begin at stage 1.

From Braunwald, E. (ed.): *Heart Disease: A Textbook of Cardiovascular Medicine,* 3rd ed. Philadelphia, W.B. Saunders, 1988, with permission.

TABLE 11–4. Indications for Terminating Graded Exercise Testing

Physical exhaustion
Excessive dyspnea or leg fatigue
Excessive chest pain or other exercise induced symptom
Excessive ST segment deviation
Ventricular tachycardia
Ventricular premature beats precipitated or aggravated by exercise (over 25% of beats)
Ectopic supraventricular tachycardia
Any intracardiac block precipitated by exercise
Peripheral circulatory insufficiency (pallor, clammy skin, drop in blood pressure)
Subject wishes to stop exercise

From Braunwald, E. (ed.): *Heart Disease: A Textbook of Cardiovascular Medicine,* 3rd ed. Philadelphia, W.B. Saunders, 1988, with permission.

Although this test has been shown to be quite effective in the diagnosis and treatment of patients with coronary artery disease, its usefulness in the diagnosis of other cardiopulmonary diseases is limited.

The Cardiopulmonary Stress Test

The equipment required to conduct this type of test includes a treadmill or cycle ergometer, a device for recording ventilation, a system for analyzing expired gases, and either an oximeter for monitoring arterial oxygen saturations or an indwelling arterial catheter for sampling blood gases. In specialized cases, Swan-Ganz catheterization may also be used if central venous blood sampling and hemodynamic monitoring are necessary.

The graded exercise testing (GXT) procedure is performed by having the patient exercise at a series of standardized work loads. Typically, the work load is increased by increments that result in an increase in oxygen uptake of approximately 3.5 ml/kg per minute (1 MET) per stage. The patient should begin the test at a low work load, such as walking on the treadmill at 0% grade and 1 to 2 miles per hour or by pedaling the cycle without any load at a rate of 50 to 60 revolutions per minute. After a 2- to 3-minute warm-up period, the work load is increased by equal increments every minute while cardiopulmonary measurements are made toward the end of each stage. The test is stopped when the patient reaches a predetermined heart rate or if he or she demonstrates any of the symptoms or signs listed in Table 11–4.

TABLE 11–5. Derived Measurement for Clinical Exercise Testing

Maximum oxygen consumption ($\dot{V}O_2$ max)
Respiratory quotient (R.Q., RER)
Oxygen pulse (O_2 pulse)
Breathing reserve (dyspneic index)
Wasted ventilation (V_D/V_T)
Anaerobic threshold ($\dot{V}O_2$ AT)

Table 11–5 lists the variables that can be derived from the measurements made during a cardiopulmonary stress test. The usefulness of each of these derived variables in assessing an individual's physical work capacity is discussed in subsequent sections of this chapter.

Test for Exercise-Induced Bronchospasm

To test individuals suspected of having exercise-induced bronchospasms, or exercise-induced asthma (EIA), baseline spirometry is obtained before the patient performs an exercise bout and then at 0, 5, 10, and 15 minutes after he or she has completed the exercise. Patients who experience exercise-induced bronchospasms show a characteristic decline in $FEV_{1.0}$ at 5 to 10 minutes after exercise is completed and then spontaneously recover to pre-exercise levels.

Emergency Procedures

All clinical exercise laboratories should be equipped to handle medical emergencies that can arise during exercise tests. Table 11–6 lists the drugs and resuscitation equipment that should be available. It is important that all laboratory personnel be familiar with these drugs and equipment as well as proper resuscitation techniques.

TABLE 11–6. Equipment and Supplies for Management of Complications*

1. Defibrillator with full tube of electrode paste
2. Assorted airways, ventilation bag, oxygen, and laryngoscope
3. Intravenous fluid (5% dextrose) with tubing, needles, and assorted syringes
4. Assorted drugs, including lidocaine, quinidine, disopyramide, procainamide, propranolol, atropine, isoproterenol, norepinephrine, metaraminol, digoxin, furosemide, dopamine, nifedipine, verapamil

* From Braunwald, E., *Heart Disease: A Textbook of Cardiovascular Medicine*, 3rd ed. Philadelphia, W.B. Saunders Co., 1988.

DATA COLLECTION

Recent advances in computer technology have made it relatively easy for the clinician to simultaneously monitor cardiovascular, respiratory, and/or metabolic changes that occur while a patient exercises. The variables measured during an exercise test depend on the questions that need to be answered about a patient and whether noninvasive or invasive methods are needed. The following section summarizes the measurements most often obtained in clinical exercise testing.

Heart Rate and Electrocardiography

It is generally agreed that electrocardiograms (ECGs) provide the most accurate measurement of cardiac frequency during exercise testing. ECGs, when obtained properly, can also provide documentation of specific cardiac arrhythmias, as well as S-T segment and T wave changes that result from cardiac ischemia.

Among the various types of electrodes available for stress testing, the silver–silver chloride electrodes, which can be attached to the skin with a circular adhesive pad, have been shown to be quite satisfactory. Remember, however, that adequate preparation, such as abrading the skin to remove cornified epithelium before attaching the electrodes, and the proper use of conducting gel, affect the quality of the ECG tracing recorded.

Although a number of electrocardiographic lead configurations have been proposed for exercise testing (Fig. 11–5) in healthy young subjects, a one-lead configuration with the active electrode in the V5 position and an indifferent electrode placed on the sternum or forehead has been shown to be sufficient for obtaining information on heart rate and ischemic electrocardiographic changes. For patients over 35 years old and those suspected of having cardiopulmonary disease, a standard 12-lead configuration yields more specific information on exercise-induced cardiac ischemia.

Arterial Blood Pressure

As discussed in Chapter 9, the direct measurement of arterial blood pressure is an invasive technique

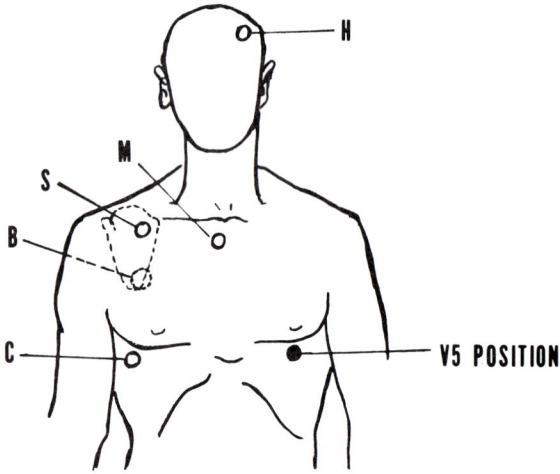

FIGURE 11–5. ECG lead configurations commonly used in exercise testing. (From Braunwald, E.: *Heart Disease: A Textbook of Cardiovascular Medicine*, 3rd ed. Philadelphia, W.B. Saunders, 1988, with permission.)

that requires arterial puncture and the placement of an indwelling arterial catheter. The catheter is connected to a pressure transducer-amplifier system that provides a continuous recording of the blood pressure.

Indirect measurements of arterial blood pressure can be obtained noninvasively with a sphygmomanometer and a stethoscope by a trained observer or automatically with a system that uses ultrasound or contact microphones interfaced with an on-line computer system. These techniques provide good estimates of systolic and diastolic pressures at rest and at low levels of work; however, at high work rates, motion artifacts can disguise the diastolic pressure, and only the systolic pressure can be recorded.

Although the direct technique provides a continuous record of arterial pressure that is more accurate than the noninvasive measurements, this technique should be limited to those patients with conditions that warrant invasion of the vascular space.

Cardiac Output

The measurement of cardiac output during exercise represents a formidable task. Three techniques commonly used in clinical exercise testing are the direct Fick, indicator dilution, and CO_2 rebreathing techniques.

The *direct Fick technique* requires the measurement of expired gases as well as the sampling of arterial and mixed venous blood. As discussed later, expired gases can be analyzed relatively easily, whereas the arterial and mixed venous blood samples require the use of indwelling arterial catheters and Swan-Ganz catheterization. Also, it is imperative that expired gas collection and blood sampling be done simultaneously. The oxygen consumption is calculated with the inspired/expired gas analysis and the arterial and mixed venous oxygen contents (Cao_2 and $C\bar{v}o_2$, respectively) derived from the blood gas measurements. The cardiac output (C.O.) is then derived using the following equation:

$$C.O. = \dot{V}o_2 \div Cao_2 - C\bar{v}o_2$$

In the *indicator dilution technique*, a radioisotope like xenon-133 or a dye like indocyanine green is injected into the circulation while blood is sampled from an artery downstream of the injection site. The *thermodilution technique*, a variation of the indicator dilution technique, requires a thermistor (attached to the distal end of the Swan-Ganz catheter) to measure the changes in blood temperature that occur when a small sample (5 to 10 ml) of cold physiologic saline is injected into the circulation.

The CO_2 *rebreathing technique* is a noninvasive method that is accomplished by having the patient breathe into and out of a 5 L polyethylene bag that contains a known concentration of carbon dioxide. By measuring the CO_2 production, and the CO_2 concentrations in the patient's expired gases at the beginning of the test and after he or she has reached equilibration, the cardiac output can be calculated with the following equation:

$$C.O. = \dot{V}co_2 \div C\bar{v}co_2 - Caco_2$$

The arterial and mixed venous carbon dioxide contents are derived from the CO_2 dissociation curve. In normal subjects, the pulmonary blood flow is assumed to equal the systemic blood flow. In patients with large intrapulmonary shunts, the measurement of pulmonary blood flow may underestimate the actual systemic blood flow because not all of the blood perfusing the lung of these patients goes through well-ventilated alveoli.

Respiratory Volumes and Flows

The measurement of expired gas volumes during exercise testing can be accomplished with a Tissot spirometer, which is simply a large water-sealed spirometer (Fig. 11–6). Alternatively, the volume of air breathed can be determined by integrating

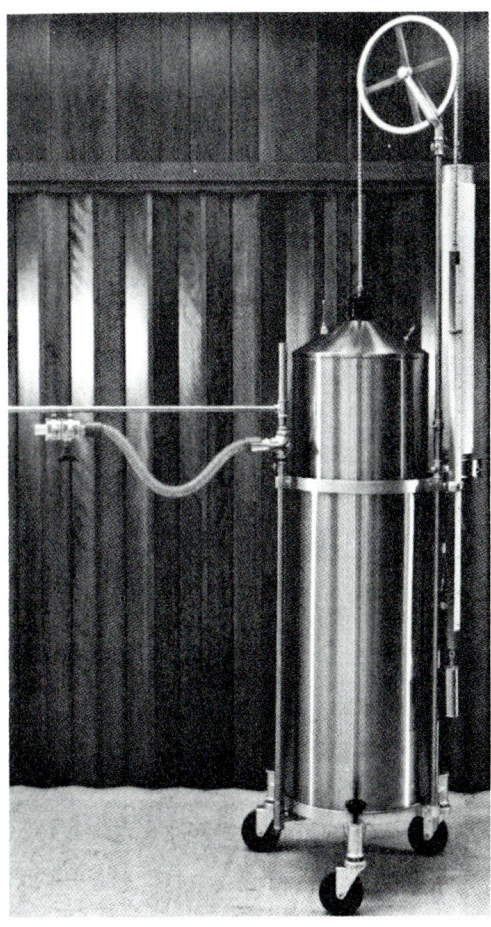

FIGURE 11–6. Tissot spirometer. (From Polgar, G., and Promadhat, V.: *Pulmonary Function Testing in Children: Techniques and Standards.* Philadelphia, W.B. Saunders, 1971, with permission.)

the flow signals obtained with turbine flowmeters or differential pressure pneumotachographs. As with all spirometers, these devices should be calibrated prior to testing.

Metabolic Measurements

The determination of oxygen consumption ($\dot{V}O_2$) and carbon dioxide production ($\dot{V}CO_2$) requires the measurements of the volume (or flow) of expired gas over time (i.e., the minute ventilation), the fractional concentrations of inspired and expired oxygen (FIO_2 and FEO_2, respectively), the fractional concentrations of inspired and expired carbon dioxide ($FICO_2$ and $FECO_2$, respectively), the barometric pressure (P_B), and the temperature of the mixed expired gas (T°C). Minute ventilation can be determined with any of the spirometers discussed in the previous section.

A number of gas analyzers that operate on physical principles can be used to determine the composition of inspired and expired gas. These include the *multiple gas* analyzers, such as mass spectometers, gas chromatographs, and thermal conductivity meters; and the *single gas* analyzers, such as paramagnetic and polarographic oxygen analyzers and nondispersive infrared carbon dioxide analyzers. Chemical methods, such as the Scholander and Lloyd-Haldane techniques, are also available for quantitation of gas mixtures. Although measurements made with chemical analyses are considered to be more accurate than those obtained with physical gas analyzers, the chemical methods are time-consuming and thus are not particularly useful when analyzing a large number of samples.

Figure 11–7 shows a typical metabolic cart used in the determination of $\dot{V}O_2$ and $\dot{V}CO_2$ during exercise. The patient breathes through a one-way

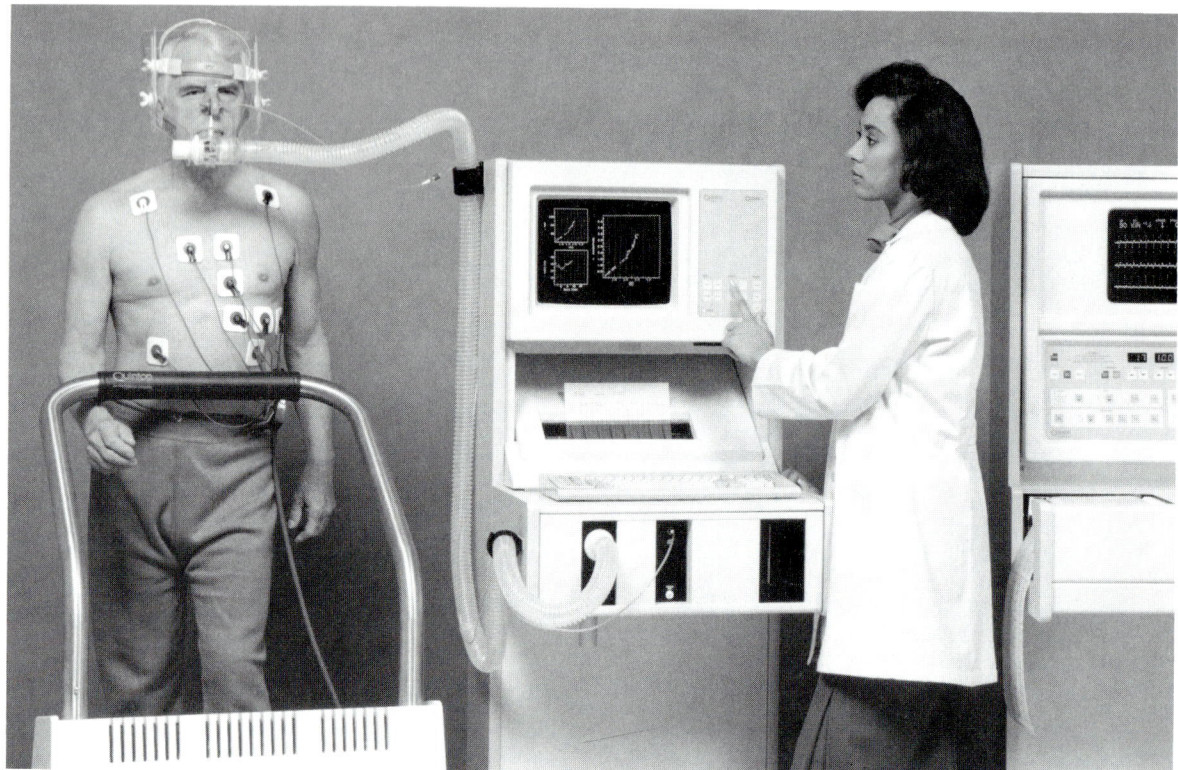

FIGURE 11–7. Metabolic measurement cart used to measure inspired and expired gas volumes and concentrations. (Courtesy of Quinton Instrument Company, Seattle, WA.)

(non-rebreathing) valve that contains a low dead-space volume, and the expired gas is directed via wide-bore corrugated tubing (with an internal diameter of 3 to 5 cm) into the system. Mixed expired gas samples are then analyzed. Calculations of $\dot{V}O_2$ and $\dot{V}CO_2$ are made with an on-line computer system that is interfaced with the gas analyzers.

DATA ANALYSIS

Maximum Oxygen Consumption

The maximum oxygen consumption ($\dot{V}O_2$ max) may be defined as the $\dot{V}O_2$ at which performance of increasing levels of exercise fails to further increase a subject's oxygen uptake. The main determinants of $\dot{V}O_2$ max include the patient's age, sex, weight, and height as well as his or her level of fitness. When expressed relative to total body weight, typical sedentary adults have $\dot{V}O_2$ max values of 20 to 30 ml/kg of body weight (if the $\dot{V}O_2$ is expressed relative to the lean body weight, which is the total body weight minus the weight of fatty tissues, these values become slightly higher).

The determination of an individual's $\dot{V}O_2$ max is usually accomplished with a maximum exercise test; however, submaximum exercise tests have also been shown to give fairly good estimates of $\dot{V}O_2$ max for individuals who cannot perform maximum tests. When using a maximum exercise test to determine the maximum oxygen consumption, $\dot{V}O_2$ max is thought to occur when the patient reaches his or her maximum predicted heart rate. A patient's maximum heart rate (HR max) can be predicted using the following equation:

$$HR\ max = 220 - age$$

For submaximal test, the $\dot{V}O_2$ max is estimated by having the subject perform a series of submaximal exercise tests for 6 minutes each. During the last minute of each exercise test, the heart rate is measured and recorded. A maximum oxygen consumption can then be derived by relating the heart rate response to a given amount of work.

Studies have shown that the $\dot{V}O_2$ max measured during arm-crank exercise is approximately 70% of that measured when the same patient performs exercise with a leg ergometer. In comparisons of leg ergometer and treadmill exercise, $\dot{V}O_2$ max measured with a leg ergometer has been shown to be about 90% of that measured when a patient performs treadmill exercise.

The maximum oxygen consumption is reduced in conditions in which the oxygen delivery to and/or utilization by the muscles is impaired. $\dot{V}O_2$ max is therefore reduced in patients with heart or peripheral vascular diseases, lung disease, endocrine disorders, and musculoskeletal disease. Additionally, it is typically reduced in patients receiving β-adrenergic blocking agents (e.g., propranolol) and in poorly motivated patients.

Electrocardiography

In the diagnosis of coronary artery disease, the degree of S-T segment displacement that occurs during exercise is considered to reflect the severity of myocardial ischemia, whereas the degree of myocardial obstruction responsible for the ischemia is directly related to the duration of S-T segment depression that occurs after exercise is concluded. Although S-T segment depression can occur in normal subjects during exercise, this depression is usually not more than 0.10 mV (1 mm) and occurs for 40 milliseconds or less. For patients with coronary artery disease, the presence of an S-T segment depression of 0.1 mV or greater for 80 milliseconds is associated with a significant narrowing of the coronary vessels.

Figure 11–8 shows three types of S-T segment displacements that can occur in patients with exertional myocardial ischemia. In Type I displacements, transient S-T segment depressions occur during exercise, but virtually disappear within 1 minute after exercise is concluded. Type II S-T segment depressions are considered to be a more serious type of response because the S-T segment depression not only occurs during exercise but also intensifies at the conclusion of exercise effort. Usually 10 to 20 minutes are required for the T wave to become fully upright and for the S-T segment to return to the pre-exercise isoelectric line. Type IIIa S-T segment elevations are characteristic of patients with *Prinzmetal's angina*, which is thought to result when a spastic occlusion of a single major coronary vessel is provoked by transmural ischemia. A second type of S-T segment elevation (Type IIIb) occurs in patients with myocardial scarring or dyskinesis that has resulted from a pre-existing disease.

Oxygen Pulse

According to the Fick principle, the total volume of oxygen that a person consumes per minute ($\dot{V}O_2$) is determined by the cardiac output (C.O.) and the volume of oxygen extracted by the tissues ($CaO_2 - C\bar{v}O_2$) or:

$$\dot{V}O_2 = C.O. \times (CaO_2 - C\bar{v}O_2)$$

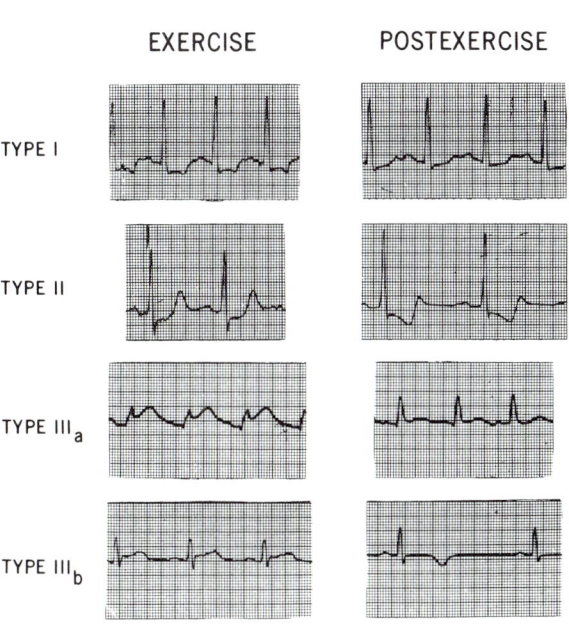

FIGURE 11–8. Classification of S-T segment displacements that commonly occur with exertional myocardial ischemia. (From Braunwald, E.: *Heart Disease: A Textbook of Cardiovascular Medicine*, 3rd ed. Philadelphia, W.B. Saunders, 1988, with permission.)

By substituting stroke volume times cardiac frequency for cardiac output, we get:

$$\dot{V}O_2 = (HR \times SV) \times (CaO_2 - C\bar{v}O_2)$$

The volume of oxygen removed from the blood with each heartbeat, or the oxygen pulse ($\dot{V}O_2/HR$), is often used as an noninvasive index of the stroke volume and the arterial-mixed venous oxygen content difference:

$$\dot{V}O_2/HR = SV \times (CaO_2 - C\bar{v}O_2)$$

In healthy subjects, the oxygen pulse is approximately 3 to 5 ml per beat at rest and increases to 10 to 15 ml per beat at maximum exercise. Trained athletes demonstrate higher oxygen pulses for any given oxygen consumption primarily from the increased amount of blood ejected with each heartbeat and increased extraction of oxygen by the tissues. In patients with reduced stroke volumes, such as those with valvular heart diseases or moderate to severe coronary artery disease, the oxygen pulse is less than 10 ml per beat. The oxygen pulse is also reduced in patients with anemia, severe hypoxemia, and high levels of carboxyhemoglobin.

Breathing Reserve (Dyspneic Index)

Earlier, the maximum voluntary ventilation (MVV) was defined as the maximum volume of air that a person can inspire and expire during a 1-minute period (remember that the MVV is only measured for 12 to 15 seconds; the ventilation per minute is then calculated by multiplying the volume measured for 12 to 15 seconds by 5 or 4). Because the MVV is determined by the strength of the respiratory muscles, the elastic recoil properties of the lungs and chest wall, and the patency of the airways, it is thought that this measurement is a reflection of a person's *maximum ventilatory capacity*. Conversely, the maximum ventilation that a person achieves during steady state exercise is determined by the requirements of gas exchange and acid-base balance.

The breathing reserve can be defined as the difference between the MVV and the maximum minute ventilation achieved during a maximum exercise effort or as the ratio of the minute ventilation that a person achieves during a maximum exercise effort to the MVV. Normal healthy subjects use only about 60% of their maximum ventilatory capacity during a maximum exercise effort. Patients with increased ventilatory requirements, such as those with ventilation perfusion imbalances, or those who demonstrate reductions in maximum ventilatory capacity, such as those with airway obstruction or restriction, demonstrate a characteristic decrease in breathing reserve and may be forced to use 90% to 100% of their maximum ventilatory capacity. (It should be noted that well-trained athletes also utilize high percentages of their maximum ventilatory capacity.)

Wasted Ventilation ($\dot{V}_D/\dot{V}_T$)

In a typical adult at rest, the physiologic deadspace ventilation represents approximately one third of the total minute ventilation (i.e., $\dot{V}_D/\dot{V}_T = 0.3$). During a maximum exercise effort, healthy subjects demonstrate a decrease in their $\dot{V}_D/\dot{V}_T$ to approximately 0.2 to 0.25, with the largest decrement in $\dot{V}_D/\dot{V}_T$ occurring at light work loads (see Fig. 11–1). In patients with pulmonary vascular disease (either primary or secondary to obstructive or restrictive lung disease), the $\dot{V}_D/\dot{V}_T$ may be only slightly elevated at rest, but it remains constant or even increases instead of decreasing during exercise. (Because exercise makes ventilation/perfusion mismatching more evident, this abnormal finding is sometimes the only gas exchange abnormality evident during exercise testing.)

Anaerobic Threshold

When the oxygen requirements of the exercising muscles cannot be met by an adequate oxygen delivery, aerobic oxidative mechanisms must be supplemented by anaerobic mechanisms. This increase in anaerobic oxidation is reflected by an increase in lactate and the lactate-pyruvate ratio in muscle and arterial blood. Clinically, the work rate at which anaerobic oxidation becomes evident, or the *anaerobic threshold*, can be determined by observing changes in expired volumes and the concentration of expired gases or by arterial blood gas analyses.

As Figure 11–9 shows, during the early phase of exercise, the $\dot{V}O_2$, $\dot{V}CO_2$ and $\dot{V}E$ increase proportionately. At approximately 50% to 60% of the maximum oxygen consumption, $\dot{V}CO_2$ and $\dot{V}E$ begin to increase out of proportion to the $\dot{V}O_2$ because of the requirement for increasing amounts of anaerobic oxidation. (The higher minute ventilation occurs as a result of stimulation of the arterial chemoreceptors by increases in hydrogen

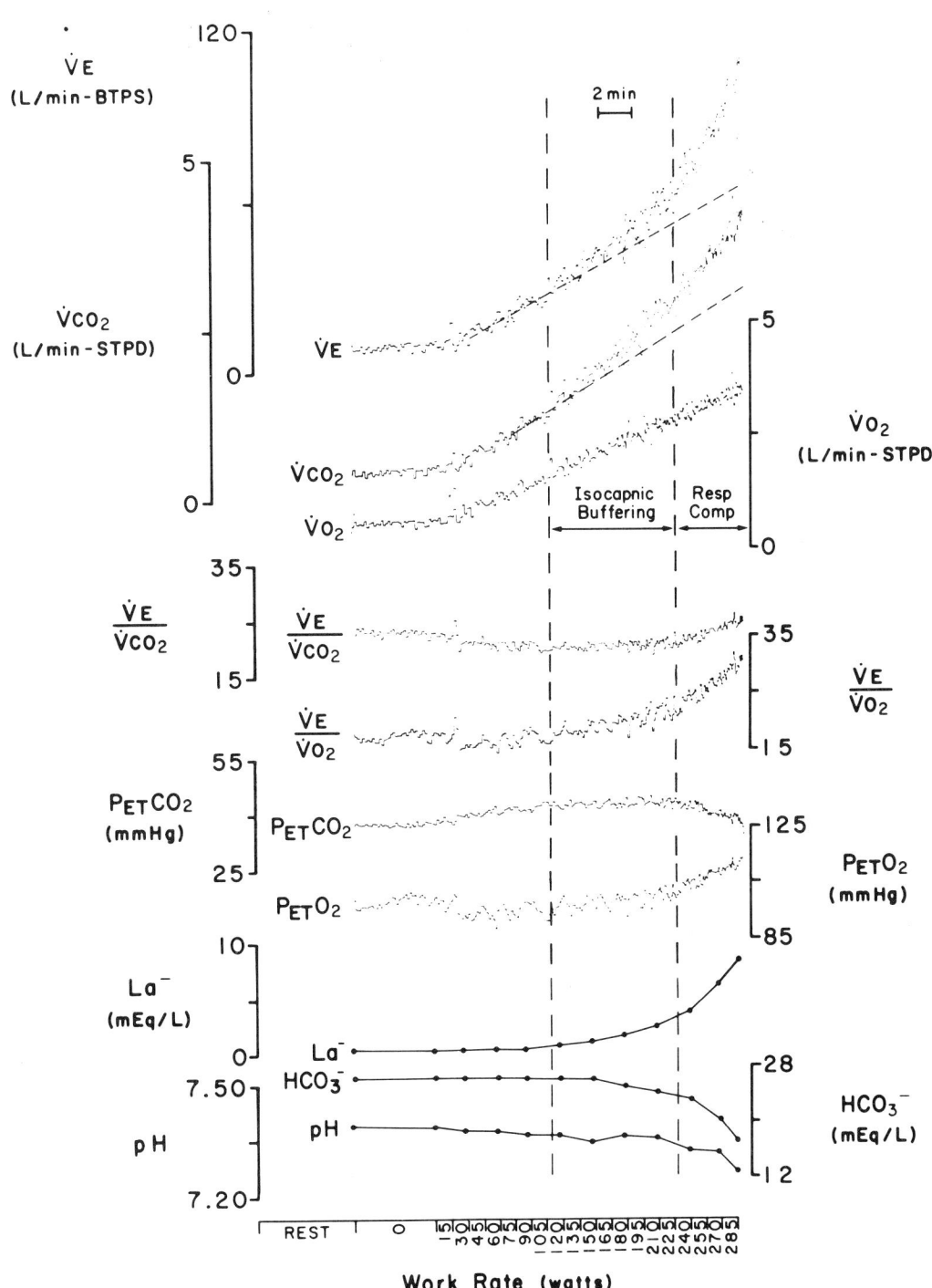

FIGURE 11–9. Graph showing gas exchange and arterial blood gas changes that occur in a healthy subject during a maximum exercise effort. The anaerobic threshold occurs in the area between the two vertical lines. (From Wasserman, K., Hansen, J.E., Sue, D.Y., and Whipp, B.J.: *Principles of Exercise Testing and Interpretation.* Philadelphia, Lea & Febiger, 1988, with permission.)

ions that are formed from lactic acid and from increases in carbon dioxide that result from the buffering of lactic acid.) Thus, one method of determining the anaerobic threshold is to note the point at which there is an increase in end-tidal P_{O_2}, while the end-tidal P_{CO_2} remains relatively constant. As the work rate is increased beyond this point, the patient is unable to protect his or her arterial pH through respiratory compensation and an uncompensated metabolic acidosis results.

A second method of determining the anaerobic threshold is to observe the work rate at which the respiratory exchange ratio (RER) rises above 1.0. The increase in RER occurs because the $\dot{V}_{CO_2}$ increases to a greater extent than the $\dot{V}_{O_2}$ primarily from isocapnic buffering of lactic acid (i.e., $H^+ + HCO_3^- \rightleftharpoons H_2CO_3 \rightleftharpoons CO_2 + H_2O$, with the resultant carbon dioxide being exhaled).

A third method of determining the anaerobic threshold is to monitor the ventilatory equivalents for oxygen and carbon dioxide ($\dot{V}_{E_{O_2}}$ and $\dot{V}_{E_{CO_2}}$, respectively). The ventilatory equivalents for oxygen and carbon dioxide represent the minute ventilation that a person must achieve to attain a certain oxygen consumption or carbon dioxide production. At the anaerobic threshold, the $\dot{V}_E/\dot{V}_{O_2}$ increases considerably while the $\dot{V}_E/\dot{V}_{CO_2}$ stays relatively constant, thus indicating that ventilation exceeds the amount required for oxygen uptake but not for carbon dioxide excretion.

The anaerobic threshold occurs at approximately 50% to 60% of the $\dot{V}_{O_2}$ max in normal subjects. (It may be 70% to 80% of $\dot{V}_{O_2}$ max in well-trained athletes.) It is lower for arm-crank exercise than for bicycle ergometry or treadmill exercise. The reasons for this discrepancy are not known but may be related to the size of the muscle groups, the recruitment patterns of the motor units used during arm-crank tests compared to those used during leg tests, or the distribution of fast- and slow-twitch muscle fibers in the arms and legs.

As with the maximum oxygen consumption, the anaerobic threshold is reduced in conditions in which the oxygen flow to the tissues or utilization of oxygen by the tissues is impaired. Thus, it is reduced in patients with coronary artery disease and aortic stenosis as well as in those with peripheral vascular disorders, such as atherosclerosis and systemic hypertension.

EXERCISE PRESCRIPTIONS

Recommendations for exercise in patients with cardiopulmonary disease should be based on exercise testing results and on the patient's willingness to participate in a structured exercise regimen. The exercise prescription should include specifications for (1) the type of exercise to be performed, (2) the intensity of the effort, (3) the frequency at which the exercise should be performed, and (4) the duration of training. Additionally, the clinician should always consider whether the patient will be able to accomplish the prescription without experiencing dyspnea, light-headedness, chest pain, arrhythmias, or simply feeling exhausted. Specific guidelines should be developed for patients who have experienced a myocardial infarction or who have chronic pulmonary disease.

Bibliography

American College of Sports Medicine: *Guidelines for Exercise Testing and Prescription,* 3rd ed. Philadelphia, Lea & Febiger, 1986.

Astrand, P.O.: Human physical fitness with special reference to sex and age. *Physiol. Rev.* 36:307–335, 1956.

Astrand, P.O., and Rodahl, K.: *Textbook of Work Physiology.* New York. McGraw-Hill, 1970.

Beaver, W., Wasserman, K., and Whipp, B.J.: On-line computer analysis and breath-by-breath graphical display of exercise function tests. *J. Applied Physiol.* 34:128–137, 1973.

Braunwald, E.: *Heart Disease. A Textbook of Cardiovascular Disease.* Philadelphia, W.B. Saunders, 1984, pp 258–278.

Davis, J.A., Frank, M.H., Whipp, B.J., and Wasserman, K.: Anaerobic threshold alterations caused by endurance training in middle aged men. *J. Applied Physiol.* 46(6):1,039–1,046, 1979.

Davis, J.A., Odak, P., Wilmore, J.H., and Kurtz, P.: Anaerobic threshold and maximal aerobic power for three modes of exercise. *J. Applied Physiol.* 41(4):544–550, 1976.

Eggleston, P.A., and Guerrant, J.L.: A standardized method of evaluating exercise induced asthma. *J. Allergy Clin. Immunol.* 58(3):414–425, 1976.

Franklin, B.A., Hellerstein, H.K., Gordon, S., and Timmis, G.C.: Exercise prescription for the myocardial infarction patient. *J. Cardiopulmonary Rehabil.* 6:62–79, 1986.

Jones, N.L., and Campbell, E.J.M.: *Clinical Exercise Testing,* 2nd ed. Philadelphia, W.B. Saunders, 1982.

Jones, N.L., Jones, G., and Edwards, R.H.T.: Exercise tolerance in chronic airway obstruction. *Am. Rev. Resp. Dis.* 103:477–491, 1971.

Jones, N.L., McHardy, G.J.R., Naimark, A., and Campbell, E.J.M.: Physiological deadspace and alveolar-arterial gas pressure differences during exercise. *Clinical Science* (31):19–29, 1966.

Kattus, A.A.: (Chairman). *Exercise Testing and Training of Apparently Healthy Individuals: A Handbook for Physicians.* Dallas, American Heart Association, 1972.

Kattus, A.A.: (Chairman). *Exercise Testing and Training of Individuals with Heart Disease or At High Risk for Its Development: A Handbook for Physicians.* Dallas, American Heart Association, 1975.

Kozlowski, J.H., and Ellestad, M.H.: The exercise test as a guide to management and prognosis. *Clinics in Sports Medicine* 3(2):395–411, 1984.

Leff, A.R. (ed.): *Cardiopulmonary Exercise Testing*. New York, Grune & Stratton, 1986.

McHenry, P.L.: Risk of graded exercise testing. *Am. J. Cardiol.* 39:935–937, 1977.

Owles, W.H.: Alterations in the lactic acid content of the blood as a result of light exercise, and associated changes in the CO_2-combining power of the blood and in the alveolar CO_2 pressure. *J. Physiol.* 69:214–237, 1937.

Sidney, K.H., and Shephard, R.J.: Maximum and submaximum exercise tests in men and women in the seventh, eighth, and ninth decades of life. *J. Applied Physiol.* 43(2):280–287, 1977.

Wasserman, K., Hansen, J.E., Sue, D.Y., and Whipp, B.J.: *Principles of Exercise Testing and Interpretation*. Philadelphia, Lea & Febiger, 1987.

Wasserman, K., and Whipp, B.J.: Exercise physiology in health and disease. *Am. Rev. Resp. Dis.* 112:219–249, 1975.

Wasserman, K., Whipp, B.J., Koyal, S.N., and Beaver, W.L.: Anaerobic threshold and respiratory gas exchange during exercise. *J. Applied Physiol.* 35(2):226–243, 1973.

OBJECTIVES

AFTER READING THIS CHAPTER, THE STUDENT WILL BE ABLE TO:

1. Describe the different body fluid compartments and give their approximate volumes and electrolyte compositions.
2. List some clinical causes of dehydration and overhydration.
3. Discuss the rationale for administering intravenous fluids.
4. Explain the different techniques for obtaining material for bacterial culture and identification.
5. Identify the characteristic shapes, staining characteristics, and grouping patterns observed for different types of bacteria.
6. Discuss ways of determining which antibiotics should be useful in treating an infection by a particular organism.
7. Define nosocomial infection, and contrast the most common organisms causing pneumonia in hospitalized versus nonhospitalized patients.
8. Describe the role of respiratory care equipment in transmission of nosocomial infections. List methods for reducing this form of disease transmission.
9. Indicate the importance of universal blood and body fluid precautions.
10. Contrast antisepsis, disinfection, and sterilization. List chemical antimicrobials commonly used clinically. Describe steam sterilization, gas sterilization, pasteurization, and gamma irradiation.
11. List commonly used antibiotics and the microorganisms usually sensitive to them.
12. Discuss the two ways in which the immune system acts to protect the body from microbial infection. List some causes of immunodeficiency.
13. List and discuss methods for evaluating nutritional status.
14. Describe indirect calorimetry and the importance of determining respiratory quotient.

12
CLINICAL CHEMISTRY AND MICROBIOLOGY

CHAPTER OUTLINE

FLUIDS AND ELECTROLYTES
　Fluid Compartments
　Disturbances of Fluid Balance
　Electrolyte Levels
　Electrolyte Imbalances
　Basis of Fluid and Electrolyte Management
MICROBIOLOGY
　Obtaining Culture Material
　Microbial Identification
　　Staining and Microscopic Evaluation
　　Culture Techniques
　　Determining Antibiotic Sensitivity
　Antibiotics
　Microorganisms of the Respiratory Tract
Immunopathology
Respiratory Therapy Equipment and Transmission of Nosocomial Infections
Physical Decontamination Techniques
Chemical Disinfectants
Disposable Supplies
NUTRITIONAL ASSESSMENT
　Anthropometric Measurements
　Biochemical Measurements
　Indirect Calorimetry
　Assessing Caloric Requirements

FLUIDS AND ELECTROLYTES

Fluid Compartments

The human body is about 60% water, so an individual weighing 70 kg contains about 40 L of water (*total body water*) (Fig. 12–1). Approximately two thirds of the total body water is inside cells (25 L of *intracellular water*), and one third is outside of cells (15 L of *extracellular water*). Furthermore, extracellular water is subdivided into *interstitial fluid* (about 12 L), *intravascular fluid* (plasma, about 3 L), and fluid in special compartments, such as cerebrospinal fluid, intraocular fluid, and joint (synovial) fluid (about 1 L total). The fluid in these special compartments is called *transcellular fluid*. The interstitial fluid composition is more like plasma than intracellular fluid.

Each of these fluid compartments has a role in the functioning of the body. Most cells are about 80% water, and the organelles and chemicals that the cells utilize while carrying on metabolism are suspended or dissolved in it. The cells are bathed and surrounded by interstitial fluid, which provides nutrients and oxygen to the cells, while removing carbon dioxide and other waste products of cellular metabolism.

The interstitial fluid is therefore in equilibrium with the intracellular fluid across the cell membrane. The interstitial fluid is also in equilibrium with and constantly replaced by fluid from the blood vessels (see Chapter 2). Plasma is filtered through pores in the capillary walls to constantly form new interstitial fluid. Excess interstitial fluid is eliminated by reuptake into the plasma through the capillary walls or by lymphatic drainage, which returns the excess interstitial fluid (lymph) to the veins.

The exchange between plasma, interstitial fluid, and intracellular fluid serves to deliver oxygen and nutrients into the cells while removing waste products from them. The waste products are then carried to the excretory organs where they are eliminated from the body. The exchange between plasma, interstitial fluid, and intracellular fluid also serves to maintain the volume of each compartment.

Disturbances of Fluid Balance

The volume of the fluid compartments is maintained relatively constant by the same factors that increase or decrease fluid elimination to match fluid intake. Furthermore, thirst can modify fluid intake when increased fluid is needed. However, the sensation of being thirsty may not occur until moderate dehydration is present. Conditions that result in fluid imbalance initially affect plasma volume, but then, because the fluid compartments are in equilibrium, interstitial and finally intracellular fluid volume are affected. *Dehydration* has many causes, including prolonged vomiting, inability to drink, protracted diarrhea, excessive diuresis (urinary excretion), water loss caused by sweating, inadequate intravenous fluid administration, blood loss, and interstitial fluid loss from burns (Table 12–1). Certain endocrine abnormalities can also produce dehydration. Diabetes insipidus causes excessive urine formation if the posterior pituitary gland fails to secrete normal levels of antidiuretic hormone (ADH). Adrenal insufficiency (Addison's disease) results in low levels of the adrenal hor-

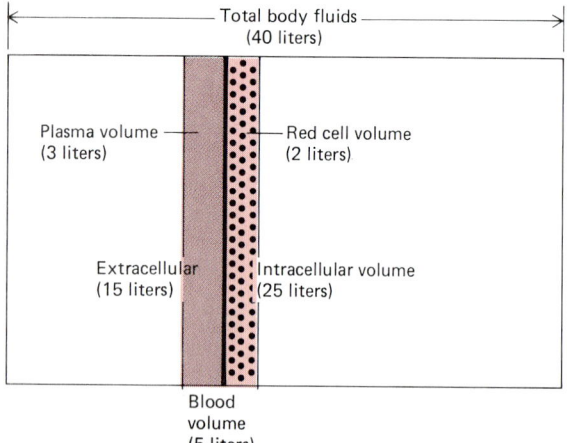

Figure 12–1. Diagram of the body fluid compartments. (From Guyton, A.C.: *Textbook of Medical Physiology*, 7th ed. Philadelphia, W.B. Saunders, 1986, with permission.)

TABLE 12–1. Causes of Fluid Imbalance

Dehydration
Prolonged vomiting
Inability to drink
Protracted diarrhea
Diaphoresis (sweating)
Excessive urinary excretion
Insufficient intravenous fluid administration
Blood loss
Interstitial fluid loss (as from burns or sepsis)
Endocrine abnormalities

Overhydration
Near drowning
Overtransfusion
Renal insufficiency
Endocrine abnormalities

mone aldosterone. This causes urinary loss of sodium and water and can result in dehydration.

Dehydration can have profound effects on the cardiopulmonary system and can also seriously influence many different modalities of cardiopulmonary therapy. Severely decreased intravascular volume can lower blood pressure (hypotension) resulting in cardiovascular collapse and death. Diminished cardiac output can interfere with carbon dioxide elimination by increasing alveolar deadspace in the lung. Metabolic (lactic) acidosis can result from cardiac outputs reduced to the point of inadequate oxygen delivery and resultant anaerobic metabolism. Positive pressure ventilation is poorly tolerated in the presence of inadequate blood volume; life-threatening hypotension can result. Dehydration also dries airway secretions, making them more adherent and difficult to remove, which may result in airways obstruction and atelectasis.

Causes of *overhydration* (see Table 12-1) include excessive intake (such as near-drowning, or overtransfusion with intravenous fluids) as well as inadequate excretion (as from renal insufficiency). Endocrine abnormalities that produce excessive levels of ADH cause fluid retention and overhydration. Conn's syndrome (excessive aldosterone levels) causes edema (excessive retention of salt and water).

Overhydration affects cardiac function and frequently results in pulmonary edema, which interferes with gas exchange. The increased fluid in the lungs also makes them less compliant and more difficult to ventilate. Severe overhydration can also result in cerebral edema, coma, and seizures.

Determination of a patient's fluid volume status is usually made from the patient's history, skin turgor (tenseness and recoil), moistness of mucous membranes, and in neonates, condition of the fontanelles ("soft spots" of the head where the cranial bones haven't yet fused). The clinical laboratory can measure the osmolarity (concentration of dissolved particles) of body fluids, such as blood or urine, to help determine the patient's degree of hydration. A high plasma or urine osmolarity may suggest dehydration. Clinically, daily patient weights are routinely used to assess fluid balance. Additional information is obtained from an accurate record of the patient's oral and intravenous intake as well as output, such as urine or blood loss.

Clinical laboratory tests usually do not give direct information concerning fluid volume status but can do so indirectly. Elevated metabolic waste products in the plasma, such as urea nitrates and creatinine, suggest renal disease, which affects volume status. Decreasing plasma volume sometimes elevates the blood cell concentration (hematocrit). However, the most meaningful information concerning fluid volume status is obtained mainly by measuring the quantity of urine output along with central venous pressure and pulmonary artery occlusion (pulmonary capillary wedge) pressure. This is because appropriate intravascular fluid volume is more important clinically than total body fluid volume status.

Electrolyte Levels

The composition of the substances dissolved in intracellular water is quite different from that of the substances dissolved in extracellular water (Fig. 12-2). In general, intracellular water contains high levels of potassium, protein, phosphates, and magnesium, while extracellular water is high in sodium and chloride and low in potassium and protein. Clinical laboratory tests are commonly performed on plasma to determine its electrolyte concentrations. The electrolyte compositions of the different

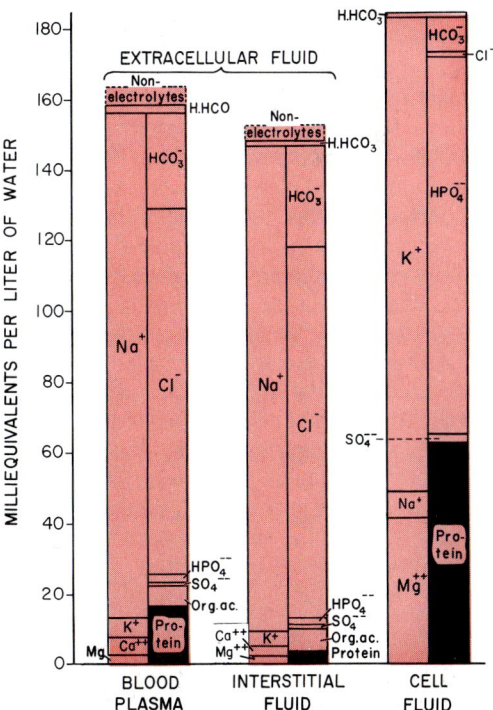

Figure 12-2. The constituents of plasma, interstitial fluid, and intracellular fluid. (From Guyton, A.C.: *Textbook of Medical Physiology*, 7th ed. Philadelphia, W.B. Saunders, 1986, with permission.)

extracellular compartments (e.g., interstitial fluid, plasma, and cerebrospinal fluid) are approximately equivalent.

Intracellular fluid electrolyte concentrations cannot be easily measured but fortunately are much less variable than those of extracellular fluid. Relative concentrations of electrolytes in the intracellular and extracellular compartments are crucial for the maintenance of resting membrane potentials and development of action potentials in excitable tissues, including the heart. Electrolyte concentrations also influence the contractility of muscle cells.

Electrolyte Imbalances

There are many critical interactions between the respiratory system and electrolyte levels. Changes in the acid-base status promote shifts in electrolytes across cell membranes and thus alter the concentrations of certain electrolytes inside and outside the cell. Acidosis raises extracellular potassium because the increased extracellular hydrogen ions (H^+) enter cells, causing potassium ions (K^+) to leave the cells to maintain electrochemical neutrality. Conversely, alkalosis lowers plasma and interstitial K^+ concentration. Alkalosis favors the binding of calcium to protein and so reduces the concentration of ionized calcium in the plasma. Extracellular ionized calcium levels are crucial for myocardial cell contractility.

Inappropriate intake or excretion of electrolytes can result in imbalances that can be life-threatening. Abnormalities in extracellular potassium levels can produce serious cardiac dysrhythmias. Very low extracellular potassium makes heart muscle cells depolarize very easily; high extracellular potassium decreases myocardial excitability. Abnormal calcium levels also affect myocardial contractility and excitability. This is important to remember during procedures that frequently produce dysrhythmias, such as airway suctioning. Individuals with electrolyte imbalances are even more prone to dysrhythmias during suctioning or hypoxia, so added care and vigilance in monitoring the ECG are needed.

Basis of Fluid and Electrolyte Management

The patient unable to take fluids orally depends upon the judicious administration of intravenous fluids to maintain the volume of the different body fluid compartments. Fluid and electrolyte intake must match the amount of fluid lost by urination, wound drainage, gastric suctioning, and even sweating. Body fluids are even lost because of humidification of inspired air by the patient's respiratory system if dry gases are inhaled. The fluid loss that is not easily measurable (evaporation from the airways, sweating, and loss in the feces) is called *insensible* fluid loss, but both insensible and measurable fluid losses must be replaced by adequate intake.

There are several considerations in determining the appropriate volume of intravenous fluids to administer. The patient's normal fluid losses (urination, sweating, and evaporation) must be replaced by maintenance intravenous fluids when the patient is unable to take fluids orally for an extended period. Children have a higher metabolic rate and a proportionally greater fluid requirement. Therefore, intravenous fluid administration is guided by the patient's weight. Maintenance fluid is routinely administered at 4 ml/kg/hr for the first 10 kg of the patient's weight, 2 ml/kg/hr for the second 10 kg, and 1 ml/kg/hr for every kilogram above that. For example, a patient weighing 45 kg would receive 40 ml/hr for the first 10 kg, 20 ml/hr for the second 10 kg and 25 ml/hr for the remaining 25 kg for a total IV infusion rate of 85 ml/hr. A baby weighing 8 kg would receive 32 ml/hr for IV maintenance fluid.

The type of IV fluid administered is determined by the composition of the fluid that the patient is losing and also any electrolyte abnormalities that the patient has. Most commonly, a solution containing 5% (5 gm/dl) glucose and 0.45% NaCl is administered as maintenance IV fluid. This concentration is called half normal saline, while normal saline (0.9%) is isotonic (same number of dissolved particles) to plasma.

Electrolyte abnormalities occur most frequently from either inappropriate intravenous fluid administration, prolonged diuretic use, renal disease, or endocrine abnormalities. Electrolyte deficiencies can be treated by addition of the particular substance to the patient's intake (usually intravenously). Common electrolytes administered in this way include potassium, calcium, magnesium, sodium, and chloride. Extreme care must be exercised when administering these drugs because too rapid or excessive infusion can produce severe complications, including seizures and cardiac arrest.

Fluid administered intravenously first enters the intravascular space and then the interstitial space, if the fluid contains only small particles that can pass through the pores in the capillary endothelium. Such a fluid is called crystalloid. Colloid solutions, such as albumin, contain large molecules that are retained intravascularly. These large molecules produce an osmotic gradient that also retains the fluid in the vessels.

Biological membranes (such as a cell wall or blood vessel wall) can act as a barrier to the movement of large molecules like proteins. Proteins, such as enzymes, are trapped inside the cell by the cell membrane; albumin, a plasma protein, is trapped inside the blood vessels, unable to pass through the blood vessel wall into the interstitial space. Water passes through the membrane toward the side with the greater concentration of nondiffusible substances in a process called *osmosis*.

Administration of large volumes of crystalloid tends to expand the interstitial volume producing edema of the tissues. Colloid administration does not expand the extravascular space if the endothelial membrane is intact. Trauma (such as surgery) or infection can partially disrupt the endothelial membrane, producing a leakage of plasma from the capillaries. This is called *third-space* loss of intravascular volume and requires the administration of extra intravenous fluid to maintain adequate intravascular volume.

As mentioned previously, the adequacy of the intravascular volume can be evaluated by the blood pressure, heart rate, urine output, venous pressure, and pulmonary capillary wedge pressure. When invasive monitoring is not present, it may be difficult to determine if the patient is over- or underhydrated. When urine output decreases, the intravascular volume may be depleted or excessive, causing heart failure, which decreases kidney function. Rapid administration of a moderate volume of intravenous fluid can improve vital signs if dehydration is the problem.

Excessive intravenous fluid can produce pulmonary edema and impair heart function (cardiac failure). Avoid overhumidification of inspired gases and prevent introduction of excessive water into the patient's lungs when clearing accumulated water from ventilator tubing. Large amounts of water instilled into the lungs tend to denature surfactant and decrease lung compliance. Excessive saline irrigation to mobilize airway secretions and even repeated flushing of arterial lines can produce volume overload, particularly in neonates.

MICROBIOLOGY

Obtaining Culture Material

Sputum collection is a largely unsatisfactory method of obtaining material for culture in order to identify the organism or organisms responsible for a respiratory tract infection. This is because of the contamination of the material by organisms from the teeth, mouth, and pharynx. However, sputum collection is useful for diagnosis of tuberculosis infection.

Suctioning of sputum through a tracheostomy, endotracheal tube, or bronchoscope does provide a specimen uncontaminated by the organisms of the mouth and pharynx. It is important to realize that organisms identified in this manner may only be *colonizing* (residing in) the airway but not necessarily infecting it. The use of a sterile glove, suction catheter, specimen trap and aseptic (noncontaminating) technique is important to avoid contamination of the specimen as well as to prevent spread of the organisms to other individuals. Proper suctioning technique is also mandatory to avoid hypoxia in the patient (see Chapter 17). Patients who do not have a productive cough can often be induced to produce sputum (*sputum induction technique*) by use of nebulized saline (3% to 5%).

Transtracheal Aspiration. This is another technique used to obtain material from the airways without contamination by organisms from the mouth and pharynx (Fig. 12–3). The skin of the neck overlying the cricothyroid membrane or trachea is cleaned with an iodine solution. The tip of an intravenous catheter is introduced through the

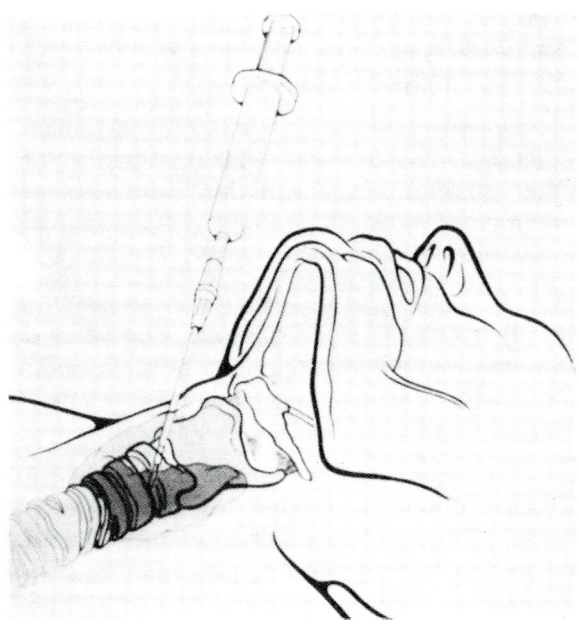

FIGURE 12–3. Transtracheal aspiration. (Reproduced with permission. © *Textbook of Advanced Cardiac Life Support*, 1987, American Heart Association.)

skin and into the lumen of the trachea as in performing transtracheal catheter ventilation (see Chapter 19). The needle is then withdrawn while the plastic catheter is left in place. The intraluminal location of the catheter tip is verified by aspiration of air through a syringe attached to the catheter. The patient is informed that he or she will cough soon and then 2 to 3 ml of preservative-free saline is injected through the catheter into the airway. This usually produces a forceful cough by the patient, and the catheter is aspirated with a syringe. It is necessary to obtain only a very small specimen for microbiological culture to be done. Complications of transtracheal aspiration include subcutaneous emphysema and injury to structures adjacent to the trachea, such as the esophagus, blood vessels, or nerves.

Bronchoscopy can be used to obtain culture material with minimal contamination from the mouth and pharynx. Most commonly, a flexible bronchoscope is used first to lavage the distal airway with saline (to loosen the secretions) and then to suction the material into a container where it can be analyzed. Bronchoscopy is discussed in greater detail in Chapter 14.

Transpleural Aspiration or Biopsy. This encompasses a variety of techniques usually performed by physicians by which pleural fluid or lung tissue is obtained to identify an infecting organism or inspect lung morphology. *Thoracentesis* is the insertion of a needle through the chest wall in order to drain pleural fluid, which can be sent for culture to determine if infecting organisms are present. Excess pleural fluid is called *pleural effusion* and is not always caused by infection but may also result from tumors, trauma, or other causes.

Occasionally, a needle is inserted through the chest wall and into an area of infected lung to obtain material for identification of infecting organisms. This is done in an area of the lung where the alveoli are *consolidated* (filled) with pneumonia organisms and fluid. Open lung biopsy is performed when the pathologic organism cannot be identified by other techniques. This is the most invasive method and requires a thoracotomy (opening of the chest cavity) and excision of a portion of the diseased lung.

All of these transpleural techniques carry the risk of pneumothorax and intrathoracic bleeding, which can result in sudden dyspnea or hypoxia. A chest radiograph after these procedures can help determine if one of these complications has occurred.

Blood Cultures. Blood cultures are performed to identify organisms that may be present in the circulation. Blood is obtained by venipuncture through skin cleansed with iodine solution. Arterial lines are usually not appropriate sites for obtaining blood for culture because the stopcocks are rapidly colonized with organisms and are very difficult to adequately disinfect.

Microbial Identification

Sputum specimens should first be examined grossly (see Chapters 15 and 17). The color, smell, and quantity of the sputum can suggest the severity and even the identity of the infecting organism in certain types of lung infection. It is also important to note the patient's degree of difficulty in clearing the airway.

Staining and Microscopic Evaluation

After obtaining suitable uncontaminated material for identifying infectious organisms, a rapid evaluation for the presence of bacteria can be performed. If bacteria are present, they can be generally classified within minutes as to which types of antibiotics they may be sensitive. The most common technique is called a *Gram stain*. Some of the material to be studied is spread on a microscope slide and then stained with a series of chemicals. Depending on the color they stain, bacteria are divided into two main categories: gram-positive bacteria stain purplish, and gram-negative bacteria stain reddish. In addition to determining the staining characteristics, microscopic inspection of the slides reveals the characteristic shapes of the organisms, such as rod (bacillus), ball (coccus), or spiral (spirochete); the presence or absence of spores; and grouping characteristics, for example, pairs (diplococci), clumps, chains, or singly (Fig. 12–4). Additionally, specialized stains exist to help identify certain organisms, such as an acid-fast technique specific for tuberculosis. Different staining techniques are used to identify fungi and one-celled parasitic organisms, such as *Pneumocystis*. Electron microscopy may be necessary to evaluate material infected with viruses.

Culture Techniques

Microscopic evaluation of gram-stained material provides certain descriptive information about the characteristics and probable sensitivities of infectious bacteria. However, precise identification of an infecting organism as well as precise determination of its antibiotic sensitivities is dependent on

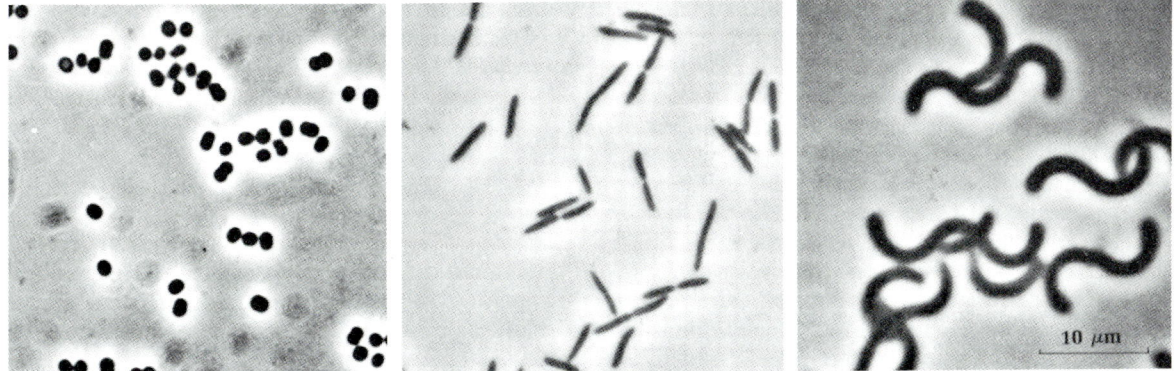

Figure 12–4. Characteristic shapes of bacteria. (From Stanier, R.Y., Doudoroff, M., and Adelberg, E.A.: *The Microbial World*, 3rd ed. Englewood Cliffs, N.J., Prentice-Hall, with permission.)

microbial culture techniques that usually require 2 to 3 days to carry out. Some slow-growing organisms, such as fungi, can require over a week. Bacteria obtained from the patient are grown in a glass Petri dish filled with a nutrient material (usually agar-based). The manner in which the material is spread out on the agar separates the bacteria into single colonies. The bacteria are usually grown in several dishes that contain different nutrients. Certain bacteria possess enzymes that allow them to metabolize specific nutrients, while other types of bacteria may lack these enzymes and so are unable to grow in these nutrients. For example, certain bacteria are able to break down blood mixed in the agar and thus are called *hemolytic*, while bacteria unable to break down the blood are called *nonhemolytic*. Some bacteria grow in the presence of oxygen (aerobic) while others can grow only in the presence of low oxygen levels (anaerobic). Facultative anaerobes can alter their metabolism in order to grow in the presence of oxygen but grow more rapidly in its absence. Based on the information from microscopic evaluation as well as the nutrients in which they are able to grow, the bacteria can usually be precisely identified.

Some viruses can be cultured and identified by expensive culture techniques called tissue culture (human cell colonies grown in bottles are infected with the culture material and then examined for disease-producing viruses). This is necessary because viruses are not true organisms and are capable of reproduction only within other living cells.

Determining Antibiotic Sensitivity

While the identification efforts described above are proceeding, the bacteria are also grown on large plates upon which are placed small discs, each containing a different antibiotic (Kirby-Bauer technique). If bacteria obtained from the patient grow near the antibiotic disc, then the organism is *insensitive* to that antibiotic. However, if the bacteria are unable to grow near the disc, then they are *sensitive* to the drug. If bacterial growth is inhibited for some distance from the disc, then the organism is very sensitive to the drug and that drug should be useful in treating the infection by that organism (Fig. 12–5).

Antibiotics

Antibiotics are useful in treating infections caused by certain sensitive organisms (Table 12–2). They must be ordered by a physician and may be ad-

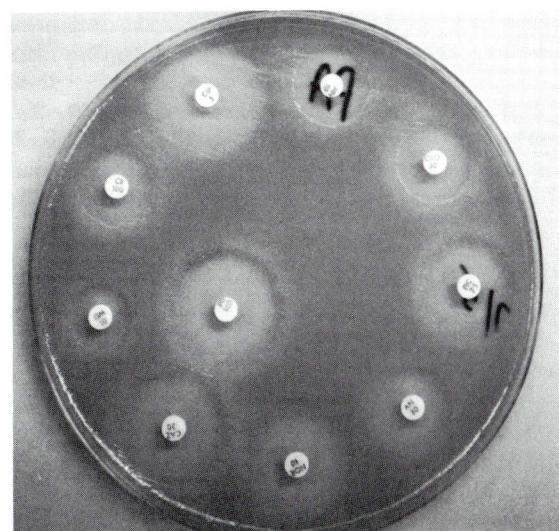

Figure 12–5. Inhibition of bacterial growth by antibiotics—Kirby-Bauer technique.

TABLE 12-2. Commonly Used Antibiotics

Antibiotic	Usually Sensitive Microorganisms	Comments
Penicillins		
Aqueous penicillin	Gram-positive (*Pneumococcus*)	Allergic reactions common
Ampicillin	Gram-positive and some gram-negative	Allergic reactions common
Methicillin and oxacillin	Gram-positive (*Staphylococcus*)	Useful against organisms that have an enzyme (penicillinase) that can break down penicillin
Cephalosporins		
Cephalothin sodium and cephalexin monohydrate	Gram-positive (*Staphylococcus*) and some gram-negative	Useful in some penicillin-resistant organisms
Tetracycline	Gram-positive and gram-negative	Broad-spectrum antibiotic
Gentamicin and tobramycin	Gram-negative	Very powerful, but can cause kidney and hearing damage
Erythromycin	Gram-positive	Useful in patients allergic to penicillin
Amphotericin B	Yeast	Allergic reactions common
Isoniazid (rifampin, ethambutol, and streptomycin are other anti-TB drugs)	*Mycobacterium tuberculosis*	Side effects include peripheral neuritis, allergic reactions, and hepatitis

ministered by different routes, depending on the clinical situation. Intravenous or intramuscular injection and oral ingestion are the most common administration routes. In certain situations, such as treatment for infected airways secretions in cystic fibrosis patients, antibiotics have been nebulized. Antibiotics are also used as ointments for topical application as well as irrigated into various infected body cavities and spaces.

Microorganisms of the Respiratory Tract

The environment, including the air, contains many different types of microorganisms. Additionally, many others reside on the skin, in the upper respiratory tract, and in the gastrointestinal tract. The presence of microorganisms in the body without the production of disease is called *colonization*. However, in susceptible individuals with diminished resistance, infection and disease may result from organisms already present or from organisms transmitted from the environment or from other individuals. If the infecting organism is derived from a hospital environment, equipment, or personnel, it is called a *nosocomial infection*. These infections involve 5% to 10% of the patients in American hospitals. Nosocomial infections are undesirable for two reasons: (1) they indicate failure to prevent cross-transmission of infecting organisms, and (2) the transmitted organisms are usually more virulent as well as more antibiotic-resistant. Nosocomial organisms are frequently more virulent because badly infected individuals are more common inside hospitals and antibiotic therapy is selective for the proliferation of resistant bacteria.

There are many nonpathogenic organisms normally found in the upper respiratory tract. The respiratory tract below the vocal cords is usually considered to be essentially free of microorganisms because of the function of the glottis and other defense mechanisms (see Chapter 3). Occasionally, microorganisms enter the lower respiratory tract by microaspiration or are carried in inspired air. These bacteria are normally engulfed by phagocytic macrophages, transported up the airways by the mucociliary escalator, and coughed out. In a debilitated patient with lowered resistance, these organisms can produce pneumonia. Many different organisms can produce pneumonia, which is actually a nonspecific name for any disease process that results in alveoli filled with microorganisms, fluid, and white blood cells. Aspiration of gastric contents can also infect the lung with several organisms that are normally nonpathogenic, but in this situation, they may produce pneumonia or lung abscesses.

Respiratory tract infection is the most common reason that people seek medical assistance. Bronchiolitis in small children is most commonly associated with an infection by respiratory syncytial virus. This disease does not usually occur after early childhood because of changes in airway size and host resistance. Pediatric patients also are susceptible to acute epiglottitis. This massive swelling of the epiglottis is almost always caused by *Haemophilus influenzae* and is a life-threatening emergency.

About 90% of respiratory tract infections occur

in previously healthy individuals and are viral in origin. There is no specific therapy for these viral infections. Of the remaining 10%, a bacterial infection responsive to antibiotic therapy is most common in an individual with one or more causes of decreased resistance. Chronic debilitation, malnourishment, presence of underlying chronic pulmonary diseases, excessive tissue damage or resection, use of immunosuppressive drugs, and administration of prophylactic antibiotics increase the risk of respiratory tract infection. Pneumonia can also be caused by fungi or protozoans. The most common protozoan cause of pneumonia is *Pneumocystis carinii*.

The most common cause of pneumonia acquired outside of the hospital but resulting in hospital admission (50% to 80%) is *Streptococcus pneumoniae* (pneumococcus). This gram-positive coccus is quite sensitive to penicillin and usually responds well to therapy, resolving (healing) with little residual damage. However, nosocomial pneumonia is most commonly caused by gram-negative bacilli (*Serratia, Klebsiella, Escherichia, Proteus, Haemophilus,* and *Pseudomonas*). *Staphylococcus,* a nonmotile, nonspore-forming, gram-positive bacterium arranged in grape-like clusters, is also a frequent cause of nosocomial infection. The bacteria producing nosocomial pneumonia frequently cause necrotizing (tissue destroying) lung damage and also are more frequently antibiotic resistant. These pathogenic organisms are most commonly introduced by inhalation of contaminated aerosols or particulate matter into the lower respiratory tract of the debilitated patient who is already hospitalized. Nosocomial pneumonia is an extremely frequent occurrence among patients in intensive care units.

Immunopathology

Viral infections are not responsive to antibiotic treatment. In most cases, however, the body's immune system is able to overcome a viral infection. The immune system acts to remove from the body almost all foreign molecules, except those too small for it to recognize. The protective function of the immune system is provided in two ways (Table 12–3): 1. *cellular immunity* mediated by the T-lymphocytes, which act with other white blood cells to devour (phagocytize) and remove foreign particles; 2. *humoral immunity* mediated by B-lymphocytes, which produce *antibodies* (globulin proteins that chemically combine with foreign par-

TABLE 12–3. Immune System's Functions

Cellular Immunity	Humoral Immunity
T-lymphocytes: phagocytosis	B-lymphocytes: antibody production (immunoglobulins)

ticles and either inactivate, destroy, or else render the particles easier for the T-lymphocytes to phagocytize).

Immunodeficiency renders an individual extremely susceptible to infection. On rare occasions, infants are born with an absence of T-lymphocytes, B-lymphocytes, or both. These individuals usually die rapidly of infection unless they are raised in an essentially sterile environment. *Acquired immunodeficiency* can afflict individuals, rendering them susceptible to infection by opportunistic organisms (those that prey on weakened individuals). Malignancies, particularly leukemias and lymphomas, replace normal lymphocytes with cancer cells. Chemotherapy for cancer can also destroy lymphocytes, decreasing the effectiveness of the immune system. Patients receiving organ transplants are given immunosuppressive drugs to prevent transplant rejection but are thus also prone to infection. Cortisone and other glucocorticoid drugs have wide use in medicine, but unfortunately, they depress the immune system. Infection with human immunodeficiency virus (HIV) can virtually destroy the immune system, resulting in acquired immunodeficiency syndrome (AIDS).

The modern pathology laboratory can determine if an individual is lacking all or part of his or her immune defenses by using tests that measure the amounts of the different antibodies or by assessing the activity of the lymphocytes. These tests are commonly performed on patients suffering from repeated respiratory tract infections. Extra care must be given to immunodeficient or immunosuppressed individuals, including protective isolation from healthcare personnel and other patients as well as using impeccable aseptic technique.

An overactive immune system can also be a problem, resulting in allergies or asthma. Hypersensitivity can be immediate (acute) or delayed. Acute hypersensitivities usually involve interactions with antibodies attached to histamine-containing mast cells (see Chapter 15). Delayed hypersensitivity usually involves T-lymphocytes that migrate to the affected area, as occurs in a positive tuberculin (purified protein derivative, PPD) skin test. An individual suspected of being acutely hypersensitive is tested by cutaneous exposure to different types of foreign particles (scratch test). If sensitivity to a certain substance is discovered, *desensitization* can be performed to make the individual tolerate that substance.

Respiratory Therapy Equipment and Transmission of Nosocomial Infections

Respiratory therapy equipment frequently plays a role in the development of nosocomial respiratory tract infections. Within 22 hours of endotracheal intubation, gram-negative microorganisms can usually be cultured from secretions obtained from the lower respiratory tract. Aerosols produced by respiratory therapy equipment can transport organisms into the lower airway. Contamination of the tracheostomy or endotracheal tube during intubation or suctioning also bypasses normal pulmonary defense mechanisms.

Nebulizers and humidifiers contain water, which can act as a reservoir for microorganisms, especially *Pseudomonas*. Nebulizers entrain (aspirate) room air during their operation and thus are frequently contaminated. The small water particles produced, carrying the contaminating organisms, are transported to the small airways.

Current standards dictate changing ventilator breathing circuits at 48-hour intervals to reduce the risk of bacterial contamination. Bacterial filters inserted into the inspiratory limb of the breathing circuit have not been shown to decrease the incidence of respiratory tract infections in the intensive care setting. However, use of ensheathed suction catheters reduces endotracheal tube contamination and also inhibits transmission of organisms to healthcare personnel.

The importance of handwashing with antiseptic solutions cannot be overstressed. The most common route for transmission of nosocomial infection is by hand contact. Careful handwashing before and after patient care prevents transmission of microorganisms from patient to patient. Breakdown of this simplest isolation technique has resulted in several hospital epidemics. Also, strict aseptic technique must be followed when performing diagnostic and therapeutic procedures on hospitalized patients. Patient-to-patient spread of infection has been well documented following the use of a Wright spirometer on several patients without proper disinfection technique.

Recommendations for prevention of HIV transmission in healthcare settings emphasize the need to treat tissue, blood, and body fluids from *all* patients as *potentially infective* (universal blood and body fluid precautions).

In addition to gowns, use gloves and masks during all procedures when exposure to blood or body fluids is possible. Also, the use of masks and protective eyewear or a face shield is recommended. Additionally, the availability of mouthpieces, resuscitation bags, and other ventilation devices is strongly recommended in areas where patients may require ventilatory resuscitation in order to reduce the need for mouth-to-mouth ventilation.

Handwashing is mandatory following exposure to *each* patient and whenever the hands are soiled. All supplies and equipment contaminated with blood, secretions, or excretions should be double-bagged for removal from the patient care area if appropriate. Disposable supplies are usually then incinerated; reusable equipment is disinfected according to hospital policy. Table 12–4 lists isolation precautions when direct patient contact or contact with body fluids and blood is not expected, such as during a ventilator adjustment.

Wound and skin isolation precautions are used when the patient has an open or infected break in the skin. Dysentery and other gastrointestinal infections may require enteric isolation precautions. The spread of virulent pneumonias or respiratory contagion can be reduced through respiratory isolation precautions. Strict isolation precautions are used when the patient has a life-threatening, contagious disease. When a patient is immunocompromised, protective precautions (reverse isolation) are taken to protect him or her from acquiring nosocomial or other infections.

Microbiological surveillance of respiratory care equipment and personnel is a necessary component of quality assurance of medical care. The microbiology lab may periodically perform spot checks by obtaining cultures from respiratory therapy equipment as well as from the nasopharynxes of healthcare personnel. However, routine testing of effluent gases, swabbing, and rinsing equipment on a weekly basis are no longer recommended. Instead, the hospital infection control team should coordinate an intensive investigation whenever there is an outbreak of nosocomial infection.

Physical Decontamination Techniques

Preparing equipment and supplies for patient use involves not only ascertaining proper function but

TABLE 12–4. Isolation Procedures When Contact Is Not Expected With Blood, Body Fluids, or the Patient Directly

Type	Gowns	Gloves	Mask	Closed Doors	Private Room
Wound and skin	0	0	During dressing changes	0	0
Enteric	0	0	0	0	For pediatric patients
Respiration	0	0	+	+	+
Strict	+	+	+	+	+
Protective	+	0	+	+	+

0 = not needed; + = needed.

also preventing the spread of infection. Certain types of supplies (such as endotracheal tubes) are checked for *sterility* (complete destruction of both spores and vegetative organisms), while other equipment (ventilators) is inspected for cleanliness. After equipment has been used, it must be appropriately decontaminated before subsequent use on another patient.

Physical decontamination consists of mechanical methods, such as scrubbing and filtration, as well as nonmechanical agents, such as heat and irradiation.

Equipment is first disassembled to allow more thorough cleaning. Scrubbing with soap, water, and chemical antimicrobial agents removes dirt and debris which contain many microbes. This first step of cleaning greatly increases the effectiveness of later *disinfection* (killing vegetative bacteria but not spores) or sterilization techniques. This also increases the aesthetics of reusing equipment. If equipment has undergone sterilization but still appears dirty, it will be poorly tolerated by the patient.

Filters are commonly placed between the ventilator and breathing circuit in order to disinfect the inspired gas. These filters can be designed with pore sizes small enough to remove even large viruses. If the patient has an especially virulent infection, an additional filter is sometimes placed on the expiratory limb of the breathing circuit to reduce equipment and environmental contamination (double-filtering).

Other physical methods for decontamination of equipment include (in order of increasing temperature) pasteurization, boiling, steam sterilization, and dry heat. *Pasteurization* techniques involve a machine that washes equipment for at least 30 minutes in a detergent-water mixture heated to 62°C. This method does not effectively eliminate spores and so is considered disinfecting rather than sterilizing. Immersion in boiling water (100°C) for 3 minutes destroys vegetative organisms but does not kill resistant spores. Alkalinizing the solution with sodium bicarbonate or sodium hydroxide enhances the destruction of spores. Increasing altitude decreases the temperature at which water boils so the duration of the boiling should be increased 5 minutes per 1,000 feet of elevation above sea level.

Pressurized steam (autoclaving) at 2 atmospheres of pressure attains a temperature of 121°C and rapidly destroys microorganisms. Autoclaving denatures protein, producing *sterilization* within 15 minutes.

Raising the pressure to 3 atmospheres produces steam at 134°C, which accomplishes sterilization within 3 minutes. Moisture enhances the conduction of heat and the rate of microbial destruction. Verification of sterilization requires monitors that measure the temperature and duration of heating (thermometer, thermocouples, or heat-sensitive tapes). Although autoclaving is the most common sterilizing technique, its use is limited for respiratory care because much of the equipment is composed of rubber or plastic which tends to melt at high temperatures.

Dry heat is occasionally used for materials that cannot withstand moist heat methods. Dry heat is conducted less well than moist; bacterial spores tolerate fairly high temperatures. Therefore, very high temperatures (160 to 180°C) for prolonged times (1 to 2 hours) are applied.

Gamma irradiation (exposure to a radioactive material, such as cobalt-60) is gaining popularity as a sterilization technique. Although there are cost and space constraints, there is no risk of retained radioactivity.

Decontamination techniques can chemically alter the equipment that is being disinfected, which can predispose the equipment to breakdown, alter its physical characteristics, or even make the equipment toxic to the patient. Steam sterilization can cause rupture of equipment with closed air-containing spaces. Chemical disinfectants can be quite adherent to certain materials. Gamma irradiation can make plastics less pliable. Interactions between the decontaminating agents, the equipment, organisms, and the patient make it essential to follow approved decontamination procedures.

Chemical Disinfectants

Antiseptics are chemicals used for handwashing or preparing the skin for aseptic procedures and so must not be harmful or irritating to skin or mucous membranes. Thus, antiseptic agents are usually only *bacteriostatic* (prevent or delay microorganism reproduction). *Chemical disinfectants*, on the other hand, are used for decontamination of equipment. By definition, disinfectants produce an irreversible, lethal effect on the vegetative forms of microorganisms but are not necessarily sporicidal. Some chemicals are effective antiseptics and, at increased concentrations, also serve as disinfectants. However, not all antiseptics can act as disinfectants; conversely, many disinfectants are too caustic or irritating to act as antiseptics (Table 12–5). Chemical disinfectants can be used during the

TABLE 12–5. Chemical Antimicrobial Agents

Type	Example	Disadvantages	Description
Alcohol	Ethyl or isopropyl	Not sporicidal; can damage equipment	Colorless, bactericidal, inexpensive
Mercurial preparations	Thimersol (Merthiolate)	Ineffective antiseptic and disinfectant; inactivated by organic material	Bacteriostatic only
Iodine preparations	Tincture of iodine	Causes tissue necrosis at high concentrations, allergenic, and stains	Broad-spectrum bactericide and kills fungus, certain viruses, and spores
Iodophors ("tamed iodine")	Povidone-iodine (Betadine) and Wescodine	Not as effective as tincture of iodine	Iodine carried by surface active solvent; nonstaining, nonallergenic, relatively nonirritating
Phenolic compounds	Lysol, hexachlorophene, and O-syl	Hexachlorophene is neurotoxic; not sporicidal or virucidal	Good bactericide, prolonged residual effect
Cationic quaternary ammonium compounds	Benzalkonium chloride (Zephiran)	Bacteristatic only against some organisms; neutralized by soap	Nontoxic to tissues, nearly odorless, partially effective as antiseptic and disinfectant
Chlorine preparations	Chloropactin and Clorox	Corrodes metal in high concentrations; inactivated by organic material	Weak disinfectant, inexpensive, effective against HIV
Chlorhexidine	Hibiclens	Causes deafness (like many other antimicrobials) when instilled in the middle ear; rarely, dermititis and photosensitivity	Persistent antimicrobial effects against wide range of microorganisms; good handwashing agent
Aldehyde solutions:			
Acid glutaraldehyde	Sonacide	Toxic residue; causes contact dermatitis; less sporicidal than alkaline	Low pH liquid immersion; high level of disinfection; bactericidal, sporicidal, and virucidal
Alkaline glutaraldehyde	Cidex	Toxic residue; causes contact dermatitis	High pH liquid immersion, high level disinfectant
Ethylene oxide (ETO)	Oxyfume	Fumes and residue are toxic and irritating; mutagenic and carcinogenic; requires aeration	Odorless, poisonous, explosive gas with broad antimicrobial action used in combination with Freon or CO_2 to reduce flammability; very useful for heat- or moisture-sensitive equipment

scrubbing of equipment or the supplies can be soaked in the chemical disinfectants to destroy microbes. With gas sterilization, the supplies are placed in an airtight chamber, which is then filled with lethal gas.

Chemical antimicrobials can be useful for disinfecting respiratory therapy equipment, either for soaking the equipment component in or for use in a washer-sterilizer machine. It is important to follow the supplier's instructions and recommendations for specific agents.

Some of the most commonly used antimicrobials in respiratory care practice are aldehydes. Glutaraldehyde is clinically related to formaldehyde but has stronger antimicrobial action. Glutaraldehyde can be buffered to produce either an acid or alkaline solution.

Acid glutaraldehyde is bactericidal and virucidal within a few minutes. Spores are resistant to this disinfectant, but if the solution is heated to 60°C, sterilization occurs in one hour. Alkaline glutaraldehyde, buffered by a 0.3% bicarbonate agent, does not require heating to produce sterilization. Equipment disinfected and sterilized with glutaraldehyde must be thoroughly rinsed and dried before use because these chemicals are quite toxic and irritating to mucous membranes. Personnel handling these solutions should wear rubber gloves to avoid contact dermatitis.

Gas sterilization utilizes the active chemical ethylene oxide (ETO), mixed with carbon dioxide or Freon gas to reduce flammability. ETO is a very toxic chemical that is most effective in the presence of water. Therefore, a humidity of 50% should be maintained. After exposure to the gas for a sufficient time to destroy all organisms, adequate aeration time must be allowed to ensure complete removal of the residual ethylene oxide, which is quite caustic and irritating. Aeration cabinets utilize warmed (50°C), rapidly circulating filtered air which greatly reduces the time required for aeration. At temperatures above 60°C, polymerization of ETO occurs, which halts its sterilizing action.

Disposable Supplies

The advent of inexpensive plastics has resulted in respiratory equipment that is prepackaged, sterilized, and disposable for single-patient use. This type of equipment has reduced the risk of patient cross-contamination and has also diminished the necessity for disinfection or sterilization of equipment by respiratory care departments. Disposable endotracheal tubes, suction catheters, laryngoscopes, and ventilator circuits are a few examples of prepackaged, sterile respiratory care supplies available. However, some types of equipment, such as ventilators and Wright spirometers, are too expensive for single-patient use, so disinfection or sterilization is necessary. Occasionally, disposable equipment is disinfected and reused on other patients, but these types of supplies do not usually hold up well under repeated washing.

NUTRITIONAL ASSESSMENT

Cardiopulmonary clinicians are playing an increasingly active role in the clinical evaluation of nutritional status. It is easy to understand that critically ill patients can be undernourished because of an inadequate nutritional intake as well as the increase in metabolic demands caused by their illness. It may be less apparent that malnutrition can also result from overnutrition in the form of excessive enteral (utilizing the gastrointestinal tract) or parenteral (bypassing the gastrointestinal tract, usually administered intravenously) nutrition. Thus, malnutrition can be from either under- or overnutrition caused by (1) lack or excess of food, (2) a deficiency or excess of certain essential elements in the diet, and/or (3) abnormal assimilation.

Undernutrition affects many systems of the body. Cardiovascular effects include decreased myocardial muscle mass, causing less forceful heart contraction. Wasting of the ventilatory muscles decreases vital capacity and mucociliary clearance, worsening pulmonary function. The hepatic effects of undernourishment include decreased liver metabolism and biliary excretion of drugs and reduced plasma protein synthesis. The immune system is less able to fight infection. The skeletal muscles weaken and atrophy, and wound healing may be delayed. The tissue breakdown caused by undernourishment is called catabolism.

Overnourishment causes fat deposition, especially in the liver, interfering with normal liver function. This increase in the abdominal content pushes up the diaphragm, reducing the FRC and increasing the work of breathing at a time when the patient may already be weakened from the effects of the illness. If overnutrition is mostly in the form of excessive carbohydrates, the pulmonary complications are even worse. The detrimental effects of elevated blood glucose are apparent from the multiple complications associated with diabetes mellitus. Excessive blood sugar levels impair white blood cell function and increase susceptibility to infection. Also, excess dietary carbohydrates are turned into fat (lipogenesis) by a metabolic pathway (pentose shunt) that produces a molecule of carbon dioxide for every molecule of glucose that is stored as fat. This carbon dioxide is produced without any concomitant ATP production or oxygen consumption. The increased carbon dioxide production without increasing oxygen consumption causes an elevation of the respiratory quotient (carbon dioxide production/oxygen consumption). The increased carbon dioxide production combined with the effects of an enlarged liver can make weaning from mechanical ventilation difficult, if not impossible (see Chapter 19).

Nutritional support in the form of enteral and parenteral alimentation must be judiciously administered to avoid under- or overnourishment. There are several useful methods to help determine the nutritional status and dietary requirements of an individual. Table 12–6 gives the Harris-Benedict equation for estimating basal energy expenditure. There are also techniques to determine if nutritional support therapy is adequate or in excess of the body's metabolic demands. Table 12–7 lists the components of a nutritional assessment.

Anthropometric Measurements

A test used to determine nutritional status is *skinfold measurement*, which estimates the fat mass of a body. About 50% of the body's fat mass is in the subcutaneous tissue. Measurement of the *midarm muscle circumference* can be used to evaluate the muscle component of the fat-free body mass.

TABLE 12–6. Harris-Benedict Estimation of Basal Energy Expenditure

Male:	$66 + (13.7 \times W) + (5 \times H) - (6.8 \times A)$
Female:	$665 + (9.6 \times W) + (1.7 \times H) - (4.7 \times A)$
Child:	$22.1 + (31.1 \times W) + (1.2 \times H)$

W is weight in kilograms, H is height in centimeters, and A is age in years

TABLE 12–7. Components of a Nutritional Assessment

Clinical Assessment
1. Medical history
2. Physical examination

Dietary Assessment
1. Intake-output record

Anthropometric Measurements
1. Age (years); total body weight (kg); height (cm); body surface area (m^2)
2. Body fat mass
   a. Triceps skinfold measurement
3. Fat-free muscle mass
   a. Midarm circumference

Biochemical Measurements
1. Total muscle mass
   a. Creatinine-height index
   b. Urinary nitrogen
2. Visceral protein
   a. Serum albumin
   b. Serum transferrin

Immune Function
1. Total white blood cell count
2. Total lymphocyte count
3. Delayed hypersensitivity

Indirect Calorimetry and Gas Exchange
1. Direct measurements of $\dot{V}_{O_2}$, $\dot{V}_{CO_2}$, RQ (R.E.R.), and $\dot{V}_E$
2. Arterial and mixed venous blood gases

Biochemical Measurements

Measurement of the total amount of creatinine excreted in 24 hours is an index of total muscle mass. The degree of body muscle depletion can be estimated by comparing the patient's height and creatinine excretion to standard values. This so-called *creatinine-height index* is widely used clinically but ignores the wide normal values in healthy body habitus (shape).

The degradation of all amino acids gives rise to ammonia, which is transported from peripheral sites to the liver. In the liver, the ammonia is detoxified by incorporation into urea, which is excreted by the kidneys. Urinary nitrogen constitutes the major excretory route for the products of protein breakdown.

When an individual's protein intake is deficient or when protein catabolism is accelerated by tissue trauma or disease, urinary nitrogen exceeds intake of nitrogen as protein, and the individual is said to be in *negative nitrogen balance*. This represents the loss of tissue proteins. The use of amino acids labeled with isotopic tracers provides greater insight into the dynamic internal equilibria between protein synthesis and protein degradation, but this has not gained widespread clinical application.

Recently, measurements of specific serum proteins have been evaluated for their correlation with hepatic protein synthesis and the functional protein mass of other viscera, such as the heart, lungs, kidneys, and intestines. Serum proteins, including albumin, transferrin, free albumin, fibronectin, fibrinogen, haptoglobin, and C-reactive protein, have been studied to determine if a relationship exists between malnutrition and decreased serum concentration of these molecules. These studies seem to indicate that low levels of these serum proteins may be caused by disease, but the protein depletion does not appear to be the cause of the disease.

Changes in body weight as well as correlation of the patient's weight to height also give information concerning nutritional status. Nutritional imbalances produce more subtle changes in the body that affect subcellular, cellular, and organ functions, including the immune system and its ability to resist infection. With malnutrition, the total lymphocyte count becomes decreased, and cell mediated immunity is lost (anergy). Table 12–8 lists a range of values used in determining the degree of malnutrition.

Indirect Calorimetry

The development of machines that accurately analyze expired gases allows for the determination of oxygen consumption and carbon dioxide production, which is necessary for accurate estimation of caloric expenditure and the respiratory quotient. This technique, called indirect calorimetry, is based on the premise that the amounts of oxygen consumed and carbon dioxide produced during oxidation of protein, carbohydrate, and fat are characteristic and constant for each fuel.

Assessing Caloric Requirements

The prediction equations of Harris, Benedict, and others are good estimates of caloric requirements for normal populations but are inaccurate for individuals with metabolic abnormalities caused by injury, disease, or therapeutic intervention. Indirect calorimetry is an accurate determination of a patient's metabolic rate at the time of the test. Metabolism of the different substrates (carbohydrate, fat, and protein) produces different respiratory quotients (RQ) (Table 12–9). Additionally, every gram of urinary nitrogen represents 6.25 gm of protein catabolized. The contribution of protein is subtracted from the minute oxygen consumption and carbon dioxide production, and the remaining ratio is the nonprotein RQ. Dietary intake is tailored to meet the nutritional requirements of a patient in order to (1) restore or maintain nitrogen balance with protein supplementation and (2) adjust the balance of dietary carbohydrate and fat to meet the nonprotein caloric requirements of the patient while avoiding the complications of an undesirably elevated RQ.

TABLE 12–8. Range of Values Used in Determining Degree of Malnutrition

Category	Impairment		
	Mild	Moderate	Severe
Percent ideal weight	80%–90%	70%–79%	<70%
Percent usual weight	85%–95%	75%–84%	<75%
Creatinine excretion index	60%–80%	40%–59%	<40%
Albumin, gm/dl	2.8–3.4	2.1–2.7	<2.1
Transferrin, mg/dl	150–200	100–149	<100
Total lymphocyte count	1,200–2,000	800–1,199	<800
Cell-mediated immunity	Reactive	Reactive	Anergic

(From Grant, J. P.: *Handbook of Total Parenteral Nutrition.* Philadelphia, W. B. Saunders, 1980, with permission.)

TABLE 12-9. Metabolic Values of Nutrients

	Protein	Carbohydrate	Lipid
kcal/gm	4.3	4.1	9.3
RQ	0.8	1.0	0.7

Energy expenditure (EE) is defined by the Weir equations:

$$EE = (3.9[\dot{V}_{O_2}] + 1.1[\dot{V}_{CO_2}])1.44$$

or

$$EE = (3.941[\dot{V}_{O_2}] + 1.106[\dot{V}_{CO_2}])1.44 - 2.17\ (UN)$$

where $\dot{V}_{O_2}$ is oxygen consumption (in milliliters per minute), $\dot{V}_{CO_2}$ is carbon dioxide production (in milliliters per minute), UN is total urinary nitrogen (in grams per day), and EE is energy expenditure (in kilocalories per day). Thus, by accurately measuring energy expenditure, the calories and components of the diet can be appropriately administered. Variations in a patient's stability, test conditions, instrument function, and interpretation can affect the measurements in indirect calorimetry. Familiarity with the technique and equipment helps assure reliable measurements to avoid the serious complications of over- and undernutrition.

High glucose intake increases carbon dioxide production, which necessitates increased alveolar ventilation. Increased ventilatory load is seen when the RQ exceeds 0.85 and increases directly as the RQ rises beyond 1.0. An elevated RQ is therefore a warning sign suggesting the development of a fatty liver and increased ventilatory requirements, which can complicate the weaning of a mechanically ventilated patient. When carbohydrate calories are replaced by lipids, the RQ drops toward 0.7 as ventilatory requirements and carbon dioxide production fall. Several hours are required for changes in the proportion of dietary fats and carbohydrates to be manifested as changes in the RQ.

In summary, certain chemical laboratory studies are used to determine an individual's nutritional status. This may be necessary for patients who are unable or unwilling to eat normally for long periods. Measurement of the daily excretion of nitrogen waste products in the urine indicates the level of protein metabolism. These measurements determine the adequacy of the protein content in the diet and help to ensure that the patient is not excessively breaking down his or her own tissue proteins (catabolism). Evaluation of nitrogenous waste excretion, oxygen consumption, carbon dioxide production, respiratory quotient, and measurements of dietary intake of carbohydrates, fats, and proteins together establish the patient's nutritional status as well as suggest dietary inadequacy or excess.

Bibliography

Askanazi, J.R., and Hyman, S.H.: Respiratory changes secondary to the high carbohydrate loads of T.P.N. *JAMA* 243:1,444, 1980.
Blodgett, D.: *Manual of Respiratory Care Procedures*. Philadelphia, J.B. Lippincott, 1980.
Boyd, R.F., and Hoerl, B.G.: *Basic Medical Microbiology*, 3rd ed. Boston, Little, Brown, 1986.
Carroll, H.J., and Oh, M.S.: *Water, Electrolyte and Acid-Base Metabolism, Diagnosis and Management*. Philadelphia, J.B. Lippincott, 1978.
Darin, J.: Respiratory therapy equipment in the development of nosocomial respiratory tract infections. *Curr. Rev. Respir. Ther.* 4:83, 1985.
Finegold, S.M., and Baron, E.J.: *Bailey and Scott's Diagnostic Microbiology*, 7th ed. St. Louis, C.V. Mosby, 1986.
Fischbach, F.T.: *Annual of Laboratory Diagnostic Tests*, 2nd ed. Philadelphia, J.B. Lippincott, 1984.
Foster, G.D., Knox, L.S., Dempsey, D.T., et al.: Caloric requirements in total parenteral nutrition. *JACN* 6(3):231–253, 1987.
French, S.N. *Nutritional Assessment via Indirect Calorimetry*. Saint Paul, Medical Graphics, 1987.
Garner, J.S., and Favero, M.S.: CDC guidelines for the prevention and control of nosocomial infections. *Am. J. Infect. Control* 14:110–129, 1986.
Grant, J.P.: *Handbook of Total Parenteral Nutrition*. Philadelphia, W.B. Saunders, 1980.
Guyton, A.C.: *Textbook of Medical Physiology*, 7th ed. Philadelphia, W.B. Saunders, 1986.
Harris, J.A., and Benedict, F.G.: *A Biometric Study of Basal Metabolism in Man*. Washington, D.C. Carnegie Institute, Publication No. 279, 1919.
Henry, J.B.: *Todd-Sanford-Davidsohn Clinical Diagnosis and Management by Laboratory Methods*, 17th ed. Philadelphia, W.B. Saunders, 1984.
Hyde, E.A., Moore, G.S., and Higgins, B.D.: A survey of fungal flora in respiratory therapy equipment. *Resp. Care*. 24:921–927, 1979.
Irwin, R.S., Demers, R.R., Pratter, M.R., et al.: An outbreak of *Acinetobacter* infection associated with the use of a ventilatory spirometer. *Resp. Care*. 25:232–237, 1980.
Jawetz, E., Melnick, J.L., and Adelberg, E.A.: *Review of Medical Microbiology*, 12th ed. Norwalk, CT., Lange Medical Publications, 1976.
McLaughlin, A.J.: *Manual for Infection Control*. Boston, Little, Brown, 1983.
Perkins, J.J.: *Principles and Methods of Sterilization in Health Sciences*. Springfield, IL, Charles C Thomas, 1978.
Centers for Disease Control: Recommendations for prevention of HIV transmission in health-care settings. *MMWR* 36(2S), August 21, 1987.

Spaulding, E.H.: Chemical disinfection and antiseptics in the hospital. *J. Hosp. Res.* 9:7–27, 1972.

Volk, W.A., Benjamin, D.C., Kadner, R.J., and Parsons, J.T.: *Essentials of Medical Microbiology,* 3rd ed. Philadelphia, J.B. Lippincott, 1986.

Weir, J.B.: New methods of calculating metabolic rate with special reference to protein metabolism. *J. Physiol.* 109:1–9, 1949.

Westenskow, D., Cutler, C.A., and Wallace, W.D.: Instrumentation for monitoring gas exchange and metabolic rate in critically ill patients. *Crit. Care Med.* 12(3):183, 1984.

OBJECTIVES

AFTER READING THIS CHAPTER, THE STUDENT WILL BE ABLE TO:

1. Discuss therapeutic and clinical applications of radiology.
2. Discuss physical principles involved in taking a radiograph.
3. State the risks and precautions for healthcare professionals exposed to radiation.
4. Interpret chest radiographs in an organized manner.
5. Recognize certain pathologic conditions of the chest, such as pneumonia, masses, improper position of tubes, foreign bodies, and fractures.
6. Describe the use of special radiologic procedures including tomography, fluoroscopy, angiography, and CT and MRI scans.

13
RADIOLOGY

CHAPTER OUTLINE

RISKS OF EXPOSURE TO RADIATION
PRINCIPLES OF RADIOGRAPHY
METHOD FOR INTERPRETING CHEST RADIOGRAPHS
  Body Orientation
  Bony Tissues
  Soft Tissues
  Heart and Mediastinum
  Lung Lobes and Segments
RADIOGRAPHIC APPEARANCE OF CHEST PATHOLOGY
  Normal Chest Radiograph
  Rotated Patient
  Subcutaneous Emphysema
  Right Mainstem Bronchus Intubation
  Cardiomegaly
  Prosthetic Heart Valve
  Thymus
  Tension Pneumothorax
  Fluid in the Pleural Cavity
  Pneumothorax
  Elevated Diaphragm
  Depressed Diaphragm
  Foreign Body
  Diseases of the Pulmonary Parenchyma
  Phrenic Pacemakers
ADDITIONAL RADIOLOGIC TECHNIQUES
  Bronchography
  Angiography
  Fluoroscopy
  Tomography
  Nuclear Medicine Scans
  Computed Tomography
  Ultrasonography
  Magnetic Resonance Imaging
RADIOGRAPHIC UNKNOWN

Radiology is a specialty with techniques used for both diagnosis and therapy. Clinically, the most common use of radiation is *radiography,* accomplished by means of a diagnostic tool commonly called an x-ray machine. However, this is not the only diagnostic use of radiation.

For certain types of tests called *nuclear scans,* radioactive chemicals called isotopes are ingested, inhaled, or injected. These are important to respiratory therapists involved in pulmonary function tests, such as determining FRC. Ventilation-perfusion scans are useful clinically for evaluating pulmonary emboli. Scans also are important in other specialties, notably thyroid scans, bone scans, or liver-spleen scans. The isotope is localized in the organ under study, and the amount and distribution of radiation emitted give information on the tissue structure and the presence of disease.

Radiation may also be used therapeutically because its ionizing characteristics break molecular bonds that are necessary for cellular function. If administered in high intensity, it kills cells, particularly cells in the process of dividing. Therapeutic radiology is most commonly used for treating tumors that have a high rate of cellular division, especially cancerous. High-intensity radiation may be produced by a machine similar to those used for taking radiographs or may come from an isotope, such as cobalt, whose radiation is focused from outside the body onto a particular part of the body. Therapeutic radiation may also be administered by means of isotopes that are injected or otherwise placed inside the body, such as radium implants for uterine cancer. Administration of an isotope of iodine decreases thyroid gland activity in hyperthyroidism.

RISKS OF EXPOSURE TO RADIATION

The multiple and frequent clinical applications of radiation, both for diagnosis and treatment, attests to the usefulness of these techniques. However, frequent exposure to radiation is a definite health risk to clinicians, including respiratory therapists. For hospital-based personnel, therefore, a *film badge* must be worn for monitoring the dosage of exposure to radiation. Clinicians who work for years in a hospital may be subjected to a sizeable cumulative dose of radiation and may suffer radiation-induced illnesses, such as cancer, cataracts, or arthritis. Furthermore, their offspring are at increased risk for having birth defects. With modern equipment, however, even radiologic technologists and radiologists show no increased incidence of radiation-induced disease, or increased genetic disorders.

PRINCIPLES OF RADIOGRAPHY

The basic principles of radiography are easily understood. X-rays, which are high-energy beams, can chemically change the sensitive coating on film. If your camera and film have ever been scanned by an x-ray monitor at an airport, for example, you may have later found that the film was ruined. The amount of x-ray energy reaching the film determines the amount of chemical change on the radiographic plate, just as the amount of light reaching the film in your camera determines the degree of exposure on the film when you take a picture. Objects placed between the source of an x-ray beam and the radiographic film block the path of the beam and result in a decreased exposure to that portion of the film. The density and thickness of a material determines the amount of penetration by the x-ray beam. Bone is one of the densest materials in the body, and air is the least dense. Water and fat have intermediate densities, and most tissues of the body have about the same density as water. When the x-ray beam passes through air-containing structures, such as the lung, it is unimpeded and passes through easily, exposing that portion of the radiographic film. Thus, radiographs of normal lungs look black when the film is developed. On the other hand, bone or dense materials, such as metals, put between the beam and the film may result in an unexposed portion of the film, which appears white or clear when the radiograph is developed. Fluid-filled tissue, such as the heart as it pumps blood or lungs affected by pneumonia, appears intermediately gray or only slightly dark, depending on the thickness and density of the tissue and the intensity of the x-ray beam. Furthermore, high-contrast material may be placed inside an organ to outline its structure when it is radiographed. These contrast studies include angiograms, which involve placing a dense liquid into blood vessels and taking a radiograph that then shows the structure, integrity, and distribution of the vessels.

The intensity of the x-ray beam varies directly with the amount of voltage to the cathode tube, the part of the machine that produces the beam. Other factors that affect the amount of exposure of the radiographic film are the duration of the beam, which is similar to the shutter speed on the camera, and the size opening or aperture through which the beam passes before going through the object and striking the photographic plate.

The radiologic technician determines the approximate beam duration and intensity and the focus aperture for the x-ray machine to produce a good contrast between the air-containing, fluid-containing, and bony structures on the radiographic film for a person of a given size, weight, and shape. Subsequent radiographs are usually taken at the same settings and at maximal lung inflation so that variations in the lightness or darkness on the film represent differing amounts of fluid or air in the tissues, as occurs in certain diseases, and are not just differences in technique.

When examining an x-ray film, keep in mind that it is a two-dimensional representation of a three-dimensional body. Thus, radiographs taken from several angles, such as *anteroposterior* (AP), *lateral*, or *oblique*, can give information about the location and characteristics of a lesion inside the body. Additionally, the farther an object is from the radiographic film the larger the object tends to appear on the film because the x-rays diverge as they leave the cathode tube. This explains why the heart, which is in the front of the thoracic cavity, looks large when the x-ray plate is against the patient's back and the beam passes first through the front (called an anteroposterior film). The heart appears smaller in the posteroanterior (PA) film because the heart is closer to the film; therefore, a posteroanterior film is most appropriate for determining the presence of cardiomegaly.

METHOD FOR INTERPRETING CHEST RADIOGRAPHS

There are five basic steps involved in interpreting a chest radiograph to ensure that all the available information can be gleaned from it:
1. Body orientation
2. Bony tissues
3. Soft tissues
4. Heart and mediastinum
5. Lung lobes and segments

If you remember to follow these five steps in examining the parts of a chest radiograph, you won't be blinded by the obvious abnormality on one part of the film from seeing the more subtle, but possibly more important, abnormality on another part of the film.

Body Orientation

First, ascertain which is the patient's right side and which is the left. Usually, these are designated on the film. Also, the arch of the aorta and the gas bubble in the stomach are both usually on the left side (except in rare cases, such as dextrocardia). Specifying "sideness" correctly is crucial, if only to ensure that chest physical therapy for pneumonia is delivered to the appropriate area.

Bony Tissues

Second, examine the images of the bony structures. Those of the vertebrae, ribs, clavicles, and scapulae should all be studied for fractures or abnormalities. Rib fractures may preclude the administration of chest physical therapy over the affected area and also may increase the risk of pneumothorax, especially for the patient on mechanical ventilation. A vertebral fracture should alert you to the risk of neurologic injury and possible paraplegia if the patient is moved before the fracture is stabilized. The bony structures also show how much the film was exposed. The distinctiveness of the spinous processes of the vertebrae, marking the midline, indicates the degree of exposure, an important fact to know when comparing films. With proper exposure, the spinous processes in the first three thoracic vertebrae should be apparent, but those behind the heart should be obscured. Overexposure, although showing more spinous processes, may eliminate the subtle shadings of an abnormality, whereas underexposed films may give the impression of congestion or of lesions where there are none.

For a routine chest radiograph, the relation of the patient, the film, and the beam should be symmetric. That is, the patient's chest must be parallel to the x-ray film while the x-ray beam should be exactly perpendicular to both the patient and film. If the patient and the film do not directly face the beam, the resulting radiograph shows the effects of rotation, which may be misinterpreted as abnormal. The manner in which the heads of the clavicles relate to the midline is important in determining the angle to which the patient is rotated. Other chest x-ray positions, such as oblique, lateral, or lordotic, use other relations for the x-ray beam, photographic plate, and patient in order to more accurately locate the depth of a structure in the chest as well as change the relationships of objects within the chest. For instance, a tumor hidden behind a bone in one position might be revealed when the objects "move" in relation to each other with a different position.

Third, study the soft tissues that lie outside the thorax for abnormalities. Each breast contour should be noted to determine the probable position of the nipple, which overlies the lung and may be confused with a density in the lung. Subcutaneous air in the tissue of the neck and thorax gives these areas the appearance of light and dark stripes. They normally appear to be homogeneous. The presence of bullets, pacemakers, and catheters should also be noted in the soft tissues at this time. All tubes should be traced for their entire length to determine their location. Nasogastric tubes should be traced to assure that they end in the stomach and not the trachea. Endotracheal tubes should end about 2 to 3 cm above the carina, at the interspace between the second and third thoracic vertebrae, to help prevent both extubation and bronchial intubation.

Central venous lines should be traced from their origins to the vena cava because sometimes they do not thread correctly and may go up the jugular veins into the head. Swan-Ganz catheters should be traced through the heart and into the pulmonary vessels. If the tip of the Swan-Ganz catheter remains in the heart, it irritates the heart muscle, producing potentially lethal arrhythmias. On the other hand, if the Swan-Ganz catheter is advanced too far, then several complications are possible. The catheter tip can migrate distally into a pulmonary vessel and occlude it, producing a pulmonary infarction. A catheter tip that has migrated distally into a small vessel can produce pulmonary artery rupture when the balloon at the catheter tip is inflated. Insertion of an excessive length of Swan-Ganz catheter can produce loops and knotting that can injure the heart and vessels when the catheter is withdrawn. ECG wires and ventilator tubing lying outside the patient should also be evaluated.

Heart and Mediastinum

Fourth, study the heart and mediastinum. The widest diameter of the heart should normally fill only one side of the thoracic cavity. If the heart is wider than this, it suggests cardiomegaly. However, remember that the film should have been taken posteroanteriorly in order to make the determination of cardiomegaly.

Cor pulmonale indicates hypertrophy or dilation of the right ventricle as a consequence of a primary disorder that affects either the structure or function of the lungs. In severe cases with long-standing pulmonary hypertension, the chest radiograph has a moderately widened cardiac shadow as well as dilated pulmonary outflow tract and main vessels. However, the peripheral markings are attenuated.

In infants, the superior mediastinum is normally widened by the thymus gland, which is one of the lymphoid glands (as are the tonsils). The thymus normally decreases in size with age so that only remnants remain in adults. Enlargement of the superior mediastinum in adults suggests the person may have a malignancy, such as lymphoma. Calcification of the pericardium causes the heart to be outlined with a thin rim of bone density. Likewise, the arch of the aorta may calcify from atherosclerosis and sometimes metal density from artificial heart valves may be seen. The wire sutures used to close the sternum after heart surgery may also be seen on a patient's radiograph.

Lung Lobes and Segments

Finally, look at the lung lobes and segments. The temptation is to look there first, but doing so may cause one to overlook abnormalities in the other parts of the chest. In examining this portion of the chest radiograph, again, a plan is helpful to avert omissions. First, examine the general outline of the lungs at the pleural interface. Careful attention to this step can reveal fluid or air in the potential space between the lung and chest wall (pneumothorax, hemothorax, or pleural effusion). The normal slight elevation of the right diaphragm should be noted as well as any irregularities of the mediastinum and cardiopleural interface. Next, the lobes should be examined to observe shifting of the tissues or lobar bronchi, which would indicate overinflation or collapse (atelectasis). Finally, the lung tissue itself should be examined and the segmental distribution of any abnormalities ascertained. Noting whether a lesion has a focal or uniform distribution helps determine its cause. Masses, fluid infiltration (either alveolar or interstitial), emphysematous blebs, or cavities may be noted in the lung tissue.

RADIOGRAPHIC APPEARANCE OF CHEST PATHOLOGY

Normal Chest Radiograph

You now have the means to systematically examine a normal chest radiograph (Fig. 13–1). First, note the gas bubble in the stomach and the location of the heart and aortic knob on the left. Then, note the symmetry and regularity of the bones. The irregularity on the left clavicle correlates with the patient's medical history, which shows that bone was fractured in a fall from a horse. The spinous processes are apparent in the first three thoracic vertebrae but are hidden on the vertebrae behind the heart. This confirms correct exposure. Note that the heads of the clavicles are the same distance from the spinous processes, indicating no rotation of the patient. Now note the homogeneity of the soft tissues of the chest wall and contours of the breasts, which indicate that this radiograph is most likely that of woman. No catheters are present.

Next, note the narrowness of the superior mediastinum. The heart is on the left and its size is less than half of the thoracic cavity, ruling out cardiomegaly. The pulmonary vessels radiate symmetrically from the mediastinum like the roots of a plant, decreasing in size and apparently in number as they fan out. Some individuals are born with a normally functioning heart abnormally located in the right side of the chest *(dextrocardia)*. When this is found, the clinician should investigate the possible presence of a pathologic condition called *situs inversus* (malrotation of the abdominal viscera) because the two conditions are frequently associated.

Last, examine the pleural interface of the lung, chest wall, mediastinum, and diaphragm to see that no fluid or air is in this potential space. The right side of the diaphragm is higher than the left because of the presence of the liver. The pulmonary vessels and airways appear symmetric, which would rule out collapse or overinflation. The lung itself appears fairly homogeneous, without focal densities or lucencies that might depict masses or cavities.

Rotated Patient

Note that although most of the heart is on the right side, we know left from right because the right side of the diaphragm is elevated and the knob of the aorta is on the left (Fig. 13–2). The reason that the heart appears mostly on the right is evident by the heads of the clavicles: the unequal distances from the spinous processes clearly show the patient was in a rotated position. The radiograph also is overexposed, causing the detail of the lungs and ribs to be lost.

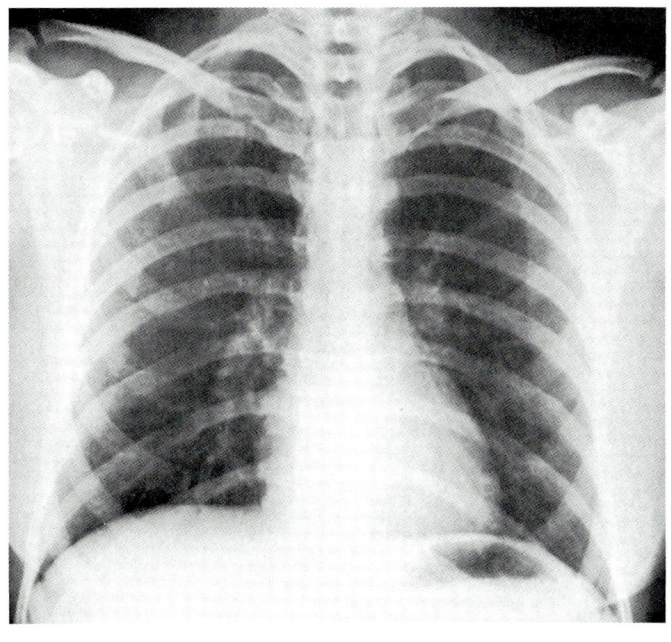

FIGURE 13–1. Normal chest radiograph. (From Squire, L.F., Colaiace, W.M., and Strutynsky, N.: *Exercises in Diagnostic Radiology*, vol. 1. Philadelphia, W.B. Saunders, 1981, with permission.)

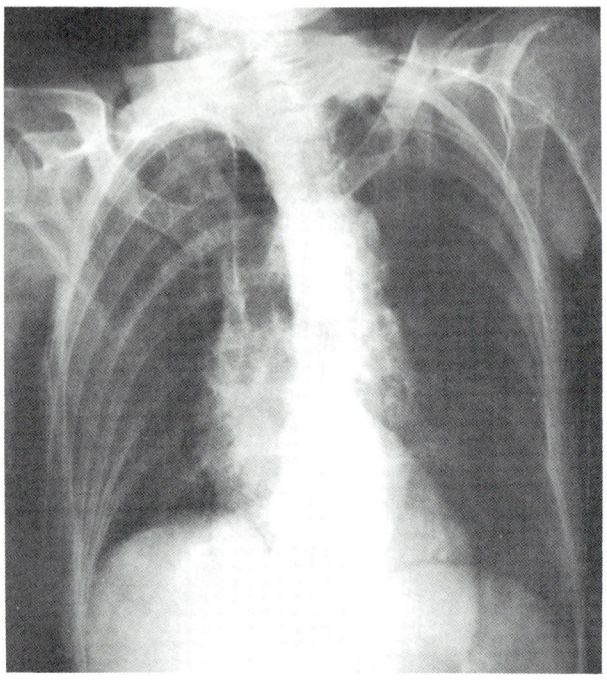

FIGURE 13–2. Overexposed radiograph of a rotated patient. (From Squire, L.F., Colaiace, W.M., and Strutynsky, N.: *Exercises in Diagnostic Radiology*, vol. 1. Philadelphia, W.B. Saunders, 1981, with permission.)

Subcutaneous Emphysema

The small chest and thin bones of this radiograph help in identifying it as that of a neonate (Fig. 13–3). The black areas (air) in the soft tissues of the right lateral chest wall and neck indicate subcutaneous emphysema. This condition is common with chest tube placement, especially in the presence of high intrathoracic pressure because of ventilator therapy and other factors. On palpation, it would feel like crisped rice cereal *(crepitus)*. The arrows denote a thin line of the pericardium affected by pneumopericardium (air in the pericardium).

Right Mainstem Bronchus Intubation

This radiograph shows right mainstem bronchus intubation in a child (Fig. 13–4). The carina is indicated by the arrowhead. This condition may be life-threatening for two reasons. Any blood flow through the nonventilated left lung is not aerated, resulting in $\dot{V}/\dot{Q}$ mismatch (shunt). Additionally, the right lung is subjected to high airway pressure because the entire tidal volume is delivered to only one lung if a volume-cycled ventilator is used. Barotrauma may result. Breath sounds over the collapsed left lung will be absent or decreased. The radiodensity to the left of the spine is that of a dislodged tooth in the esophagus. This suggests that the intubation was difficult and that when the endotracheal tube was finally placed in the larynx, it was advanced too far. Dislodged teeth may also wind up in the airway, which usually necessitates bronchoscopic removal.

Cardiomegaly

This posteroanterior chest radiograph (Fig. 13–5A) shows a patient with a transvenous cardiac pacemaker. The heart is slightly enlarged and fills more than half of the thoracic cavity, indicating cardiomegaly; remember, however, that a PA radiograph is more diagnostic of this than an anteroposterior radiograph because of the magnification of the heart by an AP radiograph. Cardiomegaly and prominent pulmonary vasculature are usually apparent in radiographs of patients with left ventricular failure. Upper lobe vessels become more prominent than lower vessels and interstitial edema accompanies pulmonary venous congestion. There is a diffuse increase in the interstitial markings (Fig. 13–5B), usually in a linear fashion (Kerley's B-lines). Increased pulmonary edema produces alveolar flooding characterized by diffuse bilateral consolidation (Fig. 13–5C).

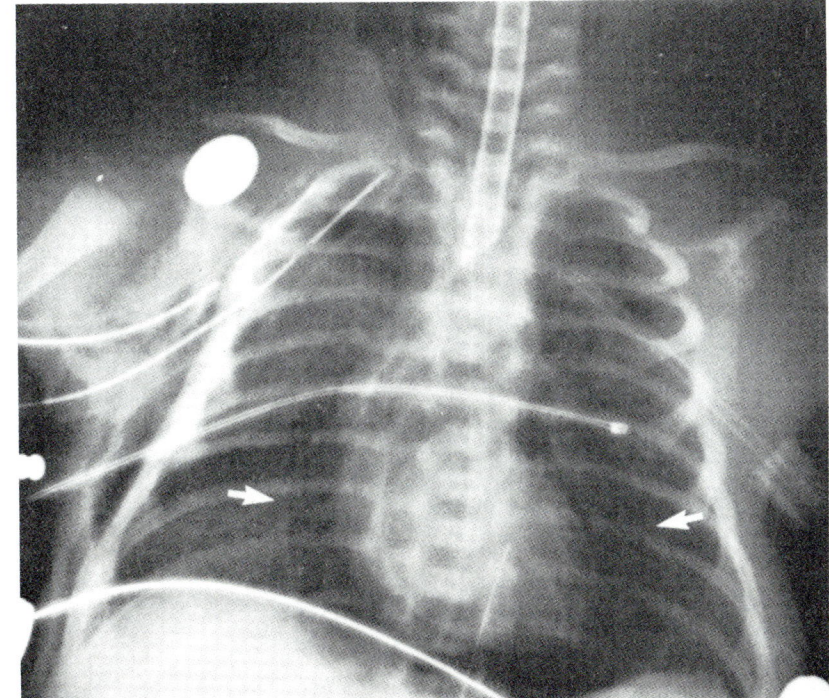

FIGURE 13–3. Cervical and right chest wall subcutaneous emphysema in a neonate. Arrows indicate thin pericardium with a halo of pneumopericardium outlining a small heart. The small heart suggests tamponade. (From Goodman, L.R., and Putman, C.E.: *Intensive Care Radiology: Imaging of the Critically Ill.* Philadelphia, W.B. Saunders, 1983, with permission.)

Prosthetic Heart Valve

This radiograph also shows cardiomegaly (Fig. 13-6). The patient had undergone mitral valve surgery. The artificial valve is seen near the center of the heart. The endotracheal tube and pericardial drainage tubes are in proper position. A surgical needle, inadvertently left in the left atrium, is indicated by the curved arrow. It eventually embolized to the abdominal aorta. Note the course of the central venous pressure catheter inserted via the left jugular vein. It was mistakenly threaded into the right jugular vein (white arrow).

Thymus

Note the widening of the superior mediastinum in this radiograph of a newborn (Fig. 13-7). The thymus, which is normally enlarged in the neonate, usually atrophies, becoming replaced by fat in adolescence. Were this the radiograph of an adult, a widened superior mediastinum would be more suggestive of a lymphoma if the mass were anterior, or of a neural tumor if the mass were posterior. Note also the nearly horizontal arrangement of the neonatal ribs. This shows why the intercostal muscles are ineffective for increasing intrathoracic volume, making neonates diaphragm breathers.

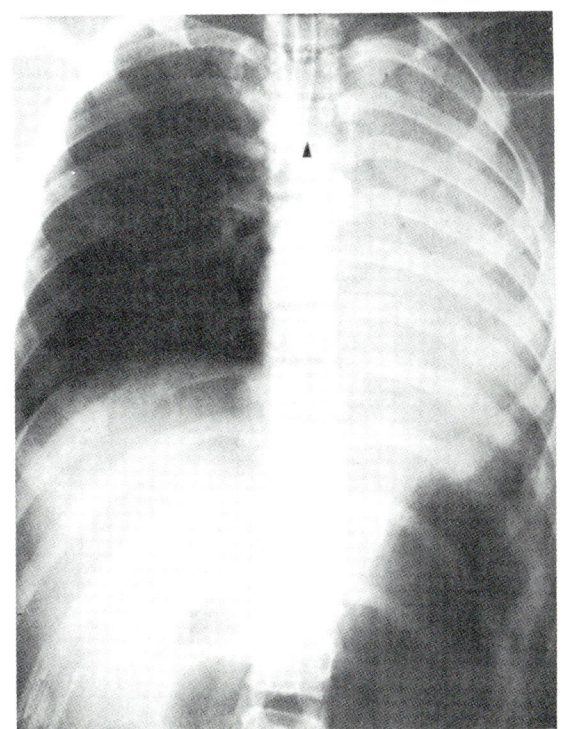

FIGURE 13–4. Right mainstem bronchus intubation. Arrowhead indicates carina. The radiodensity to the left of the spine represents a dislodged tooth in the esophagus. (From Goodman, L.F., and Putman, C.E.: *Intensive Care Radiology: Imaging of the Critically Ill.* Philadelphia, W.B. Saunders, 1983, with permission.)

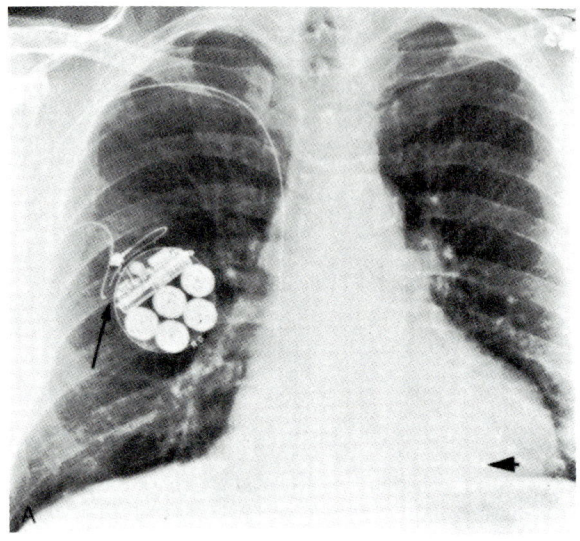
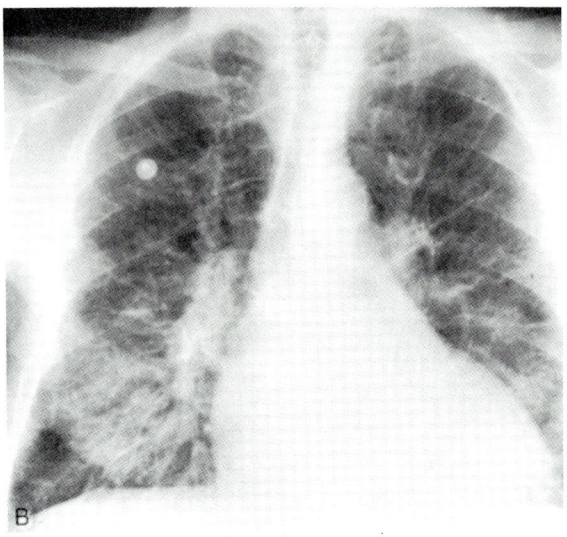
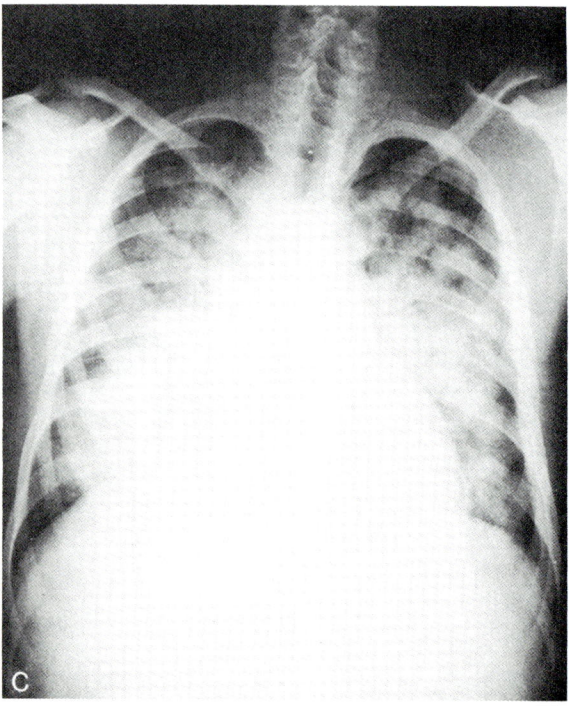

FIGURE 13–5. *A*, Cardiomegaly in a patient with a transvenous cardiac pacemaker (long arrow). Short arrow indicates the tip of the pacing electrode in the right ventricle. (From Goodman, L.F., and Putman, C.E.: *Intensive Care Radiology: Imaging of the Critically Ill.* Philadelphia, W.B. Saunders, 1983, with permission.) *B*, Early pulmonary edema, showing increased interstitial marking in a linear arrangement (Kerley's A and B lines). (From Fraser, R.G., and Paré, J.A.: *Diagnoses of Diseases of the Chest*, 2nd ed., vol. 1. Philadelphia, W.B. Saunders, 1977, with permission.) *C*, Diffuse bilateral alveolar consolidation resulting from severe pulmonary edema. (From Fishman, A.P.: *Pulmonary Diseases and Disorders*. New York, McGraw-Hill, 1980, with permission.)

We have examined radiographs with pathology in the subcutaneous tissues, bones, heart, and mediastinum. Now let's look at some radiographs of lung pathology, starting with a problem at the pleural interface.

Tension Pneumothorax

Although a normal lung would collapse to a small dense mass at the hilum, severe pulmonary consolidation from pneumonia prevents complete collapse of this right lung (Fig. 13–8). Note the absence of lung markings outside of the collapsed lung; this is a finding that rules out skinfolds, which sometimes are mistaken for pneumothorax because they produce lines parallel to the chest wall. The depression of the diaphragm and the shift of the trachea and mediastinum to the left confirm the diagnosis of a right-sided tension pneumothorax. A tension pneumothorax is a condition in which an air leak from the lung or airway acts as

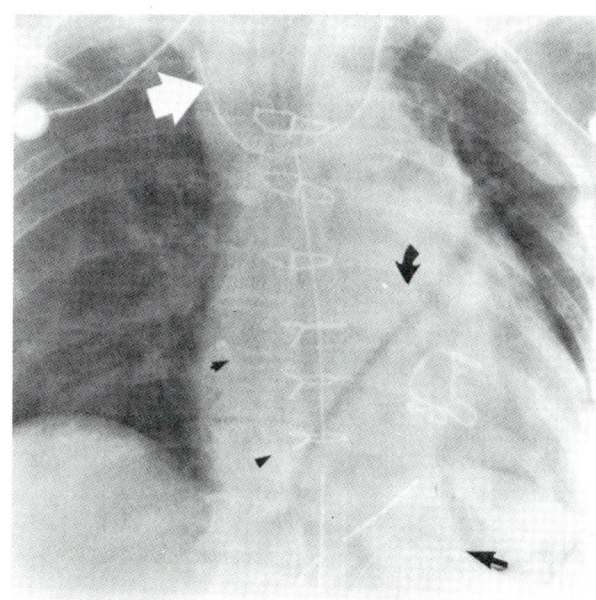

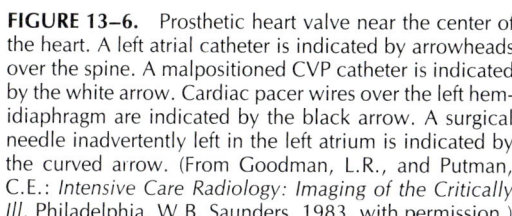

FIGURE 13-6. Prosthetic heart valve near the center of the heart. A left atrial catheter is indicated by arrowheads over the spine. A malpositioned CVP catheter is indicated by the white arrow. Cardiac pacer wires over the left hemidiaphragm are indicated by the black arrow. A surgical needle inadvertently left in the left atrium is indicated by the curved arrow. (From Goodman, L.R., and Putman, C.E.: *Intensive Care Radiology: Imaging of the Critically Ill.* Philadelphia, W.B. Saunders, 1983, with permission.)

a one-way valve, allowing gas to enter the pleural cavity but not to leave it. This action can greatly elevate intrapleural pressure. Thus, this condition is a medical emergency because the patient can die quickly unless the tension is released by inserting a chest tube or needle. The increasing intrathoracic extrapulmonary pressure impedes venous return and may lead to cardiopulmonary arrest.

Fluid in the Pleural Cavity

Figure 13-9 shows fluid in the left pleural cavity and some subcutaneous emphysema near the left shoulder. The patient had a left pneumonectomy 6 days previously, and fluid has filled the left hemithorax. The type of fluid cannot be ascertained from the radiograph but can usually be determined from the history. An excess of pleural secretions is called a pleural effusion and may result from inflammation, infection, pulmonary embolus, congestive heart failure, or malignancy. If blood fills the pleural cavity, a hemothorax occurs, which may result from trauma or surgery. Lymph may also fill the pleural cavity after injury to the thoracic duct, which is called chylothorax. In this radiograph, extrapulmonary air fills the top of the pleural cavity. Because no lung is present on the

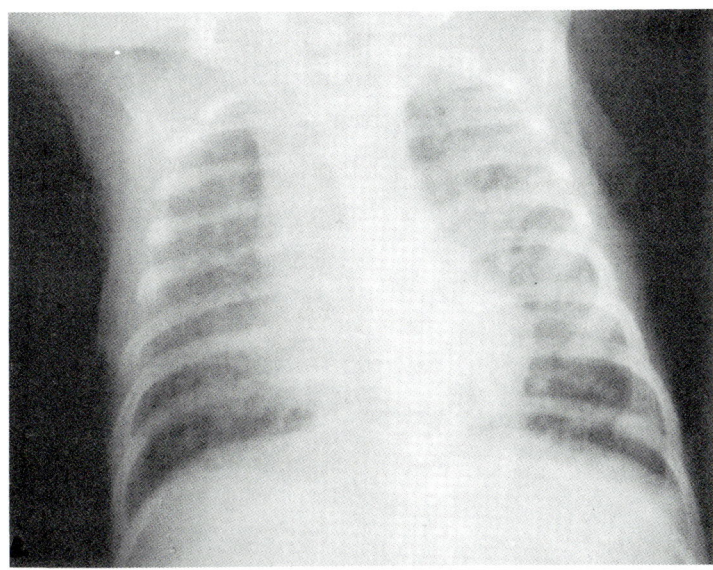

FIGURE 13-7. Superior mediastinal widening in the newborn caused by the presence of the thymus. (From Meschan, I.: *Analysis of Roentgen Signs in General Radiology*, vol. 2. Philadelphia, W.B. Saunders, 1973, with permission.)

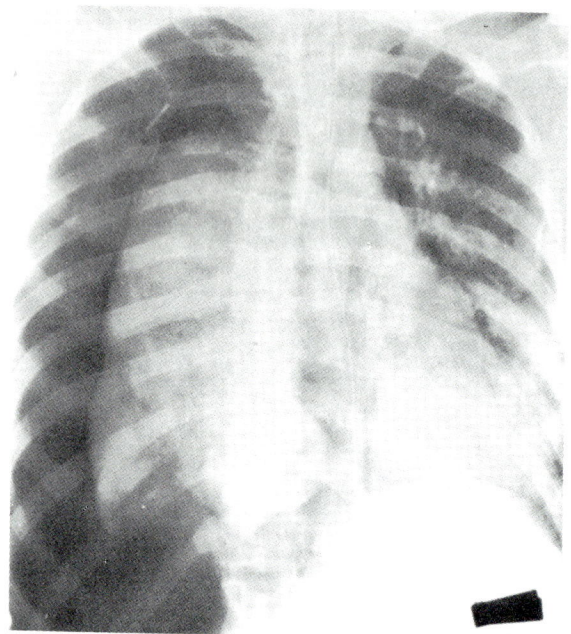

FIGURE 13-8. Tension pneumothorax with incomplete collapse due to consolidation in the right lung. The diaphragm is markedly depressed on that side, and the mediastinum is shifted to the left. (From Goodman, L.R., and Putman, C.E.: *Intensive Care Radiology: Imaging of the Critically Ill*. Philadelphia, W.B. Saunders, 1983, with permission.)

left side, no lung markings are visible. When fluid partially fills the pleural cavity, the lung on that side is compressed, producing atelectasis. If the radiograph is taken with the patient standing or sitting, then the fluid occupies the bottom of the hemithorax. A radiograph taken with the patient in the lateral position (lying on his side) causes the fluid to shift and occupy the lateral portion of the chest cavity. Figure 13-9B shows an upright chest radiograph of a patient with a pleural effusion. The effusion becomes more obvious when the patient is placed in the lateral position (Fig. 13-9C).

Pneumothorax

Figure 13-10A is an inspiratory film. This technique is usually desired in a chest radiograph because it produces the greatest contrast between normal lung tissue and consolidated or atelectatic lung tissue. However, it is not as useful for determining the presence of a limited pneumothorax. Figure 13-10B, an expiratory film, shows the extrapulmonary air, with the margin of the collapsed lung indicated by the black arrows.

Elevated Diaphragm

Normally, the right diaphragm is about 1 or 2 cm higher than the left because of the presence of the liver. In Figure 13-11A, the right diaphragm is decidedly higher than the left because the patient had an enlarged, cancerous liver pushing the diaphragm up. A hemidiaphragm may also be pulled upward by a collapsed, atelectatic lung.

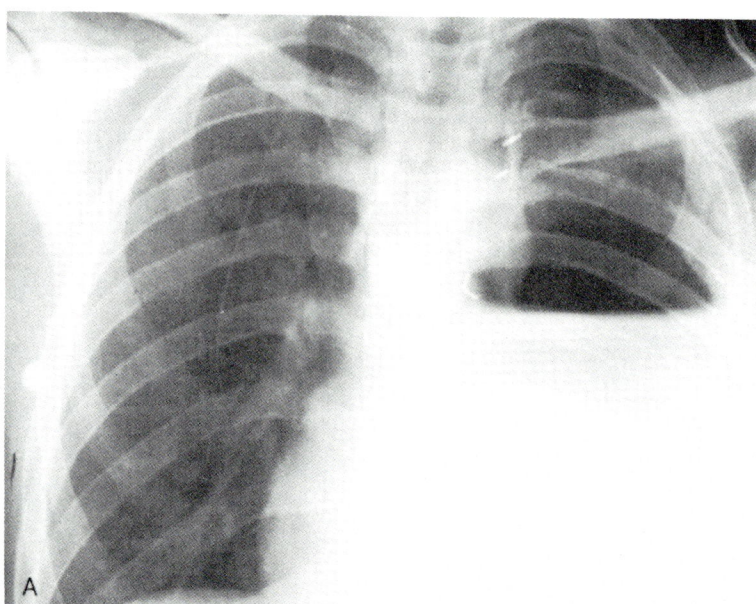

FIGURE 13-9. *A*, Fluid in the pleural cavity 6 days after a left pneumonectomy. The patient must have been sitting or standing to produce the horizontal air-fluid interface. Note the surgical clips near the hilum and superior mediastinum. (From Goodman, L.R., and Putman, C.E.: *Intensive Care Radioiology: Imaging of the Critically Ill*. Philadelphia, W.B. Saunders, 1983, with permission.)

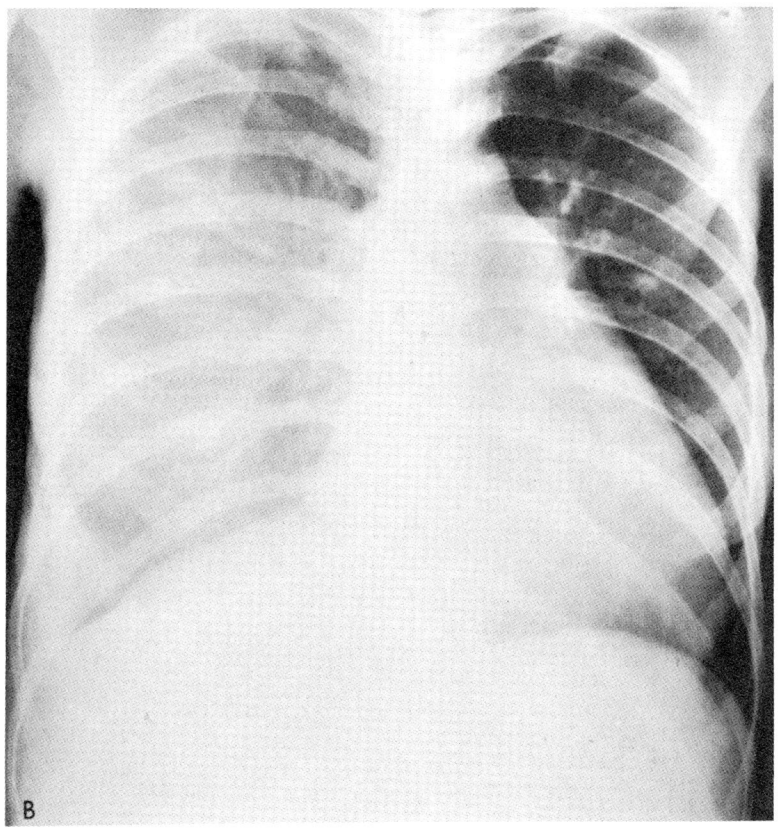
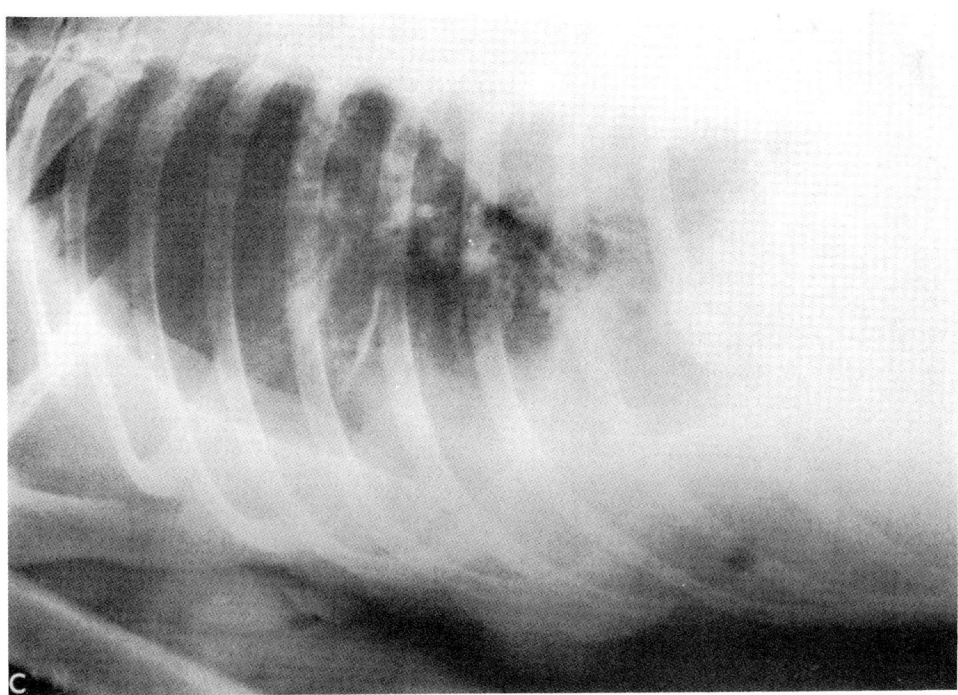

FIGURE 13–9. Continued B, A pleural effusion causing a decreased amount of air in the lung on that side and blunting of the right angle formed by the ribs and diaphragm (costophrenic angle). C, When a radiograph is taken with the patient lying with the right side down, the effusion fluid "layers out" below the air-filled lung. (From Fraser, R.G., and Paré, J.A.: *Diagnoses of Diseases of the Chest*, 2nd ed., vol. 1. Philadelphia, W.B. Saunders, 1977, with permission.)

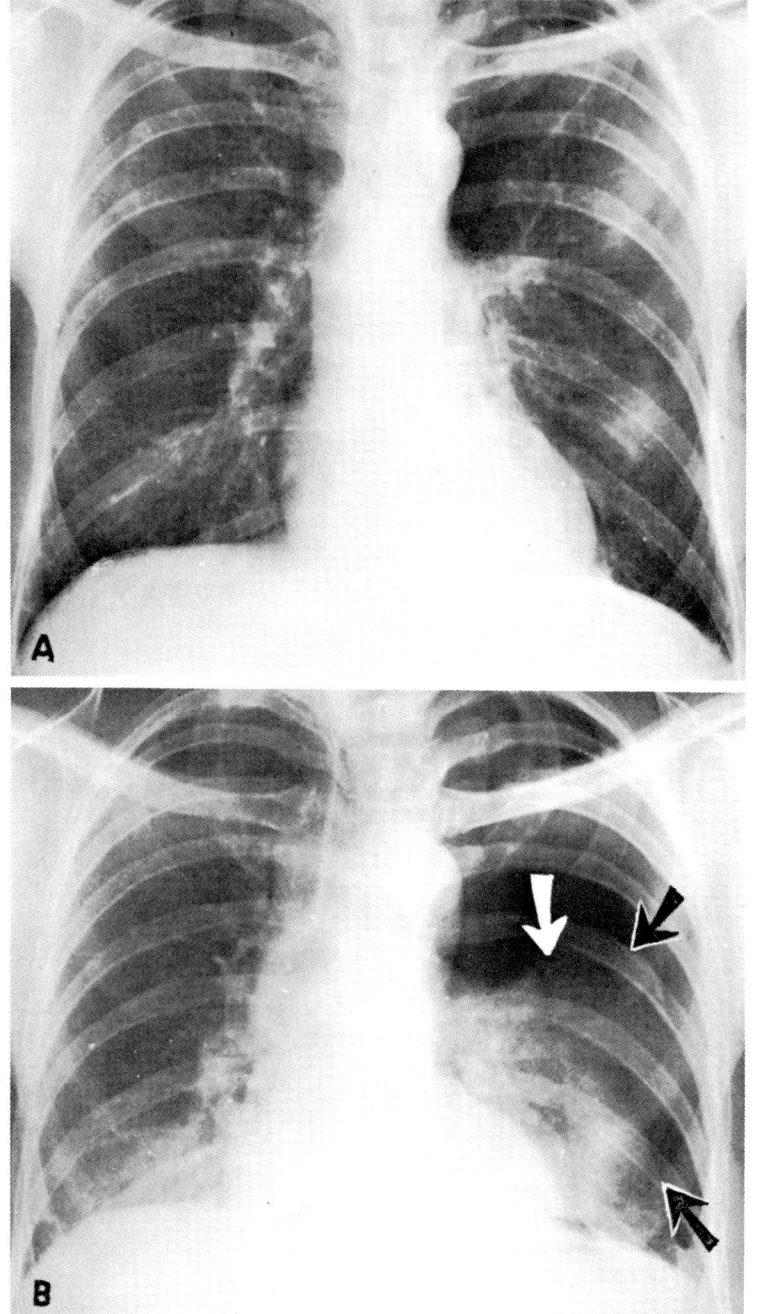

FIGURE 13–10. A, An inspiratory film with no apparent pneumothorax. B, An expiratory film with obvious left pneumothorax. The lung outline is indicated by arrows. (From Felson, B., Weinstein, A.S., and Spita, H.B.: *Principles of Chest Roentgenology. A Programmed Text.* Philadelphia, W.B. Saunders, 1965, with permission.)

Diffuse loss of air volume in the lungs is called *microatelectasis* but may be difficult to differentiate from a film taken during exhalation. Atelectasis of one or more lung lobes (Fig. 13–11B) not only elevates the diaphragm on that side but can also produce other indirect signs, including shifts of the mediastinum and lung fissures (anatomic divisions between lobes) toward the area of collapse. The areas of lung surrounding the opacified area of collapse may be hyperinflated and appear hyperlucent on the radiograph. Recognition of atelectasis on the chest radiograph is important because the causes are frequently easily treatable (excessive and retained secretions or foreign bodies). Inadequate treatment of atelectasis often results in postobstruction pneumonia.

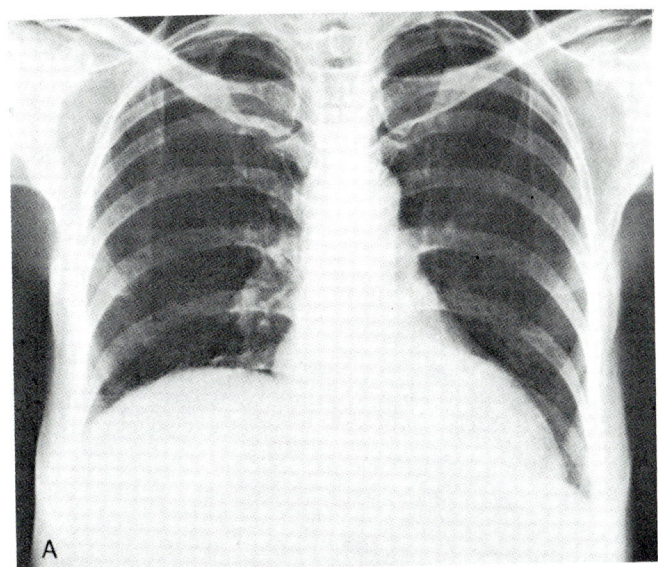

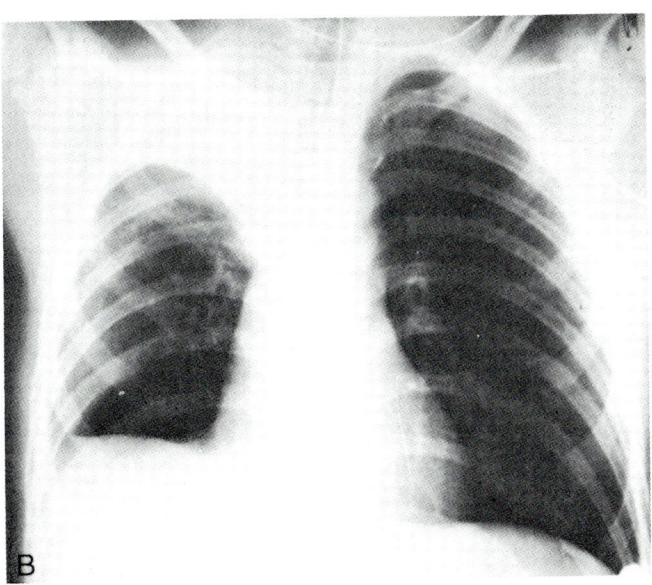

FIGURE 13–11. *A*, Elevated right diaphragm in a patient with an enlarged liver. (From Squire, L.F., Colaiace, W.M., and Strutynsky, N.: *Exercises in Diagnostic Radiology*, vol. 1. Philadelphia, W.B. Saunders, 1981, with permission.) *B*, Atelectasis of the right upper lobe, producing shift of the diaphragm, heart, horizontal fissure (between lobes), and trachea. (From Hinshaw, H.C., and Murray, J.F.: *Diseases of the Chest*, 4th ed. Philadelphia, W.B. Saunders, 1980, with permission.)

Splenomegaly may result in an elevation in the left side of the diaphragm. A paralyzed hemidiaphragm, which may result from phrenic nerve injury, would be elevated on an inspiratory film by virtue of the paradoxical movement of the paralyzed hemidiaphragm during spontaneous ventilation.

Depressed Diaphragm

Both hemidiaphragms are considerably depressed in this patient with emphysema, gas trapping, and greatly distended lungs (Fig. 13–12A). The heart becomes long and narrow. The patient usually appears barrel-chested. A lateral chest radiograph would also show a depressed diaphragm as well as increased retrosternal air space. Bullae (large, circumscribed, air-filled cavities in the lung) are also common findings in patients with emphysema (Fig 13–12B). Remember that a tension pneumothorax can also produce a severely depressed diaphragm.

Foreign Body

Figure 13–13 is of a 2-year-old boy. A foreign body is seen at the level of the cricopharyngeal muscle,

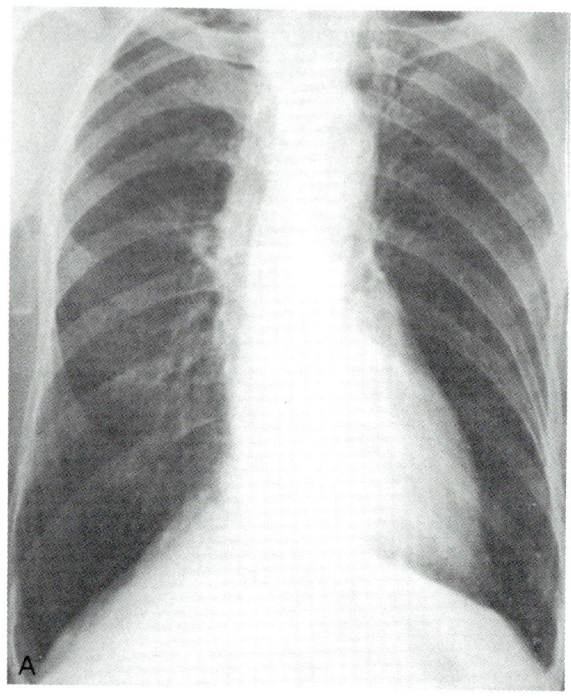
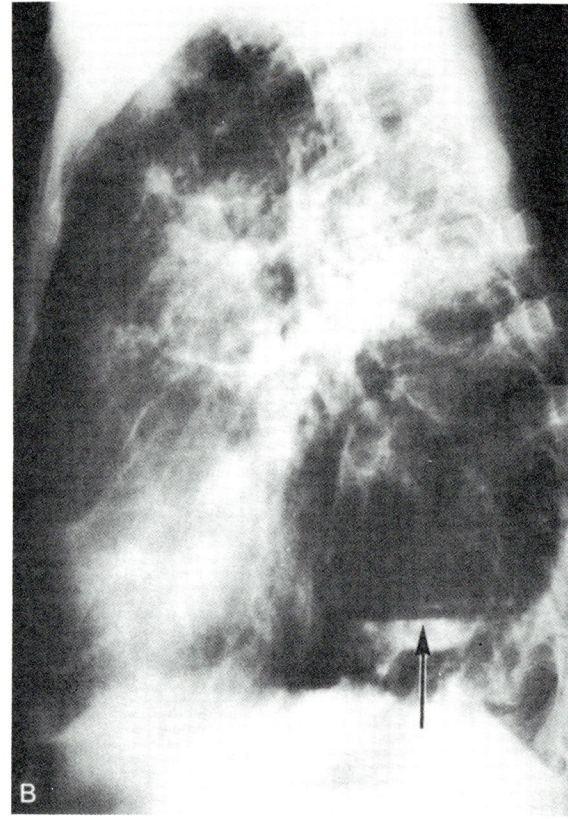

FIGURE 13–12. *A,* Bilateral depressed diaphragms in a patient with COPD. (From Squire, L.F., Colaiace, W.M., and Strutynsky, N.: *Exercises in Diagnostic Radiology,* vol. 1. Philadelphia, W.B. Saunders, 1981, with permission.) *B,* Lateral chest radiograph of a patient with severe emphysema, showing retrosternal (between the sternum and mediastinum) air. There is also an air-fluid level in an infected bulla behind the heart (arrow). (From Fishman, A.P.: *Pulmonary Diseases and Disorders.* New York, McGraw-Hill, 1980, with permission.)

which marks the bottom of the pharynx and the top of the esophagus. It is right behind the larynx but may produce airway obstruction. This radiograph should also help remind you to be careful around the airway. If a tooth is dislodged during an intubation attempt, try to retrieve it before ventilating the patient, because otherwise the tooth may be forced down the airway necessitating bronchoscopic removal.

Diseases of the Pulmonary Parenchyma

Pulmonary Masses. Scattered nodular densities in the lung usually suggest metastatic cancer to the lung (Fig. 13–14). Cancer often metastasizes to the lungs, as noted in Chapter 3, because of the venous blood filtration function of the pulmonary circulation. This patient also had calcification of the aortic arch. The presence of a solitary density in the lung is more suggestive of a primary (still in the site of origin) lung cancer, usually a bronchogenic carcinoma.

Focal Pulmonary Infiltrates. Objects of the same radiographic density in anatomic contact obscure each other's borders. Pneumonia in a portion of lung contacting the heart, aorta, or diaphragm obliterates the distinct outlines. This loss of outlines is called the *silhouette sign.* Figure 13–15A shows the border on the left side of the heart obliterated by lingular pneumonia. Right middle lobe pneumonia obliterates the right heart border because of contact, although the diaphragm is not obliterated (Fig. 13–15B). Right middle lobe opacification may be due to pneumonia, but this is also a frequent site of accumulation of aspirated material because of the configuration of airways in the supine patient (see Chapter 17). Right lower lobe pneumonia does not obliterate the right heart border but may obliterate the diaphragm.

Diffuse Pulmonary Infiltrates. Figure 13–16A

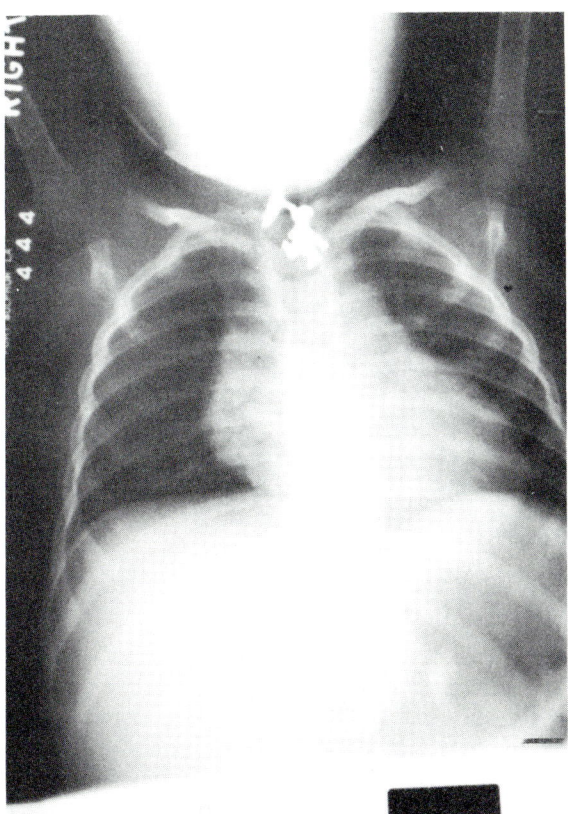

FIGURE 13–13. Foreign body at the level of the cricopharyngeal muscle.

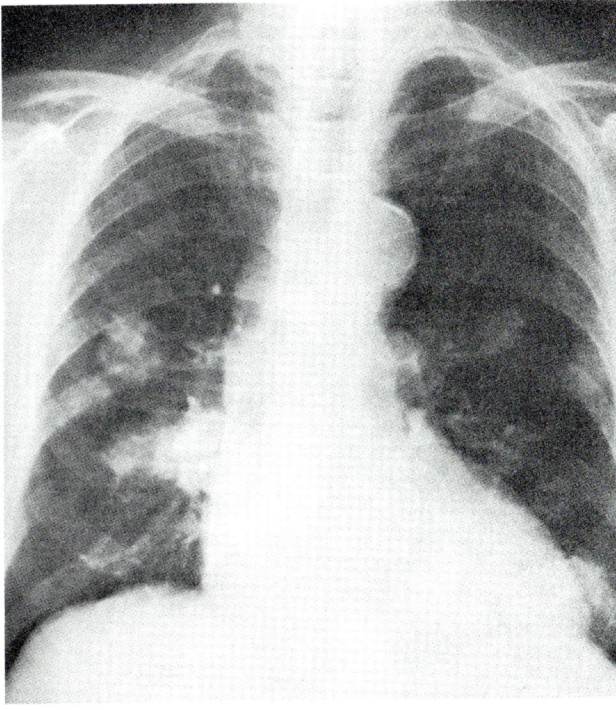

FIGURE 13–14. Pulmonary masses due to metastatic carcinoma. (From Squire, L.F., Colaiace, W.M., and Strutynsky, N.: *Exercises in Diagnostic Radiology*, vol. 1. Philadelphia, W.B. Saunders, 1981, with permission.)

demonstrates a bilateral diffuse accumulation of fluid in the air spaces. The diagnosis in this patient was ARDS, but similar radiographic findings would result from congestive heart failure, pulmonary edema, massive aspiration, pneumonia, severe infection, lung contusion, pulmonary embolism, fat embolism, or any other condition that produces widespread accumulation of fluid in the alveoli. This radiograph also shows a Swan-Ganz catheter in the main pulmonary artery. Also, the endotracheal tube cuff is overinflated. Its external pressure reservoir may be seen over the right lung (arrows). It simulates a bulla or bleb (air-containing cavity in the lung).

A similar-appearing radiograph is obtained from an infant with infant respiratory distress syndrome (IRDS). This syndrome was formerly called hyaline membrane disease but has since been appreciated as a complex interaction between immature lung physiology and the stresses of the transition to extrauterine life. Figure 13–16B, obtained from a baby with this common syndrome, shows a dense, so-called ground-glass appearance to the lungs (reticulogranular pattern). Typically, the radiograph also shows air bronchograms, which are greatly dilated intrapulmonary upper airways contrasting with the background of diffuse, finely nodular densities. The treatment of IRDS includes prolonged mechanically assisted ventilation which occasionally produces the persistent lung disorder *bronchopulmonary dysplasia,* which shows widespread linear infiltrates on a chest radiograph (Fig. 13–16C).

Phrenic Pacemakers

The phrenic nerve electrodes are seen over the transverse processes of T-1 (Fig. 13–17). A fine wire leads to each pacer from the electrode. Note also the presence of a tracheostomy. Patients with high cervical spinal cord injuries or other neurologic diseases, such as poliomyelitis, may benefit

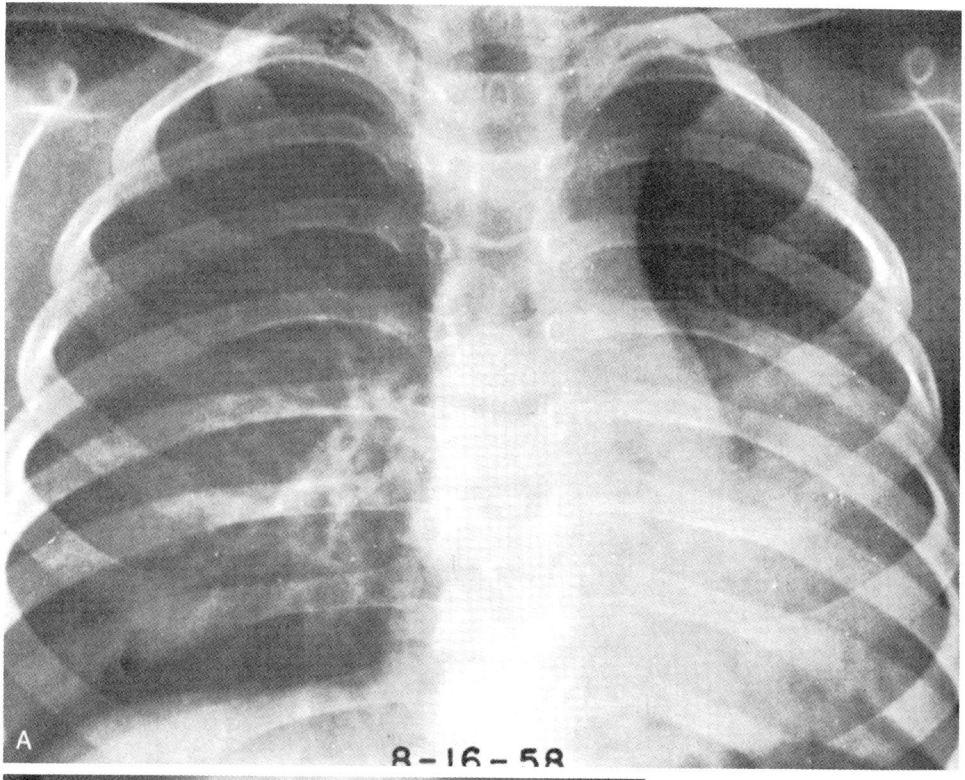
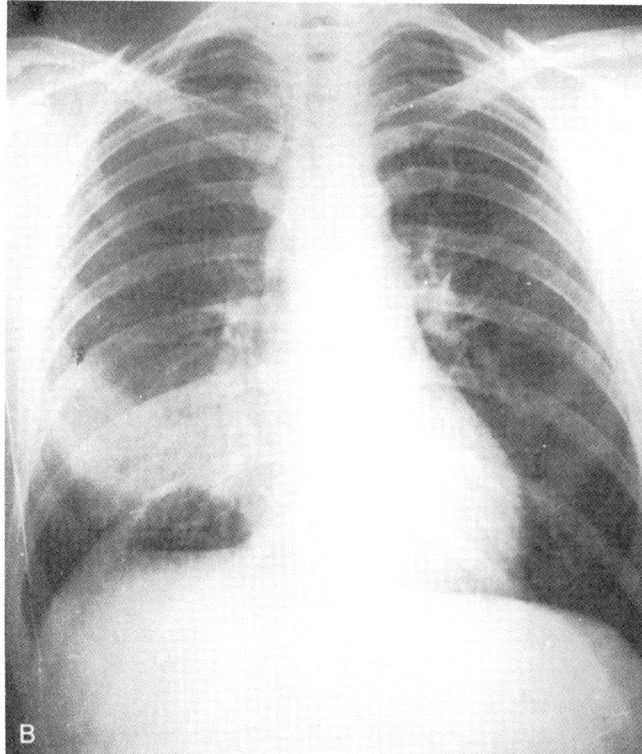

FIGURE 13-15. *A*, Lingular pneumonia obscuring the left heart border. Loss of the normal radiologic outline is called "the silhouette sign." *B*, Right middle lobe pneumonia obliterating the right heart border. (From Felsen, B., Weinstein, A.S., and Spita, H.B.: *Principles of Chest Roentgenology. A Programmed Text.* Philadelphia, W.B. Saunders, 1965, with permission.)

FIGURE 13–16. *A*, Diffuse pulmonary infiltrates due to ARDS. The endotracheal tube cuff is overdistended. Its external pressure reservoir is indicated by the arrows. (From Goodman, L.R., and Putman, C.E.: *Intensive Care Radiology: Imaging of the Critically Ill.* Philadelphia, W.B. Saunders, 1983, with permission.) *B*, Infant respiratory distress syndrome, showing diffuse infiltrates and air bronchograms.

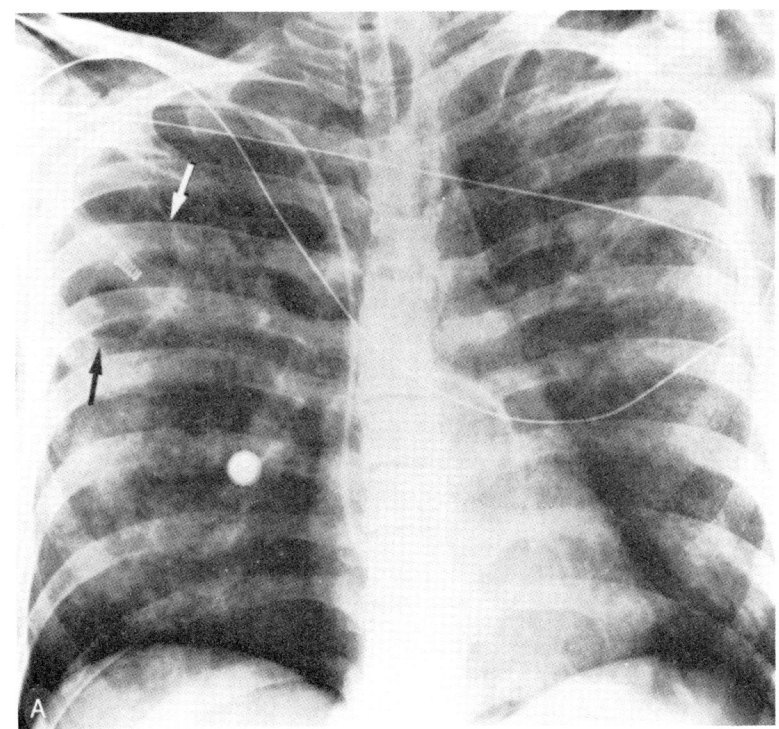

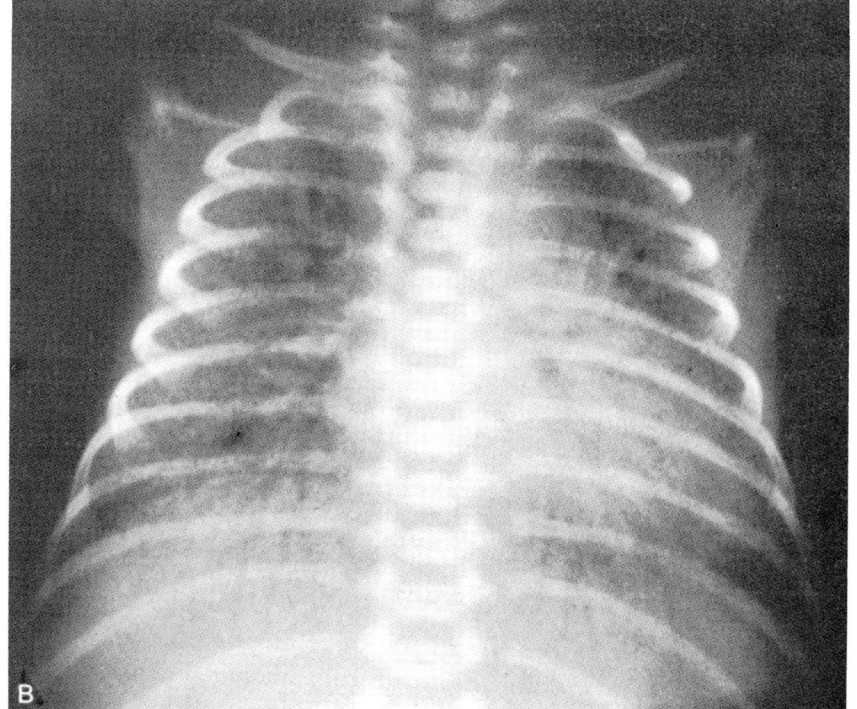

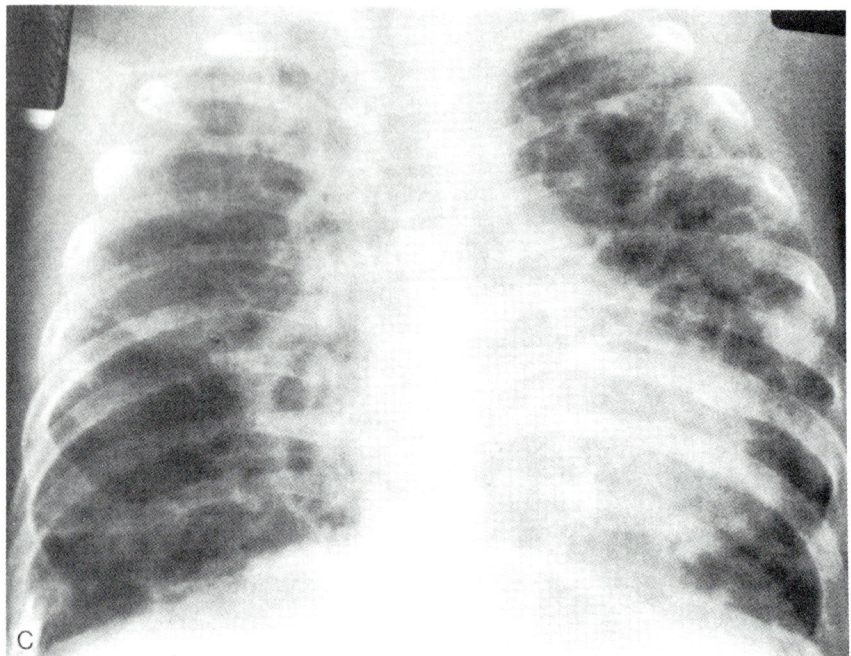

FIGURE 13–16. *Continued C,* Widespread linear infiltrates of bronchopulmonary dysplasia in an infant following prolonged mechanical ventilation. (From Hinshaw, H.C., and Murray, J.F.: *Diseases of the Chest,* 4th ed. Philadelphia, W.B. Saunders, 1980, with permission.)

from phrenic pacemakers to help keep them from being ventilator-dependent.

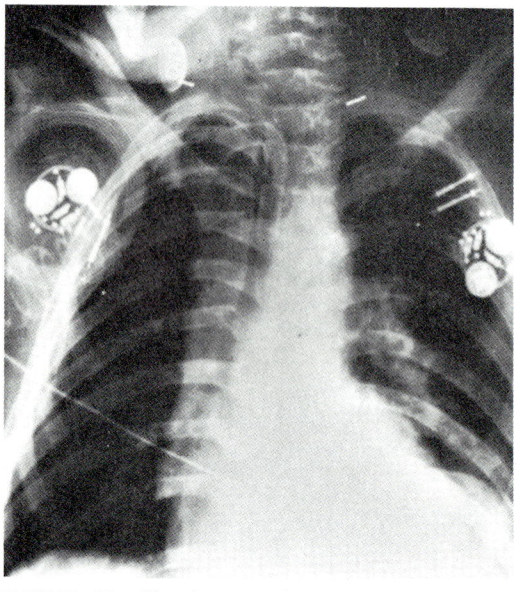

FIGURE 13–17. Phrenic pacemakers in a patient with a tracheostomy. The electrodes are seen over the transverse processes of T-1. (From Goodman, L.R., and Putman, C.E.: *Intensive Care Radiology: Imaging of the Critically Ill.* Philadelphia, W.B. Saunders, 1983, with permission.)

ADDITIONAL RADIOLOGIC TECHNIQUES

Bronchography

Injection of a radiodense contrast substance into the bronchi during bronchoscopy outlines the bronchi when a radiograph is taken (Fig. 13–18). The arrows indicate mucous plugs obstructing the airway. Bronchograms are also used in the diagnosis of bronchiectasis (pathologic extreme dilation of a bronchus, usually as a result of infection).

Angiography

If a radiodense material is injected into a blood vessel and a radiograph is taken, the material will outline the course of the vessels in the tissue. Figure 13–19 shows a pulmonary angiogram revealing multiple bilateral intraluminal clots and abrupt cutoff of the right upper and middle lobe pulmonary arteries, consistent with massive pulmonary embolism.

Fluoroscopy

Fluoroscopy is a radiographic technique that allows continued observation of the radiographic image on a screen like that of a television. Paradoxical movement of the diaphragm may be observed during breathing by means of fluoroscopy if the patient has phrenic nerve damage. Fluoroscopy can also be used to guide the placement of catheters and to follow the distribution of dye after its injection into blood vessels. These procedures may last for some time, and accumulated dosage of radiation should be monitored in exposed healthcare professionals.

Tomography

A tomograph consists of an apparatus in which the x-ray tube and film move synchronously but in opposite directions. The fulcrum of movement is set to the plane of the lesion to be studied. Structures above and below the level of the lesion are blurred, but the plane of the fulcrum remains in sharp focus. Thus, an x-ray "slice" is made through the patient at the level of the lesion.

Nuclear Medicine Scans

Ventilation and perfusion of the lungs can be evaluated by techniques called nuclear scanning, which use radioactive isotopes (Fig. 13–20). Ventilation is determined by scanning (measuring the distribution of radioactivity) for inhaled xenon-133

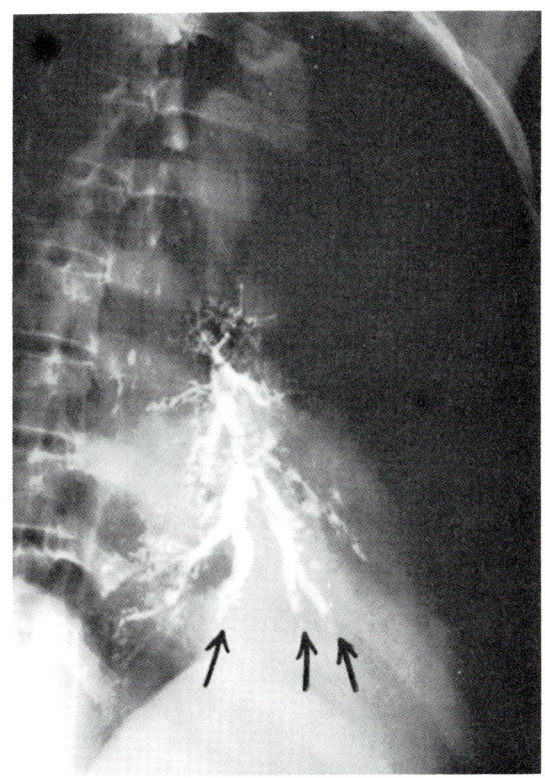

FIGURE 13–18. Bronchogram of airways with mucous plugging. (From Felson, B., Weinstein, A.S., and Spita, H.B.: *Principles of Chest Roentgenology. A Programmed Text*. Philadelphia, W.B. Saunders, 1965, with permission.)

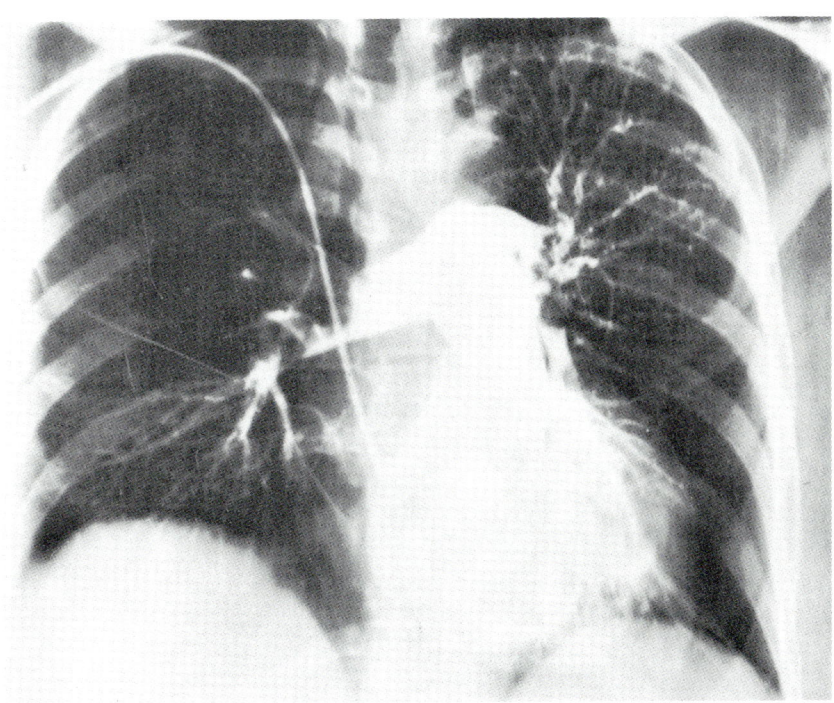

FIGURE 13–19. Pulmonary artery angiogram shows multiple bilateral intraluminal clots and abrupt cutoff of the right upper and middle lobe pulmonary arteries caused by multiple large pulmonary emboli. (From Goodman, L.R., and Putman, C.E.: *Intensive Care Radiology: Imaging of the Critically Ill*. Philadelphia, W.B. Saunders, 1983, with permission.)

133XE VENTILATION-PERFUSION

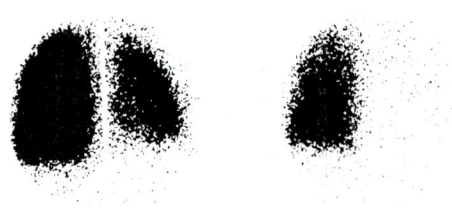

PERFUSION   VENTILATION

FIGURE 13-20. Ventilation and perfusion scans with xenon-133 viewed **posteriorly** from a patient with a tumor in the right mainstem bronchus. The ventilation scan shows no ventilation of the right lung while the perfusion scan shows persistent right lung perfusion. Thus, the right lung is the site of pulmonary shunt and the cause for arterial hypoxemia. (From Tisi, G.M.: Preoperative evaluation of pulmonary function, *American Review of Respiratory Disease* 119:293-310, 1979, with permission.)

gas. Distribution of perfusion is determined by measuring the distribution of radioactivity in the lungs' circulation by intravenously injecting radioactive particles (macroaggregated albumin labeled with iodine-131), which are embolized into the areas of the pulmonary circulation being perfused. Intravenous injection of xenon-133 that has been dissolved in a liquid is another technique that shows the distribution of perfusion.

Computed Tomography

Computed tomography involves rotating an x-ray emitter and an x-ray receiver around the patient, and feeding the images into a computer, which then constructs serial images of horizontal slices through the patient. The technique, like fluoroscopy, requires that the subject be still, and if ventilatory support is necessary for the patient, the respiratory therapist may be subjected to radiation if not properly shielded.

The radiograph in Figure 13-21A shows a right-sided effusion, but pneumonia of the lung in the area could not be ruled out. The CT scan of the same person in Figure 13-21B demonstrates a loculated (compartmentalized) effusion at the base. The lung that could not be seen on the radiograph because it was hidden by the effusion can be seen on the CT scan and is unaffected by pneumonia.

Ultrasonography

Ultrasonography is an imaging technique that utilizes high-frequency sound waves reflected by the differing densities of the body's tissues. This technique is very popular for visualizing the function of the heart muscle and valves (echocardiography). Because ultrasound does not use ionizing ra-

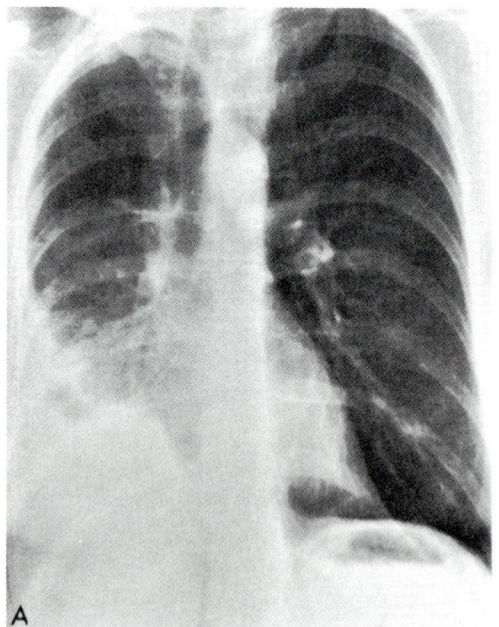
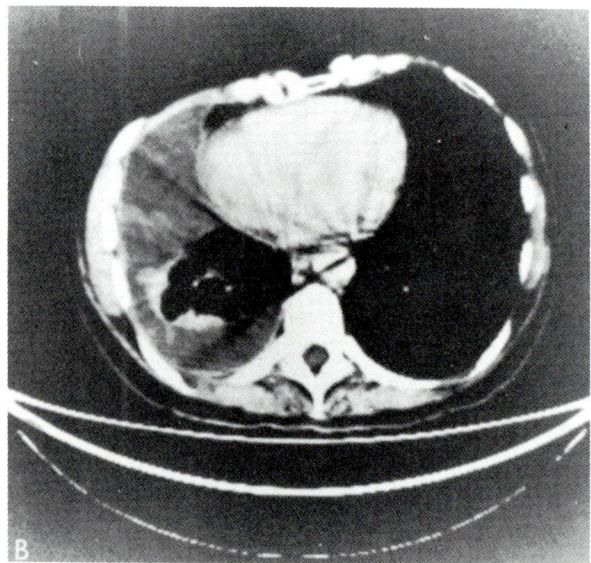

FIGURE 13-21. *A*, Chest radiograph of a patient with unexplained fever. There is a right-sided effusion, but pneumonia in the concealed lung cannot be ruled out. *B*, CT scan of the same patient showing the effusion but also the relatively uninvolved adjacent lung. (From Goodman, L.R., and Putman, C.E.: *Intensive Care Radiology: Imaging of the Critically Ill*. Philadelphia, W.B. Saunders, 1984, with permission.)

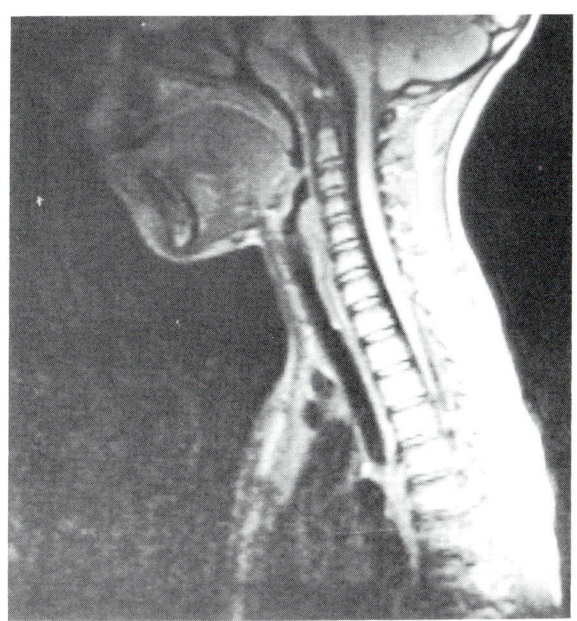

FIGURE 13–22. Magnetic resonance imaging scan shows the fine resolution of the cerebellum and spinal cord that can be obtained.

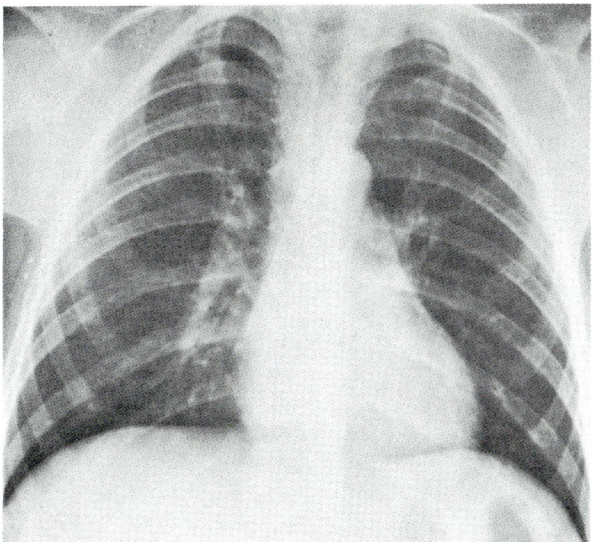

FIGURE 13–23. Radiologic unknown. (From Squire, L.F., Colaiace, W.M., and Strutynsky, N.: *Exercises in Diagnostic Radiology*, vol. 1. Philadelphia, W.B. Saunders, 1981, with permission.)

diation (such as x-rays or gamma rays), it can be used to study a developing fetus without causing birth defects. However, ultrasonography is not very useful for studying the lungs and chest because the large amount of air in the lungs scatters the ultrasonic waves.

Magnetic Resonance Imaging

Magnetic resonance imaging (MRI) is a recently developed technique gaining wide clinical use because of its high resolution images (Fig. 13–22). Like ultrasonography, it does not use ionizing radiation. The patient is placed in a constant high-intensity magnetic field which causes the nuclei of the atoms in the body to become aligned. A pulse of radio frequency energy is directed toward the tissue. When this pulse ends, the energy is emitted from the tissue as a weak radio frequency signal.

In clinical usage, this technique requires that the patient remain very still for intervals of about 2 minutes. This may be very difficult for children or patients who are ill or disoriented. At times, this technique may be used on patients requiring mechanical ventilation. Cardiopulmonary clinicians may be needed to ventilate these patients with self-inflating resuscitation bags. Although there is no danger from the radiation used in this technique, the presence of the intense magnetic field requires that no metallic objects are allowed in the vicinity.

RADIOGRAPHIC UNKNOWN

If you said that Figure 13–23 was a normal radiograph you were mostly right, but you failed to follow the sequence for examining chest radiographs because you missed the absent clavicles.

Bibliography

Felson, B., Weinstein, A.S., and Spita, H.B.: *Principles of Chest Roentgenology. A Programmed Text*. Philadelphia, W.B. Saunders, 1965.

Fishman, A.P.: *Pulmonary Diseases and Disorders*. New York, McGraw-Hill, 1980.

Fraser, R.G., and Paré, J.A.: *Diagnoses of Diseases of the Chest*, 2nd ed., vol. 1. Philadelphia, W.B. Saunders, 1977.

Goodman, L.R., and Putman, C.E.: *Intensive Care Radiology: Imaging of the Critically Ill*. Philadelphia, W.B. Saunders, 1983.

Hilton, S.W., Edwards, D.K., and Hilton, J.W.: *Practical Pediatric Radiology*. Philadelphia, W.B. Saunders, 1984.

Hinshaw, H.C., Murray, J.F.: *Diseases of the Chest*, 4th ed. Philadelphia, W.B. Saunders, 1980.

Jacobson, H.G., (ed.): Fundamentals of magnetic resonance imaging, JAMA 258:3417–3423, 1987.

Meschan, I.: *Analysis of Roentgen Signs in General Radiology*, vol. 2. Philadelphia, W.B. Saunders, 1973.

Shanks, S.C., and Kerley, P. (eds.): *A Textbook of X-Ray Diagnosis by British Authors*, vol. 3. Philadelphia, W.B. Saunders, 1973.

Squire, L.F., Colaiace, W.M., and Strutynsky, N.: *Exercises in Diagnostic Radiology*, vol. 1. Philadelphia, W.B. Saunders, 1981.

Tisi, G.M.: Preoperative evaluation of pulmonary function. Am. Rev. Resp. Dis. 119:293–310, 1979.

OBJECTIVES

AFTER READING THIS CHAPTER, THE STUDENT WILL BE ABLE TO:

1. Describe the tests used during pregnancy and labor to monitor the development and well-being of the unborn baby.
2. List the factors evaluated to formulate an Apgar score and summarize the use of neonatal and pediatric tests and monitors, such as umbilical cord blood gases, and umbilical artery catheterization.
3. Discuss the value of monitoring growth and development during childhood.
4. Explain how the evaluation of adult cardiopulmonary disease symptoms is used to form differential diagnoses and flow diagrams.
5. Compare diagnostic with monitoring techniques and give examples of assessment tests that do both.
6. Compare flexible and rigid bronchoscopy and discuss the clinical use of bronchoscopy and mediastinoscopy.

14
INTEGRATED APPROACH TO PATIENT ASSESSMENT

CHAPTER OUTLINE

PERINATAL ASSESSMENT
    Alpha-fetoprotein
    Ultrasound
    Amniocentesis
    Chorionic Villus Biopsy
    Inhibition of Labor
    Fetal Heart Rate
    Fetal Scalp Blood Sampling
    Induction of Labor
    Apgar Score
    Umbilical Cord Blood Gases
    Umbilical Artery Catheterization
    Capillary Blood Gases
    Neonatal Case Presentation

PEDIATRIC ASSESSMENT
    Developmental Milestones
    Electromyography
    Sweat Test
    Assessment for Foreign Bodies
    Pediatric Case Presentation

ADULT ASSESSMENT
    Evaluation of Symptoms
    Special Diagnostic Techniques
        Bronchoscopy
        Mediastinoscopy
    Adult Case Presentation

An evaluation of a patient's health is initiated either as a routine screening examination or in response to a patient seeking assistance for a specific complaint. Routine screening examinations begin with the perinatal assessment performed on nearly all infants at the time of their delivery. Scheduled routine checkups are done at specific ages to evaluate the growth and development of children, administer immunizations, and recognize any disease present at an early stage. Medical evaluation for employment or periodic checkups, such as women's annual Pap smears, are times when abnormalities are commonly discovered.

Concern over a specific health problem can also cause an individual to undergo a medical evaluation. When someone comes to a healthcare provider for routine screening or for treatment of a specific complaint, the entire patient should be evaluated. It is easy to become focused on a specific task or problem and miss other possibly more important problems. Obtaining the patient's medical history and performing a careful physical examination are basic and essential tools for initial patient assessment that determine whether further evaluation is necessary and also what tests should be done.

Additionally, assessment means more than just identifying what particular disease the patient has. A more important role of assessment is monitoring the patient's condition. This can help to determine if the patient is responding favorably to treatment or if complications or new problems have arisen.

PERINATAL ASSESSMENT

Assessment of fetal growth and development ideally begins fairly soon after conception. Routine prenatal care by an obstetrician includes recording the rate of maternal weight gain and predicting the date when delivery of the baby is expected (term or due date). Factors such as extremes of maternal age or maternal disease (e.g., hypertension or diabetes) are used by the obstetrician to determine if the pregnancy has a high risk of developing a greater-than-normal chance of fetal or maternal complications. There are several diagnostic tests available if the obstetrician suspects that there may be a problem with fetal development.

Alpha-fetoprotein

Tests that measure the levels of alpha-fetoprotein or hormones in the maternal blood can help assure that the pregnancy is progressing normally. Elevations of alpha-fetoprotein in the amniotic fluid suggest abnormalities in the development of the fetal brain or spinal cord, such as anencephaly or meningomyelocele.

Ultrasound

The structure and position of the developing fetus and placenta can be determined by ultrasound, a sensitive technique that gives an extensive picture of the tissues without the damaging radiation effects associated with x-rays. Ultrasound is also useful to give a fairly precise determination of fetal age.

Amniocentesis

Amniocentesis can also be used to help determine if the baby is mature enough for delivery. During amniocentesis, a long needle is inserted through the skin and wall of the mother's abdomen, through the wall of the uterus, and into the uterine cavity in order to obtain a sample of amniotic fluid (the fluid that surrounds the fetus). The insertion of the needle is directed by ultrasound in order to avoid contact and injury to the fetus and placenta. The amniotic fluid is analyzed to determine the phosphatidylglycerol (PG) level, which is a rather specific indicator of lung maturity. The presence of PG in the amniotic fluid indicates adequate surfactant levels. When the fetal lungs are mature enough for delivery, the development of infant respiratory distress syndrome (IRDS) is unlikely.

A less specific indicator of lung maturity is the lecithin-sphingomyelin (L/S) ratio of the fluid obtained by amniocentesis. The lecithin measured by this technique represents mature surfactant (mainly dipalmitoyl lecithin), and the sphingomyelin is a chemical metabolic precursor in surfactant formation. When the L/S ratio is two or more (this means that there is at least twice as much mature surfactant as precursor present), then the fetal lungs are probably mature enough for delivery (see Chapter 3).

The amniotic fluid obtained during amniocentesis is studied for the presence of infectious organisms. Cells shed from fetal tissues into the amniotic fluid are prepared for chromosomal studies, which can reveal such abnormalities as Down's syndrome. Amniocentesis may also reveal several other diseases known as *inborn errors of metabolism* (such as phenylketonuria), in which the developing fetus lacks certain enzymes necessary for metabolic processes. Genetic counseling is given to the parents when amniocentesis indicates a severe defect, so the parents can make informed decisions about the current pregnancy as well as future ones.

Chorionic Villus Biopsy

In another technique called chorionic villus biopsy, a portion of the placenta is extracted for laboratory analysis. This type of biopsy provides more material for analysis than amniocentesis, so a more thorough evaluation can be performed.

The extensiveness of prenatal assessment depends on the degree of risk of complications to the mother or fetus. The perinatal period is when problems frequently occur, so the extent and frequency of assessment are increased at this time. Therefore, the frequency of maternal visits to the obstetrician increases as the due date approaches.

Inhibition of Labor

Certain maternal conditions require that the fetus must be delivered prematurely, usually by cesarean section (incision through the abdominal and uterine walls). However, if the baby is delivered too early, it suffers the complications of prematurity, such as intraventricular hemorrhage (bleeding into the immature brain) or respiratory distress (from immature lungs with inadequate surfactant levels). Ultrasound, amniocentesis, and the date of conception (as determined by the last menstrual period) reliably determine the fetal age to help avoid premature delivery when possible.

When labor begins prematurely, certain drugs given to the mother can inhibit labor (tocolytics) and delay delivery. This allows more time for the fetus to develop in the uterus. The two main drugs for inhibition of labor are ritodrine, a beta$_2$ catecholamine (see Chapter 15), and magnesium sulfate. When the labor cannot be stopped or other causes (infection or maternal illness) require premature delivery, the mother is given glucocorticoids, such as cortisone. Maternal administration of glucocorticoids speeds the maturation of the fetal lung by increasing production of surfactant in the fetus.

Fetal Heart Rate

When the mother goes into labor, the intensity of monitoring greatly increases. Maternal vital signs (heart rate, blood pressure, ventilatory rate, and temperature) are recorded in addition to the frequency and duration of uterine contractions, dilation of the cervix (size of the opening of the mouth of the womb), and how far the baby has descended in the birth canal (effacement). Many hospital labor and delivery units use machines that continuously monitor uterine contractions and the fetal heart rate (normally 120 to 160 beats per minute).

The relationship of the fetal heart rate and the uterine contractions is important. Normally, the fetal heart rate fluctuates a small amount independently from the uterine contractions. If the fetal heart rate becomes constant (loss of variability), fetal distress may be the cause. Slowing of the fetal heart rate (deceleration) may be an ominous sign, depending on the relationship to uterine contractions:

1. Early decelerations are considered benign and begin soon after the onset of uterine contractions. They are due to fetal head compression when delivery is imminent.
2. Late decelerations are a danger sign, beginning later during the uterine contractions, sometimes with prolonged duration. They suggest uteroplacental insufficiency (inadequate blood flow to the uterus or placenta).
3. Variable decelerations can occur at any time, usually from umbilical cord compression.

Variable or late decelerations strongly indicate fetal distress (hypoxia). In addition to bradycardia, the response of the fetus to hypoxia is to make ventilatory efforts and to empty the bowels. This is the cause of *meconium aspiration* (when the fetal bowel movement, called meconium, is drawn into the fetal lungs). If the hypoxia is not relieved, the fetus can die inside of the uterus. When the fetus begins to show signs of distress (loss of heart rate variability or malignant decelerations), an emergency cesarean section is usually performed to reduce the risk of meconium aspiration or death.

Fetal Scalp Blood Sampling

Blood gases obtained from a sample of blood from the fetal scalp taken through the birth canal before the delivery are sometimes helpful to confirm the presence of fetal distress (see Chapter 10). Hypoxia or, more significantly, severe acidosis (a pH less than 7.2) indicated by blood sampling, strongly suggests a dangerous situation for the fetus. Prompt delivery by emergency cesarean section may be necessary to permit treatment for fetal asphyxia.

Induction of Labor

Occasionally, a pregnancy persists past the normal duration. If delivery has not occurred by 2 weeks after the estimated due date, this condition is called *postmaturity*. Increasing postmaturity is associated with increased risk of complications. For this reason, delivery is carried out by *induction* (labor stimulated by intravenous administration of the hormone *oxytocin*) or by cesarean section to prevent excessive postmaturity.

Apgar Score

Following delivery, either vaginally or by cesarean section, the newborn (neonate) is immediately assessed to determine the necessary intensity of care. The system of neonatal assessment most commonly used is the Apgar score (Table 14–1). It is determined at 1 and 5 minutes after birth.

For an Apgar score of 7 to 10, no treatment is necessary, except to keep the neonate warm. An infant with a rating of 4 to 6 (moderate depression) should be stimulated by slapping its feet while ventilating with oxygen administered by bag and mask. An Apgar score of 0 to 3 indicates cardiac arrest or severe depression. Initial treatment should be positive-pressure ventilation with 100% oxygen by bag and mask. If the neonate does not respond, endotracheal intubation or more agressive resuscitation is performed. Note that the initial assessment determines whether or not treatment is necessary. After the administration of the therapy, the neonate is again assessed to determine if the treatment has been effective and whether more or different therapy is needed.

Umbilical Cord Blood Gases

Umbilical cord blood gases are useful to determine the extent of fetal distress before delivery. Their results are similar to but more reliable than fetal scalp blood gases. Obviously, the value of scalp blood gases is that they can be obtained before delivery. Umbilical cord blood gases are more valuable to verify that an emergency (cesarean section) was justified. Also, cord blood gas findings correlate well with the 1- and 5-minute Apgar scores, thus providing some prognostic information.

Normal values for blood gases from the umbilical cord artery are a pH of 7.23, plus or minus 0.05, and a base deficit of 10.9, plus or minus 3.5. Values from the umbilical cord vein are a pH of 7.34, plus or minus 0.06, and a base deficit of 8.1, plus or minus 3.5. Notice that the umbilical cord vein has a higher pH than the artery because the artery delivers deoxygenated blood to the placenta while the vein carries oxygenated blood from the placenta to the fetus.

Umbilical Artery Catheterization

It is important to differentiate umbilical cord blood gases from blood gases obtained via a catheter placed into the neonate's umbilical artery. The umbilical artery catheter is threaded into the baby's systemic circulation while umbilical cord blood gases are taken from the portion of umbilical cord that remains attached to the placenta after it is separated from the baby.

A catheter is routinely placed into one of the two

TABLE 14–1. Neonatal Assessment Using the Apgar Score

Apgar	Sign	Action to Assign Score	Number of Points		
			0	1	2
Appearance	color	visual assessment	blue, pale	body pink, extremities blue	completely pink
Pulse	heart rate	count cord pulse; feel precordium or auscultate heart	absent	<100	>100
Grimace	reflex irritability	flick sole of foot	no response	some motion	cry
Activity	muscle tone	manipulate extremity	limp, flaccid	some flexion of extremities	well-flexed
Respiration	respiratory effort	visual assessment	absent	slow, irregular hypoventilation	good strong cry

(From Apgar, V.: A proposal for a new method of evaluation of the newborn infant. *Anesth. Analg.* 32:260–267, 1953, with permission.)

umbilical arteries of an infant who is very ill perinatally. An umbilical artery catheter is a convenient site for continuously monitoring blood pressure and for obtaining arterial blood for blood gas analysis in these very small patients. In this manner, repeated arterial and venous punctures to obtain blood samples are avoided. The umbilical vein can also be cannulated to provide access for intravenous administration of drugs and fluid. Care must be observed in positioning arterial and venous catheters because if they are inserted too far they may occlude the circulations of certain organs, resulting in infarction. Overhydration is also a risk from repeated flushing of these catheters. Usually, the continuous flushing of these catheters is provided by an infusion pump at a rate of 1 ml/hour or less.

Capillary Blood Gases

Capillary blood gases (usually obtained from a heel puncture in neonates) are much less precise than arterial blood gases due to the possibility of venous contamination as well as exposure to air. However, capillary gases are easier to obtain than arterial blood gases when no arterial line is present. Capillary blood gases provide some meaningful information on the baby's acid-base status, oxygenation, and carbon dioxide elimination. Capillary blood gases, pulse oximetry, exhaled P_{CO_2}, or transcutaneous oxygen and carbon dioxide can be more easily measured when it is too difficult to obtain arterial blood. Methods of monitoring the respiratory system are more fully described in Chapter 10.

Although normal P_{O_2} levels are lower in neonates than in adults, if the P_{O_2} falls below the normal range for the neonate, hypoxic injury can occur. Unfortunately, higher-than-normal P_{O_2} levels can also be hazardous to newborns, resulting in pulmonary damage (oxygen toxicity) or eye damage (retinopathy of the premature), or possibly bronchopulmonary dysplasia (BPD), although recent studies implicate elevated airway pressures more than high oxygen concentration.

Neonatal Case Presentation

Baby X was delivered at term by emergency cesarean section with general anesthesia when the fetal monitor detected severe and prolonged bradycardia during the mother's labor. During surgery, the amniotic fluid was found to contain thick meconium and the umbilical cord was tightly wrapped three times around the baby's neck.

What needs to be done to begin care for this newborn?

After delivery, the first step in caring for a neonate is to evaluate it. This determines the degree of further therapeutic intervention. The loops of umbilical cord around the baby's neck could easily restrict blood flow between the baby and the placenta (the site of fetal gas exchange with the mother's blood). This produces fetal hypoxia that causes fetal bradycardia, release of meconium into the amniotic fluid, and fetal ventilatory efforts that result in meconium being drawn into the lungs. The fetal heart rate can be most rapidly determined by palpating the umbilical cord where it is attached to the baby's navel. Frequent reassessment determines the extent of monitoring and additional treatment.

At delivery, Baby X was flaccid (poor reflexes), cyanotic, and apneic but had a heart rate of 40. The infant's mouth and nose were rapidly suctioned to remove thick meconium, and the vocal cords were visualized with a laryngoscope while meconium was suctioned from the trachea. A size 3.0 endotracheal tube was rapidly inserted and 100% oxygen administered during ventilation by self-inflating resuscitation bag.

Should the baby have been ventilated before the meconium was suctioned from the airway?

There is some controversy on this issue, but many clinicians feel that, whenever meconium is in the amniotic fluid, the mouth and nose should be suctioned first. Next, the larynx is exposed with a laryngoscope and a suction catheter passed between the vocal cords before making any attempts at ventilation.

Suctioning of the trachea should be performed before ventilation in order to prevent meconium from being pushed farther down the airways. The fact that the meconium is thick or thin does not seem to influence the development of meconium pneumonitis, so all neonates with meconium in the amniotic fluid should be treated this way.

The patient's heart rate returned to normal and the patient's color, activity, and reflexes improved. Respiratory effort was still absent, so the Apgar score was 1 at 1 minute and 5 at 5 minutes. Umbilical artery blood gases at delivery showed a pH of 7.08, P_{CO_2} of 48 mmHg, P_{O_2} of 16 mmHg, and a base excess of -9.8. The endotracheal tube was taped in place, and bilateral breath sounds were auscultated. Mechanical ventilation by self-inflating resuscitation bag with an F_{IO_2} of 100% was maintained, and the neonate was kept warm during the trip to the neonatal intensive care unit.

What parameters should be monitored during this baby's stay in intensive care?

In intensive care, an umbilical artery catheter was inserted to monitor the baby's blood pressure and arterial blood gases. Transcutaneous P_{O_2} and P_{CO_2} were also continuously monitored to determine the adequacy of ventilation. A chest radiograph revealed that the endotracheal tube and umbilical artery catheter were in good position, with both lungs showing areas of haziness probably due to atelectasis. On the 2nd day following delivery, the patient suddenly began to require increasing positive-pressure ventilation while the transcutaneous and arterial blood gases showed progressing hypercapnea and hypoxemia.

What are some of the likely causes of this patient's sudden deterioration? What should be done?

Possible causes for the patient's worsening respiratory status include ventilator malfunction, endotracheal tube obstruction, inadvertent extubation, and pneumothorax. The patient should immediately be removed from mechanical ventilation and ventilated with oxygen by a self-inflating resuscitation bag. This should be initiated while the chest is auscultated in order to rapidly determine the cause of the problem. In this patient, breath sounds could be auscultated well only over the left hemithorax, and a chest radiograph revealed a right-side pneumothorax. The pneumothorax (which is commonly seen in babies on PEEP) was treated with a chest tube, after which ventilation was easier and the blood gases improved. The baby did well and was weaned and extubated after about 8 days of mechanical ventilation. Neonates who respond poorly may require conventional ventilation for much longer periods, tracheostomy, high-frequency ventilation (see Chapter 19), or extracorporeal membrane oxygenation (ECMO). During ECMO, blood is taken out of the body from a large vein, and passed through a heart-lung machine where it is oxygenated and carbon dioxide is removed. The blood is then returned to the body via a large artery. However, ECMO is extremely costly, with a high risk of complications.

Summary. Pulmonary aspiration of meconium can be easily diagnosed by first seeing meconium in the amniotic fluid and then suctioning it from the baby's pharynx and trachea. However, the effect of aspirated meconium on the newborn requires diligent monitoring and evaluation.

PEDIATRIC ASSESSMENT

Hospital admission is frequently quite psychologically traumatic to children, so the majority of pediatric evaluations are done in the pediatrician's office. Babies are usually examined by a pediatrician within 24 hours of birth and then at scheduled intervals as they develop. Most birth defects are apparent at birth or shortly thereafter, although certain inherited diseases (such as Huntington's chorea) are not expressed until adulthood. Evaluation of children is quite different from the assessment of adults. Very young children may be unable to talk or to discuss their condition. Additionally, certain childhood diseases kill their victims at an early age, so disease such as cystic fibrosis and some muscular dystrophies do not appear in adults.

Developmental Milestones

Children develop at their own rate, but there are developmental milestones (Scanlon neurobehavioral score) that children are supposed to achieve by certain ages. If the child is unable to perform certain tasks by a given age, then he or she may be suffering from developmental delay, and further evaluation may be necessary. For example, a child who is very late at beginning to crawl may also have poor head control (weak neck muscles). If the child later shows muscular weakness and inability to stand or walk, then certain tests might be performed.

Electromyography

In addition to an evaluation by a neurologist, an electromyograph (EMG) can evaluate problems in neuromuscular transmission. A muscle and nerve biopsy may also be performed on the child to obtain tissues for microscopic evaluation and biochemical testing. These diagnostic techniques are useful in identifying the different types of inborn errors of metabolism (usually caused by an absence or abnormality of certain cellular enzymes), neuromuscular dystrophies, and other neuromuscular diseases. These are frequent diagnoses for children showing progressive weakness and developmental delay. These children commonly require therapy to help mobilize airway secretions because they are too weak to clear them by coughing. The use of tracheostomy and ventilatory assistance by a mechanical ventilator for the young patient with an eventually lethal condition are controversial ethical issues.

The respiratory tract is a common source of complaints in children. The problems with this system are so frequent that they are usually treated empirically, that is, wide-spectrum treatment is given without certainty as to the precise diagnosis. The basis for this type of treatment is that most problems are viral in origin and resolve without treatment in about 2 weeks. Antibiotic coverage for most common bacterial infections has a fairly low risk of complications, and most childhood conditions that produce wheezing resolve as the patient gets older. The common dual therapy of antibiotics and bronchodilators is effective for a variety of childhood pulmonary problems that are usually outgrown eventually.

Sweat Test

Certain pulmonary problems are unresponsive to standard treatments. If a child suffers from repeated or worsening pulmonary problems, a more aggressive evaluation is done. Children with cystic fibrosis are subject to repeated respiratory tract infections, among other problems. In addition to other tests performed during evaluation of repeated pulmonary complaints, a sweat test may be conducted. During the sweat test, a portion of the patient's skin is enclosed in plastic wrap and the sweat (ideally, over 100 mg) is collected. The sodium and chloride levels, measured in a clinical chemistry laboratory, are characteristically elevated in a patient with cystic fibrosis. In children, a chloride concentration of 60 mEq/L or more indicates the presence of cystic fibrosis, while a value of less than 50 mEq/L suggests the absence of the disease. Values for sodium and chloride concentrations in sweat increase with age.

Assessment for Foreign Bodies

Aspiration of a foreign body is another common cause of pediatric pulmonary symptoms. Foreign bodies composed of certain dense materials may be apparent in the lungs on a chest radiograph. Less dense particles, such as an aspirated peanut, cannot be seen on a radiograph but can be observed and removed by bronchoscopy. Recurrent pneumonia in the same portion of the lung strongly suggests the presence of an aspirated, radiolucent foreign body.

Pediatric Case Presentation

Jimmy K. is now a 13-year-old boy who was born by normal spontaneous vaginal delivery. Although he appeared to be normal at birth, when feedings were started, he immediately exhibited choking, coughing, and cyanosis.

What are some possible causes for these problems?

Abnormalities of laryngeal or esophageal anatomy can cause pulmonary aspiration, but a more common cause is a birth defect called tracheoesophageal (TE) fistula. This is a congenital connection between the trachea and esophagus that is a life-threatening condition usually requiring surgical correction. There are several anatomic variations of TE fistulas (see Fig. 6–12). This patient had the type in which the upper end of the esophagus ended in a blind pouch. The lower esophageal portion communicated with the trachea near the carina. Many types of TE fistulas greatly complicate airway management. The unrepaired patient often has chronic pulmonary aspiration and pneumonia. When the patient receives positive-pressure ventilation, the stomach and intestines are inflated. This elevates the diaphragm and makes lung inflation increasingly more difficult. The blindly ending esophagus results in pulmonary aspiration of saliva and oral feedings.

How can a patient with a TE fistula be mechanically ventilated safely?

It is helpful to know the anatomy of the defect before attempting mechanical ventilation. This may be accomplished by putting a small amount of radiopaque dye down the esophagus to determine on a radiograph the location of the fistula and the anatomy of the trachea and esophagus. Usually, the fistula is 1 to 2 cm above the carina, so placement of the endotracheal tube at the carina allows adequate ventilation of the lungs while occluding the passageway to the esophagus. In certain situations, the formation of a gastrostomy (an opening into the cavity of the stomach through the abdominal wall) prevents the inflation of the bowels by allowing an escape route for gas that enters the esophagus.

Four days after birth, this child had surgery to close his TE fistula and to place a gastrostomy for feeding. The child was then unable to take anything by mouth. At 18 months of age, the child had a segment of his colon grafted between the stomach and esophageal pouch to form a complete esophagus (called colonic interposition). This surgery is an extensive procedure requiring an incision in the abdominal (laparotomy) and thoracic (thoracotomy) cavities. Incisions of the abdominal or thoracic wall interfere with the mechanics of ventilation by causing pain, swelling, and injury to the muscles of ventilation. This child required several days of ventilation postoperatively but subsequently improved rapidly. Oral feeding was then successful. There was one episode of pneumonia when he was 4 years old.

At 8 years of age, the child was noted to have a slight curvature of his spine in his chest. The patient's pediatrician recommended observation of the curve to see if it worsened. The curve remained fairly stable until the child reached his 12th birthday, when the growth spurt produced progressing spinal asymmetry. It was diagnosed as idiopathic thoracic scoliosis unrelated to the TE fistula. The child was admitted to the hospital for surgery to straighten and fuse the spine. As part of the preoperative evaluation, a pulmonary function test was performed. The patient was cooperative and showed good effort. He wore a noseclip to perform the test and was on no medications. The patient was 143 cm tall, weighed 31.1 kg, and had the pulmonary function test results shown in Table 14-2.

What is your interpretation of these results?

The patient has severe restrictive lung disease but with inspiratory and expiratory force adequate for a productive cough. The patient had preoperative blood gases of a pH of 7.44, P_{CO_2} of 44 mmHg, P_{O_2} of 81 mmHg, and bicarbonate of 31 mEq/L while breathing room air (21% oxygen). Except for the scoliosis and scars from previous surgery, the patient's physical exam and laboratory studies were essentially normal.

The patient underwent surgery in the prone position for fusion and insertion of a metal rod from the 2nd to the 12th thoracic vertebra. An arterial line, two intravenous lines, urine output, pulse oximeter, and capnograph were used for intraoperative management.

What is the value of capnographic monitoring intraoperatively?

A capnograph is an extremely valuable intraoperative monitor. The end-tidal P_{CO_2} is usually a good approximation of arterial P_{CO_2}. If no carbon dioxide is measured in the exhaled gas, then accidental extubation or esophageal intubation are the usual causes. End-tidal P_{CO_2} is also useful to detect the presence of air embolism. Whenever the surgical field is above the level of the heart, there is a risk that air can enter the veins and embolize to the lungs. The presence of air bubbles in the pulmonary blood vessels obstructs pulmonary capillary blood flow resulting in increased alveolar deadspace. According to Bohr's method, increased alveolar deadspace results in a decrease in end-tidal P_{CO_2} and an arterial-alveolar P_{CO_2} gradient. A certain percentage of patients have intracardiac shunts (ventricular septal defects or atrial septal defects) that allow venous air to enter the arterial circulation where it is then embolized causing tissue infarction. If the arterial air goes to the brain, a stroke may result.

In view of the patient's pulmonary status and the extent of surgery, would you expect that prolonged postoperative intubation and ventilation were necessary for tracheobronchial hygiene in this patient?

The patient was stable throughout surgery but lost 1,200 ml of blood and was transfused with two units of blood. At the end of surgery, the patient had good gas exchange with a tidal volume of 350 ml and a 25 cm H_2O negative inspiratory pressure. The patient was extubated in the operating room and taken to the recovery room where ABGs on 40% oxygen by aerosol mask showed a pH of 7.30, P_{CO_2} of 53, P_{O_2} of 120, and bicarbonate of 24. The patient remained extubated postoperatively with adequate blood gases when receiving supplemental oxygen by nasal cannula. On the 4th postoperative day, the chest radiograph revealed an area

TABLE 14-2. Jimmy K.'s Pulmonary Function Test Results

	Predicted	Observed	% Predicted
FVC (L)	2.5	.92	37
FEV_1 (L)	2.28	.84	37
FEV_1/FVC (%)	91	91	100
FEF_{25-75} (L/sec)	2.79	1.09	39
FEF_{max} (L/sec)	5.4	3.34	62
Maximum expiratory pressure (torr)	60-120	60	—

of pneumonia. Culture of airway material grew *Pseudomonas*, which responded to the appropriate antibiotic therapy. The patient received frequent chest physical therapy and nebulization. The remainder of the recovery was uneventful.

ADULT ASSESSMENT

Evaluation of the adult is based on the patient's medical history and physical examination. Patients most frequently seek medical assistance for problems with the respiratory tract.

The patient's chief complaint or reason for seeking medical evaluation is defined by his or her symptoms (subjective findings reported by the patient) and signs (physical findings observed by the examiner). The possible causes for a patient's complaints that correspond to the patient's signs, symptoms, and initial laboratory findings are listed in order from the most likely cause to decreasingly likely causes. Such a list is called the *differential diagnosis*. The most likely diagnosis is also considered to be the working diagnosis, and appropriate treatment for this diagnosis is frequently started while further evaluation is in progress. More specific tests to confirm or rule out the diagnosis are then performed.

Lung diseases constitute a well-studied field, and several references are available that include differential diagnoses in the form of flow diagrams. A flow diagram for lung disease usually starts with the patient's x-ray findings and signs and symptoms. This is followed by the most likely diagnosis compatible with those findings. Specific tests that would confirm or rule out that diagnosis are then given.

A characteristic of many pulmonary diseases is that they can be episodic, that is, symptoms fluctuate in severity (as in asthma). The careful observations of healthcare personnel are essential both for diagnosing the illness and also for determining its severity.

Patients seek medical assistance for several symptoms referable to the cardiopulmonary system, such as shortness of breath, cough, the sensation of a foreign body in the airway, wheezing, and chest pain. Careful evaluation of a patient's medical history, physical exam, and laboratory tests is useful in diagnosing the cause of the patient's symptoms. However, once the diagnosis has been made, many of these same diagnostic techniques continue to be used in order to determine the severity of the disease, and the response to treatment. Cardiopulmonary clinicians are routinely concerned with disease of the cardiopulmonary system but frequently are involved with problems in other body systems that affect cardiopulmonary function.

Evaluation of Symptoms

The presence of certain symptoms suggests cardiac or pulmonary disease. When a symptom or collection of symptoms can be caused by only one specific disease, these characteristic symptoms are said to be *pathognomonic* for that disease. For example, after a fall, shortening of the leg with the foot turned out and pain over the thigh are pathognomonic for a hip fracture. However, the majority of symptoms can be the result of several different diseases and are then said to be *nonspecific*. Nonspecific symptoms include cough, foreign body sensation, dyspnea, and cyanosis.

Cough. Characteristics of a cough and accompanying sputum production can sometimes suggest the identity and severity of a disease that is causing it. Heavy coughing with much sputum production upon awakening suggests *bronchitis*, which is a common disease among smokers. Distinctive aspects of a cough include its frequency, force, and the presence or absence of sputum mobilization (*productive* or *nonproductive* cough). Furthermore, the sputum is described by its color, amount, odor, and stickiness as well as the presence or absence of blood flecks (*blood-tinged*). A cough that produces material that is almost entirely blood is called *hemoptysis* and may suggest dire illness. Massive hemoptysis is caused by rapid bleeding into the airway, which may be due to pulmonary artery rupture, and is an occasional complication of pulmonary artery catheterization. Methods for proper collection and study of sputum are discussed in Chapter 12.

Foreign Body Sensation. The presence of a foreign object in the airway is extremely irritating and commonly stimulates coughing and attempts at clearing the throat. The sensation of a foreign body in the airway can also occur as a result of an irritation, tumor, or nerve injury without a foreign object actually being present. This sensation can produce much anxiety, especially following aspiration of food or other objects. Some aspirated foreign bodies appear on the radiograph, but many are not visible. Their presence or absence must be determined by direct visualization using such techniques as bronchoscopy, described later in this chapter.

Dyspnea. Difficult breathing may result from a

wide variety of conditions. Any condition in which the patient states that breathing is difficult is called dyspnea, which also includes conditions in which observers detect labored or dysfunctional breathing. By itself, the symptom of dyspnea is so nonspecific that it is almost meaningless, but in the presence of other signs and symptoms, it can suggest the type and severity of disease. The feeling of shortness of breath can be caused by airways obstruction, decreasing compliance of the lung, fatigue of the respiratory muscles, hypoxemia, or hypercapnia. Dyspnea may also suggest a problem with the cardiopulmonary system (such as angina), but further evaluation is necessary to determine the exact cause. Several noncardiopulmonary conditions, such as severe indigestion, exercise, or pregnancy, can produce dyspnea.

Chest Pain. Localization of the pain to the external chest wall or inside the thorax can help suggest its cause. Dyspnea with tenderness over the chest wall can suggest rib fractures or arthritis. Worsening of localized pain during deep breaths or coughing without tenderness of the chest wall may be caused by pleuritis (inflammation of the pleura).

Cyanosis. A bluish appearance of the skin, usually of the lips and nail beds, is highly suggestive of cardiopulmonary disease producing hypoxemia. The presence of deoxyhemoglobin in a concentration of 5 gm/dl in the arterial blood usually produces this bluish color. Many conditions can result in low oxygen level in the blood (such as shunt, apnea, and hypoxia). A bluish skin color can also result from methemoglobinemia (the presence of reduced hemoglobin, see Chapter 3), cold environment, and poor heart function. Like dyspnea, cyanosis in itself does not tell you what is wrong, but it strongly indicates the presence of a potentially lethal problem. Rapid action to determine the cause of the cyanosis and prompt treatment (such as increased inspired oxygen concentration) should rapidly follow when this alarming sign is discovered.

Other Symptoms Caused by Cardiopulmonary Disease. Cardiopulmonary diseases that produce chronic hypoxemia also frequently produce *clubbing* (rounding and elevation) of the fingernails. *Paradoxical breathing* (expansion of an area of the chest wall while the remainder of the chest contracts and vice versa) suggests instability of the chest wall caused by rib fracture or paralysis of the diaphragm. *Retractions* (excessive contraction of the accessory muscles of ventilation) suggest labored breathing and dyspnea. Of course, cardiopulmonary diseases can produce even less specific symptoms, such as fever and rapid heart rate.

Other Symptoms Caused by Noncardiopulmonary Diseases. As previously mentioned, noncardiopulmonary diseases can produce symptoms that are commonly associated with cardiopulmonary diseases. This is because most diseases are not isolated in a specific part of the body, but involve multiple organ systems. Additionally, diseases may affect the functioning of the nervous system, which can then affect the function of the respiratory system. For example, many diseases of the abdominal cavity, such as subphrenic (subdiaphragmatic) abscess, affect the intra-abdominal pressure and diaphragmatic action. Renal failure can cause increased blood volume, affecting heart function while also producing metabolic acidosis (because of the loss of the kidney's ability to excrete fluid and acid). Hyperventilation results as the body compensates for the metabolic acidosis.

Cirrhosis (scarring) of the liver results in increased pressure in the vessels delivering blood to the liver (hepatic portal vein hypertension). This portal hypertension is the cause of swollen blood vessels in the esophagus (esophageal varices, which frequently rupture and bleed). These esophageal veins are connected to the hepatic portal veins. Because blood flow through the liver is obstructed, the pressure in the hepatic portal vein increases. The blood escapes from the hepatic portal vein by entering the esophageal veins, which then become swollen. The esophageal veins are connected to the bronchial veins, and the bronchial veins are connected to the pulmonary veins. These connections between the bronchial and pulmonary veins are one of the causes of anatomic shunt (see Chapter 3). Thus, the increased pressure in the portal vein in a patient with cirrhosis causes increased pressure in the esophageal veins and bronchial veins, which causes increased desaturated blood to enter the pulmonary veins. For this reason, patients with cirrhosis have an increased pulmonary shunt.

Special Diagnostic Techniques

When the patient's medical history, physical exam, and radiographs indicate the presence of certain types of lung or chest disease, further diagnostic tests are useful to identify the disease more precisely. Biopsy material obtained during bronchoscopy and mediastinoscopy can identify the exact tissue type and extent of spread of chest tumors. It is important to identify the exact type of tumor to determine which therapy is most likely to be effective. Some types of tumors are more sensitive to drugs (chemotherapy), while others respond better to radiation therapy, surgery, or a combination of therapies.

Bronchoscopy

Most diagnostic techniques have little or no therapeutic value except for making the patient feel better because something is being done. In other words, most tests which are used to determine the identity or the severity of a disease are not useful in treating or curing the disease. However, bronchoscopy is an exception because it can be used for treatment as well as diagnosis.

There are two types of bronchoscopes commonly used. A *rigid bronchoscope* is a straight, hollow tube, usually made of metal, with a light on the end that is inserted down the airway. The rigid bronchoscope enters through the mouth, passes through the larynx and down the trachea while the patient is under general anesthesia. By turning the patient's head to one side or the other, the tube can then be inserted down the mainstem bronchus to visualize the openings for the lobar bronchi. The rigid bronchoscope is most useful for removal of large aspirated foreign bodies but is also useful for clearing thickened airway secretions and obtaining samples for laboratory analysis.

A *fiber-optic* bronchoscope consists of a collection of flexible fiber-optic filaments that can be inserted through the nose or mouth, down the larynx and into the more distal airways. The fiber-optic filaments are composed of thin strands of glass of a specific thickness so that light carried by the filament is reflected back into the filament and not lost. These filaments can be curved around corners so this type of bronchoscope is flexible, but severe bending may snap the glass fibers and distort the image seen through the bronchoscope.

The flexibility of the fiber-optic bronchoscope allows it to be advanced farther down the airways than is possible with a rigid bronchoscope. A fiber-optic bronchoscope can usually be inserted into the lobar bronchus, which permits some of the segmental bronchi to be visualized. The fiber-optic bronchoscope is not as useful as a rigid bronchoscope for retrieval of large aspirated foreign bodies. However, the fiber-optic bronchoscope is very useful for removal of thick airway secretions by directed suctioning and retrieval of foreign bodies beyond the reach of a rigid bronchoscope. Also, the fiber-optic bronchoscope allows visualization of more of the conducting airways than the rigid bronchoscope does. Biopsy forceps (tweezers) and brushes can be passed through the flexible bronchoscope to obtain tissue samples from the more distal airways. The flexible bronchoscope is also useful in facilitating endotracheal intubation in certain situations (see Chapter 18). Fiber-optic bronchoscopy can often be done with local anesthesia and sedation, without subjecting the patient to general anesthesia, because it is much less injurious if the patient moves during fiber-optic bronchoscopy than during rigid bronchoscopy.

Mediastinoscopy

When certain types of tumors are found in a patient's lung or mediastinum, a technique called mediastinoscopy can be useful to determine the type of tumor and if it has metastasized. During mediastinoscopy, an incision is made in the skin of the suprasternal notch while the patient is under general anesthesia. With careful dissection, the surgeon creates a space behind the sternum. The mediastinoscope, like the rigid bronchoscope, is a hollow metal tube with a light on the distal end. The tip of the mediastinoscope is passed through the incision and into the space behind the sternum. The surgeon looks through the scope to visualize mediastinal structures. Tissue samples from mediastinal tumors or lymph nodes can be taken through the mediastinoscope. Hemorrhage is an obvious complication if a vascular structure is inadvertently biopsied. For this reason, most tissues are aspirated with needle and syringe before a biopsy is taken.

Adult Case Presentation

Harold G. is a 53-year-old street vendor who sells hot dogs from a cart. His medical history is essentially unremarkable except that he has smoked two packs of cigarettes a day for 42 years. He has frequent colds and a productive cough especially in the morning. He has noticed a weight loss of 20 pounds during the past few months. For the last few days, his cough has been worse, producing foul-smelling sputum. He has also had a fever and felt poorly. Upon physical examination, this emaciated man had a respiratory rate of 28. Auscultation of an area over the right upper thorax revealed diminished breath sounds. Percussion over that area was dull compared to percussion over the rest of the thorax, which suggests consolidation (alveolar filling) in that area. Laboratory studies revealed an elevated white blood cell count, which is consistent with an infectious process. A chest radiograph showed opacification of the right upper lobe with the remainder of the lungs and other chest structures appearing normal. Arterial blood gases revealed a pH of 7.32, P_{CO_2} of 50 mmHg, and a P_{O_2} of 61 mmHg.

What are some likely disease processes that might cause these problems?

Pneumonia, tuberculosis, and empyema (infection in the pleural cavity) are but a few of the diseases that could cause these symptoms. Sputum specimens were obtained for a Gram stain and bacterial culture with determination of antibiotic sensitivity of pathologic organisms. The test for acid-fast bacillus was negative, which suggests that tuberculosis was not the cause. However, the Gram stain of the sputum was loaded with white blood cells and gram-positive diplococci, most likely *Streptococcus*.

The patient was admitted to the hospital and started on intravenous antibiotics and supplemental oxygen by nasal cannula. His temperature returned to normal, and the sputum became less foul-smelling but was still abundant. His chest radiograph showed resolution of the pneumonia with lessening of the lung opacification except for a fairly discrete circular area near the hilum.

What are some of the possible diagnoses for this discrete area of opacification near the hilum, and what is its relationship to the pneumonia?

Likely causes of a discrete intrapulmonary mass include tumor, abscess, or bronchogenic cyst. When a lesion such as this one involves a lobar or segmental bronchus, it is fairly common for the distal lobe or segment to develop pneumonia. The mass may compress or obstruct the conducting airways so that the naturally occurring mechanisms for clearing the airway (the mucociliary escalator) are ineffective. Mucus and microorganisms become trapped in the distal lung, producing pneumonia.

After this lesion was detected, fiber-optic bronchoscopy was performed to help determine its cause. Through the bronchoscope, the mucosal (luminal) surface appeared irregular near the bifurcation to the right upper lobe. Biopsy of the area taken at that time revealed a bronchogenic carcinoma. The patient was put on a high-calorie diet and scheduled for mediastinoscopy 2 days later. During this interval, the patient underwent a CT scan to delineate the extent of the tumor and possibly to detect metastases. Tests using injected isotopes (a bone scan and a liver-spleen scan) were also performed to help determine if the cancer had spread to these organs. The increased metabolic activity of the cancer cells causes isotopes to accumulate in them. Cancer cells do not bind to one another in the same way that normal cells do, so they are more likely to break off from the tumor and be carried by the blood or lymph system to distant tissues and begin other tumors there. This patient's scans revealed no evidence of metastases.

Other tests performed before the mediastinoscopy were arterial blood gases and pulmonary function tests (Table 14–3). Arterial blood gases on room air showed a pH of 7.36, P_{CO_2} of 48 mmHg, P_{O_2} of 71 mmHg, and bicarbonate of 29 mEq/L. The patient's flow-volume loop is shown in Figure 14–1.

What is your interpretation of the patient's blood gases and pulmonary function tests?

The patient has mild hypercapnia and moderate hypoxia in room air. He also has obstructive airway disease, as evidenced by the decreased FEF_{25-75} and by the concavity of the expiratory effort–independent portion of the flow volume loop. The difference in residual volumes measured by helium dilution and body plethysmograph suggests trapped gas consistent with emphysema. His improvement in pulmonary function following bronchodilators indicates reversible bronchoconstriction. A significant improvement with bronchodilators is usually considered to be >15% improvement in FEV_1 (see Chapter 9). Following these tests, mediastinoscopy was performed to help rule out spread of the tumor to the hilum and mediastinal structures. Tumor in these locations is usually unresectable. However, mediastinoscopy revealed no apparent metastasis. The patient was scheduled for surgery to resect the lung tumor. Preceding surgery, the patient continued to receive the high-calorie diet. He was also started on mucolytic and bronchodilating medications as well as chest physical therapy to loosen and remove airway secretions.

The patient underwent surgery to remove the tumor along with the right upper lobe of the lung (lobectomy). The patient tolerated the procedure fairly well, requiring no blood transfusion. Intraoperative blood gases on 100% inspired O_2 and controlled ventilation showed a pH of 7.36, P_{CO_2} of 40 mmHg, P_{O_2} of 101 mmHg, and bicarbonate of 23 mEq/L. Copious amounts of mucus and blood were suctioned from the endotracheal tube intraoperatively.

Should the patient be allowed to breathe spontaneously and be extubated after surgery?

Patients should be allowed to breathe spontaneously and therefore are extubated as soon as

INTEGRATED APPROACH TO PATIENT ASSESSMENT

TABLE 14-3. Harold G.'s Pulmonary Function Test Results

	Unit of Measurement	Predicted	Prebronchodilators		Postbronchodilators	
			Actual	% Predicted	Actual	% Predicted
Spirometry (BTPS)						
FVC	Liters	4.54	4.50	99	4.46	98
FEV_1	Liters	3.57	2.59	72	3.14	88
FEV_1/FVC	Percent	78	57	—	70	—
FEF_{25-75}	Liters/second	3.64	1.35	37	2.05	56
FET_{25-75}	Seconds	0.53	1.66	308	1.34	253
Lung Volume (BTPS)						
VC	Liters	4.54	4.50	99	4.46	98
TLC	Liters	6.61	8.27	125	8.25	125
RV (body plethysmograph)	Liters	2.09	3.77	180	3.14	150
RV/TLC	Percent	31	45	—	38	—
FRC	Liters	3.90	5.32	136	4.37	112
ERV	Liters	1.81	1.55	85	1.68	93
IC	Liters	2.70	2.95	109	2.94	109
RV (helium dilution)	Liters	2.09	3.27	156	2.67	128
Diffusion (STPD)						
$D_{L_{CO}}$	ml CO/min/mmHg	31	22	71	—	—

they no longer meet the criteria for intubation and mechanical ventilation (see Chapters 18 and 19). The blood gases revealed an abnormally low Po_2 for 100% inspired oxygen. This patient's abundant airway secretions required an adequate cough mechanism for their removal. However, thoracotomy interferes with these mechanisms by causing pain and muscle injury. Weaning a patient from mechanical ventilation is based on arterial blood gases and vital signs. Tests to evaluate a patient's ability to tolerate extubation also include the forced vital capacity and maximal spontaneous negative inspiratory pressure, which can be easily measured at the patient's bedside. The patient's vital capacity should be at least 10 ml/kg and negative inspiratory pressure of -20 cm H_2O before extubation is contemplated.

This patient had a vital capacity of 400 ml and a negative inspiratory pressure of -15 cm H_2O, so he was left intubated and placed on mechanical ventilation. Postoperatively, the patient was able to be gradually weaned, partially because of agressive treatment to remove airway secretions. However, on the 3rd postoperative day, a brisk flow of bright red blood began coming from the endotracheal tube and the patient became hypotensive and tachycardic.

What should be done at this time?

The first thing to do is call for help from a surgeon or intensive care doctor. The patient should be placed on 100% inspired oxygen. Intravenous fluids should be administered rapidly, and the blood bank called for emergency blood. If the chest tube is in place and clamped, it should be temporarily unclamped to check for the presence of blood or tension there. A procedure that is sometimes helpful in a situation like this is to attempt to advance the endotracheal tube into the mainstem bronchus of the unaffected lung. This protects and continues ventilation of the good lung while acting as a tamponade to stop the bleeding in the operated lung. A return to surgery may be necessary.

However, none of the these maneuvers were successful, and this patient proceeded to have a

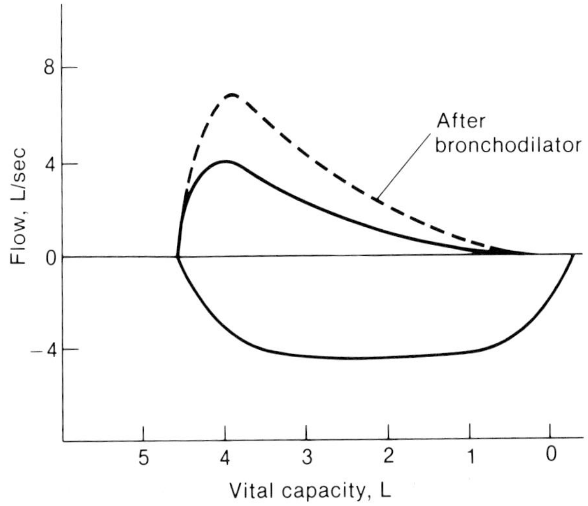

FIGURE 14-1. Harold G.'s flow-volume loop.

cardiac arrest and was unable to be resuscitated. Autopsy revealed that a staple on the pulmonary artery had eroded through the stump of the upper lobe bronchus and then dislodged when the patient coughed, causing a fatal hemorrhage.

Bibliography

Apgar, V.: A proposal for a new method of evaluation of the newborn infant. *Anesth. Analg.* 32:260–267, 1953.

Brown, B.L., and Gleicher, N.: Intrauterine meconium aspiration. *Obstet. Gynecol.* 57:26–29, 1981.

Brown, D.R., Fenton, L.J., and Tsang, R.L.: Blood sampling through umbilical catheters. *Pediatrics* 55:257–260, 1975.

Fishman, A.P.: *Pulmonary Diseases and Disorders*. New York, McGraw-Hill, 1980.

Fraser, R.G., and Paré, J.P.: *Diagnosis of Diseases of the Chest*, 2nd ed. Philadelphia, W.B. Saunders, 1977.

Gordon, A., and Johnson, J.: Value of umbilical blood acid-base studies in fetal assessment, *J. Reprod. Med.* 30:329–336, 1985.

Haight, L.: The esophagus. In Rautch, M.M., et al. (eds.): *Pediatric Surgery*, vol 1, 3rd ed. Chicago, Year Book, 1979, p 446.

Hinshaw, H.C., and Murray, J.F.: *Diseases of the Chest*, 4th ed. Philadelphia, W.B. Saunders, 1980.

Mellins, R.B.: Pulmonary physiotherapy in the pediatric age group. *Am. Rev. Respir. Dis.* 110:137, 1974.

Ostheimer, G.W.: Resuscitation of the newborn. In Ostheimer, G.W. (ed.): *Manual of Obstetric Anesthesia*. New York, Churchill Livingstone, 1984, pp 319–344.

Polgar, G., and Weng, T.R.: The functional development of the respiratory system from the period of gestation to adulthood. *Am. Rev. Respir. Dis.* 120:1979.

III
TREATMENT OF CARDIOPULMONARY DISEASE

OBJECTIVES

AFTER READING THIS CHAPTER, THE STUDENT WILL BE ABLE TO:

1. Describe how certain characteristics of a drug can determine the patient's response to its administration.
2. Discuss the advantages and disadvantages of the different routes by which drugs can be administered.
3. Calculate mg/ml dosages of drugs from percent solutions or from drug concentrations given as a ratio such as 1:1,000 epinephrine.
4. Compare the mechanism of action of drugs that are structurally specific (receptor dependent) and those that are nonspecific.
5. List the causes of retained secretions in the airway and how medications promote mobilization of secretions.
6. Contrast the characteristics of the sympathetic and parasympathetic systems.
7. Classify the adrenergic receptors into alpha, beta$_1$ and beta$_2$ types and describe their main effects.
8. Discuss the pathophysiology of bronchospasm and note the sites where bronchodilating drugs, such as catecholamines, methylxanthines, glucocorticoids, and cromolyn, act to relieve airway obstruction.
9. Discuss medications that affect the control of breathing and include indications and risks associated with the use of ventilatory depressants and stimulants.
10. Contrast depolarizing and nondepolarizing muscle relaxants and give considerations for their appropriate use.
11. Describe the causes of coughing and how treatments can be used to stimulate or suppress coughing.
12. Define upper airway congestion and its causes and define the actions of the two main types of decongestants and give examples.
13. List drugs that affect the strength of contraction of cardiac muscle and give their side effects.
14. Discuss medications used to control cardiac dysrrhythmias as well as to increase or decrease the heart rate.
15. List the determinants of myocardial oxygen consumption and explain the actions of medications for myocardial ischemia.
16. Discuss vasodilating and vasoconstricting drugs, their indications, and their mechanisms of action.
17. Explain the indications for different intravenous fluid solutions, such as parenteral hyperalimentation, electrolyte solutions, blood, and blood fractions.
18. Recognize the clinical uses of procoagulant and anticoagulant drugs.
19. Discuss the dynamics of body water and explain the actions of medications that enhance diuresis.

15
PHARMACOLOGY

CHAPTER OUTLINE

PHARMACOLOGIC PRINCIPLES
DRUG-RECEPTOR INTERACTIONS
   Routes of Administration
      Intravenous Administration
      Intramuscular Administration
      Subcutaneous Administration
      Oral and Rectal Administration
      Inhalation Administration
   Metabolism and Excretion
   Drug Interactions
MUCOKINETIC AGENTS
AUTONOMIC NERVOUS SYSTEM
BRONCHODILATORS
   Sympathomimetics
   Parasympatholytics
   Methylxanthines
   Glucocorticoids
   Cromolyn
   Other Bronchodilators

ANTIMICROBIALS
AGENTS THAT AFFECT CONTROL OF BREATHING
   Respiratory Depressants
   Paralyzing Agents
   Stimulants for Breathing
COUGH TREATMENTS
DECONGESTANTS
CARDIOVASCULAR DRUGS
   Cardiac Medications
      Cardiac Inotropes
      Antiarrhythmia Drugs
      Medications for Cardiac Ischemia
   Vasoactive Drugs
   Other Agents Used on the Circulatory System
DIURETICS

This chapter is intended to be an overview of the entire field of pharmacology pertinent to the treatment of cardiopulmonary disease. Detailed descriptions of medications used in cardiopulmonary care may be found in other texts. A cardiopulmonary clinician must understand basic pharmacologic principles in order to provide safe and effective drug therapy.

A *drug* is a chemical substance used to affect physiologic and biochemical processes in order to diagnose, prevent, or treat disease. A *medication* is a drug used to treat disease (therapeutically). Drugs such as helium and radioactive xenon are used to diagnose pulmonary diseases but are not therapeutic. For example, bronchodilators may be used as a diagnostic drug during pulmonary function testing to reveal the presence of bronchospasm, but asthma may require the use of bronchodilators therapeutically as a life-saving medication. Occasionally, radioactive drugs are given for treatments, especially for cancer (see Chapter 13). The gamma rays emitted by the radioactive molecules are destructive to cells with a high rate of reproduction (like cancer cells).

PHARMACOLOGIC PRINCIPLES

Certain characteristics of a drug determine a patient's response to its administration. Drugs produce their biochemical and physiologic effects depending on their (1) site and mechanism of action, (2) absorption, (3) distribution, (4) structure-activity relationships, (5) metabolism, and (6) excretion.

Drugs are administered in the hope of achieving a specific desired action in a particular tissue or organ. A desired action or therapeutic effect may be achieved in a number of ways. The tissue or organ location where a drug acts to produce its therapeutic effect is called the *site of action*. *Mechanism of action* describes the manner by which the drug affects the target tissue or organ to produce the desired effect.

The *absorption* and *distribution* of a drug depend on its chemical and physical characteristics. The size of the drug molecule, its fat solubility, and its degree of ionization and route of administration determine a drug's uptake and distribution in the body. A drug's *structure* determines whether its activity depends on interaction with certain cellular receptors as well as the intensity of any drug receptor interaction that occurs. The *action* of a drug usually diminishes when its concentration decreases in the target tissue. Drug activity decreases when the drug is *metabolized* or broken down into inactive compounds. *Excretion* of a drug (usually in the urine or feces) also terminates its action.

Generally, drugs affect living systems by stimulating or depressing cellular activity. Only responses that are genetically endowed functions of the responding cells may occur. Drugs do not impart new or original functions to cells but depend on existing metabolic pathways.

DRUG-RECEPTOR INTERACTIONS

Pharmacologic agents that combine and interact with specific cellular membrane sites (*receptors*) are classified as structurally specific drugs (e.g., the catecholamines). The chemical interactions between certain drugs and their receptors are extremely specific. Although the chemical structures of two drugs may be only slightly different, significant differences in the drug-receptor responses (and therefore their activities) may occur. Other pharmacologically active substances, such as inhalational anesthetics, osmotic diuretics, or even water, are considered to be structurally nonspecific. For example, mucokinetic drugs do not interact with specific receptor sites but instead affect the tenacity and adhesiveness of mucus after it has been secreted.

Structurally specific drugs influence the activities of some cells but not others. These substances initiate their activity at some site or receptor that is unique to responding cell populations. Drug-receptor interactions may trigger responses by modifying cell membrane permeability, altering normal cellular transport mechanisms, modifying genetic template transcription or influencing cellular enzyme activity.

Some tissues or organs have more receptors or more sensitive receptors than the cells of other tissues. The drug may produce a greater effect in these organs. If the drug produces the desired effect in the *target organ*, it is said to be therapeutic. The actions of a medication other than those specifically desired are termed *side effects*. A drug is useful therapeutically if its beneficial actions outweigh the hazards and deleterious side effects (adverse reactions) of the drug. The severity of adverse or harmful side effects vary from individual to individual and may contraindicate the use of a drug in those sensitive to the drug.

The intensity of the physiologic response elicited by a structurally specific drug depends on the total concentration of drug-receptor complexes. The degree of attraction between a drug and a cellular receptor is an important factor determining the total number of drug-receptor complexes formed, and, hence, the intensity of the response. The degree of receptor attraction between a drug and the cellular receptor is called *affinity*. The forces most frequently active in the attraction of a drug to a receptor include Van der Waals forces, hydrogen bonding, and ionic bonding (see Chapter 1).

In addition to affinity, a drug must also turn on receptor function in order to initiate a response. The ability of a drug to induce the necessary sequence of cellular reactions required for a response is termed *intrinsic activity* or *efficacy*. A drug that has both receptor affinity and intrinsic activity is called an *agonist*. A drug that has affinity for a cellular receptor but no intrinsic activity is called an *antagonist* or *blocking agent*. It occupies a receptor site but is unable to induce an effect.

Note that receptors frequently are enzymatic proteins. Factors affecting protein structure, such as pH, ion concentration, and temperature, participate in determining enzyme conformation, stability, and optimal receptor performance. This is one of the reasons that in a prolonged cardiac arrest, sodium bicarbonate is given to correct the severe metabolic acidosis caused by the persistent hypoperfusion. This must be done before administering the epinephrine to stimulate the cardiac receptors because the cardiac receptors are not responsive to epinephrine in an acid environment. Note that sodium bicarbonate is not for use except in pre-existing metabolic acidosis or prolonged hypoperfusion (more than 10 minutes) according to the American Heart Association's guidelines.

Routes of Administration

Many drugs must first enter the circulation to reach their site of action. Others, such as mucolytic aerosols or topical antibiotics, act locally at the site of their application. Drugs may be introduced directly into the circulation by intravenous administration, or they may be absorbed into the blood stream from the muscles, skin, oral mucosa, subcutaneous tissues, digestive tract, or lungs. The perfusion of the tissue into which the drug is administered affects the rate of absorption, as does the solubility of the drug in the tissue. Upon entering the circulation, the drug is delivered to the target tissues at a rate determined by the blood flow.

Intravenous Administration

This method of administration has the obvious advantage of fastest delivery of the drug to the circulation. It is usually the best route when speed is essential. During a severe bronchospasm, intravenous administration of catecholamines or xanthines is more prompt and effective than administration of inhaled drugs because sometimes the ventilatory obstruction may be so great that the drug cannot reach the site of action.

There are multiple disadvantages to intravenous (IV) administration that may carry considerable risk. Obtaining intravenous access is often painful and may be difficult, particularly in obese or uncooperative patients or those who have had multiple previous IVs. Once placed in a vein, catheters are frequently dislodged or migrate out of the vein so that drugs and fluids are unintentionally delivered extravascularly. When this happens, the IV is said to be *infiltrated* or "blown." Drugs inadvertently given via an infiltrated IV can produce edema or necrosis of the overlying skin or even the entire extremity. Furthermore, although arteries are sometimes cannulated for monitoring blood pressure, they are sometimes entered unintentionally while trying to gain venous access. Many drugs given intra-arterially can produce severe arteriospasm and even lead to necrosis of an extremity. Arterial lines should be clearly marked and injection ports covered to prevent their accidental injection with drugs.

When drugs are administered intravenously, the response is rapid but may be of short duration as the drug is removed from the circulation. This initial decrease in the concentration of drug in the circulation is called *redistribution* and is due to the drug entering other body compartments, such as fat or interstitial fluid. This is different from *elimination* or *excretion* by which the drug is removed from the body (for example, exhalation of volatile anesthetic gases or biliary or urinary excretion).

Continuous intravenous administration with a pump (*IV infusion*) holds the rate of administration constant for indefinite periods, allowing the establishment, maintenance, and adjustment of optimal plasma levels when necessary. Intravenous injection is also a useful route of administering drugs that cannot be absorbed well from tissue depots or the gastrointestinal tract. When the intestines are not functioning because of surgical trauma or disease, fluids, nutrients, and drugs normally administered orally may have to be delivered intravenously. Some drugs may be chemically or enzymatically destroyed before appreciable absorption can occur from these sites. Insulin, for example, cannot be taken orally because it is a polypeptide drug broken down by enzymes in the stomach and intestines.

The rapidity of response to drugs given intravenously requires that injections be given slowly, over at least a minute and for some drugs even more gradually. Side effects and adverse reactions also occur rapidly with IV drugs, so slow administration may allow these bad effects to be recognized and the injection halted before the whole dose has been administered.

Other problems associated with IV catheterization include inflammation of the vein (phlebitis), venous thrombosis (clot formation), venous emboli that can travel to the lungs, and infection by bacterial contaminants.

Intramuscular Administration

Drugs given intramuscularly (IM) are usually injected into the large skeletal muscles, taking care to avoid nerves and blood vessels. The usual sites are gluteal (the upper and outer quadrant of the buttocks), quadriceps (the anterior middle third of the thigh), or deltoid (the lateral upper third of the shoulder). These areas are very vascular and absorption is fairly rapid, usually within 10 to 30 minutes. The tissues also may function as a depot, allowing drug uptake to be somewhat sustained. For example, narcotics given intramuscularly have a fairly rapid onset of action and then a continued duration as absorption from the tissues occurs, in contrast to narcotics given IV, which have almost immediate analgesia and respiratory depression with fairly rapid decrease in effect as the drug is removed from the circulation.

Subcutaneous Administration

Drugs administered subcutaneously (SC) are absorbed more slowly than via the IM route because the subcutaneous tissues are more poorly perfused than the muscles. Pain on injection, local necrosis, and sterile abscesses are complications of SC injections.

Oral and Rectal Administration

Perhaps the least complicated and best tolerated route of drug administration is orally (*PO*, Latin for *per os*, which means "by mouth"). Chemical characteristics of the drug determine whether it is absorbed more in the acid environment of the stomach or the more neutral pH environment of the intestines. An empty stomach facilitates the rate of absorption. Some drugs may chemically combine with certain foods making the drugs unable to be absorbed. For example, if tetracycline is given with milk, the calcium in the milk binds with the drug, reducing its absorption. However, certain drugs are so irritating to the inner lining (mucosa) of the GI tract that they are recommended to be taken with meals. Drug absorption across the GI tract is fairly rapid because of its high vascularity.

Drugs taken orally are absorbed across the stomach or intestinal lining and are taken up by the blood vessels supplying these tissues. Blood leaving the stomach and intestines is carried to the liver by veins that are part of the hepatic portal system (see Fig. 2–1). Because of this, drugs that are rapidly metabolized by the liver may not be effective if administered orally.

The portal circulation may be bypassed if the drug can be absorbed by a part of the alimentary tract that is not drained by the portal veins. Certain drugs may be absorbed rapidly if placed under the tongue (sublingually). Nitroglycerin tablets used for the treatment of angina are usually administered sublingually because the medication is inactivated by the liver if it is swallowed and absorbed in the stomach.

Drugs administered rectally also bypass the hepatic portal circulation. Additionally, the suppository route is effective in a patient who is nauseated or vomiting. Aminophylline is a pulmonary drug that can be administered rectally. Its use is occasionally accompanied by vomiting, which would limit its uptake if administered orally. All drugs administered rectally (PR—per rectum) should be isotonic with plasma to avoid irritation of the rectal mucosa.

Inhalation Administration

Drugs may be aerosolized, instilled, or inhaled into the respiratory tract. This route of administration provides a rapid effect because of the high vascularity and huge surface area of the respiratory system.

Aerosol therapy involves delivering drugs in the form of airborne particles into the airway for the treatment of localized disease processes, usually obstructive bronchopulmonary disease. This form of drug administration places effective concentrations of the drug at the site of desired action while minimizing extrapulmonary or systemic effects that may be associated with these drugs when they are administered by other routes. The production, administration, and distribution of aerosols is described in detail in Chapter 16. Many of the drugs used in the treatment of asthma are available in multidose inhalers (MDI) that deliver a metered dose when the inhaler is compressed.

The use of *inhalation anesthetics* takes advantage of the rapid absorption and high vascularity of the lungs to reliably produce general anesthesia. *Intranasal sprays* of the pituitary hormone drugs oxytocin or antidiuretic hormone may effectively deliver them via this portion of the respiratory system.

The abundant vascularity and large surface area for absorption also permit the lungs to be used as a route for emergency administration of drugs. During a cardiopulmonary arrest in a patient without intravenous access, drugs such as epinephrine and atropine may be instilled down the endotracheal tube to obtain their systemic effects. Other drugs, such as calcium chloride or sodium bicarbonate, should not be administered undiluted via the endotracheal tube during emergency situations because they are very damaging to the respiratory mucosa and destroy pulmonary surfactant. Also, sodium bicarbonate is not administered endotracheally because of the large volumes required.

Several different respiratory gases are used for the diagnosis and treatment of respiratory disease. Oxygen is used diagnostically for Fowler's method of calculating the anatomic deadspace and in determining the closing volume, as described in Chapter 9. Therapeutically, oxygen is used to treat a great variety of potentially lethal diseases (see Chapter 16). Inhalation of elevated carbon dioxide concentrations has been used to stimulate breathing but is usually avoided because it causes catecholamine release and increases respiratory work. Because of its low density, helium is used for flow studies in patients with obstructive pulmonary disease. The airway's resistance to breathing a helium-oxygen mixture is much less than for breathing room air, so a helium-oxygen mixture is also occasionally beneficial for the management of severe airways obstruction. However, it is much more commonly used by divers to make breathing easier at great pressures (and to decrease the possibility of decompression sickness). A diagnostic use for helium is in density-dependent flow tests to differentiate upper and lower airways obstruction.

Carbon monoxide and xenon are also used for certain diagnostic pulmonary function tests but only low concentrations with no pharmacologic effects are utilized. Anesthetic gases, on the other hand, have profound physiologic effects but are not in the intended scope of this book. However, it is important to note that several anesthetic gases, such as halothane, enflurane, and isoflurane, are potent bronchodilators, depress breathing, and diminish sensitivity to increased arterial carbon dioxide concentrations.

The route of administration is one of the determinants of a drug's effect on an individual. The patient's willingness to go along with the therapy (or *patient compliance*) also affects the response. If the patient refuses to take the treatment (noncompliance), then the therapy is a failure from the start. The attitude and personality of the cardiopulmonary clinician may spell the difference between success and failure. Time and effort spent explaining a treatment, enthusiasm, and above all compassion are as much a part of a successful treatment as the drugs and equipment.

Metabolism and Excretion

Dosages of medication are usually given on a time schedule because the concentration of drug in the tissues decreases as the drug is metabolized and excreted. The *half-life* of a drug is the length of time for the body to reduce the concentration of a drug to half its initial peak level. The half-life determines the frequency at which a drug should be administered in order to maintain an appropriate therapeutic level in the body. The rates of metabolism and excretion are the main determinants of a drug's duration of action. However, certain drugs are excreted from the body in the same form as they were administered. Inhalational anesthetic gases are mostly exhaled from the lungs unchanged, and penicillin is excreted in the urine with its molecular structure unaltered.

The molecular structures of many drugs are altered by metabolism to terminate their action and/or to promote their removal from the body. Enzymes in the cells or plasma can inactivate or modify drug structure. Also, the liver is a site of enzyme conversion of drugs to less active forms. These enzymes may decrease the fat solubility of a drug, rendering it more water-soluble so that it can be more easily excreted in the urine. Diseases that decrease liver or kidney function can prolong the half-life of many drugs. This may result in the accumulation of the drug and the risk of attaining toxic drug levels if the interval between doses is not increased. Kidney and lung disease can also affect the body's acid-base status, which influences a drug's activity and excretion. The body's pH helps determine the degree of ionization of a drug. It is more difficult for highly ionized drugs to cross biological membranes.

The dosage of a medication is prescribed by a physician. However, it is the responsibility of all nonphysician cardiopulmonary clinicians who administer drugs to know if the dosage prescribed is appropriate, as well as the drug's contraindications, precautions, warnings, adverse reactions, and interactions. If the medication or dosage called for seems excessive or inappropriate, it is the responsibility of the cardiopulmonary clinician to check with the physician to make sure there has been no error in transcription. This information is contained in the *Physicians' Desk Reference* (PDR) as well as other pharmacology reference books. The dosage of drugs is usually given on a per weight basis, that is, a certain amount of drug is given for each kilogram of the patient's body weight. Following this principle, an approximate dose can be calculated for any size patient. Several factors must be considered, however, to determine the optimal dosage. The distribution, handling, and metabolism of most drugs in children differ significantly from those in adults. The very young and the elderly metabolize most drugs more slowly. Pregnancy may also affect drug metabolism, and possible drug effects on the unborn fetus must be considered. Cigarette smoking is associated with a more rapid metabolism of theophylline. Drug interactions, discussed later, can also alter a drug's effects.

When a drug is repeatedly administered over a period of time, use of the same dosage may result in a decreased response. This is known as *tolerance* and is common with prolonged narcotic usage.

When preparing to administer a drug, always check that the correct drug is being administered. Many drugs have similar names and spellings that may be confused when trying to decipher handwritten orders. If you are not sure of the drug or dosage, don't be afraid to ask for confirmation. Syringes and containers of drugs must be clearly labelled with the drug name and concentration. Drug concentrations are usually written as mg/cc but occasionally as percent solution. Conversion to mg/cc from percent solution is easily done. For example, a 2% solution would have 20 mg/cc. Drug concentrations are also sometimes given as a ratio such as 1:1,000 epinephrine. This converts to 1 mg/cc (1 mg of epinephrine in 1,000 mg solvent). Remember that 1 cc (ml) of water equals 1,000 mg.

A 1:200,000 epinephrine solution would have 0.005 mg of epinephrine per cc of solvent.

Drug Interactions

Patients frequently receive several medications simultaneously. A person receiving two or more drugs may be subject to drug interactions that can affect the intensity or duration of action as well as increase the risk of side effects. Some drugs, such as barbiturates and phenytoin, induce liver enzymes that accelerate metabolism of other drugs, such as corticosteriods. A patient who has been receiving the anticoagulant warfarin (Coumadin) may develop excessive bleeding if he or she starts taking digitalis because the digitalis decreases warfarin binding, resulting in a greater anticoagulant effect. Other drug interactions are discussed later in the section on methylxanthines. There are entire books devoted to drug interactions, and this information is also contained in drug package inserts and prescribing information of the *Physicians' Desk Reference*.

When one drug interacts with another possessing similar activity, an *additive* response may result, which is the sum of the individual effects. *Synergism* is when one drug increases the effect of another drug that possesses a different main action. Barbiturates as well as ethanol have a synergistic effect on the ventilatory depressant effects of narcotics. *Potentiation* is when the combined effect of two or more drugs is greater than the sum of their individual effects. Catecholamines and aminophylline have a potentiating effect when used together for the treatment of asthma.

Administration of a drug may result in an undesirable interaction with other drugs that are being administered concurrently. Additionally, drugs used to treat pathology in one organ system can produce unwanted effects in other organ systems, particularly if they also are diseased. While administering a drug or treatment, careful monitoring of the patient's vital signs and mental status can frequently alert the clinician to the development of potentially dangerous side effects.

MUCOKINETIC AGENTS

One of the most common therapeutic interventions by a cardiopulmonary clinician involves clearing the airways of respiratory secretions. The mucosa lining the conducting airways performs a dual function of producing mucus to trap airborne particulate matter and then carrying it to the pharynx where it can be expectorated or swallowed (see Chapter 3). The particles trapped in the mucus can be transported by the motion of the cilia, which are active extensions of the cells that line the conducting airways, or by coughing or sneezing. The respiratory (gas exchanging) airways have no cilia.

Mucus is normally produced from viscous secretions of goblet cells in the airway epithelium, watery secretions from bronchial glands that reside under the epithelium, and transudate from the tissue vasculature. In the presence of infection, exudate and cellular debris are also contained in the mucus.

The normal mucus blanket that lines the conducting airways has been described as having two layers: the more watery sol layer in which the cilia beat, and the overlying viscous gel layer in which the airborne particles become trapped. The sol layer may be more liquid because the mucus is produced by the adjacent goblet cells and bronchial glands, and then secreted onto the ciliated cells. The gel layer, because it is more superficial, becomes more viscous as it loses water to the dry inspired air.

The cilia beat at about 1,000 times per minute in a coordinated manner to move the mucus. On their forward stroke, they straighten up vertically on the columnar epithelial cells of the respiratory tract. They make contact with the viscous gel layer and propel it toward the pharynx. On the return stroke, they bend and move back to their original positions through the watery sol layer without touching the gel layer and then begin their next stroke. Thus they contact and move the gel layer only during the forward portion of their stroke (Fig. 15–1).

The consistency of mucus depends on the proportions of mucoprotein, water and cellular debris. Mucoproteins consist of protein and sugar subunits bound together in very long molecules called mucopolysaccharide chains. The subunits are bound by amino acid (peptide) and sulfur (disulfide) bonds to form the long, adherent molecules.

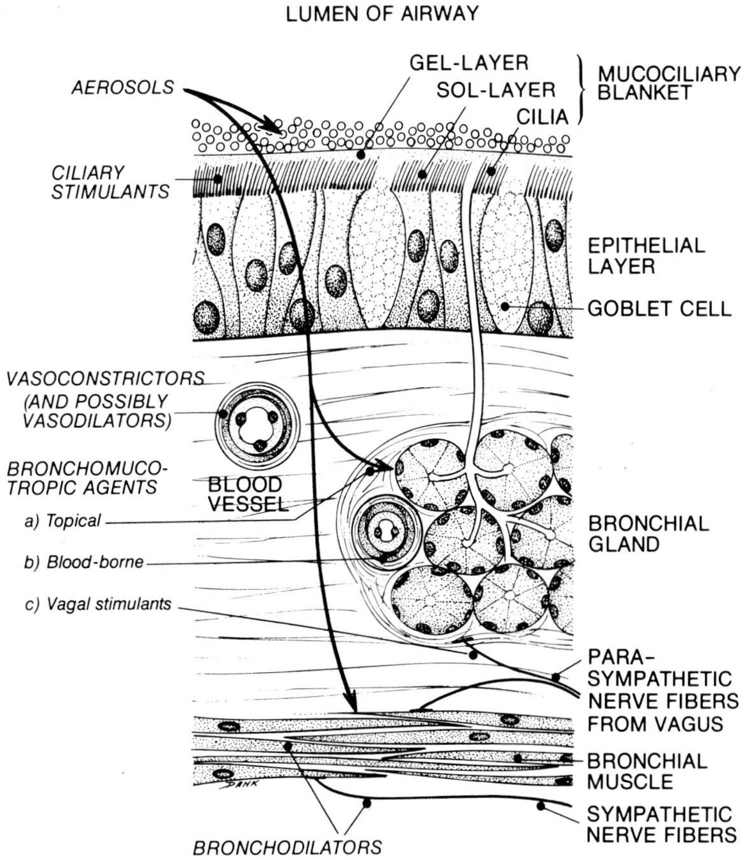

FIGURE 15–1. Major components of the mucokinetic system. (From Ziment, I.: Secretions of the Respiratory Tract: Physiology and Pharmacology, New York, Projects in Health, Inc., 1976, with permission.)

Elevated sputum calcium levels are believed to increase the strength of mucoprotein bonds and sputum viscosity.

Illness can produce retained secretions in a number of ways. Retained secretions in the airways may be the result of overproduction of mucus, increased viscosity, and/or ineffective ciliary and cough mechanisms to remove the secretions. Overproduction of mucus may result from infection or irritation of the respiratory tract. Vagal stimulation that results from airway instrumentation, such as bronchoscopy or laryngoscopy, promotes copious watery secretions by the bronchial mucus glands, which are under vagal control. Cigarette smoking, with its accompanying bronchitis and respiratory tract irritation, increases sputum production. Pneumonia causes alveolar filling and increased airway secretions due to irritation and the breakdown of bacteria and leukocytes. The infected sputum is yellow and very thick because of the addition of cellular debris. The capillary endothelium also becomes more permeable with increased leakage of plasma filtrate into the tissues.

Thick, tenacious secretions are difficult to remove even with normal ciliary and cough mechanisms. In cystic fibrosis, very thick secretions with elevated calcium ion levels develop. Breathing cold, dry gases (as usually occurs during general anesthesia) also tends to produce thickened, viscous secretions.

Ineffective ciliary and cough mechanisms allow secretions to build up in the airways. Besides drying and thickening airway mucus, general anesthesia tends to cause retained secretions by decreasing ciliary motility. Nonpulmonary disease may weaken the individual so that he or she cannot cough effectively and clear the conducting airways. Conditions producing a distended abdomen (such as intestinal obstruction, severe cirrhosis, or marked obesity) decrease an individual's ability to take deep breaths and therefore to cough effectively. The ability to cough is vital not only to clear secretions but also to clear the airway of material aspirated when swallowing. Table 15-1 lists the causes of retained secretions.

Whatever the cause of retained secretions, the result is increased work of breathing from decreased airway diameter and increased airway resistance. The retained secretions can also obstruct airways, producing areas of low ventilation/perfusion (shunt) and decreased PaO_2. Alveoli distal to an obstruction tend to collapse (atelectasis) and are difficult to reinflate because of surface tension forces.

Therapeutic measures taken to remove retained secretions are usually aimed at decreasing mucus thickness and enhancing coughing and ciliary transport. Mucus transport may be enhanced by increasing the depth of the watery sol layer, allowing the cilia to beat more freely, or by decreasing the viscosity and adhesiveness of the gel layer. Breaking the peptide or disulfide bonds of the long mucopolysaccharide chains makes them into smaller molecules that are less viscous.

The simplest way to promote mobilization of secretions is to liquify them with *wetting agents*. Humidifying inspired gases and nebulized saline treatments are the most common ways to decrease mucus plugging (see Chapters 16 and 17). Water and saline solutions act to dilute the mucus, making it less viscous. Hydration of mucus decreases its adhesiveness and also allows the cilia to beat more effectively. Systemic hydration is also important in mobilizing secretions. Patients with bronchospasm usually reduce their intake of fluids and can become dehydrated.

Hypertonic saline has been used as a nebulized mucokinetic agent. It produces an osmotic gradient that draws fluid from the mucosal blood vessels and tissues into the airway, inducing dilute secretions and augmenting expectoration. Hypertonic saline is also used in the induced sputum technique described in Chapter 12 for obtaining specimens for microbial culture. However, it is ir-

TABLE 15-1. Causes of Retained Secretions

Increased Sputum Production	Increased Sputum Viscosity	Decreased Sputum Removal
Cystic fibrosis	Cystic fibrosis	General anesthesia
Bronchitis	General anesthesia	Debilitating illness
Vagal stimulation	Bronchitis	Decreased vital capacity
Pneumonia	Pneumonia	Cigarette smoke
Cigarette smoke		Endotracheal intubation
Insecticide poisoning		Chronic tracheostomy
Allergies		Surgery

ritating to the airways and may create electrolyte imbalances.

Sodium bicarbonate has been used as a mucokinetic wetting agent. Sputum may be less adherent in an alkaline medium because the peptide bonds are less stable. The hypertonic solutions used produce an osmotic gradient and bronchorrhea. However, bronchodilators, which are frequently used concurrently, undergo a more rapid breakdown in an alkaline solution.

Sodium bicarbonate may be nebulized into the airway or directly instilled into areas of viscous secretions via bronchoscope. The usual concentration is 1.4% to 2.5%, but concentrations up to 25% have been used. The usual aerosol dosage for adults is 2 to 5 ml every 6 hours. Concentrations greater than 2.5% are irritating to the respiratory mucosa and may induce bronchospasm.

Alcohol has also been used to increase mucus flow (bronchorrhea) by irritation of the airway. However, agents that promote mucokinesis by irritation are not usually well tolerated as means of mobilizing secretions. The main therapeutic use of ethyl alcohol aerosolized into the airway is foam dispersal by alteration of surface tension in pulmonary edema. The usual volume nebulized is 1 to 3 ml of a 20% to 50% solution, which greatly reduces the volume of the foam. There are several causes of pulmonary edema, and definitive treatment (supplemental oxygen, continuous positive airway pressure, or vasodilators) must be based on accurate assessment of the cause. Nebulized alcohol only treats the symptoms of pulmonary edema.

Wetting agents are not the only drugs that reduce mucus stickiness. Mucus viscosity is also decreased by agents that break down mucoprotein and other molecules found in mucus. The acetylcysteine (Mucomyst) molecule contains a strong sulfhydryl portion that breaks the disulfide bridges of the mucoprotein molecules in the mucus, rendering them into smaller, less viscous molecules. Acetylcysteine is usually administered by bronchoscopic lavage or nebulization, but some research is being done with oral administration. Bronchoscopic administration is very successful at dislodging mucous plugs but is traumatic to the airways. Nebulization is much better tolerated by the patient, but the medication goes to airways that are unobstructed and not to plugged airways. Therefore, the mucokinetic effect is much less. The dosage for direct instillation is 1 to 2 ml of 10% to 20% solution as often as every hour. The nebulizer dosage is 2 to 20 cc of 10% solution every 2 to 6 hours. Acetylcysteine, especially in higher concentrations (20% solution), is irritating to the respiratory tract and may cause bronchospasm. It is frequently used in conjunction with a bronchodilator.

Nebulized enzyme solutions have been used to decrease the size of the molecules and the viscosity of the sputum. Deoxyribonuclease breaks down DNA from cellular debris and has been used in patients with thick, purulent sputum. Other enzymes digest the peptide bonds of the mucoprotein. However, enzymes are very irritating, expensive, and frequently produce allergic reactions. For these reasons, they have fallen from common usage.

The preceding drugs are mostly administered by inhalation to produce mucokinesis. Other drugs called *expectorants* are administered orally to promote mobilization of mucus by irritation of the respiratory mucosa or by stimulation of vagal reflexes, which promotes watery secretion by the bronchial mucus glands. Expectorants include potassium iodide, glyceryl guaiacolate, ipecac syrup, and terpin hydrate. Parasympathomimetic drugs induce mucokinesis but are also prone to cause bronchospasms. The effectiveness of expectorants as mucokinetic agents is controversial. They are primarily given for mild self-limiting diseases to help soothe inflamed airways. Many are available in over-the-counter preparations, but clinical indications for the use of these drugs are few. Dosages are available from the package inserts.

Mucokinetics are usually administered by inhalation techniques and generally act in a nonspecific manner. That is, they do not need to interact with any cellular receptor but instead act directly on mucus to render it less viscous and adherent. Expectorants, on the other hand, are mostly administered orally and act on irritant receptors. They can stimulate vagal reflexes that cause the bronchial mucous glands to produce watery, less adherent secretions that can wash out retained tenacious mucous plugs.

After decreasing the viscosity of secretions, they must be mobilized. Postural drainage, coughing techniques, and suctioning (discussed in Chapter 18) are necessary adjuncts to pharmacologic interventions when attempting to mobilize secretions.

AUTONOMIC NERVOUS SYSTEM DRUGS

As previously mentioned, drugs that act on the cellular receptors in certain tissues are called specific-acting. An area of great importance to cardiopulmonary clinicians is the treatment of bronchospasm in which many potent specific-acting drugs are used. However, to understand the pharmacology of the treatment of bronchospasm and many other cardiopulmonary diseases, some knowledge of the autonomic nervous system is essential.

The autonomic nervous system is the portion of the nervous system that automatically and unconsciously controls the nonvoluntary functions of the body necessary to maintain a constant internal environment (homeostasis).

The nervous system is divided into a central and peripheral portion. The central portion consists of the neural tissues of the brain and spinal cord that integrate information coming in and direct responses going out via the peripheral nerves.

The central nervous system (CNS) receives stimuli from the internal and external environment by afferent (sensory) peripheral nerve fibers. The CNS responds to stimuli by sending nerve impulses via efferent (effector) peripheral nerve fibers that innervate essentially all the organs of the body. The efferent nerve fibers are either *somatic* or *autonomic*. The somatic nerves go only to skeletal muscles and are under voluntary control. The autonomics go to essentially all the tissues of the body except the skeletal muscles. However, the blood vessels in the skeletal muscles possess autonomic innervation. The hypothalamus and medulla oblongata are the areas of the brain most directly involved in controlling the autonomics. The *synapses* (junctions between two nerve cells) of the somatic efferent nerves (to skeletal muscles) are entirely within the CNS. The most distal synapses of autonomic nerve fibers are located in ganglia that are entirely outside of the cerebrospinal axis. Neurons that conduct impulses from the CNS to an autonomic ganglion are called *preganglionic fibers*. Neurons carrying an impulse from an autonomic ganglion to the target or effector organ are called *postganglionic fibers*. The transmission of a nerve impulse from one nerve cell to another or from a nerve cell to a target organ is mediated by a chemical called a *neurotransmitter*. A neurotransmitter is released at the synapse from the presynaptic neuron in response to an action potential in that nerve cell. An *excitatory* neurotransmitter interacts with the postsynaptic neuron's cell membrane and can evoke an action potential in that cell. An *inhibitory* neurotransmitter would hyperpolarize the cell membrane of the postsynaptic neuron and make it harder to depolarize. The neurotransmitter in all autonomic ganglia is acetylcholine (ACh). Hydrolyzing enzymes called *cholinesterases* inactivate acetylcholine at the synapse.

The autonomic nervous system is composed of two usually antagonistic systems of nerves: the sympathetic and the parasympathetic. The sympathetic (adrenergic) system often is thought of as causing the "fight-or-flight" response of the body to stress. It is the body's rapid-acting protective system that stimulates the consumption of a great deal of energy. The parasympathetic (cholinergic) system mediates the "feed-or-breed" states of the body. It is reparative, conserves energy, and opposes the actions of the sympathetic system. However, it is not mandatory for either system to act in an all-or-none manner. In day-to-day life, portions of the two systems can act completely independently.

The peripheral extensions (outside the CNS) of the autonomic nervous system are composed of a two-neuron connection. A neuron with its nucleus (cell body) in the CNS has a cell process (axon) that extends peripherally from the CNS to the autonomic ganglion and is called the preganglionic fiber. The preganglionic fiber synapses in the ganglion with the postsynaptic neuron. The cell body of the postsynaptic neuron resides in the ganglion, and its axon extends to the effector organ (Fig. 15–2).

The sympathetic or thoracolumbar outflow has ganglia located very close to those portions of the spinal cord and so has short preganglionic and long postganglionic fibers. The parasympathetic or craniosacral outflow has long preganglionic fibers and short postganglionic fibers because parasympathetic ganglia are located in or very near the effector organs.

As mentioned previously, the neurotransmitter released at the autonomic ganglia by the preganglionic fibers in both the sympathetic and parasympathetic systems is acetylcholine. The postganglionic fibers of the parasympathetic system also release ACh, but the postganglionic fibers of the sympathetic system usually release norepinephrine (noradrenaline). For this reason, the parasympathetic system is called *cholinergic*, and the sympathetic system is called *adrenergic*. In the medulla of the adrenal gland, release of ACh by preganglionic sympathetic neurons stimulates an outpouring of epinephrine. However, this epinephrine comes from cells of the adrenal medulla and not from postganglionic neurons.

The cellular receptors for the different neurotransmitters are very specific. Both sympathetic and parasympathetic ganglia have ACh receptors

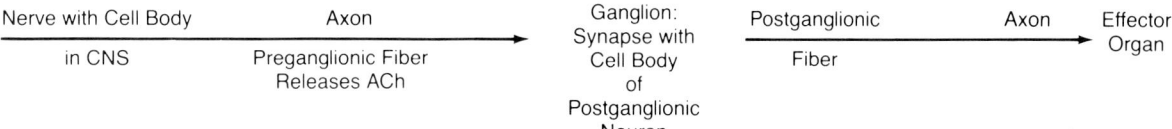

FIGURE 15–2. Generalized anatomy of the autonomic nervous system. (Adapted from Rarey, K.P., and Youtsey, J.W.: *Respiratory Patient Care.* Englewood Cliffs, N.J., Prentice-Hall, 1981.)

called *nicotinic receptors* (because they can be stimulated by the drug nicotine). Additionally, somatic motor neurons release ACh to stimulate the nicotinic receptors of skeletal muscle, but the receptor structure is slightly different from ganglionic nicotinic receptors. Postganglionic parasympathetic neurons release ACh, which stimulates receptors at the parasympathetic effector site called *muscarinic receptors* (named after the drug muscarine). Acetylcholine is the neurotransmitter for both the nicotinic and muscarinic locations, but the receptors are slightly different. Drugs that selectively work at one site or the other allow us to achieve a specific effect.

Drugs such as nicotine that stimulate the autonomic ganglia have no therapeutic use but would tend to vasoconstrict while increasing heart rate and blood pressure. Other effects can be variable because both sympathetic and parasympathetic activity are enhanced. Likewise, ganglionic blockers, such as trimethaphan camsylate (Arfonad), depress both the sympathetic and parasympathetic systems but have some therapeutic use as vasodilators. Table 15–2 lists the characteristics of the sympathetic and parasympathetic systems.

Parasympathomimetic drugs are sometimes called cholinergic, but muscarinic is more specific. Conversely, atropine is called an anticholinergic drug, but its parasympatholytic action is more correctly called antimuscarinic.

Target tissue receptors for the sympathetic system are of two basic types, alpha and beta. A third but less important type, the dopaminergic, has been found to increase blood flow to the intestines and kidney and to increase urine formation. Alpha receptors have been subdivided into $alpha_1$ and $alpha_2$. Drugs that stimulate $alpha_1$ receptors produce slight bronchoconstriction, vasoconstriction, hypertension, and a decreased heart rate mediated by the baroreceptor reflex. $Alpha_1$ stimulants are also used to decrease congestion of the nasal and airway mucosa. Less well known are the $alpha_2$ receptors that act mostly as presynaptic inhibitors, that is, they act by negative feedback to decrease the release of norepinephrine. Additionally, stimulation of $alpha_2$ receptors in the CNS reduces central sympathetic outflow. The beta receptors have been differentiated into two groups: $beta_1$ receptors, which primarily affect the heart, and $beta_2$ receptors, which when stimulated, produce vasodilation and bronchodilation.

Table 15–3 demonstrates the specific actions of

TABLE 15–2. Divisions of the Autonomic Nervous System

	Sympathetic (Adrenergic)	Parasympathetic (Cholinergic)
Main Action*	Fight-or-flight	Feed-or-breed
Origin	Thoracic and lumbar spinal segments T1 to T12 and L1 to L3	Cranial nerves III, VII, IX, and X and sacral spinal segments S2 to S4
Preganglionic fiber length	Short	Long
Ganglia location	Near spinal cord	On or near target sites
Neurotransmitter at ganglia	ACh	ACh
Receptor at ganglia	Nicotinic	Nicotinic
Postganglionic fiber length	Long	Short
Neurotransmitter at target sites	Norepinephrine (ACh at sweat glands)	ACh
Receptor at target sites	Alpha, beta, or dopaminergic	Muscarinic
Neurotransmitter action terminated by	Enzymes (monoamine oxidase or catechol-O-methyl-transferase) or by reuptake by nerve terminal	Enzyme (cholinesterase)

* See Table 15–3 for specific actions.

TABLE 15–3. Sympathetic and Parasympathetic Receptor Effects

System Receptor	Alpha	Sympathetic Beta$_1$	Beta$_2$	Parasympathetic Muscarinic
Blood vessels	Vasoconstriction	—	Vasodilation	Slight vasodilation or no action
Heart rate	(Reflex decrease)	Increased	—	Decreased
Force of contraction	—	Increased	—	Decreased
Bronchial muscle	Slight bronchoconstriction	—	Bronchodilation	Bronchoconstriction
Bronchial glands	Decreased secretions	—	—	Increased secretions
Pupils	Dilation	—	—	Constriction
Digestive and urinary tracts	Sphincter contraction	—	Decreased peristalsis and secretions	Sphincter relaxation, increased peristalsis and secretions

the sympathetic and parasympathetic systems and indicates the type of receptor site utilized to achieve those effects.

As previously mentioned, acetylcholine is inactivated by cholinesterase enzymes. Thus, drugs that are cholinesterase inhibitors (such as neostigmine or edrophonium) enhance the action of ACh. Catecholamine (epinephrine and norepinephrine) action is terminated in several ways:

1. The chemical may be taken up by adrenergic neurons.
2. The chemical may be deactivated at the synapse by the enzyme monoamine oxidase (MAO).
3. The chemical may be deactivated in the circulation or the liver by the enzyme catechol-*O*-methyl transferase (COMT).

Understanding the autonomic nervous system permits a more rational approach to the pharmacology of the cardiopulmonary system.

BRONCHODILATORS

The posterior wall of the trachea, where the C-shaped cartilage is open, contains a layer of smooth muscle called the tracheal muscle. The walls of the bronchi also contain a smooth muscle layer between the plates of cartilage. Strips of smooth muscle encircle the bronchioles and alveolar ducts, as noted in Chapters 3 and 5. The smooth muscle of the airways is under sympathetic and parasympathetic control. Most drugs used in the treatment of bronchospasm are believed to act on specific mechanisms that regulate airway smooth muscle tone. Adenosine 3′,5′-monophosphate (*cyclic AMP*) appears to work in the bronchial smooth muscle cells to produce relaxation and bronchodilation, and guanosine 3′,5′-monophosphate (*cyclic GMP*) seems to be required intracellularly for bronchoconstriction. To relieve bronchospasm, levels of intracellular cyclic AMP are increased either by augmenting the production or inhibiting the breakdown of cyclic AMP. Stimulation of the enzyme *adenyl cyclase* catalyzes the conversion of adenosine triphosphate (ATP) to produce cyclic AMP. Inhibition of the enzyme *phosphodiesterase* halts the rapid breakdown of cyclic AMP. Conversely, inhibiting the formation of cyclic GMP tends to diminish bronchoconstriction.

Catecholamines and other sympathomimetics acting at beta$_2$ receptor sites on bronchial smooth muscle cells stimulate adenyl cyclase to produce cyclic AMP. Catecholamine stimulation of the alpha receptor on bronchial smooth muscle seems to decrease cyclic AMP and produce slight bronchoconstriction. *Methylxanthines* inhibit phosphodiesterase, blocking the breakdown of cyclic AMP. Anticholinergic drugs decrease the concentrations of intracellular cyclic GMP, relaxing bronchial tone. *Corticosteroids* potentiate beta agonists and have a delayed, but prolonged, bronchodilating effect of their own, probably by directly increasing the intracellular concentration of cyclic AMP (Fig. 15–3).

Bronchodilation may also be produced indirectly by inhibiting the release of chemicals mediating bronchoconstriction from leukocytes. Mast cells are a type of leukocyte that are fixed in the connective tissue of the body, including the lungs. They contain cytoplasmic granules of such substances as heparin, histamine, slow-reacting substance of anaphylaxis (SRS-A), proteolytic enzymes, and eosinophilic chemotactic factor. As discussed in Chapter 5, the mast cells of sensitized individuals carry membrane-bound, allergen-spe-

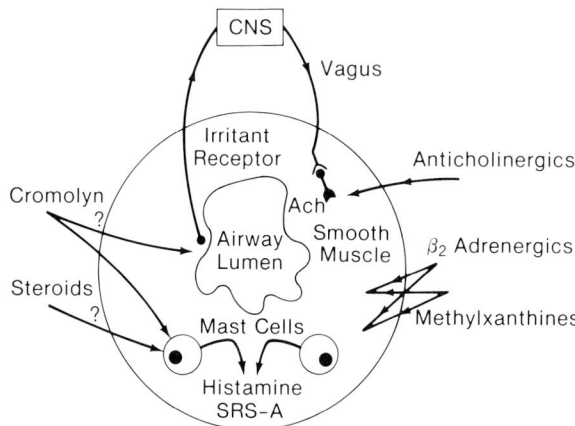

FIGURE 15–3. Factors affecting the tone of bronchial smooth muscle. Double arrows from B_2 adrenergics and methylxanthines indicate synergism. (From Leitch A.G.: Asthma—Mechanisms and management. *Clin. Notes Respir. Dis.* 21(1):3–9, 1982, with permission.)

cific immunoglobulin (antibody) molecules. When an allergen (antigen) combines with the membrane-bound antibody, cells are activated, resulting in the release of the previously mentioned chemical mediators of anaphylaxis. These substances, particularly histamine and SRS-A, stimulate lung irritant receptors promoting vagal bronchoconstricting reflexes. Also, direct action of these mediators on bronchial smooth muscles promotes bronchoconstriction. Corticosteroids and cromolyn inhibit degranulation of mast cells, thereby blocking bronchoconstriction. A person who is allergic to a drug (such as penicillin) may develop an anaphylactic reaction when he or she is inadvertently administered that drug. In addition to bronchospasm, symptoms of anaphylaxis include flushing, hypotension (due to vasodilation), and urticaria (hives).

SRS-A produces a slowly increasing and sustained contraction of bronchial smooth muscle and has long been considered a mediator of primary importance in asthma. SRS-A consists of three members of a group of compounds collectively called the *leukotrienes* because they originated from leukocytes and had a conjugated triene as a structural characteristic. Leukotrienes are derived from arachidonic acid by the catalytic action of the 5-lipoxygenase enzyme (see Fig. 5–14). Arachidonic acid is a free fatty acid derived from cell membrane phospholipids by the action of phospholipases (which, interestingly, are inhibited by corticosteroids). Arachidonic acid is converted by the cyclo-oxygenase enzyme in an alternative pathway to the prostaglandin family and the thromboxanes. Aspirin inhibits the action of cyclo-oxygenase on arachidonic acid. Excess leukotrienes produced from arachidonic acid by the unblocked 5-lipoxygenase pathway may be the explanation for aspirin-induced bronchospasm. Leukotriene antagonists or lipoxygenase inhibitors may be of value in the clinical management of asthma in the future.

Sympathomimetics

The drugs most frequently used for the treatment of bronchospasm interact with the beta$_2$ receptor on the cell membrane of bronchial smooth muscle to stimulate adenyl cyclase and enhance cyclic AMP formation. In addition, beta adrenergic agents reduce the release of mast cell components, decrease mucous gland secretion, and increase cilia motility. Catecholamines can be administered orally as tablets, intravenously injected, or inhaled. Inhaled catecholamines have reduced systemic effect, but some of the drug is absorbed by the airway circulation.

Systemic stimulation of alpha receptors produces vasoconstriction and hypertension. Beta$_1$ receptor stimulation may produce tachycardia and arrhythmias. Systemic beta$_2$ stimulators affect the nervous system, causing nervousness, sleeplessness, and tremor. A drug that is a selective agonist for the beta$_2$ receptor would have fewer undesirable side effects. Additionally, the CNS side effects of nervousness and tremor may be reduced by aerosolization because this route delivers the drug directly to the desired site of action while minimizing systemic effects. However, as mentioned previously, *severe* airway constriction may prevent delivery of inhaled drugs to the desired site of action, so the drug must be administered IV.

Many sympathomimetic drugs are suitable for inhalation therapy for bronchoconstriction. *Epinephrine* used to be popular as an aerosol or metered-dose inhalant (MDI) bronchodilator, but its marked beta$_1$ effects on the heart and blood vessels have curtailed its use. Also, its effectiveness as a bronchodilator is somewhat limited because it stimulates alpha receptors that tend to bronchoconstrict weakly. *Racemic epinephrine* is a synthetic mixture of dextro- and levo-epinephrine, whereas the natural hormone exists only as the levo form. The racemic mixture is claimed to have adequate beta$_2$ activity but less beta$_1$ and alpha effect when compared with epinephrine. The alpha receptor activity also makes racemic epinephrine a useful drug for treatment of mucosal edema, as occurs in croup. *Isoproterenol* (Isuprel) was once the most popular inhalational bronchodilator, but its marked beta$_1$ activity risks dangerous cardiac inotropic and chronotropic stimulation. Isoproterenol is unfortunately one of the shortest-acting bronchodilators when given by inhalation. *Isoetharine* (Bronkosol), although it has less beta$_2$ effect than isoproterenol, has much less beta$_1$ activity, making it less likely to cause serious cardiac side effects than isoproterenol. *Metaproterenol* (Alupent) has comparable potency to isoproterenol, but because it is not inactivated by COMT, the effect is more sustained. Fewer doses (10 to 20 mg three times daily for adults) are needed, and fewer cardiac side effects are likely.

Terbutaline (Brethine) is a selective, long-acting beta$_2$ agonist but still has some beta$_1$ side effects. Terbutaline is also used as a tocolytic agent. *Albuterol* (Ventolin) is very similar to terbutaline but appears to be slightly more potent.

Many of the sympathomimetics used for the inhalational treatment of bronchospasm may also be administered by alternate routes (intramuscularly, intravenously, subcutaneously, or orally). The route of administration greatly affects the ratio of bronchodilation to cardiostimulating effects. Inhalation favors airway dilation with fewer systemic effects. *Ephedrine* (0.3 to 0.5 mg/kg every 4 hours) is the longest established oral agent for the treatment of bronchospasm but is not suitable for inhalational use.

Excessive use of sympathomimetics can cause nervousness, tremor, and excitation. Catecholamines should be used with caution in patients with hypertension, heart disease, diabetes, or hyperthyroidism.

Parasympatholytics

Drugs that antagonize the parasympathetic nervous system would decrease cyclic GMP levels inside bronchial smooth muscle cells, reducing bronchoconstriction. Such drugs are called anticholinergic but are more specifically designated *antimuscarinic* or *parasympatholytic*.

Atropine (administered by inhalation or by other routes) and related antimuscarinic drugs have been used for years to treat airway obstruction caused by bronchiolar smooth muscle constriction and glandular secretions. Parasympatholytic drug action is twofold—reduction of secretions and bronchodilation. Atropine also appears to be effective in treating vagally mediated bronchospasm initiated by airway irritants. Atropine also inhibits airway secretions but increases mucus viscosity. Atropine or other muscarinics are routinely given as preoperative medications to decrease airway secretions and vagal reflexes associated with laryngoscopy and endotracheal intubation. However, if the patient already has thick airway mucus, then the use of atropine may aggravate the obstruction and airway plugging. The dose of nebulized atropine for bronchodilation is 0.05 mg/kg in children and 0.025 mg/kg in adults. Newer antimuscarinic agents, such as ipratropium (Atrovent), are being investigated for use alone or with catecholamines for the treatment of bronchospasm. Usually ipratropium is administered from a metered-dose inhaler that delivers 20 mcg per puff. The adult dosage is 40 to 80 mcg, but up to 500 mcg have been used with few side effects. Ipratropium is poorly absorbed, so it has few systemic effects. Untoward side effects include tachycardia, dry mouth, and delirium.

Methylxanthines

Drugs of this class inhibit the breakdown of cyclic AMP by the naturally occurring enzyme *phosphodiesterase*, thereby increasing levels of cyclic AMP in the bronchial smooth muscle cells. Phosphodiesterase inhibitors are therefore potent bronchodilators. The major methylxanthines used for treatment of bronchospasm are *theophylline, aminophylline*, and their derivatives.

Aminophylline in solution is quite alkaline and irritating to the tissues, so several neutral salts of theophylline have been developed. Theophylline is a frontline drug for:

1. Acute treatment of reactive airways disease.
2. Continuous treatment of chronic asthma.
3. Prevention of recurrent apnea of the newborn.

However, theophylline has a narrow margin of safety (the effective dose is near the toxic dose). Additionally, there are multiple conditions (smoking, diet, age, disease, or other drugs) that can alter theophylline metabolism (Table 15–4). Therefore, therapeutic drug monitoring for theophylline blood levels is very important to insure that plasma theophylline concentrations are adequate but not excessive.

Certain drugs, including barbiturates, phenytoin, and rifampin are called enzyme inducers because they can induce changes in the liver so that more liver enzymes are produced and drug metabolism is increased. Aminophylline elimination

TABLE 15-4. Conditions or Medications Affecting Theophylline Metabolism

Increased Elimination	Decreased Elimination
Enzyme inducers	Enzyme inhibitors
Barbiturates	Cimetidine
Phenytoin	Allopurinol
Rifampin	Hepatotoxic agents
Smoking	Oral contraceptives
Diet	Propranolol
High-protein	Erythromycin
Charcoal-broiled foods	Liver disease
	Conditions that decrease liver perfusion
	Heart failure

Adapted from Saefler, S. J.: Practical considerations in the safe and effective use of theophylline. *Ped. Clin. North Am.* 30(5):949, 1983.

is increased by these drugs. Other drugs called enzyme inhibitors (cimetidine, allopurinol) as well as hepatotoxic agents (oral contraceptives, propranolol, or erythromycin) can decrease theophylline breakdown.

In addition to bronchodilation, the methylxanthines have many other systemic effects, some of which may be beneficial. They increase cardiac output and decrease venous pressure. They improve renal perfusion and act as a diuretic. They cause cerebral stimulation and increased phrenic nerve activity. They also provide skeletal muscle stimulation as well as coronary and pulmonary vasodilation. The most common adverse reactions from methylxanthines are increased gastric secretions, nausea, vomiting, and gastric bleeding. Agitation, nervousness, seizures, and adverse cardiovascular effects, such as vasodilation, tachycardia, or bradycardia, are also related to administration of large doses of methylxanthines. The adverse reactions from large doses of methylxanthines as well as the rapid metabolism of the drug necessitate frequent oral dosages. Sustained release forms such as Theo-Dur and Theo-24 require less frequent administration.

For acute treatment of severe bronchospasm, therapeutic blood levels of theophylline can be rapidly attained by intravenous administration. A patient who has not been receiving theophylline previously would receive a loading dose of approximately 5 to 6 mg/kg over 10 to 30 minutes and then continue to receive 0.5–0.6 mg/kg/hr until the symptoms were relieved. The patient would then be converted to an oral methylxanthine at a dosage that would maintain appropriate blood levels.

Athletes, students, and others have long been familiar with the mental stimulation and respiratory benefits of coffee, tea, and colas, which provide theophylline and other methylxanthines, such as caffeine and theobromine. These drugs are administered orally, rectally, and intravenously but not usually by aerosol because their relative insolubility prevents production of a potent aerosol. However, research with nebulized methylxanthines is progressing. Theophylline is also available in combination drugs, such as Elixophyllin, Quibron, and Tedral, which also contain mucolytics, sedatives, and/or catecholamine bronchodilators.

Glucocorticoids

Bronchospasm is frequently caused by allergies that provoke mast cell release of irritant substances, such as histamine and slow-reacting substance of anaphylaxis (SRS-A), as discussed in Chapter 5 (see Fig. 5-13). Glucocorticoids are potent antiallergy drugs that reduce antibody formation, thereby preventing antigen-antibody reactions and activation of mast cells. Glucocorticoids are corticosteroid, anti-inflammatory agents that reduce tissue swelling and airway resistance. Furthermore, glucocorticoids bronchodilate directly by increasing intracellular cyclic AMP and, indirectly, by potentiating catecholamine action at the beta$_2$ receptors. Glucocorticoids are probably the most effective bronchodilators, but their onset of action is slow and their use almost always leads to dependence.

Besides their use in treating bronchospasm, glucocorticoids are used to diminish acute inflammatory responses (glottic edema from traumatic airway instrumentation). Systemically, glucocorticoids are used to treat inflammation and autoimmune diseases, such as rheumatoid arthritis and myasthenia gravis. Long-term side effects of glucocorticoid use include edema, easy bruisability, truncal obesity, and striae (stretch marks). More serious side effects also include psychosis, hypertension, impaired ability to fight infection, peptic ulceration, diabetes, potassium loss, and osteoporosis. Furthermore, the patient becomes dependent on the drug. Rapid discontinuation of the drug may reveal inadequate adrenal and pituitary function while the disease process rebounds with increased severity.

Glucocorticoids have been administered orally, intravenously, and by inhalation for the treatment of bronchospasm. Occasionally, if a patient has status asthmaticus and does not adequately respond to bronchodilator therapy, systemic glucocorticoids may be necessary. Prednisone is the glucocorticoid most commonly used systemically, but it requires activation by the liver. Thus, this drug may have unreliable therapeutic effect in patients with severe liver disease.

Beclomethasone (Vanceril), triamcinolone acetonide (Azmacort), and flunisolide (AeroBid) are widely used in aerosol form with decreased need for systemic steroids and fewer systemic side effects. Numerous other glucocorticoids are being investigated for their use in the treatment of bronchospasm.

Cromolyn

Cromolyn is not a bronchodilator but is only of prophylactic value for bronchospasm. It does not relieve bronchospasm but rather interferes with the antigen-antibody reaction on tissue mast cells. This inhibits the release of histamine and SRS-A. It is administered as an inhaled powder or solution. Although somewhat irritating to the airways, it has few side effects other than occasionally causing an allergic rash. Its use can help glucocorticoid-dependent asthmatics to decrease or discontinue their steroid dose.

Other Bronchodilators

Prostaglandins, which have been previously mentioned as derivatives of arachidonic acid, have been studied for their use in treatment of bronchospasm. The six primary prostaglandins (PG), designated PGE_1, PGE_2, PGE_3, PGF_{1a}, PGF_{2a}, PGF_{3a}, elicit various physiologic responses in the body. Prostaglandins PGE_1 and PGE_2 produce bronchodilation; PGF_{2a} is a bronchoconstrictor. The use of PGE_1 and PGE_2 by aerosol is being evaluated.

Calcium channel blockers, such as verapamil and nifedipine, can alleviate bronchoconstriction when given orally or by inhalation. Ketotifen, an antihistamine and mast cell stabilizer, has shown promise as an oral bronchodilator but causes drowsiness as a side effect. *Leukotriene blockers* and *inhibitors of 5-lipoxygenase* (see Fig. 5–14), the enzyme necessary for leukotriene production, are also being studied for their use in decreasing the formation of SRS-A. New agents are constantly being studied for use in the treatment of bronchospasm.

Although histamine has been isolated in mast cells and associated with allergic processes leading to bronchospasm, antihistaminic drugs have not been shown to be effective in the treatment of bronchospasm. Antihistamines are discussed later under treatment for colds and coughs.

ANTIMICROBIALS

The effects of infection on the cardiopulmonary system have been discussed in Chapter 12, as were medications specific for sensitive infections. Administration of specific antimicrobial agents by inhalation is a technique that has been in and out of favor. In the case of respiratory infections, toxic antimicrobial medications may be delivered directly to the area desired in small enough doses to reduce the risk of systemic side effects. However, injudicious administration of these drugs may eliminate nonpathogenic organisms (so-called natural flora) in the airway and promote the development of resistant strains. The usual treatment for infection is by systemic antimicrobials administered orally, intramuscularly, or intravenously. The drug type and dosage depend on the location and severity of the infection and the sensitivity of the microorganism (see Chapter 12).

Mucokinetics can be loosely included here as nonspecific antimicrobials. By enhancing the action of the mucociliary escalator, mucus and the infectious agents trapped in mucus are mobilized from the airway, decreasing the risk of infection. Conversely, retained secretions and the resultant atelectasis provide an excellent site for the development of infection. Surgeons frequently blame early postoperative fever on atelectasis resulting from the diminished vital capacity and decreased coughing associated with anesthesia and surgery.

The most important measure for prevention of infection during the care of patients with cardiopulmonary disease involves the use of disinfectants and aseptic technique. Hospital-acquired infections are called *nosocomial*. In addition to potentially lethal complications, nosocomial infections frequently involve resistant organisms, the survival of which is favored in a hospital environment. Infections caused by health-care personnel are termed *iatrogenic* and frequently result from the failure to use aseptic technique.

AGENTS THAT AFFECT THE CONTROL OF BREATHING

The normal rhythmic cycle of inspiration and expiration is automatically produced by neurons located in the medulla and pons of the brain (brain stem). The tidal volume and ventilatory rate are normally controlled by the number and frequency of nerve impulses from these portions of the brain stem. These nerve impulses direct the action of the muscles of respiration. Drugs that depress the activity of the respiratory centers in the brain stem tend to decrease breathing. On the other hand, drugs that antagonize these depressants and drugs that stimulate the brain tend to increase ventilation.

Respiratory Depressants

Drugs that depress CNS activity, such as tranquilizers, hypnotics (sleeping pills), anesthetics, and analgesics, also tend to decrease breathing as a side effect. Respiratory depression is almost always an undesirable side effect, so patients receiving these types of drugs must be carefully monitored. *Tranquilizers* include the powerful antipsychotic medications such as the phenothiazines (e.g., Thorazine). Although they do not depress ventilation much themselves, the major tranquilizers increase the respiratory depression of the other CNS depressants. *Hypnotics* usually produce sedation at low doses and sleep at higher doses; they have little pain-relieving activity (analgesia). The barbiturates are the most familiar group of hypnotics. *General anesthetics* include inhalational agents, such as halothane, that produce hypnosis and analgesia but also depress ventilation.

Narcotics are the most effective analgesics but usually relieve pain at the cost of decreased sensitivity of the respiratory centers to retained carbon dioxide. Other adverse reactions from narcotics include addiction, nausea and vomiting, constipation, biliary colic, urinary retention, bronchospasm, and reduced mucociliary clearance. Morphine is one of the most commonly used narcotics for pain relief, but it causes histamine release, which is responsible for itching and flushing in addition to the problems listed above. Meperidine (Demerol) causes little histamine release but has antimuscarinic properties that produce tachycardia and dry mouth. There are many narcotics, naturally occurring, semisynthetic, or totally synthetic, that have been developed to provide adequate pain relief while attempting to reduce adverse reactions.

Many of the new synthetic narcotics combine the potent analgesic action of the opiates with some narcotic antagonist effect to diminish the respiratory depressant effect. These so-called agonist-antagonists, such as pentazocine lactate (Talwin), nalbuphine (Nubain), buprenorphine tartrate (Stadol), take advantage of selective stimulation or inhibition of the recently discovered Mu, Sigma, and Kappa narcotic receptors (Table 15–5).

A situation in which depression of breathing may be desirable is for the mechanically ventilated patient who is opposing the ventilator breaths ("bucking the ventilator"). Sedatives and analgesics allow the patient to tolerate mechanical breaths, probably by blunting the Hering-Breuer inflation reflex. This may decrease airway pressures and also diminish the risk of inadvertent extubation. Sedatives may also be helpful for the treatment of hysterical hyperventilation. Nonproductive coughing due to airway irritation, such as after a tracheostomy, may be depressed by narcotics, especially codeine. Compared with an equal cough-supressing (antitussive) dose of morphine, codeine has less analgesic, euphoric, and respiratory depressant effect on respiration and is thus a safer drug with less risk of addiction.

Paralyzing Agents

Although they may be euphemistically called muscle relaxants, this group of potent drugs can dras-

TABLE 15–5. Major Opiate Receptor Subtypes

Effect	Receptor/Response		
	Mu	*Kappa*	*Sigma*
Analgesia	Yes	Yes	No
Respiration	Depression	Depression	Stimulation
Behavior	Euphoria	Sedation	Dysphoria
Pupil	Miosis	Miosis	Mydriasis
Morphine withdrawal	Suppression	No suppression	No suppression

Adapted from Martin, W. R., Eades, C. G., Thompson, J. A., Huppler, R. E., and Gilbert, P. E.: The effects of morphine- and nalorphine-like drugs in the non-dependent and morphine-dependent chronic spinal dog. J. Pharmacol. Exp. Ther. 197:517–532, 1976.

tically reduce or abolish skeletal muscle (voluntary) strength. The cardiopulmonary clinician must be acutely aware of the action of these drugs in two critical situations. Patients sometimes are unable to be mechanically ventilated because they attempt a Valsalva maneuver whenever the machine tries to deliver a breath (bucking). If sedation and analgesics fail to resolve this problem, paralyzing agents are sometimes required. When adequate paralyzing agents have been administered, the patient becomes dependent on the ventilator, and ventilator disconnection can result in death.

During anesthesia for certain types of surgery, paralyzing agents are used to prevent muscular contraction in response to painful stimuli. At the end of surgery, the muscle relaxants are reversed in a manner that is described later. Postoperatively, the patient must be closely observed for a certain interval because paralysis may recur resulting in respiratory arrest (usually because the muscle relaxant reversal drug wears off before the muscle relaxant). Additionally, low temperatures, certain antibiotics (particularly aminoglycosides), and drugs such as respiratory depressants or magnesium sulfate can augment the effects of incompletely reversed paralyzing agents, resulting in ventilatory failure.

Paralyzing drugs are divided into two main categories—*depolarizing* and *nondepolarizing muscle relaxants*. The nondepolarizing muscle relaxants are competitive blocking agents that inhibit neuromuscular transmission by competing with acetylcholine for the receptors on the motor endplate. Nondepolarizing agents are antagonists to ACh, occupying the cholinergic receptors but not activating them. Pancuronium, curare, and gallamine are examples of nondepolarizing or competitive blocking agents.

Nondepolarizing muscle relaxants can have their action terminated or reversed by administration of anticholinesterase drugs, such as neostigmine or edrophonium. Anticholinesterase drugs block the breakdown of acetylcholine at the nerve terminal. The increased levels of acetylcholine compete with the nondepolarizing muscle relaxants for receptors on the skeletal muscles. When the paralyzing agents are displaced from the cell membrane receptors, muscle strength returns.

Depolarizing muscle relaxants are agonists to ACh and combine with the cholinergic receptor sites producing endplate depolarization at the myoneural junction. However, depolarizing agents are not rapidly metabolized and removed from the skeletal muscle endplate, in contrast to the rapid breakdown of ACh. Thus, in the presence of depolarizing muscle relaxants, the endplate remains occupied, and subsequent impulses to the muscles do not produce contractions. *Succinylcholine* is the most commonly used depolarizing muscle relaxant. It causes muscle twitching and contractions (fasciculations) before producing paralysis. Administration of depolarizing muscle relaxants also produces increased extracellular potassium, which can be extreme in the presence of certain types of pathology, such as some neuromuscular diseases or extensive burns. Depolarizing muscle relaxants do not usually have to be reversed due to their relatively short half-lives.

Stimulants for Breathing

Some drugs increase breathing by opposing the action of respiratory depressants. *Narcotic antagonists*, such as naloxone (Narcan), displace narcotics from their opiate receptors in the brain. This specifically reverses the respiratory depressant effect of narcotics but unfortunately also abolishes their analgesia. Studies with narcotic agonist-antagonists have been carried out in the hopes of finding potent analgesics without respiratory depressant effects or opiate-receptor blockers with the ability to reverse the respiratory depression of previously administered narcotics without ablating analgesia.

A less specific reversal of respiratory depression occurs with *physostigmine* (Antilirium), a drug that blocks the action of the enzyme cholinesterase to break down acetylcholine in the CNS. ACh is the principal neurotransmitter in the reticular activating system. By augmenting CNS cholinergic traffic, the patient's level of wakefulness increases while breathing tends to increase. Physostigmine has been used to reverse such diverse drugs as phenothiazines, general anesthetics, and sedatives.

Amphetamines, which are catecholamines with considerable CNS activity, can increase the level of consciousness, stimulate the respiratory centers, and augment breathing. Similarly, *methylxanthines* (the bronchodilating and diuretic effects of which have already been mentioned) increase CNS and respiratory center activity. *Analeptics*, drugs that specifically stimulate the central nervous system, have been used for combating depressed respiration. This diverse group of drugs includes doxapram, picrotoxin, and lobeline. All CNS stimulants may cause convulsions as a side effect.

Progesterone and other progestational agents have been used successfully on patients with hypoventilation syndromes, especially obesity hypoventilation (pickwickian) syndrome. Progesterone levels are high during pregnancy and are believed to result in the fall of $PaCO_2$ to about 30 mmHg normally observed during the third trimester. Thyroid hormone has been used to stimulate breathing in the hypoventilating myxedematous hypothyroid patient.

Carbonic anhydrase inhibitors, such as acetazolamide (Diamox), inhibit renal reabsorption of bicarbonate resulting in alkalinization of the urine and decreased blood pH. For the patient hypoventilating from severe metabolic alkalosis, carbonic anhydrase inhibitor administration can rapidly and effectively restore ventilatory drive. Similarly, infusion of acid or acidic buffers can also correct ventilatory depression caused by severe metabolic acidosis.

The tricyclic antidepressant *protriptyline* has been used to improve respiratory patterns in patients with obstructive sleep apnea. The proposed mechanisms include alteration of airway tone and decreased REM sleep (the stage of sleep in which the most severe apnea occurs).

Almitrine stimulates peripheral chemoreceptors and is undergoing clinical evaluation as a ventilatory stimulant, especially in patients with COPD. It increases the ventilatory response to hypoxia and possibly improves ventilation–perfusion matching in patients with COPD.

COUGH TREATMENTS

The irritant receptors in the respiratory tract are of major importance in the cough reflex. These irritant receptors have been divided into two types: *mechanoreceptors*, which are mainly in the airways above the carina, and *chemoreceptors*, which are mainly in the smaller airways and lung parenchyma. Airway mechanoreceptors can be stimulated by aspirated material or airway instrumentation, such as bronchoscopy, suctioning, or endotracheal intubation. Chemoreceptors in the lungs can be stimulated by inhalation of irritating aerosols, such as the mucolytic acetylcysteine, by smoke, or by industrial chemical inhalation. Stimulation of the irritant receptors can produce coughing as well as bronchospasm. Coughing can interfere with normal breathing and result in vomiting. Airway mucus production and salivation also increase with coughing. Severe coughing may produce fractured ribs and chest, back, or abdominal pain.

A certain amount of coughing to help clear the airways of secretions and microaspiration after swallowing is normal. Frequent coughing is annoying and painful and may be symptomatic of pulmonary disease. Many treatments to decrease excessive coughing have been developed. Some treatments directly desensitize the irritant receptors with local anesthesia. Local anesthetics can be instilled or nebulized into the airway to help reduce the coughing associated with bronchoscopy or endotracheal intubation. Sensation to the larynx can also be blocked by injecting local anesthetic at the superior laryngeal nerve as it passes under the thyroid cartilage. Some cough formulas, especially the narcotics, act on the central nervous system to diminish the cough response. Bronchospasm and coughing are both components of obstructive airways disease and some coughs appear to be initiated by bronchospasm. Bronchodilators, mucokinetics and hydrating agents have all been used for different types of coughs. Mucokinetics and hydrating agents can help convert a dry, hacking, nonproductive cough into a productive cough that removes the stimulus to the irritant receptors.

Although cough suppression is desirable in some situations, patients with retained secretions and decreased ability to cough may require stimulation of the cough reflex. Although inhalation of irritant substances has been attempted, the most reliable cough production comes from mechanical stimulation of the airway by suction catheters. Verbal cough-coaching by cardiopulmonary clinicians also stimulates coughing in motivated patients. Chest physiotherapy and postural drainage helps make coughing more productive in clearing the airways.

DECONGESTANTS

The nasal and conducting airway mucosa are very vascular areas. Irritation and infection produce vasodilation and vascular congestion that causes these tissues to swell. This tissue swelling results from more blood in the vessels and increased interstitial fluid (edema) caused by increased blood pressure in the capillaries. Depending on its location, mucosal swelling can cause nasal obstruction and/or increased airways resistance.

There are two main types of decongestants: *alpha-adrenergic drugs*, which cause vasoconstriction and thereby decrease blood flow and fluid transudation (edema formation) into the area, and *antihistamines*, which antagonize histamine-mediated allergic diseases of the respiratory tract and which may also have some anticholinergic mucosal drying effects.

Several kinds of catecholamines stimulate the alpha-adrenergic receptors in the respiratory mucosal blood vessels, shrinking the mucosal surface. Some of these catecholamines, such as racemic epinephrine, are useful treatments for epiglottitis and postextubation laryngotracheal edema. Racemic epinephrine is usually nebulized, which helps reduce undesired cardiac beta receptor stimulation. Other catecholamine mucosal vasoconstrictors, such as *phenylephrine* (Neo-Synephrine), are primarily alpha receptor stimulants with little or no beta activity. Phenylephrine is a very popular nose drop for treating nasal congestion associated with colds or allergy. Phenylephrine is also very beneficial when administered to shrink the nasal mucosa in preparation for a nasal intubation. This greatly helps reduce the frequency and severity of associated nose bleeds but systemic hypertension is an occasional undesirable side effect that must be anticipated with alpha-adrenergic stimulation. Less hypertension and more prolonged decongestion are obtained from another alpha-agonist, *oxymetazoline* (Afrin), but with a different side effect, rebound congestion when the drug effect wears off.

The body has two types of receptors that are stimulated by histamines. The H_1 receptor mediates most of the responses to histamine. Activation of the H_2 receptors stimulates gastric secretion. The great variety of antihistaminic drugs used to treat the respiratory effects of allergy and histamine release are inhibitors of H_1 receptors. Recently, blockers of H_2 receptors have been developed to treat peptic ulcers. H_2 blockers (cimetidine, for example) have essentially no effect on respiratory mucosal swelling.

CARDIOVASCULAR DRUGS

Many of the drugs that are used to diagnose, prevent, or treat pulmonary disease have been noted to have cardiovascular effects. Similarly, many drugs used on the cardiovascular system have effects on the pulmonary system. Adequate cardiovascular function is necessary to deliver gas-exchanging blood to the tissues; inadequate cardiovascular function leads to heart failure, increases in venous pressure, and pulmonary edema. Decreased pulmonary function can produce low oxygen concentration in arterial blood, which decreases oxygen delivery to the heart. Myocardial ischemia can decrease the heart's contractility and also lead to heart damage (myocardial infarction). The two systems are obviously strongly linked.

Oxygen therapy has been mentioned as a treatment for lung disease. Increased oxygen tension is infrequently therapeutic to the lungs and, at high concentrations, may even be toxic to lung tissues. However, lung disease frequently decreases systemic arterial blood oxygen content, which can damage organs, such as the heart, that have high metabolic rates. In most lung diseases, oxygen is given not so much to treat the lungs as to prevent damage to other organs.

Cardiac Medications

Medications for the treatment of heart disease can be considered in three classes: cardiac inotropes affect the strength of myocardial contraction (contractility), antiarrhythmics affect the rate and rhythm of cardiac depolarizations, and anti-ischemia medications can preserve the function of stressed heart muscle cells. Some medications may fit into more than one category or have beneficial actions in one category but detrimental effects in another.

Cardiac Inotropes

Positive inotropic (cardiotonic) *drugs* increase the strength of contraction of cardiac muscle; *negative inotropic drugs* decrease myocardial contractility. The catecholamines that stimulate beta$_1$ receptors increase the strength of myocardial contraction and are also *positive chronotropes*; that is, they increase the heart rate as well. Not all drugs that are positive inotropes are also positive chronotropes. Digitalis and calcium increase myocardial contractility, but both also decrease heart rate.

The sympathomimetic amines (catecholamines) are used to produce short-term increases in the contractility of cardiac muscle. Because of the fairly short half-life of these drugs, continuous intravenous infusion techniques can be utilized when the drug is given for a prolonged period. Dopamine and dobutamine are cardiac inotropes that are commonly used by continuous infusion in the intensive care unit. They are used to strengthen heart contractions and improve cardiac output. Dopamine infusions are also given sometimes at very low levels to stimulate dopaminergic receptors in the renal and mesenteric vessels. This can increase renal blood flow and urine output, which are frequently diminished in critically ill patients. However, the side effects of adrenergic medications (hypertension, arrhythmias, and increased myocardial oxygen demand) limit their usefulness in long-term treatment of cardiac patients.

Drugs that block the beta$_1$-adrenergic receptors in the heart are called *beta blockers*. They decrease the contractility of the heart, slow the heart rate, and also decrease myocardial work and oxygen demand, reducing cardiac ischemia. *Propranolol* is the classic beta blocker; however, it also blocks beta$_2$ receptors in the lungs and may produce bronchospasm. Newer beta blockers, such as *metoprolol* and *practolol*, are specific for beta$_1$ receptors with little or no action at the beta$_2$ sites.

Digitalis belongs to a group of inotropic drugs called *cardiac glycosides* that are unrivaled for the long-term treatment of congestive heart failure (see Chapter 5). The increased myocardial contractile force is responsible for the beneficial effects of digitalis in congestive heart failure: increased cardiac output, decreased heart size, decreased venous pressure and blood volume, diuresis (increased urine output), and relief of edema. Digitalis also tends to slow the heart rate during normal sinus rhythm but drastically decreases the ventricular rate in atrial fibrillation.

Digitalis is one of the most commonly prescribed drugs in the world, but its therapeutic dosage is very near its toxic dose range. The toxic side effects of digitalis overdose include nausea, vomiting, visual disturbances, and arrhythmias, including life-threatening bradycardia. Hypokalemia (low blood potassium concentration) increases the risks of digitalis toxicity. As discussed later, certain diuretics have the unfortunate side effect of reducing blood potassium. Liver and kidney disease can decrease excretion of digitalis, increasing the risk of toxicity.

Intravenous administration of *calcium salts*, such as calcium chloride, has a positive inotropic effect. If administered too rapidly, intravenous calcium chloride may produce bradycardia, vasodilation, and hypotension. According to recent American Heart Association recommendations, calcium is no longer routinely used during resuscitation, except for the treatment of acute hyperkalemia, hypocalcemia, or calcium channel blocker toxicity. Rapid administration of blood anticoagulated with citrate may reduce circulating ionized calcium levels, decreasing myocardial contractility. *Calcium channel blockers*, such as verapamil and nifedipine, are primarily used as coronary vasodilators and antiarrhythmics, but they also possess negative inotropic and chronotropic activity.

Hypoxia, vagal stimulation, and cholinergic drugs all have negative inotropic effects. Antimuscarinic medications, such as atropine, slightly increase myocardial contractility while greatly increasing heart rate.

Antiarrhythmia Drugs

Arrhythmia is a misleading term because it means no cardiac rhythm. Dysrhythmia is perhaps a better term because it means an abnormal heart rhythm with potentially detrimental physiologic consequences. A sinus rhythm that is too fast (sinus tachycardia) or too slow (sinus bradycardia) can be life-threatening.

The electrical activity of the heart, normal conduction pathways and the electrocardiogram were discussed in Chapter 2. Dysrhythmia occurs when the heart rate is too fast or too slow, when the action potential originates at some location other than the sinoatrial node, or when the normal sequence and interval of first atrial then ventricular depolarization does not occur.

The three objectives of antiarrhythmia therapy are to slow down a fast heart rate, to speed up a slow heart rate, or to decrease the frequency of *ectopic beats*, which originate in some site other than the sinoatrial node. Ectopic beats usually diminish stroke volume by not allowing adequate time for ventricular filling and/or by loss of effective atrial contractions so that the ventricles have less volume when they begin to contract.

An excessively fast heart rate (tachycardia) does not allow enough time for ventricular filling to occur. As a result, stroke volume and cardiac output decrease. In addition, tachycardia increases the oxygen demand of the heart but diminishes oxygen delivery because of the decreased cardiac output and diminished time for coronary perfusion. The coronary vessels are better perfused during diastole than during systole. High heart rates usually decrease the amount of time the heart is in diastole more than the amount of time the heart is in systole. The heart rate can be slowed by nonselective beta blockers (propranolol), by selective beta$_1$ blockers (metoprolol), and by calcium channel blockers (verapamil). As mentioned previously, digitalis tends to slow ventricular heart rate, especially when atrial fibrillation or flutter is present. Increased blood pressure in the carotid sinus triggers the baroreceptor reflex, which slows sinus tachycardia. The baroreceptor reflex can be stimulated by carotid massage, Valsalva maneuvers, or administration of vasopressors, such as the alpha agonist phenylephrine. *Anticholinesterase* drugs, such as edrophonium (Tensilon), affect the heart by the peripheral action of accumulated acetylcholine, resulting in decreased heart rate. Drugs to slow heart rate must be administered with care because drug interactions and overdosage may produce life-threatening bradycardia.

A rapidly decreasing heart rate is a frequent life-threatening emergency that requires prompt and appropriate action by a cardiopulmonary clinician. Severe hypoxia causes a progressive and rapidly fatal bradycardia. When confronted with bradycardia, hypoxia is the first cause that must be ruled out. The importance of first assuring adequate oxygenation and ruling out hypoxia as the cause of bradycardia before proceeding to other treatments cannot be overemphasized. When bradycardia is not caused by hypoxia, antimuscarinic drugs, such as atropine, are most commonly used to increase heart rate. For profound bradycardia or bradycardia unresponsive to antimuscarinics, beta agonist drugs are used to increase heart rate and contractility. However, they also increase the frequency of ectopic beats and myocardial oxygen demand, thus increasing the risk of myocardial ischemia. Antimuscarinics also increase cardiac oxygen demand but are less likely to induce ectopic beats.

Depolarization of ectopic foci causes premature atrial contractions (PACs), atrial flutter, atrial fibrillation, premature ventricular contractions (PVCs), ventricular flutter, and ventricular fibrillation. In addition to reducing the effectiveness of cardiac contractions, ectopic beats, such as PVCs, may increase in frequency and seriousness to worse types of dysrhythmias. Ectopic beats may be caused by excessive catecholamines from painful stimulation, fear, and psychological states, such as those associated with trauma or surgery. PVCs frequently limit the amount of catecholamines that can be administered in the treatment of bronchospasm. Hypoventilation and hypercapnia (elevated blood carbon dioxide) stimulate the sympathetic nervous system, producing catecholamine release and ectopic beats. Central venous and pulmonary artery catheters, such as Swan-Ganz catheters, may produce dysrhythmias by striking the inner surface of the heart.

Intravenous *lidocaine* is commonly used in the emergency treatment of ventricular dysrhythmias. Its onset of action is very rapid but terminates quickly when its infusion is halted. *Quinidine* and *procainamide* can both be administered orally and both are effective for long-term treatment of ventricular dysrhythmias. *Phenytoin* is effective in the treatment of ventricular ectopic rhythms, including those associated with digitalis toxicity. *Bretylium* is a newer agent that has proved to be useful in the treatment of ventricular fibrillation by enhancing pacemaker activity in the myocardial conducting system. This increases the activity of the normal conducting system, which decreases the incidence of ectopic beats.

Medications for Cardiac Ischemia

Cardiac ischemia poses a dual risk to the heart. The ischemia can injure or kill heart muscle cells as well as decrease the ability of the heart to pump blood, which increases the severity of the ischemia. Cardiac ischemia decreases contractility, and ischemia of the conducting system can also provoke dysrhythmias and ectopic beats. The result of cardiac ischemia may be injury or death (infarction) of heart cells. Myocardial oxygen delivery can sometimes be improved by increasing a low cardiac output, dilating coronary arteries that are in spasm, or increasing the oxygen content of the coronary blood. Once oxygen delivery has been assured, cardiac ischemia is treated mainly by decreasing myocardial oxygen demand.

Cardiac oxygen requirements depend on how hard the heart is working. Myocardial oxygen consumption is determined by three factors: systolic wall tension, heart rate, and contractility. Systolic wall tension is affected by the length of the heart muscle cells when they begin to contract and the pressure that the chamber must attain to eject the blood. The length of the heart muscle cells before systole is determined by the volume in the chamber at the end of diastole (the preload). A heart cell that is stretched consumes more oxygen when it contracts. For the right side of the heart, the amount of stretch or preload is reflected by the central venous pressure. The preload of the left side of the heart is reflected in the left atrial pressure. This is approximated by the pulmonary capillary wedge pressure. Decreasing the volume in a dilated chamber greatly reduces its oxygen demand. Preload can be reduced by venodilation, especially with *nitroglycerin*. Diuretics decrease intravascular water by promoting urine formation, which also decreases preload.

To eject blood, a contracting chamber of the heart must overcome the pressure and resistance of the vessels downstream (the afterload). Increased vascular pressure and resistance require the heart to work harder to squeeze blood into the arteries. *Arterial dilators*, such as alpha blockers, ganglionic blockers, or direct vascular smooth muscle relaxants, reduce vascular resistance and decrease oxygen demand of the heart. When using arterial dilators, decreased oxygen demand must not be outweighed by decreased oxygen delivery because of lowered myocardial perfusion pressure.

The contractility or inotropic state of the heart can be thought of as the speed at which a contraction occurs (how fast the pressure increases in the chamber). The contractility also determines the amount of tension that the chamber attains before it begins to relax. *Inotropic drugs*, such as digitalis, calcium, and beta$_1$ agonist drugs, increase contractility and frequently increase myocardial oxygen demand. *Myocardial depressants*, such as beta blockers (propranolol), and calcium channel blockers (verapamil) and volatile inhalational anesthetics (halothane) decrease myocardial oxygen consumption.

Increased heart rate increases the oxygen demand of the heart but provides less time for coronary perfusion. When the heart rate is too fast to allow for complete ventricular filling, cardiac output and coronary perfusion both diminish. Many drugs used for the treatment of bronchospasm (beta agonists and methylxanthines), produce a rapid heart rate and possible cardiac ischemia. Drugs that are used for tachycardic dysrhythmias can also be used to reduce the ischemia caused by rapid heart rate.

Vasoactive Drugs

The resistance in a blood vessel is determined by the tone of its smooth muscle. This vascular resistance affects the distribution of perfusion, so that more blood goes to areas of less resistance. As mentioned previously, vascular resistance (after-load) is also a determinant of myocardial oxygen demand.

Treatments for high blood pressure may act at many different target sites: decreased effect of the CNS on the sympathetic nervous system (clonidine), blockade of autonomic ganglia (trimethaphan), depletion of catecholamines from postganglionic sympathetic neurons (reserpine), blockade of alpha receptors in the vessels (phentolamine), or direct relaxation of vascular smooth muscle (nitroprusside). A recently developed antihypertensive, captopril, is of particular interest to cardiopulmonary clinicians because it blocks the formation of the potent vasoconstrictor angiotensin II by inhibiting the action of the lung enzyme angiotensin converting enzyme. Diuretics, drugs that increase urine production, are very important in the long-term medical control of hypertension.

Alpha agonist drugs can be used to elevate low blood pressure. Vasoconstricting drugs have also been used to reduce vascular absorption of local anesthetics from tissues, which prolongs the numbing effect while decreasing the systemic toxicity of the local anesthetics. Vasopressin (ADH) is a posterior pituitary hormone with potent vasoconstricting actions that has been used clinically to stop certain types of bleeding.

Other Agents Used on the Circulatory System

In addition to agents that act on the heart and the smooth muscle of blood vessels, other common substances are frequently used to insure perfusion of the tissues with blood. The maintenance of an adequate circulating blood volume is pharmacologically enhanced by the administration of intravenous fluids, procoagulants, and anticoagulants.

A tremendous variety of *intravenous fluids* has been developed for administration to patients to assure adequate circulating blood volume with appropriate levels of nutrients, electrolytes, proteins (clotting factors), and formed elements (blood cells and platelets). Glucose is the most common nutrient included in intravenous solutions, usually as 5% dextrose. However, the entire body's nutritional requirements can be met by intravenous administration of carbohydrates, fats, amino acids, vitamins, and trace elements (*parenteral hyperalimentation*). Care must be taken to avoid administration of more carbohydrates than metabolic demands require because the excess carbohydrates are converted to fat. This fat production greatly increases carbon dioxide production, respiratory quotient, ventilatory work, and size of the liver. As the liver increases in size, diaphragmatic excursions are limited at a time when increased ventilation is needed to remove the excess carbon dioxide. In this manner, hyperalimentation with excessive carbohydrates can lead to respiratory failure and ventilator dependence. Carbon dioxide production studies are frequently performed on patients receiving parenteral hyperalimentation to see if excessive carbohydrates are being administered.

Ringer's lactate solution and *Ringer's lactate with 5% dextrose* are two of the most common intravenous solutions administered because they closely approximate plasma electrolyte concentrations. These solutions are administered to replace plasma that has leaked through the walls of the blood vessels following trauma, dehydration, sweating, or evaporation. This type of loss of blood volume to the tissues surrounding the blood vessels is called third-space loss. The other two "spaces" where fluid is lost are urine and hemorrhage. Fluid lost from the circulation to form urine is commonly replaced by hypotonic solutions, such as 5% dextrose in water or 5% dextrose in one quarter or one half normal saline. *Normal saline* is 0.9% saline solution, which has the same tonicity (concentration of osmotically active dissolved particles) as plasma. Normal saline is most commonly used to dilute packed blood cells before administration.

Blood loss is replaced with the appropriate fraction from whole blood. A unit of blood donated at a blood bank may be separated by centrifugation into its components: packed red blood cells, platelets, and plasma. The plasma may be stored at room temperature or frozen, which better preserves the clotting factors. The standard principle of blood replacement is to treat blood loss by giving packed red blood cells to maintain at least a 30% hematocrit in the patient. As mentioned previously, plasma loss is treated by administration of isotonic electrolyte solutions, such as Ringer's lactate. When plasma loss is excessive, it is sometimes replaced by *colloid solution*, such as albumin, or synthetic colloids, such as hetastarch (Hespan) and dextrans (Dextran). Ringer's lactate, albumin solutions, and synthetic colloids are much safer to use for the replacement of plasma loss because unlike donor plasma, they carry no risk of infection to the recipient by hepatitis or AIDS.

The plasma removed from donor blood during the formation of packed red blood cells is either frozen or processed to form special blood products. Fresh frozen plasma is given to treat certain clotting abnormalities because plasma removed from the body rapidly loses the activity of the labile clotting Factors V and VIII unless it is frozen. Plasma not stored as fresh frozen may be processed to form certain factors used for the treatment of hemophiliacs or to produce antibody concentrates (RhoGam or immune globulin). Plasma may also be processed to form albumin solutions in a manner that kills viruses, eliminating the risk of hepatitis and AIDS. A fraction from whole blood that is rich in platelets can be administered to patients with clotting abnormalities caused by low platelet levels (*thrombocytopenia*).

Administration of electrolyte and blood product solutions is frequently necessary to insure adequate circulating blood volume. In addition, the administration of fresh frozen plasma, calcium, and platelets can treat an ineffective clotting mechanism (coagulopathy). In certain situations, such as cardiac or vascular surgery or when excess clot formation is present, the blood's ability to clot can be diminished by the administration of anticoagulant drugs, such as heparin. Heparin can be used to keep blood liquid during conditions that usually would promote clot formation. Low flow or exposure to collagen or roughened surfaces enhances clot formation. This explains the formation of clots in the large-diameter leg veins of bedridden patients. These clots can break free and travel in the vessels through the heart and finally lodge in the pulmonary blood vessels as pulmonary emboli. Anticoagulant therapy decreases the formation of thrombi that are potential pulmonary emboli. Heparin is also essential to prevent clotting of blood in blood gas machines, which would interfere with their use. When the anticoagulant effect of heparin is no longer desirable in a patient, it can be allowed to wear off or the heparin can be rapidly antagonized by a drug called *protamine*. Heparin is a polypeptide and therefore can only be administered by injection. For long-term anticoagulant administration, an oral medication, such as coumadin, is frequently used. These oral anticoagulants are essentially anti–vitamin K, which is necessary for the liver to produce the clotting factors prothrombin and Factors VII, IX and X. The action of coumadin can be terminated by administration of extra vitamin K.

DIURETICS

Normal functioning of the heart and lungs depends on the presence of an appropriate circulating blood volume. Inadequate blood volume may be the result of blood loss, which is best treated by intravenous fluid therapy. Vasodilation can also cause hypoperfusion by producing a hypovolemia relative to the increased vascular space. Substances such as general anesthetics or histamine (released by anaphylaxis) can produce profound vasodilation, relative hypovolemia, and hypoperfusion (cardiovascular collapse), which is best treated with intravascular fluid administration and vasopressors.

Excessive fluid volume can have a detrimental effect on the cardiovascular and pulmonary systems as well. Blood volume overload can fill the pulmonary interstitial space initially and eventually can spill into the alveoli, producing the clincal condition known as pulmonary edema, which greatly impedes the diffusion of oxygen from the alveoli into the blood. The circulatory effects of excess body water can include hypertension, edema, cardiac dilation, and heart failure. Excess fluid volume can be treated by restricting salt and intravenous fluid intake. Furthermore, excretion of excess body water can be augmented by the use of diuretics, which enhance glomerular filtration or reduce the kidney's ability to reabsorb electrolytes and water. *Methylxanthines* increase urine formation by enhancing glomerular filtration.

Carbonic anhydrase inhibitors, such as acetazolamide (Diamox), tend to acidify the blood while producing a copious alkaline urine. Hydrochlorothiazide (Diazide) and *loop diuretics*, such as furosemide (Lasix), promote urine formation but cause electrolyte loss, particularly of potassium. *Osmotic diuretics*, such as mannitol or urea, promote water excretion because they are freely filterable in the glomerulus, their reabsorption is limited, and their osmotic presence in the filtrate holds electrolytes and water there. *Aldosterone antagonists*, such as spironolactone (Aldactone), increase sodium and water excretion but promote potassium retention. It should be remembered that aldosterone is a naturally occurring adrenal cortical steroid hormone that acts to promote sodium and water retention and potassium loss. The potassium-sparing effects of the aldosterone antagonists have been combined with the potassium-wasting effects of the diazides to produce drugs such as Aldactazide, a combination of spironolactone and hydrochlorothiazide, which maintain potassium near normal while promoting diuresis.

Bibliography

Beal, J.M. (ed.): *Critical Care for Surgical Patients*. New York, Macmillan, 1982.
Burton, G.G., Gee, G.N., and Hodgkin, J.E.: *Respiratory Care*. Philadelphia, J.B. Lippincott, 1977.
Conn, P.F.: *Diagnosis and Therapy of Coronary Artery Disease*. Boston, Little, Brown, 1979.
Divertie, M.B., and Brass, A. (eds.): *The CIBA Collection of Medical Illustrations*, Vol. 7. CIBA Pharmaceutical Company, Summit, New Jersey, 1979.
Goodman, L.S., Gilman, A., Rall, T.W., and Murad, F. (eds.): *The Pharmacologic Basis of Therapeutics*, 7th ed. New York, Macmillan, 1985.
Guenter, C.A., and Welch, M.H.: *Pulmonary Medicine*. Philadelphia, J.B. Lippincott, 1977.
Kafer, E.R., and Marsh, H.M.: The effect of anesthetic drugs and disease on the chemical regulation of ventilation. *Int. Anesthesiol. Clin.* 15:1–38, 1977.
Lehnert, B.E., and Schachter, E.N.: *The Pharmacology of Respiratory Care*. St. Louis, C.V. Mosby, 1980.
Leitch, A.G.: Asthma—Mechanisms and management. *Clin. Notes Respir. Dis.* 21:3–9, 1982.
Martin, W.R., Eades, C.G., Thompson, J.A., Huppler, R.E., and Gilbert, P.E.: The effects of morphine- and nalorphine-like drugs in the non-dependent and morphine-dependent chronic spinal dog. *J. Pharmacol. Exp. Ther.* 197:517–532, 1976.
Rarey, K.P., and Youtsey, J.W.: *Respiratory Patient Care*. Englewood Cliffs, N.J., Prentice-Hall, 1981.
Saefler, S.J.: Practical considerations in the safe and effective use of theophylline. *Ped. Clin. North Am.* 30(5):949, 1983.
Shapiro, B.A., Harrison, R.A., Kacmarek, R.M., Cane, R.D., and Trout, C.A.: *Clinical Application of Respiratory Care*, 3rd ed. Chicago, Year Book, 1985.
Shepherd, J.T. and Vanhoutte, P.M.: *The Human Cardiovascular System: Facts and Concepts*. New York, Raven Press, 1979.
Spearman, C.B., and Sheldon, R.L. (eds.): *Egan's Fundamentals of Respiratory Therapy*, 4th ed. St. Louis, C.V. Mosby, 1982.
Young, J.A., and Crocker, D.N. (eds.): *Principles and Practice of Respiratory Therapy*, 2nd ed. Chicago, Year Book, 1976.
Ziment, I.: *Respiratory Pharmacology and Therapeutics*. Philadelphia, W.B. Saunders, 1978.

OBJECTIVES

AFTER READING THIS CHAPTER, THE STUDENT WILL BE ABLE TO:

1. Describe the physical properties of oxygen.
2. Describe several techniques used to purify oxygen.
3. Discuss agencies and codes regulating the manufacture, storage, and transport of medical gases.
4. Describe the devices used to regulate the flow of gas from bulk storage and cylinder storage systems used in medical gas therapy.
5. Discuss the indications and contraindications for oxygen therapy.
6. Describe the physiologic response to hypoxia.
7. Describe how oxygen can be administered with low-flow systems, such as nasal cannulas and catheters, and simple oxygen masks.
8. Describe the administration of oxygen through high-flow oxygen devices, such as air-entrainment masks.
9. Describe various types of environmental oxygen therapy devices, such as oxygen tents, croupettes, oxyhoods, incubators, and hyperbaric chambers.
10. Discuss the use of helium-oxygen mixtures in the treatment of patients with airway obstruction.
11. Discuss the complications of oxygen therapy.
12. Define absolute humidity, relative humidity, and humidity deficit.
13. Describe several devices used in humidity and aerosol therapy.

16
ADMINISTRATION OF OXYGEN AND OTHER THERAPEUTIC GASES

CHAPTER OUTLINE

MANUFACTURE, STORAGE, AND TRANSPORT OF OXYGEN
  Physical Properties of Oxygen
  Preparation of Oxygen
  Storage of Oxygen
    Bulk Storage Systems
    Cylinder Storage
  Regulators
  Flow Meters
  Safety Systems for Administering Medical Gases
INDICATIONS FOR OXYGEN THERAPY
  Types of Hypoxia
  Physiologic Response to Hypoxia
ADMINISTERING ENRICHED OXYGEN MIXTURES
  Nasal Catheters
  Nasal Cannulas
  Simple Oxygen Masks
  Face Tents
  Partial Rebreathing Masks
  Nonrebreathing Masks
  Rebreathing Masks
  Air-Entrainment Devices
  T-Tubes and Tracheostomy Masks
  Environmental Oxygen Therapy Devices
COMPLICATIONS OF OXYGEN THERAPY
HELIUM-OXYGEN THERAPY
CARBON DIOXIDE–OXYGEN THERAPY
HUMIDIFICATION OF MEDICAL GASES
  Evaporating Devices
  Aerosol-Generating Devices
COMPLICATIONS OF HUMIDITY AND AEROSOL THERAPY

ADMINISTRATION OF OXYGEN AND OTHER THERAPEUTIC GASES

In Chapters 2 and 3, we discussed how the amount of oxygen delivered to the tissues depends on:

1. The fractional concentration of oxygen in the inspired air (FIO_2).
2. The individual's ability to move air into and out of the lungs (ventilation).
3. The uptake and transport of oxygen by the blood (hemoglobin, diffusion, and cardiac output).
4. The uptake and utilization of oxygen by the tissues (internal respiration).

We then described how various stresses and diseases can adversely affect oxygen transport and lead to hypoxia or a deficiency of oxygen at the tissue level (see Chapters 4 and 5). In this chapter, we discuss how administering medical gases (e.g., enriched oxygen mixtures) can be used effectively to treat spontaneously breathing patients with impaired cardiovascular and pulmonary function.

MANUFACTURE, STORAGE, AND TRANSPORT OF OXYGEN

Physical Properties of Oxygen

Oxygen is a colorless, odorless, and tasteless gas that makes up about 21% (by volume) of the atmosphere, 90% (by weight) of water, and 50% (by weight) of the earth's crust. It is produced in nature through the process of photosynthesis, in which green plants use chlorophyll to trap radiant energy and convert carbon dioxide and water into carbohydrates and molecular oxygen.

Elemental oxygen contains 8 protons and can contain 8, 9, or 10 neutrons in its nucleus. Approximately 99% of the oxygen atoms in the atmosphere contain 8 neutrons; thus the major isotope of oxygen has an atomic mass of 16. Fewer than 1% of the oxygen atoms in the atmosphere contain 9 or 10 neutrons in their nuclei, and these isotopes are referred to as O^{17} and O^{18} respectively. These latter two isotopes are often used as tracers in biological assays. (Remember that the atomic mass equals the number of protons plus the number of neutrons in the nucleus of an atom.)

Oxygen is more dense than air—at 0°C and 1 atm of pressure (760 torr), it has a density of 1.429 gm/L, whereas under the same conditions, air has a density of 1.293 gm/L. (At 20°C and 1 atm, oxygen has a density of 1.33 gm/L.) Oxygen is slightly soluble in water and has a solubility coefficient of 0.03 ml/L of water at 37°C and 1 atm. In the liquid state, oxygen has a pale blue color; its boiling point is −183°C. Solid oxygen is also pale blue and melts at −218.4°C.

Ambient oxygen is a diatomic molecule, that is, it consists of 2 oxygen atoms covalently bonded together. Ambient oxygen has a molecular weight of 32 daltons, and it possesses the property of paramagnetism (being attracted into a magnetic field) because of the presence of 2 unshared electrons.

Oxygen is classified as a nonflammable gas that supports combustion. It combines with most metals slowly at room temperature to form metal oxides; however, certain metals, such as sodium and calcium, burn readily when heated in the presence of oxygen. Nonmetals react more readily with oxygen to form oxides, such as water and carbon dioxide. In animals, carbon dioxide is a by-product of *aerobic* metabolism (i.e., enzyme-mediated oxygen-dependent metabolism).

Preparation of Oxygen

Enriched oxygen can be prepared from air or from several oxygen-containing compounds, such as water and sodium peroxide. Table 16–1 lists six methods commonly used to manufacture purified oxygen. For practical reasons, the primary means of preparing oxygen for commercial use involves either the fractional distillation of air or the use of oxygen concentrators.

In the fractional distillation process, gaseous air is first compressed and condensed into a liquid and then slowly heated until all of the gases except oxygen are boiled off. Figure 16–1 illustrates the production of oxygen using the fractional distillation process.

Oxygen concentrators are electrically powered devices that produce enriched oxygen mixtures by filtering air either through a specially designed molecular sieve or through a series of polymeric membranes. For devices that use molecular sieves, room air is filtered through an inorganic silicate (zeolite). Nitrogen, carbon dioxide, and other gases, as well as water vapor, are removed as the gas passes through the sieve, leaving an enriched

TABLE 16–1. Methods of Obtaining Purified Oxygen

1. Fractional distillation of air.
2. Heating of metal oxides.
3. Electrolysis of water.
4. Action of water on sodium peroxide.
5. Heating oxygen-containing salts.
6. Oxygen concentrators.

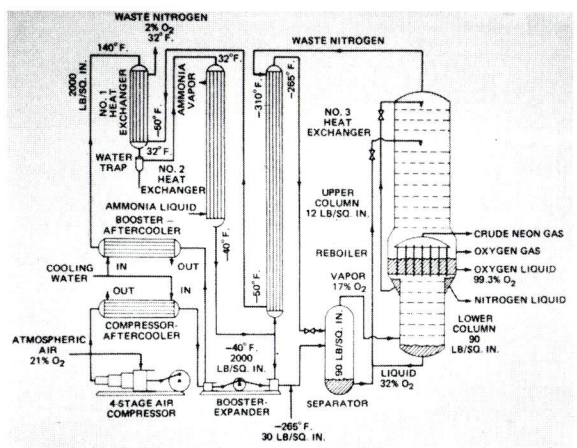

FIGURE 16–1. Apparatus used in the fractional distillation of air to produce purified oxygen. (Courtesy of Union Carbide Corporation, Linde Division, Indianapolis.)

oxygen mixture. Oxygen concentrators typically produce oxygen mixtures containing 50% to 90% oxygen, depending on the flow rate used. Generally, the oxygen concentration produced is inversely proportional to the flow rate used. For example, at a flow rate of 1 to 2 L per minute, fractional concentrations of oxygen of 0.9 can be produced. At flow rates of 8 to 10 L per minute, the fractional concentration falls to 0.3 to 0.5. For oxygen concentrators that rely on polymeric membranes, air is filtered across a membrane of about 1 mm thickness that is permeable to oxygen and water vapor. As a result, these devices produce humidified oxygen mixtures that have fractional concentrations of 0.3 to 0.4 when the gas flow is between 1 and 10 L per minute.

Storage of Oxygen

Purified oxygen that is produced, for example, by fractional distillation of air is stored as a liquid in bulk reservoir containers or as a gas in individual steel cylinders for use in medical gas therapy.

Bulk Storage Systems

Figure 16–2 shows a schematic of a typical hospital bulk storage system for liquid oxygen. A primary reservoir containing oxygen is connected via a reducing valve to a piping system, which carries oxygen to various zones within the hospital. A secondary bank of oxygen cylinders connected to the primary system functions as a backup when the primary system is empty or not functioning. The bulk oxygen supply can be tapped at a number of wall outlets located throughout the hospital using quick-connect, plug-in adaptors like those shown in Figure 16–3. Note that each zone contains a cut-off valve that allows for isolation of a zone without the interruption of gas flow to any of the other zones in the system. A pressure ma-

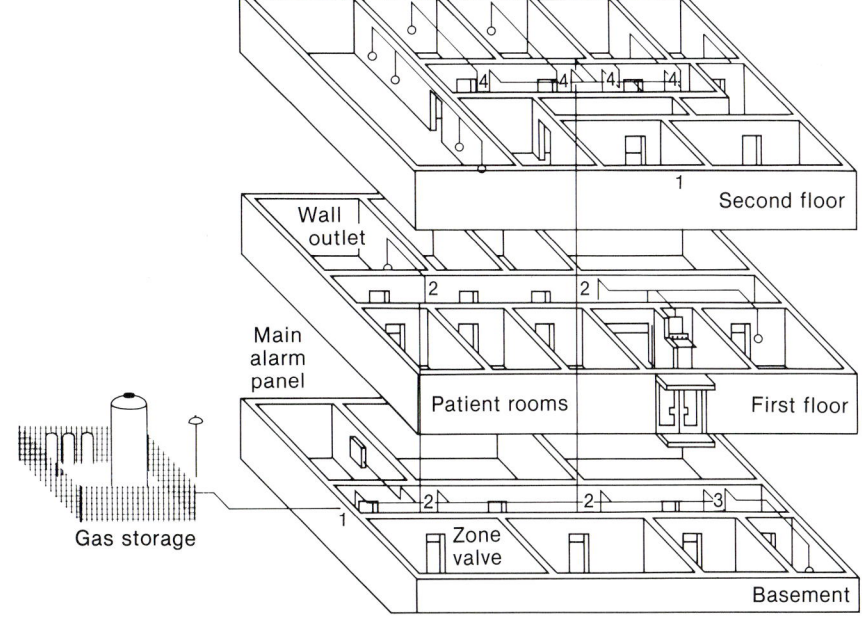

FIGURE 16–2. Bulk storage oxygen system. (Reproduced by permission from: McPherson, S.P.: *Respiratory Therapy Equipment*, 3rd ed. St. Louis, 1985, The C.V. Mosby Co.)

444 ADMINISTRATION OF OXYGEN AND OTHER THERAPEUTIC GASES

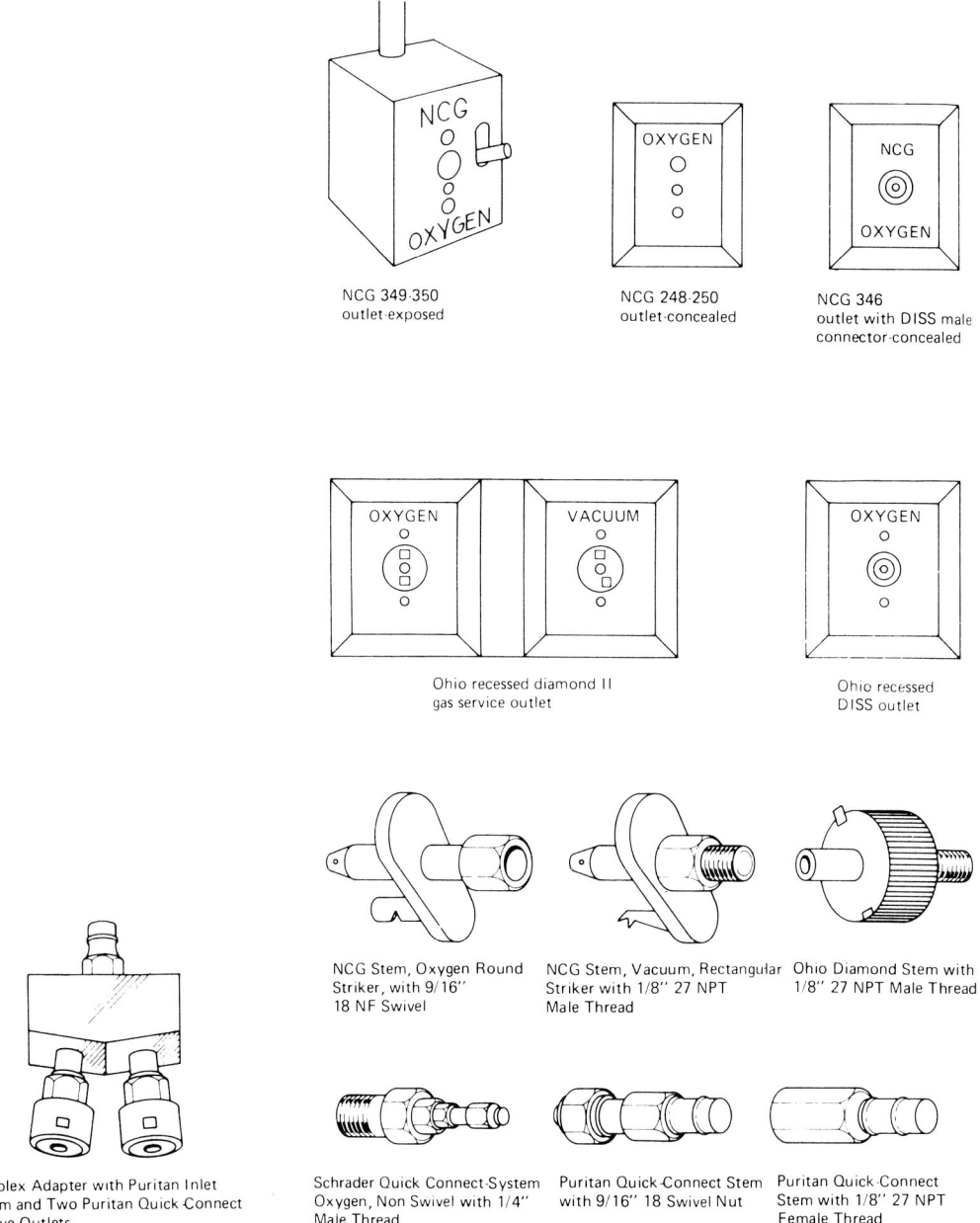

FIGURE 16–3. Quick-connect, plug-in types of adaptors commonly used in medical gas therapy. (From Husinger, D.L., Lisnerski, K.L., Maurizi, J.J., and Philips, M.L.: *Respiratory Technology Procedures and Equipment Manual.* Reston, Va., Reston Publishing Co., 1980, with permission.)

nometer is usually located in each zone so that the operating pressure of the system can be easily monitored. (For hospital systems, the working pressure is typically 50 pounds per square inch.)

Cylinder Storage

Cylinders used for the storage of oxygen and other medical gases are constructed of seamless steel (or in some cases aluminum). Each cylinder must comply with a set of standards that have been established by the U.S. Department of Transportation (DOT) (before 1970, the standards were set by the Interstate Commerce Commission) and the Board of Transport Commissioners (BTC) of Canada, with the assistance of the National Fire Protection Association (NFPA), the Compressed Gas Association (CGA), and the American Society of

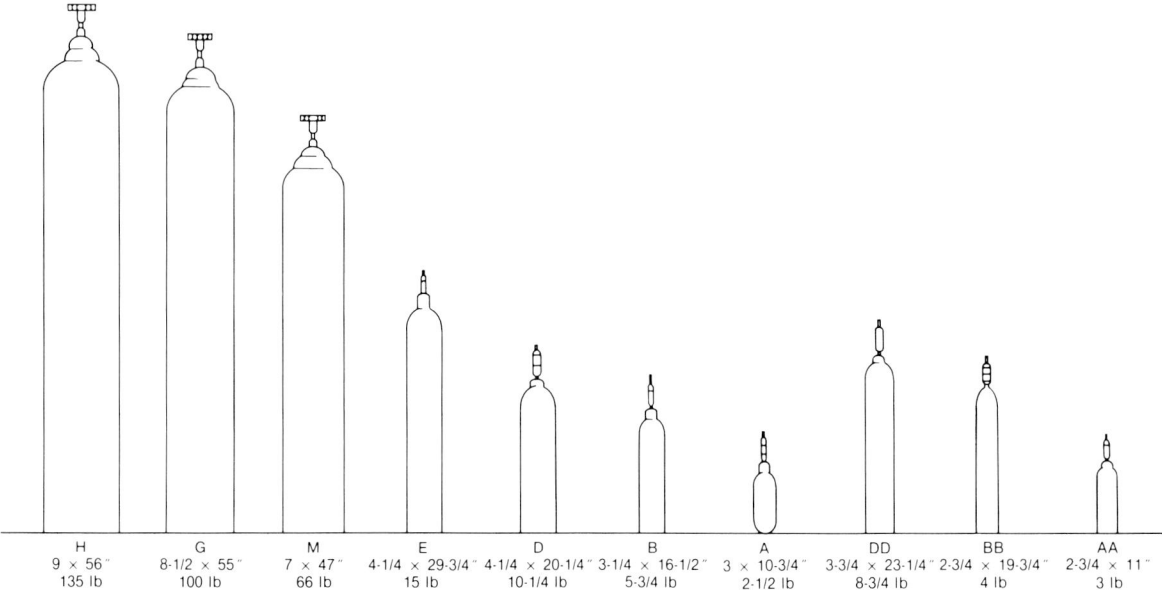

FIGURE 16–4. Various types of cylinders used in medical gas therapy have diameter-indexed valves. The volume capacities of the major cylinders used in respiratory care are as follows: for Cylinder H, 244 cu ft/6900 L; for Cylinder G, 186 cu ft/5260 L; for Cylinder M, 21.9 cu ft/1337 L; for Cylinder E, 22 cu ft/622 L; and for Cylinder D, 12.6 cu ft/12.6 L. (Modified from Garrett, D.F., and Donaldson, W.P.: *Physical Principles of Respiratory Therapy Equipment*, Madison, WI, Ohio Medical Products, 1975.)

Mechanical Engineers (ASME). These regulations include specifications for the manufacture, filling, labeling, transport, and testing of cylinders. Additionally, these agencies require that all cylinders be inspected every 5 to 10 years.

Figure 16–4 shows the various types of cylinders that are used to store medical gases. Each type of cylinder is designated with a letter code, which denotes its diameter and height. The most frequently used cylinders are the E, G, and H cylinders. E cylinders are most often used for portable emergency oxygen and for anesthetic gases, whereas the G and H cylinders are used for long-term gas therapy.

As Figure 16–5 shows, each cylinder is permanently labelled with a set of engravings, which

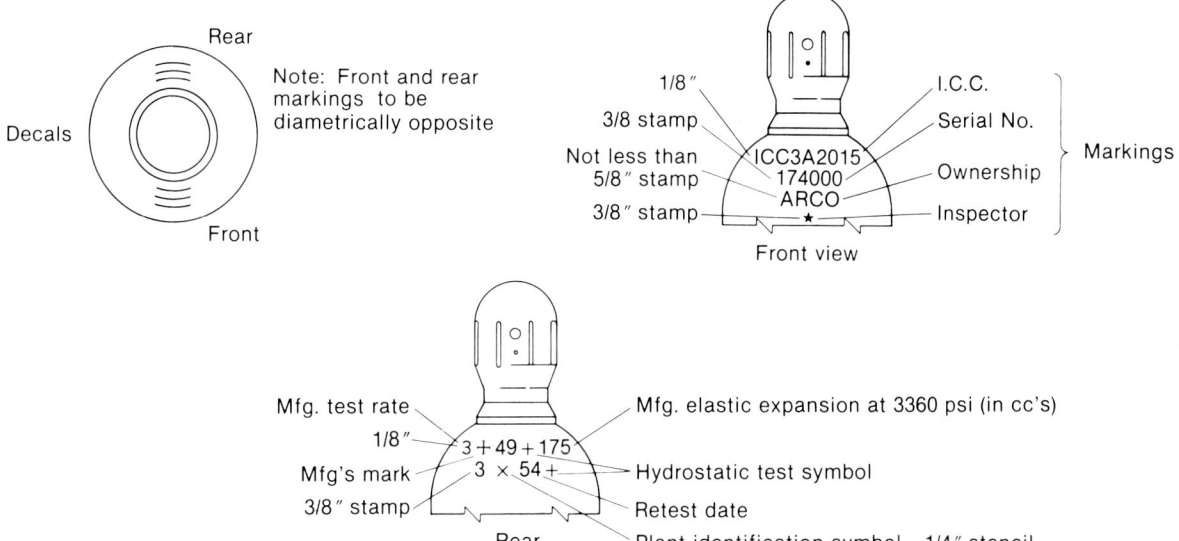

FIGURE 16–5. Cylinder engravings used to identify cylinder contents. (Courtesy of Compressed Gas Association; from Burton, G.G., and Hodgkin, J.E. (eds.): *Respiratory Care: A Guide to Clinical Practice*, 2nd ed. Philadelphia, J.B. Lippincott, 1984.)

are located on the side of the cylinder. These engravings contain information on the manufacturer of the cylinder, the material used to construct the cylinder, the process used to make the cylinder, the maximum filling pressure at which it can operate, the serial number of the cylinder, the owner of the cylinder, and the date and marking of the inspecting agency.

A cylinder color code is also used for easy identification of contents of gas cylinders. This color code is endorsed by the American Society of Anesthesiologists and the Compressed Gas Association (CGA); it is also recommended by the U.S. Bureau of Standards (Table 16–2). It should be remembered that although this color code can serve as a guide for identifying the contents of gas cylinders, each cylinder should bear a label that lists the gas(es) contained in the cylinder and stating whether it meets the purity standards set by the Food and Drug Administration and the U.S. Pharmacopeia.

Federal regulations require that cylinders be inspected every 5 to 10 years. Cylinders are checked every 5 years unless marked with a star that is engraved on the tank specifications, in which case the cylinder is checked every 10 years (see Fig. 16–5). Generally, cylinder retesting involves immersing the cylinder in a special water jacket, like the one in Figure 16–6.

Regulators

A regulator serves to reduce the gas pressure at the tank outlet from about 2,000 pounds per square inch (psi) to approximately 50 psi, which is the operating pressure required for flow meters and other gas therapy devices, such as IPPB machines.

Regulators can be classified as either nonadjustable or adjustable as well as by whether they have a single reduction chamber or multiple reduction chambers. Nonadjustable regulators deliver a preset pressure when the cylinder is turned on (typically 50 psi). Adjustable regulators can be adjusted to deliver pressures between 0 and 100 psi. Figure 16–7 shows diagrams of both single-stage and double-stage regulators that are routinely used in medical gas therapy.

By reading the pressure in the cylinder from the regulator meter and knowing the flow rate at which the gas is being delivered, one can calculate the duration of flow until the tank empties (Table 16–3).

Flow Meters

These devices control and indicate the flow rate of gas from an oxygen source, such as from a cylinder or from a wall outlet of a bulk storage oxygen system. Generally, flow meters are classified as either fixed-orifice (Bourdon gauge) or variable-orifice (Thorpe tube).

As Figure 16–8 shows, the Bourdon gauge contains a hollow movable arm that straightens under pressure. A needle attached to the arm indicates the flow of gas on a dial that is calibrated in liters per minute. In the Thorpe tube, a floating ball within a tapered plastic tube is used to register gas flow. Because the tube's diameter increases from

TABLE 16–2. Color Code Used to Identify Gas Cylinder Contents

Gas Mixture	Color Code
Oxygen	green (or white)
Carbon dioxide	gray
Nitrous oxide	light blue
Cyclopropane	orange
Helium	brown
Ethylene	red
CO_2-O_2	gray-green
Helium-oxygen	brown-green

TABLE 16–3. Calculation of the Duration of Cylinder Gas Flow

To determine how long a cylinder of gas will provide gas flow:
1. Convert the number of cubic feet of gas in the cylinder into liters of gas.

$$1 \text{ cubic foot} = 28.3 \text{ L}$$

$$\text{Conversion factor} = \frac{\text{cubic feet of gas in the cylinder* } \times 28.3}{\text{pounds per square inch of pressure in a full cylinder}}$$

2. Compare flow required with the volume of gas in the cylinder. The result is the amount of time that the cylinder will provide a given gas flow.

$$\text{Duration} = \frac{\text{cylinder pressure} \times \text{conversion factor}}{\text{flow rate required}}$$

Example: How long will a half-full H cylinder provide gas flow to a patient using a nasal cannula at 4 L per minute?

$$\text{Conversion factor} = (244 \text{ cu ft/L} \times 28.3 \text{ L}) \div 2,200 \text{ psi}$$

$$= 3.14$$

$$\text{Duration} = 1,100 \text{ psi} \times 3.14 \div 4 \text{ L/min}$$

$$= 863.5 \text{ minutes or } 14.4 \text{ hours}$$

* See Figure 16–4 for volume capacities of commonly used cylinders.

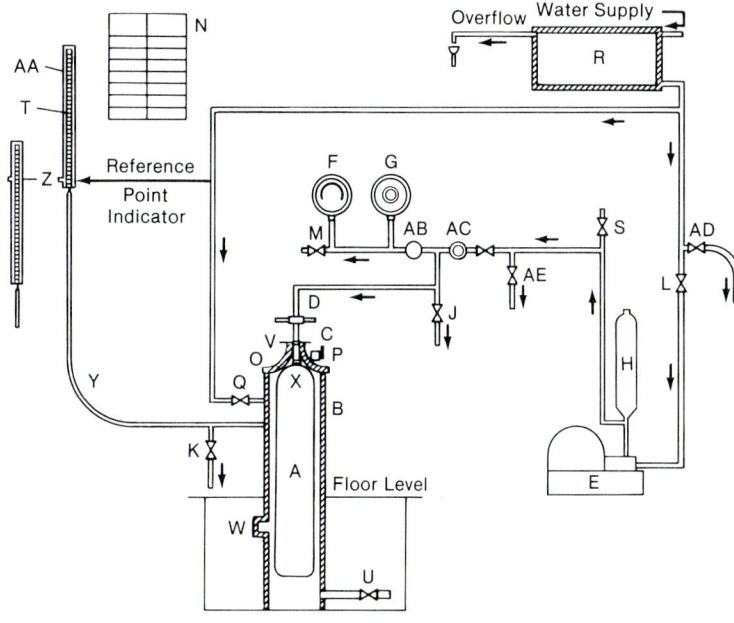

FIGURE 16–6. System for hydrostatic testing of gas cylinders used in medical gas therapy. The cylinder is immersed and filled with water and the water displacement in the surrounding jacket is measured. The pressure inside the tank is then raised to 3,000 pounds per square inch and the amount of water displaced in the water jacket is again measured. The compliance of the tank is then calculated. Loss of compliance in the metal casing of the tank indicates excessive wear and a possible hazard. (Courtesy of Compressed Gas Association: *Handbook of Compressed Gases*, 2nd ed., New York, VanNostrand Reinhold Co., 1981.)

A Cylinder
B Water Jacket
C Cylinder Connection
D Detachable Pressure Connection
E Hydraulic Pressure Source
F Pressure Indicating Gage**
G Pressure Recording Gage*
H Pressure Surge Chamber (Optional)
I, J, K, L, Q Valves
M Valve (for Master Gage In-Line Testing)
N Test Data Sheet
O Water Jacket Cover
P Pet Cock
R Water Reservoir (Optional)
S Safety Relief Device
T Burette, Reading in cc
U Clean-out Valve (Optional)
V Wing Nut
W Safety Port or Other Suitable Means of Relief or Containment
X Water Jacket Cover Gasket
Y Flexible Water Line
Z Reference Point Indicator
AA Movable Burette Panel
AB Pressure Snubber
AC Check Valve
AD Valve for Filling Cylinder Prior to Test
AE Pressure Control Valve

*Optional for manufacturers when testing new cylinders
**Must be capable of being read to a 1% accuracy. Suggested increments for corresponding test pressure.

Test Pressure	Increments
To 899	10 psi
900–2999	25 psi
3000–4100	50 psi
4500–10,000	100 psi

the bottom to the top of the tube, a greater pressure, and therefore flow, is required to raise the ball. The flow can be determined by using a calibrated scale attached or engraved on the face of the tube.

Flow meters can also be classified as either *uncompensated* or *compensated*. Restriction of gas flow from an uncompensated flow meter causes the indicated flow to be *lower* than the actual gas flow from the flow meter. Bourdon gauges and Thorpe tubes that have a needle valve distal to the floating ball are examples of uncompensated flow meters. In a compensated Thorpe tube, the needle valve is located before the floating ball, and thus, restrictions after the floating ball affect the ball in the same way as closing the needle valve. In these devices, the indicated flow equals the actual flow from the flow meter.

Safety Systems for Administering Medical Gases

A number of safety systems have been developed by the Compressed Gas Association to help insure the proper attachment of equipment, such as regulators, to gas cylinders. These include the American Standard Safety System (ASSS), Diameter Index Safety System (DISS), and Pin Index Safety

448 ADMINISTRATION OF OXYGEN AND OTHER THERAPEUTIC GASES

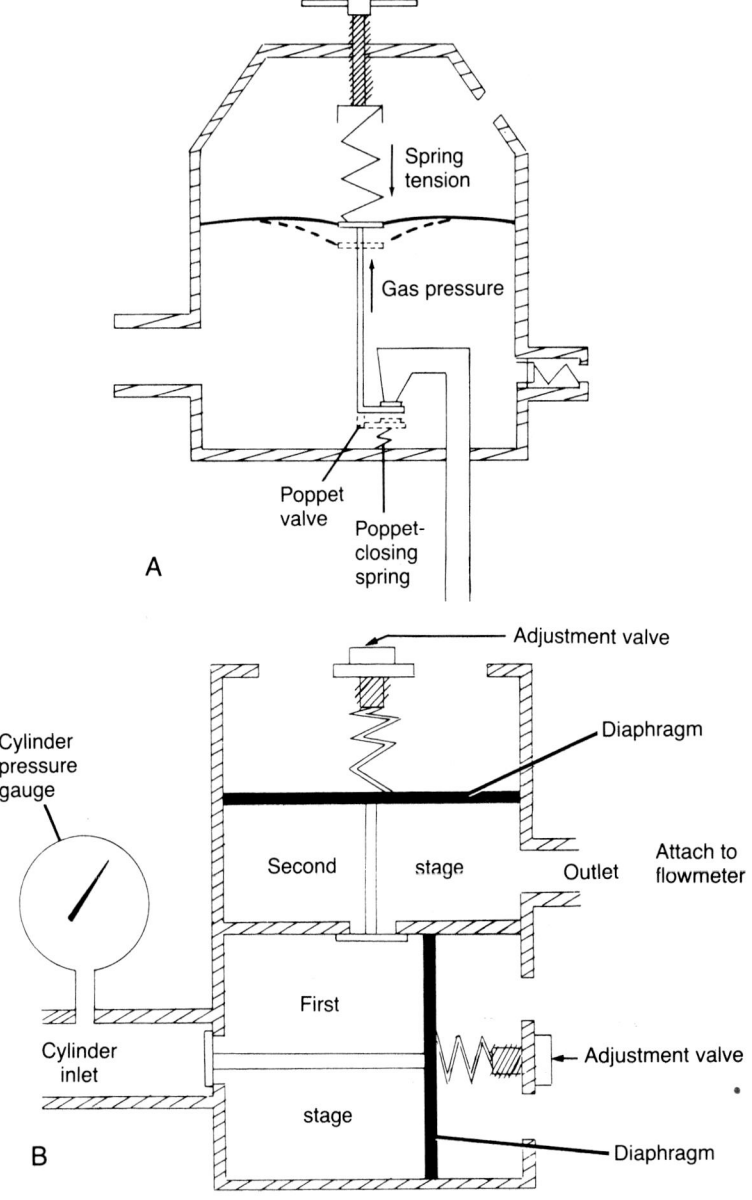

FIGURE 16–7. Medical gas regulators: *A*, Single-stage regulators. *B*, Multistage regulator. Note that the number of reduction chambers can be determined by counting the number of pop-off valves. (From McPherson, S.P.: *Respiratory Therapy Equipment*. 3rd ed. St. Louis, 1988, The C.V. Mosby Co.)

System (PISS). The following is a summary of each system.

American Standard Safety System regulates the connections between compressed gas cylinders and attached equipment, such as regulators. These connections involve threaded outlets that are indexed by thread type, thread size, right- or left-handed threading, external or internal threading, and nipple-seat design. Left-handed threads are reserved for gas mixtures that cannot sustain life (e.g., those containing less than 20% oxygen, or enriched carbon dioxide, hydrogen, or helium).

Diameter Index Safety System includes regulations for removable threaded connectors that are subjected to pressures of 200 psi or less. Connections between gas pressure regulators, flow meters, oxygen proportionators, and threaded connectors are examples of equipment that follows DISS regulations.

Pin Index Safety System governs gas flow from the smaller cylinders like the E type cylinders. In this system, a post-type valve connects to a yoke fitting which compresses a washer against the flat valve face outlet. The yoke contains pins that are

ADMINISTRATION OF OXYGEN AND OTHER THERAPEUTIC GASES

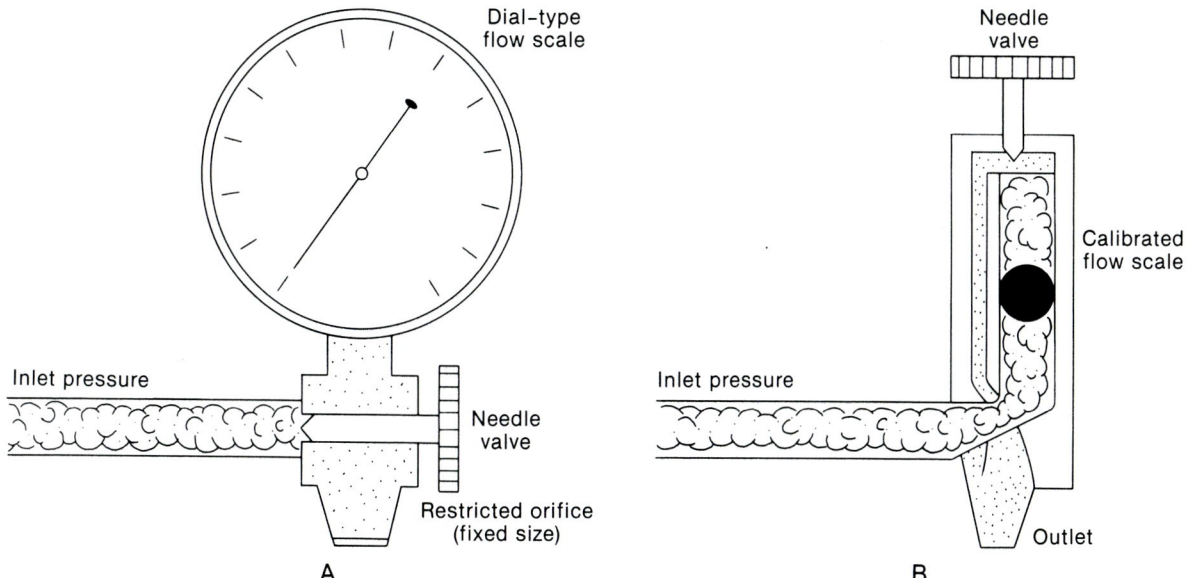

FIGURE 16–8. Oxygen flow meters: *A*, Bourdon gauge (uncompensated). *B*, Thorpe tube (compensated). (From Husinger, D.L., Lisnerski, K.L., Maurizi, J.J., and Philips, M.L.: *Respiratory Technology Procedures and Equipment Manual.* Reston, Va., Reston Publishing Co., 1980, with permission.)

placed in such a way as to be specific for a particular gas. Figure 16–9 shows examples of the safety systems.

INDICATIONS FOR OXYGEN THERAPY

In a recent report released by the American College of Chest Physicians (ACCP) and the National Heart, Lung, and Blood Institute (NHLBI), it was suggested that the primary indication for the initiation of oxygen therapy is the prevention and/or reversal of hypoxia, which can be defined as a deficiency of oxygen at the cellular level. Because present technology does not make it feasible to measure cellular oxygen tensions directly, the clinician must therefore rely on assumptions derived from the evaluation of oxygen delivery to the tissues (i.e., arterial Po_2, denoted by PaO_2), mixed venous oxygen tension ($P\bar{v}O_2$), and vital organ

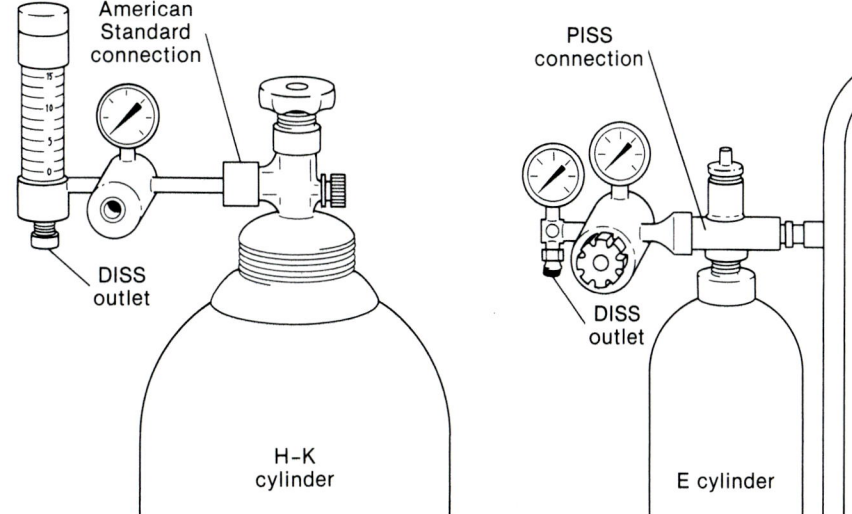

FIGURE 16–9. Safety systems for medical gas cylinders: *A*, American Standard Safety System. *B*, Diameter Standard Safety System. *C*, Pin Index Safety System. (From Spearman, C.B., Sheldon, R.L., and Egan, D.F.: *Egan's Fundamentals of Respiratory Therapy,* 4th ed. St. Louis, C.V. Mosby, 1982.)

function, particularly the brain, heart, and kidneys.

Generally, supplemental oxygen is indicated in acute situations in which there is laboratory documentation of a PaO_2 less than 60 torr or an oxygen saturation (SaO_2) less than 90% when a patient is breathing room air. Furthermore, initiation of oxygen therapy is appropriate prior to the documentation of hypoxemia whenever cellular hypoxia is suspected on clinical grounds, such as acute dyspnea or shock, or following a myocardial infarction.

The following is a brief review of the major types of hypoxia and how each of these states can affect oxygen delivery and utilization. It should be remembered that although our understanding of the scientific basis of oxygen therapy is increasing, it is still incomplete. Thus, the following recommendations for oxygen therapy are based on current knowledge.

Types of Hypoxia

As discussed in Chapter 4, hypoxia is generally classified into four categories: hypoxemic, anemic, hypoperfusion, and histotoxic.

Hypoxemic Hypoxia is associated with conditions in which the partial pressure of oxygen in arterial blood (PaO_2) is abnormally low, such as hypoventilation, diffusion impairments, ventilation-perfusion imbalances, and intracardiac and absolute intrapulmonary shunts, or during ascent to high altitudes. Hypoxemic hypoxia caused by hypoventilation, diffusion impairments, ventilation-perfusion mismatch, or ascent to high altitudes can be treated quite effectively with enriched oxygen mixtures. Oxygen therapy is not effective in treating intracardiac and absolute intrapulmonary shunts. Also, it is not able to correct the *hypercapnia* (increased $PaCO_2$) that is associated with hypoventilation. In fact, administering oxygen to someone who has a reduced sensitivity to carbon dioxide, such as a patient with severe chronic bronchitis, can lead to problems because breathing enriched oxygen would raise the PaO_2 and lessen the "hypoxic drive."

Anemic Hypoxia. Conditions in which hemoglobin is unable to combine effectively with oxygen lead to anemic hypoxia. As discussed in Chapter 4, carbon monoxide intoxication, methemoglobinemia, and sulfhemoglobinemia are examples of anemic hypoxia that are commonly encountered by the cardiopulmonary specialist. In anemic hypoxia, the PaO_2 and PaO_2 are normal, but the arterial oxygen content, the $P\bar{v}O_2$, and the $C\bar{v}O_2$ are reduced. Although it is possible that breathing 100% oxygen mixtures can aid in the treatment of anemic hypoxia, the most effective therapy involves blood replacement. Carbon monoxide poisoning can also be treated effectively by placing the patient in a hyperbaric chamber so that an increased amount of oxygen can be dissolved in the patient's plasma. Although this therapy is quite effective in carbon monoxide poisoning, it has been used on only a limited scale owing to the high cost of purchasing and maintaining these devices.

Hypoperfusion Hypoxia occurs when the cardiac output is severely reduced, such as during septic shock. Mixed venous PO_2's and oxygen contents are reduced in this form of hypoxia while the PaO_2, PaO_2, and CaO_2 remain normal. Generally, oxygen therapy is ineffective in treating hypoxia caused by a reduction in cardiac output.

Histotoxic Hypoxia occurs when the amount of oxygen delivered to the tissues is sufficient, but because of abnormal cellular chemistry, the tissue cells are unable to utilize oxygen for energy metabolism. Cyanide poisoning is an example of histotoxic hypoxia because cyanide blocks the reaction of cytochrome oxidase with oxygen in oxidative phosphorylation. The PaO_2, PaO_2, and CaO_2 are all normal and the $P\bar{v}O_2$ and $C\bar{v}O_2$ are high. As one would expect, oxygen therapy is not effective in the treatment of histotoxic hypoxia because any oxygen delivered to the cells cannot be utilized.

Physiologic Response to Hypoxia

The cardiopulmonary response to hypoxia depends on the type and severity of hypoxia, the ra-

TABLE 16–4. Physiologic Effects of Hypoxia

Body System	Signs and Symptoms
Cardiovascular system	Hypotension
	Bradycardia
	Sudden hypertension
	Tachycardia
	Arrhythmias
	Cyanosis
Pulmonary system	Tachypnea
	Dyspnea
Central nervous system	Depressed mental activity
	Headache
	Paranoia
	Nausea
	Increased CSF pressure

pidity of its onset, the duration of the hypoxic episode, and the patient's physiologic reserve capacity.

The physiologic effects of hypoxia are shown in Table 16–4. Acute hypoxia results from a relatively rapid decrease in oxygen availability, such as occurs during ascent to altitude, central hypoventilation due to depressant drugs or anesthetics, carbon monoxide poisoning, or cyanide intoxication, or following myocardial infarction. Chronic hypoxia occurs in persons living at high altitude for prolonged periods and in patients with chronic obstructive pulmonary diseases or congenital cardiac defects.

ADMINISTERING ENRICHED OXYGEN MIXTURES

As noted earlier, oxygen therapy is effective in the treatment of most types of hypoxemic hypoxia and, to some extent, can aid in the treatment of anemic hypoxia; it cannot, however, reverse the effects of hypoperfusion or histotoxic hypoxia. The aim of oxygen therapy, therefore, is to provide a sufficient amount of oxygen in the inspired air to fully utilize the oxygen-carrying capacity of arterial blood. In most cases, this can be accomplished by maintaining the patient's PaO_2 between 60 and 90 torr. At PaO_2's below 60 torr, the patient must be functioning on the steep portion of his or her oxyhemoglobin dissociation curve, and small decreases in PaO_2 result in very large decreases in SaO_2 and CaO_2. At PaO_2's greater than 90 torr, hemoglobin is almost fully saturated with oxygen and very large changes in PaO_2 result in only small changes in SaO_2 and thus CaO_2. (For patients with chronic obstructive pulmonary disease, the PaO_2 is usually maintained between 50 and 70 torr because higher PaO_2's depress the patient's hypoxic drive and may lead to respiratory arrest.)

A number of devices are available for administering enriched oxygen mixtures to spontaneously breathing subjects. Generally, they are divided into low-flow and high-flow systems. *Low-flow devices* do not provide all of the patient's inspiratory volume, and thus, the patient must entrain room air to make up for this deficit. The FiO_2 varies with the amount of air entrained by the patient. *High-flow devices* have either fixed air-oxygen entrainment ratios or reservoir capacities that are adequate to provide all of the patient's inspired volume and flow needs. The FiO_2 in high-flow systems remains fairly constant and is not affected by the patient's ventilatory pattern.

Nasal catheters, nasal cannulas, simple oxygen masks, face tents, and partial rebreathing masks are examples of low-flow systems. Air-entrainment devices are examples of high-flow systems.

Nasal Catheters

One of the first devices used to administer enriched oxygen was the nasal (oropharyngeal) catheter. As Figure 16–10 shows, these devices are made of soft rubber or plastic and have multiple holes at their terminal end. Oxygen catheters are available in 8 to 10 French sizes for children and 12 to 14 French sizes for adults. At flow rates of 4 to 15 L per minute, nasal catheters can provide FiO_2's of 0.24 to 0.5 depending on the ventilatory pattern of the patient.

The following is a brief description of the procedure for inserting a nasal catheter:

1. Before inserting the catheter, the distance between the patient's nose and earlobe is measured and marked on the catheter with a piece of surgical adhesive tape. This approximates the distance that the catheter should be inserted into the patient's nose.

2. The terminal end of the catheter is coated with a water-soluble lubricant and the flow rate of oxygen is set at 4 to 6 L per minute to insure that the catheter is patent. Note that oxygen delivered through a nasal catheter should be humidified before it is administered to the patient because administering dry gases can irritate the mucosa of the respiratory tract.

3. Using the natural contour of the catheter, the catheter is slowly advanced into one of the nares until it appears in the oropharynx just below the uvula. The catheter is then retracted slightly until it is no longer seen. If resistance is met when inserting the nasal catheter, it should be withdrawn, and insertion through the other naris should be attempted. If obstruction is encountered in both nares, an alternative means of oxygen administration should be used.

4. The catheter is taped to the patient's nose and face to avoid inadvertent dislodging, and the flow rate is adjusted to meet the ventilatory and oxygenation demands of the patient.

The major complications encountered when administering oxygen via nasal catheters include irritation of the nasal mucosa and gastric distention. Mucosal irritation occurs when high oxygen flow rates are used (flow rates greater than 8 L per minute) and if the gas is not humidified adequately.

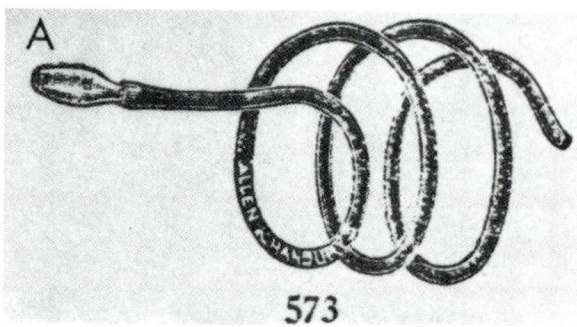 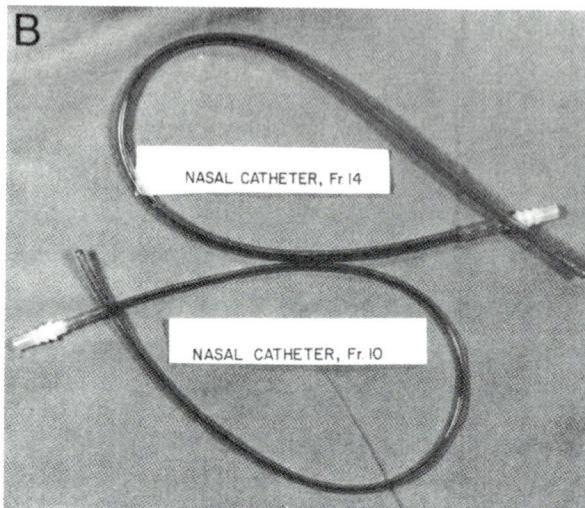

FIGURE 16-10. *A,* A vintage oxygen inhaler with glass mouthpiece. (From Leigh, J.M.: The evolution of the oxygen therapy apparatus. *Anaesthesia* 29:462–485, 1974, reproduced with permission). *B,* Nasal catheter. (From Barnes, T.A.: *Respiratory Care Practice.* Chicago: Year Book Medical Publishers, 1988.)

Gastric distention occurs if the catheter is inserted too far, so that it presses against the epiglottis. Nasal catheters should be used with caution in comatose or debilitated patients because loss of epiglottal reflexes in these patients can also lead to gastric distention.

Nasal catheters are not used extensively in oxygen therapy because they are uncomfortable for patients to wear for prolonged periods and because they should be changed about every 8 hours. They are useful, however, for patients who have experienced facial trauma and are thus unable to use other oxygen delivery systems, such as a nasal cannula or a face mask.

Nasal Cannulas

Nasal cannulas (prongs) represent an another means of delivering enriched oxygen mixtures through the nose. These devices have two hollow soft plastic prongs, which are positioned about ½ inch inside the external nares (Fig. 16–11). Nasal cannulas can deliver $F_{I}O_2$'s between 0.24 and 0.50, depending on the flow rate used and the patient's ventilatory pattern. Because the fractional concentration of oxygen delivered through a nasal cannula to a patient is influenced not only by the volume of oxygen delivered by the cannula per minute but also by the total ventilatory needs of the patient, the oxygen concentration varies for any given flow rate of oxygen as the patient's inspiratory flow changes. The following table summarizes average oxygen concentrations that can be delivered via a nasal cannula, assuming that the patient's inspiratory volume is stable.

Flow Rate (L/min)	Approximate $F_{I}O_2$
1–2	0.24–0.28
3–5	0.28–0.35
6–9	0.35–0.45
10–15	0.45–0.50

Generally, the oxygen concentration increases from 2% to 5% with each liter per minute increase in the oxygen flow rate. Prolonged use of high flow rates can cause irritation of the tips of the external nares and also of the frontal sinuses. For these reasons, oxygen flow rates of 2 to 4 L per minute are typically used for long-term oxygen therapy.

Simple Oxygen Masks

Figure 16–12 shows a simple oxygen mask. These devices are made of plastic and cover the nose and mouth. The patient's inspired gases are derived from the source gas and by entrainment of room air through the ports located on the sides of the mask; exhaled gases are vented through these side ports.

Simple oxygen masks are available in both adult and pediatric sizes. At flow rates of 6 to 12 L per minute, simple oxygen masks can deliver $F_{I}O_2$'s between 0.35 to 0.65. (It is important that the oxygen flow rate be sufficient to prevent carbon diox-

ADMINISTRATION OF OXYGEN AND OTHER THERAPEUTIC GASES

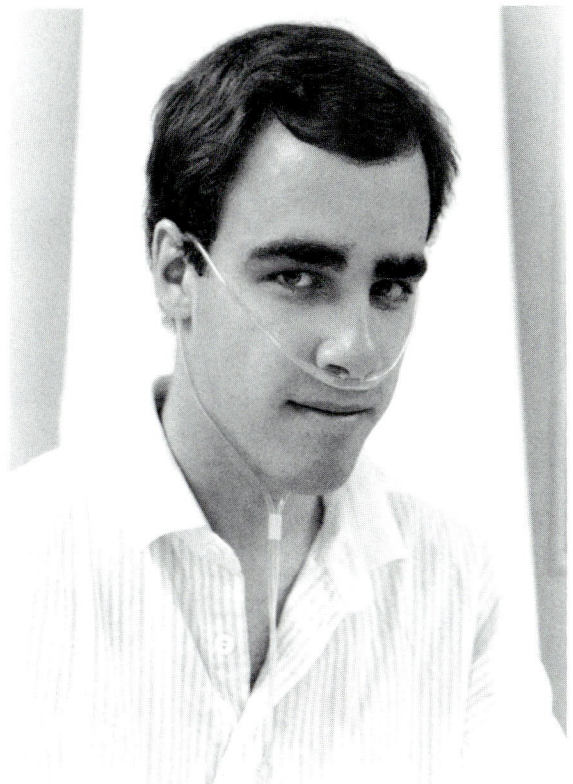

FIGURE 16–11. Nasal cannula.

ide retention within the mask—usually a flow rate of 6 L per minute prevents this from occurring.) The following is a list of approximate F_IO_2's that can be delivered via a simple oxygen mask for several oxygen flow rates:

Flow Rate (L/min)	Approximate F_IO_2
6–8	0.35–0.45
8–10	0.45–0.55
10–12	0.55–0.65

Face Tents

These devices are used to treat patients who require oxygen and high levels of humidification (Fig. 16–13). A constant flow of gas that is saturated with water vapor is administered to the patient via wide-bore tubing connected to the mask inlet. The patient's exhaled gases are vented out of the top of the face tent. Face tents can deliver F_IO_2's between 0.30 to 0.50. The F_IO_2 is set by adjusting an air entrainment port that is incorporated into the nebulizer unit (discussed later).

Partial Rebreathing Masks

Partial rebreathing masks are similar in design to the simple oxygen mask, except that they are equipped with a reservoir bag (Fig. 16–14). During a normal expiration, the reservoir bag fills with source gas and part of the patient's exhaled gases. (Usually, the first third of the exhalation enters the reservoir bag along with source gas, which is in-

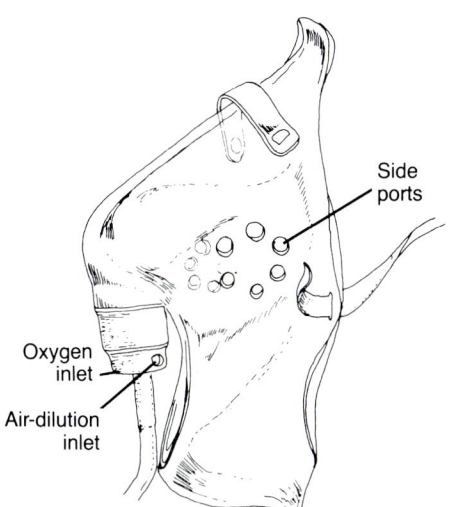

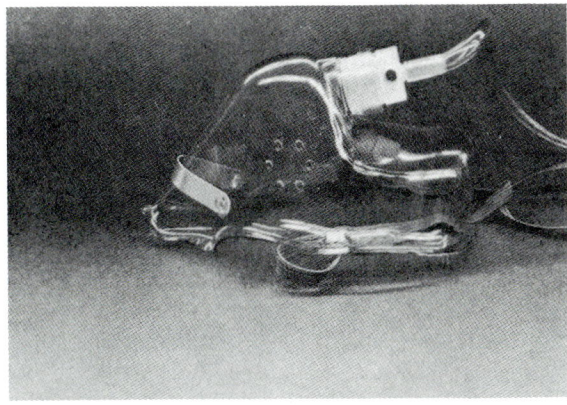

FIGURE 16–12. Simple oxygen mask. (Reproduced by permission from: McPherson, S.P.: *Respiratory Therapy Equipment*, 3rd ed. St. Louis, 1985, The C.V. Mosby Co.)

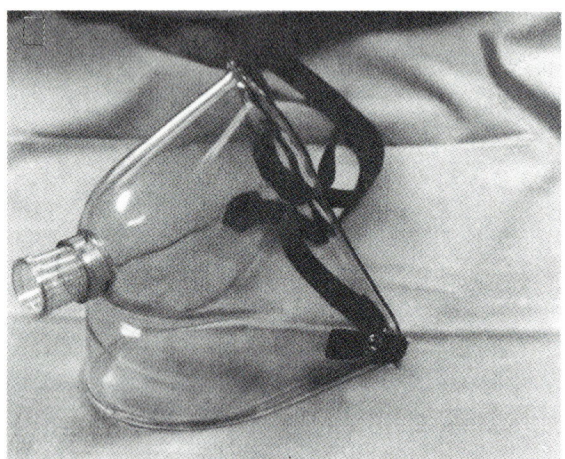

FIGURE 16–13. Oxygen face tent. (From Barnes, T.A.: *Respiratory Care Practice.* Chicago: Year Book Medical Publishers, 1988.)

troduced at a rate of 6 to 10 L per minute; the remainder of the exhalation is vented through ports located on the sides of the mask.) During the subsequent inspiration, therefore, the patient breathes a mixture containing source gas plus the part of the previous exhaled breath that entered the reservoir bag. Remember that this rebreathed gas contains a high oxygen concentration and a low carbon dioxide concentration because the exhaled gas from the previous breath was derived primarily from the anatomic deadspace.

Partial rebreathing masks can deliver F_IO_2's of 0.30 to 0.60 depending on the oxygen flow rate used and the patient's inspiratory volume. Note that the oxygen flow rate should be set high enough that the bag does not collapse on inspiration.

Nonrebreathing Masks

Nonrebreathing masks have reservoir bags like the partial rebreathing masks but in addition have a set of one-way valves located at the opening between the bag and the mask and over the side ports of the mask. (Usually, one of the valves over the side ports is removed as a safety precaution in the event that the gas flow into the reservoir bag is interrupted or that the valve between the mask and the bag fails to open during an inspiratory effort by the patient).

As Figure 16–15 shows, the valves on a nonrebreathing mask are positioned in such a way that during inspiration, the valve between the bag and mask opens while the valve over the side ports remains closed. Conversely, during expiration, the valve between the mask and the bag closes, and the side port valve(s) opens. The only gas that the patient can inspire must come from the reservoir bag because all of the exhaled gas is directed to the atmosphere and the side ports are closed during inspiration, thus preventing the entrainment of room air.

As with the partial rebreathing mask, the flow rate of source gas into the bag should be sufficient

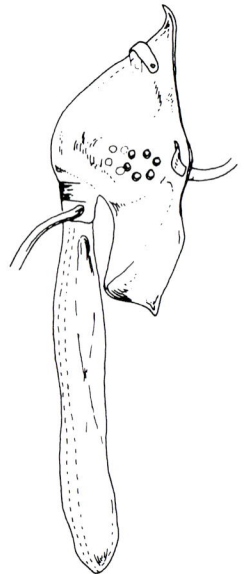

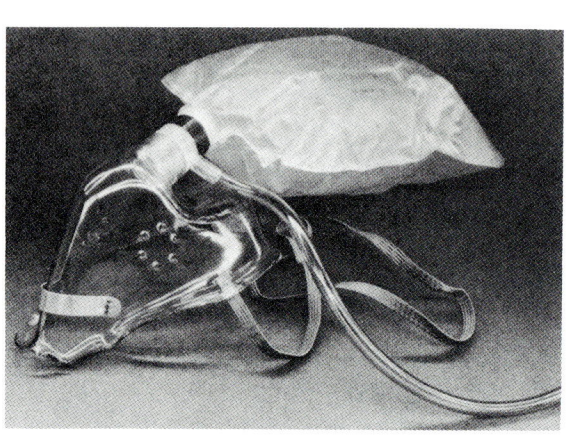

FIGURE 16–14. Partial rebreathing mask. (Reproduced by permission from: McPherson, S.P.: *Respiratory Therapy Equipment,* 3rd ed. St. Louis, 1985, The C.V. Mosby Co.)

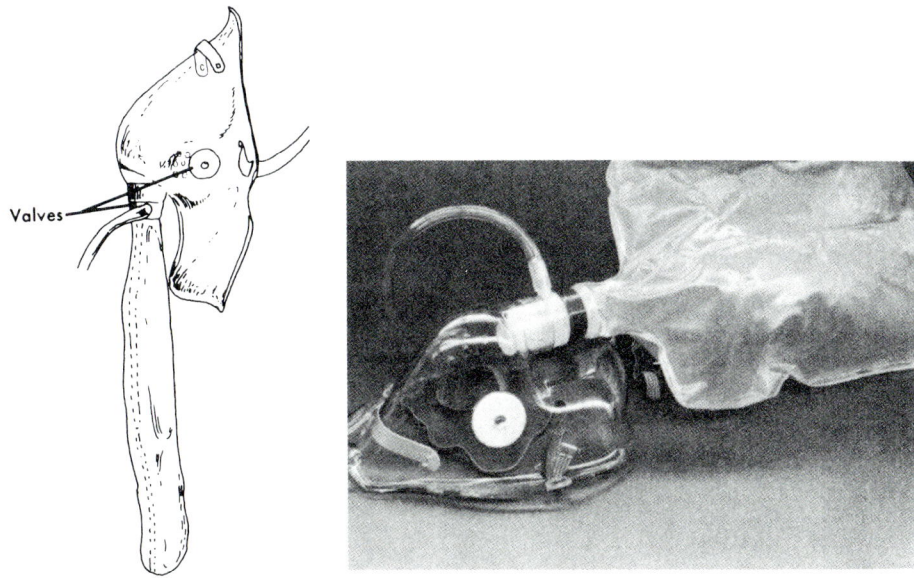

FIGURE 16–15. Nonrebreathing mask. (Reproduced by permission from: McPherson, S.P.: *Respiratory Therapy Equipment*, 3rd ed. St. Louis, 1985, The C.V. Mosby Co.)

that the bag does not completely collapse during an inspiratory effort by the patient. Theoretically, nonrebreathing masks should be able to deliver F_{IO_2}'s of 1.00 as long as the patient's entire inspiratory volume and flow demands are being provided from the reservoir bag. In practice, disposable nonrebreathing masks actually deliver F_{IO_2}'s of 0.90 ± 0.10 because of the loose fit of the mask on the patient's face.

Rebreathing Masks

Although these devices are not routinely used clinically to administer oxygen to patients, they are used in anesthesia to prevent anesthetic gases from escaping into the atmosphere. Because all of the patient's inspiratory volume is being supplied via the rebreathing device, these masks can be referred to as a high-flow oxygen system. Figure 16–16 illustrates a typical rebreathing system. Note that it contains a mask or an adaptor that connects to the patient, a reservoir bag, a source of oxygen, and a means of removing exhaled carbon dioxide. As the patient breathes into and out of the reservoir bag, carbon dioxide is removed by passing the exhaled gas through an absorbent such as calcium hydroxide while oxygen is added to replace the oxygen used by the patient. Full rebreathing systems can provide F_{IO_2}'s of 1.00.

Air-Entrainment Devices

Air-entrainment devices, which include the so-called Venturi-type masks, represent a high-flow

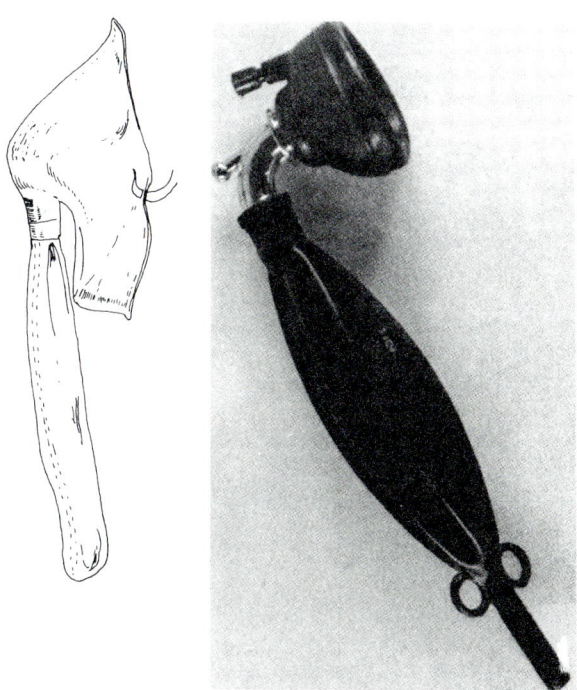

FIGURE 16–16. Rebreathing system. (Reproduced by permission from: McPherson, S.P.: *Respiratory Therapy Equipment*, 3rd ed. St. Louis, 1985, The C.V. Mosby Co.)

oxygen system because the volume and FIO_2 of the gas mixture delivered to the patient is preset and therefore controlled.

As Figure 16–17 shows, air-entrainment masks operate on the *Bernoulli* principle. As a gas flows through a tube at a high linear velocity, the lateral wall pressure of the tube can become subatmospheric, thus causing entrainment of room air through ports located along the sides of the tube. The volume of room air entrained depends on the linear velocity of the gas flowing through the tube and the size of the entrainment ports. The FIO_2 of the gas being administered can therefore be varied by changing the diameter of the jet or the diameter of the entrainment ports. Table 16–5 shows the air-oxygen entrainment ratios and the volume of gas delivered to the patient for several oxygen concentrations.

As long as the mask's total gas output meets or exceeds the patient's inspiratory volume and flow needs, the FIO_2 remains stable. For this reason, air-entrainment masks are often used to deliver oxygen to patients who require fairly constant FIO_2's, such as patients with chronic obstructive pulmonary disease. As stated earlier, the stimulus for breathing in many of these patients is hypoxia. Inadvertent administration of high FIO_2's for prolonged periods can therefore lead to respiratory arrest and eventual death.

TABLE 16–5. Air–Oxygen Entrainment Ratios

FIO_2	Air:O_2 Entrainment Ratio	Total Liter Gas Flow*
0.24	25:1	97 LPM at an oxygen flow of 4 LPM
0.28	10:1	68 LPM at an oxygen flow of 6 LPM
0.35	5:1	48 LPM at an oxygen flow of 8 LPM
0.40	3:1	32 LPM at an oxygen flow of 8 LPM
0.60	1:1	Total gas flow is twice oxygen flow

* Total liter gas flow expressed as liters per minute (LPM).

T-Tubes and Tracheostomy Masks

For patients who have an oral or nasal endotracheal tube or a tracheostomy tube in place, humidified oxygen can be administered via a T-tube or tracheostomy mask (Fig. 16–18). At flow rates of 10 to 15 L per minute, these devices can deliver FIO_2's of 0.35 to 1.0. The amount of oxygen delivered to the patient is set by adjusting an air entrainment port located on the nebulizer unit that is used to humidify the gas (discussed later).

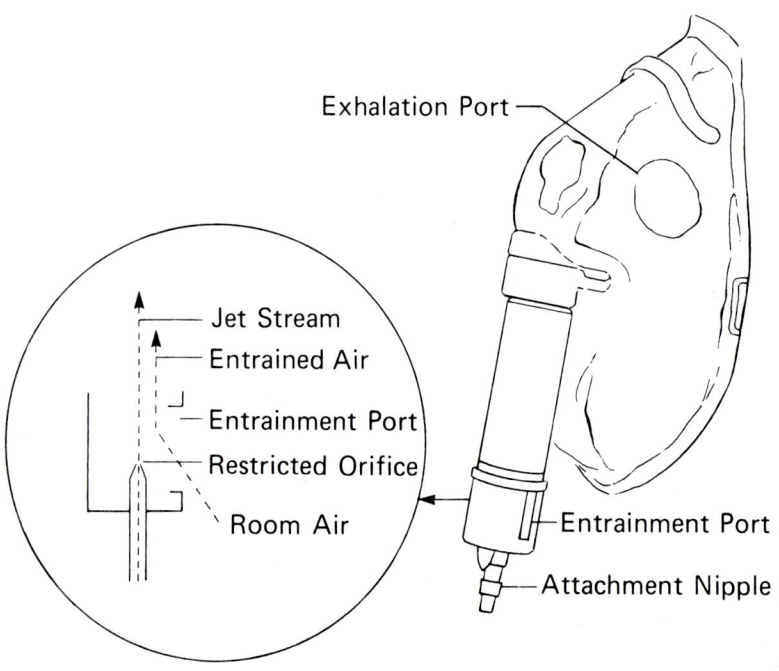

FIGURE 16–17. Air-entrainment mask. (From Epstein, J., and Gaines, J.: *Clinical Care of the Adult Patient.* Bowie, Md., Robert J. Brady Co., 1983, with permission.)

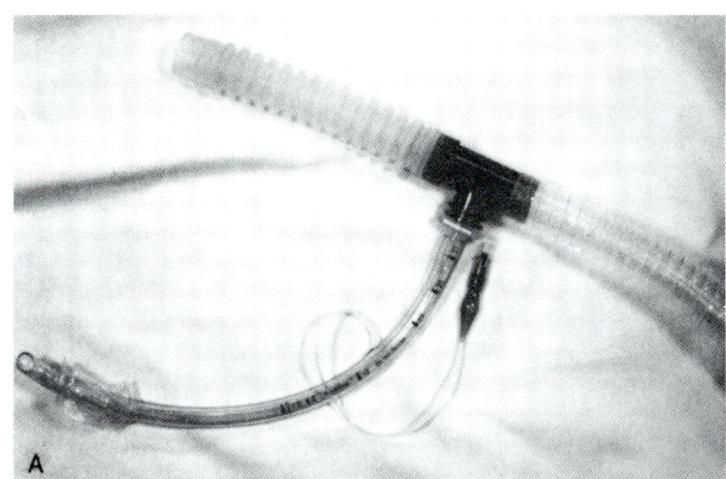

FIGURE 16–18. T-connector and tracheostomy mask used to administer aerosol therapy to patients with an endotracheal tube or tracheostomy tube in place. (Modified from Barnes, T.A.: *Respiratory Care Practice.* Chicago: Year Book Medical Publishers, 1988.)

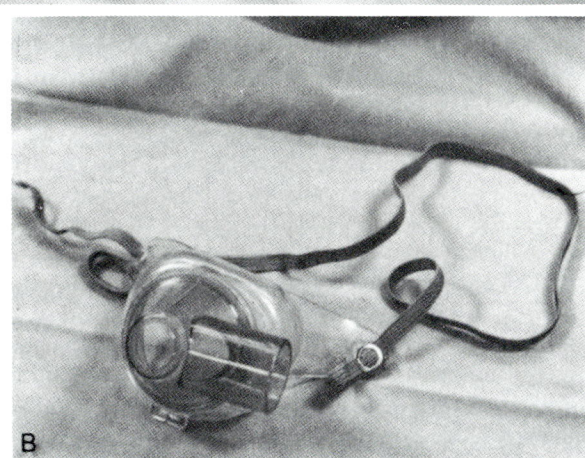

Environmental Oxygen Therapy Devices

Environmental oxygen therapy devices include oxygen tents and croupettes, oxyhoods, incubators, and hyperbaric chambers. All can provide an environment in which the concentration of oxygen as well as the environmental temperature and humidity can be partially or completely controlled.

Oxygen Tents and Croupettes (croup tents) are most often used for pediatric patients who require high humidity in an oxygen-enriched environment, but who are unable to tolerate either oxygen masks or face tents. They are also used to administer enriched oxygen mixtures with high humidity to burn patients, who also cannot tolerate standard oxygen therapy devices.

As Figure 16–19 shows, a typical *oxygen tent* is an electrically powered apparatus with a canopy that surrounds the patient. The FIO_2's that can be delivered to a patient with an oxygen tent are limited to about 0.40 to 0.50. To prevent carbon dioxide retention within the tent, the flow rate of source gas into the tent is set at 15 L per minute. The temperature of the gas flowing through the tent is controlled with a refrigeration unit, which uses Freon as a coolant fluid. Normally, the temperature in the tent is maintained at 10 to 12 degrees below room temperature to keep a cool environment. The moisture content of the gas within the tent is regulated using a humidifier or an aerosol generator.

Croupettes are miniature canopy units that are pneumatically powered by either compressed air or oxygen (Fig. 16–20). They are used to deliver oxygen therapy or humidity therapy (or both) to infants and toddlers with croup, epiglottitis, pneumonia, or atelectasis. When oxygen is used as the source gas, FIO_2's of 0.60 to 0.70 can be achieved at flow rates of 8 to 10 L per minute, as long as

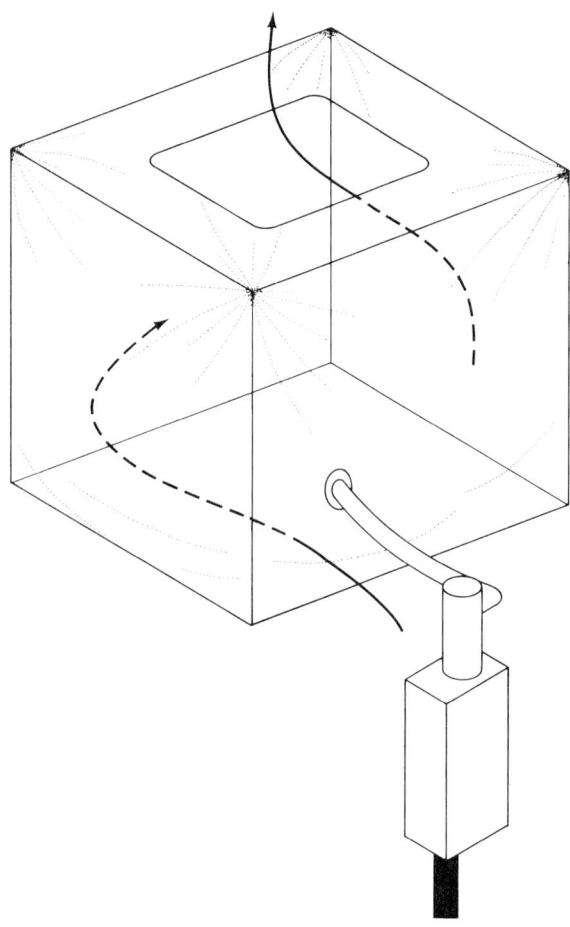

FIGURE 16–19. Oxygen tent. (Reproduced with permission from Barnes, T.A., and Lisbon, A.: *Respiratory Care Practice*. Copyright © 1988 by Year Book Medical Publishers, Inc., Chicago.)

the canopy is tucked snugly under the patient's mattress and remains closed. The temperature of the gas within the tent is usually maintained at 6 to 8 degrees below room temperature for patient comfort. This is accomplished by using a cooling panel filled with cracked ice. Gas flowing into tent is humidified by passing the source gas through a bubble humidifier before it enters the tent.

Oxyhoods are constructed with clear plexiglass (Fig. 16–21). They are particularly useful for administering enriched oxygen mixtures to neonates and infants because they cover only the head and leave the rest of patient's body available for nursing care. The concentration of oxygen delivered to the child as well as the temperature and humidity content of the gas within the hood can be controlled by using an oxygen blender along with an appropriate humidification system. Generally, using source gas flow rates of 6 to 10 L per minute prevents carbon dioxide retention within the hood. It is important that the temperature of the gas being administered to the child be maintained at a neutral thermal temperature (37°C) since blowing cool gases over an infant's face can increase the metabolic rate and thus the amount of oxygen consumed by the infant (i.e., shivering generates heat through muscle contractions).

Incubators, unlike oxygen tents and croupettes, are primarily used to provide a warm environment for premature infants (remember that tents provide an environment with a temperature lower than room air). The temperature inside the incubator is usually regulated near the neutral thermal temperature. F_IO_2's of 0.40 and greater can be administered with incubators using a compen-

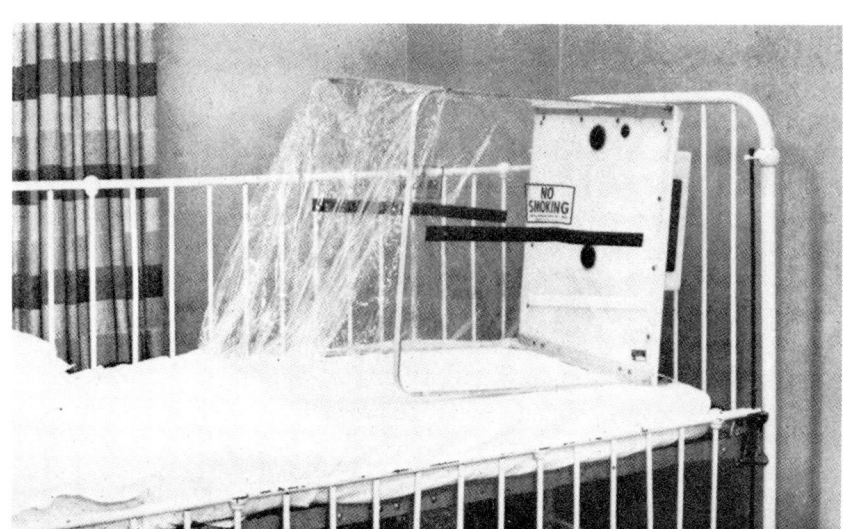

FIGURE 16–20. Croupette. (From Safar, P. (ed.): *Respiratory Therapy*. Philadelphia, F.A. Davis, 1965.)

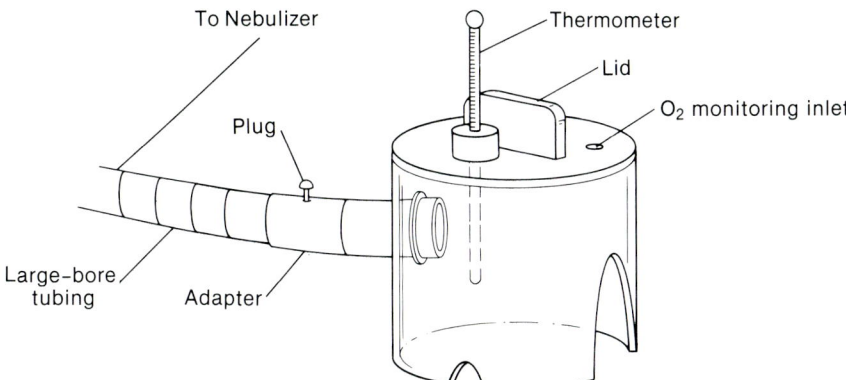

FIGURE 16–21. Oxyhood. (From Eubanks, D.H., and Borne, R.C.: *Comprehensive Respiratory Care: A Learning System.* St. Louis, C.V. Mosby, 1985.)

sated flow meter attached to the oxygen inlet of the incubator. Note that a red metal flag is attached to the oxygen inlet port of the incubator to show the F_{IO_2} being administered to the infant—in the down position, 0.40 is administered; in the up position, an F_{IO_2} greater than 0.40 is administered to the infant. Although this is a very good warning system for the therapist to check intermittently to determine what F_{IO_2} is being administered to the infant, it cannot replace the need to monitor the F_{IO_2} with an appropriate oxygen analyzer.

Hyperbaric Chambers, as the name implies, provide environments in which the ambient pressure is greater than 1 atm (14.7 psi). They are made of rigid steel and concrete. (In some cases, they are constructed with a special type of rigid plastic.) Most hyperbaric chambers used in medical gas therapy can achieve ambient pressures of 2 to 3 atm.

Hyperbaric chambers are classified as either *fixed multiplace chambers* or as *portable monoplace chambers* (Fig. 16–22). Multiplace chambers are walk-in devices that can hold three to four people comfortably; the monoplace chambers can hold only one person at a time.

The composition of the atmosphere inside the chamber is varied according to the chamber pressure being used. In most cases, a gas mixture of 80% nitrogen and 20% oxygen is used; however, 80% helium and 20% oxygen mixtures are also used.

Hyperbaric oxygen therapy has been shown to be quite effective in the treatment of carbon monoxide poisoning, burns, frostbite, gas gangrene, and decompression sickness (i.e., the bends or caisson disease). As stated previously, these devices have not been used extensively in clinical medicine because of their cost of construction and operation. Furthermore, a number of hazards are inherent in hyperbaric therapy, including:

1. Increased fire potential due to the complete saturation of materials contained within the chamber with chamber gas.
2. Increased incidence of pneumothorax because of changes in lung pressure induced by hyperbaric ambient pressures.
3. Ruptured eardrums in patients with occluded eustachian tubes.
4. Increased potential for developing oxygen toxicity.

COMPLICATIONS OF OXYGEN THERAPY

Among the complications that can occur during the administration of enriched oxygen mixtures are respiratory depression, atelectasis, circulatory depression, pulmonary oxygen toxicity, and retrolental fibroplasia. For the most part, these complications can be prevented by careful monitoring of the oxygen concentrations being delivered to the patient as well as the patient's oxygenation status. The various analytical techniques used to monitor oxygen therapy are discussed in Chapter 10.

The following is a brief review of the major physiologic complications encountered during the therapeutic administration of oxygen.

Respiratory Depression. As stated earlier, administration of enriched oxygen mixtures to patients whose major stimulus to breathing is hypoxia can lead to respiratory arrest and eventual death. Initially, somnolence or even coma occurs as a result of hypoventilation and subsequent hypercapnia (i.e., increased Pa_{CO_2}). To prevent this complication, oxygen should be administered at relatively low concentrations (less than 30%), and

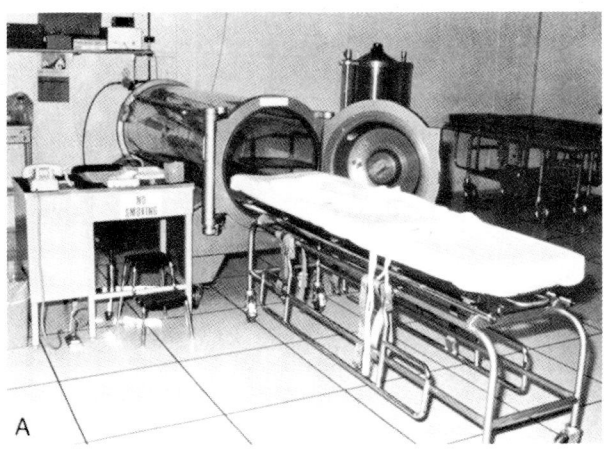
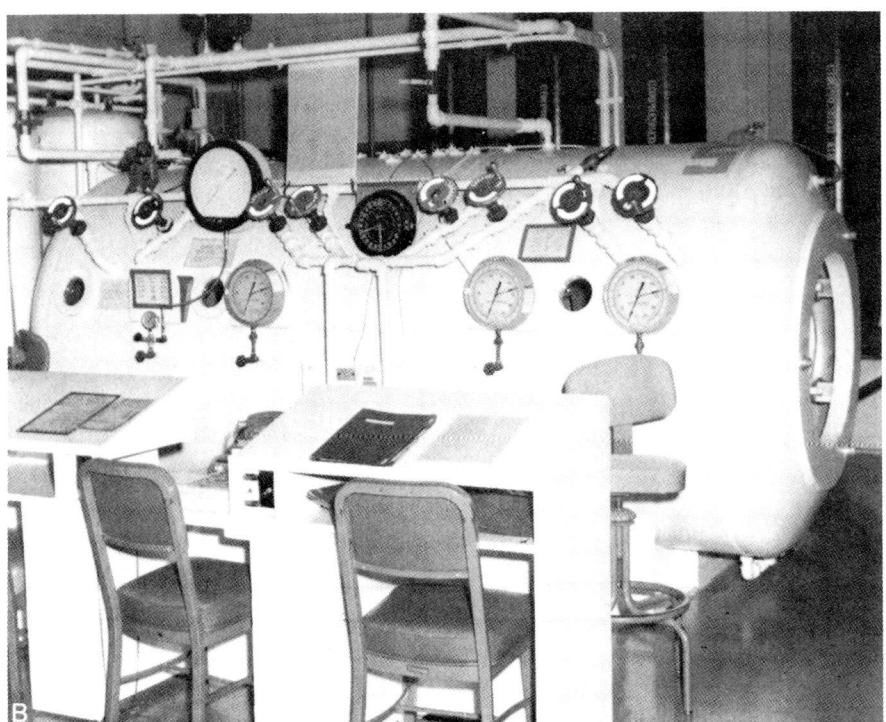

FIGURE 16–22. Hyperbaric chambers: *A,* Portable monoplace chamber. *B,* Fixed multiplace chamber. (From Davis, J.C., and Hunt, T.K.: *Hyperbaric Oxygen Therapy.* Bethesda, Md., Undersea Medical Society, Inc., 1977.)

the patient should be observed carefully for any signs of respiratory depression. Additionally, arterial blood gases should be monitored on a regular basis (e.g., daily).

Atelectasis. When high concentrations of oxygen are administered over a prolonged period, nitrogen is washed out of the patient's lungs and may lead to what is termed *absorption atelectasis.* This condition occurs because the only gases remaining in the patient's alveoli after breathing the enriched oxygen mixtures are oxygen, carbon dioxide, and water vapor. Obstruction of the airways leads to absorption of oxygen from the alveoli by the pulmonary circulation, and the total gas volume in the alveoli decreases. Atelectasis occurs with the decrease in alveolar volume.

Circulatory Depression. The cardiovascular response to hypoxia involves increased sympathetic tone and a consequent peripheral vasoconstriction. Plasma volume decreases as fluid moves into the interstitial space. With the administration of oxygen, the vasoconstriction is inhibited, and the resulting vasodilation can lead to circulatory collapse. Although this problem is not often encountered in patients requiring oxygen therapy, the clinician should not overlook it because the consequences are extremely serious or life-threatening.

Pulmonary Oxygen Toxicity. Prolonged exposure to oxygen can damage the lung; if exposure continues, the damage may prove fatal. Generally, oxygen toxicity—also known as adult respiratory distress syndrome (ARDS) or bronchopulmonary dysplasia (BPD) in neonates—is divided into two stages: an early exudative stage and a late proliferative stage. The early exudative phase is characterized by alveolar edema, pulmonary congestion, and intra-alveolar hemorrhage, along with the formation of hyaline membranes. The late proliferative phase is characterized by increased alveolar edema, pronounced hyperplasia (an increased number of cells) of the alveolar epithelial cells, and alveolar fibrosis.

Retrolental Fibroplasia (RLF) is a fibrotic lesion in the posterior chamber of the eye that can lead to permanent blindness. It is generally limited to premature infants who have been exposed to excessively high oxygen concentrations at birth. The retinal changes, which result from arteriolar vasoconstriction, appear as early as 3 to 6 weeks of age.

To date, studies have shown that RLF can be avoided by administering oxygen concentrations of 40% or less to premature infants. When higher F_IO_2's are required, arterial blood gases should be monitored routinely because the incidence of RLF is related more to excessively high PaO_2's than to high F_IO_2's.

HELIUM-OXYGEN THERAPY

Helium is a colorless and odorless gas that has an atomic weight of 4.003 daltons and a density of 0.1785 gm/L. It is classified as noncombustible and nonflammable, and it is only slightly soluble in water. Helium is chemically inert and therefore does not participate in any biochemical process within the body.

Helium-oxygen (or *heliox*) mixtures are sometimes used to treat patients with airway obstruction because they have a lower density than that of air. An 80% helium and 20% oxygen mixture has a density of 0.429 gm/L; air has a density of 1.293 gm/L, so the heliox mixture is about one third as dense as oxygen. A 70% helium and 30% oxygen mixture is also available. Remember from earlier discussions in Chapters 1 and 3 that when the density of a gas increases, the chance of generating turbulent flow becomes greater as the velocity of gas flow increases (Reynold's number). Furthermore, if the diameter of the airway is decreased, as occurs in patients with chronic obstructive pulmonary disease, the likelihood of generating turbulent airflow is even further enhanced.

By using a gas mixture that is less dense than air (typically 80% helium and 20% oxygen), it is reasonable to assume that there is a better distribution of gas within the lung because of a reduced tendency to generate turbulent airflow. Furthermore, the lower density of the heliox mixture compared with ambient air reduces the amount of driving pressure required to achieve any given airflow.

The only notable side effect of breathing a heliox mixture is that the patient's voice may be transiently distorted. Otherwise, helium-oxygen mixtures have been shown to be completely safe. Heliox mixtures can be administered through a tightly fitting mask or through an inspiratory positive-pressure breathing device. Remember that, because of a difference in the density of a helium-oxygen mixture compared with that of air or oxygen, the use of air or oxygen flow meters to deliver a helium-oxygen mixture results in inaccurate flow rate readings (the indicated flow rate on the air or oxygen flow meter is lower than it actually is for the helium-oxygen mixture). This inaccuracy can be corrected by multiplying the value read from the flow meter by 1.8 because oxygen is approximately 1.8 times more dense than a helium-oxygen gas mixture.

CARBON DIOXIDE–OXYGEN THERAPY

Carbon dioxide is an odorless, colorless gas that has a density approximately 1.5 times more than that of air. Carbon dioxide does not support combustion and cannot support life when administered alone. It makes up approximately 0.03% of the atmosphere and is the major by-product of animal metabolism and the combustion of carbonaceous fuels. Carbon dioxide is available commercially as a gas, a liquid, and a solid. Cylinders typically contain a mixture of gaseous and liquid carbon dioxide. It is relatively nonreactive and nontoxic in low concentrations. When it is combined with water, carbonic acid is formed. Carbonic acid in high concentrations is corrosive to most metals.

For medical purposes, oxygen is combined with purified carbon dioxide (99.9% purity) in a typical 95:5 ratio, that is, 95% oxygen and 5% carbon dioxide. (Mixtures of 90% oxygen and 10% carbon dioxide are also used for medical purposes and are commonly referred to as *carbogen*.) Because breathing CO_2-O_2 mixtures is a powerful respiratory center stimulant and a potent vasodilator, it is sometimes used to treat hypoventilation due to low tidal volumes and as a method to improve cerebral blood flow. It has also been used to treat singultus, or hiccups. Although the mechanism by which breathing hypercapnic mixtures can stop hiccups is uncertain, it has been suggested that this stimulates the respiratory center, which responds by sending a rhythmic discharge of impulses to the diaphragm. The increased number of impulses reaching the diaphragm overrides the spasmodic contractions associated with hiccups, and a normal ventilatory pattern may be restored.

When administering carbogen mixtures to patients, the treatment must not last longer than 10 minutes, and the patient must be observed for any side effects, such as dyspnea, elevation of arterial blood pressure, headache, dizziness, altered vision, muscle tremors, and paresthesia.

Carbon dioxide is also used in many nonmedical applications, for example, in the manufacture of carbonated beverages, in refrigeration, and as a fire-extinguishing agent.

HUMIDIFICATION OF MEDICAL GASES

Humidification of inspired gases is essential for the proper functioning of the respiratory system. As discussed in Chapter 3, the upper airways under normal circumstances provide sufficient heat and humidity to warm inspired gases to 37°C and fully saturate them with water by the time they reach the alveoli. (Alveolar air contains approximately 44 mg of water vapor per liter of gas inhaled. Water vapor exerts a pressure of 47 torr at a temperature of 37°C.)

For patients receiving medical gas therapy, it is necessary to supplement the body's normal humidification system because therapeutic gases are dry and can irritate the respiratory mucosa, reduce mucociliary transport, and cause drying and retention of lung secretions. This is especially true if the patient's upper airways are bypassed by tracheostomy or an endotracheal tube.

In the following section, two techniques commonly used to add moisture to inspired gases are discussed—evaporation and aerosol generation. Before reading this section, refer to Table 16–6, which lists several definitions necessary for a full understanding of the principles of humidity and aerosol therapy.

Evaporating Devices

Pass-over, bubble, and cascade humidifiers are typical evaporating devices (Fig. 16–23). These devices deliver humidity in the form of water vapor or what is sometimes called gaseous water.

In the *pass-over* (blow-by) *humidifier*, the inspired gas is simply passed over a heated reservoir of water and then delivered to the patient. This type of humidifier is only moderately effective in adding moisture to inspired gas because the gas contacts the water surface for such a limited amount of time. Most units have a heater incorporated to increase the evaporation of water.

The *bubble humidifier* is the type most commonly used in respiratory therapy. With this device, the source gas is conducted below the surface of the water reservoir and allowed to bubble to the top. In many bubble humidifiers, the source gas is passed through a ground stone to break the water up into smaller bubbles. Bubble humidifiers are generally more effective than the simple pass-over

TABLE 16–6. Terminology for Humidity and Aerosols

Term	Definition
ATPS	Ambient temperature and pressure saturated with water vapor (37°C, 760 mmHg)
BTPS	Body temperature and ambient pressure saturated with water vapor
Absolute humidity	Actual amount of water contained in a given volume of gas expressed in grams per cubic meter or milligrams per liter
Relative humidity	Amount of water vapor actually present in a volume of air, compared with the amount of water vapor necessary to fully saturate that volume of air at the same temperature
Percent body humidity	Amount of water in a volume of air, compared with the amount of water vapor in air saturated at body temperature
Humidity deficit	Amount of water that the respiratory mucosa must supply to the inspired air to achieve 100% saturation in the alveoli

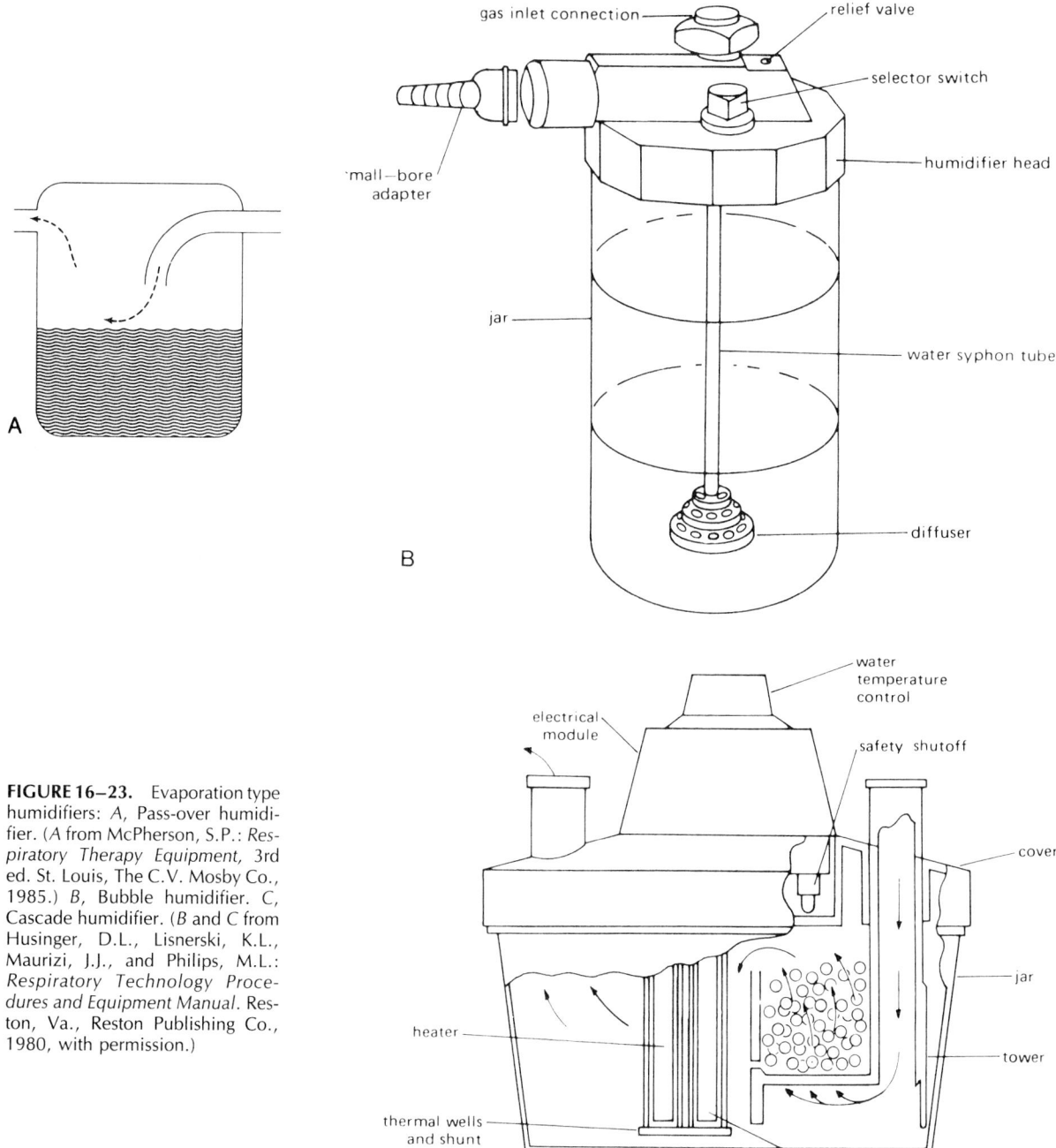

FIGURE 16-23. Evaporation type humidifiers: *A*, Pass-over humidifier. (*A* from McPherson, S.P.: *Respiratory Therapy Equipment*, 3rd ed. St. Louis, The C.V. Mosby Co., 1985.) *B*, Bubble humidifier. *C*, Cascade humidifier. (*B* and *C* from Husinger, D.L., Lisnerski, K.L., Maurizi, J.J., and Philips, M.L.: *Respiratory Technology Procedures and Equipment Manual*. Reston, Va., Reston Publishing Co., 1980, with permission.)

humidifiers because the surface area available for evaporation and the time of exposure of water to the gas are increased. Heating jackets that fit around the humidifier jar can be added to raise the temperature of the water and increase the evaporation rate of water and thus the relative humidity of the gas.

The *cascade humidifier* is similar to the bubble humidifier except that the source gas is bubbled through a reservoir tower that contains a plastic mesh floor. As Figure 16-23 shows, the mesh floor serves to increase the air-liquid interface, and thus the evaporation rate of water is augmented. The evaporation rate of water can be further enhanced by heating the water in the reservoir to temperatures up to 60°C. The gas is delivered to the patient from the cascade through large-bore corrugated tubing. The temperature drop of the gas between the cascade and the patient averages about 2°C for every foot of tubing.

Aerosol-Generating Devices

Jet humidifiers, Babington devices, and ultrasonic nebulizers are examples of aerosol-generating devices. These devices add moisture to inspired gases in the form of water droplets. Aerosol particles that range from 1 to 5 μ in diameter can be deposited in the nose, trachea, pharynx, bronchi, or alveoli, depending on the size of the particles. Aerosol particles over 5 μ in diameter are usually removed by the nasal filtering process; aerosol particles 1 to 3 μ in diameter are generally deposited in the alveoli. (A micron equals 0.000001 meter or 1/25,000 of an inch.) Aerosol distribution and deposition are also influenced by gravity, the pattern of ventilation, particle stability, and inertial impaction.

Figure 16–24 is a diagram of a *jet nebulizer*. These devices operate on the Bernoulli principle. As gas flows through a jet, the air pressure around the jet decreases, and water is drawn into the capillary tube. When the water reaches the gas stream, it is shattered into small particles. The gas stream is directed at a baffle that serves to reduce the size of the aerosol particles by removing large water droplets. A side port is incorporated into the gas inlet for the entrainment of room air.

Jet nebulizers are usually described as either mainstream or sidestream devices. In mainstream devices, the major portion of the gas being delivered to the patient passes through the nebulizer while a jet that is powered by an additional gas source controls the amount of liquid nebulized. With sidestream devices, the main gas delivered to the patient does not pass through the nebulizer, but instead, the nebulizer is positioned as a side accessory, and the nebulized liquid enters the mainstream of gas from the side. Figure 16–25 illustrates both types of nebulizers.

Jet nebulizers can provide a high relative humidity with particles ranging from 1 to 40 μ in diameter. (The relative humidity from an unheated jet averages about 60%; jet nebulizers can provide 100% relative humidity when heated to 37°C.) Jet nebulizers are available as hand-held nebulizers (volume capacity of about 15 ml) that can be used for intermittent aerosol therapy or with large reservoirs (volume capacity of 250 ml to 1 L) for long-term continuous therapy. In the large reservoir devices, a Venturi device is sometimes incorporated so that the volume of air entrained into the nebulizer unit can be controlled. (F_IO_2's of 0.35, 0.50, 0.70, and 1.00 are usually possible.) It should be noted that the water output from the nebulizer decreases as the amount of air entrained by the device decreases.

Like jet nebulizers, *Babington nebulizers* use a jet of air to break water into small droplets. As Figure 16–26 shows, the Babington device operates on the following principle: a high-pressure (usually 50 psi) gas source is supplied to the inside of a hollow sphere that has a continuous film of water covering it; gas exiting the sphere through a small port contacts the water film and forces the water droplets onto a baffle opposite the gas outlet port on the sphere. Excess water drains to a reservoir located below the sphere and then recirculates to form the film of water on the outer surface of the sphere. These devices can produce a high relative humidity, with the majority of the

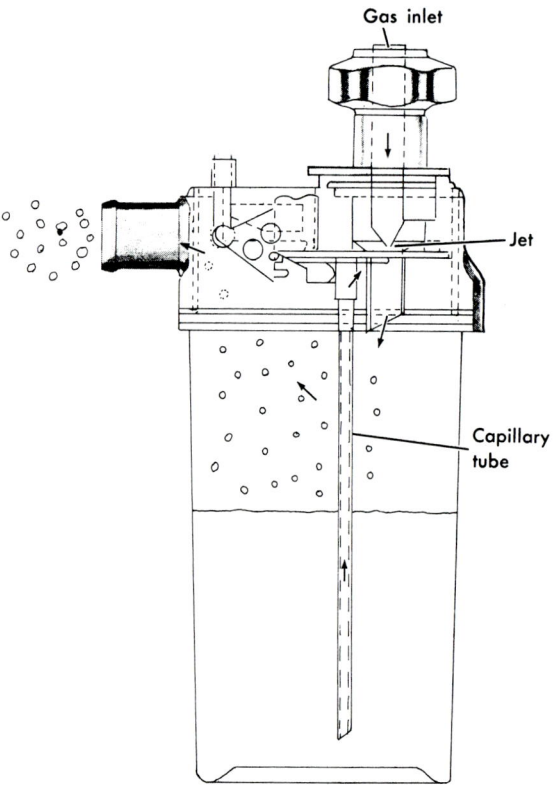

FIGURE 16–24. Jet nebulizer. (From McPherson, S.P.: *Respiratory Therapy Equipment*, 3rd ed. St. Louis, 1985, The C.V. Mosby Co.)

through an ultrasonic device using a cup that sits within a couplant fluid. The size of the particles produced by an ultrasonic nebulizer is determined by the frequency of the sound waves, and the total volume of particles generated is controlled by the amplitude. In general, ultrasonic nebulizers produce aerosol particles that average about 3 μ or less in diameter.

Ultrasonic nebulizers are most often used for intermittent aerosol therapy, but they are also used for long-term continuous therapy. (An example of the latter technique is to incorporate an ultrasonic mist into a croupette, but remember that the patient's fluid balance should be monitored in those receiving continuous aerosol therapy.)

Aerosol therapy can be provided intermittently or continuously. Intermittent aerosol therapy is used in conjunction with chest physiotherapy and postural drainage to liquify and clear excessive amounts of mucus from the lung. Intermittent aerosols are also used to deliver drugs, such as bronchodilators. Continuous aerosols are generally used to add high humidity to the inspired gases of patients who have had their upper airways bypassed with a tracheostomy or endotracheal tube.

Aerosol therapy can be administered to spontaneously breathing subjects by attaching the aerosol generator to an aerosol mask, which is similar in design to the simple oxygen mask. Patients who

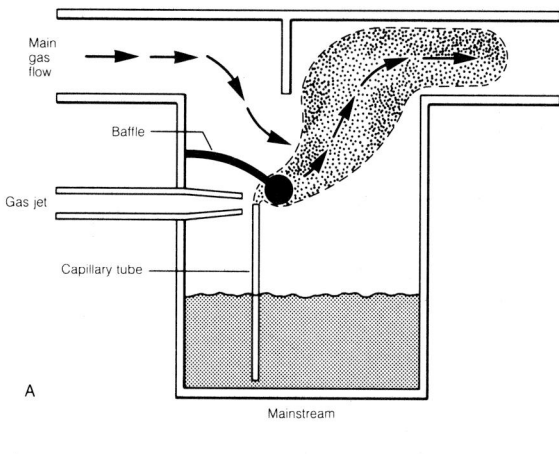
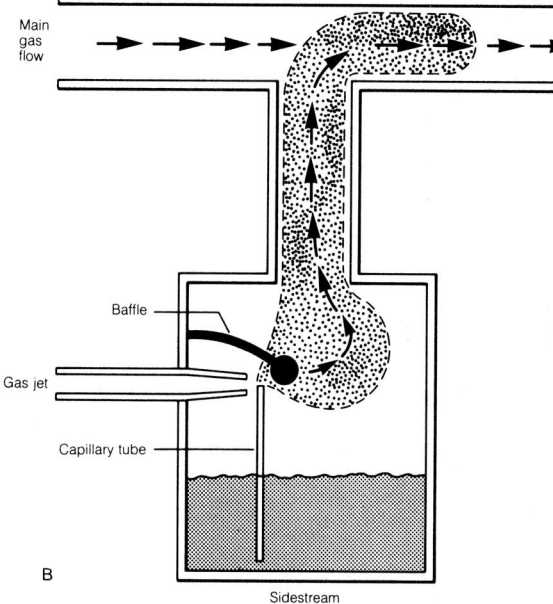

FIGURE 16–25. Two types of jet nebulizers: *A*, Mainstream device. (Courtesy of Bird Products Corporation, Palm Springs, CA.) *B*, Sidestream device (courtesy of Puritan-Bennett Corporation, Overland Park, KS.). (From Barnes, T.A.: *Respiratory Care Practice.* Chicago: Year Book Medical Publishers, 1988.)

aerosol particles produced less than 5 μ in diameter.

Figure 16–27 shows an *ultrasonic nebulizer*. These devices use high-frequency sound (typically 1.35 MHz or 1.35 million cycles per second) to break water up into an aerosol mist. The high-frequency sound waves are produced when voltage is applied to a transducer with piezoelectric characteristics. Piezoelectric materials change their shape (i.e., vibrate) when voltage is applied to them (see Chapter 1).

Sterile distilled water can be administered

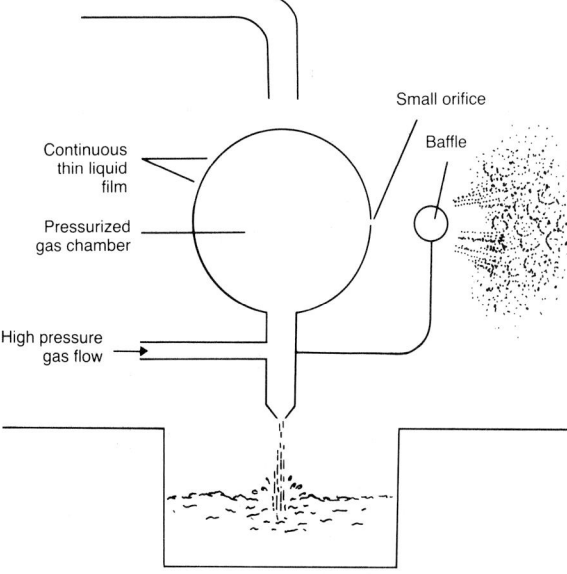

FIGURE 16–26. Babington nebulizer. (Reproduced by permission from: Eubanks, D.H., and Bone, R.C.: *Comprehensive Respiratory Care: A Learning System.* St. Louis, 1985, The C.V. Mosby Co.)

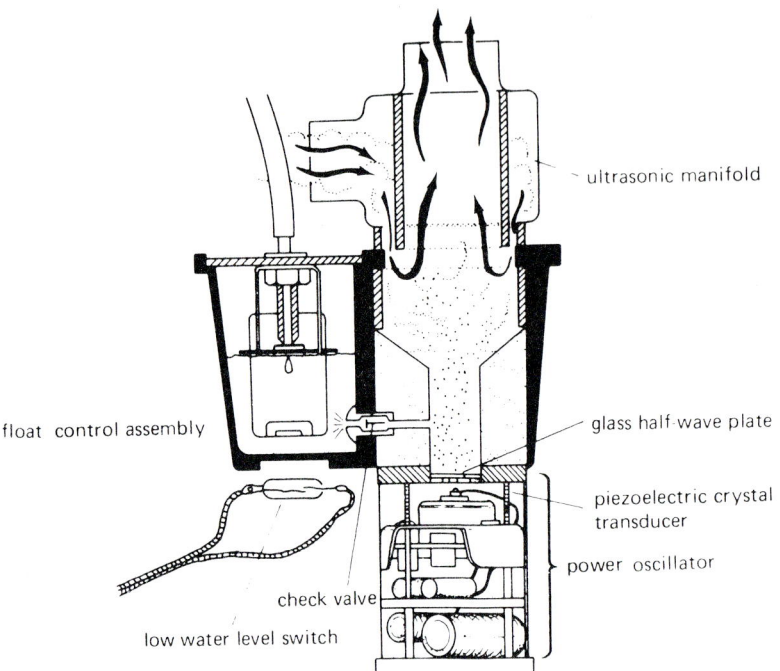

FIGURE 16–27. Ultrasonic nebulizer. (From Husinger, D.L., Lisnerski, K.L., Maurizi, J.J., and Philips, M.L.: *Respiratory Technology Procedures and Equipment Manual*. Reston, Va., Reston Publishing Co., 1980, with permission.)

have tracheostomy or endotracheal tubes in place can receive aerosol therapy via corrugated tubing with a T-connector attached directly to the tracheostomy or endotracheal tube. As discussed in Chapter 19, aerosol therapy may be administered in conjunction with mechanical ventilation. Most commercially available mechanical ventilators have an aerosol-generating device incorporated into their design. If the ventilator does not have this feature, a nebulizer can be inserted into the ventilator circuit on the inspiratory side of the circuit using a T-connector, thus not interfering with the flow of gas from the ventilator.

COMPLICATIONS OF HUMIDITY AND AEROSOL THERAPY

The most common problems encountered with humidity and aerosol therapy include overhydration with concomitant fluid and electrolyte disorders and an increased risk of developing nosocomial infections. These complications can occur particularly in neonates and severely debilitated patients. Another problem with aerosol therapy is bronchospasm caused by irritation of the bronchial mucosa from inhaling hypotonic and hypertonic solutions. Tracheal erosion and alterations in lung mechanics caused by changes in alveolar surface tension have also been reported in patients who were receiving continuous aerosolized normal saline solutions.

The problem of overhydration can be minimized by monitoring fluid and electrolyte balances and weight gain in patients receiving continuous humidity therapy. Monitoring these variables usually alerts the physician and staff to the possible effects of overhydration. With regard to preventing nosocomial infections through these devices, daily replacement of humidifiers and nebulizers should decrease their incidence. The organisms that have been mainly implicated in nosocomial infections include *Pseudomonas*, *Proteus*, *Flavobacterium*, *Herelea*, and *Alcaligenes*.

Bibliography

Anthonisen, N.R.: Hypoxemia and oxygen therapy. *Am. Rev. Respir. Dis.* 126:729–733, 1982.

American College of Chest Physicians and the National Heart, Lung, and Blood Institute: National conference of oxygen therapy. *Respir. Care* 29(9):922–935, 1984.

Arnold, W.H., Jr., and Grant, J.L.: Oxygen-induced hypoventilation. *Am. Rev. Respir. Dis.* 95:255, 1967.

Barnes, T.A. (ed.): *Respiratory Care Practice*. Chicago, Year Book, 1988.

Burton, G.G., and Hodgkin, J.E. (eds.): *Respiratory Care: A*

Guide To Clinical Practice. 2nd ed. Philadelphia, J.B. Lippincott, 1984.

Bushnell, S.S.: *Respiratory Intensive Care Nursing.* Boston, Little, Brown, 1973.

Campbell, E.J.M.: Oxygen administration. *Anesthesiology* 18:503, 1963.

Campbell, E.J.M.: Oxygen therapy in diseases of the chest. *Br. J. Dis. Chest* 58:149, 1964.

Cherniack, R.M., and Hakimpour, K.: The rational use of oxygen in respiratory insufficiency. *JAMA* 199:146, 1967.

Doershuk, C.F., Matthews, L.W., Gillespie, C.T., Lough, M.D., and Spector, S.: Evaluation of jet-type and ultrasonic nebulizers in mist tent therapy for cystic fibrosis. *Pediatrics* 41:723–732, 1968.

Dole, M.: The natural history of oxygen. *J. Gen. Physiol.* 49(Suppl.):5, 1965.

Dorsey, O.L.: The physical chemistry of the oxygen atom. *Respir. Therapy,* November/December, 1975.

Egan, D.F.: *Fundamentals of Respiratory Therapy,* 3rd ed. St. Louis, C.V. Mosby, 1977.

Eldridge, F., and Gherman, C.: Studies of oxygen administration in respiratory failure. *Ann. Intern. Med.* 68:569, 1968.

Eubanks, D.H., and Bone, R.C.: *Comprehensive Respiratory Care: A Learning System.* St. Louis, C.V. Mosby, 1985.

Forster, R.E., Dubois, A.B., Briscoe, W.A., and Fisher, A.B.: *The Lung: Physiologic Basis of Pulmonary Function Tests,* 3rd ed. Chicago, Year Book, 1986.

Frank, L., and Massaro, D.: Oxygen toxicity. *Am. J. Med.* 69:117–126, 1980.

Friedman, S.A., Weber, B., Briscoe, W.A., et al.: Oxygen therapy: Evaluation of various air-entrainment masks. *JAMA* 228:474, 1974.

Levitzky, M.G.: *Pulmonary Physiology,* 2nd ed. New York, McGraw-Hill, 1986.

Litt, M., and Swift, D.E.: The Babington nebulizer: A new principle for generation of therapeutic aerosols. *Am. Rev. Respir. Dis.* 105:308–310, 1972.

Martin, L.: *Pulmonary Physiology in Clinical Practice: The Essentials for Patient Care and Evaluation.* St. Louis, C.V. Mosby, 1987.

McPherson, S.P.: *Respiratory Therapy Equipment,* 3rd ed. St. Louis, C.V. Mosby, 1985.

Parks, C.R.: Mist therapy. Rationale and practice. *J. Pediatr.* 76:305–313, 1970.

Patz, A.: Oxygen administration to the premature infant. *Am. J. Ophthalmol.* 63:351, 1967.

Petty, T.L.: Continuous or nocturnal oxygen therapy in hypoxemic chronic obstructive lung disease: A clinical trial. *Ann. Intern. Med.* 93:391, 1980.

Petty, T.L.: *Ambulatory Oxygen.* New York, Thieme-Stratton, 1983.

Petty, T.L., and Neff, L.M.: The history of long-term oxygen therapy. *Respir. Care* 28:859, 1983.

Rau, J.L., Jr., and Rau, M.Y.: *Fundamental Respiratory Therapy Equipment: Principles of Use and Operation.* Sarasota, Fla., Glenn Educational Medical Services, 1977.

Sara, C., and Currie, T.: Humidification by nebulization. *Med. J. Aust.* 1:174–179, 1965.

Shapiro, B.A., Harrison, R.A., Kacmarek, R.M., and Cane, R.D.: *Clinical Application of Respiratory Care,* 3rd ed. Chicago, Year Book, 1985.

Stewart, B.N., Hood, C.I., and Block, A.J.: Long term results of continuous oxygen therapy at sea level. *Chest* 68:486, 1975.

OBJECTIVES

AFTER READING THIS CHAPTER, THE STUDENT WILL BE ABLE TO:

1. Explain how certain positions can facilitate the drainage of specific lung segments.
2. List the indications as well as the precautions for postural drainage treatments.
3. State the physical principle by which chest physical therapy promotes the mobilization of airway secretions.
4. Describe the techniques of percussion and vibration utilized in chest physical therapy.
5. List the sequence of events involved in producing a cough and state the adverse effects that can be produced by coughing.
6. List the various techniques utilized for breathing retraining.
7. Describe paradoxical breathing and the pathophysiology that produces it.
8. Enumerate the ways in which severe lung disease can interfere with normal activities of daily living and how exercise training can help improve exercise tolerance.
9. State the indications for airway suctioning.
10. Describe catheters utilized for airway suctioning.
11. Give the sequence of steps that should be followed during airway suctioning and explain the importance of oxygenation before, during, and after airway suctioning.
12. List the complications of airway suctioning and describe techniques to reduce their incidence or severity.
13. List the benefits that may be expected from incentive spirometry.
14. Differentiate the characteristics of a patient who should receive incentive spirometry versus a patient for whom inspiratory positive-pressure breathing would be more appropriate.
15. Describe an IPPB machine and explain how it works.
16. Discuss the contraindications for IPPB as well as its complications.

17
BRONCHOPULMONARY HYGIENE

CHAPTER OUTLINE

POSTURAL DRAINAGE
  Anatomic Basis
  Indications and Contraindications
CHEST PHYSICAL THERAPY
  Percussion
  Vibration
COUGHING AND BREATHING RETRAINING
  Coughing
  Cough Control
  Breathing Retraining

SUCTIONING PROCEDURES
  Airway Suctioning Technique
  Complications of Airway Suctioning
INCENTIVE SPIROMETRY
INSPIRATORY POSITIVE-PRESSURE BREATHING
  Administration of IPPB
  Complications of IPPB

BRONCHOPULMONARY HYGIENE

In a healthy person, normal physiologic mechanisms act to maintain bronchial hygiene and provide a clean conducting airway as well as ventilated alveoli. This requires that the bronchial glands and goblet cells produce secretions that are normal in quantity and consistency. In addition, the mucociliary escalator and cough mechanisms must function successfully to remove these secretions from the airway. An individual who is unable to clear the airway of pulmonary secretions develops airway plugging and subsequent collapse of the alveoli distal to the obstruction. In many pathologic states, certain treatment techniques to promote bronchopulmonary hygiene are utilized in order to:

1. Maintain the conducting airways clear of secretions.
2. Facilitate the drainage of alveoli that have been filled with secretions or infected material.
3. Decrease alveolar collapse and atelectasis.

The patient's ability to spontaneously clear the airway of secretions may be impaired when the production of airway secretions is increased, when the secretions have increased viscosity and tenacity, or when the patient is unable to cough effectively. The presence of secretions in the airway increases the work of breathing by increasing the resistance to airflow. If secretions totally occlude and plug the airway, then the subsequent absorption atelectasis distal to the obstruction results in pulmonary shunting. This shunting decreases the P_{O_2} of the arterial blood at a time when the patient has an increased oxygen demand due to the increased work of breathing. Bronchitis and other diseases that irritate the conducting airways result in increased secretion production. Dehydration or breathing dry gas, such as during general anesthesia, can result in tenacious, viscous secretions. Any debilitating illness or surgery (particularly of the abdomen or chest) weakens the patient's ability to produce an effective cough to clear the airway.

Certain bronchopulmonary hygiene maneuvers are utilized to help empty alveoli that have been filled with fluid (usually as a result of pneumonia). This material is called an *exudate* and is characterized by a high content of protein, inflammatory cells (white blood cells), or cellular debris. This material is not a *secretion* because secretions are the product of a gland. Drainage of exudates from the alveoli is beneficial because it removes this infected material from the body and returns the alveoli to their gas exchanging role, thus decreasing pulmonary shunt.

Patients who do not cough, sigh, or take deep breaths for prolonged periods of time develop alveolar collapse (absorption atelectasis) even without plugging of the airways by secretions. The pain and *splinting* (protecting the area of injury) following upper abdominal or chest surgery, for example, may inhibit a patient from coughing or taking deep breaths. This may produce alveolar collapse. The resulting decrease in the number of ventilated alveoli produces decreased compliance (increased elastic recoil of the lung), and increased work of breathing. The increased airways resistance caused by airway secretions also increases the work of breathing. To compensate for the pain and increased elastic work of breathing, the patient takes smaller, more rapid breaths. This cycle of decreased compliance and tidal volume and increased respiratory rate, airway resistance, and work of breathing usually results in ventilatory failure and the need for mechanical ventilation.

Bronchopulmonary hygiene techniques are utilized to break this cycle that frequently ends in ventilatory failure. These include postural drainage, chest physical therapy, suctioning procedures, coughing and breathing retraining, incentive spirometry, and inspiratory positive-pressure breathing (IPPB). These techniques may be used alone but are frequently used in combination to improve ventilation and decrease ventilation-perfusion mismatch.

POSTURAL DRAINAGE

Postural drainage is a technique that promotes the removal of secretions and fluid from the lung by taking advantage of gravity. Patients who remain supine or in a semisitting position for prolonged periods tend to pool fluid and secretions in the dependent portions of their lungs. Postural drainage and other bronchopulmonary hygiene techniques are utilized to reverse this process by mobilizing this material.

Anatomic Basis

The anatomy of the bronchial tree and its segmental organization is discussed in Chapter 3 (see Fig. 3–4). The arrangement of individual segmental bronchi determines the optimal position for drainage from a specific segment. The patient is positioned in such a way that the segment requiring drainage is directly above its segmental bronchus.

In this arrangement, gravity facilitates the movement of the secretions out of the affected portion of the lung, down the segmental bronchus, and into the large-diameter airways where they can be more easily removed. To augment the effects of gravity in mobilizing this material, percussion or vibration of the chest wall is performed. Additionally, the patient may be instructed to cough or make repeated throat-clearing efforts. Figure 17–1 illustrates several of the positions utilized for drainage of specific bronchopulmonary segments.

Indications and Contraindications

When postural drainage is ordered by a physician, the particular involved segments should be indicated. When postural drainage is included as a part of chest physiotherapy, the therapist must determine where his or her efforts should be concentrated. This can be done by determining which lobes or segments are involved by auscultation,

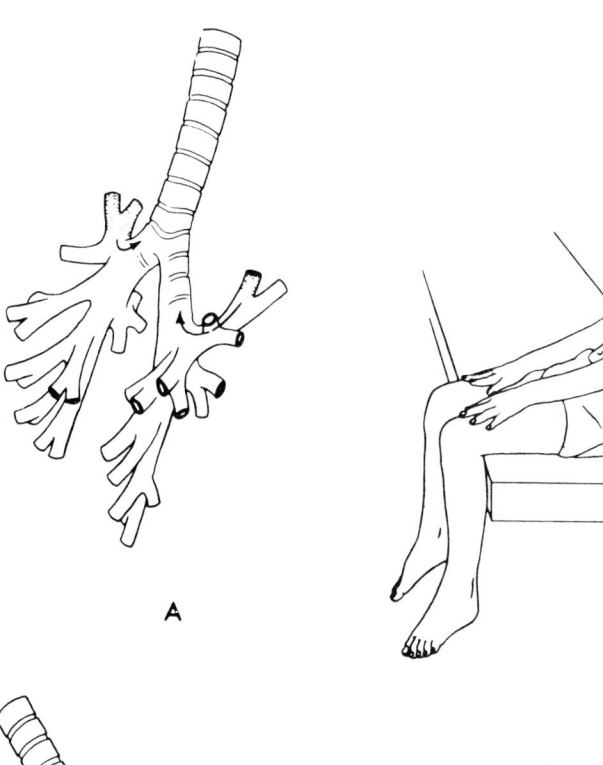

FIGURE 17–1. Postural drainage positions for specific bronchopulmonary segments. (From Kendig, E.L.: *Disorders of the Respiratory Tract in Children*. 3rd ed. Philadelphia, W.B. Saunders, 1977, with permission.)

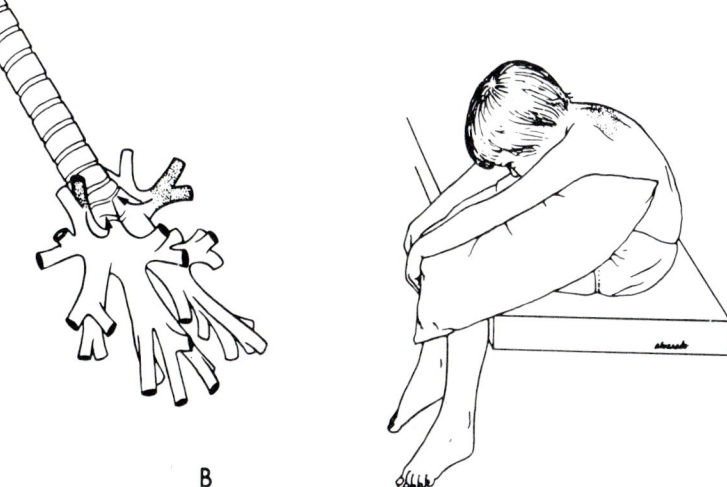

Illustration continued on following page

472 BRONCHOPULMONARY HYGIENE

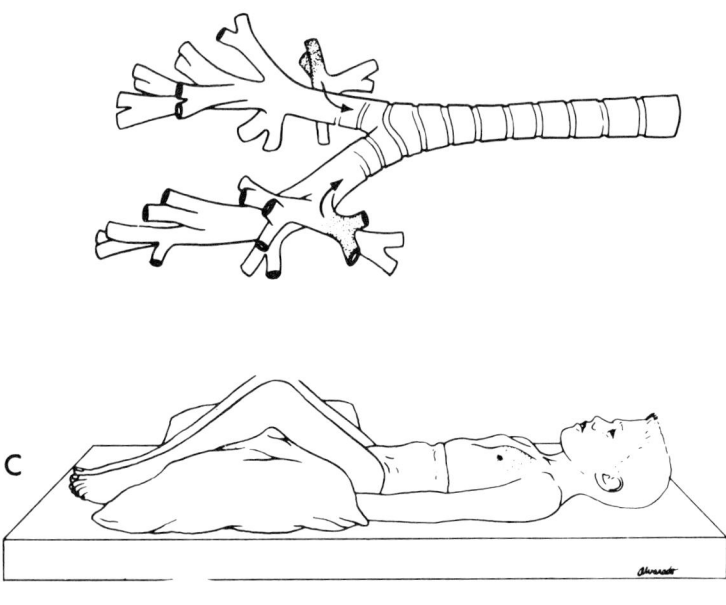

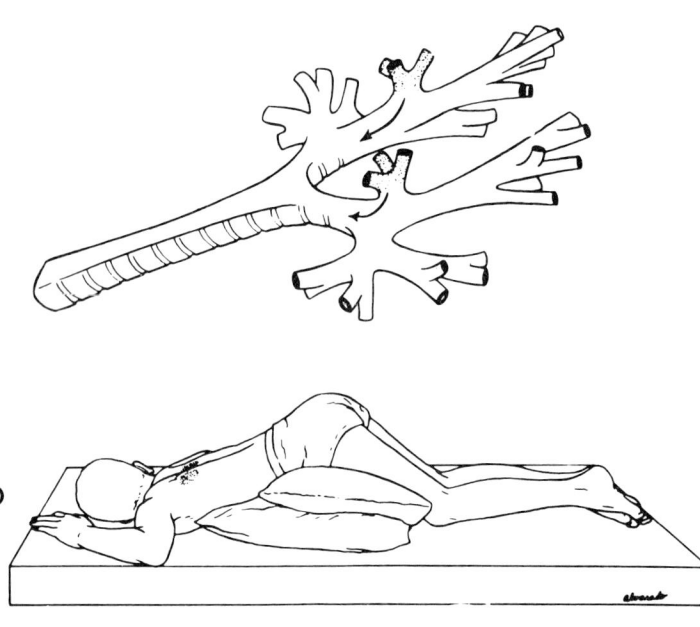

FIGURE 17–1 Continued

reviewing the patient's chart, and examining the chest radiographs.

Postural drainage is beneficial for suppurative lung diseases, such as pneumonia, bronchitis, and lung abscess (a collection of purulent material within the lung parenchyma). This technique is also useful for conditions such as bronchiectasis, cystic fibrosis, and chronic obstructive pulmonary disease in which increased sputum production or decreased mucus removal impedes airway hygiene. Postural drainage techniques are useful in patients who are paralyzed or weakened with neuromuscular disease, unconscious, or undergoing prolonged bedrest. In patients who are on prolonged mechanical ventilation, the mere presence of an endotracheal tube impedes the clearance of secretions from the airway. Additionally, patients who have experienced aspiration of gastric contents during induction of general anesthesia and those who have chronic aspiration from inadequate glottic mechanisms may benefit from postural drainage techniques.

Postural drainage should not be performed soon after the patient has eaten and is contraindicated

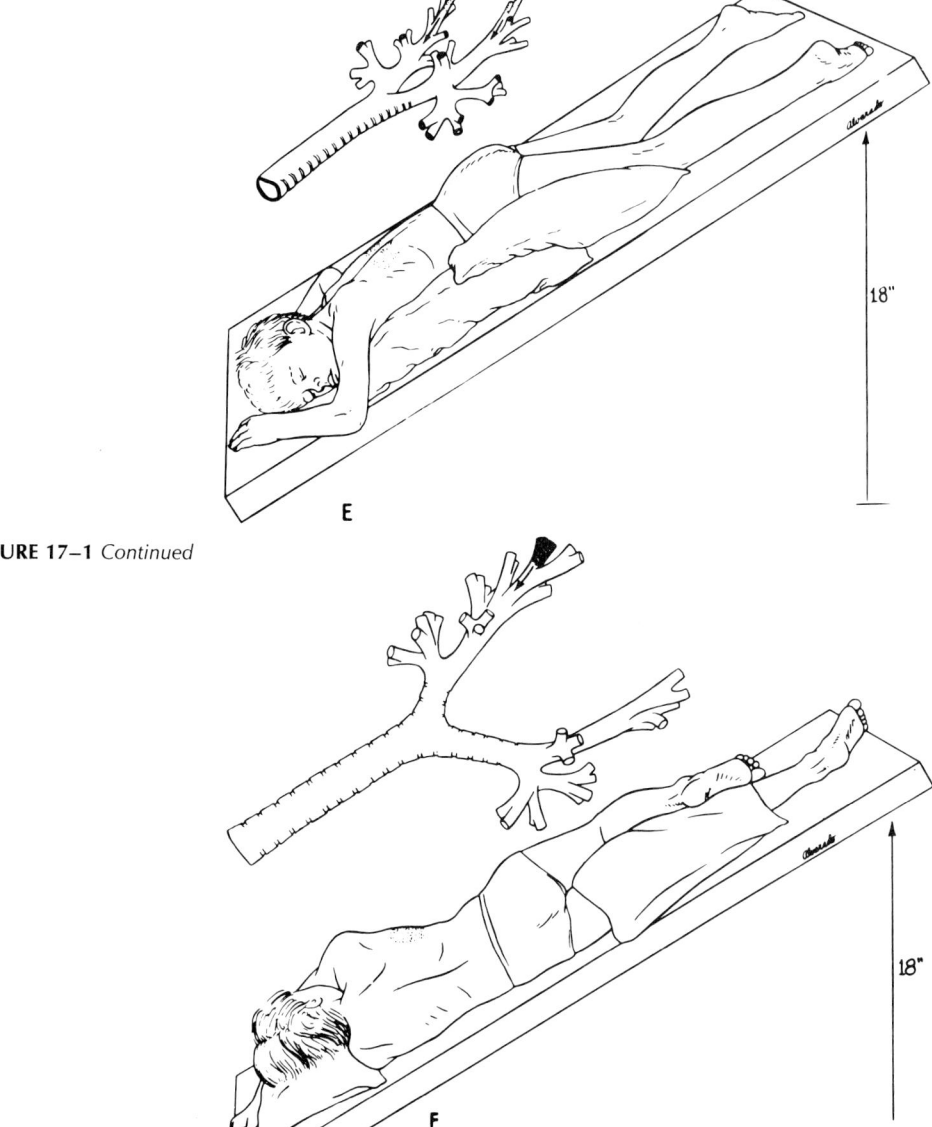

FIGURE 17–1 Continued

Illustration continued on following page

in patients in the midst of acute medical or surgical emergencies, during the immediate postoperative phase (because of the cardiovascular instability caused by anesthesia), and in patients with unstable spine injuries. Many of the positions utilized for postural drainage require that the head be below the rest of the body, which may increase intracranial pressure. For this reason, these positions are contraindicated in patients with pre-existing elevated intracranial pressure, because brain hemorrhage, herniation of brain tissue, or stroke may result. Positioning the patient with the head down and the legs elevated (Trendelenburg's position) may be contraindicated in patients with severe hypertension or congestive heart failure. Care must be taken to avoid stress on healing tissues, such as spinal fusions or skin grafts. This type of treatment may require modification in patients with shortness of breath, cardiac conditions, or obesity and in pregnant or geriatric patients.

Simply changing a patient's position for postural drainage or other clinical interventions can produce complications. Intravenous and arterial lines can be dislodged causing hemorrhage. Disconnection of central venous lines can result in venous air embolism. Movement of Swan-Ganz catheters

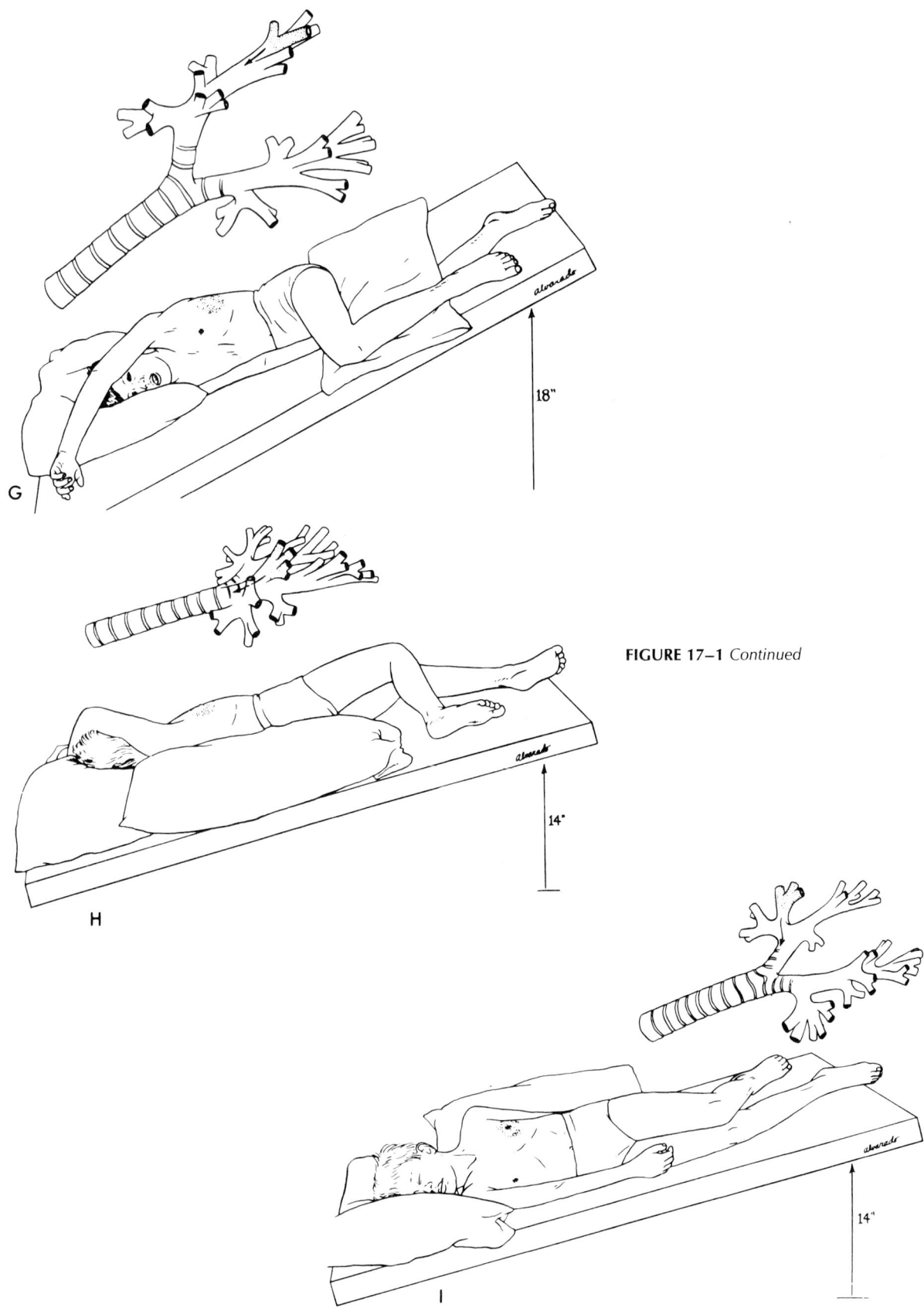

FIGURE 17–1 Continued

passing through the heart can set off life-threatening arrhythmias. Disconnection from mechanical ventilation or inadvertent extubation can follow position changes. Therefore, caution is essential when changing a patient's position.

CHEST PHYSICAL THERAPY

As mentioned in the previous section, postural drainage is commonly used with the chest physical therapy techniques of percussion and vibration. These techniques induce airway vibration in the underlying lung structures, which helps dislodge fluid from alveoli as well as mobilize viscous airway secretions. Chest physical therapy is commonly used in conjunction with mucokinetic drugs that disrupt the disulfide bonds between the mucoprotein molecules of the mucus, causing the secretions to become more liquid.

Before beginning any type of chest physical therapy, the underlying skin and tissues should be examined. This is to ascertain if any area should be avoided. It also gives a little time to interact with the patient and develop rapport before beginning the treatment. If the patient prefers being covered for the treatment, only a thin smock or sheet should be used. Thick cloth, such as a towel, decreases the impact of the therapy and lessens the effect on loosening the secretions.

Percussion

Percussion involves striking the chest wall with a cupped hand over an area of lung affected by retained fluid and secretions. It makes a hollow sound when performed properly; a slapping sound indicates incorrect technique. Both hands are alternately used in a rapid, steady rhythm. Treatment usually lasts about 2 to 3 minutes before repositioning the patient and beginning treatment again. This gives the patient time to rest and to cough up any secretions that may have been loosened before treatment over another area begins. The total percussion time should be about 10 to 20 minutes, but care should be taken not to treat small areas for a prolonged time because the skin may become irritated.

Percussion is useful to aid in the mobilization of thick secretions. Percussion may be administered during both inhalation and exhalation. Care should be taken not to percuss over bony prominences. Because of the risk of fractures, percussion should be avoided in conditions in which the bones are weak or brittle, such as osteoporosis or when cancer invades the bones. Caution should be used when percussing a patient with fractured ribs because of the pain over the area of injury as well as the risk of damaging the underlying lung with the jagged edges of the fractured bone and possibly producing a pneumothorax. Percussion is also contraindicated in patients with uncontrolled bleeding disorders or clotting problems. Patients with primary lung cancer may not be recommended for percussion because of the possibility of causing metastasis.

Vibration

Manual vibration is usually performed by placing one hand on top of the other upon the chest over the affected lung area. Rapid vibratory motions are produced by muscle contractions of the forearms and shoulders. Because this maneuver also compresses the chest, it should be timed to coincide with the patient's exhalation. This technique is especially useful for mobilizing liquid and loose secretions. In an alternative form of manual vibration, a hand is placed on the side of each hemithorax to provide bilateral vibration with increased compression.

There are many types of mechanical vibrators now available commercially for use in chest physical therapy. These instruments are less fatiguing to the therapist, require less skill, and are more relaxing to the patient. However, their usefulness is greatest when combined with postural drainage, coughing, and other techniques to improve bronchopulmonary hygiene.

COUGHING AND BREATHING RETRAINING

Coughing

Airway secretions are made less tenacious by humidification and administration of nebulized mucokinetic drugs. These less adherent secretions may then be mobilized into the larger airways by postural drainage. This movement into larger airways can often be facilitated by percussion and vibration therapy. The secretions are then removed from the large airways by coughing or suctioning (discussed later).

A cough consists first of an inspiration that is much larger than a normal tidal volume. Next, the glottis closes, and contraction of the expiratory thoracic and abdominal muscles raises intra-abdominal and intrathoracic pressure to 50 to 100 mmHg. The glottis then opens quickly, followed by a rapid expiratory flow rate of 8 to 10 L per second. Usually, a series of subsequent coughs occurs with some degree of inspiration for each one. Material in the large airways and larynx is moved into the pharynx, where it then may be either expectorated or swallowed.

Coughing is an important component of bronchopulmonary hygiene and should be utilized and encouraged whenever airway secretions accumulate and the patient is able to perform this maneuver. Weakened individuals frequently need coaching and encouragement to perform an effective cough.

Patients can usually cough most forcefully when they are in the sitting position with the trunk flexed slightly forward. This enhances the increase in intra-abdominal pressure produced by the contraction of the abdominal muscles. If the patient has recently undergone surgery, he or she should be instructed on methods of splinting (stabilizing) the incision site while making coughing efforts. The patient may hug his or her pillow, pressing it against the surgical site, which acts as an effective splint.

Coughing can be quite tiring for a patient who is weakened by surgery or illness. Certain methods can help reduce the effort required by the patient while still clearing secretions from the airways. One method requires that the patient make repeated attempts to clear his or her throat with sharp grunting sounds but with only gentle effort. Another technique, in which the patient produces rapid small coughs called *machine-gun coughing,* is less work for a weak patient. In a variation called *huffing,* the patient forcefully and repeatedly makes the sound *huh.* With this technique, high flow rates are produced through the partially opened vocal cords, carrying out airway secretions, but high airway pressures are not produced, and less effort is required of the patient. The patient with air trapping should be instructed to cough from mid inspiration instead of full inspiration because this lowers intrathoracic pressure and produces less airway collapse.

Cough coaching is most beneficial for patients with retained airway secretions. This includes individuals with surgical incisions or trauma to the thorax or abdomen. Also included are patients who are weak as a result of prolonged mechanical ventilation or neurologic or muscular disorders. The adverse effects of induced coughing include rib fractures, hernia, prolapsed vagina, and increased risk of aspiration. The increased intra-abdominal and intrathoracic pressure also produces increased blood pressure, and increased intraocular and intracranial pressures, which may damage the eyes or brain. Prolonged or vigorous coughing can decrease venous return to the heart, resulting in lowered cardiac output and fainting. Fainting as a result of coughing is called *tussive syncope.* Patients who are unresponsive or uncooperative may be induced to cough by compression and massage over the trachea at the sternal notch.

Coughing can also be induced by oral or nasal insertion of a catheter into the posterior pharynx or larynx. This is called *snogging,* in medical slang. The goal of this type of cough induction is to clear airway secretions and improve gas exchange. However, compassion and judgment must be used as well because overzealous snogging is actually patient abuse. Injudicious snogging of a patient with pre-existing hypoxemia can produce uncontrollable coughing, arrhythmias, and death.

In a similar technique for cough induction, a transtracheal catheter (see Chapter 12) is inserted through the cricothyroid membrane but is left in place. This is called a *tickle tube* in medical jargon because 2 to 3 ml of normal saline injected through the catheter directly into the patient's trachea usually elicits vigorous coughing. The same precautions apply as for snogging. Complications from tickle tubes include infection, subcutaneous emphysema, and laryngeal injury.

Cough Control

The therapist presses against the front of the patient's lower thorax, applying a slight resistance to the patient's inspiratory efforts. As the patient begins to exhale and make a coughing effort, the therapist increases the compression to augment the velocity and volume of the patient's expiratory air flow. Occasionally, patients with severe air trapping may feel that they cannot exhale after a large inspiration. In this situation, the therapist may assist the patient by applying compression to the abdomen and lower thorax, which allows some exhalation to occur so that the patient can then take in the next breath.

Breathing Retraining

Long-term control of breathing is mostly an unconscious function. However, patients with certain types of pathology may benefit from treatment instruction to modify their breathing pattern. Many different techniques of breathing training have been developed.

Diaphragmatic Breathing

Patients with severe air trapping overinflate their lungs to such an extent that the muscles of the diaphragm become flattened. This greatly diminishes the effectiveness of diaphragmatic contraction in the generation of negative intrathoracic pressure. In pathologic states in which the diaphragm has become ineffective in inspiration, the thoracic and accessory muscles of inspiration (external intercostals, scalenes, sternocleidomastoids, pectoralis, and trapezius) are increasingly utilized. Although much effort may be exerted by these muscles, they are relatively ineffective in moving a stiff, overinflated barrel chest. (Remember that at high thoracic volumes, chest wall recoil is inward instead of outward.) Ventilatory mechanics may be so severely disturbed that the patient exhibits paradoxical breathing (contracting the abdominal muscles while attempting to inspire and relaxing them during expiration).

Training patients to maximize the effectiveness of their diaphragmatic breathing is begun by focusing attention on the motion of the abdominal wall. The therapist's hands are placed on the abdominal wall beneath the costal margins, and patients are instructed to push away the therapist's hands with their abdomen when they inspire. During exhalation, the therapist's hands should move inward. By placing their own hands upon the abdomen, patients can continue these exercises when the therapist is absent. Proper diaphragmatic breathing coordinates the contraction and relaxation of the muscles of ventilation so that less energy is expended. It is easier to move the more flexible abdominal wall than it is to expand and contract a stiff, barrel chest.

Diaphragmatic strength may be increased by repeating the exercises or by performing work against increased resistance. Weights placed on the abdominal wall when the patient is in the supine position can improve the conditioning of the diaphragm and thus should also improve its effectiveness in ventilation.

Segmental Breathing

For this technique, the therapist's or patient's hands are placed on an area of the chest wall overlying a diseased lung region. The patient then makes ventilatory efforts that produce the greatest excursion of the hand from inflation to deflation. This is intended to result in increased ventilation to this lung area and improved matching of ventilation and perfusion. However, there is little evidence to indicate that this lung area actually receives a greater proportion of the tidal volume ventilation. On the other hand, this treatment may be useful in helping a patient with protective muscular splinting following trauma or surgery to overcome a fear of pain during deep breathing.

Resistance Breathing

Many patients with gas trapping from airways collapse do resistance (pursed-lip) breathing spontaneously. During exhalation, patients are instructed to purse their lips as if they were whistling. Exhalation is therefore carried out slowly but continuously. This expiratory resistance transmits backpressure to the bronchial tree to prevent early collapse of small airways, thus allowing more complete exhalation from the alveoli. Forced expiratory efforts should be discouraged during this technique because they tend to cause dynamic compression of the airways and increase gas trapping.

Exercise Training

Patients with severe lung disease may not be able to perform normal activities of daily living (ADL) because they easily become short of breath. These activities include doing housework, climbing stairs, and walking. Use of the previously mentioned breathing retraining techniques and graded exercises can help reduce shortness of breath and improve their quality of life. During exercise, breathing should be coordinated with the activity. Activity that requires contraction of the abdominal muscles or flexion of the trunk should coincide with exhalation while straightening should be coupled with inhalation. With conditioning, patients' ability to tolerate exertion improves. The feeling of breathlessness is diminished, thus relieving a major area of discomfort.

Inspiratory resistive training devices have been used for rehabilitation of patients with chronic airway obstruction, but their effectiveness is controversial. In resistive training, the patient inspires against a resistance that is increased by the therapist during subsequent efforts.

SUCTIONING PROCEDURES

Of all the techniques described for promoting bronchopulmonary hygiene, suctioning has the greatest risks for both the therapist and patient and therefore requires the greatest caution. Suctioning is necessary for patients who are unable to adequately clear the secretions from their airways. Suctioning may also be used diagnostically to obtain material for examination and culturing (see Chapter 12).

Suction catheters are soft, hollow, and smooth cylindrical tubes made of nontoxic material that is designed to cause as little trauma and friction as possible while passing over the tracheal mucosa. The distal tip must be smooth and molded with side holes to help prevent mucosal trauma. This tip may be flared or beveled. As Figure 17–2 shows, the proximal end of the catheter has a vent and fitting to attach to the connecting tubing from the vacuum source. The vent should be larger in diameter than the suction tubing, and it should be easily occluded by the therapist's thumb in order to regulate the intermittent application of suction pressure. The vacuum pressures should range from −80 to −100 mmHg because excessive negative pressure results in mucosal injury and hemorrhage.

Suction catheters are available in a variety of sizes. They must be sterile and are therefore usually disposable. The catheter should be relatively straight to facilitate directing it to the desired area. Suction catheters are most commonly used to aspirate material from the trachea, but when more distal suctioning is desired, straight catheters enter the right mainstem bronchus over 80% of the time. When suctioning of the left mainstem bronchus is necessary, a suction catheter with a curved tip (Coudé) allows easier passage into the left bronchus.

It may be necessary to suction the mouth and pharynx to obtain an unobstructed view before attempting endotracheal intubation. This area may also need suctioning after vomiting, or regurgitation. Drainage of blood or secretions into the pharynx and mouth of a semiconscious patient following nasal or oral surgery or trauma may similarly require suctioning. Suctioning of the mouth and pharynx should be done with a large-diameter soft suction catheter or a hard plastic tube called a Yankauer catheter (Fig. 17–2). These large-diameter devices allow rapid removal of viscous or particulate material from the pharynx, decreasing the risk of its movement into the lungs.

Suctioning is frequently used in combination with other techniques, such as mucokinetic drugs, postural drainage, vibration, percussion, and coughing in order to mobilize secretions.

Airway Suctioning Procedure

If a patient has an endotracheal or tracheostomy tube in place, then airway suctioning can be performed rather easily through these artificial airways. In the absence of these airways, oral or nasal tracheal suctioning must be done. Oral or nasal tracheal suctioning requires that a catheter be passed through the mouth or nose, through the larynx, and into the trachea to remove secretions in the lumen of the trachea. Although it is technically somewhat difficult to get the distal tip of the suction catheter in the desired place, attempts at passing the catheter through the larynx into the trachea frequently provoke vigorous coughing, which moves the secretions into the pharynx where they can be more easily removed. The following sequence should be followed during a suctioning procedure:

1. Explain the procedure to the patient.
2. Hyperinflate with 100% oxygen for 5 to 10 spontaneous, slow, deep breaths or with a self-inflating resuscitation bag. If the patient is on a ventilator, manual sighs can be given to hyperinflate.
3. Use a catheter that is no greater than half the diameter of the artificial airway or nostril through which it is to be inserted. Lubricate the catheter before inserting if there is no artificial airway in place.
4. The catheter should be inserted until resistance is met; then the catheter is withdrawn about 1 cm before applying suction.

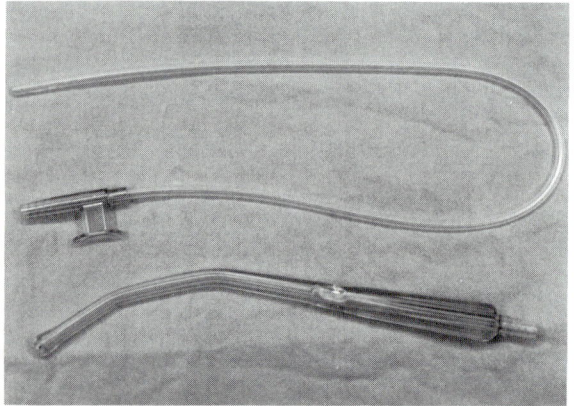

FIGURE 17–2. Catheters used for suctioning patients. *Top*, a flexible catheter. *Bottom*, a hard plastic Yankauer catheter used for removing material from the mouth and pharynx.

5. Apply suction intermittently only during withdrawal, rotating the catheter, for no longer than 10 to 15 seconds.

6. Reoxygenate and ventilate for at least 1 minute, and allow vital signs to return to baseline before repeating. The mouth and pharynx may be suctioned with the same catheter following tracheal suctioning, but the reverse order should not be used because of the increased risk of tracheal contamination.

7. Note the color, amount, and consistency of material removed as well as any problems occurring during the procedure.

When no artificial airway is in place, it is usually easier to enter the trachea via the nasal route. The first thing to do is to explain the routine to the patient, especially the coughing that it usually provokes. The patient is placed in a semi-Fowler or semisitting position. Before insertion, the catheter is coated with a water-soluble lubricant. The apex of the nose is elevated slightly, and the catheter is inserted into the nasal cavity in a direction parallel to the roof of the oral cavity (see Fig. 18-5). If repeated or frequent suctioning is necessary, then the placement of a nasopharyngeal airway may reduce trauma to the nasal mucosa.

The catheter is then passed into the pharynx; this may induce some gagging by the patient. If the catheter does not pass into the trachea after a few attempts, the patient should stick out his or her tongue, which is held in the therapist's gloved hand in order to facilitate passage through the vocal cords. Then, the patient is instructed to take slow, deep breaths or to cough gently. This opens the larynx and allows passage of the catheter through the vocal cords and into the trachea. Also during nasotracheal suctioning, one knows when the catheter is in the trachea because the patient's breathing can be heard through the side vent of the catheter. When the catheter enters the trachea, the patient begins to cough more deeply and is not able to speak normally. The catheter should be inserted until it meets an obstruction and then withdrawn a centimeter or two before applying suction. Apply suction only during withdrawal of the catheter. It should be intermittent and the catheter should be rotated to allow suctioning of the greatest area.

Complications of Airway Suctioning

As mentioned previously, suctioning poses risks to the patient. It also carries the risk of infecting other individuals in the area, including the therapists. Complications of airway suctioning include hypoxemia, arrhythmias, hypotension, atelectasis, and damage to the airway mucosa.

Hypoxemia

Patients who require suctioning often also require enriched oxygen therapy. Suctioning frequently results in the discontinuation of this supplemental oxygen. The insertion of the suction catheter into the trachea permits aspiration of the airway secretions but results in aspiration of substantial amounts of intrapulmonary air. The patient not only has his or her supplemental oxygen interrupted but also has the air sucked right out of the lungs! Pre- and postsuctioning oxygenation are beneficial in avoiding hypoxemia during suctioning. The use of certain adaptors with gaskets allows oxygenation, mechanical ventilation, and PEEP to continue while suctioning is being carried out.

Arrhythmias

Dangerous cardiac arrhythmias may be induced during suctioning. Hypoxemia may produce myocardial ischemia, resulting in premature ventricular contractions or even cardiac arrest. Suctioning may also irritate the larynx and trachea, resulting in vagal stimulation that can lead to profound bradycardia. Preoxygenation and avoidance of excessive duration of suctioning may help to avoid myocardial ischemia. Vagal stimulation may be avoided or treated by gentler suctioning technique, nebulization or instillation of local anesthetic drugs, or blocking vagal effects with drugs such as atropine. Careful cardiac monitoring is recommended during suctioning.

Hypotension

Hypotension may result from either profound bradycardia due to vagal stimulation or severe coughing that impedes venous return and may cause fainting. Suctioning attempts should be interrupted during severe coughing episodes.

Atelectasis

Suctioning removes air from the lungs and may result in atelectasis if postsuction hyperinflation isn't carried out. If too large a suction catheter is used, inadequate amounts of air may be drawn down the airway, thus resulting in distal air being removed from the lungs. This can cause total collapse of the lung. The maximum diameter of a suction catheter should therefore be no greater than half the internal diameter of the artificial airway or nostril through which it is to be inserted. Paroxysms of coughing may result in pneumothorax and collapse of the lung due to rupture of emphysematous blebs or injury to airway structures.

Airway Mucosal Injury

Some damage to the tracheal mucosa is inevitable whenever suctioning is employed. However, this should be kept to a minimum by using gentle technique and lubrication. Airways should be suctioned only when there are excessive secretions in the airway. Rough or sharp catheters should not be used. Extra caution is needed if the patient has hemophilia or other bleeding disorders.

Infection

Sterile technique must be utilized when suctioning below the vocal cords. A catheter that has been used to suction the mouth or pharynx should never be used subsequently in the trachea. After a suction catheter or Yankauer is used, it must be disposed of properly to avoid contamination of other patients or of healthcare providers. Closed tracheal suction systems (such as the Ballard) have been developed to provide a protective sheath around the suction catheter so that the outside of the suction catheter is not exposed to the environment. This allows the catheter to be reinserted into the trachea without contamination as well as providing a barrier against the airway secretions for everyone else. Universal blood and body fluid precautions are described in Chapter 12.

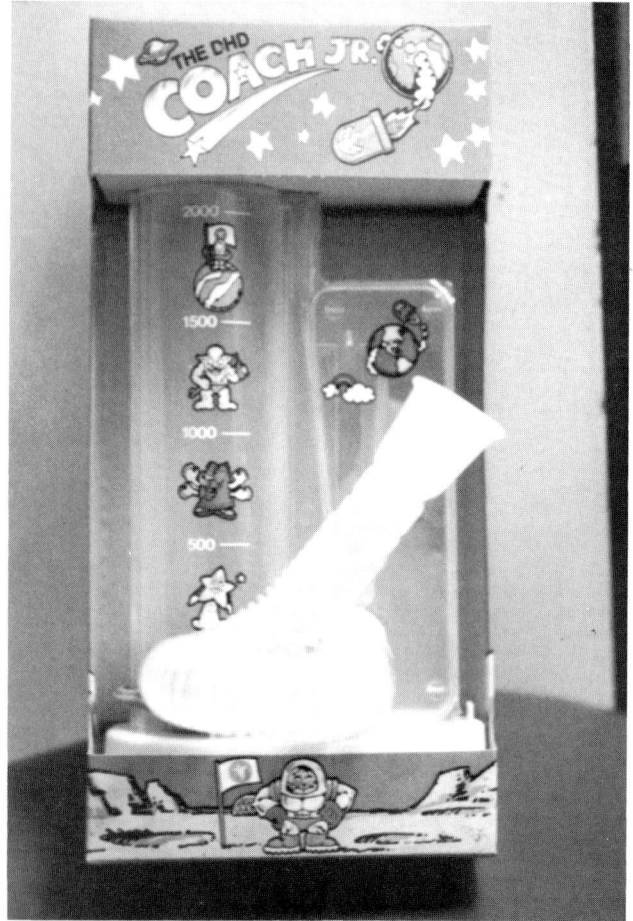

FIGURE 17–3. A pediatric incentive spirometer. Forced inspiration on the mouthpiece raises the ball to the desired goal.

INCENTIVE SPIROMETRY

Incentive spirometry (sustained maximal inspiration) is a technique that motivates patients to periodically take large breaths to help prevent atelectasis, reinflate atelectatic alveoli, train respiratory muscles, and improve the cough mechanism. Incentive spirometry is effective for individuals who are *able* to take deep breaths but do not do so spontaneously because of sedation or lethargy due to being bedridden.

An incentive spirometer is used to encourage a patient to perform a sustained maximal inspiration. The patient's goal is to raise a ball in a column or light a light that indicates that he or she has performed an adequate inhalation. The patient is requested to perform a certain number of inspirations per hour. Obviously, the therapist's ability to motivate the patient to reach the goal is vital to the success of this form of therapy.

The equipment for this form of therapy, as Figure 17–3 shows, is much less expensive than that used for IPPB treatments (discussed in the next section). It also requires less involvement by cardiopulmonary care clinicians. Incentive spirometry is as effective as IPPB for patients who are able to take deep breaths.

Other techniques have been used in the past to stimulate lung inflation and coughing. An apparatus called a blow bottle requires patients to produce forced exhalations. This technique was found to be much less effective than incentive spirometry—in fact, blow bottles were found to produce dynamic compression of the airways and gas trapping. Their use should be discouraged. Carbon dioxide inhalation has also been used to stimulate ventilation but is much less effective than incentive spirometry. In addition, carbon dioxide inhalation may produce tachycardia, hypertension, and headache.

Incentive spirometry has a lesser incidence of complications than IPPB. Infection due to contamination of the machine and tubing by other patients is probably the greatest risk from incentive spirometry, and this is decreasing because of the availability of disposable units (Fig. 17–4). Although unlikely, pneumothorax is also possible, especially in patients with emphysema. Also, patients may hyperventilate if they attempt to reach their goals too rapidly. Incentive spirometry is not useful in patients who are unconscious or unable to cooperate, and IPPB may be more useful in these situations.

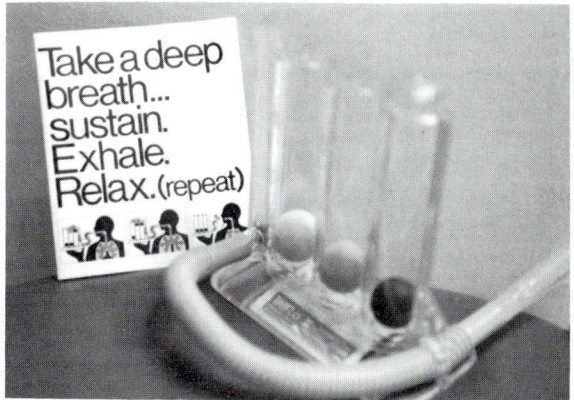

FIGURE 17–4. A disposable incentive spirometer. The goal is achieved when the ball reaches the top of the column.

INSPIRATORY POSITIVE-PRESSURE BREATHING

Inspiratory positive-pressure breathing (IPPB) is the application of positive pressure to a patient's airways, triggered by the onset of his or her inspiratory effort. When the pressure level desired by the therapist is attained, the positive pressure ceases and the lungs empty passively because of the elastic recoil of the respiratory system. IPPB is usually administered via a mask or mouthpiece attached to the IPPB machine, but it may also be delivered to a tracheostomy by using a connector tube. IPPB treatments are given to patients who are breathing spontaneously.

IPPB is appropriate in certain pathologic states in which impairment of ventilatory function results in a decreased ability to expand the lungs or chest wall. Ventilatory drive must be present. A vital capacity of less than 15 ml/kg is an indication for the use of IPPB. This means that the patient has almost no ventilatory reserve. However, the patient must not be so ill as to require mechanical ventilation because IPPB can only be administered to a spontaneously breathing patient. The patient must be able to make enough of an inspiratory effort to trigger the IPPB machine to deliver the inspiratory positive pressure.

Application of inspiratory positive pressure to the airways of patients unable to breathe deeply therefore increases their inspired volume. The increased alveolar distending pressure also helps to reverse or prevent atelectasis. This reduction in atelectasis occurs as a result of direct inflation of the alveoli through the airways or by collateral ventilation from adjacent alveoli through the canals of Lambert or pores of Kohn. Reduction of atelectasis obviously improves the distribution of ventilation and matching of ventilation and perfusion, thus improving the patient's blood gases. In addition, reduction of atelectasis increases the overall compliance of the lungs, thus reducing the work of breathing. This should increase the tidal volume and reduce the respiratory rate.

The mechanically assisted hyperinflation of the lungs should also improve coughing mechanics because there is a larger volume to exhale. This should help remove airway secretions, thus further reducing the work of breathing and decreasing atelectasis. IPPB may also be used as a means to administer bronchodilators and mucokinetic drugs. The decrease in airway resistance due to bronchodilation and mobilization of airway secretions may also decrease the work of breathing.

The cost-effectiveness of IPPB is quite controversial, apparently because many physicians feel that this treatment modality, which requires the use of expensive equipment and continuous direction by a therapist, has often been prescribed when it is not needed. Individuals who are able to take deep breaths spontaneously may be more appropriately managed with less expensive therapeutic modalities, such as incentive spirometry or cough stimulation by tracheal suctioning. IPPB should not be used routinely in prophylactic bronchial hygiene therapy.

The benefits of IPPB include:

1. Improved distribution of ventilation (reduced atelectasis).

2. Improved coughing mechanics and removal of airway secretions due to increased expiratory volumes.

3. Increased delivery of nebulized medication in patients unable to take deep breaths.

IPPB is useful in many disease states that result

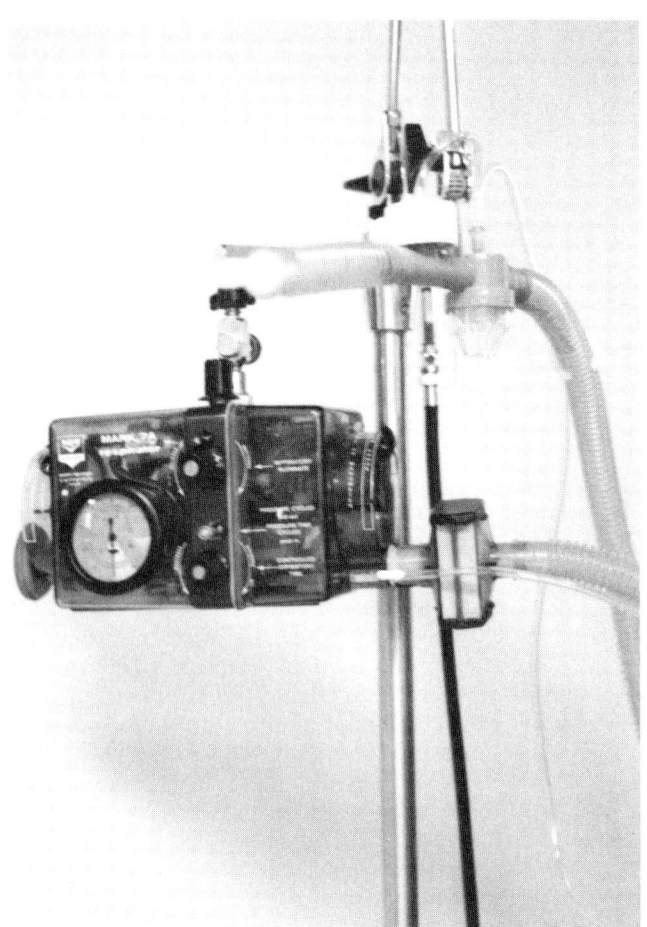

FIGURE 17–5. A machine for delivery of inspiratory positive-pressure breathing (IPPB).

in an inability to take a deep breath, such as neuromuscular disease, chronic obstructive pulmonary disease, restrictive disease, and splinting (taking shallow breaths to prevent painful movement) due to pain following upper abdominal or thoracic surgery.

Administration of IPPB

The patient must form a seal with the mouthpiece attached to the tubing from the IPPB machine (Fig. 17–5). Trying different sizes and shapes of mouthpieces usually reveals one that forms the best seal for a certain patient. A patient who is edentulous (that is, has no teeth) or has facial abnormalities may require the use of a mask. The *sensitivity* of the IPPB machine should be set so that only 1 to 2 torr of negative inspiratory pressure exerted by the patient initiates the flow of inspiratory pressure from the machine.

The pressure limits of the IPPB machine are variable but for most patients are about 10 to 15 cmH_2O. It is important to remember that the delivery of adequate volume and not the pressure of the breath makes this treatment effective. The delivery pressure limit should be adjusted so that the exhaled volume is at least 10 ml per kilogram of body weight for that patient. In patients with poorly compliant lungs, a driving pressure of 30 to 40 cmH_2O is sometimes required.

The gas delivered by the IPPB machine should always be humidified. Administration of dry gas can cause bronchoconstriction and increased airways resistance. Patients with asthma or COPD should also receive nebulized bronchodilators through the IPPB mouthpiece.

A gas mixture appropriate for the patient must also be administered through the IPPB device. If the patient is receiving supplemental oxygen, the same concentration should be delivered during the IPPB treatment. Caution must be used to prevent the use of high oxygen concentrations when treating COPD patients with carbon dioxide retention and hypoxic drive for ventilation. Inadvertent use of 100% oxygen in these patients can result in profound hypoventilation or apnea. The use of 100% oxygen should also be avoided because it leads to rapid absorption atelectasis. Although the positive pressure may inflate collapsed or partially collapsed alveoli, when the treatment is completed, the oxygen is rapidly absorbed into the pulmonary capillary blood, resulting in complete collapse of these alveoli.

The flow rate is also variable on IPPB machines. It should be adjusted so that the patient receives a slow, gradual inspiration yet still has adequate time for exhalation when receiving 6 to 10 breaths per minute. The rate of positive-pressure breaths depends on the frequency at which the patient makes inspiratory efforts. The patient must breathe slowly, approximately 10 breaths per minute. After the positive-pressure breath has been administered, the patient should relax but hold the breath in for 2 to 3 seconds to allow expansion of the slow alveoli. Then passive exhalation occurs. The patient should be allowed to rest after about 5 to 10 minutes of treatment, and the complete treatment session should last no more than 20 minutes.

Contraindications for IPPB include untreated pneumothorax, bronchopleural cutaneous fistula, and other conditions that can result in subcutaneous emphysema. It is also not recommended in patients who have recently undergone lobectomy or pneumonectomy, because some surgeons fear that the positive airway pressure may disrupt the closure of the airways stump. IPPB should be used with caution in patients who have recently received a needle biopsy of the lung, because positive airway pressure may produce a leak causing pneumothorax in these individuals. IPPB should also be used with caution in patients who have had transtracheal catheters inserted to aspirate sputum or stimulate coughing (tickle tubes), because the airway leak can produce subcutaneous emphysema over the neck. Administration of IPPB to an individual with massive hemoptysis (cough producing bloody sputum) may produce air embolus to the left ventricle and systemic arteries, but obviously, obtaining more comprehensive airway control in these patients is more important than IPPB administration.

Complications of IPPB

Hypocapnia

Too frequent delivery of large tidal volumes may rapidly lower the arterial P_{CO_2}, resulting in loss of ventilatory drive. Mild hypocapnia may produce tingling and numbness of the lips; more severe decreases in carbon dioxide may result in seizures and unconsciousness.

Elevated Intrathoracic Pressure

The increase in airway pressure may impede blood flow through the great veins and the pulmonary circulation, reducing venous return to the left ventricle and diminishing cardiac output. If the treatment is prolonged, hypotension and tissue hypoxia may result. Impeding venous return from the brain can also result in increased intracranial pressure. This may be especially hazardous in a patient who has pre-existing increased intracranial pressure from other causes. In this situation, the patient's head must be elevated during IPPB treatment. IPPB may also produce gastric distention; this occurs more commonly when it is administered by mask. Besides causing discomfort, inflation of the stomach may lead to vomiting and aspiration of gastric contents.

Barotrauma

Patients who have gas trapping and receive IPPB may be subject to distention of emphysematous blebs. Although the positive airway pressure administered by IPPB is not usually excessive, the coughing that frequently accompanies IPPB treatment may produce very high pressures. Such high pressures can rupture these blebs, resulting in pneumothorax. Patients who suddenly become dyspneic during IPPB treatment should be evaluated for the possibility of ruptured blebs and pneumothorax. IPPB should be discontinued until the pneumothorax is relieved, because further administration of IPPB results in a tension pneumothorax. Hemoptysis may also result from the coughing produced by IPPB; similarly, treatment should be suspended until the physician has been notified.

Infection

The tubing and mouthpiece should be used only by one patient, with great care taken to avoid cross-contamination between patients. Nondisposable IPPB equipment must be cleaned before re-use with another patient.

Bibliography

Ali, J., Serrette, C., Wood, L.D.H., and Anthonisen, W.R.: Effect of postoperative intermittent positive-pressure breathing on lung function. *Chest* 85:192–196, 1984.

Anesthesia Study Committee of the New York State Society of Anesthesiologists: Clinical Anesthesia Conference: Endotracheal suction and death. *N.Y. State J. Med.* 68:565–566, 1968.

Baier, H., Begin, R., and Sackner, M.A.: Effect of airway diameter, suction catheters and the bronchofiberscope on airflow in endotracheal and tracheostomy tubes. *Heart Lung* 5:235–238, 1976.

Banner, A.S.: Cough: Physiology, evaluation, and treatment. *Lung* 164:79–92, 1986.

Bartlett, R.H.: Respiratory therapy to prevent pulmonary complications of surgery. *Respir. Care* 29:667–679, 1984.

Bodai, B.I.: A means of suctioning without cardiopulmonary depression. *Heart Lung* 11:172–176, 1982.

Brown, S.E., Stansbury, D.W., Merrill, E.J., et al.: Prevention of suctioning-related arterial oxygen desaturation: Comparison of off-ventilator and on-ventilator suctioning. *Chest* 83:621–627, 1983.

Cabol, L., Devaskar, S., Siassi, B., et al.: New endotracheal tube adapter reducing cardiopulmonary effects of suctioning. *Crit. Care Med.* 77:552–555, 1979.

Demers, R.R.: Complications of endotracheal suctioning procedures. *Respir. Care* 27:453–457, 1982.

Freeman, A.P., and Goodman, L.: Suctioning the left bronchial tree in the intubated adult. *Crit. Care Med.* 10:43–45, 1982.

Frownfelter, D.L.: *Chest Physical Therapy and Pulmonary Rehabilitation.* Chicago, Year Book, 1978.

Graham, W.G., and Bradley, E.A.: Efficacy of chest physiotherapy and positive pressure breathing on the resolution of pneumonia. *N. Engl. J. Med.* 299:624, 1978.

Kigin, C.M.: Chest physical therapy for the postoperative or traumatic injury patient. *Phys. Ther.* 61:1,724–1,736, 1981.

Kubota, Y., Magaribuchi, T., Toyoda, Y., et al.: Selective bronchial suctioning in the adult using a coudé-tipped catheter with a guide mark. *Crit. Care Med.* 10:767–769, 1982.

Langrehr, E.A., Washburn, S.C., and Guthrie, M.P.: Oxygen insufflation during endotracheal suctioning. *Heart Lung* 10:1,028–1.036, 1981.

Leith, D.E., Butler, J.P., Seddon, S.L., and Brain, J.D.: Cough. In Macklem, P.T., and Mead, J. (eds.): *Handbook of Physiology,* vol. 3. Bethesda, Md., American Physiological Society, 1988.

MacKenzie, C.F., Ciesla, N., Imle, P.C., and Klemic, N.: *Chest Physiotherapy in the Intensive Care Unit.* Baltimore, Williams and Wilkins, 1981.

Peters, R.M., and Turnier, E.: Physical therapy indications for and effects in surgical patients. *Am. Rev. Respir. Dis.* 122:147–154, 1980.

Pierce, A.K., and Saltzman, H.A. (eds.): Conference on a scientific basis of respiratory therapy. *Am. Rev. Respir. Dis.* 110:1–203, 1974.

Pierson, D.J. (ed.): Perioperative Respiratory Care: Special Symposium Issues. *Respiratory Care* 29:459–549; 603–682, 1984.

Pontoppidan, H.: Mechanical aids to lung expansion in nonintubated surgical patients. *Am. Rev. Respir. Dis.* 122:109–119, 1980.

Sanders, C.V., Johanson, W.G., Jr., and Sanford, J.P.: Serratia marcescens infections from inhalation therapy medications: Nosocomial outbreak. *Ann. Intern. Med.* 73:15–21, 1970.

Schuppisser, J.P., Brandil, O., and Meili, U.: Postoperative intermittent positive-pressure breathing versus physiotherapy. *Am. J. Surg.* 104:682–686, 1980.

Shapiro, B.A.: Chest physical therapy administered by respiratory therapists. *Resp. Care* 26:655–656, 1981.

Shapiro, B.A., Peterson, J., and Cane, R.D.: Complications of mechanical aids to intermittent lung inflation. *Respir. Care* 27:467–470, 1982.

Skelley, B.F., Deeren, S.M., and Powaser, M.M.: The effectiveness of preoxygenation methods to prevent endotracheal suction-induced hypoxemia. *Heart Lung* 9:316–323, 1980.

Tyler, M.L.: The respiratory effects of body positioning and immobilization. *Respir. Care* 29:472–483, 1984.

Zadai, C.C.: Physical therapy for the acutely ill medical patient. *Phys. Ther.* 61:1,746–1,754, 1981.

Ziment, I.: Intermittent positive pressure breathing. In Burton, G.G., Gee, G.N., and Hodgkin, J.E.: *Respiratory Care: A Guide to Clinical Practice*, pp. 570–573. Philadelphia, J.B. Lippincott Co., 1977.

OBJECTIVES

AFTER READING THIS CHAPTER, THE STUDENT WILL BE ABLE TO:

1. List the indications for the use of an artificial airway.
2. Discuss the different types of artificial airways.
3. Describe proper positioning of the head and jaw for establishing a clear airway.
4. Describe the Heimlich maneuver and discuss appropriate situations for its use.
5. Describe the oropharyngeal airway and how it is used.
6. List the characteristics of a nasopharyngeal airway and describe the techniques used in its insertion.
7. Differentiate an esophageal obturator airway from an esophageal gastric tube airway and describe a situation where they may be useful in maintaining an airway.
8. Discuss the technique of laryngoscopy and compare the different types of laryngoscope blades.
9. State the characteristics of endotracheal tubes and explain the meanings of the markings on the outside of the tube.
10. Explain the techniques for orotracheal and nasotracheal intubation.
11. List the differences between pediatric and adult airway anatomy.
12. Characterize how movement of the patient's head results in migration of an endotracheal tube.
13. Explain the use and care of a cuff on an endotracheal tube.
14. Describe some of the different techniques that can be used when there is difficulty intubating a patient.
15. List the indications for endobronchial intubation. Describe the different types of double lumen endobronchial tubes.
16. Discuss clinical situations that would require the use of methods for quick access of the airway, such as cricothyroidotomy or transtracheal catheter ventilation, and characterize these techniques.
17. Contrast emergency and chronic tracheostomy techniques and discuss their indications.
18. Identify the three major groups of problems associated with the use of artificial airways.
19. List common injuries occurring during the application of artificial airways.
20. Describe mechanical or structural problems that may exist in certain types of artificial airways.
21. Describe complications associated with long-term use of artificial airways.
22. Describe how you would determine when the usage of an artificial airway is no longer necessary.
23. Explain the techniques for terminating the use of an artificial airway.

18
AIRWAY MANAGEMENT

CHAPTER OUTLINE

INDICATIONS FOR ARTIFICIAL AIRWAYS
   Relief of Airway Obstruction
   Airway Protection from Aspiration
   Facilitation of Bronchopulmonary Hygiene
   Positive Airway Pressure Adjunct

TYPES OF ARTIFICIAL AIRWAYS
   Positioning the Head and Jaw
   Oropharyngeal Airway
   Nasopharyngeal Airway
   Esophageal Obturator Airway
   Endotracheal Intubation
      Laryngoscopy
      Technique for Orotracheal Intubation

      Difficult Intubations
      Nasotracheal Intubation
   Endobronchial Intubation
   Cricothyroidotomy
   Tracheotomy

PROBLEMS ASSOCIATED WITH ARTIFICIAL AIRWAYS
   Injuries During Application of Airways
   Mechanical or Structural Problems with Artificial Airways
   Complications Associated with Long-Term Use

TERMINATING USE OF ARTIFICIAL AIRWAYS

The upper airway connects the lungs to the atmosphere outside the body. Complete occlusion of the upper airway rapidly leads to death from hypoxia and hypercapnia. The mucosa in the lumen of the upper airway is one of the most sensitive parts of the body, with many irritant receptors and protective reflexes that help maintain the passageway for airflow. These irritant receptors and protective reflexes play an important role in initiating coughing to insure the patency of the airway as well as to clear pulmonary secretions. Protective reflexes in the airway also help prevent *pulmonary aspiration* (the entry of liquid or solid material, such as upper airway secretions, food, or stomach acid, into the airways below the vocal cords). Pulmonary aspiration can be very damaging to lung tissues and can greatly diminish the gas-exchanging ability of the lungs. If the upper airways are occluded, lose their protective reflexes, or need intensive help to clear pulmonary secretions, then the use of an artificial airway may be necessary.

The patency of the upper airway depends on the normal anatomy and muscular tone of the nose, mouth, pharynx, larynx, and trachea. With injury or disease, the anatomy of the upper airway may become distorted, compressing or obstructing the passageway for air flow. Furthermore, brain injury, neuromuscular disease, or general anesthetics can result in loss of tone of the upper airway voluntary muscles with resultant obstruction. Coma or obtundation (depressed neurologic activity) can also produce a loss of upper airway reflexes, increasing the risk of aspiration. Obviously, cardiopulmonary arrest impairs neurologic function and causes loss of upper airway muscular tone, producing airway obstruction in addition to apnea. Resuscitative efforts must therefore encompass first re-establishing a patent airway and then trying to ventilate the patient. The use of an artificial airway may be needed when a patient requires prolonged positive-pressure ventilation.

The upper airway in children is predisposed to obstruction because of the narrowness of the nasal passages, the glottic slit, and the trachea. Children also have a relatively large tongue and abundant airway secretions. Pathologic conditions, such as hypertrophied tonsils and adenoids, are sometimes superimposed, further compromising the patency of the pediatric airway.

The anatomy of the upper airway of infants is different from that of adults (see Fig. 3–2). The larynx of the newborn is more superior, with the glottic slit (the space between the vocal cords) lying opposite the bottom of the third cervical vertebra. In the adult, the glottis lies opposite the inner space of the fourth and fifth cervical vertebrae. The epiglottis of the neonate is narrow and omega-shaped (Ω) and relatively immobile in relation to the vocal cords, in contrast to the broad, mobile, V-shaped adult epiglottis. The narrowest portion of the pediatric upper respiratory tract is at the cricoid ring. In older children (over 6 to 8 years old) and adults, the narrowest portion of the upper airway is the glottic slit. Many congenital anomalies and inherited metabolic disorders are associated with abnormalities of upper airway anatomy.

INDICATIONS FOR ARTIFICIAL AIRWAYS

There are four indications for the use of an artificial airway:

1. To *establish an airway* when a patient is obstructed or unable to maintain the patency of his or her own natural airway.
2. To *protect the airway from aspiration* when the patient is comatose or has lost his or her protective tracheolaryngeal reflexes.
3. For *bronchopulmonary hygiene* when the patient has an inadequate cough reflex, has excess mucus production, or is unable to clear the secretions from his airway.
4. When the patient requires *prolonged positive-pressure ventilation*, such as for respiratory arrest, for application of PEEP, or during anesthesia, particularly if paralyzing agents are used.

Relief of Airway Obstruction

There are many causes of airway obstruction that require the use of an artificial airway. If a supine patient is comatose or under general anesthesia, he or she can be so relaxed that the tongue falls back in the mouth and obstructs the airway. The airway obstruction experienced by patients who emerge from anesthesia may be considered as a severe form of snoring. Patients who are obese or who have extra folds of tissue in the airway may suffer from sleep apnea, which is caused by airway obstruction when they lose consciousness (see Chapter 5).

Compression of the airway by masses in the neck, such as tumors, fat, expanding hematomas, or infection, can require the placement of an artificial airway. There are many processes that involve the larynx and obstruct its orifice, thereby requiring alternative ways of insuring airflow. As noted in Chapter 6, epiglottitis is a bacterial infection that causes such severe swelling of the tissues immediately above the laryngeal inlet that the airway may become completely occluded. Injury to the recurrent laryngeal nerve may produce vocal cord paralysis and airway obstruction. Laryngeal spasm is a condition that may produce partial or complete airway obstruction by abnormal contractions of the laryngeal muscles caused by hypokalemia, tetany, or light levels of general anesthesia. Anaphylaxis can rapidly produce severe laryngeal edema to the point of suffocation and death unless treated. Additionally, laryngeal edema from instrumentation, such as bronchoscopy or previous endotracheal intubation, may require the use of an artificial airway to help assure the patency of the air passageway.

Airway Protection from Aspiration

Attempts at mechanical ventilation with an obstructed airway can result in inflation of the stomach. This increases the possibility of vomiting (active) and regurgitation (passive movement of stomach contents into the pharynx), which can produce potentially lethal aspiration. Protection of the airway from aspiration may also require tubes that block the esophagus or prevent material in the mouth and pharynx from entering the lungs. The presence of a cuffed tube in the trachea minimizes, but does not necessarily prevent, aspiration. Aspiration around an inflated, properly positioned cuffed endotracheal tube has been documented.

Induction of general anesthesia removes the protective reflexes of the larynx. If the patient has a full stomach or increased intra-abdominal pressure, such as from bowel obstruction or pregnancy, the airway must be protected from aspiration of stomach contents when general anesthesia is induced. Similarly, a patient who is comatose from head trauma or weakened from neuromuscular disease may have inadequate laryngeal reflexes and may be at risk for pulmonary aspiration. Surgery in the mouth, nose, and pharynx may cause accumulation of blood, secretions, or pus in the pharynx that may be aspirated if the upper airway is not protected.

Facilitation of Bronchopulmonary Hygiene

The use of artificial airways to facilitate bronchopulmonary hygiene is dependent on the type of pathology that necessitates their use. Patients who are acutely ill or recently postoperative may temporarily require the use of an artificial airway to facilitate suctioning airway secretions. Patients with chronic pulmonary disease or certain types of neuromuscular disease that cause progressive weakness, especially of ventilatory muscles, may benefit from long-term artificial airways that allow easy access for suctioning of pulmonary secretions. Suctioning of the airway is extensively discussed in Chapter 17.

Positive Airway Pressure Adjunct

Positive airway pressure with or without mechanical ventilation may require the use of an artificial airway. The presence of an artifical airway, however, does not require the use of positive-pressure ventilation. A patient may ventilate well spontaneously once the airway obstruction has been relieved. Similarly, the application of positive-pressure ventilation does not always mandate the application of an artificial airway, for example, the use of continuous positive airway pressure (CPAP) by mask. However, positive-pressure ventilation is almost always associated with the use of some type of artificial airway, particularly for prolonged applications. An artificial airway can help reduce inflation of the stomach with air and assure patency of the airway when mechanical ventilatory support is required. By relieving airway obstruction, artificial airways also reduce the amount of pressure necessary to ventilate the lungs.

TYPES OF ARTIFICIAL AIRWAYS

There are several types of artificial airways (Table 18–1), but they are not interchangeable. Some are appropriate for certain indications but may be in-

TABLE 18–1. Types of Artificial Airways

1. Extension of the neck and elevation of the jaw.*
2. Oropharyngeal and nasopharyngeal airways.
3. Esophageal obturators.
4. Orotracheal and nasotracheal tubes.
5. Endobronchial tubes.
6. Cricothyroidotomy.
7. Tracheotomy.

*Although positioning the head and jaw does not utilize a mechanical airway, this procedure is artificial in the sense that the natural airway is obstructed.

appropriate or dangerous in other situations. Problems associated with the different artificial airways are described later.

Positioning the Head and Jaw

Although positioning the head and jaw is not literally an artificial airway, it is often a very effective method of re-establishing airflow when loss of muscular tone in the natural airway causes obstruction. Fainting or general anesthesia can result in loss of tone of the upper airway voluntary muscles with resultant airway obstruction. Simple extension of the head and lift of the chin (elevation of the jaw) may clear the airway, allowing the patient to continue spontaneous breathing (Fig. 18–1).

Because of anatomic differences from the adult, the extension of the neck of a neonate may actually *produce* upper airway obstruction. To open the neonatal airway, the mandible should be elevated with the head in a relatively neutral position (sniffing position). Similarly, in young children, hyperextension of the neck may produce airway obstruction. Thus, only mild extension with jaw elevation is necessary in this age group. In all age groups, flexion of the neck produces airway obstruction and should be avoided.

Positioning of the head and chin can facilitate spontaneous ventilation in the comatose patient. This technique is a valuable initial adjunct for the administration of cardiopulmonary resuscitation (CPR) because it facilitates artificial ventilation (mouth-to-mouth) when equipment is unavailable. In a trauma victim with possible neck injury, initial attempts at opening the airway use the chin-lift or jaw-thrust method without head-tilt to reduce the chance of spinal cord injury. If the airway remains occluded, head-tilt is gradually and gently applied until the airway is open.

Clearing the airway by positioning of the head and jaw is standard procedure when general anesthesia is administered by mask. During general anesthesia, this simple technique often prevents airway obstruction that would require the insertion of a more invasive type of airway.

Perform the *Heimlich maneuver* (subdiaphragmatic abdominal thrusts) first before attempting artificial ventilation if a person collapses or has a cardiopulmonary arrest near an eating establishment or if there is evidence of foreign matter obstruction of the airway. The rescuer stands behind the victim, wraps his or her arms around the victim's abdomen, clasping the hands together, and then presses the fists into the victim's abdomen beneath the ribs to dislodge food or objects on which the victim has choked. Slapping a choking person on the back drives the aspirated object further into the victim's airway and lungs, worsening the obstruction, and is the incorrect way to handle choking.

Oropharyngeal Airway

The oropharyngeal airway is a question mark–shaped apparatus made of plastic, rubber, or metal (Fig. 18–2). It fits between the lips and teeth, curves over the top and back of the tongue, and inserts into the lower posterior pharynx. Properly positioned, the oropharyngeal airway holds the tongue away from the posterior wall of the pharynx. Metal airways are frequently associated with

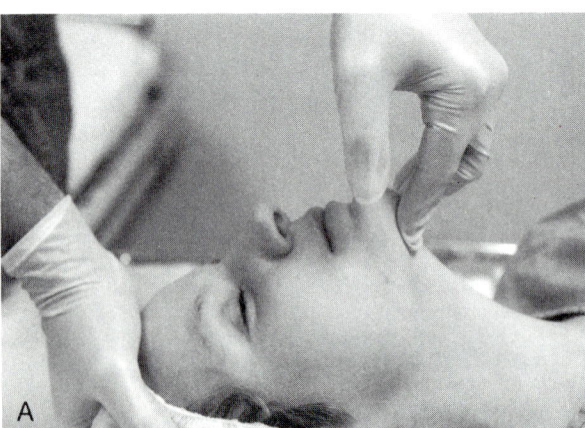 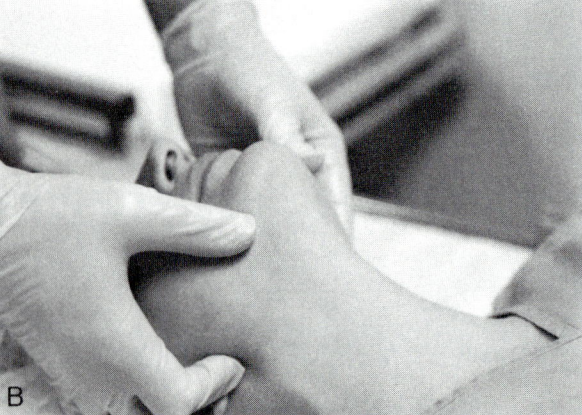

FIGURE 18–1. *A*, The head tilt-chin lift method of opening the airway. *B*, The head tilt-jaw thrust method of opening the airway. This technique can be used while holding a mask on the face for positive-pressure ventilation.

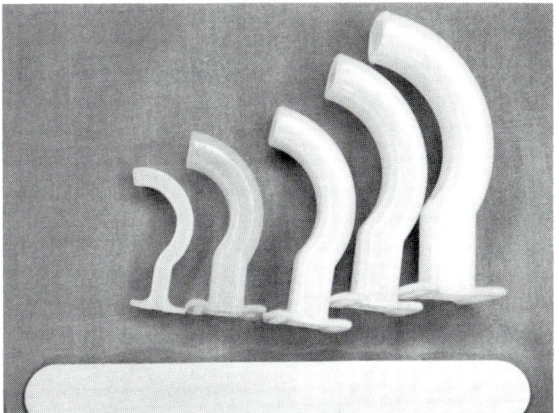

FIGURE 18–2. Oropharyngeal airways.

damage to the teeth and are no longer in common use. Oropharyngeal airways usually have a flange at the buccal (cheek) end that prevents the airway from falling back into the mouth. The bite portion of the airway fits between the teeth or gums. It must be firm enough to prevent the patient from occluding the air channel while biting hard. Oropharyngeal airways come in a variety of sizes, which are usually referred to by their length in millimeters.

The oropharyngeal airway is usually inserted after the tongue has been lifted out of the way with a tongue depressor (Fig. 18–3A). Improper placement of the oropharyngeal airway may push the tongue backward against the posterior pharynx, creating or aggravating the problem of airway obstruction. Another method of inserting the airway is to turn it so that it is inserted backward (with the outward curve facing the tongue) as it enters the mouth (Fig. 18–3B). When the airway has been inserted as far as it will go and approaches the posterior wall of the pharynx near the back of the tongue, it is rotated 180 degrees into its proper position. This technique does not require the use of a tongue depressor but risks abrasion of the roof of the mouth. Touching the back of the tongue and posterior pharynx with the oropharyngeal airway can stimulate retching and vomiting in a patient who is responsive. Insertion of the oropharyngeal airway with a tongue blade is probably the better technique because initial insertion of the tongue blade determines if the patient will tolerate the oropharyngeal airway before the airway is actually forced in. Proper head and jaw position must still be maintained with the use of this airway.

Nasopharyngeal Airway

The nasopharyngeal airway is a soft rubber or plastic tube that is inserted through the nostril into the posterior pharynx behind the tongue (Fig. 18–4). In its proper position, the nasopharyngeal airway lifts the tongue away from the posterior pharynx and allows the passage of air into the lower pharynx and larynx. It is very useful for supporting the airway in the patient who is post-ictal (the period immediately following an epileptic seizure), comatose, or emerging from anesthesia. Also, by passing a suction catheter through a nasopharyngeal airway, nasotracheal suctioning can be done relatively easily. Nasopharyngeal airways may be contraindicated in patients with coagulopathy, on anticoagulant medication, or with sepsis or deformity of the nasal cavity and nasopharynx.

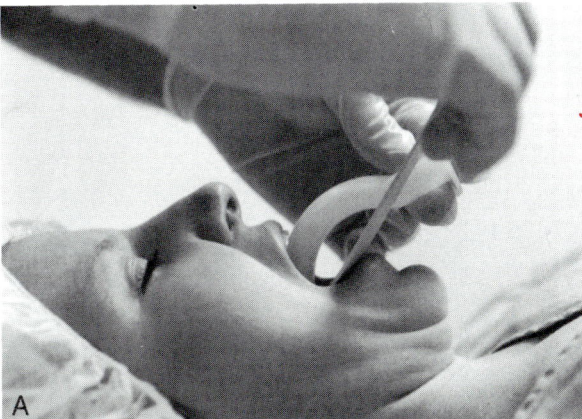
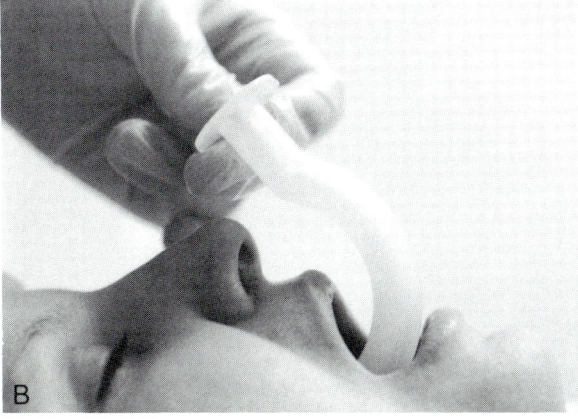

FIGURE 18–3. *A*, Inserting an oral airway using a tongue blade to displace the tongue forward. *B*, After inserting the airway in this manner, it is rotated 180 degrees into its final resting position.

492   AIRWAY MANAGEMENT

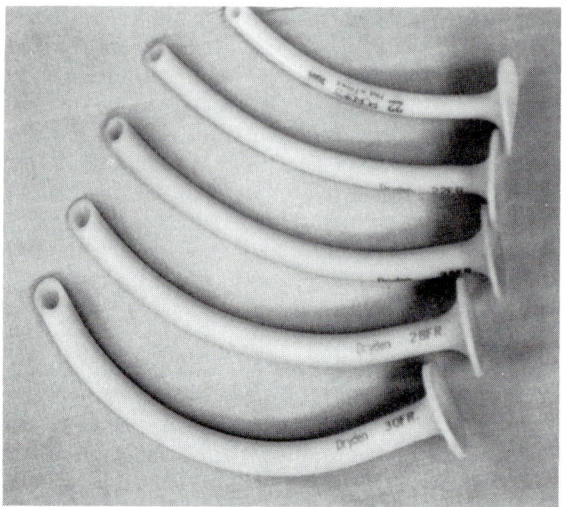

FIGURE 18–4. Nasopharyngeal airways.

Different types of nasopharyngeal airways are available, but they all have flanges at the nasal end and usually have a bevel at the pharyngeal end. Their shape follows the curvature of the nasal cavity and nasopharynx. Their size is usually measured by the French scale. The external diameter should be smaller than the external naris. A nasopharyngeal airway is much better tolerated than an oral airway in a responsive patient.

Before the tube is inserted, the nostril should be prepared with a vasoconstrictor, such as phenylephrine (Neo-Synephrine) or oxymetazoline (Afrin), to prevent nosebleed and also to facilitate the ease of passage by shrinking the nasal mucosa. The nasopharyngeal airway should be inserted gently with a lubricant. If the patient is awake, topical local anesthesia should also be utilized to facilitate insertion. The floor of the nasal cavity runs parallel to the roof of the mouth. However, the nostril opens slightly below the level of the floor of the nasal cavity. For this reason, insertion of a nasopharyngeal airway is easiest to perform if the nostril is elevated by pushing up on the tip of the nose, and the nasal airway is inserted directly toward the back of the head and directly parallel to the roof of the mouth (Fig. 18–5). Gentle steady pressure should be exerted but if excessive resistance is encountered, the other nostril or a smaller tube should be used.

Esophageal Obturator Airway

The esophageal obturator is a more invasive type of artificial airway with the benefit of ease of insertion by relatively untrained individuals. This type of airway has found the greatest use by emergency medical technicians in patients with cardiopulmonary arrest. The esophageal obturator has been developed for establishing an airway and attempting to protect the airway from aspiration of regurgitated stomach contents. It is inserted orally, and the tip lies in the esophagus. A balloon at the distal tip is then inflated to obstruct the esophageal orifice, blocking passive regurgitation (Fig. 18–6). Another lumen, which opens above the pharynx, is used to apply positive pressure to ventilate the patient. These types of airways are not effective in blocking active vomiting and may result in esophageal damage in an awakening patient who begins struggling. One type of esophageal obturator airway is a tube that is open at the

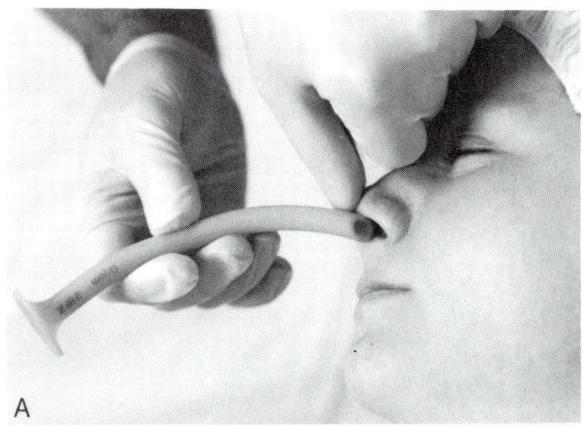 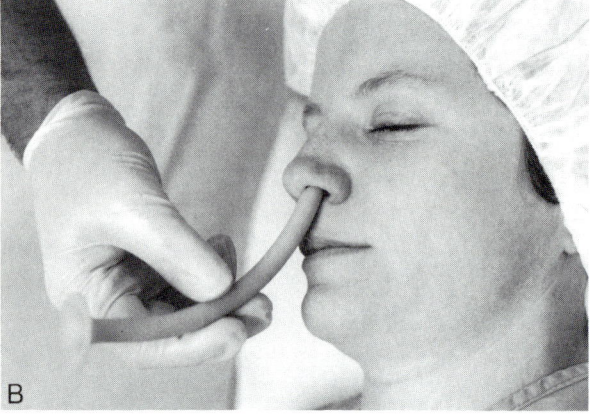

FIGURE 18–5. *A*, Correct insertion of a nasopharyngeal airway: The tip of the nose is elevated, and the airway is inserted perpendicularly, in line with the nasal passage. *B*, Incorrect insertion: The airway is being pushed into the turbinates and away from the nasal air passage.

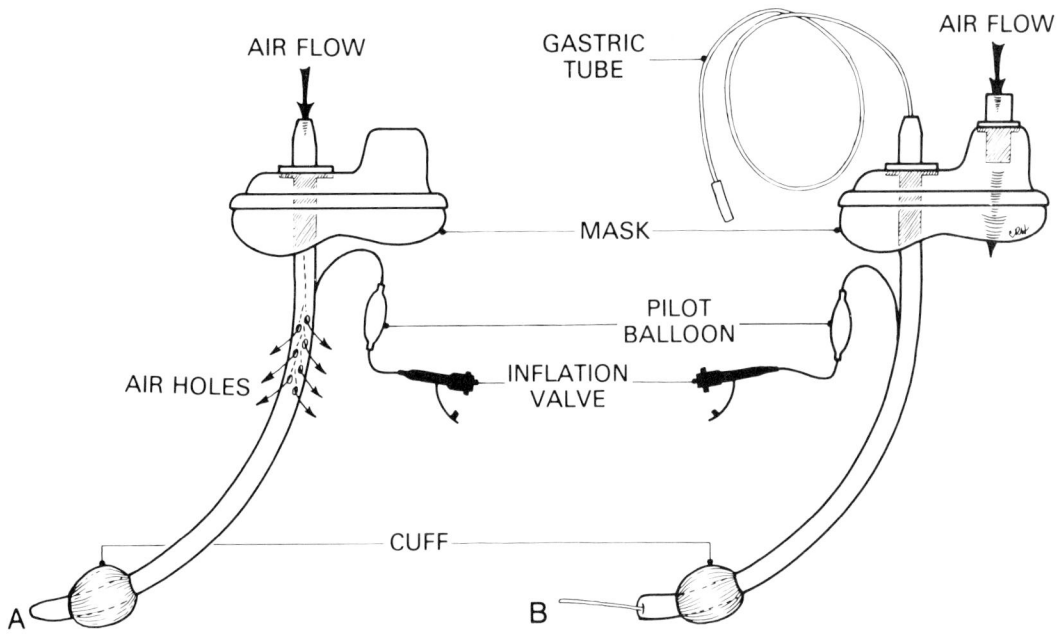

FIGURE 18–6. *A*, The esophageal obturator airway. *B*, The esophageal gastric tube airway. (From Miller, R.D. (ed.): *Anesthesia*, New York, Churchill Livingstone, 1981, with permission.)

top but has a blind end at the bottom (Fig. 18–6A). The lower blind end, which is inserted in the esophagus, has an inflatable cuff. There are several side holes located near the upper end, which allow the air to enter the pharynx from the inside of the tube. The upper end of this type of airway must be inserted through a specially designed face mask. Plastic prongs at the end of the tube project through a hole in the mask to hold the mask and tube together.

This type of tube is inserted by opening the mouth and blindly passing the tube into the mouth and pharynx (Table 18–2). With the head flexed forward and the tube in the midline, it should follow the natural curvature of the pharynx and pass directly into the esophagus. The tube is advanced until the mask is seated tightly against the face to effect an airtight seal (Fig. 18–7). When inserted in this manner, the cuff lies below the level of the carina of the trachea.

TABLE 18–2. Guidelines for Placement of an Esophageal Obturator Airway

1. Hold the mouth open with one hand while inserting the airway with the other hand.
2. Never use force while inserting the airway.
3. Flexion of the neck facilitates placement of the tube.
4. Be sure the tube remains in the midline.

Next, the person inserting the obturator blows into the airway (or uses a self-inflating resuscitation bag) and checks for chest expansion. If the tube is properly positioned in the esophagus and the nose and mouth sealed off by the face mask, air should exit from the side holes into the pharynx. Some air may pass into the stomach before the cuff on the esophageal airway is inflated, but most of it should enter the trachea. The cuff should not be inflated until correct placement in the esophagus is determined. If the chest does not rise and breath sounds cannot be auscultated over the lateral lung fields, then the airway is not in the esophagus and may be in the trachea. Auscultation over the epigastric area produces gurgling sounds, and breath sounds are not heard over the lungs if the tube is not properly placed in the esophagus. In this event, the airway should be removed immediately, and ventilation by another method should be tried.

When proper placement of the tube has been assured, the cuff should be inflated with up to 30 ml of air. With the face mask tightly sealed against the face, ventilation should be continued with a self-inflating resuscitation bag or other mechanical ventilator.

This type of airway should not be used in children under 16 years old, in cases of known esophageal disease, or when caustic poisons have been

AIRWAY MANAGEMENT

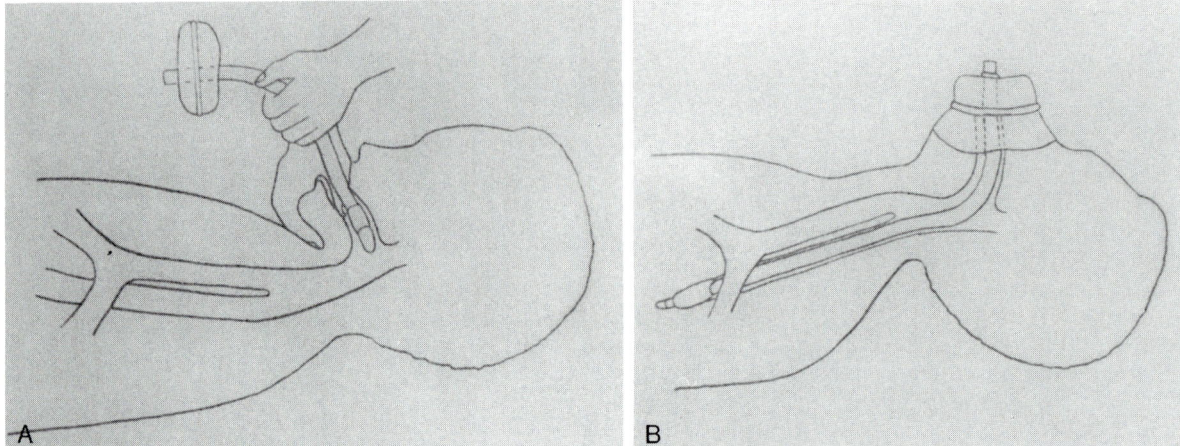

FIGURE 18–7. Insertion of an esophageal airway: With the head and neck flexed forward, the obturator is introduced into the esophagus with one hand while elevating the tongue and jaw with the other hand. The rim of the face mask must be pressed tightly against the face to form an airtight seal. (Reproduced with permission. © *Textbook of Advanced Cardiac Life Support* 1987, American Heart Association.)

ingested. It is intended for short-term use only and should be removed as soon as the patient regains airway reflexes (and only when suctioning equipment is immediately available). For patients requiring long-term ventilation and airway support, the esophageal airway is replaced by an endotracheal tube.

The method of conversion from an esophageal obturator to an endotracheal tube for airway management is controversial. Many people believe that the esophageal obturator should not be removed until the airway is secured and protected from aspiration by a cuffed endotracheal tube. Others suggest that the esophageal obturator should be removed as soon as the stomach contents have been aspirated by a gastric tube. The trachea should be intubated after the gastric tube and obturator are removed because laryngoscopy would then be least obstructed. It is important to remember that the use of an esophageal obturator for ventilation may produce distention of the stomach, and its removal can result in massive regurgitation.

The conservative approach to the conversion from an esophageal obturator to an endotracheal tube would be first to attempt laryngoscopy with the esophageal obturator in place and then, if the vocal cords can be successfully visualized, to insert the endotracheal tube. The esophageal obturator can be removed once the cuff of the endotracheal tube has been inflated. If the esophageal obturator obstructs the view of the vocal cords during laryngoscopy, then a person skilled at laryngoscopy and intubation should attempt endotracheal intubation after the stomach has been suctioned and the esophageal obturator removed.

The esophageal gastric tube airway is a modification of the esophageal obturator airway (Fig. 18–6B). In this type of tube, the distal tip is open. There is an opening in the mask through which the gastric tube can be passed to decompress the stomach. Unlike the esophageal obturator airway, there are no side holes in the tube. The lungs are ventilated via a separate opening in the mask. This modification permits the decompression of the stomach while the esophagus is still occluded.

Endotracheal Intubation

Endotracheal intubation consists of the passage of the tip of an artificial airway directly into the lumen of the trachea. The tube may enter the body either by the orotracheal route, passing first through the oral cavity and oropharynx before entering the laryngeal orifice (sometimes called the glottic slit); or by the nasotracheal route, passing through the nasal cavity, nasopharynx, then oropharynx and into the larynx. Although some tubes are specifically designed for orotracheal or nasotracheal routes, many are suitable for both. These hollow tubes are open at both ends and contain a standard 15 mm adaptor for attachment to a self-inflating resuscitation bag or mechanical ventilator tubing. Orotracheal and nasotracheal intubation is usually facilitated by laryngoscopy.

Laryngoscopy

A laryngoscope is an instrument used to visualize the laryngeal orifice (glottic slit) and surrounding structures. Some laryngoscopes have a separate light source and are designed for diagnostic evaluation of the larynx or for use during laryngeal surgery by otorhinolaryngologists. However, most laryngoscopes are used to facilitate intubation of the larynx and trachea and consist of two basic parts: the handle and the blade (Fig. 18–8). The handle is used to hold the laryngoscope and has a rough surface for traction. The handles are usually interchangeable and contain batteries for the light source. They are available in several sizes, and some have rechargeable batteries. Recently, a plastic laryngoscope with disposable blades has been developed to help reduce the risk of patient cross-contamination.

The laryngoscope blade is the part inserted into the mouth. It usually has a built-in light source, most commonly a bulb near the distal end of the blade. The laryngoscope blade is attached to the handle by inserting a U-shaped indentation on the base of the blade onto a small bar on the top of the handle (Fig. 18–9). This connection point between the handle and blade is called the fitting. The hook-on fitting is most commonly used in the United States, because it allows rapid exchange of blades. With proper alignment and complete insertion, the bar on the handle is locked into the indentation on the blade. The blade is then lifted on the handle until the light goes on. The circuit is completed when the blade is in its proper position. Most laryngoscope blades form a right angle with the handle when ready for use. However, certain types form acute or obtuse angles.

It is advisable to have laryngoscopes of several

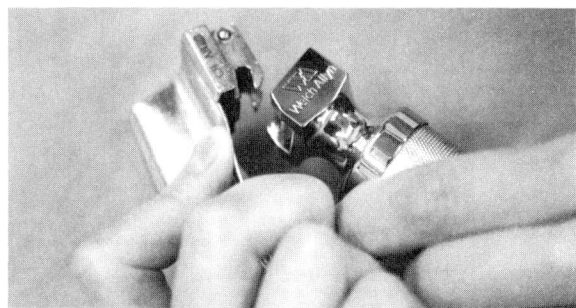

FIGURE 18–9. The bar on the laryngoscope handle fits into the U-shaped indentation on the base of the blade.

different sizes available. This is especially important for care of pediatric patients, because of wide variations in patient size, age, and underlying disease. The type and size of laryngoscope blades are usually stamped into the metal near the base. The sizes of blades generally fall within this range:

No. 0—premature infants
No. 1—term newborn to 3 years old
No. 2—3 years old to adolescents
No. 3—adults
No. 4—large adults

Although there are many types of laryngoscope blades, they are usually subdivided into two groups, according to their shape (Fig. 18–10). Curved blades, such as the MacIntosh, are advanced into the space between the base of the tongue and the pharyngeal surface of the epiglottis (vallecula). The glottic opening is exposed by lifting the blade forward and upward (Fig. 18–11A). The handle should not be pulled back because that

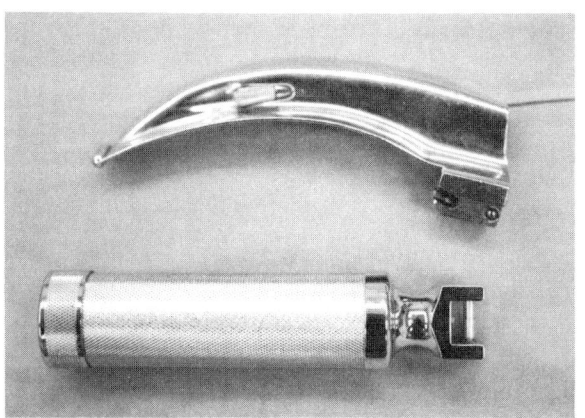

FIGURE 18–8. The laryngoscope handle and blade.

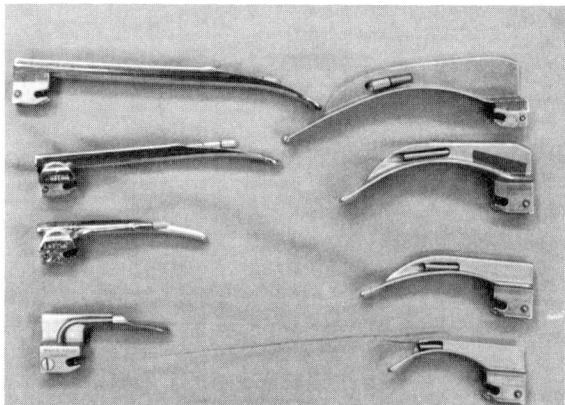

FIGURE 18–10. Examples of different sized commonly used laryngoscope blades. The blades on the right are curved (MacIntosh). The blades on the left are straight but with a curved distal tip (Miller).

496 AIRWAY MANAGEMENT

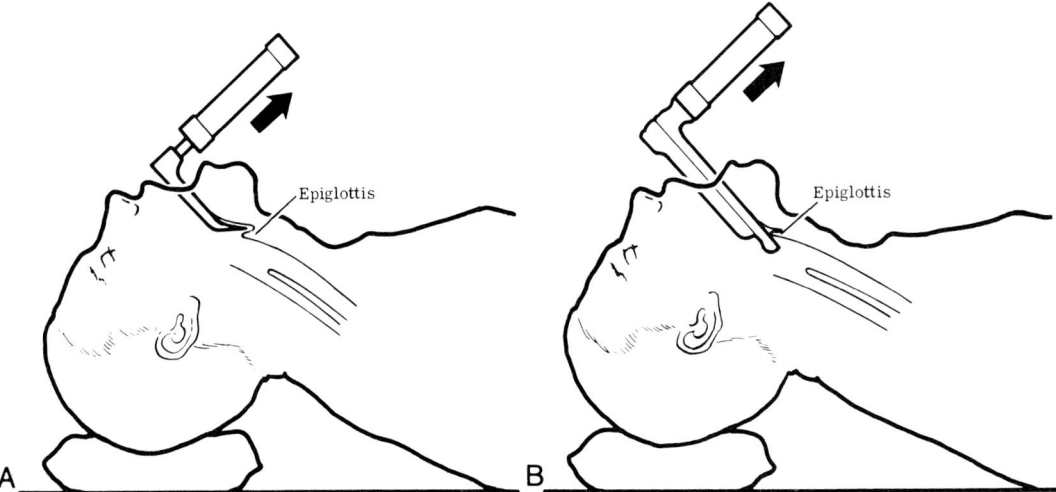

FIGURE 18-11. *A*, The distal tip of a curved blade is placed into the space between the base of the tongue and the pharyngeal surface of the epiglottis (vallecula). *B*, The distal tip of a straight blade is placed upon the laryngeal surface of the epiglottis. Forward and upward traction is exerted along the axis of the laryngoscope blade, as denoted by the arrows. Care must be taken to avoid rocking back with the laryngoscope, which may damage the teeth. (From Miller, R.D. (ed.): *Anesthesia*, New York, Churchill Livingstone, 1981, with permission.)

may damage the teeth. Straight laryngoscope blades, such as the Jackson-Wisconsin, are passed beneath the laryngeal surface of the epiglottis. Forward and upward movement of the blade by lifting the handle elevates the epiglottis and exposes the glottic slit (Fig. 18-11B). Again, the handle should not be pulled back because the teeth may be damaged. Straight blades with a curved tip, such as the Miller blade, are most commonly used in the manner of straight blades but may be occasionally used like a curved blade by inserting the tip into the vallecula.

The choice of which laryngoscope blade to use is most often based on personal preference. Many clinicians feel that a curved laryngoscope blade is less traumatic because it is placed in the vallecula and not directly upon the epiglottis as a straight blade is. The epiglottis is innervated by the superior laryngeal branch of the vagus nerve, and irritation of this area is believed to be more frequently associated with bronchospasm and coughing as well as edema of the epiglottis. For children, particularly neonates, many believe that a straight blade is more useful because of the large and relatively immobile epiglottis, which must be moved out of the way with direct compression by the straight laryngoscope blade in order to view the vocal cords (Fig. 18-11B). Curved blades may be placed directly on top of the epiglottis, and straight blades may be placed on the vallecula, so the real determinant of which type of laryngoscope blade to use is really based on the experience of the laryngoscopist. In general, the blade with which you are most experienced allows you to visualize the vocal cords most rapidly and with the least trauma.

Technique for Orotracheal Intubation

Several different types of endotracheal tubes are suitable for orotracheal insertion. Endotracheal tube sizes are indicated according to internal diameter (I.D.), which is marked on the outside of each tube. Different tube sizes are available in I.D. increments of 0.5 mm. Some endotracheal tubes are also marked in French units, which are the external diameter in millimeters multiplied by 3.14 (π). Tube length or distance from the tracheal end is also indicated on the outside of the tube by numbers that represent centimeters from the tracheal tip of the tube. These numbers permit accurate determination of the length of the tube inserted past the nares or lips. Endotracheal tubes are either radiopaque or have a stripe of radiopaque material along the outside, so the tube position can be determined on radiographs. The letters Z-79 (Committee Z-79 on Anesthesia Equipment of the U.S.A. Standards Institute) or I.T. (Implantation Tested) written on a tube indicate that evaluation of the tube material has revealed no tissue irritant or toxicity properties.

The first endotracheal tubes were made of natural rubber. Since then, endotracheal tubes have been composed of a great variety of materials, including synthetic rubber, silicon rubber, nylon, Teflon, polyethylene, and polyvinyl chloride (PVC). Some of these substances have been found to produce toxic reactions in the tissues and are no longer commonly used. The majority of endotracheal tubes now in use are disposable and composed of polyethylene or PVC, with a few varieties made of silicon rubber. A type of endotracheal tube called wire-embedded or *Anode* tube has a wire spiral embedded in the plastic or rubber for use in certain situations to help prevent kinking and obstruction of the airway.

A typical tracheal tube should have a radius of curvature of 14 cm (conforming to the curvature of the adult's natural airway structures). The cross section of the tube's internal and external walls should be circular, making them less likely to kink. The distal end of the tube, inserted into the patient's trachea, has a slanted portion called the bevel. The bevel facilitates threading the tube through the glottic slit. The distal tip should be rounded, with no sharp edges or points. There is usually a hole through the wall of the tube at the distal end opposite the bevel known as the *Murphy eye*, which allows the passage of gas through the tube even if the bevel is occluded, such as by pressing against the wall of the trachea. Tube markings are located on the beveled side of the tube near the end that protrudes from the patient's mouth (Fig. 18–12).

In adults, the use of an inflatable cuff near the distal end of the tube allows an airtight seal to be formed between the wall of the trachea and the endotracheal tube. In children, an airtight seal is accomplished by using an uncuffed tube that fits snugly inside the cricoid ring. It is therefore important to be able to predict the appropriate size of an endotracheal tube for a patient, particularly in children. This avoids the risks of reintubation if the tube is too small or if it has a large air leak when positive pressure is administered. Similarly, a tube that is too large may traumatize the airway structures or may be nearly impossible to insert.

Although several formulas and tables have been developed for determining the size and length of an endotracheal tube, the best correlation is based on the age of the patient (Table 18–3).

Although these guidelines help determine the approximate size and length of an endotracheal tube, clinical judgment and auscultation are also needed. When attempting intubation, endotracheal tubes should be available one size larger and one size smaller than the one indicated by this list. Insertion of an endotracheal tube too far into the trachea may result in inadvertent endobronchial intubation (usually into the right mainstem bronchus) and loss of breath sounds on one side. Additionally, the tube may impinge on the carina, resulting in sympathetic stimulation, coughing, and agitation of the patient.

The diameter of the natural airway is small in children. Cuffed endotracheal tubes are not recommended for routine use in children because the presence of the cuff prevents placement of the tube with the largest possible internal diameter in order to minimize airway resistance.

TABLE 18–3. Average Dimensions of Endotracheal Tubes Based on Patient Age

Age	Internal Diameter (mm)	French Unit	Distance Inserted From Lips to Place Distal end in the Midtrachea (cm)*
Premature	2.5	10–12	10
Full term	3.0	12–14	11
1–6 months	3.5	16	11
6–12 months	4.0	18	12
2 years	4.5	20	13
4 years	5.0	22	14
6 years	5.5	24	15–16
8 years	6.5	26	16–17
10 years	7.0	28	17–18
12 years	7.5	30	18–20
14 years and over:			
Females	7.5–8.0	32	20–22
Males	8.5–9.0	34–36	22–24

* Add 2 to 3 cm for nasal tubes.

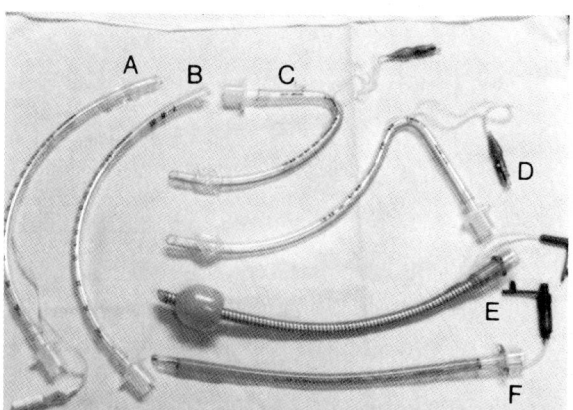

FIGURE 18–12. Different types of endotracheal tubes (note markings on the side of the tubes): *A*, A PVC cuffed tube. *B*, An uncuffed pediatric tube. *C*, An oral RAE (preformed) tube. *D*, A nasal RAE tube. *E, F,* Wire embedded nonkinking Anode tubes.

In adults, insertion of an endotracheal tube usually decreases deadspace because it contains a smaller volume of gas than the natural air passages. However, in pediatric patients, long tubes, connectors, and adaptors may result in increased deadspace and increased airways resistance.

It is important to remember that movement of the patient's head can increase the risk of malpositioning the tube. Flexing the neck usually results in migration of the tube down the airway, enhancing the likelihood of endobronchial intubation. Extension of the neck may result in extubation because the tube is drawn up the airway. Turning the head tends to slightly advance the tube downward as well as to promote preferential ventilation or even endobronchial intubation on that side. When the tip of the endotracheal tube is directed more toward one mainstem bronchus than the other (usually more toward the right), the flow of air preferentially favors that side. Gas tends to flow in a straight line because angulation produces turbulence and increased resistance.

When a cuffed endotracheal tube is used, the cuff is inflated with just enough air to produce an airtight seal when positive pressure is applied to the tube. The pressure in the cuff should be monitored with a manometer, usually at 8-hour intervals or whenever volume is added or removed from the cuff. The volume required to inflate the balloon is variable but generally in the range of 5 to 10 ml. Pressure should be maintained at 25 cmH_2O or less. The effects of cuff pressure are discussed later under complications. If high pressures are required to produce an airtight seal, the endotracheal tube may be too small for that patient, and replacement with a larger diameter tube may allow a seal to be formed at a lower cuff pressure.

The first cuffed endotracheal tubes used high pressure and low volume cuffs. This accomplished the primary objectives of cuffed tubes, that is, allowing the delivery of positive-pressure ventilation and protecting against aspiration. However, these tubes had the serious drawback of frequent tracheal damage, usually as a result of impaired mucosal blood flow. Modern endotracheal tube cuffs use high volume and low pressures, which greatly decrease the amount of pressure necessary to form a seal with the trachea and thus decrease the incidence and severity of tracheal damage.

The endotracheal tube cuff pressure is monitored by respiratory care personnel by either continuous or intermittent measurements with a manometer. This assures that the pressure remains at 25 cmH_2O, which is the capillary perfusion pressure for the tracheal mucosa. Patients who are inhaling nitrous oxide, as during general anesthesia, may develop increased cuff pressure. This is because the nitrous oxide is poorly soluble in the body's tissues and rapidly diffuses into air-containing cavities, such as the endotracheal tube cuff, which increases its volume and pressure. A pneumothorax is also susceptible to expansion for the same reason in a patient breathing nitrous oxide.

Certain types of endotracheal tubes have pressure-regulating devices to maintain low pressure against the tracheal wall (Fig. 18–13). The McGinnis pressure-regulating balloon is utilized in certain commercially available endotracheal tubes. An external pressure-regulating valve and control balloon limit the pressure developed in the tube's cuff to 20 to 25 cm H_2O as long as the control balloon is not inflated to the size of the outer cover. Overexpansion of the control balloon can cause very high cuff pressures.

Other devices to limit cuff pressure include a spring-loaded pressure-regulating relief valve (Shiley) as well as a cuff filled with soft spongy foam (Fome Cuff). The cuff is deflated, flattening the foam for placement during intubation. Once the tube is in place, air is allowed to enter the cuff, which allows the foam to attempt to resume its normal shape, thus providing an effective but low-pressure seal against the tracheal wall. These pres-

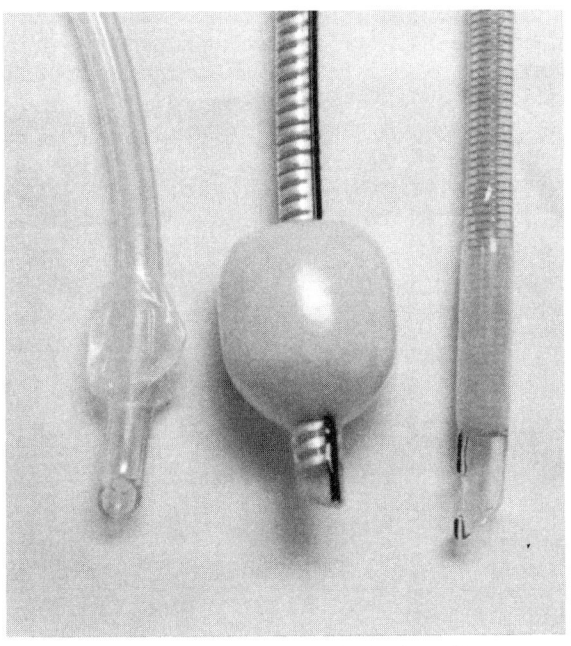

FIGURE 18–13. Endotracheal tube cuffs.

sure-regulating cuffs are also available for tracheostomy tubes.

Everything should be ready *before* an intubation attempt is begun. Table 18–4 lists all the basic materials that should be available before an intubation is attempted.

The patient should lie supine on a flat surface with the head positioned in the midline and slightly extended. Although both a head-up tilted position to reduce regurgitation and a head-down position to reduce aspiration have been suggested, positioning on a level surface facilitates ease and rapidity of intubation.

The ideal position for intubation is one in which the axes of the mouth, pharynx, and larynx are aligned (Fig. 18–14). This is accomplished by (1) extending the head and (2) flexing the neck at the cervical spine by slightly elevating the head. Because of the relatively large size of the head in infants and children, elevation of the head is not required for intubation. Hyperextension may obscure visualization and should be avoided, particularly with neck injuries.

Endotracheal intubation should be preceded by a period of ventilation with 100% oxygen. If the patient is apneic, mechanical ventilation with 100% oxygen by face mask and bag should be administered before any intubation attempt.

During intubation, the patient's ECG should be carefully monitored. The occurrence of a dysrhythmia or severe bradycardia requires the termination of intubation attempts, and the patient should again be ventilated with 100% oxygen by bag and mask.

If the patient is about to undergo general anesthesia and surgery, a sleep-inducing drug followed by a muscle relaxant is usually given at this point.

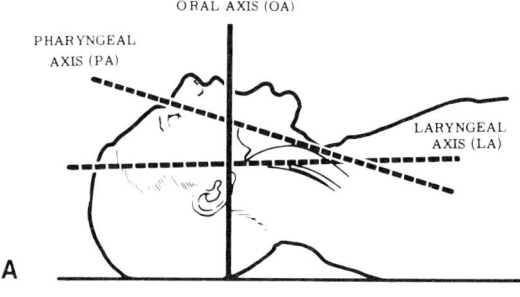
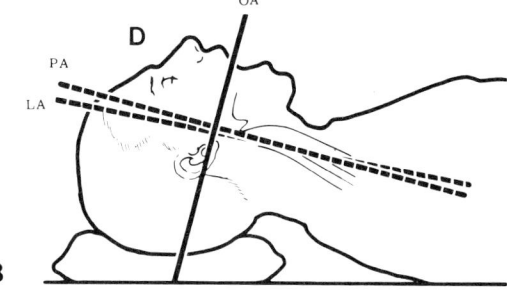
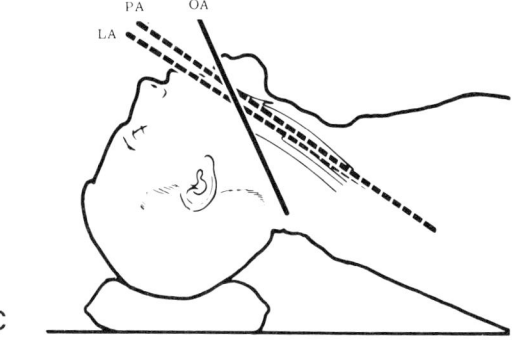

FIGURE 18–14. Correct positioning of the head and neck aligns the oral axis (OA), pharyngeal axis (PA), and laryngeal axis (LA). This is done by elevation of the occiput with a pillow while the shoulders remain on the table and by extension of the head. (From Miller, R.D. (ed.): *Anesthesia*, New York, Churchill Livingstone, 1981, with permission.)

TABLE 18–4. Preparation for Orotracheal Intubation

1. Suction device and tubing, set up and ready for immediate use.
2. Self-inflating resuscitation bag capable of administering 100% oxygen with appropriate size mask or other suitable means of mechanical ventilation with 100% oxygen.
3. Laryngoscope handle and appropriately sized and shaped blade.
4. Endotracheal tube appropriate for patient's age and tubes one size larger and one size smaller.
5. Syringe to inflate cuff if tube is cuffed (check cuff for leaks prior to insertion of the tube).
6. Stethoscope to check breath sounds and vital signs.
7. Tape to secure tube.
8. Immediate access to resuscitation drugs and equipment (code cart).
9. Stylet to provide rigidity and appropriate curvature to the endotracheal tube, when necessary.

This facilitates intubation by taking away a patient's ability to move. It is important to realize that these drugs stop spontaneous respiration and also block the laryngeal reflexes that prevent aspiration. Therefore, these drugs should only be administered by individuals experienced at intubation and mechanical ventilation. If the patient has suffered cardiopulmonary arrest and needs intubation to facilitate resuscitation, muscle relaxants are not usually necessary because these individuals are usually nonresponsive.

The patient's mouth should be opened with the intubator's right hand by pushing on the mandibular teeth with the thumb and the maxillary teeth with the fingers. This allows less traumatic insertion of the laryngoscope blade. The laryngoscope, held by the handle in the left hand, is inserted on the right side of the patient's mouth in order to avoid the incisor teeth and to deflect the tongue away from the lumen of the blade. The laryngoscope is then moved toward the midline, pushing the tongue to the left side of the mouth. The tongue should not be allowed to flop over the right side of the laryngoscope blade because this obscures the laryngoscopist's vision and inhibits insertion of the endotracheal tube. If a curved laryngoscope blade is used, its tip is positioned in the vallecula. By lifting up but not tilting the laryngoscope, the base of the tongue and epiglottis are elevated, and the glottic slit is exposed. If a straight blade or a straight blade with a curved tip is used, then the tip is placed upon the laryngeal surface of the epiglottis. Lifting the handle compresses and elevates the epiglottis, exposing the glottic slit. In neither case should the laryngoscopist lever the handle toward himself or herself because this may damage the patient's incisor teeth. Visualization of the glottis may be facilitated by slightly elevating the occiput or by gentle depression or lateral movement of the thyroid cartilage by external pressure on the neck. If the blade is inserted too deeply, the entire larynx may be elevated, exposing the esophagus.

Once the vocal cords are exposed, the endotracheal tube is passed to lie midway in the trachea. A cuffed endotracheal tube is inserted until the cuff just passes through the cords and no farther. The tips of uncuffed tubes may be colored or marked so that when the appropriate marking passes through the cords, no further insertion should be attempted (Fig. 18-15). At this point, the tube must be stabilized. The laryngoscopist then directs his or her attention to the portion of the tube protruding from the patient's mouth and determines the number marking on the side of the tube that corresponds to the patient's incisors or gums, if the patient is edentulous (toothless). This number is important to note so that when the tube is secured with tape or by other means, appropriate placement can be ascertained. Breath sounds should be auscultated before and after securing the tube with tape to assure correct placement and to rule out esophageal, pharyngeal, or bronchial placement of the distal tip of the endotracheal tube. Once the patient is intubated, his or her head should not be flexed or extended because the tip of the tube will move, as mentioned previously.

If prolonged intubation is anticipated, the tube

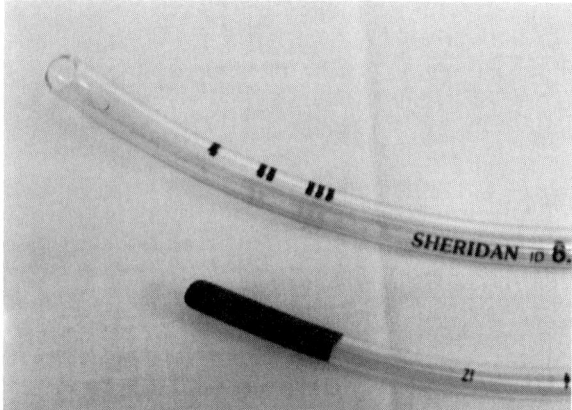

FIGURE 18-15. Endotracheal tubes with marks for assuring proper position.

may be better secured by application of a sticky substance, such as benzoin, to the patient's face before taping the tube in place. Tape or straps around the patient's head also increase the stability of the tube.

Emergency endotracheal intubation carries a great risk of regurgitation and aspiration of gastric contents. In this situation, an assistant should apply firm downward pressure over the cricoid, the only complete cartilaginous ring in the airway. This compresses the esophagus against the cervical vertebrae, preventing regurgitation (Sellick manuever, Fig. 18-16). This is maintained until intubation has been completed and the endotracheal tube cuff is inflated.

Difficult Intubations

Although the great majority of endotracheal intubations may be done in the manner just described, anatomic or pathologic alterations can make visualization of the larynx exceedingly difficult. In such instances, additional procedures may facilitate intubating difficult cases.

An endotracheal tube can be threaded over a flexible introducer. With the aid of a laryngoscope, the small-diameter introducer can be inserted into the larynx even without adequate exposure. After withdrawal of the laryngoscope, the endotracheal tube is threaded over the introducer into the trachea, and the introducer is then withdrawn.

The distal end of an endotracheal tube can be shaped using a wire stylet. An endotracheal tube with a stylet inside is usually shaped to resemble a hockey stick. The use of stylets is somewhat controversial, and many clinicians avoid them entirely. Disadvantages include tracheal or laryngeal trauma and using a tube larger than necessary. The

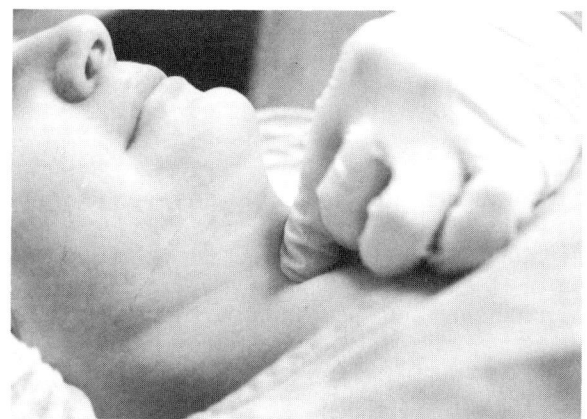

FIGURE 18–16. Compression of the esophagus between the cricoid cartilage and the vertebra (Sellick maneuver).

tip of the stylet should not extend beyond the end of the endotracheal tube, and great care must be taken to prevent this. Stylets should not be used for nasotracheal intubation because they increase the risk of nasopharyngeal injury.

Fiber-optic endoscopes are occasionally used to facilitate difficult intubations. The flexible portion of the fiber-optic endoscope is inserted through the endotracheal tube. By means of a proximal handle, the distal tip can be flexed over a wide range. Looking into the eyepiece of a flexible fiber-optic endoscope reveals the structures at the distal tip. As the laryngoscopist visualizes these structures and directs the distal tip by manipulating the proximal handle, he or she can advance the distal tip of the endoscope through the vocal cords and into the trachea. The endotracheal tube is then slid down and through the cords with the endoscope used as an introducer. The endoscope is then withdrawn. Small-diameter (pediatric) bronchoscopes are used in a similar manner. Disadvantages to using fiber-optic endoscopes are the difficulties in identifying the airway structures; secretions or condensation obscuring the field of vision; and the size of the instrument, which precludes its use with small internal diameter endotracheal tubes in children.

Retrograde intubation is a slightly more traumatic method of endotracheal intubation in a patient with a difficult airway. A catheter is introduced through the cricothyroid membrane and passed via the larynx into the mouth or nose. The tube is then threaded over the catheter into the mouth or nose and then down into the larynx and trachea. The technique for placement of the catheter is similar to that used for cricothyrotomy, which is discussed later.

Nasotracheal Intubation

When the mouth cannot be opened very wide and limited mobility of the cervical spine exists, blind nasotracheal intubation may be used. Topical anesthesia is applied to the nasal cavity, pharynx, and larynx. With the bevel facing the nasal septum, the well-lubricated endotracheal tube is introduced through the nostril along the floor of the nose into the pharynx. With the patient breathing spontaneously, the tube is advanced while the clinician listens for the sounds of air moving through the tube. Laryngoscopy is not necessary for this technique, but excessive extension or flexion of the head and neck should be avoided.

Although nasotracheal intubation is sometimes performed because the orotracheal route is not accessible, there are situations in which nasotracheal intubation is preferable to oral intubation even though the latter technique could be performed. An anesthesiologist may place a nasotracheal tube to facilitate certain types of oral or pharyngeal surgery. More commonly, nasotracheal tubes are used when the patient is expected to remain intubated for several days. This method of endotracheal intubation is more comfortable for the patient as well as being a more secure airway. Orotracheal intubation irritates the lips, tongue, and pharynx, while nasotracheal intubation is much less irritating. In addition, a nasotracheal tube is much less likely to be dislodged by patient movements. Movements of the patient's tongue and jaw can easily cause extubation with an orotracheal tube (tonguing the tube out). This is much less likely to occur with nasotracheal intubation.

Routine nasotracheal intubation is more difficult and more time-consuming to perform than routine orotracheal intubation. For this reason, nasotracheal intubation should not be the initial mode of endotracheal intubation in a patient who is hypoxic or in ventilatory failure. Orotracheal intubation should be performed initially and then converted to nasotracheal intubation once the patient is stable.

If the patient is conscious, the use of anesthetics and analgesics should be considered before attempting nasotracheal intubation. These drugs as well as muscle relaxants, which are sometimes used to facilitate intubation, should be administered only by individuals skilled at laryngoscopy and intubation because their use may produce total loss of a marginal airway. The nostrils should be examined to determine if air passage is easier on one side or the other if the patient is breathing spontaneously. The nostril with the easiest airflow is the one through which the initial intubation attempt should be done. However, both nostrils should be prepared a few minutes before attempting intubation by spraying them with 0.05% oxymetazoline or 0.25% phenylephrine. If the patient is going to be awake for the intubation, then local anesthetic should also be sprayed into the nasal cavity, pharynx, and larynx. Usually, 4% topical lidocaine is used for this purpose.

If time permits, the nasal cavity may be gradually dilated by inserting well-lubricated nasopharyngeal airways of increasing sizes. The nasotracheal tube is introduced through the nostril and nasal cavity and then into the nasopharynx.

If the patient's mouth cannot be opened, the blind nasotracheal technique is used, with the patient breathing spontaneously as described previously. In most cases, however, the mouth can be opened, so a laryngoscope is inserted to expose the tip of the nasotracheal tube in the pharynx as well as the laryngeal orifice. If the nasotracheal tube has been inserted too far, then it usually has gone into the esophagus and should be withdrawn until the tip can be seen in the pharynx. If the tip of the nasotracheal tube is not visible, then it should be advanced until it comes into view. Caution must be exercised if the nasotracheal tube is not visible because the tube may have burrowed submucosally behind the posterior pharyngeal wall, giving the appearance of a lump in the back of the throat. If this is the case, the tube should be withdrawn, which makes the lump disappear, and intubation attempts should then be made through the other nostril, or a smaller size tube should be used. When both the glottic slit and the tip of the nasotracheal tube are in view, the tip is grasped with Magill forceps (Fig. 18–17). While the laryngoscopist directs the tip of the tube toward the glottic slit with the Magill forceps, an assistant is instructed to insert the tube further by pushing gently down on the part remaining outside of the patient's nostril.

If the patient has been previously intubated with an orotracheal tube, then it should not be removed until the laryngoscopist has a good view of the glottis and the tip of the nasotracheal tube is grasped in the Magill forceps and is ready to be inserted through the glottic slit. In this way, the patient will be extubated for the shortest period of time possible, and the risk of aspiration is minimized. When the tip of the tube has passed through the cords, it is inserted until the upper end of the cuff is seen passing through the vocal cords (or until the appearance of the appropriate mark on an uncuffed tube). The cuff is then inflated, and breath sounds are auscultated bilaterally. After application of benzoin to the patient's face, the tube is then securely taped. The tape may be applied around the endotracheal tube and across the patient's upper lip or along the bridge of the nose or both for added security. Care must be taken to avoid traction or pressure on the rim of the nostril (ala) because necrosis of this thin area of the nose may result.

Endobronchial Intubation

The two main indications for deliberate endobronchial intubation are: (1) to provide independent airways and ventilation to each lung (usually in the case of unilateral lung disease) or (2) to improve surgical conditions during intrathoracic procedures by providing a quiet nonventilated lung. If deliberate endobronchial intubation is used only for improving intraoperative conditions, then at the end of the procedure, the endobronchial tube is replaced by a standard endotracheal tube. Specific indications for independent lung ventilation include unilateral lung diseases, such as lung abscess, bronchiectasis, bronchopleural fistula, or pulmonary contusion predominantly involving one lung.

Independent lung ventilation may be accomplished with a double-lumen endobronchial tube, which permits separate but simultaneous ventilation of both lungs. The Carlens double-lumen tube is introduced under direct vision laryngoscopy through the glottic slit. The thick-walled, red rubber tube is then rotated and advanced down the trachea with the tip pointed to enter the left mainstem bronchus. When the rubber hook near the end of the tube engages the carina, the tube should be

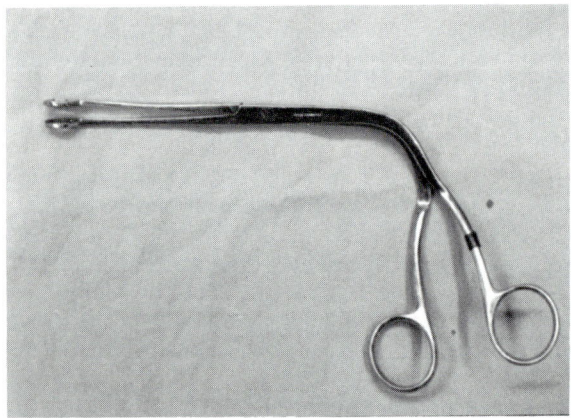

FIGURE 18–17. Placement of a nasotracheal tube is facilitated with Magill forceps.

inserted no farther. After inflation of the tracheal and left mainstem bronchus cuffs, correct placement should be verified by auscultation during independent ventilation of the tubes separately as well as together. The left lung should be ventilated through the tube lumen that lies in the bronchus, while the right lung receives ventilation through the lumen that opens above the carina (Fig. 18–18A). Effective isolation of the lungs and selective ventilation should be verified by auscultation and may be further verified by the use of a pediatric bronchoscope passed through the lumens of both tubes to verify the locations of the ends of this type of airway.

The White tube is a modification for placement in the right mainstem bronchus (Fig. 18–18B). The cuff on the bronchial tube is fenestrated to permit ventilation of the right upper lobe. This is because the distance from the carina to the right upper lobe bronchus is only about 1.5 cm. The left mainstem bronchus is about 5 cm long before it divides into the bronchi for the left upper and left lower lobes.

The Robertshaw double-lumen tube is available in a left and right sided bronchial model. Both are composed of PVC, which allows the tubing to be much thinner walled, thereby maximizing the internal diameters available. Unlike the Carlens or White double-lumen tube, the Robertshaw has no carinal hook. This increases the likelihood of incorrect placement by advancing the tube too far down the bronchus, but it is less traumatic to the carina.

Double-lumen tubes can be used to prevent spillage or contamination from a diseased to a nondiseased lung, for correction of life-threatening ventilation-perfusion mismatch, and for special procedures such as thoracoscopy or unilateral bronchopulmonary lavage. Intraoperatively, the most common indication for the use of a double-lumen endobronchial tube is to collapse a lung during intrathoracic operations to provide a quiet accessible surgical field. Hypoxemia is the greatest risk of one lung ventilation following endobronchial intubation. Although hypoxic pulmonary vasoconstriction tends to divert blood flow away from the collapsed lung, some shunting persists as some blood flow continues through the collapsed lung. To help avoid hypoxemia, 100% oxygen should be delivered to the ventilated lung during unilateral ventilation. The use of PEEP or CPAP

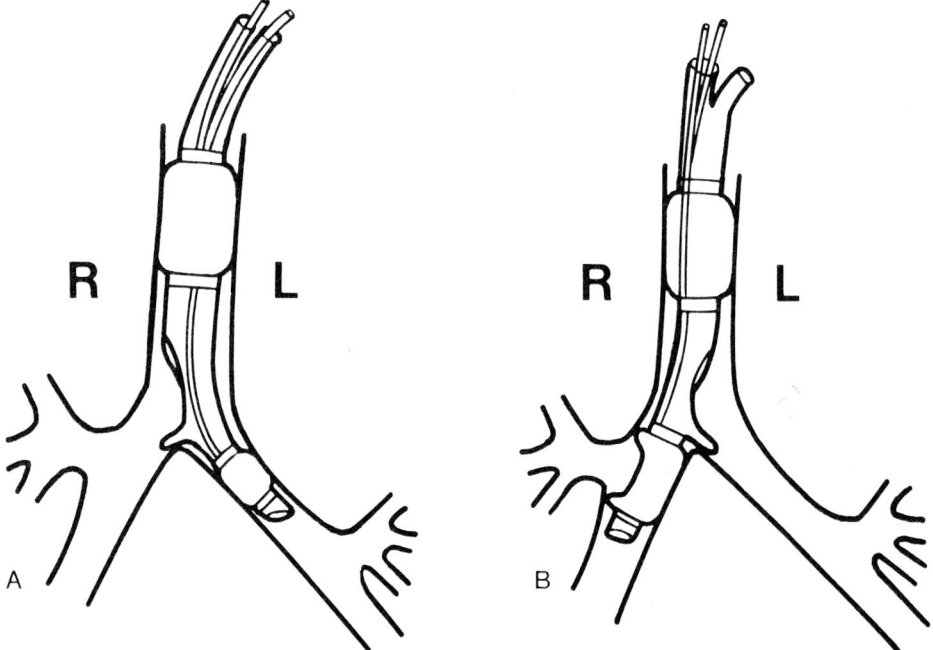

FIGURE 18–18. *A*, The Carlens double-lumen endobronchial tube is positioned with the distal end in the left mainstem bronchus when the rubber hook engages the carina. Inflation of both the tracheal and left mainstem bronchus cuffs isolates the lungs and permits selective ventilation when the tube is properly positioned. *B*, The White tube is positioned with the tip in the right mainstem bronchus when the hook engages the carina. Ventilation of the right upper lobe is accomplished via an opening through the cuffed portion of the tube opposite the right mainstem bronchus. (From Miller, R.D. (ed.): *Anesthesia*, New York, Churchill Livingstone, 1981, with permission.)

in the ventilated lung may divert blood flow from that lung to the nonventilated lung, increasing shunt.

Independent ventilation has been used for intensive care therapy of unilateral lung disease. The use of higher distending pressures in the diseased lung may divert blood flow from that lung and into the "normal" lung, improving matching of ventilation and perfusion. Independent ventilation may also be useful in the presence of a bronchopleural cutaneous fistula, which occasionally produces a leak so bad that adequate ventilation cannot be delivered via a conventional endotracheal tube because the air rushes out of the lung through the fistula without producing any ventilation.

Double-lumen endobronchial tubes are occasionally used for a surgical procedure called unilateral bronchopulmonary lavage. This is done for patients with a disease called alveolar proteinosis. In this disease, thick secretions develop on the walls of the alveoli, impairing gas exchange with the pulmonary capillary blood. The patient is anesthetized, and while ventilation is continued in one lung, the other lung is irrigated with saline several times, which washes out the protein buildup. Because the airways are separated by the double-lumen endobronchial tube, the ventilated lung is protected from spillage of the irrigation, so gas exchange can continue.

The major complications associated with double-lumen endobronchial tubes are airway trauma and malposition. These large tubes are not recommended for use in children.

Cricothyroidotomy

Cricothyroidotomy is a method for rapid access to the airway when attempts at endotracheal intubation are unsuccessful. The cricothyroid membrane is a dense fibroelastic structure immediately subcutaneous in location that is easy to identify. The area has no overlying large veins, and the posterior wall at this level is rigidly separated from the esophagus by the cricoid cartilage, making esophageal injury unlikely with cricothyroidotomy (in contrast to tracheostomy).

After careful palpation, location, and identification of the membrane between the cricoid and thyroid cartilages, a horizontal incision of less than 1/2 inch is usually made. A small endotracheal tube, tracheostomy tube, or other available cannula is then inserted to maintain the patency of the opening. Positive-pressure ventilation with high oxygen concentrations can then be delivered through these tubes. Various cricothyroidotomy kits are available commercially. This technique successfully allows rapid access of the airway by relatively untrained individuals. In cases of airway obstruction in which attempts at endotracheal intubation are unsuccessful, cricothyroidotomy can be an emergency life-saving technique (Fig. 18–19).

For an emergency in which less equipment is available, transtracheal catheter ventilation is performed by inserting a 14-gauge plastic intravenous catheter-needle assembly percutaneously through the cricothyroid membrane (Fig. 18–20). During insertion, negative pressure is applied by aspiration with a syringe; when the tracheal lumen is entered, air rushes into the syringe. The needle is then withdrawn and the catheter is advanced down into the trachea. The catheter hub is connected by a length of intravenous extension tubing to a hand-operated release valve. This, in turn, is attached by another length of tubing to a source that delivers

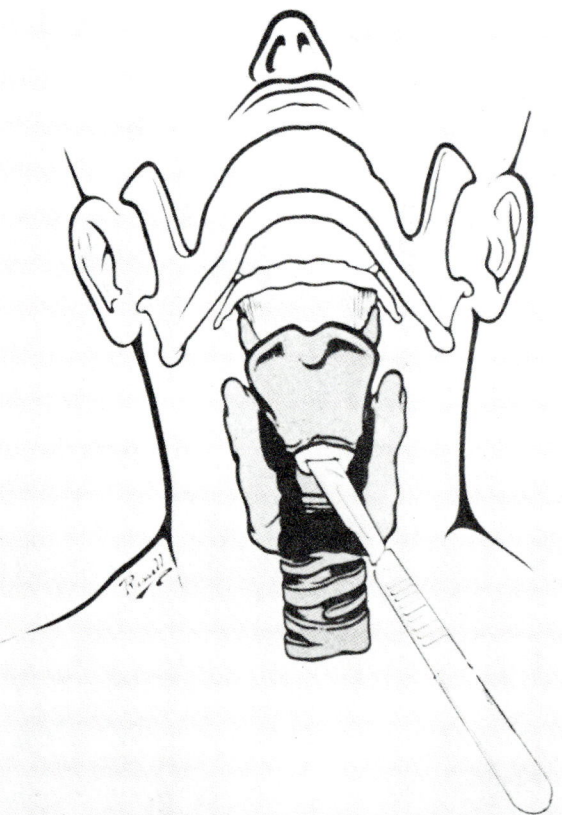

FIGURE 18–19. Cricothyroidotomy performed with a scalpel. An endotracheal tube is inserted through this opening into the lumen of the trachea. (Reproduced with permission. © *Textbook of Advanced Cardiac Life Support* 1987, American Heart Association.)

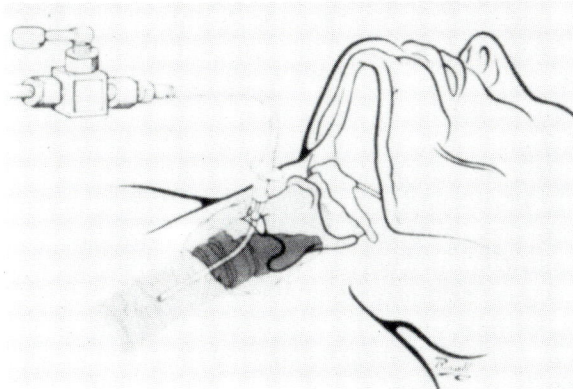

FIGURE 18–20. Transtracheal catheter ventilation. (Reproduced with permission. © *Textbook of Advanced Cardiac Life Support* 1987, American Heart Association.)

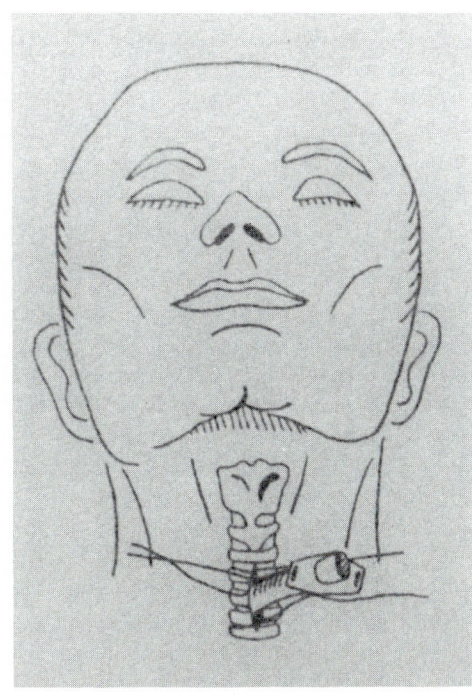

FIGURE 18–21. Insertion of tracheostomy tube through an incision made at the third and fourth tracheal rings.

oxygen at 50 psi. When the release valve is open, the oxygen flow inflates the lungs. When the patient's lungs appear inflated, the valve is then released and exhalation occurs passively. Because exhalation occurs through the upper airway, complete obstruction above the trachea prevents exhalation.

Usually, upper airway obstruction is incomplete. The retrograde gas leak may cause a partially obstructing foreign body to be expelled and also tends to expel oropharyngeal secretions, decreasing the problem of pulmonary aspiration. If a release valve and high-pressure oxygen source are not available, an adapter from a 2.5 mm diameter endotracheal tube may be inserted into the catheter hub and ventilation performed by a self-inflating resuscitation bag with 100% oxygen. However, minute ventilation by this mode is usually inadequate to maintain carbon dioxide at physiologic levels. Therefore, this mode of ventilation usually is only used to provide oxygenation while attempts at endotracheal intubation or tracheostomy are carried out. Cricothyroidotomy has also been used with high-frequency ventilation (see Chapter 19.)

Tracheotomy

Tracheotomy for the establishment of a percutaneous airway is almost always performed at the second to fourth tracheal rings (Fig. 18–21). An acute or emergency tracheostomy can prevent or bypass upper airway obstruction in patients who cannot be safely or successfully intubated endotracheally. Chronic tracheostomy, on the other hand, is more commonly performed electively because of the risk of laryngeal injury associated with prolonged oral or nasal endotracheal intubation. Tracheostomy is usually performed in the operating room by surgeons.

Tracheostomy tubes are L-shaped, and their size is determined by their internal diameter (Fig. 18–22). Indications for tracheostomy include airway obstruction above the level of the trachea that makes endotracheal intubation unsafe or unsuccessful. Tracheostomy is also indicated for patients who are unable to cough up bronchial secretions because of muscular weakness or other debility. When the pharyngeal or laryngeal reflexes are permanently lost, the lungs must be isolated from the pharynx and larynx by tracheostomy. Tracheostomy is also useful when prolonged positive-pressure ventilation is necessary. Prolonged endotracheal intubation risks injury to laryngeal structures, which is reduced by tracheostomy. Although much has been made of the 10% to 50% decrease in anatomic deadspace that tracheostomy produces, there appears to be little significance to this clinically.

Tracheostomy tubes tend to be left in place for prolonged periods, so accumulation of secretions on the tube can be a problem. Many types of tracheostomy tubes possess an inner cannula or sleeve

AIRWAY MANAGEMENT

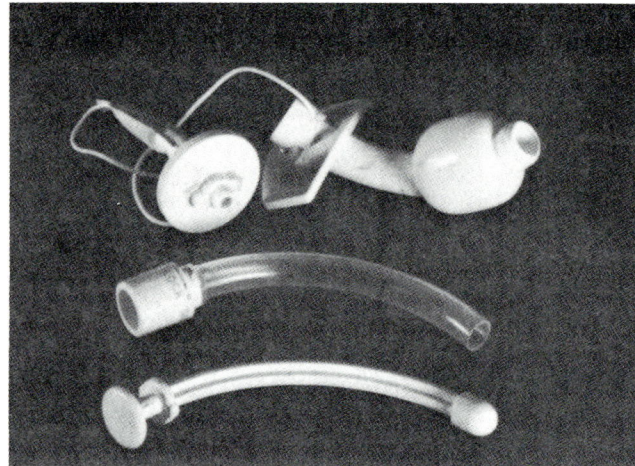

FIGURE 18–22. Shiley's tracheostomy tube with pressure-regulated valve for its low-pressure cuff. Also shown are the inner cannula (middle) and obturator (bottom). (From McPherson, S.: *Respiratory Therapy Equipment.* St. Louis, C.V. Mosby, 1985, with permission.)

that can be removed and cleaned periodically without having to remove the entire tracheostomy tube. Inadvertent total removal of the tracheostomy can result in life-threatening airway obstruction, especially if the tracheostomy was only recently performed. Chronic tracheostomy (such as following laryngectomy) results in the development of a permanent fistula in the neck with the result that no tracheostomy tube may be needed.

A *fenestrated* tracheostomy tube has an opening in the posterior wall above the cuff. The patient can inhale and exhale through the fenestration and around the tube when the inner cannula is removed. The cuff is deflated, and the normal inlet is occluded. This device is useful to assess a patient's ability to be extubated and also to allow the patient to verbalize when the tube is occluded and the cuff deflated. The inner cannula must be used when a seal is necessary.

The Pitt Speaking Tracheostomy tube allows tracheotomized patients to talk. A special modification provides a flow of gas from an external source through the patient's vocal cords, permitting vocalization.

PROBLEMS ASSOCIATED WITH ARTIFICIAL AIRWAYS

There are three major groups of problems associated with the use of an artificial airway: 1. Injuries to the patient sustained while inserting or applying an artificial airway. 2. Mechanical or structural problems. 3. Complications associated with long-term use.

Injuries During Application of Airways

Even a process as benign and noninvasive as extension of the neck and lifting the jaw can have devastating consequences if the patient has an unstable neck fracture. Traumatized patients with possible neck injuries should not be moved until the risk of spinal cord injury has been ruled out. Forceful attempts to elevate the jaw to clear the airway may result in a dislocated jaw and subsequent chewing difficulties.

The most common complication associated with the insertion of a nasopharyngeal airway is *epistaxis* (nosebleed). Nosebleed may be avoided by use of topical alpha adrenergic stimulants, such as phenylephrine (Neo-Synephrine) or oxymetazoline (Afrin), before attempting nasal intubation. A nosebleed may be extremely severe in a patient who is anticoagulated or has a coagulopathy. Unrelenting nosebleed may require treatment by surgical ligation of the maxillary artery, which provides blood flow to the lower nasal cavity. More extensive damage to structures in the nose and the nasopharynx is unlikely because of the softness of this particular airway.

A strong contraindication to the insertion of a nasopharyngeal airway or of any other object nasally (nasotracheal tube, nasogastric tube, temperature probe, or nasal suction tube) is the presence of a basilar skull fracture (usually associated with head injury). This can result in the passage of the tube directly into the brain or (more likely) the insertion of infectious organisms into the brain and meninges, producing encephalitis or meningitis. Signs of a basilar skull fracture include leakage of cerebrospinal fluid (CSF) from the nostrils or ears, bilateral hematomas under the eyes, or hematomas below and behind the external ears.

Insertion of an oropharyngeal airway may result in injury to the tongue or palate. Teeth can be damaged or dislodged if the patient bites hard on an airway, especially one of the metal types. These relatively hard devices may rupture abscesses in the mouth or orpharynx. As mentioned previously, incorrect placement of an oropharyngeal airway may push the tongue against the back of the pharyngeal wall, worsening obstruction. In a semi-awake individual, placement of an oropharyngeal airway may produce retching and vomiting with a potential of pulmonary aspiration. A semi-awake patient may also bite the person trying to insert the oropharyngeal airway.

Insertion of a long nasopharyngeal or oropharyngeal airway can precipitate coughing or laryngospasm if it touches the epiglottis or vocal cords. This usually occurs if the airway is inserted before attaining an adequate depth of general anesthesia and most frequently involves oral airways.

Hazards associated with the insertion of an esophageal obturator airway include laceration and rupture of the esophagus. Also, this tube may be inadvertently inserted into the trachea. Inflation of the large volume cuff may produce tracheal injury as well as occlude ventilation. This type of tube may also produce retching and vomiting in a patient whose airway reflexes are intact or who becomes responsive after the tube has been placed.

Complications associated with the insertion of an orotracheal tube can be caused by either laryngoscopy or placement of the tube itself. Teeth are frequently damaged or dislodged during laryngoscopy. Care must be taken to prevent dislodged teeth from entering the airway. Difficult laryngoscopy may also traumatize the tongue, pharynx, and larynx. The jaw may even be dislocated.

It is less traumatic to intubate under controlled stable conditions, that is, when you are not hurried. The main way to reduce the number of emergency intubations is to prevent accidental extubation. Some emergency intubations will always be necessary, but this is one area where experience is the best teacher. Skill at intubation (as with almost everything else) comes with experience.

If the patient has a peritonsillar or retropharyngeal abscess, airway instrumentation may cause abscess rupture and aspiration of this infected material. The risk of missed orotracheal intubation must also be included, that is, intubation of the esophagus or vallecula. Rupture of either of these structures or penetration of the wall of the larynx or trachea by the tracheal tube can produce pneumomediastinum or pneumothorax after positive-pressure ventilation has been applied.

Complications associated with nasotracheal intubation include all those associated with orotracheal intubation because laryngoscopy is frequently involved. There is also the risk of injuring nasal and nasopharyngeal structures. Additional complications include epistaxis, avulsion and aspiration of adenoids, and fracture or dislocation of the turbinates. Occasionally, nasotracheal tubes may burrow beneath the mucosa of the pharynx as they leave the nasal cavity. This makes it impossible to pass the tube through the vocal cords but is not otherwise usually associated with severe problems.

As mentioned previously, the endotracheal tube presses against the inner wall of the trachea. Nasotracheal tubes and oral tracheal tubes also press upon the vocal cords. The endotracheal tube produces irritation where it passes through the vocal cords. In addition, the contact of the endotracheal tube frequently produces a sore throat and hoarseness upon extubation. Mucosal edema associated with this irritation may partially or totally obstruct the extubated airway. Cool mist (humidified air by mask or face tent) is often used postextubation to decrease airway edema. Partial obstruction of the airway may be successfully relieved by the use of steroids or by nebulization of vasoconstrictors, such as racemic epinephrine (Vaponephrine). Total obstruction obviously requires immediate reintubation.

Placement of endobronchial tubes is associated with the same risks as orotracheal tubes. In addition, because of their shape and precise requirements for correct placement, insertion of endobronchial tubes is a time-consuming process that may result in a significant hypoxic interval. Furthermore, placement of the tube produces intense carinal stimulation, increased activity of the sympathetic nervous system, and frequently arrhythmias. Improper placement of the tube as well as movement of the tube may result in total airway obstruction or obstruction of one of the mainstem bronchi.

Acute complications of cricothyrotomy and tracheotomy are essentially the same. They include hemorrhage, esophageal injury, subcutaneous emphysema, and pneumothorax, with most of these resulting from forceful insertion of the tube.

Although artificial airways are inserted to treat airway obstruction, they themselves may become obstructed from airway secretions and blood clots. This is especially likely in tubes of narrow diameter. Kinking and external compression of the artificial airway may similarly obstruct the flow of air. Frequently, awake patients who have oral endotracheal or endobronchial tubes try to bite on them, causing obstruction. The concomitant use of a bite block or oral airway prevents this. The use of a nasotracheal tube eliminates obstruction of the tube by the patient biting it and makes untimely extubation less likely.

In addition to the periodic monitoring of respirations as part of monitoring vital signs, any changes in the patient's condition should serve as a stimulus to obtain a new set of vital signs. These include ventilatory rate and breath sounds, especially in a patient who has previously had trouble with upper airway obstruction.

Untimely extubation is a risk that you must always be prepared for. Not every patient who extubates himself or herself needs to be reintubated, but the risk of this always exists, and the equipment for reintubation should be readily accessible. At the patient's bedside should be a source of increased oxygen concentration, a mask, and a means to deliver positive-pressure ventilation. The patient's mouth should be well suctioned and the adequacy of ventilation evaluated. If the patient has severe lung disease or upper airway obstruction, then reintubation may be necessary. It is much less nerve-racking to avoid accidental extubation by carefully securing the airway with tape and headstraps or, if necessary, to sedate the patient or even to use restraints.

Mechanical or Structural Problems with Artificial Airways

Manufacturing flaws may partially or totally obstruct the inner lumen of any hollow artificial airway. Additionally, loose fragments may be aspirated into the lungs. Careful inspection of the patency and completeness of artificial airways should be carried out before insertion.

Occasionally, the valve to the injection port for the cuff of an artificial airway may become damaged. This so-called pilot valve is easily damaged by forcibly inserting a syringe tip into it when attempting to change the pressure and volume inside the cuff. If the pilot connector is broken or if the cuff becomes damaged and develops a leak, the artificial airway may need to be replaced with a new one.

The cuff portions of artificial airways are a frequent area of manufacturing flaws. A cuff may herniate through a weak spot into the inner lumen of an artificial airway, thus occluding it. The cuff may extend over the end of the artificial airway and occlude it (this was more common when cuffs were not firmly attached to the outside of artificial airways) (Fig. 18–23). Cuff rupture caused by overinflation or puncture by teeth is possible for any type of cuffed artificial airway. Although standardization of equipment has greatly decreased the incidence of airway connections failing to fit each other, the risk of this happening still exists and should be anticipated.

Complications Associated with Long-Term Use

The sites where artificial airways contact patient tissues are susceptible to injury. Airway pressure upon patient tissues may occlude blood flow, resulting in ischemic damage. Movement of the airway, which may result from patient movement, coughing, or even breathing, can abrade and irritate tissue surfaces of contact. The chemical composition of artificial airways may be irritating to some patients. For this reason, most materials used for long-term artificial airways have been tested by implantation in body tissues. Artificial airway materials that have proved to be nonreactive are marked I.T. (implant tested).

Airways that pass through the nasal cavity can press on the tissue surrounding the nostril, producing ischemia and ulceration (a condition known as alar necrosis). While passing through the nasal

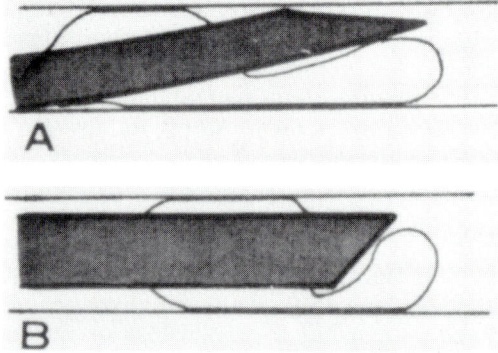

FIGURE 18–23. Occlusion of the tube lumen by compression from the cuff. (From Dorsch, J.A. and Dorsch, S.E.: *Understanding Anesthesia Equipment*, Williams and Wilkins, 1975, with permission.)

cavity, an airway may obstruct a nasal sinus, producing sinusitis and resulting systemic sepsis. Similarly, the eustachian tube may be obstructed by a nasal airway, resulting in middle ear infection. Insertion of a tube into the nose of a person with a basilar skull fracture may result in the tube entering the cranium and even the brain. Nasal leakage of cerebrospinal fluid contraindicates the use of a nasal tube because of the risk of infection.

The pressure of the endotracheal tube passing through the vocal cords may damage these structures. Long-term orotracheal, nasotracheal, or oral endobronchial intubation can produce damage to the vocal cords and larynx (ulcerations, paralysis, or nodules on the vocal cords).

Certain precautions must be taken when a cuffed artificial airway is used. The cuff is used to form a seal with the mucosa of the trachea. However, the use of excessive pressures can cause ischemia of the tracheal mucosa, which may result in necrosis of these tissues and even tracheal stenosis (narrowing). The cuff is normally inflated to approximately 25 cmH$_2$O. You may recall that the capillary hydrostatic pressure is also about 25 cm H$_2$O. Thus, if higher pressures are used to inflate the cuff, the perfusion of the underlying mucosa may be occluded. Cuff pressure must be routinely checked to help prevent the dangers of high pressure and ischemia. Monitoring cuff pressure also reduces the risk of inadequate inflation that may result in an inability to deliver the desired tidal volume because of leakage around the cuff. Pulmonary aspiration may occur around a deflated or ruptured cuff.

The proper technique for monitoring endotracheal tube cuff pressure utilizes a manometer and stopcock attached to the pilot valve so that volume can be added or taken from the cuff to produce the desired pressure. A technique that was formerly used required the cuff be inflated until there was no leak during a positive-pressure breath and then volume was removed from the cuff until a minimal leak occurred during peak inspiration. This technique should not be used because if very high airway pressures are used for ventilation, then excessively high cuff pressures can result.

Occasionally in patients with severe lung disease, very high airway pressures must be used for mechanical ventilation. These high airway pressures may be associated with a leak around the endotracheal tube cuff whenever a breath is delivered by the ventilator. In this situation, high pressures in the endotracheal tube cuff decrease the leak but may result in tracheal mucosal necrosis. Therefore, it is better to compensate for the leak by increasing the tidal volume administered until the desired *exhaled* volume is obtained. An alternative is to use a large-diameter endotracheal tube, the cuff of which would have a greater area of contact with the tracheal mucosa.

Cuffed endotracheal tubes are not routinely used in children under 6 years old because the narrowest portion of a child's upper airway is the cricoid cartilage, which forms a fairly good seal with a noncuffed endotracheal tube. If a cuffed endotracheal tube is used, a tube with a smaller internal diameter must be used because the cuff takes up space in the lumen of the airway. As dictated by Poiseuille's law, the reduction in airway diameter increases airway resistance.

Additionally, mucosal edema often develops in the area where the cuff makes contact. Following extubation, children are at much greater risk of airway obstruction from this mucosal edema because their airway diameters are smaller. The cuff increases the surface area of contact of the tube with the tracheal mucosa. It is not uncommon to get postextubation stridor in children following extubation. Some clinicians believe the incidence is increased if cuffed endotracheal tubes are used.

Endotracheal and endobronchial tubes as well as tracheostomy and cricothyroidotomy tubes may damage the tracheal mucosa and result in *tracheal stenosis* (permanent narrowing of the tracheal lumen). Occasionally, this complication is so severe that tracheal resection or permanent tracheostomy is necessary. The use of low-pressure, high-volume cuffs and careful monitoring of cuff pressure have greatly reduced the frequency of this complication.

Other complications of artificial airways (especially tracheostomy tubes) include tracheoesophageal fistula and tracheal–innominate artery fistula. Tracheal–innominate artery fistula causes patients to drown in their own blood. The tracheostomy tube can sometimes be advanced further down the trachea and the cuff temporarily overinflated to tamponade (plug or compress) the bleeding until it can be surgically repaired.

TERMINATING USE OF ARTIFICIAL AIRWAYS

Maintenance of the airway by neck extension and jaw elevation is usually a temporary measure. Its use is terminated either by the patient reviving and being able to maintain his or her own airway or by the insertion of an invasive type of airway. Similarly, oropharyngeal and nasopharyngeal airways are used primarily on a short-term basis, mostly in postanesthetic applications. As the patient awakens and the tone of the upper airway musculature returns, these devices are no longer necessary and may be removed. An esophageal obturator airway is removed when it is no longer needed. This is usually after an endotracheal tube has been placed by someone skilled at laryngoscopy and intubation. Similarly, endobronchial tubes are usually removed and replaced with endotracheal tubes when the indications for differential ventilation of the lung are resolved.

Because of the many serious complications associated with endotracheal intubation, extubation should be carried out as soon as the patient's condition allows. If the patient's airway was obstructed, then he or she should be extubated as soon as the cause of obstruction is relieved. Sometimes it is difficult to tell if the patient will tolerate extubation when swelling caused the obstruction. If the swelling was secondary to trauma, then usually 24 to 48 hours is sufficient for the swelling to subside. Acute epiglottitis also will resolve during this time if appropriate antibiotics are used. In other situations, resolution of the disease process and decreased swelling and tension in the neck would be signs indicating relief of airway compression. In any case, extubation must be performed while anticipating the possibility of an emergency reintubation. When laryngeal reflexes have returned and protection of the airway by the cuffed endotracheal tube is no longer necessary, extubation may be carried out. Remember that after a prolonged intubation, the laryngeal reflexes, such as coughing and those protecting the airway during swallowing, may be blunted for some time after extubation. Therefore, feeding and drinking should be withheld until the return of these reflexes has been confirmed. Oral feedings should progress gradually from liquids to solids following extubation.

When the patient is able to cough and clear his or her secretions, intubation for bronchopulmonary hygiene is no longer necessary. The adequacy of a patient's cough may be ascertained by measuring his or her vital capacity and negative inspiratory pressure (Table 18–5). Lastly, when the patient has been weaned from positive-pressure ventilation and is on minimal ventilatory support, discontinuation of ventilation and extubation may be carried out.

When the patient meets the criteria for extubation, the following procedures should be carried out: The patient is preoxygenated with 100% oxygen. The mouth and pharynx are carefully suc-

TABLE 18–5. Requirements for Extubation

1. Stable vital signs and cardiovascular status.
2. Causes for airway obstruction absent or resolved.
3. Upper airway reflexes intact.
4. Minimal ventilatory support.
5. Vital capacity greater than 10 ml/kg.
6. Forced negative inspiratory pressure less than -20 cm H_2O.

tioned to remove any secretions. If secretions are present in the endotracheal tube, it also should be suctioned. The patient is instructed to take a deep breath, or a breath is administered via the ventilator or self-inflating resuscitation bag, and the endotracheal tube is removed. The patient's first breath is therefore an exhalation, which helps carry any secretions out of the larynx. Careful monitoring of the patient immediately following extubation is essential in case reintubation is necessary. Supplemental oxygen may be necessary at this time. Cool mist or racemic epinephrine nebulization can reduce upper airway edema following extubation.

Some clinicians suggest that a suction catheter be placed through the endotracheal tube and suction applied during extubation to prevent pulmonary aspiration of secretions. The disadvantage of this technique is that air is removed from the lungs at a time when laryngospasm or airway edema may compromise patient ventilation. This technique is unnecessary if thorough suctioning of the mouth and pharynx is performed before attempting extubation.

Although there is considerable controversy on the subject, many clinicians believe that the complications associated with long-term cricothyroidotomy necessitate that this type of artificial airway should be promptly replaced by a surgical tracheostomy. Temporary tracheostomies are allowed to close by replacing the tracheostomy tube at intervals with one of a smaller diameter. This may take several months. Occasionally, the process of closure may be impeded by the development of a fistula that must then be surgically excised and the tracheostomy sutured closed. On the other hand, permanent tracheostomies likewise tend to heal closed, and their patency may be improved by occasionally dilating the stoma by the intermittent use of a tracheostomy tube.

Bibliography

Attia, R.R., Battit, G.E., and Murphy, J.D.: Transtracheal ventilation. *JAMA* 234:1152–1153, 1975.

Bishop, M.J., Weymuller, E.A., and Fink, B.R.: Laryngeal effects of prolonged intubation. *Anesth. Analg.* 63:335–342, 1984.

Brodsky, J.B., and Mark, J.B.: A simple technique for accurate placement of double-lumen endobronchial tubes. *Anesth. Rev.* 10(8):26–30, 1983.

Brodsky, J.B., Shulman, M.S., and Mark, J.B.: Malposition of left-sided double-lumen endobronchial tubes. *Anesthesiology* 62:667–669, 1985.

Conrardy, P.A., Goodman, L.R., Lainge, F., et al.: Alteration of endotracheal tube position. Flexion and extension of the neck. *Crit. Care Med.* 4:8, 1976.

Dorsch, J.A., and Dorsch, S.E. *Understanding Anesthesia Equipment: Construction, Care and Complications.* Baltimore, Williams and Wilkins, 1975.

Dunn, C.R., Dunn, D.L., and Moser, K.M.: Determinants of tracheal injury by cuffed tracheostomy tubes. *Chest* 65:128, 1974.

Eckenhoff, J.: Some anatomic considerations of infant larynx influencing endotracheal anesthesia. *Anesthesiology* 12:401, 1951.

Fergusson, W.V., and Fang, W.B.: Unusual problems of nasotracheal intubation. *Anesth. Rev.* 12(4):33–36, 1985.

Gregory, G.A.: Respiratory care of newborn infants. *Pediatr. Clin. North Am.* 19:311, 1972.

Harrison, E.E., Word, H.J., and Beeman, R.W.: Esophageal perforation following use of the esophageal obturator airway. *Ann. Emerg. Med.* 9:37–41, 1980.

Jastremski, M.S., Cantor, R.M., Olson, C.M., Smith, R.W., and Tyndall, G.J.: *The Whole Emergency Medicine Catalog.* Philadelphia, W.B. Saunders, 1985, pp 72–76.

Knodel, A.R., and Beekman, J.F.: Unexplained fevers in patients with nasotracheal intubation. *JAMA* 248(7):868–870, 1982.

Morain, W.D.: Cricothyroidostomy in head and neck surgery. *Plast. Reconstr. Surg.* 65(4):424–428, 1980.

Morris, F.C., Burns, D.S., and Vinson, R.: Intubation. In Levin, D.L., Morriss, F.C., and Moore, G.C. (eds.): *A Practical Guide to Pediatric Intensive Care.* St. Louis, C.V. Mosby, 1984, pp 536–541.

Salem, M.R., Mathrubhutham, M.D., and Bennett, E.J.: Difficult intubation. *N. Engl. J. Med.* 295:879–881, 1976.

Schofferman, J., Oill, P., and Lewis, A.J.: The esophageal obturator airway: A clinical evaluation. *Chest* 69:67–71, 1976.

Sellick, B.A.: Cricoid pressure to control regurgitation of stomach contents during induction of anesthesia. *Lancet* 2:404–406, 1961.

Stoelting, R.K.: Endotracheal intubation. In Miller, R.D. (ed.): *Anesthesia.* New York, Churchill Livingstone, 1981, pp 233–255.

Wagner, D.L., Gammage, G.W., and Wong, M.L.: Tracheal rupture following the insertion of a disposable double-lumen endotracheal tube. *Anesthesiology* 63:698–700, 1985.

White, R.D., Goldberg, A.H., and Montgomery, W.H.: Adjuncts for airway control and ventilation. In McIntyre, K.M., and Lewis, A.J. (eds.): *Textbook of Advanced Cardiac Life Support.* Dallas, American Heart Association, 1983, pp 39–48.

Witton, T.H.: An introduction to the fiberoptic laryngoscope. *Can. Anaesth. Soc. J.* 28(5):475–478, 1981.

OBJECTIVES

AFTER READING THIS CHAPTER, THE STUDENT WILL BE ABLE TO:

1. Review the history of mechanical ventilation and discuss the relatively recent development of modern ventilatory modalities.
2. List the indications for initiating mechanical ventilation.
3. Describe the equipment and techniques used during negative-pressure ventilation.
4. Identify functional characteristics of the breathing circuit used during positive-pressure mechanical ventilation.
5. Give examples of various power sources that are used to generate a positive-pressure breath.
6. Describe how ventilators can be classified according to mechanical and operational characteristics.
7. Define terms used in positive-pressure ventilation, such as cycling mechanism and ventilatory mode.
8. Describe four types of cycling mechanisms used in positive-pressure ventilators.
9. Describe various types of ventilatory modes that can be used with positive-pressure ventilation, including controlled ventilation, assisted ventilation, assist/control ventilation, and intermittent mandatory ventilation.
10. Discuss how synchronized intermittent mandatory ventilation and mandatory minute ventilation can be used in the management of ventilator-dependent patients.
11. Discuss special ventilator functions, such as inspiratory assist, pressure support, positive end-expiratory pressure, continuous positive airway pressure, periodic hyperinflation, and negative end-expiratory pressure.
12. List the three subdivisions of high-frequency ventilation (HFV). Contrast HFV to conventional positive-pressure ventilation. Explain the theoretical basis of gas exchange with HFV.
13. Describe the physiologic complications of mechanical ventilation on the pulmonary system.
14. Review the cardiovascular effects of mechanical ventilation and define the Traube-Hering reflex, sinus arrhythmia, and pulsus paradoxus.
15. Explain the interaction between the atria, the posterior pituitary, and the kidneys involving antidiuretic hormone. Describe the regulation of atrial natriuretic factor and its effect on the kidney.
16. Discuss the psychological effect of mechanical ventilation on critically ill patients with special regard for the care and monitoring of patients receiving paralyzing drugs.
17. Describe the process of weaning from mechanical ventilation and indicate which parameters should be reduced first.

19
MECHANICAL VENTILATION

CHAPTER OUTLINE

HISTORY OF MECHANICAL VENTILATION

INDICATIONS FOR MECHANICAL VENTILATION

TYPES OF MECHANICAL VENTILATION
  Negative-Pressure Ventilators
  Positive-Pressure Ventilators
    Methods of Generating Tidal Volume
    Mechanisms for Cycling Ventilators
    Initiation of Inspiration
    Special Functions
  High-Frequency Ventilators
    Theory of High-Frequency Ventilator Action

COMPLICATIONS OF MECHANICAL VENTILATION

Pulmonary Complications
Cardiovascular Complications
Renal Complications
Metabolic Complications
Psychologic Complications
Ventilator Malfunction

CHOOSING SPECIFIC VENTILATORY MODALITIES
  Negative-Pressure Ventilators
  Ventilator Rate and Tidal Volume Settings

WEANING FROM MECHANICAL VENTILATION

The major function of the respiratory system is gas exchange, that is, the exchange of oxygen and carbon dioxide between an organism and its environment. As discussed in Chapter 3, this is accomplished by the cyclic process of ventilation in which oxygen is brought into the lungs during inspiration and carbon dioxide is removed during expiration. During eupneic breathing, the force required to inflate the lungs during inspiration is provided mainly by contraction of the diaphragm and the external intercostal muscles, and the force required to empty the lungs during expiration is provided by the elastic recoil of the respiratory system. If a person fails to maintain this cyclic process of ventilation because of (1) a respiratory controller dysfunction, (2) a block in the transmission of impulses from the respiratory controller to the respiratory muscles, or (3) an inability to generate sufficient respiratory muscular contractile forces, the oxygen level in the arterial blood decreases, and the carbon dioxide level in the arterial blood increases.

Respiratory failure was previously defined as a state in which a patient cannot maintain his or her arterial blood gases within "normal" limits. (The clinical definition of respiratory failure is usually considered to be a Pa_{O_2} less than 50 torr and/or a Pa_{CO_2} greater than 50 torr). Additionally, respiratory failure can be acute, chronic, or both depending on the time it takes for the abnormalities of gas exchange to occur. Physiologic compensation allows gradual onset of respiratory insufficiency to be better tolerated than acute respiratory failure. However, patients with chronic respiratory insufficiency are less likely to derive long-term benefits from mechanical ventilation and these patients are often difficult or impossible to wean.

Although treatment modalities differ from one patient to another, it is generally agreed that the establishment of a patent airway, the administration of oxygen, and the maintenance of alveolar ventilation are required to effectively treat respiratory failure. Chapter 18 discussed the techniques required to establish and maintain an artificial airway, and Chapter 16 described several devices that can be used to administer oxygen to spontaneously breathing patients. This chapter discusses the use of mechanical ventilation in the treatment of patients who are unable to generate sufficient inspiratory and expiratory forces to maintain alveolar ventilation.

HISTORY OF MECHANICAL VENTILATION

There is a reference in the Old Testament (II Kings 4:34) to the use of mouth-to-mouth ventilation, which is probably the first recorded account of artificial ventilation. The first use of mechanical ventilation may have been by Paracelsus around 1530 when he used bellows to ventilate the lungs of animals. Robert Hooke in 1667 used bellows to ventilate dogs during surgery. John Hunter in 1776 advocated the resuscitative use of bellows to force air into the lungs of near-drowning victims. There are several reports in the late nineteenth century relating the use of endotracheal tubes and bellows to ventilate patients.

In the 1920s, the negative-pressure tank ventilator (the iron lung, or Drinker respirator) was in-

TABLE 19–1. Diseases Affecting the Components of Breathing

Site	Function	Disease Examples
Central nervous system	Generates ventilatory effort.	CNS depression (drug overdose), multiple sclerosis, CNS trauma.
Neural system	Transmits impulse from CNS to muscles of ventilation.	Polio, spinal cord or phrenic nerve injury.
Muscular system	Performs the work of breathing.	Paralyzing drugs (curare), muscular dystrophy.
Chest wall	Forms the rigid cage around the lungs.	Rib fractures, scoliosis.
Intrapleural	Moves lungs in unison with chest wall.	Tension pneumothorax, pleural effusion.
Airways	Conduct air to alveoli.	Upper: sleep apnea, laryngospasm, subglottic stenosis. Middle: asthma, bronchitis. Lower: emphysema.
Alveoli	Site of gas exchange from air to pulmonary capillary blood.	Pneumonia, atelectasis, late pulmonary edema, oxygen toxicity.
Interstitial space	Must be traversed by gas.	Pneumonia, early pulmonary edema.
Pulmonary capillaries	Carry gases between lungs and rest of body.	Cardiac insufficiency, pulmonary embolus.

vented and became popular because it did not require endotracheal intubation or tracheostomy. Endotracheal intubation was considered dangerous and difficult to perform at this time. In the 1930s, positive pressure was used in aviation at high altitudes. In the next decade, spontaneous positive-pressure (5 to 8 cmH$_2$O) breathing was used in the treatment of pulmonary edema.

The polio epidemic in 1952 produced a great number of patients with respiratory muscle paralysis requiring ventilatory support. There were not enough tank ventilators available, so endotracheal intubation and manual positive-pressure ventilation were performed. The success of this treatment served as an impetus for the development of mechanical positive-pressure ventilation.

Ashbaugh and colleagues introduced positive end-expiratory pressure (PEEP) for mechanical ventilation of patients with the acute respiratory distress syndrome in 1967. In 1971, Gregory and associates reported the use of continuous positive airway pressure (CPAP). Also in 1971, Kirby's group introduced intermittent mandatory ventilation (IMV). IMV allows the patient to breathe spontaneously through the ventilator circuit, and at predetermined intervals, the ventilator provides the inspiration. The clinical use of high-frequency ventilation became fairly common in the late 1970s following its description in 1967 by Sjostrand's group.

Presently, the most common applications of mechanical ventilation are in the operating room, recovery room, and intensive care unit. There has also been increasing use of home ventilation for patients requiring chronic mechanical ventilation, most commonly in patients with neuromuscular disease.

INDICATIONS FOR MECHANICAL VENTILATION

Simply put, the main indication for mechanical ventilation is inadequate spontaneous ventilation. As the patient's ability to ventilate spontaneously diminishes, oxygenation and/or carbon dioxide elimination deteriorate. Disease involving one or more of the components of breathing in Table 19–1 can impair the patient's spontaneous ventilatory effort. Some pathologic conditions can impair ventilation by affecting more than one site. A patient involved in a motor vehicle accident can have brain and spinal cord injury, rib fractures, pneumothorax, lung contusions, and pulmonary aspiration of gastric contents. Knowledge of the disease process can influence the decision concerning which type of ventilatory support is most appropriate for the patient. Disease affecting the pulmonary system can decrease a patient's spontaneous ventilation either by increasing the work of breathing, decreasing the patient's ability to perform the work of breathing, or both (Table 19–2).

Although many diseases can affect spontaneous ventilation, the pulmonary system can frequently compensate because of its large reserve and can maintain adequate alveolar ventilation. Arterial blood gases are frequently used to determine the adequacy of ventilation. An arterial PCO_2 greater than 55 torr or a PO_2 less than 55 torr suggests that mechanical ventilation *may* be necessary. Other guidelines, such as vital signs and pulmonary function tests, are helpful to determine the adequacy of the patient's ventilation (Table 19–3).

The values given in Table 19–3 are not absolute indicators for mechanical ventilation but must be correlated with the patient's clinical status and the pathophysiology of the disease. A patient who is apneic from a high spinal cord injury needs mechanical ventilation for the rest of his life. The patient paralyzed from the short-acting muscle relaxant succinylcholine (used with general anesthesia) may require mechanical ventilation for only a few minutes. An acutely elevated arterial PCO_2 strongly suggests the need for mechanical ventilation while chronic compensated elevation of the arterial PCO_2 does not.

The body may be unable to keep up with carbon dioxide elimination when ventilation is impaired, when carbon dioxide production is elevated, or when excess deadspace is present. When the breathing rate is too low (such as following narcotic overdoses) alveolar ventilation may be inadequate. On the other hand, when spontaneous ventilation is rapid, the patient may tire out from the increased work of breathing, necessitating mechanical ventilation. It is important to consider the patient's age because neonates can tolerate rates of 60 breaths per minute or more for extended periods.

TABLE 19–2. Conditions Affecting Spontaneous Ventilation

Defect	Example
Increased work of breathing	Obstructive or restrictive disease.
Decreased ability to perform the work of breathing	Starvation, neuromuscular disease, or drug overdose.
Combination of both	Severe pneumonia.

TABLE 19-3. Clinically Useful Indications of Inadequate Spontaneous Ventilation

Measurement	Normal Values	Indication for Mechanical Ventilation
Ventilatory Reserve		
Arterial P_{CO_2}, torr	35–45	>55*
Breathing frequency, per minute	12–20	<10 or >35
Vital capacity, ml/kg	65–75	<10–12
Tidal volume, ml/kg	6–8	<5
Maximum inspiratory pressure, cmH_2O	75–100	<25
V_D/V_T	0.25–0.40	>0.6
Minute ventilation, L/min	5–6	>10
Adequacy of Blood Oxygenation		
Arterial P_{O_2}, torr	70–100	<55
$P(A-a)O_2$, torr†	25–65	>450
Pulmonary shunt, %	<5	>20
Control of Intracranial Pressure		
Intracranial pressure, cmH_2O	12–15	>20

* Except in patients with chronic hypercapnia.
† While breathing 100% oxygen.

Mechanical ventilation is useful not only to replace or augment a patient's spontaneous ventilatory efforts but also to control intracranial pressure (ICP). Patients with an elevated ICP usually hyperventilate spontaneously if they are able. The reduced arterial P_{CO_2} causes cerebral vasoconstriction, decreases the volume of blood in the brain, and can result in a lower intracranial pressure. An arterial P_{CO_2} of 28 to 32 torr produces maximal cerebral vasoconstriction. An arterial P_{CO_2} below this may increase cerebral blood flow because of the shift of the oxyhemoglobin dissociation curve decreasing oxygen delivery to the brain. This causes cerebral hypoxia and vasodilation. Mechanical hyperventilation is also used during neurosurgery to reduce the size of the brain and improve surgical access.

The most important indicator for mechanical ventilation is clinical judgment. An apneic patient needs ventilation before blood gases or pulmonary function tests can be performed. On the other hand, patients who are unable to cooperate with bronchopulmonary hygiene treatments (such as those with cerebral palsy) may have acceptable arterial blood gas values immediately following surgery. However, prophylactic intubation and mechanical ventilation may be maintained for a few days to facilitate suctioning and reduce atelectasis in this type of patient until the restrictive defect induced by surgery resolves sufficiently.

Mechanical ventilation is frequently used with endotracheal intubation, so the indications may seem to be the same. However, mechanical ventilation can be carried out without endotracheal intubation, and conversely, endotracheal intubation does not mandate mechanical ventilation. The indications are different. This point is emphatically made during a cardiopulmonary arrest, for example. The patient must be mechanically ventilated with a mask and high oxygen concentration before any intubation attempt is carried out. To attempt to intubate before oxygenating the patient prolongs and worsens hypoxia to the patient's detriment. Conversely, a patient with a chronic tracheostomy following laryngectomy may spontaneously breathe quite adequately while having an endotracheal intubation.

As discussed later, mechanical ventilation includes several methods to move air into and out of the lungs. There are also modalities that supplement the patient's ventilation, affect lung volumes, or decrease the work of breathing. Mechanical ventilation can be used to totally replace a patient's spontaneous ventilation or improve the efficiency of a patient's own efforts. Mechanical ventilation encompasses several different therapeutic modes, which are discussed before the specific indications for their use.

Although mechanical ventilation provides undesirable physiologic consequences as well as life-threatening complications, there are several advantages for using mechanical ventilation early in the course of acute respiratory failure. The need for mechanical ventilation should be anticipated for patients likely to develop respiratory failure, such as individuals with chronic pulmonary disease who undergo extensive surgery. Clinical findings that suggest impending respiratory failure should trigger therapeutic intervention, which may frequently include mechanical ventilation. The patient should not be allowed to develop frank respiratory failure because the interval between the development of severe blood gas derangements and hypoxic tissue damage can be quite brief. Intervention at this time can be too late.

The development of acute respiratory failure can sometimes be avoided by insuring large tidal volumes (greater than 10 ml/kg body weight) and/or periodic artificial sighing, which helps minimize airway and alveolar collapse. The combination of endotracheal intubation and mechanical ventilation not only helps to prevent atelectasis but also facilitates suctioning to remove retained secretions. The presence of a cuffed endotracheal tube also reduces the risk of aspiration of pharyngeal contents.

The brain and heart of adult patients can be irreversibly damaged by hypoxic episodes lasting only a few minutes. Hypoxia to the immature organs of the newborn can trigger specific problems, such as intraventricular and intracerebral hemorrhage (bleeding inside the brain ventricles or the brain itself), necrotizing enterocolitis (infection and destruction of the digestive tract), and persistent fetal circulation such as patent ductus arteriosus (the fetal anastomosis between the aorta and pulmonary artery).

TYPES OF MECHANICAL VENTILATION

Mechanical ventilation is the term used to describe the process by which ventilation is maintained by artificial or extrinsic means. There are over 40 different models of mechanical ventilators available for clinical use. In the following discussion of mechanical ventilation, we have chosen to divide the various types of ventilators into two general categories: negative-pressure and positive-pressure ventilators. Within each category, we show how ventilators can be further classified according to their mechanical and operational characteristics. Because of space limitations, only examples of each of the various classes of mechanical ventilators are described. More detailed information on specific ventilators and their operational characteristics can be obtained from the Bibliography.

Negative-Pressure Ventilators

These devices attempt to mimic normal respiratory system mechanics by creating a subatmospheric pressure around the patient's lungs during inspiration to establish a negative alveolar pressure and thus the pressure gradient for airflow. This is accomplished by enclosing the patient's thorax within a sealed container that subjects the patient's chest to negative pressures. To initiate inspiration, the pressure inside the container is decreased to pressures of -5 to -15 cmH$_2$O. (As discussed in Chapter 3, all pressures are referenced to atmospheric pressure, which is arbitrarily considered to be 0 cmH$_2$O.) Expiration occurs passively as a result of elastic recoil forces of the respiratory system when the negative pressure is removed from around the thorax.

Two types of negative pressure ventilators are available for clinical use: the Drinker body tank respirator (or iron lung) and the chest cuirass.

The *body tank respirator* was introduced by Drinker and his colleagues in 1928. As Figure 19–1A shows, the patient's head is exposed to the atmosphere, and the remainder of his or her body is enclosed within an airtight chamber. An adjustable foam collar is used to provide a seal around the patient's neck. The negative pressure within the chamber is generated by an electrically driven motor that powers a bellows. (A handcrank is also provided to power the bellows in the event of an electrical power failure.) The volume of gas delivered to the patient is determined by the amount of negative pressure generated by the bellows and by the resistance and compliance characteristics of the patient's respiratory system. The ventilatory rate delivered to the patient is dependent upon the number of revolutions of the drive shaft attached to the bellows, which is controlled with a variable resistor.

A modified type of Drinker respirator has been used to provide continuous negative pressure around a patient's thorax. This increases the patient's FRC, possibly allowing for better lung compliance during spontaneous ventilation, and is comparable to PEEP (discussed later) during positive-pressure ventilation.

The *chest cuirass*, an alternative method of administering negative-pressure ventilation, was introduced by the J.H. Emerson Company in 1968. This device (Figure 19–1B) consists of a rigid shell that fits around the anterior and lateral portions of the patient's thorax. The posterior portion of the patient's thorax is sealed into the cuirass with a plastic wrap. The negative pressure generated within the shell is produced by an electrical pump, which is similar in design to a vacuum cleaner. Newer chest cuirasses have a flow sensor that is positioned at the patient's nose so that spontaneous inspiratory efforts by the patient can be used to trigger the ventilator. Thus, the chest cuirass can function as a controller, with the ventilatory rate set by the ventilator, or as an assister, in which case the ventilator cycles when the patient makes a sufficient inspiratory effort.

There are several advantages in using negative-pressure ventilation. Most important, because this type of ventilation attempts to mimic normal physiologic mechanisms, there are only minimal cardiovascular side effects in most patients.

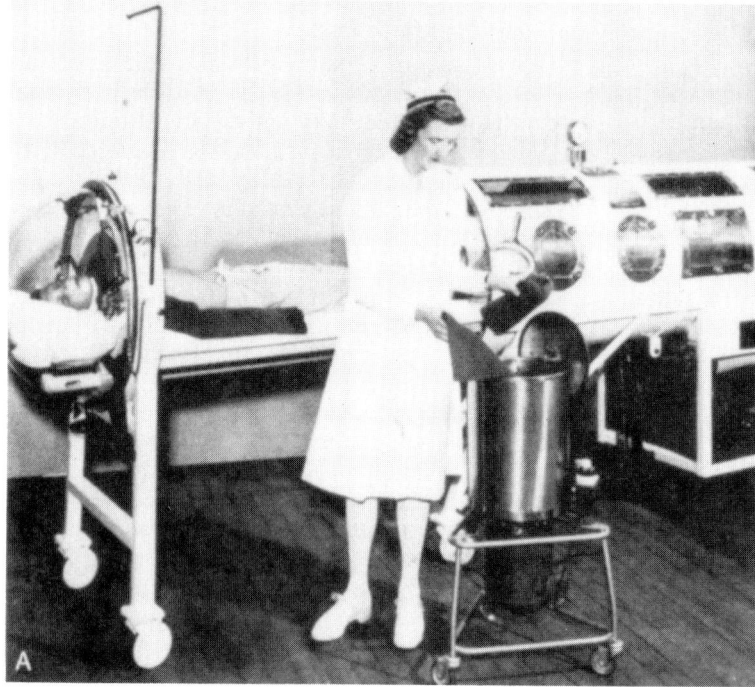

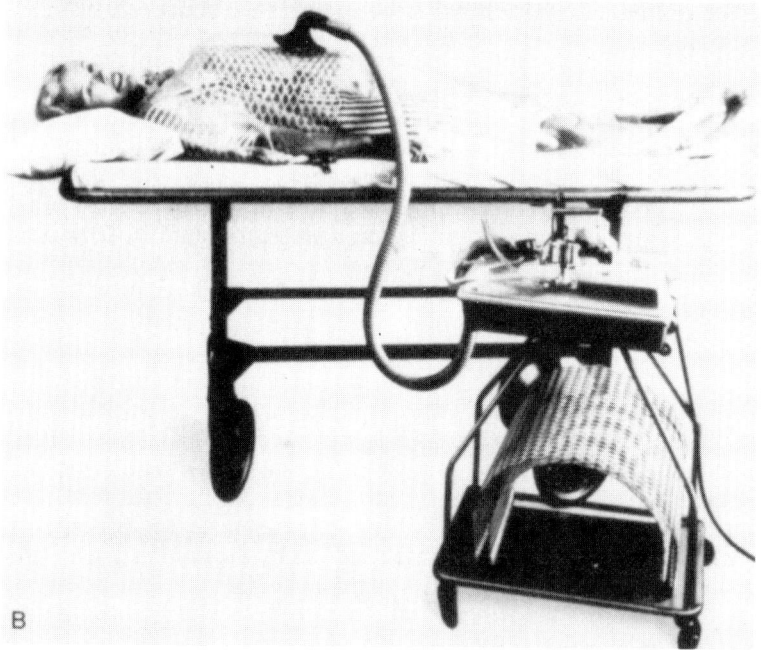

FIGURE 19–1. *A*, The Drinker body tank respirator (iron lung). *B*, Emerson chest cuirass (Courtesy J.H. Emerson Co., Cambridge, Mass.)

Additionally, because there is no need for a tracheostomy or endotracheal tube in patients who can protect their airways, they can continue to eat and talk while being artificially ventilated.

Some of the disadvantages associated with negative-pressure ventilators include:

1. Maintaining an adequate seal to prevent leaks in the system.
2. Limited access of the patient for nursing care.
3. Lack of control over the airflow rates delivered to the patient.

Furthermore, using the body tank respirator on hypovolemic patients can increase blood pooling within the abdomen with a concomitant reduction in the patient's venous return and cardiac output. This pooling occurs because the patient's abdominal vessels are subjected to the various negative pressures generated within the chamber.

The popularity of negative-pressure mechanical ventilation has declined since 1960, having reached its peak during the poliomyelitis epidemics of the 1950s. Negative-pressure ventilators are now primarily used to treat patients with spinal cord injuries and neuromuscular diseases. There has been a resurgence in the use of the chest cuirass ventilator in the home, particularly in patients who do not require a tracheostomy or endotracheal tube.

Positive-Pressure Ventilators

With this type of mechanical ventilation, positive pressure is applied at the airway opening, and air is forced into the patient's lungs. The pressure that can be generated by the ventilator is a function of the mechanical characteristics of the ventilator, whereas the pressure required to expand the patient's lungs is dependent upon the resistance and compliance characteristics of the lungs and thorax. Expiration during postve-pressure ventilation occurs passively as a result of the elastic recoil of the lungs and chest wall, and it is opposed by the resistance of the airways and the resistance offered by the expiratory limb of the ventilator circuit.

Positive-pressure ventilators are generally classified according to their operational characteristics during a respiratory cycle. These characteristics include:

1. The method used to generate the tidal volume.
2. The mechanism responsible for cycling the ventilator from inspiration to expiration.
3. The mechanism used to terminate expiration and initiate inspiration.
4. Special functions that can be performed with the ventilator, such as inspiratory plateau, continuous positive airway pressure (CPAP), positive end-expiratory pressure (PEEP), expiratory retard, and sigh (periodic hyperinflation).

High-frequency positive-pressure ventilators are usually considered separately from conventional positive-pressure ventilators. As discussed later, high-frequency ventilators are usually classified according to the respiratory frequency used to ventilate the patient and the characteristics of gas flow delivered to the patient.

The advantages of using positive-pressure ventilation in the treatment of ventilatory failure include:

1. Inspiratory pressures and airflows that can be manipulated by the therapist to achieve an optimal ventilatory pattern for a patient.
2. Easily maintained bronchial hygiene because long-term positive-pressure ventilation requires the placement of an endotracheal tube.

Complications associated with positive-pressure ventilation are primarily related to the positive pressures that occur in the airways, alveoli, and pleural space during both inspiration and expiration, including:

1. Barotrauma, such as pneumothorax, pneumomediastinum, and pneumoperitoneum.
2. Decreased venous return and cardiac output.
3. Alterations in ventilation-perfusion relationships throughout the lung.

As discussed later, the incidence and severity of these complications depend on the patient's physiologic reserve, lung and chest wall mechanics, and the amount of pressure required to effectively ventilate the patient.

Methods of Generating Tidal Volume

During the inspiratory phase of a positive-pressure breath, the ventilator can provide part or all of the force required to inflate the patient's lungs. Classification of ventilators based on the inspiratory phase usually involves descriptions of the mechanical construction of the ventilator and the pressure and flow waveforms developed by the ventilator during inspiration.

Mechanically, ventilators are classified according to:

1. Whether they are pneumatically or electrically powered.
2. The type of drive mechanism employed by the ventilator to create the tidal volume.
3. Whether a direct drive (single-circuit) or an indirect drive (double-circuit) mechanism is used to provide gas delivery to the patient.

With regard to the pressure and flow waveform developed by the ventilator during inspiration, four classes of ventilators are described: constant flow generators, constant pressure generators, nonconstant flow generators, and nonconstant pressure generators. Table 19–4 lists several commercially available ventilators.

TABLE 19–4. Commercially Available Ventilators

Ventilator	Patient application*	Power Source* I° (2°)	Cycling Mechanism* I → E	Volume Generation	IMV Capability	Fresh Gas Sources O_2	Air	Comments
Bennett MA1, MA2 7200 (CPU)**	A, P	El (Pn)	V (P)	F	Yes	40–60 psi	Ambient (MA1) 40–60 psi or Internal air compressor (MA2)	Electronic compressor produces gas drive for bellows that deliver tidal volume
Biomed MVP-10	N, P	Pn	T, V, P	F	Yes	45–55 psi	45–55 psi	Fluidic control
Bird Babybird Ventilator	N	Pn	T	F	Yes	50 psi	50 psi	Gas flow produces pressure changes that activate spring-loaded valves
Bird IMV Bird	A, P	Pn	T	P	Yes	50 psi	50 psi	Control of gas flow with spring-loaded valves
Bourns Adult Volume Ventilator Bear 1, Bear 5 (CPU)	A, P	El, Pn	V (T)†	F, P‡	Yes	32–100 psi	32–100 psi Internal air compressor	Electronic control of solenoid valves modulates flow
Bourns Infant Pressure Ventilator BP200	N	El, Pn	T	F, P§	Yes	30–75 psi	15–75 psi	Solenoid valve controls gas flow, which is modulated by needle valves
Bourns Infant Volume Ventilator LS 104-150	N	El	V ∝ T	F, P§	Yes	50 psi Ambient		Volume displacement by a piston
Emerson IMV Ventilator	A, P	El	V ∝ T	F	Yes	Flowmeter	Flowmeter	Volume displacement by a piston
Emerson Post-op Ventilator (modified)	A, P	El	V ∝ T	F	Yes	Flowmeter	Flowmeter	Volume displacement by a piston
Healthdyne Ventilator 105	N, P	El, Pn	T	F	Yes	45–65 psi	45–65 psi	Fluidic control
Monaghan Volume Ventilator 225	A	Pn	V, P, T	F	Yes	50 psi	50 psi	Fluidic control of gases that compress bellows
Ohio CCV1, CCV2	A, P	El, Pn	V (T)†	P, F‖	Yes	50 psi	Internal air compressor	Solenoid valve controls gas flow that compresses bellows
Sechrist Infant Ventilator IV-100	N, P	El	T	F	Yes	45–55 psi	45–55 psi	Fluidic control of gas flow
Siemans-Elema 900 Servo Ventilator, Servo 900C (CPU)	A, P, N	El	T	F	Yes	3–100 psi	3–300 psi	Servo flow control of gases from bellows source

From Hall, J.R.: Techniques of ventilation and oxygenation. In Kaplan, J.A., ed.: *Thoracic Anesthesia.* New York, 1983, Churchill Livingstone, Inc., with permission.

* A = adult, P = pediatric, N = neonatal. Power sources: Pn = pneumatic, El = electric. Cycling mechanism: T = time, V = volume, P = pressure. Volume generation: F = flow, P = pressure.
† If *Inspiratory hold* is employed.
‡ F or P dependent on lung-thorax conditions, airway pressure, and ventilator waveform control setting.
§ F under normal conditions; P if pressure limit is reached during inspiratory phase.
‖ F early in inspiratory phase; zero flow at end of inspiratory phase if inspiratory hold is employed.
** CPU = central processing unit (microcomputer based)

Mechanisms for Cycling Ventilators

The mechanism by which a ventilator terminates inspiration and initiates expiration is commonly referred to as the ventilator *cycling* mechanism:

- Volume cycling
- Pressure cycling
- Flow cycling
- Time cycling

Some ventilators have more than one cycling mechanism; however, only one is operational at a time. Note that the term "limiting device" is sometimes used interchangeably with cycling mechanism. Although these terms appear to be synonymous, limiting devices differ from cycling mechanisms in that they are incorporated into the ventilator design for safety purposes. These devices protect the patient from being exposed to excessive inspiratory pressures, flows, volumes, and times by terminating inspiration when a maximum value for any of these parameters has been reached.

Volume-Cycled Ventilators. With volume-cycled ventilators, inspiration ends when a preselected volume of gas is delivered to the patient (Fig. 19–2A). The duration of the inspiratory phase is primarily influenced by the ventilator flow rate achieved and the impedance offered by the ventilator-patient circuit. Traditionally, volume-cycled ventilators have been used extensively in the treatment of critically ill adult patients who are ventilator-dependent. The popularity of this type of ventilator with clinicians is related to two factors:

1. As long as the ventilator has a sufficiently high driving pressure, the preset volume is delivered to the patient regardless of changes in the resistance and compliance characteristics of the patient's respiratory system.

2. The oxygen concentration delivered to the patient can be accurately and easily controlled.

Problems commonly associated with volume-cycled ventilators include:

1. Air leaks within the ventilator or patient circuit reduce the volume of gas actually delivered to the patient.

2. For patients with increased airways resistance or decreased lung or chest wall compliance, excessively high airway and intrathoracic pressures may be generated, which can increase the incidence of barotrauma and cause signficant reductions in venous return and cardiac output.

The problems of air leaks can be minimized by monitoring the volume of exhaled gas. If the exhaled volume is significantly less than the volume delivered, an air leak is present within the ventilator-patient circuit. To avoid complications as-

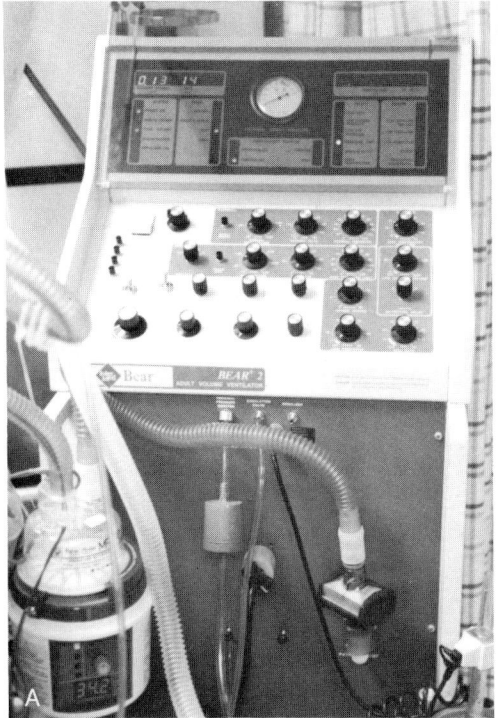
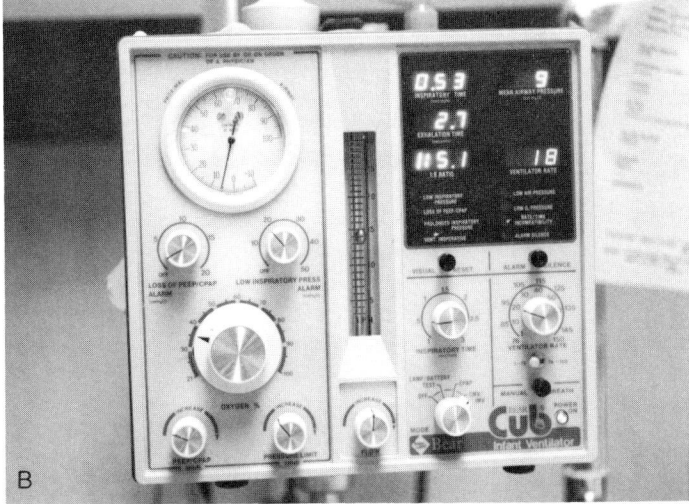

FIGURE 19–2. *A*, Volume-cycled ventilator. *B*, Pediatric pressure-limited, time-cycled ventilator.

sociated with excessive airway pressures, most volume-cycled ventilators have a pressure-limiting device incorporated into the ventilator. In some, the pressure limit is preset by the manufacturer, whereas others have an adjustable limit that can be controlled by the operator. When the pressure limit is reached, inspiration ceases, and the ventilator cycles into expiration.

Pressure-Cycled Ventilators. For pressure-cycled ventilators, inspiration ends when a preset driving pressure is attained (Fig. 19–2B). The duration of inspiration, and thus the volume of gas delivered to the patient, are determined by the driving pressure selected by the clinician and the resistance and compliance offered by the ventilator-patient breathing circuit. Pressure-cycled ventilators do not have the capability of generating high airway pressures (i.e., these devices typically are operated at pressures between 10 and 40 cmH$_2$O). Therefore, when this type of ventilator is used to treat patients with altered respiratory system mechanics (i.e., elevated airways resistance and/or reduced compliance), the volume of gas delivered to the patient and the fractional concentration of inspired oxygen (F$_I$O$_2$) may vary considerably. Because they cannot be counted on to deliver consistent ventilatory support in patients with high airways resistance or low respiratory system compliance, these devices are mainly used to ventilate patients requiring short-term ventilatory support (e.g., postoperative recovery from anesthesia) or patients in whom peak airway pressure must be limited to reduce the risk of barotrauma (i.e., in neonates).

Time-Cycled Ventilators. In time-cycled ventilators, the changeover from inspiration to expiration is brought about by a timing mechanism incorporated into the ventilator's drive mechanism. This timing mechanism may be controlled by electronic, pneumatic, electromechanical, or fluidic means. With time-cycled ventilators, the duration of the inspiratory phase is set by the clinician; the volume of gas delivered to the patient is influenced by the ventilator's driving pressure and the resistance and compliance characteristics of the ventilator-patient breathing circuit. With this type of ventilator, flow and inspiratory time determine tidal volume.

Flow-Cycled Ventilators. With flow-cycled ventilators, inspiration ends when the flow rate of gas delivered by the ventilator drops below a critical level. (Remember that the flow rate of gas into the lungs progressively decreases as lung volume increases and lung compliance decreases.) In most ventilators, this critical level is approximately 1 to 4 L per minute. The volume of gas delivered to the patient is determined by the flow rate of gas achieved and the duration of inspiration. Because the flow rate achieved is related to the driving pressure of the ventilator and the resistance of the ventilator-patient breathing circuit, inspiration may end prematurely if the driving pressure is reduced or if the resistance to airflow increases out of proportion to the ventilator's driving pressure. Table 19–5 lists the advantages and disadvantages of each of the various cycling mechanisms.

Initiation of Inspiration

The method by which a ventilator terminates expiration and initiates inspiration is commonly referred to as the *ventilatory mode*. Six modes of ventilator therapy are used clinically, including:

- Controlled ventilation
- Assisted ventilation
- Assist/control ventilation
- Intermittent mandatory ventilation
- Mandatory minute ventilation
- Pressure support

Most commercially available ventilators are also equipped with a manual control so that the operator can initiate a breath for the patient independent of these other ventilatory modes.

TABLE 19–5. Advantages and Disadvantages of Various Cycling Mechanisms

Cycling Mechanism	Advantages	Disadvantages
Volume	Gives preset volume delivered regardless of respiratory system resistance and compliance characteristics.	May cause dangerously high airway pressure.
Pressure	Limits mean pressure, reducing risk of barotrauma.	May result in inadequate alveolar ventilation, particularly if resistance becomes increased or compliance becomes decreased.
Time	Gives preset minute ventilation.	May not allow time for complete exhalation in COPD patients.
Flow	Improves dynamic compliance by reducing turbulent airflow.	May not allow time for complete exhalation in COPD patients.

Controlled Ventilation. In the control mode, the patient's ventilatory rate is set by the operator. Usually, this is accomplished either by directly choosing and setting the ventilator *firing* rate or by manipulating the inspiratory time relative to the amount of time the patient spends in expiration. Table 19–6 contains an example showing how varying I : E ratios affect the respiratory rate.

Controlled ventilation is usually only used for patients who have lost the ability to generate any inspiratory effort either because of a depressed ventilatory drive or as a result of respiratory muscle paralysis. Historically, controlled ventilation represents the oldest mode of mechanical ventilation, being introduced as a means of maintaining ventilation during thoracic surgery.

Assisted Ventilation. With assisted ventilation, the ventilator cycles into inspiration when the patient makes a sufficient inspiratory effort. The amount of effort required to trigger the ventilator can be adjusted by the operator with a *sensitivity* control. When the sensitivity is increased, only a small amount of negative pressure must be generated by the patient to cycle the ventilator from expiration to inspiration. As the sensitivity of the ventilator is decreased, the patient must make a greater effort to cycle the ventilator into inspiration. Unlike controlled ventilation in which the ventilator delivers a set minute ventilation, in assisted ventilation the patient can control his or her ventilatory rate. Note that if the patient does not make an inspiratory effort, however, the minute ventilation drops to zero. Thus, assist mode is not indicated for the treatment of patients who experience periodic apnea.

Assist/Control Ventilation. This mode of ventilation was introduced as a means of allowing the patient to provide some of the force required for ventilation, while also protecting the patient's ventilatory status in the event that he or she would experience apnea. As with assisted ventilation, the effort that the patient must exert to trigger the ventilator is adjusted by the operator by varying the sensitivity control. Additionally, a timing mechanism is incorporated into the ventilator's drive mechanism so that in the event that the patient does not make a sufficient inspiratory effort before a predetermined time, the ventilator automatically delivers a controlled mechanical breath. Assist/control ventilation has been shown to be an effective technique for weaning patients from mechanical ventilation.

Intermittent Mandatory Ventilation. With intermittent mandatory ventilation (IMV), the patient is allowed to breathe spontaneously at his or her own respiratory rate, and the ventilator periodically delivers a controlled breath at a preset time interval and tidal volume. In contrast to controlled ventilation, the rate at which mechanical breaths are delivered during IMV is usually less because patients provide some ventilation of their own. Typically, the ventilator is set to deliver a tidal volume of 12 to 15 ml/kg body weight at a rate between 1 and 10 breaths per minute, depending on the patient's ventilatory status (i.e., as determined by arterial blood gases). Figure 19–3 illustrates a typical breathing circuit that can be used to deliver IMV. In this system, a one-way valve separates the primary ventilator circuit from a continuous flow circuit that is added in parallel. During a spontaneous inspiration, the one-way valve opens, and the patient receives gas that has been heated and humidified by a humidification system that is separate from the ventilator. For a spontaneous expiration, the one-way valve closes, and the patient's exhaled gases are vented to the atmosphere through the ventilator's exhalation valve. When the ventilator cycles to deliver a mechanical breath, the one-way valve closes owing to the high pressures generated within the patient's breathing circuit, and the patient receives gas only from the ventilator. As with the spontaneous breath, exhaled gases are vented through the ventilator's exhalation valve.

Although IMV was first introduced for the ventilation of infants, it has also been used extensively for weaning adult patients from controlled mechanical ventilation. Advocates of IMV suggest that it facilitates the transition from controlled mechanical ventilation to spontaneous ventilation because:

1. The patient can adjust his or her ventilation to achieve eucapnia.

TABLE 19–6. Effects of Varying Respiratory Rate on I : E Ratios

A.	Inspiratory time (T_I)	1 sec
	Expiratory time (T_E)	2 sec
	I : E	1 : 2
	Total respiratory cycle (T_{total})	3 sec
	Respiratory rate per minute	= 60 second/total
		= 60 second/3.0 second
		= 20 breaths per minute
B.	Inspiratory time (T_I)	1 sec
	Expiratory time (T_E)	3 sec
	I : E	1 : 3
	Total respiratory cycle (T_{total})	4 sec
	Respiratory rate per minute	= 60 second/4 sec
		= 15 breaths per minute

Note that as expiratory time increases from A to B, the respiratory rate decreases.

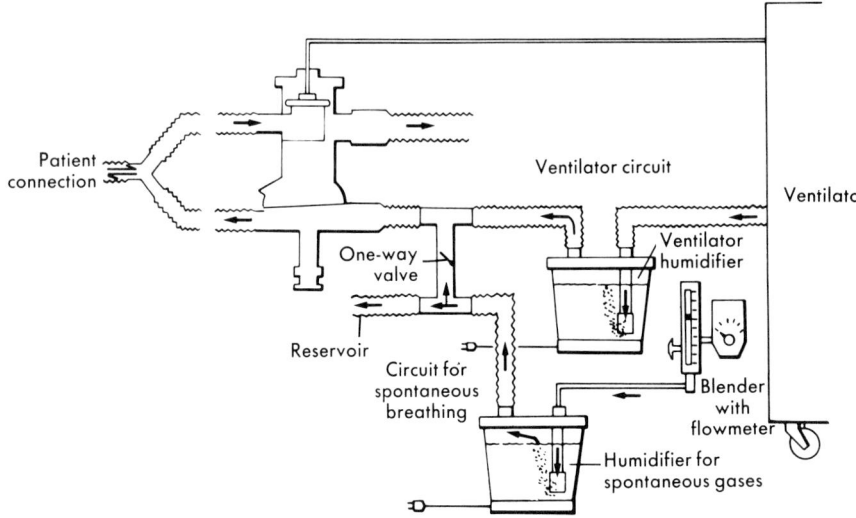

FIGURE 19-3. A typical breathing circuit used to deliver intermittent mandatory ventilation (IMV) (from McPherson, S.: *Respiratory Therapy Equipment*, 3rd. ed., St. Louis, C.V. Mosby, 1985, with permission.)

2. IMV reduces the amount of positive pressure required to effectively ventilate a patient, so the cardiovascular side effects of mechanical ventilation are minimized.

3. IMV encourages the patient to breathe spontaneously, so ventilatory muscle tone is improved.

The problem encountered with IMV is the phenomenon of "stacking breaths," in which the ventilator delivers a mechanical breath on top of the patient's spontaneous breath. This results in increased airway pressure, which can lead to barotrauma.

To avoid the problem of stacking breaths, a modification of IMV called *synchronized intermittent mandatory ventilation* (SIMV) or *intermittent demand ventilation* (IDV) incorporates an assist mode superimposed upon the spontaneous breathing pattern. Depending upon the selected frequency, a spontaneous inspiration at certain intervals triggers the delivery of a mechanical tidal volume. (Note that if the patient does not make a sufficient inspiratory effort within a set time limit, the ventilator automatically delivers a positive-pressure breath.)

Mandatory Minute Volume. Another problem encountered with IMV is the inability to regulate the patient's minute ventilation during ventilator weaning periods. Because the number of mechanical breaths is preset, changes in a patient's spontaneous ventilation directly influence the minute ventilation. Thus, as the patient's spontaneous tidal volume and breathing frequency change, his or her minute ventilation changes proportionately.

In 1977, Hewlett and his coworkers introduced the concept of mandatory minute volume (MMV), which is the delivery of a predetermined minute volume (MV) either through the patient's spontaneous ventilation or as positive-pressure breaths from the ventilator. Using microcomputer circuitry, the ventilator functions in MMV to monitor the patient's spontaneous ventilation and to provide via mechanical breaths whatever difference exists between the desired minute volume and the patient's spontaneous ventilation.

The basic concept of MMV is that the ventilator supplies a metered, preset minute volume of fresh gas into a reservoir system, from which the patient breathes (spontaneously) as much as he or she can. If the patient's spontaneous ventilation falls below the flow of fresh gas into the system, the reservoir gradually fills until at some critical level the ventilator cycles, and the gas within the reservoir is delivered to the patient by a mechanical breath. Thus, all of the fresh gas entering the reservoir enters the patient's lungs, either as a result of the patient's own spontaneous breaths or by the action of the ventilator. During MMV, a minimum level of ventilation is guaranteed, but patients with erratic, rapid, or shallow spontaneous ventilatory patterns may not benefit from MMV.

Pressure Support. With pressure support (PS), gas flow to the patient is pressurized to a preset level (e.g., 20 cmH$_2$O) at the onset of a spontaneous inspiratory effort. This pressure is maintained until the patient's flow falls to 25% of the initial peak value, at which point the ventilator cycles off and circuit flow ceases. PS reduces the work of breathing and breathing rate while increasing the patient's tidal volume, thus improving the efficiency of spontaneous ventilation. It is designed to overcome inspiratory resistance caused by the endotracheal tube and ventilator circuit. PS can be used in conjunction with MMV, IMV, CPAP, or by itself.

Airway Pressure Release Ventilation. Airway pressure release ventilation (APRV) is a recently described method of ventilatory support that has not yet become commercially available. It allows spontaneous ventilation with CPAP, but at set intervals the airway pressure drops a set level for a short period. This experimental mode of ventilatory support seems to facilitate exhalation by transiently decreasing the FRC that is maintained by CPAP. The benefit is gas exchange at lower mean intrathoracic pressures, but the clinical usefulness of APRV remains to be seen.

Special Functions

During the past 25 years, mechanical ventilator therapy has been routinely used in the treatment of patients with respiratory failure. A number of special functions have been incorporated into commercially available ventilators so that the clinician can modify the pressure, volume, and flow waveforms during both inspiration and expiration. The following briefly describes some common ventilator adjuncts available on many ventilators. Their use is discussed in greater detail in the section on management of respiratory failure.

Inspiratory Flow Patterns. During positive-pressure ventilation, a mechanical inspiration can be delivered via different flow patterns to administer the tidal volume in a way that is most appropriate for the patient and his or her disease. The most commonly used inspiratory flow patterns are called the sine wave and the square wave.

Square wave inspiratory flow delivers the peak flow almost immediately for an interval, and then it is abruptly terminated. This inspiratory mode is used to rapidly administer an inspiration but does so at high airway pressures from induced turbulence. However, the brief inspirations provide more time for expiration, which may be beneficial in conditions such as COPD.

With *sine wave* inspiratory flow, the inspiratory flow rate accelerates to a maximum and then tapers off. This mode of inspiration is believed to mimic spontaneous inspiratory patterns and provides lung inflation at lower peak inspiratory pressure.

Inspiratory flow can also be initiated in different ways during spontaneous ventilation, such as during CPAP breathing, with or without IMV. The gas for spontaneous inspiration can come from continuous flow to the circuit, or the patient may be required to exert sufficient inspiratory effort to trigger a demand valve before spontaneous inspiratory flow begins. In both cases, shortcomings in circuit design or flow delivery can dangerously increase the patient's work of breathing, which makes spontaneous ventilation more difficult. This can make weaning impossible.

Inflation Hold. With the inflation hold (inspiratory plateau) maneuver, the ventilator's exhalation valve remains temporarily closed at the end of the inspiratory phase, thus increasing the amount of time available for peripheral distribution of the inhaled gases. The benefits of using an end-inspiratory pause include an improvement in ventilation-perfusion relationships throughout the lung, a reduction in shunt and shuntlike states, and an improvement in oxygenation (assuming that right and left ventricular performance and pulmonary blood flow are adequate).

When inflation hold is applied with a volume-cycled ventilator, a preset volume of gas is delivered to the patient and then held in the ventilator-patient circuit for a predetermined time period (usually less than 2 seconds) before exhalation is allowed to occur. During the inflation hold period, the gas pressure within the ventilator circuit equilibrates with the pressure within the patient's lungs, and a pressure drop is registered on the ventilator pressure gauge. This new pressure level is called the *plateau pressure,* and it indicates the pressure required to hold the delivered volume in the ventilator-patient circuit. As discussed later, the plateau pressure can be used to monitor changes in resistance and compliance characteristics of the ventilator-patient breathing circuit.

Inflation hold has been shown to be effective in the treatment of patients with high airways resistance and/or low respiratory system compliance. Clinicians should be cautioned, however, that inspiratory hold has proved effective in most situations if the inspiratory-to-expiratory ratio is maintained above 1:2. Note that excessive levels of inflation hold can increase the mean airway pressure, which can lead to barotrauma and reductions in venous return and cardiac output.

Positive End-Expiratory Pressure (PEEP). With this form of mechanical ventilator therapy, a resistance is applied to the expiratory limb of the ventilator circuit so that a positive airway pressure is maintained throughout exhalation. The term *continuous positive-pressure breathing* (CPPB) is used to describe the use of PEEP during mechanical ventilation, whereas the application of PEEP during spontaneous breathing is referred to as *con-*

526 MECHANICAL VENTILATION

tinuous positive airway pressure (CPAP), if inspiratory positive airway pressure is maintained.

Early attempts to produce PEEP relied on flow-resistance mechanisms. Although this is effective in establishing a positive end-expiratory pressure, the level of PEEP changes with the frequency of mechanical breaths delivered by the ventilator. Modern PEEP devices utilize a threshold resistance that makes the level of PEEP independent of the rate of ventilation. Figure 19–4 illustrates various types of PEEP devices used during mechanical ventilation.

Three ranges of PEEP are presently employed in mechanical ventilator therapy: prophylactic PEEP, conventional PEEP, and high PEEP. During prophylactic PEEP, end-expiratory pressures of 1 to 5 cmH$_2$O are used; with conventional PEEP, pressures of 5 to 20 cmH$_2$O are applied, depending on the patient's cardiovascular reserve capacity. Kirby and colleagues introduced the concept of high PEEP (i.e., end-expiratory pressure levels greater than 20 cmH$_2$O) as an additional possibility in patients with adult respiratory distress syndrome (ARDS) who do not respond with increases in Pa$_{O_2}$ at a PEEP level of 20 cmH$_2$O.

The primary indications for PEEP therapy are:
1. To prevent early airway and alveolar collapse at the end of expiration by increasing the functional residual capacity.
2. To allow for improved oxygenation in pa-

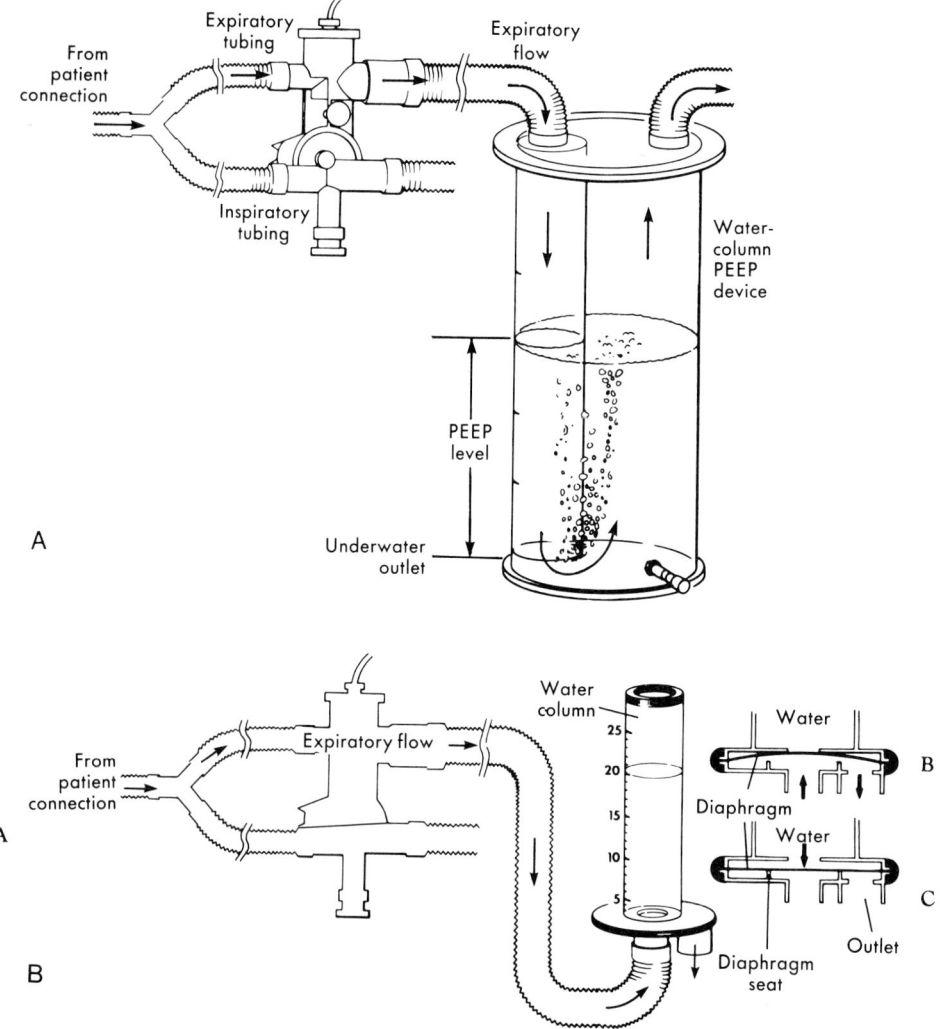

FIGURE 19–4. Various types of positive end-expiratory pressure (PEEP) devices used during mechanical ventilation. A. Immersion of expiratory limb; B. Emerson water column; C. Three methods of pressurizing the exhalation valve balloon; D. A Venturi system with an adjustable needle valve. (From Spearman, C.B., and Sanders, H.G.: Physical principles and functional designs of ventilators. In Kirby, R.R., Smith, R.A., and Desautels, D.A.: *Mechanical Ventilation.* New York, Churchill Livingstone. 1986, with permission.)

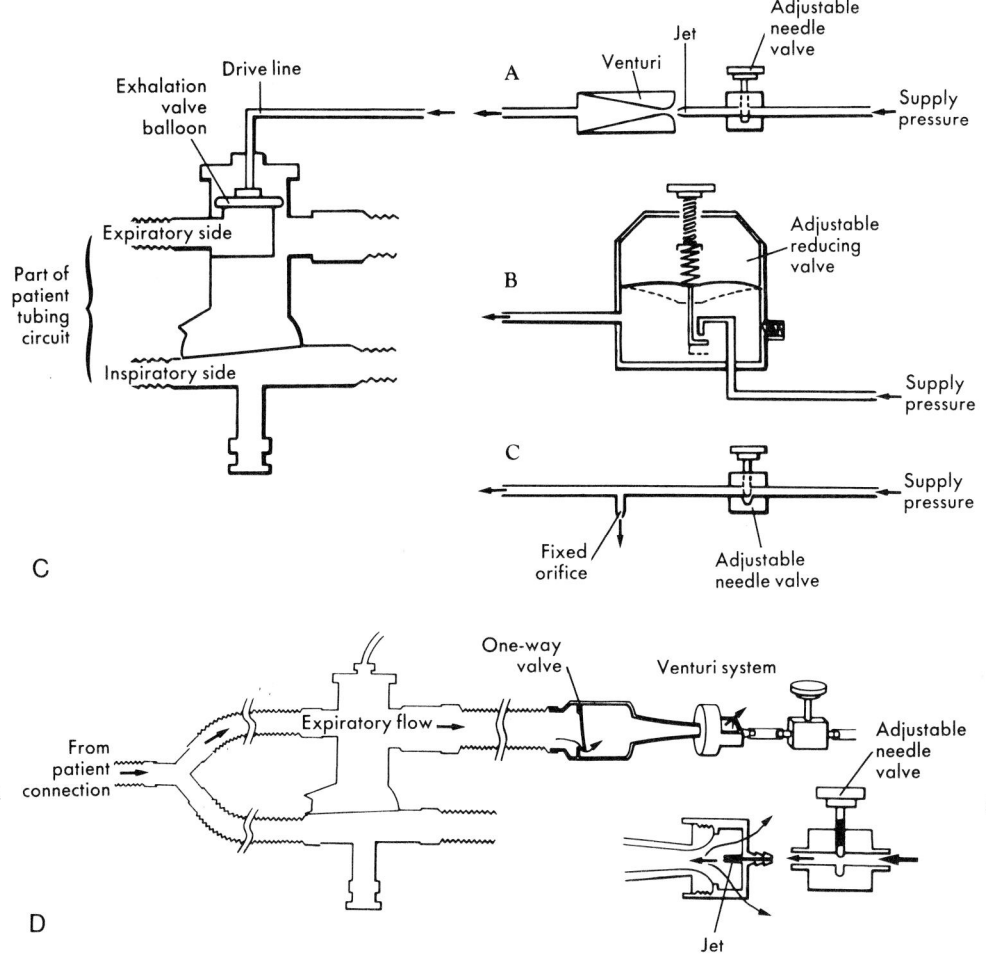

FIGURE 19-4 Continued

tients with refractory hypoxemia (i.e., Pao_2 fails to increase by 10 mmHg with increases in the fractional concentration of inspired oxygen of 0.2).

Specific indications for PEEP therapy include infant respiratory distress syndrome (IRDS), ARDS, cardiogenic pulmonary edema, and bilateral pneumonia.

Contraindications to PEEP therapy are tension pneumothorax, untreated pneumothorax, bullous emphysema, hypovolemic conditions, decreased cardiac reserve, and intracranial hypertension. The use of PEEP in patients with intracranial hypertension is a relative contraindication because careful monitoring of intracranial pressures (ICP) should make it possible to avoid a dangerous increase in ICP by titrating PEEP. PEEP therapy is also discussed in the section on management of respiratory failure.

Expiratory Retard. In patients with increased small airways resistance and evidence of air trapping, expiratory retard can be used to facilitate expiratory gas flow by reducing premature airway closure. It is produced by placing an increased expiratory resistance in line so that the patient returns to atmospheric pressure gradually rather than immediately following a positive-pressure inspiration. Note that expiratory retard differs from positive end-expiratory pressure therapy in that, with expiratory retard, the patient eventually returns to atmospheric pressure during exhalation, whereas during PEEP, the airway pressure remains above atmospheric pressure throughout exhalation.

The beneficial effects of expiratory retard in improving ventilation-perfusion relationships throughout the lung are questionable and, as such, have limited its application in the treatment of critically ill patients. When used in patients with small airways disease (e.g., emphysema), expiratory times of 4 to 8 seconds are typically used to ensure an adequate time for emptying of the lungs.

Periodic Hyperinflation (the Sigh Breath). Under normal circumstances, a person periodically takes a deep breath approximately 6 to 10 times per hour. Although the reasons for these deep breaths are not completely understood, most pulmonologists agree that this probably helps to reduce atelectasis, which can occur with shallow breathing, and thus improves ventilation-perfusion ratios throughout the lungs.

On most commercially available ventilators, an automatic sigh can be preset by the clinician so that the patient is periodically hyperinflated with a volume that corresponds to 1.5 to 2 times his or her tidal volume setting. Typically, the ventilator is set to deliver two to three sigh breaths every 6 to 10 minutes. Although recent studies have shown that patients receiving high tidal volumes (i.e., 10 to 15 ml/kg) may not benefit from periodic hyperinflation, many clinicians continue to use it prophylactically to prevent atelectasis, particularly during controlled ventilation.

Negative End-Expiratory Pressure (NEEP). With this ventilator maneuver, a subatmospheric pressure is applied to the proximal airway during the expiratory phase of a positive-pressure breath. Although theoretically NEEP should minimize the effects of positive-pressure ventilation by enhancing venous return and reducing mean airway pressure, its actual effectiveness is questionable. A number of studies have failed to demonstrate significant improvement in cardiac output or arterial pressure in spite of substantial reductions in mean airway pressure with the addition of negative end-expiratory pressures. Furthermore, the application of NEEP to patients with chronic airflow obstruction, particularly those with emphysema, can result in premature airway closure and air-trapping.

Ventilator Monitors and Alarms. The presence of several monitors and alarms on mechanical ventilators has increased the safety of this equipment by reducing the risk of patient complications. An essential monitor is for the airway pressure, with alarms for excessively high or low pressures. These alarms can indicate obstruction or disconnection, respectively. The advent of microprocessors and light-emitting diode (LED) displays have increased the parameters that can be monitored. Modern ventilators can display the ventilatory rate, tidal volume, and minute volume.

The respiratory care clinician who is monitoring the ventilator periodically checks the settings on the ventilator dials and measures the inspired oxygen concentration and the endotracheal tube cuff pressure. Airway compliance can be evaluated by measuring the airway pressure during inspiratory hold and then dividing the tidal volume by that pressure.

High-Frequency Ventilators

High-frequency ventilators (Fig. 19–5) use very high rates (60 to 7,600 cycles per minute) and low tidal volumes (5 to 300 ml). This unconventional mode of ventilation began to see clinical use in the late 1970s based on the work of the Swedish researchers Sjostrand and colleagues in 1967. Conventional positive-pressure ventilation utilizes tidal volumes and ventilatory rates similar to those of spontaneous ventilation. Airway pressure is considerably higher with conventional positive-pressure ventilation (20 to 30 cmH_2O) than with spontaneous ventilation (1 to 2 cmH_2O). High-frequency ventilation uses very high ventilatory rates and very low tidal volumes, but it more closely approximates the airway pressures of spontaneous ventilation than does conventional ventilation.

The ventilatory rates for high-frequency ventilation (HFV) range from 60 to several thousand cycles per minute (Table 19–7). Tidal volumes are usually less than the anatomic deadspace and may be as small as 5 to 15 ml per cycle. The traditional concept of deadspace strongly suggests that no alveolar ventilation would result from such small tidal volumes. Therefore, HFV must depend upon principles other than the bulk convection of conventional ventilation in order to derive adequate alveolar gas exchange.

Certain characteristics of high-frequency ventilators are quite different from those of conventional ventilators. High-frequency ventilators have low internal compliance and negligible compressible volume. Low internal compliance means that energy is not lost stretching the walls of the ventilator components. Conventional ventilators have high system compliance. Consider how the walls of the corrugated delivery tubes of a conventional ventilator expand like an accordion when the ventilator delivers a breath, particularly to a patient whose lungs have low compliance. This large-diameter tubing, as well as the humidifier, nebulizer cups, and traps, also contains a large volume of gas that is compressed when the ventilator delivers a breath. The high internal compliance and large

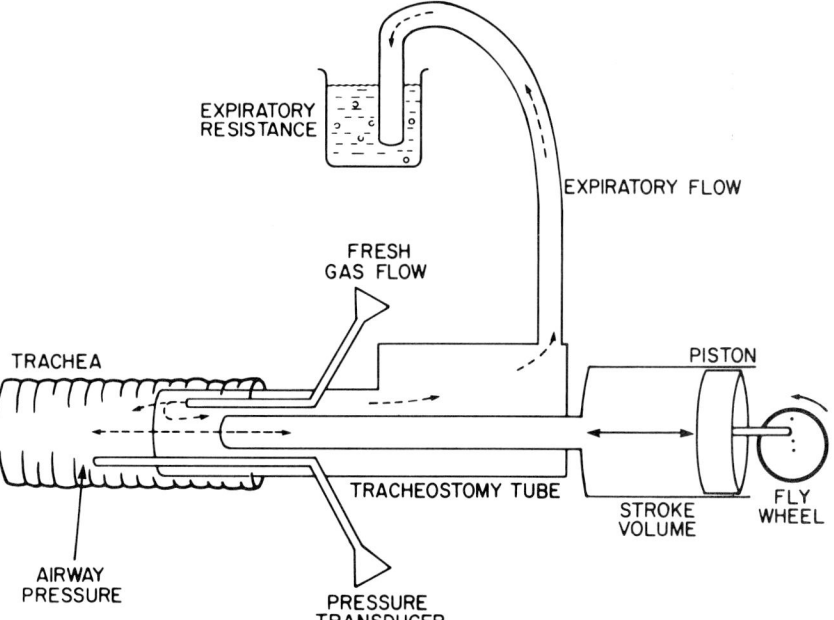

FIGURE 19–5. A high-frequency ventilator. (From Wright, K.: Ventilation by high frequency oscillation in rabbits with oleic acid lung disease. *J Appl Physiol* 50(5): 1057, 1981, with permission.)

compressible volume of conventional ventilators result in diminished tidal volumes delivered to patients with very noncompliant lungs. Measurement at the endotracheal tube would show that less gas is delivered than the ventilator settings indicate. To compensate for these factors, a conventional ventilator can be set for a higher volume in order to deliver the desired amount.

High-frequency ventilators use thick-walled, small-diameter tubing and have negligible compressible volume and a low internal compliance of the system. These characteristics enable the high-frequency ventilator to eject gas into the airways at very high flow rates but for very brief intervals. Conventional positive-pressure ventilators usually deliver gas to the patient's airways at peak pressures of about 20 to 30 cmH_2O. The gas in a high-frequency ventilator is delivered at 20 to 30 psi (1,400 to 2,100 cmH_2O). However, this pressure is administered for only a fraction of a second per breath, so only a small amount of this pressure actually arrives at the distal airways.

Theory of High-Frequency Ventilator Action

Several theories have been proposed to help explain the basis of gas exchange by HFV. HFV is believed to provide gas exchange by a combination of decreased deadspace, apneic oxygenation, coaxial flow, and augmented diffusion.

Decreased Deadspace. Most delivery tubes used for HFV bypass about a third of the anatomic deadspace while adding minimal mechanical deadspace (Fig. 19–6). A channel for the fresh gas jetted from the high-frequency ventilator is incorporated in the wall of the endotracheal tube. Furthermore, HFV produces lower mean airway pressures than conventional ventilation and thus produces less alveolar deadspace (Zone 1).

Apneic Oxygenation. Providing a continuous flow of 100% oxygen to an endotracheal tube in an apneic individual maintains hemoglobin saturation for a fairly long time by the process of apneic oxygenation. Oxygen delivery to the alveoli continues, but alveolar carbon dioxide also accumulates. Increasing P_{CO_2} dilutes the alveolar P_{O_2}. This technique is used with general anesthesia and paralyzing drugs when the patient is required to be motionless, as during lithotripsy (pulverizing kidney stones with sound waves). Adequate ar-

TABLE 19–7. High-Frequency Ventilation

Type	Rate/Minute
High-frequency positive-pressure ventilation (HFPPV)	60–120
High-frequency jet ventilation (HFJV)	120–600
High-frequency oscillation (HFO)	600–7,600 or greater

530 MECHANICAL VENTILATION

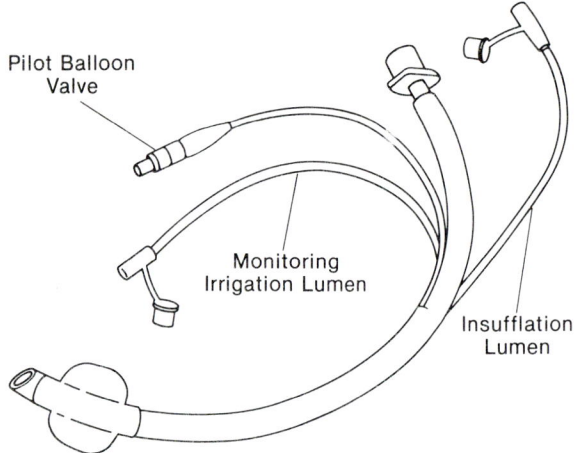

FIGURE 19–6. High-frequency ventilation tubing minimizes mechanical dead space (Courtesy Mallinckrodt, Inc. Argyle, N.Y.).

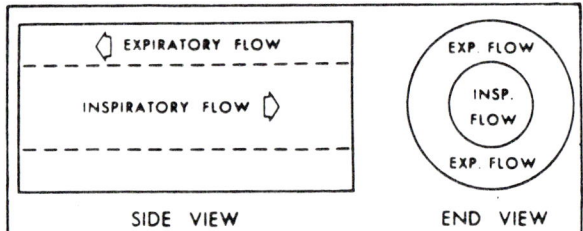

FIGURE 19–7. Coaxial flow during high-frequency ventilation. (From DeHaven, C.B.: Newer techniques: High frequency positive pressure ventilation. *Current Reviews in Respiratory Therapy* 2:174, 1986, with permission.)

terial oxygenation can be maintained for over 15 minutes of apnea, but the accumulating carbon dioxide causes a $Paco_2$ greater than 100 torr. This hypercapnia severely stimulates the sympathetic nervous system, causing elevated circulating catecholamines, tachycardia, and hypertension, and this may injure the heart tissue.

Coaxial Flow. Conventional ventilation produces a laminar flow of gases at low flow rates and turbulent flow at higher flow rates. HFV is believed to produce a different pattern of gas flow called coaxial flow by injecting gas into the airway at extremely high flow rates. Using smoke-filled tubes as models, the jet of gas shoots down the center of the tube (conducting airway) where the friction is lowest. Simultaneously, eddy currents are produced in the opposite direction at the periphery of the tube. In this way, gas enters and leaves the airway concurrently (Fig. 19–7). Functionally, anatomic deadspace is greatly reduced with HFV because inspiration can occur using just the centers of the conducting airways.

Augmented Diffusion. Exchange of gas between the alveoli and pulmonary capillaries depends on diffusion. This is based on the random movement of molecules in all directions and other forces described in Fick's law of diffusion (see Chapter 1). The molecular velocity and temperature also affect diffusion rates. Cardiac pulsations are believed to enhance diffusion across the alveolar-pulmonary capillary interface by increasing molecular movement. In the same way, the frequent pulsations of HFV increase diffusion in the airway and alveoli by vibrating the molecules. HFV can provide adequate gas exchange at lower mean airway pressure than conventional ventilation. HFV can be administered via a very small-diameter delivery tube and produces less movement of the lungs and thoracic structures than conventional positive-pressure ventilation. Indications and complications of HFV are discussed later.

COMPLICATIONS OF MECHANICAL VENTILATION

The most common types of mechanical ventilators used clinically are positive-pressure ventilators. The physiologic consequences and complications associated with their use are frequently the result of the increased intrathoracic and elevated airway pressure. Additionally, positive-pressure ventilation can worsen complications from other causes. For example, insertion of an artificial airway may perforate the trachea. Subsequent administration of positive-pressure ventilation can result in the additional complication of subcutaneous emphysema as air is forced into the tissues of the chest through the tracheal defect.

Many complications have been described with the use of high-frequency ventilation related to faulty equipment (kinked catheters for delivery of the jet of gas, flecks of metal shot down the airway). Additionally, there are problems with the humidification of the compressed gas used for high-frequency ventilation as well as loss of auscultation as a monitor for adequate distribution of ventilation.

Pulmonary Complications

Mechanical ventilation can interfere with ventilation/perfusion matching in the lungs. The lung tissue itself can be traumatized by high airway pressures. A frequent complication of high airway pressure is pneumothorax as well as other conditions associated with air leak from the lungs: subcutaneous emphysema, interstitial air in the lung, pneumomediastinum, pneumopericardium, pneumoperitoneum, and bronchopleural fistulas (see Chapter 20).

As discussed in Chapter 3, the airway pressures generated during mechanical ventilation can produce Zone 1 (alveolar deadspace) in the lung. Similarly, an inappropriate I:E ratio can result in gas trapping (especially in patients with COPD) or inadequate ventilation of "slow" alveoli. Slow alveoli require extended time for inflation to occur and are commonly associated with conditions resulting in increased airways secretions or airway narrowing.

Mechanical ventilation decreases the work of breathing that the patient is required to perform. This reduces the physiologic stress on the patient, but sometimes the patient subsequently allows the ventilator to do all the ventilatory work. Atrophy of the muscles of breathing then occurs, which makes weaning more prolonged and difficult.

Neonatal lungs are exquisitely sensitive to the effects of high airway pressure. Neonatologists become increasingly concerned when neonates require airway pressures above 25 cmH_2O for adequate ventilation. Neonates requiring prolonged positive-pressure ventilation due to infant respiratory distress syndrome may also develop bronchopulmonary dysplasia (BPD) as discussed in Chapter 6. In this condition, the lungs are characterized by hyperinflation and a mixture of over- and underinflated areas due to overdistended alveoli and fibrosis. In the infants who survive, these symptoms require several weeks to months to slowly resolve. Most infants who survive the first year become asymptomatic by age 2 and have nearly complete resolution by age 5 or 6.

Cardiovascular Complications

Intravascular pressure increases when airway pressure is elevated, which reduces venous return of blood to the heart because the great veins are exposed to extravascular compression by the positive intrapleural pressure. The decreased venous return decreases cardiac output and tissue perfusion. This can be prevented if blood volume is increased. High airway pressures associated with mechanical ventilation can also increase pulmonary vascular resistance by compression of intraalveolar vessels. This elevates pulmonary vascular pressure and may produce dilation of the right ventricle. As the right ventricle dilates, the intraventricular septum (the wall between the right and left ventricles) is shifted into the left ventricle, producing some obstruction of the left ventricular outflow tract (the path that the blood follows as it is ejected from the left ventricle during systole). This resistance may act as an additional cause of the decrease in cardiac output associated with high airway pressure.

The Traube-Hering (lung inflation) reflex (heart rate increases during inspiration and decreases during expiration) produces the so-called sinus arrhythmia on ECG. Mechanical ventilation can also evoke this ECG change as well as produce transient shifts in the electrical axis of the heart. The configuration of the heart in the chest changes with ventilation. The heart becomes elongated and shifted rightward during inspiration.

Mechanical ventilation can also produce effects on the blood pressure similar to those caused by *pulsus paradoxus,* especially when high airway pressure is used to ventilate a hypovolemic patient (Fig. 19-8). Pulsus paradoxus is caused by an alternating increase and decrease in cardiac output with each breath. During spontaneous inspiration, the increased negative pressure in the thorax causes blood to collect in the lungs with resultant decrease in the stroke volume output and pulse strength. Opposite effects occur during spontaneous expiration. This is a normal phenomenon, but it becomes markedly pronounced in some conditions such as obstructive lung disease or cardiac tamponade (compression of the heart by fluid in the pericardial sac or by a constricted pericardium).

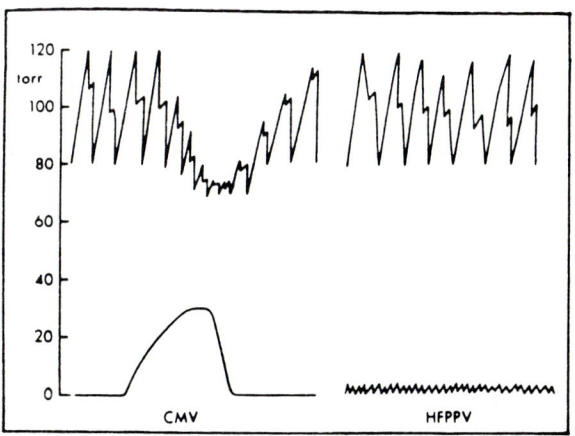

FIGURE 19-8. The effect of high airway pressure ventilation on arterial pressure. (From DeHaven, C.B.: Newer techniques: High frequency positive pressure ventilation. *Current Reviews in Respiratory Therapy* 2:174, 1986, with permission.)

Negative-pressure ventilators (especially Drinker respirators) may lower intra-abdominal pressure and can cause venous pooling there. This decreases venous return to the heart and cardiac output. This is less of a problem with the chest cuirass.

Renal Complications

Positive-pressure ventilation tends to produce retention of water and sodium while resulting in sparse concentrated urine output. The effects of positive-pressure ventilation to decrease cardiac output can also diminish renal blood flow. Additionally, the carotid and aortic baroreceptors signal the posterior pituitary to increase antidiuretic hormone (ADH) production when blood pressure falls. Perhaps more importantly, atrial stretch receptors also stimulate ADH release when venous return to the heart decreases. ADH causes the kidneys to decrease urine output by retention of water and sodium. Atrial natriuretic factor (ANF) is released from the atria when they are distended and it promotes sodium loss. ANF production is inhibited by the decreased venous return and reduced atrial stretch caused by positive-pressure ventilation. High airway pressures are also transmitted to increase both intrathoracic and intra-abdominal pressure. The increased intra-abdominal pressure counteracts the Starling forces favoring glomerular filtration. There is some evidence that even without decreases in renal blood flow, positive-pressure ventilation tends to shift the intrarenal distribution of blood flow away from the cortical nephrons that are mainly responsible for dilute urine formation.

Metabolic Complications

Patients requiring mechanical ventilation are commonly in a catabolic state from conditions such as trauma, infection, or neoplasm. Oral intake of nutrition is impeded by endotracheal intubation. This results in starvation, poor wound healing, and breakdown of normal tissues. The increased metabolic demands may require the use of enteral (using the gut) or parenteral (intravenous) hyperalimentation.

The work of breathing in normal, healthy individuals is only about 5% of the total caloric expenditure. But in pulmonary disease, the metabolic expenditure of the work of breathing can require nearly half the total calories consumed. Mechanical ventilation can reduce the work of breathing by either performing the ventilation or by making spontaneous ventilation easier by improved lung compliance. This reduces the amount of calories consumed by the ventilatory muscles and increases the energy available for healing the tissues and other metabolic functions. Medical conditions that necessitate mechanical ventilation also affect endocrine systems. Circulating hormones that are commonly elevated include adrenocorticotropic hormone (ACTH), thyrotropin-releasing hormone (TRH), cortisol, aldosterone, renin, and catecholamines.

Psychologic Complications

Endotracheal intubation and positive-pressure ventilation are usually uncomfortable for the patient. Lack of sleep, medications, and the effects of disease frequently result in a condition called ICU psychosis in the critically ill. Discomfort and ICU psychosis can cause the patient to fight the mechanical inspirations. When the patient resists mechanical ventilation by contracting his expiratory muscles, this is called "bucking the ventilator" and produces dangerously high airway pressure that can damage the lungs and may even result in ineffective and inadequate ventilation.

Different modes of ventilation may be used to find the one that is best tolerated by an individual while still providing appropriate ventilation. Occasionally, a patient must be paralyzed with a muscle relaxant, such as pancuronium, to stop fighting the ventilator.

A patient's control over his life is diminished with hospitalization and mechanical ventilation, and drug-induced paralysis makes the patient totally dependent, which can be psychologically devastating. Healthcare providers must be extremely vigilant to respect the dignity of the patients under their care. Additionally, patients paralyzed with muscle relaxants appear to be unresponsive, but they may be completely alert mentally. They cannot move in response to painful procedures, but without adequate sedation and analgesia, they will feel and remember everything done to them. The presence of increased heart rate and blood pressure or tears in the eyes of a paralyzed patient during a painful procedure should alert you to the possible need for more sedation or analgesia.

The stress associated with illnesses requiring mechanical ventilation can result in gastric ulceration and bleeding. This is especially common in patients receiving glucocorticoids, such as hydrocortisone. Gastric ulceration may be prevented by administration of antacids and drugs such as cimetidine, which reduce gastric acid secretion.

Patients who require mechanical ventilation can

become quite psychologically dependent on their ventilator. Attempts to wean these individuals may produce extreme anxiety, even in the face of adequate gas exchange. Reassurance, mild sedation (heavy sedation impedes weaning), and more gradual weaning techniques may be necessary for these individuals.

Ventilator Malfunction

The preceding sections detailed physiologic complications of properly functioning mechanical ventilators. Improper maintenance or malfunction of a ventilator can produce catastrophic sequelae. Maintenance and trouble-shooting guides for particular ventilators are available from the manufacturer and should be rigorously followed.

A partial list of complications include airway infection from contaminated humidifiers, airway burns from heater malfunctions, and loss of ventilator function from disconnection, tube fracture, elevated deadspace, rebreathing, or loss of driving pressure. Familiarity with the brands of ventilators present in your hospital will reveal which specific breakdowns are most likely.

Most ventilators have built-in alarms for early detection of elevated airway pressures, inadvertent disconnection of the patient from the ventilator, or the development of air leaks. Monitoring the ventilator and the patient is essential to avoid and detect complications.

CHOOSING SPECIFIC VENTILATORY MODALITIES

This section discusses the factors involved in determining the type of ventilator that best produces adequate gas exchange and is least likely to cause complications for the particular patient.

There are many considerations when trying to match a patient to a specific ventilatory modality. Many different types of ventilators are commercially available. A knowledge of the patient's physiology and the pathophysiology of the disease provides a rationale for choosing an appropriate ventilator.

Neonates requiring mechanical ventilation routinely receive time-cycled, pressure-limited, positive-pressure ventilation. A time-cycled ventilator delivers an inspiration to the patient for a certain interval until a certain adjustable peak airway pressure is reached. A neonate's fragile, immature lungs are readily damaged by high airway pressure. A major drawback to this type of ventilator is that a decrease in compliance in the patient's lungs produces a decrease in the tidal volume delivered. This can produce inadequate ventilation. A major consideration for ventilation in a newborn is adequate ventilation with low airway pressure. High-frequency ventilation has been used for neonates with poorly compliant lungs in an attempt to keep airway pressure low. Drawbacks to using high-frequency ventilation include difficulty in monitoring due to the loss of breath sounds, and humidification problems. For neonates, extracorporeal membrane oxygenation (ECMO), or the heart-lung machine, provides extra–pulmonary oxygenation and carbon dioxide removal, reducing the dependence on mechanical ventilation for gas exchange. ECMO permits the use of diminished airway pressure and can be used for several days while the diseased lungs heal.

Adult lungs are much more tolerant of higher airway pressures. Barotrauma to the adult lung is unlikely when peak airway pressures are below 40 cmH_2O. Routinely, maximal airway pressures are set to 60 cmH_2O, but several volume-cycled ventilators can be set at a peak airway pressure of up to 120 cmH_2O, especially for use in patients with extremely low lung compliance.

Negative-Pressure Ventilators

Negative-pressure ventilators are usually most effective on patients with normal compliance of the lungs and chest wall and with normal airways resistance (such as patients with neuromuscular disease). The ventilators enclose the chest, restricting access to the patient, but they do not require endotracheal intubation. Use of this type of ventilator is uncommon except in the occasional patient with neuromuscular disease but intact laryngeal reflexes. These patients require chronic ventilation because of the weakness of the ventilatory muscles but can avoid endotracheal intubation or tracheostomy.

Ventilator Rate and Tidal Volume Settings

The negative physiologic consequences of increased intrathoracic pressure on the heart, lungs, and kidneys as well as the risk of barotrauma have already been discussed. The philosophy guiding the choice of ventilator rate and tidal volume settings is to provide adequate alveolar ventilation at the lowest airway pressure. In general, patients suffering from primary cardiac or pulmonary diseases tend to have lungs that are poorly compliant. Use of small tidal volumes in these patients results in much lower airway pressures than if large tidal volumes are used. However, fairly rapid rates must be used to assure adequate ventilation of the alveoli. On the other hand, postoperative patients more commonly have extrathoracic problems but relatively compliant lungs. Using large tidal volumes in these patients does not excessively increase peak airway pressure. If large tidal volumes can be used, then fewer breaths per minute are required. The use of a low ventilatory rate is beneficial because:

1. It tends to result in relatively low mean airway pressure.
2. Expiratory times are prolonged.
3. Ventilation of anatomic deadspace is minimized.

In general, tidal volume is set as high as possible (up to 15 ml/kg) without causing excessive amounts of peak airway pressure. In the patient with noncompliant lungs, small increases in tidal volume produce large increases in peak airway pressure. These patients do not tolerate large tidal volumes and do better with smaller volumes at higher rates. After determining the most suitable tidal volume, the rate is set so that alveolar ventilation is about 70 ml/kg per minute for adults, 100 to 110 ml/kg per minute for children, and up to 130 ml/kg per minute for newborns.

Choosing other ventilator settings is based on the same principles of providing adequate gas exchange with the least risk of complications for the patient. Thus, the FIO_2 (see Chapters 10 and 16) is chosen to provide adequate oxygenation while avoiding oxygen toxicity and retinopathy of prematurity. Inspiratory flow settings, discussed earlier, are chosen to produce the lowest possible peak airway pressure while allowing adequate time for exhalation. The sensitivity used to trigger a mechanical breath during synchronized intermittent mandatory ventilation or assist/control ventilation is set so that overventilation is avoided but excessive patient effort is not required either.

The relationship between the I : E ratio and ventilatory rate is shown in Table 19–6. This may be a consideration in patients requiring excessive expiratory time. Similarly, interrelationships between tidal volume, minute volume, respiratory rate, and gas flow can produce combinations that a ventilator is unable to deliver. Limitations depend on specific ventilators or circuit design.

WEANING FROM MECHANICAL VENTILATION

Weaning from mechanical ventilation usually begins as soon as the patient attains acceptable blood gas values. The goal is to maintain alveolar ventilation without causing excessive stress to the patient. Decreasing the amount of mechanical ventilation reduces the risk of complications. Decision of what to wean first depends both on the type of ventilator and the physiologic response of the patient.

Before the development of intermittent mandatory ventilation, patients were weaned from controlled ventilation by progressively increasing the time off the ventilator. Development of assist/control ventilation and then intermittent mandatory ventilation made the weaning process more gradual and better tolerated. In general, the longer the patient has been on mechanical ventilation, the more gradual the weaning process. The tidal volume is usually not altered, but the rate is decreased in increments of usually 2 or only 1, depending on how the patient tolerates weaning. When the ventilator settings are minimal (0 to 1 breath every 2 minutes), the patient is evaluated for extubation.

Recently, mandatory minute ventilation (MMV) and pressure support (PS) have gained popularity as weaning techniques. Patients undergoing weaning from long-term ventilation often assume a tachypneic pattern during spontaneous ventilation. Respiratory muscle fatigue secondary to inadequate nutrition, excessive carbon dioxide production due to lipogenesis from surplus carbohydrate intake (see Chapters 10 and 12), or the presence of underlying pulmonary disease (such as increased alveolar deadspace) may predispose these patients to assume a less-than-desirable breathing pattern. In these situations, the spontaneous volume achieved by the patient may satisfy the set minute volume requirements, but the rapid, shallow breathing does not provide for effective alveolar ventilation. To help avoid this problem, PS can be used in conjunction with MMV during weaning to ensure larger tidal volumes and more uniform distribution of the inspired gas. After the ventilator breaths have reached a minimal level, the PS is reduced in increments of 2 to 5 cmH_2O, if tolerated by the patient, until a level of 5 cmH_2O is reached. When the PS reaches its minimal level, the patient is evaluated for extubation. A minimal level of PS is usually maintained to assist the patient in overcoming the resistance offered by the endotracheal tube.

Weaning of inspired oxygen concentration (FIO_2) and PEEP or CPAP usually follows a set pattern. As a patient's oxygenation of arterial blood improves, usually the FIO_2 is reduced until reaching 40% or lower. Then the PEEP or CPAP is reduced to 5 cmH_2O before attempting extubation. Extubation from higher levels of PEEP can result in atelectasis, hypoxemia, and emergency reintubation. Rarely, the PEEP is weaned before the FiO_2, especially if the patient does not tolerate the elevated airway pressures. Usually, PEEP or CPAP is weaned late because it maintains the FRC at a level that makes the lungs more compliant and makes spontaneous ventilation easier.

In certain situations, a patient is placed on a T-piece prior to extubation. A T-piece attaches to the patient's endotracheal tube and usually provides both a reservoir and fresh humidified gas with an increased oxygen concentration. In this way, there is no mechanical ventilation but the patient is still endotracheally intubated. If the patient does not tolerate spontaneous breathing in this manner, then the endotracheal tube is reattached to the ventilator and mechanical ventilation is resumed. If on the other hand, the patient maintains good vital signs and blood gases on the T-piece, then extubation is usually performed. The T-piece is very frequently used in the recovery room when patients are not quite ready for extubation following general anesthesia but rapidly come around.

As stated earlier, indications for endotracheal intubation are different from those for mechanical ventilation. When the patient no longer has the indications for mechanical ventilation, weaning should take place. When the indications for intubation are no longer met, the patient should be extubated (see Chapter 18).

Bibliography

Ashbaugh, D.G., Bigelow, D.B., Petty, T.L., and Levine, B.E.: Acute respiratory distress in adults. *Lancet* 2:319–323, 1967.

Baker, A.B., Thompson, J.B., Turner, J., and Hansen, P.: Effects of varying inspiratory flow waveform and time in intermittent positive pressure ventilation: Emphysema. *Br. J. Anesth.* 54:547–554, 1982.

Barach, A., Bickerman, H., and Petty, T.: Perspectives in pressure breathing. *Respir. Care* 20:627–642, 1975.

Burton, G.G., Gee, G.N., and Hodgkin, J.E.: *Respiratory Care: A Guide to Clinical Practice.* Philadelphia, J.B. Lippincott, 1982.

Comroe, J.H. Inflation-1904 Model. *Retrospectoscope. Insights to Medical Discovery.* Menlo Park, Calif., VonGehr Press, 1977, pp 110–113.

Cournand, A., Motley, H.L., Werko, L., et al.: Physiological studies of effects of intermittent positive pressure breathing on cardiac output in man. *Am. J. Physiol.* 152:162, 1948.

DeHaven, C.B.: New techniques: High frequency positive pressure ventilation. *Current Reviews in Respiratory Therapy* 2:171–175, 1986.

Demers, R.: Mechanical ventilation wave patterns. *Current Reviews in Respiratory Therapy* 1:81–88, 1980.

Desautels, D.: Ventilator classification: A new look at an old subject. *Current Reviews in Respiratory Therapy* 1:81–88, 1979.

Downs, J.B.: Ventilatory patterns and modes of ventilation in acute respiratory failure. *Respir. Care* 28:586–591, 1983.

Drinker, P., and McKhann, C.: The use of a new apparatus for the prolonged administration of artificial respiration: I. A fatal case of poliomyelitis. *JAMA* 92:1658–1660, 1929.

Forrette, T.L., and Cairo, J.M.: Mandatory minute volume: A conceptual approach. *Current Reviews in Respiratory Therapy* 10:163–167, 1988.

Geer, R.T.: Mechanical ventilation. In Fishman, A.P. (ed.): *Pulmonary Disease and Disorders,* vol. 2. New York, McGraw-Hill, 1980, pp 1607–1617.

George, B., Jerurski, W., and Plummer, A.: A physiological approach to patients requiring mechanical ventilation. *Respir. Care* 23:71–74, 1978.

Gibson, R.L., Jackson, J.C., Twiggs, G.A., et al.: Bronchopulmonary dysplasia: Survival after prolonged mechanical ventilation. *Am. J. Dis. Child.* 142:721–725, 1988.

Gregory, G.A., Kitterman, J.A., Phibbs, R.H. et al.: Treatment of the idiopathic respiratory distress syndrome with continuous positive airway pressure. *N. Engl. J. Med.* 284:1333–1340, 1971.

Grenvick, A.: Optimal PEEP. *Acta Anesth. Scand.* 70 (Suppl.):165–171, 1978.

Hewlett, A.M., Platt, A.S., and Terry, V.G.: Mandatory minute volume. *Anaesthesia* 32:163, 1977.

Kirby, R.R.: Positive airway pressure: System design and clinical application. In Shoemaker, W.C. (ed.): *Critical Care: State of the Art.* Fullerton, Calif., Society of Critical Care Medicine, 1985, pp 1–52.

Kirby, R.R., Robinson, E.J., Schultz, J., et al.: Continuous flow ventilation as an alternative to assisted or controlled ventilation in infants. *Anesth. Analg.* 51:871–875, 1972.

MacIntyre, N.R.: Pressure support ventilation: Effects on ventilatory reflexes and ventilatory muscle workloads. *Respir. Care* 32:447, 1987.

McPherson, S.: *Respiratory Therapy Equipment.* St. Louis, C.V. Mosby, 1983.

Morch, E.T.: History of mechanical ventilation. In Kirby, R.R., Smith, R.A., Desautels, D.A. (eds.): *Mechanical Ventilation.* New York, Churchill Livingstone, 1986, pp 1–58.

Mushin, M.W., Rendell-Baker, L., Thompson, P.W., and Mapleson, M.W.: *Automatic Ventilation of the Lungs.* Philadelphia, F.A. Davis, 1980.

Schacter, E.N., Tucker, D., and Beck, G.J.: Does intermittent mandatory ventilation accelerate weaning? *JAMA* 246:1210–1214, 1981.

Shapiro, B.A., Cane, R.D., and Harrison, R.A.: Positive end-expiratory pressure therapy in adults with special reference to acute lung injury. A review of the literature and suggested clinical correlations. *Crit. Care Med.* 12:127–141, 1984.

Shapiro, B.A., Harrison, R.A., Kacmarek, R., and Cane, R.D.: *Clinical Applications of Respiratory Care.* Chicago, Year Book, 1985.

Stock, M.C., and Downs, J.B.: Airway pressure release ventilation: A new approach to ventilatory support during acute lung injury. *Respir. Care* 32:517, 1987.

Sjostrand, U.: High-frequency positive pressure ventilation (HFPPV): A review. *Crit. Care Med.* 8:345–364, 1980.

Zarins, C.K., Bayne, C.G., Rice, C.L., et al.: Does spontaneous ventilation with IMV protect from PEEP-induced cardiac output depression? *J. Surg. Res.* 22:299–304, 1977.

Zwillich, C.W., Pierson, D.J., Creagh, C.E., Sutten, F.D., Schatz, E., and Petty, T.L.: Complications of assisted ventilation. *J. Am. Med.* 57:161–170, 1974.

OBJECTIVES

AFTER READING THIS CHAPTER, THE STUDENT WILL BE ABLE TO:

1. Discuss the principles of cardiopulmonary resuscitation and, if possible, enroll in a program to become certified in both basic and advanced cardiac life support.
2. List precautions for transporting unstable or ventilator-dependent patients.
3. List material that can accumulate in the pleural cavity and give the medical name for each condition.
4. Define tension pneumothorax and describe the emergency treatment for this life-threatening condition.
5. Define clinical algorithms and explain the goals of therapeutic planning.
6. Compare and contrast intensive care monitoring of adults and neonates.
7. Discuss the pathophysiology of diaphragmatic hernia and describe the diagnosis and treatment of this condition.
8. Explain the relationship of hyperventilation to intracranial pressure.

20
INTEGRATED APPROACH TO PATIENT THERAPEUTICS

CHAPTER OUTLINE

EMERGENCY CARE
  Cardiopulmonary Resuscitation
  Transport of the Unstable Patient
PLEURAL DRAINAGE SYSTEMS
THERAPEUTIC PLANNING
  Goals of Therapeutic Planning
  Interventions and General Patient Care
  Perioperative Care
  Intensive Care
  Neonatal Intensive Care
  Chronic Care and Rehabilitation
CASE PRESENTATIONS
  Neonatal Case Presentation
  Pediatric Case Presentation One
  Pediatric Case Presentation Two
  Adult Case Presentation One
  Adult Case Presentation Two

As we have seen in previous chapters, the first step in patient care is to assess the patient before starting any therapeutic intervention. Even in an emergency situation, such as a potential cardiopulmonary resuscitation, the first step is to attempt to arouse the victim (shaking him or her while shouting, "Are you all right?") and then feeling for a carotid pulse if he or she does not respond. This initial assessment determines the necessity, urgency, and aggressiveness of further therapeutic intervention.

Cardiopulmonary clinicians may be consulted by other healthcare providers to intubate a patient in respiratory distress. However, the cardiopulmonary clinician would be shirking responsibility and serving merely as a technician if he or she performed the intubation without an initial assessment. It may be discovered that intubation is unnecessary or even contraindicated, such as in a DNR (do not resuscitate) patient.

Patient therapeutics are guided by information obtained by patient assessment. Most assessment techniques have little therapeutic effect other than a possible placebo effect. A diagnostic test may also help reduce a patient's anxiety over not knowing what is wrong. Certain assessment modalities, such as bronchoscopy, may have great therapeutic value.

Caution is essential in the use of assessment and therapeutic techniques. The modern proliferation of tests and treatments can make us lose sight of the fact that we are trying to benefit the patient and not just get the procedure finished. Everything that we do to a patient carries some risk, even if the risk is as seemingly minor as upsetting the patient's peace of mind.

The age-old warning for healthcare providers, *primum non nocere* (first do no harm), is still applicable today. However, because every act in patient care carries some risk, we may feel that the best way to do no harm is to do nothing. Realize that failure to act may also be harmful to the patient. An appropriate awareness of the risk-benefit ratio for a procedure should guide our actions. We are willing to use techniques that are more invasive and aggressive with greater risk of complications on patients who are more critically ill. However, no patient should be exposed to risks unnecessarily. The risks must be outweighed by the probability of benefit to the patient.

The question of risk versus benefit is quite complex and raises questions of medical ethics in care of such patients as the terminally ill. Requests or orders from other healthcare providers should not be blindly followed but questioned when they seem inappropriate. Indiscriminately following requests or orders does not relieve you of your ethical or legal responsibility.

EMERGENCY CARE

The key to optimal care in emergency situations is *preparation*. The necessary supplies and personnel must be immediately available. Furthermore, the personnel must be prepared to respond in a rapid, intelligent, and appropriate manner. Hospital or departmental programs of mock emergencies can identify problems and coordinate the responses of different departments.

Equipment and supplies for emergencies must be kept in a designated location for each patient care area. These supplies are usually kept on a *code* or *crash cart*, which can be easily moved to the patient's bedside. The materials that must be present on the cart are fairly standard. However, they may be modified to suit the clinical situation, based on a cooperative decision by the hospital's physicians, nurses, and respiratory therapists. Usually, it is a nursing duty to check that the cart actually contains all the necessary supplies and the equipment is in good working order.

Cardiopulmonary Resuscitation

Every healthcare provider should know how to properly perform cardiopulmonary resuscitation (CPR). The basic principles of CPR are quite simple and effective. CPR has saved countless lives.

The American Heart Association (AHA) provides instruction in both basic cardiac life support (BCLS) and advanced cardiac life support (ACLS). BCLS can be performed by any person who has received this instruction and requires no special equipment.

The initial activity when performing BCLS is to evaluate the patient to determine the degree of unresponsiveness, ventilatory arrest (apnea), and/or circulatory arrest (pulselessness). After it is determined that the patient needs resuscitation, then mechanical ventilation (artificial respiration) and chest compressions can temporarily provide gas exchange in the lungs and perfusion of the vital organs until the patient responds and can spontaneously carry on these activities or else is pronounced dead. Cardiopulmonary resuscitation uses three basic rescue skills, the ABCs of CPR— airway, breathing, and circulation. CPR can be performed by one or two rescuers. When one rescuer is performing CPR on an adult, first determine the unresponsiveness of the victim. Summon help, if possible. Position the victim flat on his or her back. If necessary, turn the victim while supporting the head and neck. Open the airway with the head-tilt and chin-lift technique described in Chapter 18. Determine the ventilatory status of the victim. If the person is apneic, give two full breaths with 1 to 1½ seconds per breath. Determine pulselessness of the victim. Activate the Emergency Medical System (EMS), usually by dialing 911. If the patient is pulseless, begin rescue breathing while giving 15 chest compressions for every two ventilations. At the end of four cycles of compression and ventilation, check the carotid for return of pulse for 5 seconds. Guidelines for two rescuers for CPR on infants and children or for victims with obstructed airways are all contained in a certified CPR course.

Risks of CPR include blowing air into the stomach, which can result in vomiting and pulmonary aspiration, while chest compressions can cause rib fractures and injury to the underlying heart and lungs. A machine called an automatic resuscitator can provide chest compressions and/or ventilations during CPR. Devices currently available consist of a compressed oxygen–powered plunger mounted on a backboard (which is strapped onto the patient) and a time-pressure–cycled ventilator.

ACLS involves more complex therapeutic interventions, such as endotracheal intubation and administration of emergency drugs. Cardiopulmonary clinicians are routinely included in hospital code teams for resuscitating patients. Therefore, certification in BCLS and ACLS is strongly recommended for all cardiopulmonary clinicians and may be a requirement for employment.

Transport of the Unstable Patient

Cardiopulmonary clinicians are frequently enlisted to assist in transporting unstable or ventilator-dependent patients. Certain precautions are required for the transport of these patients. Patients suffering trauma or who have recently undergone anesthesia frequently have cardiovascular instability. Abrupt acceleration, deceleration, or turns can produce hypotension. Care must be taken not to dislodge catheters or endotracheal tubes. To ventilate a patient during transportation for short distances, one normally uses the right hand to squeeze the self-inflating resuscitation bag while using the left hand to hold the endotracheal tube in a fixed position on the patient's face. This helps reduce the chance of inadvertent extubation or endobronchial intubation. The little finger of the left hand may be used to palpate the carotid pulse at the same time. Additional monitors (such as a precordial stethoscope, portable ECG, arterial pressure monitor, or pulse oximeter) are strongly recommended. Changing the patient's position can bring the central venous or pulmonary artery catheter in contact with the myocardium and produce dysrhythmias. This is another reason for careful monitoring during transport.

During transport the need to ventilate the patient at a rate, tidal volume, and inspired oxygen concentration at settings comparable to those before moving is easily appreciated. Small transport ventilators are available for longer distance transportation. Equally important, a patient who is on PEEP should have the same level of PEEP during transport, even though this may require the use of a special gauge and apparatus. Discontinuation of PEEP for only a few minutes can rapidly produce atelectasis and hypoxemia. Special systems for transport with PEEP are available. PEEP levels and tidal volume must also be determined while moving the patient.

A portable suction apparatus is necessary when transporting patients more than a short distance in order to remove vomit or airway secretions that accumulate.

A situation requiring special precautions is transport in unpressurized aircraft. Rapid increases in altitude result in decreased atmospheric pressure and a proportional decrease in P_{O_2}. Increased inspired oxygen concentration may be required. Additionally, air-filled cavities increase in size when barometric pressure is rapidly decreased. This means an unrelieved pneumothorax may increase in size, possibly compromising ventilation. Venous air bubbles from intravenous lines will likewise increase in size with sudden increase in altitude in an unpressurized aircraft. Similarly, an endotracheal tube cuff can become overinflated and compromise circulation to the tracheal mucosa following a drop in atmospheric pressure.

The weight of the equipment can also be a problem when transporting a patient by aircraft. Compact and lightweight equipment is designed for this situation. Aircraft vibrations, particularly in helicopters, can make patient treatment and monitoring (auscultation, for instance) very difficult. A summary of precautions for transporting an unstable or ventilator-dependent patient is given in Table 20–1.

TABLE 20–1. Precautions for Transporting an Unstable or Ventilator-Dependent Patient

1. Stabilize the endotracheal tube to avoid accidental extubation.
2. Maintain ventilation.
3. Monitor vital signs.
4. Avoid quick turns, accelerations, or decelerations.
5. Consider the effects of changes in atmospheric pressure if using aircraft.

PLEURAL DRAINAGE SYSTEMS

The presence of gas or liquid in the pleural cavity interferes with expansion of the lung on that side. Material that can accumulate in the pleural space and the medical terms for those conditions are listed in Table 20–2.

Normally, there is only a small amount of serous fluid and no air in the pleural space. However, there are several ways in which a pneumothorax can occur. A *spontaneous pneumothorax* usually results from rupture of alveoli near the pleural surface of the lung following a forceful sneeze or cough. This is more common in an individual with a long narrow chest or with emphysema.

Piercing the surface of the lung with a needle, knife, gunshot, or sharp object, such as the jagged edge of a broken rib, can cause a pneumothorax. Physicians occasionally produce a pneumothorax when they try to insert a catheter into the subclavian vein, during thoracentesis or during transcutaneous lung biopsy. If the hole in the chest wall is large enough, the air will move in and out of the pleural cavity during the patient's ventilatory efforts, which is called a sucking chest wound.

The conducting airways can be perforated during endotracheal intubation or bronchoscopy, which can cause a pneumothorax, pneumomediastinum (air in the mediastinum), or subcutaneous emphysema (air under the skin) of the neck, chest, or abdomen. Lung surgery, such as lobectomy (removal of the lung lobe) or open lung biopsy, can produce an air leak into the pleural space. The use of high airway pressures during mechanical ventilation can also produce an air leak and pneumothorax. If the lung continues to leak air into the pleural space, the lung collapses, and pressure becomes elevated in that hemithorax. When the pressure becomes high enough, the mediastinal structures become compressed, and venous return to the heart is impaired. Cardiac output and blood pressure fall while central venous pressure becomes quite elevated in this condition, called *tension pneumothorax*. Chest radiographs reveal a collapsed, compressed lung but hyperlucent hemithorax on the affected side with the diaphragm pushed down (see Fig. 13–8). The heart and mediastinum are pushed away from the side of the tension pneumothorax and toward the normal lung. Another clinical sign of tension pneumothorax is tracheal shift away from the affected side. The hemithorax with a tension pneumothorax may appear overinflated and sounds hyperresonant to percussion.

Tension pneumothorax requires emergency treatment to relieve the pressure. This is accomplished by inserting a needle, drain, or chest tube into the affected side. This releases the pressure with a rush of air out of the chest. Failure to recognize and treat a tension pneumothorax can result in a patient's death within minutes.

Excessive amounts of serous fluid can accumulate in the pleural cavity as a result of inflammation (such as pleurisy), malignancy, or trauma. Increased serous fluid in the abdominal cavity (ascites) can also produce a pleural effusion. This fluid may be withdrawn from the thoracic cavity by inserting a needle through the chest wall into the fluid-containing space and then aspirating it, which is called *thoracentesis* (see Chapter 12). Effusions commonly resolve on their own, but a thoracentesis is frequently done for diagnostic purposes. As noted previously, care must be taken because thoracentesis can produce a pneumothorax.

When liquid is noted in the pleural space on a chest radiograph taken after chest trauma or surgery, the most likely diagnosis is a hemothorax. This is usually caused by bleeding into the pleural space from damaged intercostal vessels. A chest tube should be inserted at that time to remove the blood as well as to determine the volume of blood loss and ascertain if the bleeding is continuing. It is necessary to remove the blood from around the lung to allow inspiration and because the blood will clot and organize into a thick rind on the surface of the lung, which can later interfere with inflation. If the blood is not drained and a rind forms, it may

TABLE 20–2. Material That May Accumulate in the Pleural Space

Material	Medical Name
Air	Pneumothorax
Air under pressure	Tension pneumothorax
Serous fluid	Pleural effusion
Blood	Hemothorax
Lymph	Chylothorax

have to be removed later with a difficult surgical procedure called *decortication* of the lung. Air leaks from the surface of the denuded lung are frequently produced by this procedure.

A chylothorax almost always occurs only on the left side secondary to injury to the thoracic duct. The thoracic duct runs through the left hemithorax and drains lymph from all the structures below the diaphragm, from the left arm, and from the left side of the head. Lymph is a milky liquid rich in white blood cells. The thoracic duct drains into the left subclavian vein near its junction with the left jugular vein. The lymph ducts in the right chest are much smaller and are less likely to be injured.

Chest (intrapleural) tubes are connected to a drainage system that traps the liquid that drains from the pleural cavity. The volume and rate of drainage are measured. The drainage system also acts as a one-way valve so that liquid or air can leave the pleural space through the chest tube but cannot flow in the opposite direction if the system is intact. Obviously, if the system is not intact, air or contaminated material can enter the pleural space, resulting in a collapsed lung or infection. Additionally, suction can be applied to most pleural drainage systems to promote the removal of liquid or air from the pleural space and to facilitate the re-expansion of the lung. Usually, fairly low levels of suction (up to -25 cmH_2O pressure) are applied to chest tubes. If excessive negative intrapleural pressure is applied, lung trauma may be produced. Also, pulmonary edema may result from too rapidly re-expanding a collapsed lung.

THERAPEUTIC PLANNING

There are many textbooks on the subject of emergency care and critical care medicine. Clinical algorithms (decision trees) for assessment and treatment of specific common problems are usually included in these texts. An algorithm usually consists of a series of questions that can be answered yes or no and that eventually lead to the diagnosis and appropriate treatment (Fig. 20–1). Clinical algorithms are sometimes referred to as protocols, which suggests a certain set of responses to a clinical problem. Algorithms or protocols are used for several reasons, such as to help assure a complete and appropriate response in emergency situations. These tools are useful for clinicians who are inexperienced or in training to diagnose and treat a life-threatening problem quickly. Algorithms are also useful in clinical research to help assure consistent treatments in certain clinical situations.

One disadvantage of algorithms is that they focus on one problem and may neglect coexisting problems. Comprehensive, individualized care may suffer when "cook-book" algorithms are used. For this reason, in nonemergency situations, care plans should include the subjective and objective findings of a patient's evaluation, a list of all the patient's diagnoses, and a plan of treatment that addresses each of the patient's problems. At intervals, the patient must be reassessed to determine whether the care plan is meeting its objectives or requires changing.

Goals of Therapeutic Planning

The first goal in patient care is to be sure that the risk of the procedure is outweighed by the possible benefit to the patient. Also, patients must be made aware of the prognosis of their disease. Many cardiopulmonary diseases are chronic or progressive in nature. However, honest and straightforward discussion with the patient can help avoid unrealistic expectations of complete recovery and return to health. The patient should be prepared for the worst, but their hope should not be destroyed. Mature professionals have respect, dignity, and caring for all patients with whom they deal. As healthcare professionals, we are constantly reminded that we are mortal. Our patients do not all get better, but we can always try to make them feel better. Patients need to know that someone cares.

Interventions and General Patient Care

This book discusses many different treatments that cardiopulmonary clinicians use. It should be apparent that some treatments, such as antibiotics or immunizations, are useful to cure or prevent diseases. More commonly, therapeutic interventions treat the symptoms of the disease so that the patient can more comfortably tolerate the disease process. For example, decongestants do not help cure a cold but instead make the patient more comfortable while the body heals itself.

An understanding of the dynamics of patient-clinician interactions can improve the results of patient treatments. This may be possible by acting enthusiastic and optimistic, by improving patient understanding of the disease and treatment, and by making the patient involved in his or her own care. It is easier to care for a patient who is cooperative. Sometimes, considerable interpersonal

542 INTEGRATED APPROACH TO PATIENT THERAPEUTICS

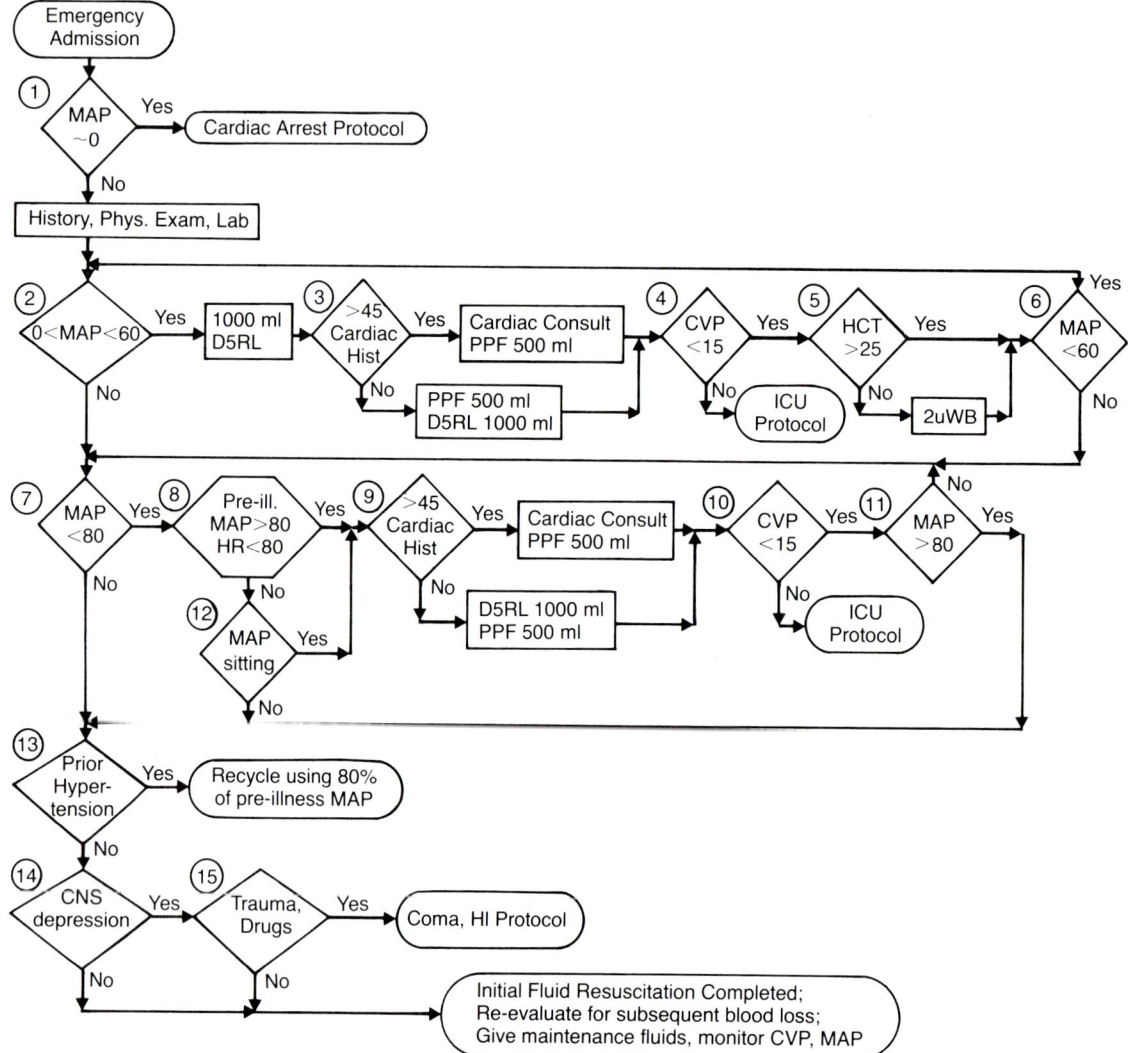

FIGURE 20–1. Clinical algorithm for the initiation of cardiopulmonary resuscitation (From Shoemaker, W.C., Thompson, W.L., and Holbrook, P.R. (eds.): *Textbook of Critical Care,* Philadelphia, W.B. Saunders, 1984, with permission.)

and psychological skills are necessary to make an uncooperative patient cooperative.

Perioperative Care

Cardiopulmonary clinicians frequently play a role in the preoperative evaluation of the patient with heart or lung disease. Preoperative pulmonary function tests are good predictors of whether a patient will require postoperative ventilation or can even survive certain types of surgery (such as pneumonectomy). Preoperative mucolytic nebulization and chest physical therapy is frequently used to "tune-up" COPD patients before surgery. These tune-ups help remove thickened secretions and improve pulmonary functions so that the patient better tolerates the physiologic stresses of anesthesia and surgery. These treatments also provide patient instruction so that they can better cooperate after the surgery. As previously mentioned, transport of a ventilator-dependent patient to the operating room may require the assistance of a cardiopulmonary clinician.

Supplemental inhaled oxygen is routinely given in the postanesthesia recovery room. In surgery, patients frequently become cold and are unable to regulate body temperature while under general anesthesia. During recovery, shivering to produce body heat is quite common, and this increases the body's oxygen demand. At the same time, the patient's ventilation may be impaired. Anesthesia relaxes the muscles of the pharynx and tongue and may result in airway obstruction. Narcotics for relief of surgical pain decrease the ventilatory drive. The combination of increased oxygen demand and decreased ventilation in the postoperative patient can be life-threatening, but the risk is decreased with the administration of supplemental oxygen.

Administration of nebulized drugs in the recovery room is another common intervention. This is helpful in the treatment of perioperative asthma. Nebulized racemic epinephrine is frequently quite effective for the treatment of airway edema secondary to the trauma of endotracheal intubation, bronchoscopy, or airway surgery.

Incentive spirometry is one of the most common postoperative therapeutic interventions by cardiopulmonary clinicians. This inexpensive treatment modality requires enthusiasm and persistence on the part of the therapist. Incentive spirometry is useful for cooperative patients who have a vital capacity of more than 15 ml/kg but less than normal levels. This includes the great majority of postoperative patients. Lower abdominal surgery (such as appendectomy or hysterectomy) usually produces a 30% reduction from the preoperative vital capacity. Upper abdominal surgery (such as cholecystectomy, gastrectomy, or splenectomy) or thoracic surgery produces a 60% or greater reduction in preoperative vital capacity. In addition, general anesthesia decreases the motility of the airway cilia, thickens airway secretions (from the use of atropine and dry, inhaled gases), and may result in airway obstruction. Incentive spirometry helps these patients take deep breaths so that they can cough better, clear their airways, and reduce atelectasis.

Intermittent positive-pressure breathing (IPPB) produces no greater benefit than incentive spirometry in patients who are cooperative and whose vital capacity is more than 15 ml/kg. However, the apparatus for administering IPPB is much more expensive than for incentive spirometry. A small group of patients whose vital capacity is more than 8 ml/kg but less than 15 ml/kg or those who are not very cooperative may benefit more from IPPB than incentive spirometry. Patients with vital capacities less than 10 ml/kg almost always require some mechanical ventilation.

Intensive Care

Intensive care units improve the outcome for critically ill patients. These units provide a high level of patient monitoring, such as indwelling pulmonary artery catheters (Table 20–3). There is a high

TABLE 20–3. Monitors Used in an Adult Intensive Care Unit

Frequent determination of vital signs
   Heart rate
   Ventilatory rate
   Blood pressure
   Temperature
Physical and neurologic evaluation
Electrocardiograph
Intra-arterial catheter
   Systemic blood pressure
   Arterial blood gases
   Other blood tests (e.g., electrolytes and hematocrit)
Central venous catheter (for infusion or measurement of central venous pressure)
Pulmonary artery catheter (Swan-Ganz)
   Pulmonary artery pressures and pulmonary capillary wedge pressure
   Mixed venous blood gases
   Thermodilution cardiac output
Pressure-limited volume ventilator with monitors and alarms
Pulse oximetry

nurse-to-patient ratio with one nurse constantly attending to the needs of only one or two patients. These units also have a high level of ancillary help. A cardiopulmonary clinician may be assigned exclusively to the patients of an intensive care unit. Many patients in intensive care units are on mechanical ventilation or require frequent blood gas analyses. Metabolic studies are also beneficial to evaluate the nutritional status of these critically ill patients. These patients often receive hyperalimentation (intravenous nutrition). Appropriate nutrition is crucial for tissue healing, hemostasis, and immunocompetence. A diet with an excessive amount of carbohydrates can make it impossible to wean a patient from the ventilator. If there is too much glucose in the diet, the excess glucose is converted and stored as fat (lipogenesis). Lipogenesis produces carbon dioxide without consuming oxygen. This makes the respiratory quotient (carbon dioxide production divided by oxygen consumption) rise. A patient is in lipogenesis when the respiratory quotient is greater than 1, and the amount of glucose in the diet must be reduced. Lipogenesis produces fat, which is stored in the liver and increases the size of the liver. The fatty liver pushes up the diaphragm, decreasing ventilatory mechanical efficiency at a time when lipogenesis is increasing carbon dioxide production. The level of dietary carbohydrate can determine whether or not a patient can adequately breathe spontaneously. Although the advantages of an intensive care unit include the proximity to supplies, monitors and specially trained personnel, the disadvantages include the risk of contamination with virulent organisms from other critically ill patients (nosocomial infections). These infections are usually resistant to antibiotics and are a common cause of death in critically ill patients.

Neonatal Intensive Care

This type of intensive care unit also has intensive monitoring, a high nurse-to-patient ratio, and extensive pulmonary support. However, different types of monitors and ventilators may be used (Table 20–4). In addition, the ventilatory status of a neonate can be evaluated by transcutaneous oxygen and carbon dioxide monitors. Pressure-cycled ventilators are commonly used on neonates to help reduce the barotrauma of fragile, underdeveloped lungs.

Neonates are not just the equivalent of very small adults but possess a different physiology. Neonates are very susceptible to injury from administration of hyperosmolar solutions (such as sodium bicarbonate), which can rupture their fragile cerebral vessels causing intracerebral hemorrhage and permanent brain damage.

Neonates have a large amount of surface area for a relatively small mass. For this reason, they are very susceptible to temperature loss if they are in a cold room. Much of the body's heat is lost via the skin, and neonates are unable to shiver to generate heat. In caring for neonates, avoid exposure to cool environments for prolonged periods because it can cause a severe metabolic strain, decreased perfusion, and lactic acidosis.

Neonates have about 100 ml of blood volume per kilogram of body weight. Therefore, blood samples for laboratory tests and blood gases must be as small as possible. Neonatal blood gases require 1/3 ml of blood or less. Indwelling arterial catheters used in neonates are continuously flushed with heparin solution, but the volumes must be measured and carefully limited because these patients are extremely sensitive to intravascular volume overload.

Premature infants have underdeveloped organs and are more susceptible to complications. Their nutritional status and liver function are poor, which increase their risk of hypoglycemia, jaundice, and drug toxicity (caused by immature metabolism and excretion by the liver).

Chronic Care and Rehabilitation

Many chronic diseases affect pulmonary function. Patients may require hospitalization for acute care, but patients requiring long-term care are frequently admitted to a nursing home or other chronic care facility. Some individuals require permanent placement in such facilities. For others, these facilities provide rehabilitation to prepare for discharge home. Rehabilitation uses a multidisciplinary approach involving physicians, nurses, occupational therapists, physical therapists, and social workers. The role of the occupational therapist is to use work-related skills to treat or train disabled persons to help restore their independence. Physical therapists use exercise, heat, cold, electricity, ultraviolet radiation, and massage to improve circulation and strengthen muscles to train an individual to perform the activities of daily living (ADL). Social workers provide counseling and try to help the patient in identifying sources of funding and support (government assistance programs or groups coping with the same disease). Respiratory care clinicians teach the patients about their disease and how to perform their own treatments, if possible. Rehabilitation in the form of coughing and breathing training are discussed in Chapter 17.

One of the goals of rehabilitation is to make the patient as independent as possible. Patients who know the course of their disease, warning signs, and home interventions can increase their participation in their own care and reduce costly hospitalizations. There are several programs for ventilatory care, airway suctioning, and tracheostomy care in the home. The patients and their families can give excellent care if they are properly trained and motivated. The home environment is usually more pleasant for the patient and less expensive, and there is less chance of acquiring an infection from an antibiotic-resistant organism.

TABLE 20–4. Monitors Used in a Neonatal or Pediatric Intensive Care Unit

Frequent determination of vital signs
Physical and neurologic evaluation
Electrocardiograph
Apnea monitors
Umbilical artery catheter
    Arterial blood gases
    Systemic blood pressure
    Blood tests
Transcutaneous P_{CO_2} and P_{O_2} monitors
Central venous catheter
Pressure-cycled or high-frequency ventilator with monitors and alarms
Pulse oximeter

CASE PRESENTATIONS

Neonatal Case Presentation

Baby Z was born at term after an unremarkable pregnancy. Almost immediately after delivery, the baby began showing signs of respiratory distress—an absence of crying, poor color, and ineffective ventilatory efforts. The baby was manually ventilated with 100% oxygen with a self-inflating resuscitation bag and mask. The neonate's color improved slightly, the heart rate was appropriate, and motor activity increased. However, the baby's spontaneous ventilatory attempts remained inadequate.

In order to deliver continued mechanical ventilation, the baby's larynx was visualized and the trachea was intubated with a 3.0 oral endotracheal tube using a Miller-0 laryngoscope blade. A viscous white material was seen oozing between the vocal cords during laryngoscopy and also in the endotracheal tube following intubation. This thick material was removed from the endotracheal tube with some difficulty using intermittent suctioning. Auscultation of breath sounds during mechanical ventilation revealed coarse, loud breath sounds on the right and distant breath sounds on the left.

What are some possible causes of these findings?

An endobronchial intubation (endotracheal tube inserted down a mainstem bronchus), pneumothorax, agenesis (failure to develop embryologically) of the left lung, or diaphragmatic hernia are possible causes of unilateral absence of breath sounds.

The baby was maintained on mechanical ventilation by a self-inflating resuscitation bag and taken to the neonatal intensive care unit. There the baby was ventilated on 100% oxygen using a Baby Bird ventilator.

What ventilator parameters should be set with this type of ventilator?

Because of the baby's poor color, the inspired oxygen concentration should be continued at 100% until blood gases indicate that it is safe to reduce it. The initial ventilator rate is commonly set at 40 for a neonate, with a peak inspiratory pressure of 23 to 25 cm H_2O. Some cardiopulmonary clinicians also start the infant on continuous distending pressure (PEEP) of 3 cmH_2O. These are initial settings only, and they are then altered based on the blood gas results.

An umbilical artery catheter was inserted in this patient and an arterial sample drawn for blood gas analysis. A chest radiograph was also taken, but before it was developed, the arterial blood gas results were found to be a pH of 7.24, P_{CO_2} of 63 mmHg, and P_{O_2} of 52 mmHg.

What should be done based on these blood gas results?

Although the blood gas results are distinctly abnormal, they do not reveal an immediately life-threatening problem. Therefore, further information should be obtained before changing ventilator settings. The breath sounds were essentially unchanged. The endotracheal tube was taped at the 9 cm mark on the tube, which is a normal distance for insertion in the neonate (see Chapter 18). The patient's vital signs were stable, and the chest wall on the left was not distended, so a tension pneumothorax was unlikely. When the chest radiograph was available, the endotracheal tube was seen to be in good position, but the left hemithorax was noted to be filled with intestines, which confirmed the diagnosis of diaphragmatic hernia (Fig. 20-2).

Diaphragmatic hernia in the newborn occurs most commonly on the left side and is a life-threatening emergency. The abdomen appears shrunken from the shift of the abdominal contents into the thorax. The presence of the intestinal contents in the thoracic cavity inhibits the growth and development (hypoplasia) of the lung on that side.

The viscous white material coming from this patient's airway is a common finding in patients with diaphragmatic hernia and is probably produced by the hypoplastic lung.

What treatment is necessary for this lesion?

Prompt surgical repair is recommended, but up to 50% of infants with this defect still die. The hypoplastic lung has a decreased number of alveoli and increased pulmonary vascular resistance. The patients with more severe hypoplasia are more likely to succumb. The diaphragm is repaired through an abdominal incision after pulling down the abdominal organs from the thoracic cavity.

What postoperative pulmonary treatment is likely?

The patient usually requires a few days of mechanical ventilation, depending on the degree of lung hypoplasia. Care must be taken to avoid high airway pressures because a pneumothorax in the lung opposite the side of the defect can be lethal. For this reason, neonates with this lesion are usually ventilated with small tidal volumes at rapid rates. Alternatively, high-frequency ventilation or extracorporeal membrane oxygenation (ECMO), may be used to reduce the amount of positive pressure needed for mechanical ventilation. Baby Z's condition gradually improved, but he required two

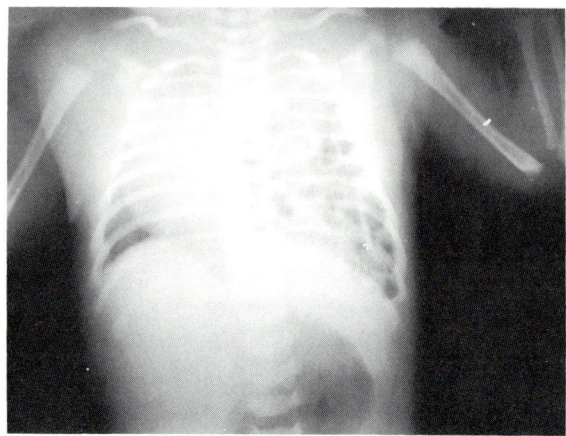

FIGURE 20-2. Baby Z's diaphragmatic hernia with intestines seen in the chest.

weeks of mechanical ventilation following the surgery.

Pediatric Case Presentation One

Willie G. is an 8-year-old boy with a long history of asthma. He has suffered numerous attacks of wheezing that usually respond to treatment with an isoetharine (Bronkosol) inhaler. On five occasions, he was treated in hospital emergency rooms for particularly severe attacks and then released. For several years, he has been taking a combination drug of theophylline, ephedrine, and phenobarbital (Tedral) orally to help prevent asthma attacks.

Willie felt feverish and tired for the past few days. His older brother had the flu a few days before with the same symptoms. Last night, Willie felt a rattling in his chest when he breathed. It responded somewhat to treatment with the inhaler, and he was able to sleep. Upon awakening this morning, however, the rattling was much worse and repeated use of the inhaler did not improve his condition. As he became more concerned about his difficult breathing, his condition worsened, and his parents took him to the emergency room.

Willie's chest appears overinflated (barrel chest), and musical wheezes that are loudest upon expiration can be auscultated over both hemithoraces. His heart rate is 120 beats per minute, and his temperature is 39.2°C.

What is the most likely diagnosis?

Very commonly, a respiratory tract infection can provoke an asthma attack in a susceptible individual. The history and elevated temperature suggest an infection, but the type of infection must be determined before appropriate treatment can be initiated. A blood count and chest radiograph were obtained while the patient was given a nebulization treatment with albuterol (Ventolin), a beta$_2$ agonist drug.

The chest radiograph showed hyperinflated lungs without any specific sites of consolidation (alveolar filling). The white blood cell count was not elevated, which suggests that Willie has a viral rather than a bacterial, upper respiratory tract infection.

The patient was also given water to drink. Asthma patients frequently become dehydrated because of their hyperventilation and decreased oral intake of fluids. The albuterol nebulization did not appear to help much, and the patient's heart rate is now 140.

What is the next therapeutic step in this situation?

The first thing is to determine if the patient's ventilatory status is worsening. If a flow-volume loop was performed before treatment, a repeat flow-volume loop will rapidly show how the patient is responding to treatment. A simple monitor of acute asthma is measuring peak air flows (see Chapter 9).

Obtaining arterial blood gases may be indicated if the patient is severely distressed. Sympathomimetic or other bronchodilating drugs should be used cautiously because the patient already has tachycardia. Further increases in heart rate could produce cardiac ischemia. However, cardiac ischemia is less likely in a pediatric patient than in an adult. Use of sympathomimetics that specifically stimulate beta$_2$ receptors, such as albuterol or terbutaline, usually causes less tachycardia than nonspecific beta agonists like isoproterenol and epinephrine (see Chapter 15).

Endotracheal intubation and mechanical ventilation are usually best avoided unless the patient is quite fatigued. The airway irritation caused by endotracheal intubation and mechanical ventilation can cause a bronchospasm to worsen. Although asthma patients are usually quite anxious, sedation is contraindicated because it can cause a respiratory arrest. Arterial blood gases drawn at this time showed a pH of 7.25, PCO_2 of 58 mmHg, and PO_2 of 68 mmHg with the patient breathing room air.

What is your interpretation of these blood gases?

The patient has an uncompensated respiratory acidosis and moderate hypoxemia. Breathing a gas mixture of helium and oxygen can improve gas flow through restricted airways because it is less dense than room air (Poiseuille's law). This should increase oxygenation and carbon dioxide elimination. Improved ventilation should reduce the patient's anxiety, which may partly cause the bronchoconstriction.

Methylxanthine medications are bronchodilators that complement the action of catecholamines. This patient was receiving an oral medication containing a catecholamine and a methylxanthine. Obtaining a further history from the patient's mother revealed that the patient reliably took his oral medication. However, the dosage had not been changed for 2 years, even though the patient had grown significantly during that time. A blood sample was drawn so that the blood levels of the drug could be determined, and it was later found that the concentration was subtherapeutic. The patient was administered aminophylline (a drug similar to methylxanthine and theophylline) intravenously and had significant reduction in bronchospasm. The patient was admitted for continued nebulization and observation overnight and was discharged the next day with an increased dosage of his oral medication. There is no specific therapy for many viral infections, which usually resolve when the body's immune system overcomes them.

What is the role of steroid medications and volatile inhalational anesthetic agents in the treatment of bronchospasm?

Steroid medications are reserved for especially severe asthma that is poorly responsive to other medications. Steroids (glucocorticoids) used in treating asthma have many side effects and take about 30 minutes before showing any effects. Nebulized or inhaled steroids have fewer side effects (see Chapter 15).

Inhaled volatile anesthetics, such as halothane, are very potent bronchodilators but are not commonly used in the treatment of asthma because they have potentially lethal vasodilating and cardiac depressant effects.

Pediatric Case Presentation Two

Yvonne B., 16 years old, was diagnosed as having cystic fibrosis, a disease characterized by abnormal glandular secretions, when she was 6 years old. She had suffered from repeated bouts of pneumonia, and a sweat test confirmed the diagnosis.

What is the basis of the sweat test?

An area of the subject's skin is enclosed in plastic wrap to form a watertight seal. The perspiration that accumulates under the plastic wrap is tested for chloride content. Individuals with cystic fibrosis have increased chloride concentrations in the secretions of their sweat glands (see Chapter 14).

Cystic fibrosis is an inherited disorder that is carried by 4% of whites in this country. It impairs the secretions of many glands in the body, such as the sweat glands, digestive glands (pancreas), and most or all mucus-producing glands, especially those in the airways.

The tenacious mucus that accumulates in the airway is a favorable environment for the growth of bacteria. In addition to promoting pulmonary infection, the thick mucus can obstruct and even completely block some airways, resulting in the collapse (atelectasis) of alveoli distal to the obstruction. Other airways may be only partially obstructed by the thick mucus in the lumen. Alveoli distal to partially obstructed airways are difficult to ventilate. Intrathoracic airway obstruction impedes both alveolar inflation and deflation. However, the airway obstruction is a greater impediment to exhalation than to inspiration because, during inspiration, the airway diameter tends to increase from increased transmural pressures and more traction by alveolar elastic recoil. During expiration, airway diameter decreases and may even be compressed during forced exhalation. This can cause accumulation of alveolar gas (gas trapping). Thus, in cystic fibrosis, as in other obstructive pulmonary disease, the completely obstructed airways have distal atelectasis, and partially obstructed airways can have overinflated, poorly ventilated alveoli distally. This ventilation/perfusion mismatch results in both increased shunt and shunt-like areas and more deadspace. Overinflation of an alveolus impedes blood flow through its pulmonary capillaries because of increased alveolar pressure.

After Yvonne was diagnosed as having cystic fibrosis, she was encouraged to begin an exercise program to increase her cardiopulmonary reserve and improve the strength of her cough to promote mucus mobilization. Daily, she received a nebulized mixture of bronchodilator (isoetharine) and mucolytic (sodium bicarbonate solution) drugs and chest physiotherapy to loosen especially adherent secretions. Additionally, pancreatic digestive enzymes were prescribed for her to mix with her food before eating it. Cystic fibrosis obstructs the secretion of digestive enzymes by the pancreas, which results in incomplete digestion of the food. This poorly digested food cannot be absorbed through the wall of the intestines and may result in malnutrition. Supplemental pancreatic enzymes promote digestion of the food and can improve the patient's nutritional status. Good nutrition is essential for the strength of the patient's respiratory muscles and also the ability to fight infection.

Despite exercise, mucolytic mobilization, and chest physical therapy, accumulation of airway secretions gradually worsened until Yvonne required fiber-optic bronchoscopy every few months to loosen and remove the thickened secretions. The thick mucus was located by the bronchoscope and sodium bicarbonate solution was instilled through the bronchoscope directly on the mucus to loosen it. The mucus was then removed by suction through the bronchoscope. These treatments effectively removed the mucus until it accumulated again. However, the treatments produced tremendous coughing, headaches, and emotional distress for Yvonne.

As Yvonne's problem with airway secretions worsened, her exercise tolerance decreased until she became short of breath following only slight exertion. She developed broadening and thickening of the distal ends of her fingers (clubbing), which is commonly seen in chronic pulmonary disease. The pulmonary shunting caused by the ventilation/perfusion mismatch produced hypoxemia. The hypoxemia gave a bluish appearance (cyanosis) to her lips, nail beds and conjunctiva (skin on the inner surface of the eyelid).

What cardiac problems are commonly associated with cystic fibrosis?

The airway obstruction produces hypoxemia and hypoxic pulmonary vasoconstriction (see Chapter 3). This increases pulmonary vascular pressure and also increases the work of the right ventricle. The increased work causes the wall thickness of the right ventricle to increase (hypertrophy). As the airway obstruction and hypoxia worsen, the pulmonary vasoconstriction and pulmonary artery pressure also increase until the right ventricle fails (cor pulmonale). Severe gas trapping can also cause pulsus paradoxus (an exaggerated drop in systemic systolic arterial pressure during inspiration). Pulsus paradoxus occurs more frequently with asthma and other forms of chronic obstructive pulmonary disease than with cystic fibrosis.

After an episode of strenuous coughing at home, Yvonne suddenly became very short of breath with rapid ventilations and marked cyanosis. She was taken to the hospital emergency room where she was given supplemental oxygen to breathe. Her condition improved only slightly and a physical exam revealed her barrel chest had only minimal ventilatory excursions. Chest auscultation revealed course rhonchi and expiratory wheezes bilaterally with breath sounds slightly decreased on the left.

What needs to be done in the care of this patient?

Further assessment and monitoring are essential to determine the cause and severity of her present problem and also to serve as a baseline for observing whether she responds favorably to any therapeutic measures. Arterial blood gases were a pH of 7.23, P_{O_2} of 43 torr, P_{CO_2} of 63 torr, and bicarbonate of 33 mEq/L. These blood gases show severe hypoxemia and partially compensated respiratory acidosis, which suggest that the patient had pre-existing respiratory acidosis with metabolic compensation until a recent event further impaired ventilatory mechanics.

What is hypoxic drive, and what is the risk of administering oxygen to a patient who is dependent on hypoxic drive to ventilate?

When chronic pulmonary disease impairs carbon dioxide elimination, arterial carbon dioxide levels become elevated (so-called carbon dioxide retention), and the patient becomes less sensitive to arterial carbon dioxide levels as a stimulus for ventilation. Such individuals are usually hypoxemic because of their lung disease, and the low arterial oxygen levels become the most important stimulus for ventilatory drive. When an individual is insensitive to arterial carbon dioxide and hypoxemia is the predominant stimulus for breathing, the patient is said to have hypoxic drive for ventilation. Hypoxic drive is a bit of a misnomer because the patient has a low arterial tension (hypoxemia) but is not necessarily hypoxic (inadequate levels of oxygen for tissue metabolism). If such an individual is given an increased inspired oxygen concentration, hypoventilation to the point of apnea may occur as the hypoxic drive for ventilation is abolished. The individual can then become very acidotic, resulting in a cardiac arrest.

Obviously, oxygen should not be withheld from a hypoxic individual in severe respiratory distress, but the possibility of blunted hypoxic drive must be recognized. Susceptible individuals should be carefully monitored, and a method of mechanical ventilation should be readily available. Furthermore, when mechanical ventilation and supplemental oxygen are required for patients dependent on hypoxic drive for ventilation, weaning can be very difficult until the inspired oxygen level is lowered to such a level that the patient's hypoxemia can then resume acting as a stimulus for ventilation.

Yvonne had minimal improvement in her dyspnea while breathing an elevated inspired oxygen concentration. A chest radiograph at that time revealed a hyperinflated right lung and pneumothorax on the left side with incomplete collapse of the left lung. Most likely, the left lung did not collapse completely because of an airway obstruction and gas trapping, which prevented complete emptying of the lung. A partial pneumothorax may also occur if the air leak into the pleural space is small, but this was not likely in this patient.

What is the treatment for a pneumothorax?

If the pneumothorax is very small (less than 15% of the pleural cavity) and is not enlarging, it may simply be monitored by daily chest radiographs and usually resolves spontaneously in a few days. If the pneumothorax is large or interferes with venous return to the heart (tension pneumothorax), a pleural vent (chest tube) must be inserted. Chest tubes and pleural drainage systems are discussed in an earlier section. A chest tube was inserted into this patient's left hemithorax, and the subsequent chest radiograph showed the pneumothorax was greatly reduced. The patient had less difficulty breathing, and her blood gases improved. However, chest radiographs taken over the next few days showed persistence of some pneumothorax. When the chest tube was clamped, the pneumothorax increased in size. A second chest tube was then inserted with further reduction of the pneumothorax. Some residual pneumothorax still persisted after several days, and the physicians decided to perform a sclerosing procedure to make the lung adhere to the chest wall. This is done by introducing a drug into the pleural space (usually via the chest tube) that produces an inflammatory reaction on the outer surface of the lung and on the inner surface of the chest cavity, which makes them adherent to each other. Drugs, such as nitrogen mustard or tetracycline, have been used for this purpose, but this is a very painful procedure. Following the sclerosing technique, Yvonne's pneumothorax resolved and did not recur. Her condition gradually improved until she was able to be discharged. However, the prognosis is still quite bleak for patients with cystic fibrosis, who usually die in their early twenties.

A recently utilized alternative is a complete heart and lung transplant, which is technically easier to perform than transplanting the lungs only. This is still a tremendously complex procedure and also requires the use of immunosuppressant drugs to prevent rejection of the transplanted tissues.

Adult Case Presentation One

Ellen P. is a 34-year-old mother of three who was loudly scolding her misbehaving children when she was stricken with a terrible headache. She lay down to rest and was later found by her husband to be unresponsive. She was taken to the hospital by ambulance where she was examined by the emergency room physician. Her blood pressure was 190/110 and her heart rate, 40 beats per minute. Her respiratory rate was 40 breaths per minute. Her left pupil was slightly larger than the right but both reacted to light.

What do these findings suggest?

This information suggests an elevated intracranial pressure (ICP) in this patient. The combination of increased blood pressure, elevated intracranial pressure, and slow heart rate is called Cushing's triad and is a very common finding in patients with brain pathology. The brain is enclosed in bone (cranium). The intracranial space also contains blood and cerebrospinal fluid (CSF) in addition to the brain. Changes in the intracranial volume of the brain, blood, or CSF affect the ICP. An increase in CSF production or a blockage in its resorption, as occurs in hydocephalus, can produce increased ICP. When the brain is injured, it tends to swell, which also increases ICP. The patient with increased ICP reflexively hyperventilates, which lowers arterial carbon dioxide and constricts the cerebral blood vessels. This vasoconstriction reduces the blood volume in the brain and tends to reduce ICP.

What is the hazard involved in increased intracranial pressure?

The risks of increased ICP include decreased cerebral perfusion pressure, which can produce brain ischemia and death, and herniation of the brain stem, in which the medulla of the brain is pushed down through the opening in the base of the skull (foramen magnum). Herniation of the brain stem corresponds with loss of all brain stem functions including loss of spontaneous ventilation.

This patient was taken for an emergency computed tomography (CT) scan of her head, which revealed swelling of the left cerebral hemisphere consistent with an intracerebral hemorrhage. The ventricles (fluid-containing cavities) of the brain were also compressed, which indicates elevated ICP. The patient was taken from the radiology department to the intensive care unit, but moments after her arrival, large amounts of pink frothy material began to flow from her mouth and nose while her breathing became more labored.

What is the problem and how should it be treated?

A fairly common complication in patients with elevated ICP is neurogenic pulmonary edema. The elevated ICP affects areas in the brain stem that control the cardiovascular system. In ways not fully understood, this produces an intense vasoconstriction in the pulmonary vessels, which elevates pulmonary vascular pressure resulting in pulmonary edema. Treatments for this condition include reduction of ICP, decreasing pulmonary vasospasm, and increasing intra-alveolar pressure to decrease edema formation.

This patient's trachea was intubated and hyperventilated with a pressure-limited volume ventilator. Mannitol, an osmotic diuretic, was given to decrease brain water and help lower ICP. Low levels of positive end-expiratory pressure were administered by the ventilator to decrease the fluid leak from the pulmonary capillaries.

What is the problem with using PEEP in patients with elevated ICP?

High levels of PEEP impede venous return to the heart but also produce elevated venous pressures. Increased venous pressures elevate intracranial blood volume and also ICP. The effect of PEEP to elevate ICP can be partially overcome by inclining the patient so that the head is elevated above the heart. This facilitates venous drainage from the brain and thus tends to lower ICP.

How much hyperventilation is optimal for reducing ICP?

Ideally, the patient's arterial $P{CO_2}$ should be between 28 and 32 mmHg for maximum cerebral vasoconstriction. Hyperventilation to a lower carbon dioxide level is deleterious because no further vasoconstricting effect occurs from the hypocapnia, but oxygen delivery to the brain can be impeded. Severe hypocapnia shifts the oxyhemoglobin dissociation curve so that the blood is less likely to give up the oxygen to the brain tissues. Furthermore, the increased mechanical ventilation needed to reduce carbon dioxide to this level produces a high intrathoracic pressure. This impedes venous return to the heart, reduces cardiac output, and decreases blood flow to the brain. Thus, cerebral hypoxia can result from excessive hyperventilation. The cerebral hypoxia is a potent cerebral vasodilator, which increases ICP.

The constriction of cerebral vessels caused by hypocapnia persists for less than a day. This is because the kidneys increase their excretion of bicarbonate, which returns blood pH to near normal (renal compensation). Thus, the tone of the cerebral blood vessels returns to normal. However, the hyperventilation is usually maintained for 3 to 5 days, and then the patient is slowly weaned because quick discontinuation produces a rebound dilation of the cerebral vessels. Unfortunately, 1 day after admission, both of Ellen's pupils became fixed and dilated. She was totally unresponsive even to painful stimuli, and her electroencephalograph (EEG) showed no brain activity. She was disconnected from the ventilator and allowed to die after her family and physicians had conferred and agreed that this was the most appropriate course of action. An autopsy showed a ruptured cerebral aneurysm.

Adult Case Presentation Two

John J. was a healthy 40-year-old until he was involved in a motor vehicle accident in which he fractured both femurs and struck his chest against the steering wheel. He lost consciousness for a few minutes after the accident and vomited. He was placed in spinal support for transport. His blood pressure dipped slightly before arrival at the hospital but returned to normal following administration of intravenous fluid. He was awake but disoriented and combative when he arrived at the hospital.

Physical exam revealed a blood pressure of 110/80, heart rate of 130, and respiratory rate of 40 breaths per minute. He had clear breath sounds bilaterally, but there were large hematomas on the skin of both anterior chest walls. He had paradoxical breathing (his chest wall moved in during inspiration and out during expiration). This condition is called *flail chest* when associated with rib fractures. The patient was given supplemental oxygen by mask (FIO_2 of 40%) while blood gases were drawn and a chest radiograph was taken. The chest radiograph revealed essentially clear lung fields but also three rib fractures on the left side. On the right side, there were four fractured ribs associated with an area of opacified lung. The arterial blood gas results were a pH of 7.30, $P{CO_2}$ of 53 mmHg, $P{O_2}$ of 55 mmHg, and bicarbonate of 27 mEq/L.

Based on the alveolar air equation, an alveolar $P{O_2}$ of 219 mmHg is expected for a patient breathing 40% oxygen. Normally, the arterial $P{O_2}$ should be only slightly lower than the alveolar $P{O_2}$. However, this patient has an arterial $P{O_2}$ of 55 mmHg. This wide alveolar–arterial $P{O_2}$ gradient suggests pulmonary shunting.

What are some reasonable explanations for the patient's respiratory problems? How are these problems diagnosed, and what is appropriate treatment?

Aspiration of gastric contents is a common complication in unconscious patients who vomit. The radiographic changes associated with aspiration may take a few hours to become apparent, but the hypoxia and lung damage occur very rapidly. It is standard procedure to assume that aspiration has occurred in an unconscious patient who has vomited. These patients require careful monitoring of the respiratory system and timely intervention, when necessary. An interval of 4 to 6 hours following a suspected aspiration is usually sufficient for radiographic changes to become apparent. Usually, the right middle lobe is the one involved in the unconscious patient who vomits while supine because that is the one most directly in the line of flow caused by gravity. However, this patient was sitting up when he aspirated, so the material would go to the basal portions of the lung. If the patient is lying on one side, the aspirated material goes to the lateral and posterior portions of the upper lobe of the dependent lung. Of course, prevention of further aspiration is essential in a patient who remains unconscious or obtunded (poorly responsive). Liquid should not be administered orally, and endotracheal intubation with a cuffed tube may be necessary to avoid further aspiration.

Rib fractures and paradoxical breathing produce inefficient alveolar ventilation, which may lead to hypoventilation, elevated carbon dioxide levels, and progressive alveolar collapse from failure to take deep breaths. Rib fractures and flail chest are usually apparent on chest radiographs and from physical exam in a patient with a history of chest trauma. It can be quite painful for patients with an injury to the chest wall to take a deep breath. These patients tend to take rapid, shallow breaths if they have inadequate pain relief. However, excessive narcotics cause respiratory depression, so pain management in these patients is a delicate matter. Other techniques for pain control to aid deep breathing include intercostal nerve block (with local anesthetic), epidural anesthesia, or epidural narcotics. Incentive spirometry can help reduce the development of atelectasis in patients with rib fractures, but IPPB and percussion techniques are discouraged because of the risk of pneumothorax caused by the jagged fracture edges. Within 2 weeks, healing of the fracture usually reduces the pain on deep inspiration.

Lung contusion injures areas of the lung that lie under the portion of the chest wall that has received a severe blow. These injured lung areas suffer edema and alveolar filling from the traumatized capillaries. Lung contusions usually occur with rib fractures, but rib fractures can occur without lung contusions. A chest radiograph reveals a localized area of increased density in the contused lung. The contused area creates intrapulmonary shunting that may be so severe that hypoxemia results. Hypoxemia from a lung contusion can be poorly responsive to PEEP because the increased alveolar pressure in the ventilated alveoli can divert blood flow to the nonventilated contused alveoli and increase the shunt and hypoxemia. Intensive ventilatory support may be required for these patients. Lung contusions usually resolve gradually like a bruise elsewhere on the body.

Fat embolism is a complication associated with fractures of long bones (such as the femur). Fatty marrow from the injured bone enters the circulation and is embolized to the lungs. These fat particles release free fatty acids, which are quite toxic and can produce a leak in the pulmonary capillary endothelium. This leads to a widespread nodular-appearing alveolar filling on a chest radiograph. However, the clinical picture associated with fat embolism usually does not appear until 1 or 2 days after the long bone fracture. This condition may be fatal and is treated like ARDS from other causes, although steroid administration may also be useful in this situation.

Cardiovascular injuries can result from trauma to the chest. The rapid increase in intrathoracic pressure caused by the chest wall striking a steering wheel can damage the heart valves, blood vessels, or heart tissue (cardiac contusion). Cardiovascular injuries can cause heart failure, which can cause fluid accumulation in the lungs as well as respiratory distress. Injury to a heart valve produces murmurs that are easily detectable on auscultation. Cardiac contusion produces elevation of cardiac enzymes in the blood serum that are quite specific for cardiac injury. Vessel injury may show up as an unusual opacity on the chest radiograph, which can be definitively evaluated by injecting contrast dye into the vessel (angiography). The findings in this individual indicated rib fractures, possible lung contusion on the right, possible aspiration of gastric contents, and possible fat embolism.

In view of the patient's severe diagnoses, poor blood gases, and ventilatory difficulty, he was orally intubated with an 8.0 mm endotracheal tube and placed on mechanical ventilation with a tidal volume of 1 L, intermittent mandatory ventilation (IMV) rate of 10, inspired oxygen concentration (FIO_2) 100%, and 5 cmH_2O CPAP. After this, the arterial blood gases showed a pH of 7.38, PCO_2 of 39 mmHg, PO_2 of 65 mmHg, bicarbonate of 25 mEq/L, and SO_2 of 93%.

A Swan-Ganz (pulmonary artery) catheter was placed in this critically ill patient to help monitor his cardiopulmonary system. A mixed venous blood gas analysis revealed a pH of 7.35, P_{CO_2} of 44 mmHg, P_{O_2} of 34 mmHg, bicarbonate of 27 mEq/L, and venous S_{O_2} of 64%. The patient's hemoglobin was 13 gm/dl, and the pulmonary artery pressure was 53/27 mmHg. The patient's shunt ($\dot{Q}_S/\dot{Q}_T$) was calculated to be 37%, which is much higher than normal (3% to 5%). The high pulmonary artery pressure is consistent with hypoxic pulmonary vasoconstriction and possible pulmonary embolism.

What should be done for this patient's persistent, severe hypoxemia?

The F_{IO_2} cannot be increased because it is already 100%. The IMV rate and tidal volume appear to be providing adequate alveolar ventilation, and so changing these settings would not be expected to produce much change in oxygenation. Techniques that can reduce pulmonary shunting are more likely to improve oxygenation in this patient. These include PEEP to diminish atelectasis, checking endotracheal tube placement to rule out endobronchial intubation (a cause of massive shunting), or removal of airway secretions by bronchoscopy or other suctioning techniques.

What is the risk of receiving a high concentration of oxygen for a prolonged period?

Oxygen toxicity develops when high oxygen concentrations are breathed for several hours. Breathing 100% oxygen for only 8 hours can begin the pathologic changes associated with oxygen toxicity. Oxygen toxicity is unlikely to develop if the inspired concentration is less than 60%.

Breathing 100% oxygen can also produce absorption atelectasis in alveoli that are poorly ventilated. When nitrogen from room air is replaced by oxygen in poorly ventilated alveoli, the pulmonary capillary blood can rapidly absorb the oxygen, resulting in collapse of that alveolus. In this way, breathing 100% oxygen results in the loss of the so-called nitrogen splint and promotes alveolar collapse.

This patient's chest radiograph showed proper endotracheal tube placement and no significant atelectasis. Therefore, the use of increased PEEP was chosen as a treatment to improve oxygenation of the blood so that the inspired oxygen concentration could be reduced. The patient's PEEP was increased in increments of 2 cmH$_2$O without significant improvement in the patient's arterial oxygenation.

Increasing levels of PEEP are administered to a patient with intrapulmonary shunting in order to improve matching of ventilation and perfusion. However, high levels of PEEP are also associated with increased intrathoracic pressure, decreased venous return, and decreased cardiac output. Pulmonary injury (barotrauma) can also result from mechanical ventilation with high airway pressure.

When the level of PEEP reached 25 cmH$_2$O, the patient became hypotensive, cyanotic, and more tachycardic. Auscultation revealed diminished breath sounds on the right. A chest tube was inserted in the right chest with a rush of air outward when the pleural cavity was entered. This suggests the presence of a tension pneumothorax that may have resulted from the high airway pressure, the rib fractures, or the interaction of these two conditions. When the chest tube was attached to a water-sealed chest drainage unit, a persistent air leak from the pleural cavity was noted. This is most likely caused by a bronchopleural fistula (communication between a conducting airway of the lung and the pleural cavity). Despite the stepwise addition of PEEP, the arterial blood gases continued to show severe hypoxemia on 100% inspired oxygen. This is quite ominous because the patient needs the high inspired oxygen concentration to maintain oxygenation of the blood, yet oxygen toxicity is inevitable. The patient remained fairly stable, and the PEEP was weaned to 10 cmH$_2$O with arterial P_{O_2} of 83 torr. The F_{IO_2} was decreased to 90% to delay the onset of oxygen toxicity. Arterial P_{O_2} fell to 73 torr.

At this point, it was noted that, when the patient was turned with his right side elevated, the arterial blood gases had better oxygenation, and when the left side was elevated, the oxygenation was worse.

What is the explanation for the changes in oxygenation when different sides were elevated?

Pulmonary blood flow goes to dependent portions of the lung because of the effects of gravity. When the body is turned so that the injured area of lung is more dependent (lower), more blood flow passes through the injured area, resulting in more shunt. When the body is turned so that the injured area is more elevated while the normal lung is more dependent, less blood flows to the area of injury, more blood flows to the normal lung, and shunt decreases while oxygenation improves.

Changes in oxygenation associated with changes in position suggest a localized disease process in the lungs which may not be responsive to treatment by PEEP. In fact, increasing PEEP can sometimes decrease the arterial P_{O_2} because the increased airway pressure can reduce blood flow to ventilated alveoli and increase blood flow to the injured area, increasing the shunt as discussed previously.

This patient seemed to have a focal lung injury, which was probably a lung contusion. Additionally, the air leak through the chest tube persisted and required an increase in the minute ventilation delivered by the ventilator. The patient was not stable enough to transport to a larger hospital, so a critical care expert was consulted. After careful evaluation of the patient, it was decided that independent ventilation of the two lungs might be helpful. First, the patient was totally paralyzed with the muscle relaxant pancuronium, and a double-lumen endobronchial (Carlen's) tube was inserted. Separation of ventilation of the two lungs was verified by auscultation. Two ventilators were used to provide independent ventilation. The right lung was ventilated with a tidal volume of 300 ml, IMV of 10, and 10 cmH$_2$O PEEP, while the left lung was ventilated with a tidal volume of 500 ml, IMV of 10, and 5 cmH$_2$O PEEP. The arterial blood gases showed improvement in the amount of oxygenation, and the inspired oxygen concentration was weaned to below toxic levels. The leakage from the bronchopleural fistula persisted, however.

In this case, after allowing a few days for the lung contusion to resolve and for the patient to stabilize, the following efforts were made to reduce the chest tube leakage. The ventilation to the right lung was switched to high-frequency positive-pressure ventilation (HFPPV), and conventional ventilation was continued with the left lung. The HFPPV provided adequate ventilation and low airway pressures, which greatly reduced the leak through the fistula. After 3 days of unilateral HFPPV, the leak stopped. The next day, the double-lumen tube was removed, and a single-lumen endotracheal tube was inserted without reopening the fistula. The arterial blood gases were acceptable with an FIO_2 of 40%. The muscle relaxant was allowed to wear off and ventilatory support was gradually weaned over the next 3 days. The patient was extubated and, 7 days later, was discharged from the hospital.

For treatment of bronchopleural fistula, various modalities are useful, including:
1. Terminating suction on the chest tube.
2. Raising the water level in the chest tube bottle to provide back pressure.
3. Intermittent chest tube occlusion, which blocks the chest tube when the ventilator gives a breath.
4. High-frequency ventilation.
5. Surgery to close the site of the leak.

Intensive care of critically ill patients requires massive effort and innovation. All systems of the critically ill patient can be involved, but intensive respiratory care frequently provides the most dramatic effect on the patient's hospital course.

Bibliography

Agostoni, E.: Mechanics of the pleural space. *Physiol. Rev.* 52:57, 1972.

Ali, J., Serrette, C., Wood, L.D.H., and Anthonisen, W.R.: Effect of postoperative intermittent positive-pressure breathing on lung function. *Chest* 85:192–196, 1984.

American Heart Association: *A Manual for Instructors of Basic Cardiac Life Support.* Dallas, American Heart Association, 1981.

Arms, R.A., Dines, D.E., and Tinstman, T.C.: Aspiration pneumonia. *Chest* 65:136–139, 1974.

Ashbaugh, D.G., Peters, G.N., Halgrimson, C.G., et al.: Chest trauma: Analysis of 685 patients. *Arch. Surg.* 95:546–555, 1967.

Askanazi, J., Weissman, C., Rosenbaum, S.H., et al.: Nutrition and the respiratory system. *Crit. Care Med.* 10:163–172, 1982.

Bierman, C.W.: Pneumomediastinum and pneumothorax: Complications of asthma in children. *Am. J. Dis. Child.* 114:42, 1967.

Burger, E.J., and Macklem, P.: Airway closure: Demonstration by breathing 100% oxygen at low lung volumes and by N$_2$ washout. *J. Appl. Physiol.* 25:139–148, 1968.

Cullen, P., Modell, J.H., Kirby, R.R., et al.: Treatment of patients with flail chest by intermittent mandatory ventilation and PEEP. *Crit. Care Med.* 3:45, 1975.

Eisenberg, M.S., and Copass, M.K.: *Emergency Medical Therapy.* Philadelphia: W.B. Saunders, 1982.

Fishman, A.P.: Cor pulmonale: General aspects. In Fishman, A.P. (ed.): *Pulmonary Diseases and Disorders*, vol. 1. New York, McGraw-Hill, 1980, pp 853–863.

Fleisher, G., and Ludwig, S.: *Textbook of Pediatric Emergency Medicine.* Baltimore, Williams and Wilkins, 1983, pp 494–496.

Gallagher, T.J., Banner, M.J., and Smith, R.A.: A simplified method of independent lung ventilation. *Crit. Care Med.* 8:396–398, 1980.

Hopkins, J.A., Shoemaker, N.C., Chang, P.C., et al.: Clinical trial of emergency resuscitation algorithm. *Crit. Care Med.* 11:621–629, 1985.

Jaffe, A.S. (ed): American Heart Association: *Textbook of Advanced Cardiac Life Support.* Dallas, American Heart Association, 1987.

Jastremski, M.S.: Hemodynamic monitoring: Concepts every clinician should know. *Consultant* 22:96–111, 1982.

Jastremski, M.S. (ed.): *The Whole Emergency Medicine Catalog.* Philadelphia, W.B. Saunders, 1985.

Johnson, M.C., and Fassett, B.A.: Bronchopulmonary hygiene in cystic fibrosis. *Am. J. Nurs.* 69:320–324, 1969.

Kaste, M., and Palo, J.: Criteria of brain death and removal of cadaveric organs. *Ann. Clin. Res.* 13:313–317, 1981.

Kelsen, S.G., and Fishman, A.P.: Clinical assessment of the regulation of ventilation. In Fishman, A.P. (ed.): *Pulmonary Diseases and Disorders*, vol. 2. New York, McGraw-Hill, 1980, pp 1,787–1,795.

Larken, P.N., and Fishman, A.P.: Clubbing and hypertrophic osteoarthropathy. In Fishman, A.P. (ed.): *Pulmonary Diseases and Disorders*, Vol. 1. New York, McGraw-Hill, 1980, pp 84–92.

Lulla, S., and Newcomb, R.W.: Emergency management of asthma in children. *J. Pediatr.* 97:346–350, 1980.

McNeil, E.L.: *Airborne Care of the Ill and Injured.* New York, Springer Verlag, 1983.

Montgomery, W.M., Herrin, T.J., and Lewis, A.J. (eds.): *Basic Life Support for Physicians.* Dallas, American Heart Association, 1982.

Rehder, K., Sessler, A.D., and Marsh, H.M.: General anesthesia and the lung. *Am. Rev. Respir. Dis.* 112:541–563, 1975.

Rowe, P.C. (ed): *The Harriet Lane Handbook.* 11th ed. Chicago, Year Book, 1987.

Safar, P. (ed.): Special Symposium Issue: Brain resuscitation. *Crit. Care Med.* 6:199, 1978.

Shackford, S.R., Smith, D.E., Zarins C.K., et al.: The management of flail chest, a comparison of ventilatory and non-ventilatory treatment. *Am. J. Surg.* 132:759–762, 1976.

Shoemaker, W.C., Thompson, W.L., and Holbrook, P.R. (eds.): *Textbook of Critical Care.* Philadelphia, W.B. Saunders, 1984.

Sublett, J.L., Pollard, S.J., Kadlec, G.J. and Karibo, J.M.: Non-compliance in asthmatic children: A study of theophylline levels in a pediatric emergency room population. *Ann. Allergy* 43(2):95–97, 1979.

Woolf, C.: A rehabilitation program for improving exercise tolerance of patients with chronic lung disease. *Can. Med. Asso. J.* 106:1,289–1,295, 1972.

Wray, W.P., and Nicotra, M.B.: Pathogenesis of neurogenic pulmonary edema. *Am. Rev. Respir. Dis.* 118:783, 1978.

Appendix 1

PULMONARY TERMS AND SYMBOLS

A Report of the American College of Chest Physicians—American Thoracic Society Joint Committee on Pulmonary Nomenclature (Reprinted, with permission, from *Chest* 67:5, May 1975. Copyright © American College of Chest Physicians)

CONTENTS
I. Terms Used in Classification of Diseases
   A. General Principles
   B. Recommendations
   C. Diseases Producing Diffuse Pulmonary Infiltration
   D. Diseases Associated with Airways Abnormality
II. Terms Used in Physical Examination
   A. Auscultation and Palpation
   B. Percussion
III. Terms Used in Respiratory Therapy
IV. Terms and Symbols Used in Respiratory Physiology
   A. General Use of Symbols
   B. Gas Phase
   C. Blood Phase
   D. Ventilation and Mechanics
   E. Diffusing Capacity
   F. Blood Gases
   G. Pulmonary Shunts
   H. Pulmonary Dysfunction

I. TERMS USED IN CLASSIFICATION OF DISEASES

A. *General Principles*
   In this statement, the following principles have been followed:
   1. Standardization of terms used for classification of illnesses is desirable. Such terms are called *diagnoses* in this statement. The selection of terms which are acceptable as diagnoses is necessarily arbitrary.
   2. A clear distinction should be made between *defining characteristics* which define an acceptable diagnostic category and *diagnostic criteria* which permit use of a diagnosis by allowing the inference that defining characteristics are also present.[1] Other *descriptors* of an illness may be used even though not acceptable as a basis for primary diagnosis.
   3. No attempt should be made to provide standardized diagnostic criteria in this type of statement, since such criteria change with new medical knowledge and vary with circumstance.
   4. A priority for defining characteristics should be recognized, with a descending order of preference, as follows: (a) etiology; (b) anatomic abnormality; (c) physiologic or biochemical abnormality; (d) signs and symptoms. A combination of terms, each with its own defining characteristics, is often appropriate as a diagnosis.

B. *Recommendations*
   The following recommendations are made in regard to the use of diagnostic terms in medical publications:
   1. The definition of each term or a reference to such a definition should be given and diagnostic criteria clearly indicated. Where possible, criteria should be stated in quantitative terms. Honesty may require use of low priority general diagnostic terms for groups of individuals.
   2. When the process of case selection does not assure that the study group is representative of all patients in an accepted diagnostic category, the selectivity should be indicated by an appropriate modifier to the diagnostic term. For example, patients with sarcoidosis who were originally selected on the basis of an abnormal chest radiograph may not be representative of the universe of sarcoidosis patients. A group of such patients might be designated as "radiographically detected sarcoidosis."
   3. Diagnostic terms, symbols, and descriptors employed should be related to other terms in common use, noting pertinent differences or similarities. Authors should justify a proposed new diagnostic term by noting clearly why existing terminology cannot be used.

C. *Diseases Producing Diffuse Pulmonary Infiltration*
   A variety of terms has been used to describe non-neoplastic infiltrative lesions in the respiratory portion of the lung. These have stressed one or another feature of a particular lesion while neglecting other features. For example, "interstitial pneumonia" has been used to refer to reactions which also have significant intra-alveolar components. "Interstitial fibrosis" has been applied to lesions without much cellular exudation. The term *alveolitis* is used here, since it implies no such anatomic or histopathologic limitation.[2] Modifiers should be used to supply additional information such as etiology, associated systemic disease, stage of the disorder, or a partic-

ular anatomic feature of the disease. *In the following classification, previously used terms considered synonymous with proposed diagnoses are included in brackets.*

1. *Diagnostic Terms Based on Etiology:*
    a. *Pneumoconiosis:* A non-neoplastic structural alteration of the lung resulting from the accumulation of inorganic dust. The causative dust should be indicated in the diagnosis. Commonly used terms such as silicosis or asbestosis are preferred to silicotic pneumoconiosis or asbestos pneumoconiosis.
2. *Diagnostic Terms Based on Anatomic Findings:*
    a. *Alveolitis* [Interstitial Pneumonia]: Inflammation of the lung distal to the terminal non-respiratory bronchiole. Unless otherwise indicated, it is assumed that the condition is diffuse. Arbitrarily, the term is not used to refer to exudate in air spaces resulting from bacterial infection of the lung. The term alveolitis may be modified by words or phrases to indicate its duration, its etiology, or its predominant histopathologic feature. For example:
    Allergic Alveolitis [Hypersensitivity Pneumonia, Organic Dust Pneumoconiosis]: Alveolitis caused by an immunologic response to an inhaled organic dust.
    Fibrosing Alveolitis [Usual Interstitial Pneumonia, Diffuse Interstitial Fibrosis]: Alveolitis accompanied by the production of fibrous tissue.
    Alveolitis with Honeycombing: Alveolitis accompanied by a revision of lung architecture with formation of abnormal thick-walled air spaces of a size easily seen macroscopically.
    Alveolitis with Hyaline Membrane: Alveolitis accompanied by layers of acellular eosinophilic material applied against the walls of air spaces.
    Desquamative Alveolitis: [Desquamative Interstitial Pneumonia]: Alveolitis characterized by uniformity of pattern with alveolar epithelial hyperplasia and intra-alveolar exudate of large mononuclear cells. A modest degree of interstitial widening, edema, fibrosis, and hyperplasia of smooth muscle is often present.
    Lymphoid Alveolitis [Lymphoid Interstitial Pneumonia]: Alveolitis characterized by diffuse interstitial accumulation of lymphocytes and plasma cells and the absence of appreciable intra-alveolar exudate.
    b. *Pulmonary Hemosiderosis:* The presence in the lung of macrophages containing hemosiderin, of any cause. Intra-alveolar hemorrhage which accompanies systemic disease (e.g., Goodpasture's syndrome) should be classified according to the systemic disease.
    Idiopathic Pulmonary Hemosiderosis [Idiopathic Brown Induration, Ceelen's Disease] is a disease confined to the lung, characterized by intra-alveolar hemorrhage or hemosiderosis, for which other accepted causes have been excluded.
    c. *Pulmonary Alveolar Proteinosis:* A chronic or recurrent disease characterized by the filling of alveoli with an insoluble exudate, usually poor in cells, rich in lipids and proteins, and accompanied by minimal histologic alteration of the alveolar walls.
    d. *Sarcoidosis:* A systemic disease characterized by the presence in tissues of noncaseating granulomas, in which no causative agent can be demonstrated.
    e. *Pulmonary Alveolar Microlithiasis:* A disease in which calcified spherules develop in air spaces.
    f. *Pulmonary Histiocytosis* [Eosinophilic Granuloma, Histiocytosis X]: Interstitial infiltrates of well-differentiated cells resembling histiocytes accompanied by variable numbers of eosinophils. Similar lesions may or may not be present in other organs.
3. *Diagnostic Terms Based on Clinical Findings:*
    a. *Diffuse Pulmonary Infiltration:* A radiographic appearance suggesting the presence within the lung of widespread tissue proliferation or exudate, where the specific etiology and anatomic findings are unknown. Modifiers such as acute, chronic with eosinophilia, etc, may be applied.
    b. *Respiratory Distress Syndrome:* A disorder of the lung characterized by the development of acute respiratory failure in the absence of airways obstruction. If the etiology is known, this should be stated. The condition may be accompanied by diffuse pulmonary infiltration and a tendency to patchy atelectasis. The term *infant respiratory distress syndrome* [hyaline membrane disease] should be restricted to disorders occurring during the first day of life and considered to be associated with altered surfactant function.

D. *Diseases Associated with Airways Abnormality*
There have been a number of efforts to standardize diagnostic terminology applied to these disorders.[3-6] A few generally accepted definitions have emerged and these are retained. However, to avoid using signs and symptoms to define a term which has acquired etiologic implications and which has anatomic meaning, "chronic bronchitis" has been redefined in etiologic terms. This does not preclude the use of clinical findings, such as sputum production, as diagnostic criteria for the disease.

1. *Diagnostic Terms Based on Etiology:*
    a. *Bronchitis:* A non-neoplastic disorder of structure or function of the bronchi resulting from infectious or noninfectious irritation. The term bronchitis should be modified by ap-

propriate words or phrases to indicate its etiology, its chronicity, the presence of associated airways dysfunction, or type of anatomic change. The term *chronic bronchitis,* when unqualified, refers to a condition associated with prolonged exposure to nonspecific bronchial irritants and accompanied by mucous hypersecretion and certain structural alterations in the bronchi. Anatomic changes may include hypertrophy of the mucus-secreting apparatus and epithelial metaplasia, as well as more classic evidences of inflammation. In epidemiologic studies, the presence of cough or sputum production on most days for at least three months of the year has sometimes been accepted as a criterion for the diagnosis.[4,6]

2. *Diagnostic Terms Based on Anatomic Findings:*
   a. *Pulmonary Emphysema:* An abnormal enlargement of the air spaces distal to the terminal nonrespiratory bronchiole, accompanied by destructive changes of the alveolar walls.[4] The term emphysema may be modified by words or phrases to indicate its etiology, its anatomic subtype, or any associated airways dysfunction.
   b. *Bronchiolitis:* Inflammation of the bronchioles which may be acute or chronic. If the etiology is known, it should be stated. If permanent occlusion of the lumens is present, the term *bronchiolitis obliterans* may be used.

3. *Diagnostic Terms Based on Clinical Findings:*
   a. *Asthma:* A disease characterized by an increased responsiveness of the airways to various stimuli and manifested by slowing of forced expiration which changes in severity either spontaneously or as a result of therapy.[4] The term asthma may be modified by words or phrases indicating its etiology, factors provoking attacks, or its duration.
   b. *Chronic Obstructive Pulmonary Disease (COPD):* This term refers to diseases of uncertain etiology characterized by persistent slowing of airflow during forced expiration. It is recommended that a more specific term, such as chronic obstructive bronchitis or chronic obstructive emphysema, be used whenever possible.

II. TERMS USED IN PHYSICAL EXAMINATION

A. *Auscultation and Palpation*
   1. *Quality of Breath Sounds:*
      Sounds heard over normal distal lung areas while breathing through the mouth are best described simply as *normal.* The character of these sounds varies somewhat from area to area even in normal individuals. In abnormal states, a localized *decrease or absence of breath sounds* may be noted.

      Bronchial breath sounds may be heard over distal lung areas in disease. These are abnormally loud breath sounds audible throughout the respiratory cycle, resembling sounds normally heard only over large airways.

   2. *Transmission to the Chest Wall of Voice-Generated Sounds or Vibrations:*
      Transmission of voice-generated sounds or vibrations to the surface of the chest is altered in a variety of chest diseases. Different terms such as increased fremitus, bronchophony, pectoriloquy, and egophony, have been used to describe altered transmission of spoken or whispered voice although these findings have essentially the same significance. The notation should be a simple description of the findings indicating decrease or increase in intensity or clarity of transmitted, whispered, or spoken voice.

   3. *Adventitious Sounds or Vibrations:*
      a. *Abnormal Sounds or Vibrations Produced by Movement of Air in the Lungs:*
         There is considerable confusion in the use of the terms *râle* and *rhonchus* to describe adventitious (not normally occurring) sounds heard over the chest. Laennec used *râle* as a generic term to include all abnormal sounds produced by movement of air in the bronchi or pulmonary tissue. In translating this into Latin, he used the word *rhonchus,* later translated into English as *wheeze.* Some continue to use *rhonchus* and *râle* as general terms for all abnormal lung sounds. However, *rhonchus* is used by others to describe only a continuous sound (wheeze) and *râle* to describe only short, interrupted, explosive sounds (crackles) heard usually during inspiration. The simplest way to resolve the confusion is to select the two most commonly used words, *rhonchus* and *râle,* and arbitrarily define the term *râle* to indicate only crackling or bubbling (discontinuous) sounds or vibrations and *rhonchus* to define only musical (continuous) sounds or vibrations, usually of longer duration. Alternative acceptable terminology substitutes *crackles* for râles and *wheezes* for rhonchi.[7] *Rhonchi* or *wheezes* may vary in pitch, quality, and intensity. *Râles* or *crackles* may also vary considerably in intensity and quality, but little is gained by their subclassification. In patients with rhonchi or wheezes, *noisy breathing* may be audible at the mouth.

      b. *Other Adventitious Sounds or Vibrations:*
         Mediastinal Crunch: A coarse crackling sound or vibration synchronous with systole, heard over the precordium in the presence of mediastinal emphysema.
         Pleural Rub: A grating sound or vibration associated with breathing and unaffected by cough.

Pericardial Rub: A regular to and fro grating sound or vibration associated with the heart beat which persists in the absence of breathing and is unaffected by cough.

Pleuropericardial Rub: A term used to describe a sound or vibration with some features of both pleural and pericardial rubs.

B. *Percussion*

Percussion notes are sounds produced by the fingers striking the chest directly or indirectly. They vary considerably in quality in different subjects and over different parts of the chest. The sounds generated over a normal lung are best described simply as *normal*. Abnormal notes of short duration and low intensity without the low pitched resonance of the normal percussion sound are called *dull*. Sounds with abnormally high pitched resonance are called *tympanitic*.

III. Respiratory Therapy Terms

In publications, specific apparatus, as well as time, volume, pressure, and concentration variables should be indicated when appropriate.

Inspiratory Positive Pressure Breathing (IPPB): Pressure above atmospheric at the airway opening during inspiration employed to assist ventilation, regardless of apparatus used.

Positive End-Expiratory Pressure (PEEP): A residual pressure above atmospheric maintained at the airway opening at the end of expiration. This may be used during spontaneous or mechanical ventilation.

Constant Positive Pressure Breathing (CPPB)—(constant positive airway pressure—CPAP): A pressure above atmospheric maintained at the airway opening throughout the respiratory cycle during spontaneous breathing.

Negative End-Expiratory Pressure (NEEP): A pressure below atmospheric maintained at the airway opening at the end of expiration.

Assisted Ventilation: Manual or mechanical ventilation in which the patient initiates inspiration and establishes the frequency of breathing.

Controlled Ventilation: Manual or mechanical ventilation in which the frequency of breathing is determined by a ventilator according to a pre-set cycling pattern without initiation by the patient.

Assist-Control Ventilation: Manual or mechanical ventilation in which the minimum frequency of breathing is predetermined by the ventilator controls but the patient has the option of initiating inspiration to give a faster rate.

Intermittent Mandatory Ventilation (IMV): Periodic controlled ventilation with inspiratory positive pressure, with the patient breathing spontaneously between controlled breaths.

Expiratory Retard (Resistance): A device providing expiratory resistance sufficient to slow expiration.

Inspiratory Hold (Plateau): A technique for holding end inspiratory pressure for some period of time during mechanical ventilation.

Mainstream Aerosol: A system for administering an aerosol which directs the mainstream of inspired air flow through the aerosol generator.

Sidestream Aerosol: A system for administering an aerosol which adds the aerosol through a side connection to the mainstream of inspiratory air flow.

Resuscitator: A portable device used in emergency situations to provide ventilation.

Ventilator: A device designed to augment or replace the patient's spontaneous ventilation.

Volume Ventilator: A device for delivering a pre-set inspired volume which, within specified limits, is irrespective of the pressure required to deliver that volume.

Pressure Ventilator: A device designed to deliver inspired gas until a pre-set level of pressure is reached.

Compressible Volume: That volume of gas contained in the apparatus external to the patient which is subject to compression during inspiratory positive pressure breathing.

Rebreathing Volume (Mechanical Dead-Space): That volume of exhaled gas which is re-inhaled on inspiration as a result of any breathing apparatus.

Simple Mask: A face mask in which there is free mixing of both inspired and expired air.

Partial Rebreathing Mask: A face mask and a reservoir bag permitting a portion of the exhaled gas to enter the bag for mixing with source gas.

Non-Rebreathing Mask: A face mask designed to separate flow of inspired and expired gases.

Venturi Mask: A face mask designed to entrain atmospheric air in order to provide a constant fractional dilution of a pressurized gas, most commonly oxygen. Within limits, the concentration of the gas delivered is independent of the gas flow.

IV. Terms and Symbols Used in Respiratory Physiology

The American Physiological Society Committee, under the Chairmanship of Pappenheimer[8] (1950) provided the basis for most of the existing systems of physiology symbols. A number of revisions[9-14] have been suggested over the years. At times, the recommended changes were not clearly justified and may even have contributed to the confusion in physiologic symbols.

In this section, a system of symbols is proposed, based upon the original recommendations of the Pappenheimer Committee. The fewest possible changes in existing conventions have been made, while attempting to ease the problem of symbol presentations for typists and typesetters. Writing of symbols as superscripts and subscripts is recommended only when the meaning of the total symbol would be otherwise ambiguous.

Several terms commonly used in describing abnormalities in lung function are also defined.

A. *General Symbols*

1.	P	Pressure (blood, or gas)
2.	$\bar{X}$	A mean value, indicated by a dash over the symbol
3.	$\dot{X}$	A time derivative indicated by a dot above the symbol

4. $\ddot{X}$ (rate). This symbol is used for both instantaneous flow and volume per unit time. The second time derivative indicated by two dots above the symbol. Example: $\ddot{V}$ = Volume expressed as liters per second squared (acceleration)

5. %X   Percent sign *preceding* a symbol indicates percentage of the predicted normal value

6. X/Y%   Percent sign *following* a symbol indicates a ratio function with the ratio expressed as a percentage. Both components of the ratio must be designated; eg $FEV_1/FVC\% = 100 \times FEV_1/FVC$

7. X_A or Xa   A small capital letter or lower case letter on the same line following a primary symbol is a qualifier to further define the primary symbol. When *small* capital letters are not available on typewriters or to printers, large capital letters may be used as subscripts; eg XA = X_A

8. X_{AB} or XAB   Additional qualifiers of the primary symbol may be identified as shown

B. *Gas Phase Symbols*
1. Primary Symbols (large capital letters):
   a. V   Gas volume. The particular gas as well as its pressure, water vapor conditions, and other special conditions must be specified in text or indicated by appropriate qualifying symbols
   b. F   Fractional concentration of a gas
2. Common Qualifying Symbols
   a. I   Inspired
   b. E   Expired
   c. A   Alveolar
   d. T   Tidal
   e. D   Dead-space or wasted ventilation
   f. B   Barometric
   g. L   Lung
   h. STPD   Standard conditions: Temperature 0°C, pressure 760 mm Hg and dry (0 water vapor)
   i. BTPS   Body conditions: Body temperature, ambient pressure and saturated with water vapor at these conditions
   j. ATPD   Ambient temperature and pressure, dry
   k. ATPS   Ambient temperature and pressure, saturated with water vapor at these conditions
   l. an   Anatomic
   m. p   Physiologic
   n. rb   Rebreathing
   o. f   Respiratory frequency per minute
   p. max   Maximal
   q. est   Estimated
   r. t   Time

C. *Blood Phase Symbols*
1. Primary Symbols (large capital letters):
   a. Q   Blood volume
   b. $\dot{Q}$ Blood flow, volume units and time must be specified
   c. C   Concentration in the blood phase
   d. S   Saturation in the blood phase
2. Qualifying Symbols (lower case letters):
   a. b   Blood in general
   b. a   Arterial
   c. c   Capillary
   d. ć   Pulmonary end-capillary
   e. v   Venous
   f. $\bar{v}$ Mixed venous

D. *Ventilation and Lung Mechanics Tests and Symbols*
1. Lung Volume Compartments: (Primary compartments are designated as volumes. When volumes are combined they are designated as capacities. All are considered to be at BTPS unless otherwise specified.)
   a. RV   Residual volume; that volume of air remaining in the lungs after maximal exhalation. The method of measurement should be indicated in the text or, when necessary, by appropriate qualifying symbols
   b. ERV   Expiratory reserve volume; the maximal volume of air exhaled from the end-expiratory level
   c. TV   Tidal volume; that volume of air inhaled or exhaled with each breath during quiet breathing, used only to indicate a subdivision of lung volume. When tidal volume is used in gas exchange formulations, the symbol V_T should be used

560 PULMONARY TERMS AND SYMBOLS

- d. IRV — Inspiratory reserve volume; the maximal volume of air inhaled from the end-inspiratory level
- e. IC — Inspiratory capacity; the sum of IRV and TV
- f. IVC — Inspiratory vital capacity; the maximum volume of air inhaled from the point of maximum expiration
- g. VC — Vital capacity; the maximum volume of air exhaled from the point of maximum inspiration
- h. FRC — Functional residual capacity; the sum of RV and ERV (the volume of air remaining in the lungs at the end-expiratory position). The method of measurement should be indicated as with RV
- i. TLC — Total lung capacity; the sum of all volume compartments or the volume of air in the lungs after maximal inspiration. The method of measurement should be indicated, as with RV
- j. RV/TLC% — Residual volume to total lung capacity ratio, expressed as a percent
- k. CV — Closing volume;[15] the volume exhaled after the expired gas concentration is inflected from an alveolar plateau during a controlled breathing maneuver. Since the value obtained is dependent on the specific test technique, the method used must be designated in the text and, when necessary, specified by a qualifying symbol. Closing volume is often expressed as a ratio of the VC, *ie* (CV/VC%)
- l. CC — Closing capacity; closing volume plus residual volume, often expressed as a ratio of TLC, *ie* (CC/TLC%)
- m. V_L — Actual volume of the lung, including the volume of the conducting airways
- n. V_A — Alveolar gas volume

2. Forced Spirometry Measurements: (All values are BTPS unless otherwise specified.)
   - a. FVC — Forced vital capacity; vital capacity performed with a maximally forced expiratory effort
   - b. FIVC — Forced inspiratory vital capacity; the maximal volume of air inspired with a maximally forced effort from a position of maximal expiration
   - c. FEVt — Forced expiratory volume (timed). The volume of air exhaled in the specified time during the performance of the forced vital capacity; *eg*, FEV_1 for the volume of air exhaled during the first second of the FVC
   - d. FEVt/FVC% — Forced expiratory volume (timed) to forced vital capacity ratio, expressed as a percentage
   - e. FEFx — Forced expiratory flow, related to some portion of the FVC curve. *Modifiers refer to the amount of the FVC already exhaled when the measurement is made*
     - $FEF_{75\%}$ — Instantaneous forced expiratory flow *after 75% of the FVC has been exhaled*
     - $FEF_{200-1200}$ — Mean forced expiratory flow between 200 ml and 1200 ml of the FVC [formerly called the maximum expiratory flow rate]
     - $FEF_{25-75\%}$ — Mean forced expiratory flow during the middle half of the FVC [formerly called the maximum mid-expiratory flow rate]
     - FEFmax — The maximal forced expiratory flow achieved during an FVC
   - f. PEF — The highest forced expiratory flow measured with a peak flow meter
   - g. $\dot{V}maxX$ — Forced expiratory flow, related to the total lung capacity or the actual volume of the lung at which the measurement is made. *Modifiers refer to the amount of lung volume remaining when the measurement is made*. For example:
     - $\dot{V}max75\%$ = Instantaneous forced expiratory flow when the lung is at 75% of its TLC
     - $\dot{V}max3.0$ = Instantaneous forced expiratory flow when the lung volume is 3.0 liters

h. MVVx — Maximal voluntary ventilation. The volume of air expired in a specified period during repetitive maximal respiratory effort. The respiratory frequency is indicated by a numerical qualifier; *eg*, MVV_{60} is MVV performed at 60 breaths per minute. If no qualifier is given, an unrestricted frequency is assumed

i. FETx — The forced expiratory time for a specified portion of the FVC; *eg*, $FET_{95\%}$ is the time required to deliver the first 95% of the FVC and $FET_{25-75\%}$ is the time required to deliver $FEF_{25-75\%}$

j. FIFx — Forced inspiratory flow. As in the case of the FEF, the appropriate modifiers must be used to designate the volume at which flow is being measured. Unless otherwise specified, the volume qualifiers indicate the volume inspired from RV at the point of the measurement

3. Measurements of Ventilation (Unless otherwise specified, conditions are as indicated in parentheses).

a. $\dot{V}_E$ — Expired volume per minute (BTPS)
b. $\dot{V}_I$ — Inspired volume per minute (BTPS)
c. $\dot{V}_{CO_2}$ — Carbon dioxide production per minute (STPD)
d. $\dot{V}_{O_2}$ — Oxygen consumption per minute (STPD)
e. $\dot{V}_A$ — Alveolar ventilation per minute (BTPS)
   V_{TA} — Alveolar tidal volume (BTPS)
f. $\dot{V}_D$ — Ventilation per minute of the physiologic dead-space (wasted ventilation), BTPS, defined by the following equation:
   $\dot{V}_D = \dot{V}_E(PaCO_2 - P_ECO_2)/(PaCO_2 - P_ICO_2)$
   V_D — The physiologic dead-space volume defined as: $\dot{V}_D/f$
g. $\dot{V}_{Dan}$ — Ventilation per minute of the anatomic dead-space, that portion of the conducting airway in which no significant gas exchange occurs (BTPS)
   V_{Dan} — Volume of the anatomic dead-space (BTPS)
h. $\dot{V}_{DA}$ — Ventilation of the alveolar dead-space (BTPS), defined by the following equation: $\dot{V}_{DA} = \dot{V}_D - \dot{V}_{Dan}$
   V_{DA} — The alveolar dead-space volume defined as: $\dot{V}_{DA}/f$
i. $\dot{V}_{Aeff}$ — Effective alveolar ventilation defined as: $\dot{V}_{Aeff} = \dot{V}_E - \dot{V}_D$
j. $\dot{V}_{Drb}$ — Rebreathing ventilation. Ventilation per minute of the rebreathing volume of any external respiratory apparatus (ATPS)
   V_{Drb} — The rebreathing volume of any external respiratory apparatus

4. Measurements of Distribution of Ventilation:[16,17] Due to the variability in methods which have been used to determine mixing indices, it is impractical to offer symbols. Authors should explain their technique fully and define normal limits for their specific method.

5. Measurements of Mechanics of Breathing (All pressures are expressed relative to ambient pressure and gases are at BTPS unless otherwise specified.)

a. Pressure terms
   Paw — Pressure in the airway, level to be specified
   Pawo — Pressure at the airway opening
   Ppl — Intrapleural pressure
   P_A — Alveolar pressure
   P_L — Transpulmonary pressure
   Pbs — Pressure at the body surface
   P(A-awo) — Pressure gradient from alveolus to airway opening
   Pw — Transthoracic pressure
   Ptm — Transmural pressure pertaining to an airway or blood vessel
   Pes — Esophageal pressure used to estimate Ppl

b. Flow-pressure relationships. (Unless otherwise specified, the lung volume at which all resistance measurements are made is assumed to be FRC.)
   R — A general symbol for resistance, pressure per unit flow
   Raw — Airway resistance
   Rti — Tissue resistance
   R_L — Total pulmonary resistance, measured by relating flow-

562 PULMONARY TERMS AND SYMBOLS

	dependent transpulmonary pressure to airflow at the mouth
Rus	Resistance of the airways on the alveolar side (upstream) of the point in the airways where intraluminal pressure equals Ppl, measured under conditions of maximum expiratory flow[18]
Rds	Resistance of the airways on the oral side (downstream) of the point in the airways where intraluminal pressure equals Ppl, measured under conditions of maximum expiratory flow
Gaw	Airway conductance, the reciprocal of Raw
Gaw/V_L	Specific conductance, expressed per liter of lung volume at which G is measured

c. *Volume-pressure relationships*

C	A general symbol for compliance, volume change per unit of applied pressure
Cdyn	Dynamic compliance, compliance measured at point of zero gas flow at the mouth during active breathing. The respiratory frequency should be designated; *eg,* Cdyn40
Cst	Static compliance, compliance determined from measurements made during conditions of prolonged interruption of air flow
C/V_L	Specific compliance
E	Elastance, pressure per unit of volume change, the reciprocal of compliance
Pst	Static transpulmonary pressure at a specified lung volume; *eg,* PstTLC is static recoil pressure measured at TLC (maximal recoil pressure)
PstTLC/TLC	Coefficient of lung retraction expressed per liter of TLC
W	A general symbol for mechanical work of breathing which requires use of appropriate qualifying symbols and description of specific conditions

E. *Diffusing Capacity Tests and Symbols*

1. Dx — Diffusing capacity of the lung expressed as volume (STPD) of gas (x) uptake per unit alveolar-capillary pressure difference for the gas used. Unless otherwise stated, carbon monoxide is assumed to be the test gas: *ie*, D is Dco. A modifier can be used to designate the technique: *eg*, Dsb is single breath carbon monoxide diffusing capacity and Dss is steady state CO diffusing capacity

   $\dfrac{1}{D}$ — Diffusion resistance

2. Dm — Diffusing capacity of the alveolar capillary membrane (STPD)

3. Θx — Reaction rate coefficient for red cells; the volume STPD of gas (x) which will combine per minute with 1 unit volume of blood per unit gas tension. If the specific gas is not stated, Θ is assumed to refer to CO and is a function of existing O_2 tension

4. Qc — Capillary blood volume (usually expressed as Vc in the literature, a symbol inconsistent with those recommended for blood volumes). When determined from the following equation, Qc represents the effective pulmonary capillary blood volume, *ie*, capillary blood volume in intimate association with alveolar gas:

$$\frac{1}{D} = \frac{1}{Dm} + \frac{1}{\Theta \cdot Qc}$$

5. D/V_A — Diffusion per unit of alveolar volume with D expressed as STPD and V_A expressed as liters BTPS. This method is preferred to the occasional practice of expressing both values STPD.

6. Dk — Diffusion coefficient or permeability constant as described by Krogh.[19] It equals $D \cdot (P_B - P_{H_2O})/V_A$

F. *Blood Gas Measurements*

Symbols for these values are readily composed by combining the general symbols recommended earlier. Some examples include:

1. $PaCO_2$ — Arterial carbon dioxide tension

2. SaO_2 — Arterial oxygen saturation
3. $Cc'O_2$ — Oxygen content of pulmonary end-capillary blood
4. $P(A-a)O_2$ — Alveolar-arterial oxygen pressure difference. The previously used symbol, A-aDO_2 is not recommended.
5. $C(a-v)O_2$ — Arteriovenous oxygen content difference

G. *Pulmonary Shunts*
  1. $\dot{Q}sp$ — Physiologic shunt flow (total venous admixture) defined by the following equation when gas and blood data are collected during ambient air breathing:
  $$\dot{Q}sp = \frac{Cc'O_2 - CaO_2}{Cc'O_2 - C\bar{v}O_2} \cdot \dot{Q}$$
  2. $\dot{Q}san$ — A special case of $\dot{Q}sp$ (often called anatomic shunt flow) defined by the above equation when blood and gas data are collected after sufficiently prolonged breathing of 100% O_2 to assure an alveolar N_2 less than 1%. It can be estimated conveniently with the following equation:
  $$\dot{Q}san = \frac{.0031 P(A-a)O_2}{.0031 P(A-a)O_2 + C(a-\bar{v})O_2} \cdot \dot{Q}$$
  3. $\dot{Q}srel$ — Relative shunt flow. The portion of shunt flow which cannot be attributed to $\dot{Q}san$
  $$\dot{Q}srel = \dot{Q}sp - \dot{Q}san$$

H. *Pulmonary Dysfunction*
  1. *Terms Related to Altered Breathing:* There are many terms in use, such as tachypnea, hyperpnea, hypopnea, etc. Simple descriptive terms, such as rapid, deep, or shallow breathing should be used instead.
      a. *Dyspnea:* A subjective sensation of difficult or labored breathing.
      b. *Overventilation:* A general term indicating excessive ventilation. When unqualified, it refers to *alveolar overventilation*, excessive ventilation of the gas exchanging areas of the lung manifested by a fall in arterial CO_2 tension. The term *total overventilation* may be used when the minute volume is increased regardless of the alveolar ventilation. (When there is increased wasted ventilation, total overventilation may occur when alveolar ventilation is normal or decreased.)
      c. *Underventilation:* A general term indicating reduced ventilation. When otherwise unqualified, it refers to alveolar underventilation, decreased effective alveolar ventilation manifested by an increase in arterial CO_2 tension. (Over- and under-ventilation are recommended in place of hyper- and hypo-ventilation to avoid confusion when the words are spoken.)
  2. *Terms Describing Blood Gas Findings:*
      a. *Hypoxia:* A term for reduced oxygenation
         Hypoxemia: A reduced blood oxygen content or tension
         Hypocarbia (hypocapnia): A reduced arterial carbon dioxide tension
         Hypercarbia (hypercapnia): An increased arterial carbon dioxide tension
  3. *Terms Describing Acid-Base Findings:*
      a. *Acidemia:* A pH less than normal; the value should always be given
      b. *Alkalemia:* A pH greater than normal; the value should always be given
      c. *Hypobasemia:* Blood bicarbonate level below normal
      d. *Hyperbasemia:* Blood bicarbonate level above normal
      e. *Acidosis:* A clinical term indicating a disturbance which can lead to acidemia. It usually is indicated by hypobasemia when metabolic (nonrespiratory) in origin and by hypercarbia when respiratory in origin. There may or may not be accompanying acidemia. The term should always be qualified as metabolic (nonrespiratory) or respiratory
      f. *Alkalosis:* A clinical term indicating a disturbance which can lead to alkalemia. It usually is indicated by hyperbasemia when metabolic (nonrespiratory) in origin and by hypocarbia when respiratory in origin. There may or may not be accompanying alkalemia. The term should always be qualified as metabolic (nonrespiratory) or respiratory
  4. *Other Terms:*
      a. *Pulmonary Insufficiency:* Altered function of the lungs which produces clinical symptoms, usually including dyspnea
      b. *Acute Respiratory Failure:* Rapidly occurring hypoxemia or hypercarbia due to a disorder of the respiratory system. The duration of the illness and the values of arterial oxygen tension and arterial carbon dioxide tension used as criteria for this term should be given. The term *acute ventilatory failure* should be used only when the arterial carbon dioxide tension is increased. The term *pulmonary failure* has been used to indicate respiratory failure due specifically to disorders of the lungs
      c. *Chronic Respiratory Failure:* Chronic hypoxemia or hypercapnia due to a disorder of the respiratory system. The duration of the condition and the values of arterial oxygen tension and arterial carbon dioxide tension used as criteria for this term should be given
      d. *Obstructive Pattern* (Obstructive ventilatory

defect): Slowing of air flow during forced ventilatory maneuvers
  e. *Restrictive Pattern* (Restrictive ventilatory defect): Reduction of vital capacity not explainable by airways obstruction
  f. *Small Airway Dysfunction:* There are tests which purport to test function of small airways (closing volume, frequency dependence of compliance, flow-volume curves). When isolated abnormalities of these tests are found, the term "small airway dysfunction" is appropriate.
  g. *Impairment:* A measurable degree of anatomic or functional abnormality which may or may not have clinical significance. *Permanent impairment* is that which persists after maximum medical rehabilitation has been achieved.
  h. *Disability:* A legally determined state in which a patient's ability to engage in a specific activity under a particular circumstance is reduced or absent because of physical or mental impairment. *Permanent disability* exists when no substantial improvement of the patient's ability to engage in the specific activity can be expected.

ACKNOWLEDGMENT: The Committee thanks the many authorities from the United States and Canada who contributed suggestions and criticisms. We especially wish to acknowledge the assistances of Drs. Fletcher, Scadding, Sykes, Forgacs, and Hughes from the United Kingdom who met with the Committee to review a draft of the statement. Finally, this effort would not have been possible without the support of Breon Laboratories, Inc., New York, New York.

REFERENCES

1. Scadding JG: Diagnosis: The clinician and the computer. Lancet 2:877–82, 1967
2. Scadding JG: Fibrosing alveolitis. Br Med J 2:686, 1964
3. Terminology, definitions, and classification of chronic pulmonary emphysema and related conditions. Thorax, 14:286–99, 1959
4. American Thoracic Society: Chronic bronchitis, asthma, and pulmonary emphysema. Am Rev Resp Dis 85:762–68, 1962
5. American Thoracic Society: Definitions and classification of noninfectious reactions of the lung. Am Rev Resp Dis 93:965–81, 1966
6. Medical Research Council Committee on the Aetiology of Chronic Bronchitis: Definition and classification of chronic bronchitis for clinical and epidemiological purposes. Lancet 1:775–79, 1965
7. Forgacs P: Crackles and wheezes. Lancet 2:203–205, 1967
8. Standardization of definitions and symbols in respiratory physiology. Fed Proc 9:602–605, 1950
9. Gandevia B, Hugh-Jones P: Terminology for measurements of ventilatory capacity. Thorax 12:290–3, 1957
10. Committee on Pulmonary Physiology, American College of Chest Physicians: Clinical spirometry: Recommendations of the Section on Pulmonary Function Testing. Dis Chest 43:214–219, 1963
11. Mead J, Milic-Emili J: Theory and methodology in respiratory mechanics with glossary of symbols. In Handbook of Physiology-Respiration, Washington, D.C., American Physiological Society, 1965, Section 3, Vol 1, Chap 11, p 363
12. Hyatt RE: Dynamic lung volumes. In Handbook of Physiology-Respiration, American Physiological Society, 1965, Section 3, Vol 2, Chap 54
13. Glossary on respiration and gas exchange: J Appl Physiol 34:549–58, 1973
14. Piiper J, Dejours P, Haab P, et al: Standardization of units and nomenclature in respiration physiology. Bull de Physio-Pathologic Resp 9:512–14, 1973
15. Anthonisen NR, Danson J, Robertson PC, et al: Airway closure as a function of age. Resp Physiol 8:58–65, 1969
16. Becklake MR: A new index of the intrapulmonary mixture of inspired air. Thorax 7:111–16, 1952
17. Brody AW, Navin JJ, Stoughton RR, et al: Standards and significance for three tests of distribution of ventilation. Am J Med 48:424–33, 1970
18. Mead J, Turner JM, Macklem PT, et al: Significance of the relationship between lung recoil and maximum expiratory flow. J Appl Physiol 22:95–108, 1967
19. Krogh A, Krogh M: Rate of diffusion of CO into lungs of man. Skand Arch f Physiol 23:236–47, 1910

Appendix 2

PREDICTION NOMOGRAM OF NORMAL VALUES FOR PULMONARY FUNCTION TESTING IN FEMALES AND MALES

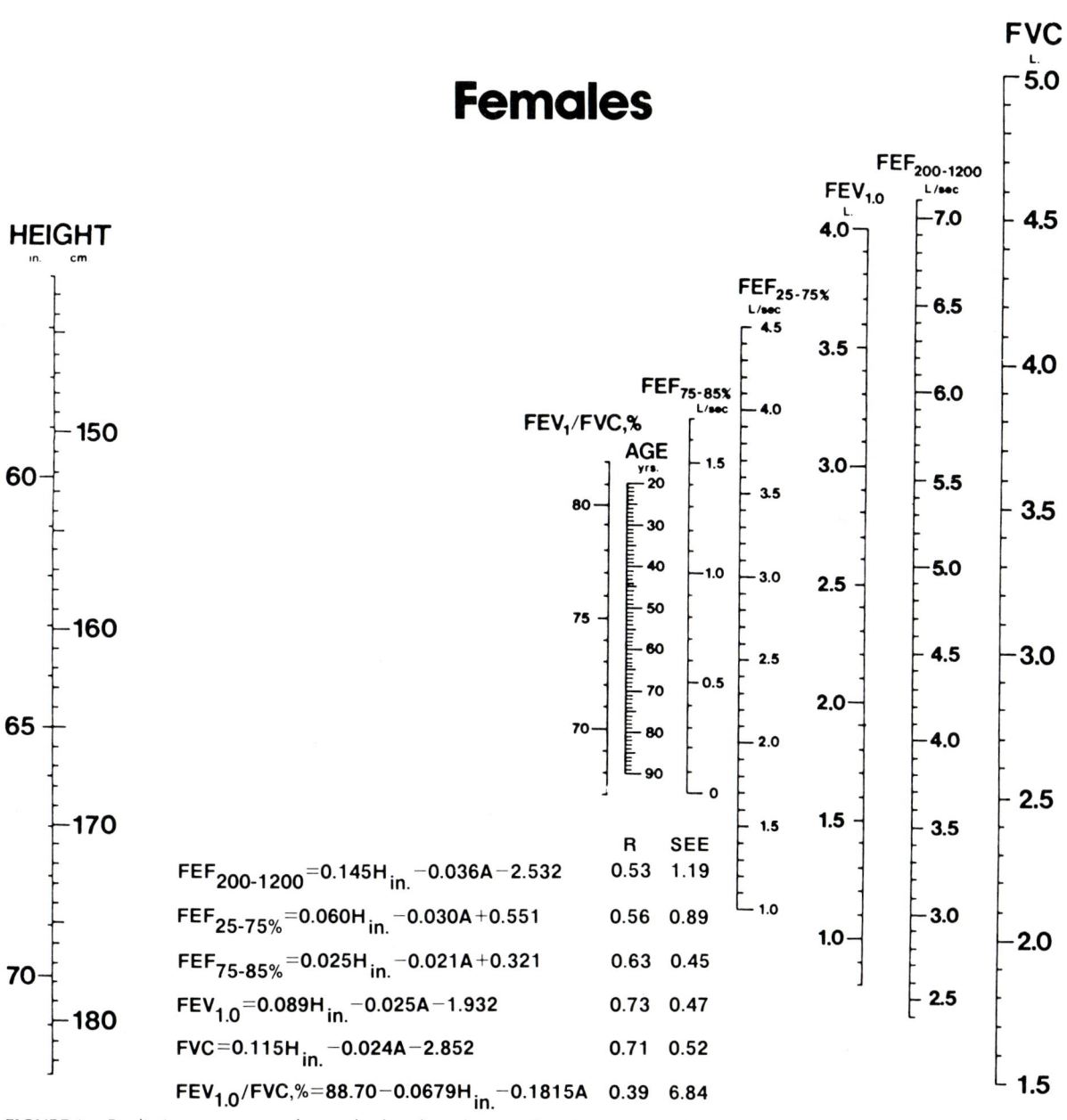

FIGURE 1. Prediction nomogram of normal values for pulmonary function testing in females and males. (From Morris, J.F.: Spirometry in the evaluation of pulmonary function. West. J. Med. 125: 110–118, 1976.)

Illustration continued on following page

Males

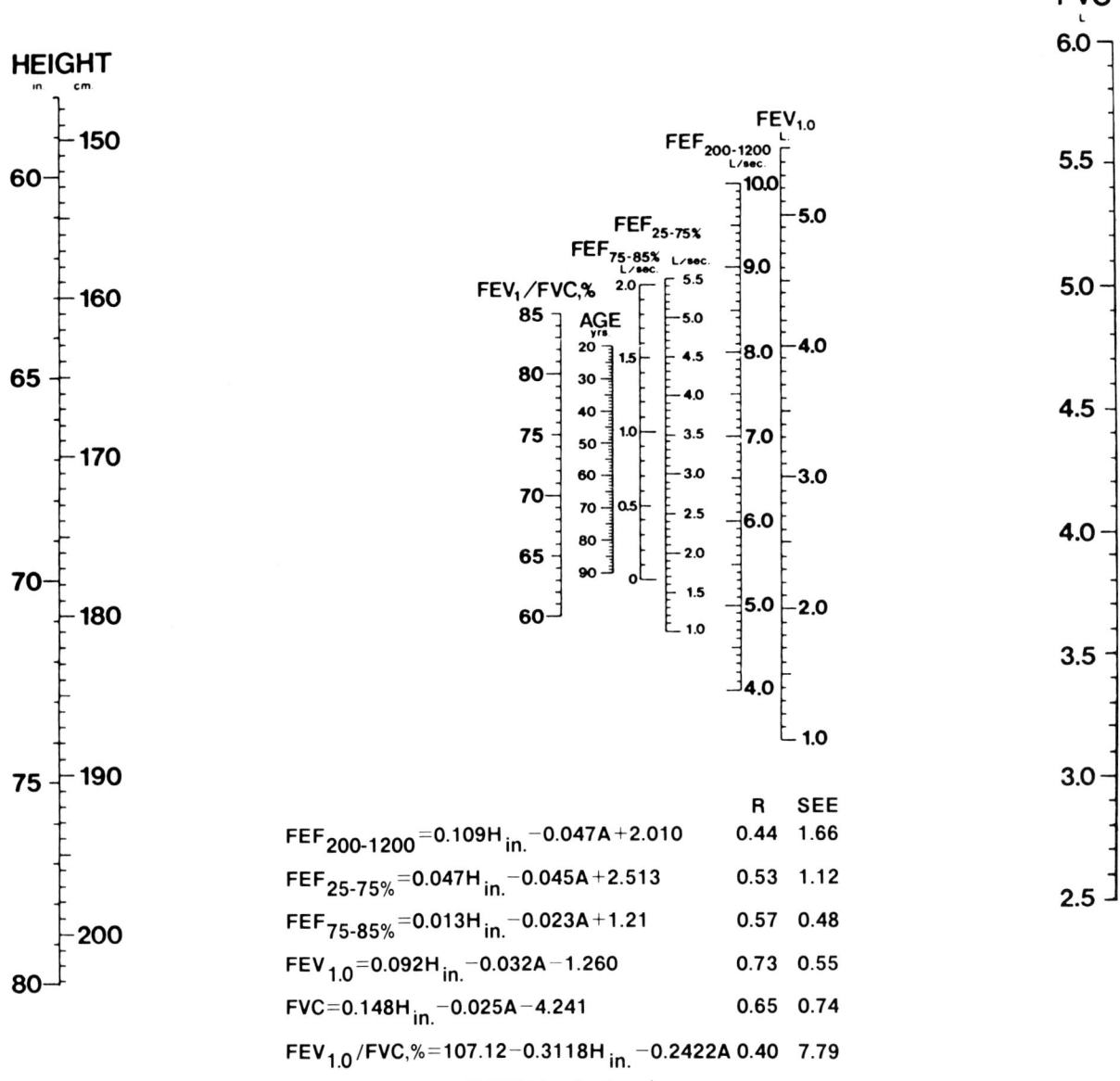

$FEF_{200-1200} = 0.109H_{in.} - 0.047A + 2.010$ R 0.44   SEE 1.66

$FEF_{25-75\%} = 0.047H_{in.} - 0.045A + 2.513$ 0.53   1.12

$FEF_{75-85\%} = 0.013H_{in.} - 0.023A + 1.21$ 0.57   0.48

$FEV_{1.0} = 0.092H_{in.} - 0.032A - 1.260$ 0.73   0.55

$FVC = 0.148H_{in.} - 0.025A - 4.241$ 0.65   0.74

$FEV_{1.0}/FVC,\% = 107.12 - 0.3118H_{in.} - 0.2422A$ 0.40   7.79

FIGURE 1 *Continued*

Appendix 3
NORMAL CLINICAL LABORATORY VALUES

Measurement	Normal Values
Urine	
Creatinine	Depends upon sex, body frame, and height.
Total nitrogen	11.0 gm/24 hr.
Serum	
Sodium	133–143 mEq/L
Potassium	3.9–5.0 mEq/L
Chloride	95–105 mEq/L
Calcium	4.5–5.7 mEq/L
Phosphate	1.8–2.6 mEq/L
Magnesium	1.5–2.4 mEq/L
Total protein	6.0–7.8 gm/dl
Albumin	>3.5 gm/dl
Transferrin	170–250 mg/dl
Total iron-binding capacity	225–400 µg/dl
Blood urea nitrogen	20–40 mg/dl (adults)
Creatinine	0.9–1.7 mg/dl
Glucose	70–120 mg/dl (fasting)
Hematology	
Blood volume	4–6 L
Erythrocytes	4.5–5.0 million/mm^3
Hemoglobin	14–16 gm/dl
Hematocrit	42%–47% of volume
Leukocytes	5,000–10,000/mm^3
Lymphocytes	25%–35% of leukocytes
Neutrophils	60%–70% of leukocytes
Monocytes	2%–6% of leukocytes
Eosinophils	1%–3% of leukocyes
Basophils	<1% of leukocytes
Platelets	250,000–350,000/mm^3

Values refer to a 70 kg adult male subject.

Appendix 4
NORMAL VALUES FOR CARDIAC PROFILES

Measurement	Normal Values
Cardiac output ($\dot{Q}$)	4–6 L/min
Stroke volume (SV)	60–70 ml/beat
Stroke index (SI)	40–50 ml/m^2
Systemic vascular resistance (SVR)	770–1,500 dyne-sec cm^{-5}
Systemic vascular resistance index (SVRI)	1,900–2,400 dyne-sec cm^{-5}/m^2
Pulmonary vascular resistance (PVR)	100–250 dyne-sec cm^{-5}
Pulmonary vascular resistance index (PVRI)	225–315 dyne-sec cm^{-5}/m^2
Left cardiac work index (LCWI)	3.4–4.2 kg-m/m^2
Left ventricular stroke work index (LVSWI)	50–62 gm-m/m^2
Right cardiac work index (RCWI)	0.54–0.66 kg-m/m^2
Right ventricular stroke work index (RVSWI)	7.9–9.7 gm-m/m^2
Arterial oxygen content (CaO_2)	17–20 ml O_2/dl blood
Mixed venous oxygen content (C$\bar{v}O_2$)	12–15 ml O_2/dl blood
Arterio-mixed-venous oxygen difference (A-$\bar{v}$ difference)	4.2–5.0 ml O_2/dl blood
Oxygen consumption ($\dot{V}O_2$)	195–285 ml/min
	3.0–3.5 ml/min/kg
	115–165 ml/min/m^2
Carbon dioxide production ($\dot{V}CO_2$)	150–200 ml/min
Respiratory Quotient (R.Q.)	0.7–1.0
Alveolar-arterial oxygen difference P(A-a)O_2	10–15 mmHg for subjects breathing room air; 10–65 mmHg for subjects breathing 100% oxygen
Shunt fraction ($\dot{Q}_S/\dot{Q}_T$)	3%–5%

Values refer to a 70 kg adult male subject.

Appendix 5
NOMOGRAM FOR CALCULATION OF BODY SURFACE AREA

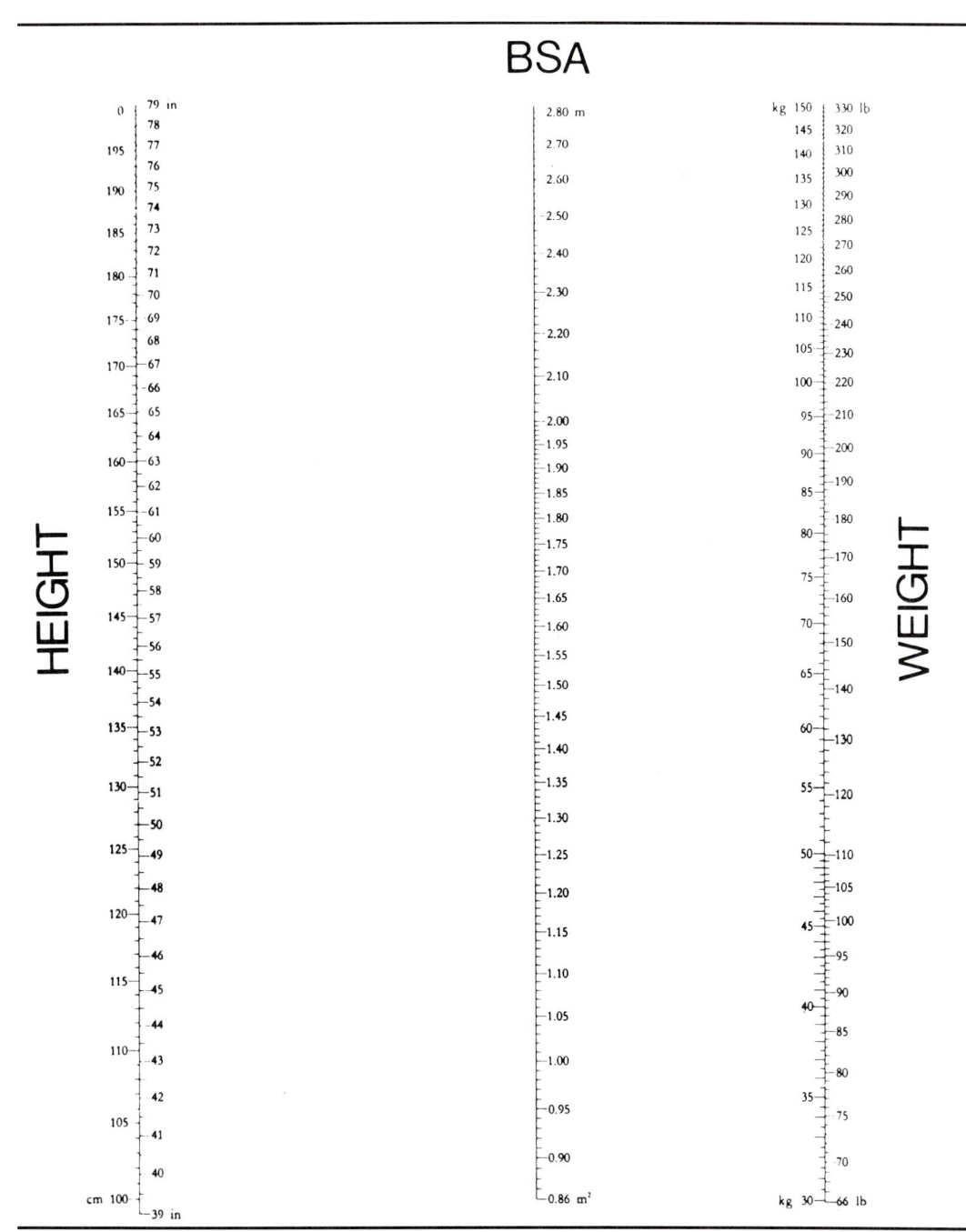

From Dubois, E.F.: *Basal Metabolism in Health and Disease.* Philadelphia, Lea and Febiger, 1936, with permission.

INDEX

Note: Page numbers in *italics* indicate illustrations; those followed by t indicate tables.

A-a oxygen gradient, 318, 331
  age-related changes in, 244
Absolute shunt, calculation of, 317–318
Absolute temperature scale, 14, *14*
Absorption, capillary, 72–73
Absorption atelectasis, 209, 332
Accessory airspaces, 90
Acclimatization, 170
Acetylcholine, as neurotransmitter, 424–425
  in cardiac regulation, 45–46, 61
Acetylcysteine, as mucokinetic, 423
Acid, 420
  fatty, 26, *28*
  fixed (nonvolatile), 138
  nucleic, 26–30, *29*, *30*
  sources of in body, 137–138
  strong, 137
  volatile, 138
  weak, 137
Acid glutaraldehyde, as disinfectant, 370t, 371
Acid-base balance, and electrolyte levels, 362
  and oxyhemoglobin dissociation curve, *132*, 132–133
  evaluation of, by blood gas analysis, 332–336
  mechanism of, 332–334, 333t
  respiratory, 88–89
Acid-base physiology, 137–143
Acidity, and hydrogen ion activity, 137
Acidosis, and electrolyte levels, 362
  metabolic, 141
    causes of, 142t
    compensated, 141–143, *143*, 333–334, 333t
    sodium bicarbonate for, 417
    uncompensated, 333t, 334
  mixed, 334
  respiratory, 140–141
    causes of, 142t
    compensated, 141–143, *143*, 333, 333t
    uncompensated, 333t, 334
Acinus, 94

Acquired immunodeficiency syndrome, 367
Actin, 53, 55, *55*
Actinoid elements, 9
Action potential, *44*, 44–46, *45*
Acute mountain sickness, 168
Adaptors, gas therapy, 443, *444*
Adenosine 3′, 5′-monophosphate, and bronchodilation, 426, *427*
Adenosine triphosphate, *30*, 30–31, 324
Adrenergic nervous system, 424–425, 425t
Adrenergic receptors, 67–68
Adult respiratory distress syndrome, 212–213, 212t, 461
  radiography in, 390–391, *393*
Advanced cardiac life support, 538–539
Adventitious sounds, *265*, 266–267, 557–558
Aerobic metabolism, 324
Aerosol therapy, 418–419
  complications of, 466
  devices for, 464–466, *464*–*466*
  in mechanical ventilation, 466
    mainstream, 558
    sidestream, 558
Affinity hypoxia, 167
Afterload, 59–60
  and stroke volume, 75, 292–293
Aging, physiologic consequences of, 241–245
AIDS, 367
Air, filtration of, 151–152
  warming and humidification of, 151
Air transport, 539
Air-entrainment mask, *455*, 455–456, *456*, 456t
Airway. See also *Bronchi; Lung;* under *Tracheal.*
  artificial. See also *Intubation.*
    esophageal gastric tube, *493*, 494
    esophageal obturator, 492–494, *493*, 493t, *494*
    indications for, 488–489
    insertion of, 490–506
      complications of, 506–509, *508*

Airway (*Continued*)
  artificial, insertion of, long-term use of, 508–509
    malfunction of, 508
    nasopharyngeal, 491–492, *492*
    obstruction of, 507–508
    oropharyngeal, 490–491, *491*
    removal of, 509–510
      accidental, 508
    types of, 489–490, 489t
Airway compression, 108–110, *109*
Airway conductance, 311
Airway constriction, 107
Airway management, 488–501. See also *Airway, artificial; Intubation.*
Airway mucosal injury, and suctioning, 480
  in humidity and aerosol therapy, 467
Airway obstruction, artificial airway for, 488–489. See also *Airway, artificial.*
  causes of, 488
  during intubation, 507
  head and jaw positioning for, 490, *490*
  Heimlich maneuver for, 490
  in asthma, 202
Airway pressure release ventilation, 525
Airway resistance, 106–110
  assessment of, 310–311, *311*
Albumin, 36
  in nutritional assessment, 372–373, 373t
Albuterol, 428
Alcohol, as mucokinetic, 423
Aldehyde disinfectants, 370t, 371
Aldose, 24, *26*
Aldosterone antagonists, 439
Aldosteronism, primary, 188
Algorithms, clinical, 541
Alkaline glutaraldehyde, as disinfectant, 370t, 371
Alkalinity, 137
Alkalosis, and electrolyte levels, 362
  metabolic, 141
    causes of, 142t

571

Alkalosis (*Continued*)
    metabolic, compensated, 141–143, *143*, 333t, 334
        uncompensated, 333t, 334
    mixed, 334–335
    respiratory, 140–141
        causes of, 142t
        compensated, 141–143, *143*, 333, 333t
        uncompensated, 333t, 334
Allen's test, 328
Allergic alveolitis, 209, 536
Allergic bronchospasm, 349, 349t, 426–427
Allergic pneumonitis, 209
Allergic reaction, 254–255, 367–368
    type I, *200*, 200–202, *201*, 201t
Almitrine, 433
Alpha receptors, 67–68, 425–426, 426t
Alpha-adrenergic decongestants, 433–434
Alpha-fetoprotein, in fetal assessment, 400
Alpha$_1$-antitrypsin, deficiency of, in emphysema, 205–206
Altitude, and hypoxia, 166, 168, 170
Alveolar air equation, 115, 331
Alveolar cells, 94–95
Alveolar dead space, determinants of, 317
Alveolar exudate, drainage of, 470
Alveolar fibrosis, diffuse, 209
Alveolar macrophages, 152, *152*
Alveolar plateau, *313*, 314
Alveolar pressure, 100–101, *101*
Alveolar proteinosis, bronchopulmonary lavage in, 504
Alveolar ventilation, 111–116
    and hypoxia, 169
    and oxygen and carbon dioxide levels, 113–115
    during exercise, 161–162, *162*
    during hemorrhage, 166
    in anesthesia, 176
    in pregnancy, 174
    regional distribution of, 115–116
Alveolar-arterial oxygen gradient, 318, 331
    age-related changes in, 244
Alveolar-capillary unit, 95–97, 497–985
Alveoli, 34–35
    age-related changes in, 242t, 243
    in children, 240
    in emphysema, 205, 206
    structural interdependence of, 101, *101*, 105
    surface tension in, 103–105, *104*
Alveolitis, 555, 556
    idiopathic fibrosing, 209
American Standard Safety System, 447–448, *449*
Amino acids, structure and composition of, 23–24, *24*
Aminophylline, 428–429
Ammeter, 19, *19*
Ammonium ions, in acid-base regulation, 142–143, *143*

Amniocentesis, 236, 400–401
Amphetamines, 432
Amphipathic, 26
Amyotrophic lateral sclerosis, 210–211
Anabolism, 23
Anaerobic metabolism, 324
Anaerobic threshold, 354, *355*, 356
Analeptics, 432
Analgesics, 431
Anatomic dead space, 93, 113
    determinants of, 317
Anatomic shunt, 167, 317–318
Anemia, and hypoxia, 167, 450
    of pregnancy, 173
    oxygen transport in, 133
Anemometer, hot-wire, 299, *301*
Anesthesia, cardiopulmonary response to, 175–176
    inhalation, 419
    paralyzing agents in, 432
    respiratory depression in, 148, *148*
Aneurysm, 182–183
Angina, 183, 184
    assessment of, 250–253, 408
    Prinzmetal's, exercise testing for, 353, *353*
Angiography, cardiac, 290
    pulmonary, 394, *395*
Angiotensin, 69–70, 70t, 165
    in pregnancy, 173
Anion, 4
Anion gap, 333
Ankylosing spondylitis, 210
Anode, 19
Anode tube, 497, *497*
Antagonist, pharmacologic, 417
Anthropometric measurements, 372
Antiarrhythmic drugs, 435–436
Antibiotic therapy, 365, 365–366, 366t, 430
    empirical, in children, 405
Antibodies, 367
Anticholinergics, as bronchodilators, 428
Anticoagulants, 438
Antidiuretic hormone, 69–70, 70t
    as vasoconstrictor, 437
    during hemorrhage, *164*, 165
Antihistamines, 433–434
Antimicrobial agents, chemical, 370–371, 370t
    pharmacologic, 365–366, 366t, 430
Antimuscarinics, as bronchodilators, 428
Antiproteolytic enzymes, 205–206
Antiseptics, 370
Aorta, 35, *36*, 39, *39*, *40*
Aortic arch arteries, 221–225, *224*
Aortic coarctation, 188, 232–233
Aortic insufficiency, 190–191, *191*
Aortic regurgitation, 190–191, *191*
    murmur in, *294*, 295
Aortic stenosis, 189–190, *190*
    murmur in, *294*, 295
Aortic valve, 35, *36*
Apgar score, 402, 402t

Apnea, of infancy, 237–238
    sleep, 148, 211, 215–216
        assessment of, 319–321, *320*
Apneusis, 145
Apneustic center, 145
Arachidonic acid, and bronchospasm, 427
Arm circumference, measurement of, 372
Arm span–height conversion table, *303*
Arrhythmias, and suctioning, 479
    drugs for, 435–436
    electrocardiography in, 279–283, *280–282*. See also *Electrocardiography*.
    in ischemic heart disease, 184, *185*, 187
    pacemaker for, 284, *284*
Arterial baroreceptors, 82–83, 147, 164
Arterial blood gases. See *Blood gas analysis; Ventilation*.
Arterial branches, aortic, 39, *39*
Arterial catheterization, flushing in, 329
    for blood gas analysis, 329–330. See also *Blood gas analysis*.
    for blood pressure monitoring, 286, 286t
    pulmonary artery, 287–290, *287–290*, 329–330
    technique for, 286t, 328–329, *329*, 329t
Arterial chemoreceptors, 82–83, 146, 149–150
Arterial dilators, for myocardial ischemia, 436–437
Arterial puncture, complications of, 328
    technique of, 328, *328*
Arterial-venous oxygen content difference, 335
Arteries. See also specific arteries.
    structure and function of, 39, *39–41*
Arteriography, 394, *395*
Arterioles, 36, 39, *42*
Arteriosclerosis, and hypertension, 187–189. See also *Hypertension*.
    and ischemic heart disease, 182–187. See also *Heart disease, ischemic*.
Arteriovenous anastomoses, cutaneous, 81
Arteriovenous shunt, 39–40, *42*
Arytenoid cartilages, 91, *91*
Asbestosis, 208
Ascites, 74
    in right heart failure, 199
Aseptic techniques, 368
Aspiration, accidental, 206–207, 405
    bronchosopy in, 409
    prevention of, airway for, 489
    radiography in, 389–390, *391*
    sensation of, 407
    meconium, 236–237, 401, *402*
    transpleural, 364
    transtracheal, 213, *363*, 363–364
Assist-control ventilation, 523, 558
Assisted ventilation, 523, 558

Asthma, 199–203, *200*, *201*, 201t, 557
  treatment planning for, case presentation for, 546–547
Ataxic respiration, 216
Atelectasis, 209–210
  absorption, 209, 332
  and oxygen therapy, 460
  and suctioning, 479–480
  radiography of, 388, *389*
Atheroma, 182, *183*
Atherosclerosis, and ischemic heart disease, 182–187. See also *Heart disease, ischemic.*
Atmospheric pressure, and zero reference level, 62
Atom, structure of, 4–9, 455
Atomic mass (weight), 4
Atomic number, 4
ATPase, sodium-potassium, 44
Atrial contractions, premature, 281, *282*
Atrial depolarization, 46–47, 47t
Atrial fibrillation, 282, *282*
Atrial flutter, 282, *282*
Atrial septal defects, 231–232
Atrial systole, 38, *56*, 57
Atrioventricular block, 279–280, *281*
Atrioventricular canal, 220, *221–223*
Atrioventricular node, 42
  in conduction pathway, 46, 47t
Atrium, 34, 35, *36*, 38
  embryologic development of, 220, *220–222*
Atropine, 428
Augmented leads, electrocardiogram, 49, *50*
Auscultation, 261–268, *263–265*, *267*, 557
  of heart sounds, *264*, 264–265
  of lung sounds, 263–264, *264*, *265*, 265–268, *267*, 557–558
  stethoscope in, 262–264, *263*
Autoclaving, 369
Autonomic nervous system, in cardiac control, 61
  in circulatory control, 66–68, *67*
  structure and function of, 423–425, *425*, 425t
Autoregulation, circulatory, 70–71
Autotransfusion, during hemorrhage, 165
Avogadro's law, 15
Avogadro's number, 18

B cells, 38
Babington nebulizer, 464–466, *465–466*
Bachmann's bundle, 46, *47*
Bacteria, antibiotic sensitivity of, 365, *365*
  identification of, 364–365, *365*
Bacterial pneumonia, 366–367
Bainbridge reflex, 83
Balloon catheter, 287–290, *287–290*
Baroreceptors, 82–83, 147, 164
Barotrauma, 172
  and inspiratory positive-pressure breathing, 484

Barotrauma (*Continued*)
  iatrogenic, and bronchopulmonary dysplasia, 236
  in mechanical ventilation, 531, 533
Basal energy expenditure, Harris-Benedict equation for, 373t
Base, 20. See also *Acid-base balance; pH.*
  conjugate, 137
  excess of, calculation of, by blood gas analyzer, 327
Basic cardiac life support, 538–539
Basilar skull fracture, and nasotracheal intubation, 506–507
Basophils, 37
Bellows spirometer, 299, *300*
Bends, 172
Bernoulli principle, 64, *65*
Beta blockers, 435
Beta receptors, 67–68, 425–426, 426t
Bicarbonate, as mucokinetic, 423
  carbon dioxide transport as, 135
  for metabolic acidosis, 417
  serum, measurement of, 327, 332–336, 333t
Bicarbonate buffer system, 138–139, *139*
Bicuspid valve, 35, *36*, 38
Biochemical processes, 22–31
Biochemistry, definition of, 22
Biopsy, chorionic villus, 401
  transpleural, 364
Biot's respiration, 216
Black lung disease, 207, 208
Bleeding. See also *Hemorrhage.*
  nasal, in nasotracheal intubation, 506
Blocking agent, 417
Blood, components of, 36–38
  culture of, 364
  increased volume of, in pregnancy, 173
  oxygen content of, 130, 131
  units of, 129
  oxygen-carrying capacity of, 130, 131
Blood cells, types of, 37–38
Blood flow. See also *Circulation; Flow.*
  and thoracoabdominal pump, 76, *76*
  control of, autonomic, 66–68
    humoral, 68–70
    local, 70–71
  distribution of, during exercise, 158–160
  and hemodynamics, 61–66
  regulation of, 84
  resistance to, 61–63, *63*
Blood gas analysis, 324–339
  calculations in, 326–327
  capillary, 330, 336, 403
  capnography in, *338*, 338–339
  fetal scalp, 401
  in neonates, 330, 402–403
  instrumentation for, 324, 327–327
  mixed venous, 335–336
  normal values for, 330–331
  oximetry in, *337*, 337–338
  perioperative, 406–407
  results of, interpretation of, 331–336

Blood gas analysis (*Continued*)
  sample collection for, 327–330
  transcutaneous, 336
  umbilical, 330, 336, 402
Blood gas analyzer, 324, 325–327
Blood gas monitoring, transcutaneous, 336
Blood gas syringe, 327–328
Blood pressure. See also *Hypertension; Hypotension.*
  determinants of, 66
  during exercise, 158–160
  in children, 239
  in mechanical ventilation, *531*, 531–532
  in pregnancy, 173
  maintenance of, 39, *40*. See also *Hemodynamics.*
  measurement of, in exercise testing, 349–350
    invasive methods of, 285–286, *286*, 286t
    noninvasive method of, *285*, 285–286
  regulation of, 57–58, 82–83
Blood transfusion, 438
Blood volume, control of, 84
Blow bottle, 480
Blow-by humidifier, 462, *463*
Blue bloaters, 203
Body plethysmography, for airway resistance determination, 310–311, *311*
  for functional residual capacity determination, 305–307, *306*
  for lung compliance determination, 307–308
Body surface area, calculation of, 569
Body tank respirator, 517–519, *518*, 533
Bohr effect, 135
Bohr equation, 113
Boiling point, 17
Bond, chemical, 9–10, *10*, *11*
  covalent, 9–10, *10*
  in protein molecule, 24, *25*
  ionic, 9
  peptide, 23, *25*
Bounding pulse, 259
Bourdon gauge, 446–447, *449*
Boyle's law, *12*, 12–13
Brachiocephalic artery, 39, *39*
Bradycardia, 279, *280*
  drug therapy for, 436
Bradykinin, 69–70, 70t
Brain, in breathing control, 144–145
Breath sounds, *265*, 266–267, 557–558
  diminished, 267
Breathing, apneustic, 145
  ataxic, 216
  Biot's, 216
  Cheyne-Stokes, 216
  constant positive-pressure, 558
  components of, diseases affecting, 514t
  continuous positive-pressure, 525–526

Breathing (*Continued*)
  control of, 144–150
    age-related changes in, 245
    assessment of, 318–321, *319*, *320*
    chemical, 147–150
    disorders of, 215–216
    during exercise, *160*, 160–161, *161*
    muscular, 120–121
    neural, 99, 144–147
    pharmacologic, 430–433
    reflex, 146–147
    voluntary, 147
  diaphragmatic, training in, 477
  eupneic, 100
  in asthma, 202–203
  inspiratory positive-pressure, 90, 481–484, *482*, 543, 558
  instruction in, 476–477
  mechanics of, 99–111
    age-related changes in, 244
  negative-pressure, 99
  paradoxical, 408
  patterns of, abnormal, 216
    assessment of, 255–257, *257*
  perinatal, 230
  positive-pressure, 99, 481–484, *482*, 489, 558
  pressure-flow relationships in, 99–102
    and compliance, 102–106
  pursed-lip, 477
    in emphysema, 206
  resistance, 477
    in emphysema, 206
  rhythmicity of, generation of, 144–145
  segmental, 477
  spontaneous automatic, 99
  work of, 110–111
    and exercise, 162
    and hypoxia, 169
    and respiratory rate, 255–257, *257*
    during diving, 171–172
Breathing reserve, 354
Bretylium, 436
Bronchi, constriction of, in asthma, 201–202
  embryologic development of, 225, *226*
  obstruction of. See *Airway obstruction*.
  structure and function of, 94
Bronchial arteries, 39, *39*
Bronchial breath sounds, *265*, 266
Bronchial circulation, 95, 116–117
Bronchial intubation, 502–504, *503*
  radiography of, 382, *383*
Bronchial smooth muscle, innervation of, 201–202
  regulation of, 426–427
Bronchial tone, and airways resistance, 107
Bronchiectasis, 241
  sputum in, 253
Bronchioles, structure and function of, *93*, 93–94
Bronchiolitis, 240–241, 557

Bronchitis, 556–557
  chronic, 203–205, 204t, 557
  sputum in, 253
Bronchoconstrictors, bronchoprovocation with, 312
Bronchodilation, regulation of, 426–427
Bronchodilators, 426–430
  bronchoprovocation with, 312
Bronchography, 394, *395*
Bronchophony, 267
Bronchopleural fistula, 553
Bronchoprovocation, 312
Bronchopulmonary bud, 225, *226*
Bronchopulmonary dysplasia, 236, 461
  and oxygen therapy, 172, 236
  radiography of, 391, *394*
Bronchopulmonary hygiene, 470–483
  artificial airway for, 489
  chest physical therapy for, 475
  coughing and breathing retraining for, 475–477
  incentive spirometry for, 480–481
  postural drainage for, 470–475, *471–474*
  structure and function of, 94
  suctioning for, *478*, 478–480
Bronchopulmonary lavage, 504
Bronchopulmonary segments, 94, *94*, *262*
Bronchoscopy, 409
  for culture material collection, 364
Bronchospasm, exercise-induced, test for, 349, 349t. See also *Exercise testing*.
  relief of, 426–430
Bronchovesicular breath sounds, *265*, 266
Brönsted-Lowry definition, 20
Bubble humidifier, 462–463, *463*
Bucking the ventilator, 532
Buffer, 137
  in human body, 138–140
Buffy coat, 36
Bulbus cordis, 220, *220–223*
Bullae, pulmonary, 389, *390*
Bundle branch block, 280–281, *281*
Bundle branches, 46, *47*
Bundle of His, 46, *47*

Caisson disease, 172
Calcium channel blockers, 435
  as bronchodilators, 430
Calcium ions, in cardiac contraction, 54–56, *55*
Calcium levels, 361–363
Calcium salts, for heart disease, 435
Caloric requirements, assessment of, 372, 374
Calorimetry, indirect, 372, 373t
Cancer, of lung, 214
  case study of, 409–412
  radiography of, 390, *391*
Cannula, nasal, 452, *453*
Capacitance, and pressure, 75–76

Capillary(ies), 34, 39–40, *42*
  continuous, 71
  pulmonary, 34–35, *36*, 41–42, 95–97, *97–98*, 117
  recruitment and distention of, 119–120
  structure of, 71–72
Capillary blood gas analysis, 330, 336, 403
Capillary blood gas sampling, 330
Capillary density, 71
Capillary exchange, mechanisms of, 72–74
Capillary filtration coefficient, 72–73
Capillary hydrostatic pressure, 73
Capnography, *338*, 338–339
  intraoperative, 406
Carbamino compounds, 135
Carbohydrate, excess, respiratory consequences of, 339, 371–372, 437, 543
  structure and composition of, 24–26, *26*
Carbon dioxide, diffusion of, 129
  during exercise, 163
  excessive. See *Hypercapnia*.
  in alveolar gas, 114–115
  inhalation of, 480–481
  measurement of. See also *Blood gas analysis*.
    capnographic, 338–339
    in exercise testing, 351, *352*
  partial pressure of, 114
    and oxyhemoglobin dissociation curve, *132*, 132–133
    evaluation of, 332–333, 333t, 335–336
    normal values for, 330
  solubility of, 126
  transcutaneous monitoring of, 336
  transfer of, maternal-fetal, 228, *230*
  transport of, *134*, 134–136, *136*
    during exercise, 163
  ventilatory equivalents of, and anaerobic threshold, 354
  ventilatory response to, 147–149, *148*
Carbon dioxide rebreathing technique, for cardiac output measurement, in exercise testing, 350
Carbon dioxide–oxygen therapy, 461–462
Carbon monoxide, and oxygen transport, 133–134
  transfer of, diffusion-limited, 127
Carbonic acid, 135, 137–138
Carbonic acid reaction, 88–89
Carbonic anhydrase inhibitors, 433
Cardiac angiography, 290
Cardiac arrhythmias, and suctioning, 479
  drugs for, 435–436
  electrocardiography in, 279–283, *280–282*. See also *Electrocardiography*.
  in ischemic heart disease, 184, *185*, 187
  pacemaker for, 284, *284*

INDEX 575

Cardiac catheterization, left-sided, 290, *291*
  right-sided, 287–290, *287–290*
Cardiac cells, action potential of, *44*, 44–45
  myocardial, 53, *54*
Cardiac conduction disturbances, 279–281, *280*, *281*
  pacemaker for, 284, *284*
Cardiac contractility, 53, *55*, 55–56, 60, 461, 625
  and Frank-Starling relationship, 59
  and stroke volume, 75, 292–293
  and ventricular function, 58–60, *59*
Cardiac cycle, *56*, 56–58
Cardiac drugs, 434–437
Cardiac function, control of, 60–61
Cardiac glycosides, 435
Cardiac life support, 538–539
Cardiac monitoring, fetal, 401
Cardiac output, and heart rate, 74–75
  and hypoxia, 169
  and stroke volume, 75
  assessment of, 291–292, 291t, *292*
  in exercise testing, 350
  determinants of, 74–75
  during anesthesia, 175
  during exercise, 158, *159*
  during hemorrhage, 164
  in children, 239
  in pregnancy, 173
Cardiac pacemaker, 284, *284*
Cardiac profiles, normal values for, 568
Cardiac stress test, 348, 348t. See also *Exercise testing.*
Cardiac tamponade, 180, *181*
Cardiac valves, 34–35, *36*, 38
  disorders of, and hypertension, 188
    and left heart failure, 189–192, *190–193*
    and right heart failure, *197*, 197–198, *198*
  left heart catheterization in, 290
  prosthetic, radiography of, 383, *385*
Cardiac work, 293
Cardiogenic shock, 194
Cardiomegaly, radiography of, 382, 383, *384*, *385*
Cardiomyopathy, 180–182
Cardiopulmonary assessment, adult, 407–412
  pediatric, 404–407
  perinatal, 400–404
Cardiopulmonary reflexes, 82–83
Cardiopulmonary resuscitation, 538–539
Cardiopulmonary stress test, 348–349, 349t. See also *Exercise testing.*
Cardiopulmonary system, perinatal alterations in, 230–231
Cardiovascular complications, of mechanical ventilation, *531*, 531–532
Cardiovascular disease, 180–199
Cardiovascular disorders, neonatal, 231–234
Cardiovascular drugs, 434–438

Cardiovascular injuries, in chest trauma, 551
Cardiovascular system, age-related changes in, 241–242
  during anesthesia, 175
  during diving, 170–173
  during exercise, 158–160, *159*
  during hemorrhage, *164*, 164–165
  during hypoxia, 167–170
  during pregnancy, 173–174
  during surgery, 175
  embryologic development of, *220–224*, 220–227, *226*, *227*
  functions of, 34
  integrated control of, 82–84
  postnatal development of, 238–239
  structure of, 34–42, *35*, *36*, *39–43*
Carlens endobronchial tube, 502–503, *503*
Cascade humidifier, *463*, 463–464
Catabolism, 23
Catalysis, 22
Catecholamines, as bronchodilators, 427–428
  as decongestants, 434
  in cardiac regulation, 61
  for cardiac disease, 434–435
Catheterization, arterial, for blood pressure monitoring, 286, 286t
  pulmonary artery, 287–290, *287–290*, 329–330
  technique of, 286t, 328–329, *329*, 329t
  umbilical artery, 330, 336, 402–403
  balloon, 287–290, *287–290*
  cardiac, left-sided, 290, *291*
  right-sided, 287–290, *287–290*
  flushing procedure for, 329
  for drug administration, 417–418
  for blood gas analysis, 329–330. See also *Blood gas analysis.*
  nasal, 451–452, *452*
  radiography in, 380
  suctioning, *478*, 478–479
  Swan-Ganz, 287–290, *288–290*, 289t
  transtracheal, emergency, 504–505, *505*
  for cough induction, 476
Cathode, 19
Cation, 4
Cell, action potential of, *44*, 44–46, *45*, 47t
Cell membrane, myocardial, 53, *54*
  permeability of, 42–43, *44*
  resting potential of, 42–44, *44*
Cellular immunity, 367, 367t
Cellular metabolism, *30*, 30–31
Centigrade temperature scale, 14, *14*
Central chemoreceptors, 149
Central nervous system, and autonomic nervous system, 424
  in cardiac control, 66–68, *67*
  in circulatory control, 66–68, *67*
  in respiratory control, 99
  structure and function of, 423–425, *425*, 425t
Central nervous system ischemia response, 83

Central sleep apnea, 148, 215
  assessment of, 319–321, *320*
Central venous pressure, 75–76
Cerebral circulation, 77–78
Cerebrospinal fluid, acid-base balance in, 149, 150
  and chemical control of breathing, 149, 150
Cervical lymph nodes, palpation of, 259–261, *261*
Charles' law, 13, *13*
Chemical bonding, 9–10, *10*, *11*
Chemical compounds, 4
  symbols for, 485
Chemical disinfectants, 370–371, 370t
Chemical equilibrium, and law of mass action, 22
Chemical reactions, 21–22, 21t
Chemoreceptors, 146, 149–150
  arterial, 82–83
  in breathing control, 146
Chest, flail, 257
  treatment of, case presentation for, 550–553
Chest cuirass, 517–519, *518*
Chest pain. See also *Angina.*
  assessment of, 250–253, 408
Chest physical therapy, 475
Chest radiography. See *Radiography.*
Chest trauma, treatment of, case presentation for, 550–553
Chest tube, 540–541
Chest wall, age-related changes in, 242t, 243
  and lung, mechanical interdependence of, *100*, 105–106, *106*
  and muscles of respiration, 97–99, *99*
  compliance of, 102–103
  contours of, inspection of, 255, *256*
  elastic recoil of, assessment of, 307–308
  movements of, palpation of, 259, *260*
  pain in, assessment of, 253
  restriction of, 210–211
Cheyne-Stokes respiration, 216
Children. See also *Neonate.*
  antibiotic therapy in, 405
  assessment of, 404–407
  cardiovascular development in, 238–239
  developmental milestones for, 404
  pulmonary development in, 239–240
Chin lift, for airway obstruction relief, 490, *490*
Choanal atresia, 234
Chokes, 172
Cholinergic nervous system, 424–425, 425t
Cholinesterases, 424, 426
Chorionic villus biopsy, 401
Chronic bronchitis, 203–205, 204t
  sputum in, 253
Chronic obstructive pulmonary disease, 199, 557. See also *Asthma; Chronic bronchitis; Emphysema.*
Chronotropic drugs, 434–435
Chylothorax, 541

Cilia, 421, *421*
Cine angiography, 290
Circulation. See also *Blood flow*.
  bronchial, 95, 116–117
  capillary (microcirculation), 71–74
  cerebral, 77–78
  coronary, 77
  cutaneous, 81
  fetal, 227–230, *229*, *230*
    perinatal alterations in, 230–231
    persistent, 234
  gastrointestinal, 81–82
  hepatic, 82
    perinatal alterations in, 230–231
  peripheral, control of, 66–71
  physical principles of. See *Hemodynamics*.
  pulmonary, 95, 117–123
    age-related changes in, 242t, 243
    anatomy of, *35*, 35–36, *36*, 41–42
    nonrespiratory functions of, 152–153
    vs. systemic circulation, 117, *118*
  renal, 78–80, *79*
  splanchnic, 81–82
  systemic, 39–41, 439–435
Circulatory autoregulation, 70–71
Circulatory depression, and oxygen therapy, 460–461
Circulatory failure, 180
Circulatory hypoxia, 167. See also *Hypoxia*.
Cirrhosis, and hepatic portal vein hypertension, 408
Clavicle, radiography of, 379
Clinical algorithms, 541
Clinical laboratory measurements, normal values for, 567
Closing volume, age-related changes in, 244
  determination of, 314
Clubbing, of digits, 257, *257*, 408
Coal worker's pneumoconiosis, 207, 208
Coarctation, aortic, 188, 232–233
Coefficient of retraction, 308
Collateral ventilation, 97
Colloid, 18, 362–363, 438
Colloid osmotic pressure, 72, 123
Common carotid artery, 39, *39*
Compliance, age-related changes in, 242
  and pressure-volume relationships, 102–106
  definition of, 102
Compounds, chemical, 4
  symbols for, *8*, *9*
Compressible volume, 558
Computed tomography, 396, *396*
Conduction disturbances, cardiac, 279–281, *280*, *281*
Congenital abnormalities, prenatal diagnosis of, 400–401
Congenital heart disease, 231–234
Cogestive heart disease, 194
Conjunctival blood gas monitoring, 336
Conn's disease, 188

Constant positive-pressure breathing, 558
Continuous positive airway pressure, 525–526
  weaning from, 534–535
Continuous positive-pressure breathing, 525–526
Contractile proteins, myocardial, 53
Contractility, cardiac, 53, *55*, 55–56, 60, 461, 625
  and Frank-Starling relationship, 59
  and stroke volume, 75, 292–293
  and ventricular function, 58–60, *60*, *61*
Controlled ventilation, 523, 523t, 558
Contusion, pulmonary, 551
Co-oximetry, 337
Cor pulmonale, and pulmonary hypertension, 196–197
  radiographic appearance of, 380
Corner vessels, 119, *120*
Coronary arteries, 39, *39*
Coronary circulation, 77
Coronary reserve, 183
Corticosteroids, as bronchodilators, 429–430
  in infant respiratory distress syndrome, 236
  structure of, 26, *29*
Cough, 151–152
  and inspiratory positive-pressure breathing, 481
  as bronchopulmonary hygiene technique, 475–476
  assessment of, 253, 407
  incentive spirometry for, *480*, 480–481, *481*
  induction of, 476
  instruction in, 476
  machine-gun, 476
  stimulation of, 433
  treatment of, 433
Cough control, 476
Covalent bonds, 9–10
Crackles, 265, 267, 557
Creatinine-height index, 372, 373t
Crepitus, 382
Cricoid cartilage, 90, 91, *91*
Cricothyroidotomy, *504*, 504–505, *505*
  replacement of, by tracheostomy, 510
Critical opening pressure, 120
Cromolyn, 430
Cross bridges, 53, *55*, 55–56
Croup, 240
Croupette, 457–458, *458*
Crystalloid, 18, 362–363, 438
Cuff, endotracheal tube, *498*, 498–499, 509
Culture, microbial, techniques for, 364–365
  sample collection for, 363–364
Cushing response, 78
Cutaneous circulation, 81
Cyanosis, 168, 257, 408
  in tetralogy of Fallot, 233

Cycle ergometer, 344, *347*. See also *Exercise testing*.
Cylinders, gas, 444–446, *445*, 446t, *447*
Cystic fibrosis, 405
  sweat test for, 405
  treatment planning for, case presentation for, 547–549

Dalton's atomic theory, 4
Dalton's law, 14–15
Dead space, alveolar, determinants of, 317
  anatomic, 317
  mechanical, 558
  physiologic, calculation of, 339
    determination of, 316–317
Decompression sickness, 172
Decongestants, 433–434
Decontamination, of equipment and supplies, 368–370
Dehydration, 360–361, 360t
Deoxyhemoglobin, 130, 135
Deoxyribonucleic acid (DNA), 26–30, *29*, *30*
Depolarization, cardiac, *44*, 44–47, *45*, 47t
  of pacemaker cells, 45–46
Depressor area, vasomotor, 66, *67*
Desquamative alveolitis, 556
Developmental milestones, 404
Dextrocardia, 381
Diameter Index Safety System, 448–449, *449*
Diaphragm, 100
  assessment of, by palpation, 259
  depression of, radiography of, 388–389, *390*
  elevation of, 386–388, *389*
  herniation of, 237
    case presentation of, 544–545
  in obstructive pulmonary disease, 202–203
  in pregnancy, 174
  pain in, 253
Diastasis, *56*, *57*, 58
Diastole, 38, *56*, 56–57
Diastolic murmur, phonocardiographic assessment of, *294*, 294–295
Dicrotic notch, 58
Diet, excess carbohydrate in, 339, 371–372, 437, 543
Differential diagnosis, 407
Differential pressure pneumotachograph, 299, *301*
Diffuse alveolar fibrosis, 209
Diffusing capacity, determination of, 314–316, 317t
Diffusion, 72
  capillary, 72
  Fick's law of, 125–126
  gas, 16–17, *17*, 125–129, *128*
  Henry's law of, 126
  of carbon dioxide, 129
    during exercise, 163

Diffusion (*Continued*)
  of oxygen, 127–129, *128*
  during exercise, 129, 163
Digitalis, 435
Digits, clubbing of, 257, *257*, 408
Dilution, calculation of, 20–21
2,3-Diphosphoglycerate, and oxyhemoglobin dissociation curve, *132*, 132–133
Dipole, 10
Direct Fick method, for cardiac output determination, 291, 291t
Disaccharide, 24–26, *27*
Disinfection, of equipment and supplies, 368–371, 370t
Disposable supplies, 371
Dissociation constant, 138
Distensibility, age-related changes in, 242
  and pulmonary vascular resistance, 120
Disulfide bond, 24, *25*
Diuretics, 438–439
Diving, cardiopulmonary alterations in, 170–172
  hazards of, 172–173
Diving reflex, 171
DNA, 26–30, *29*, *30*
Dobutamine, 434–435
Dopamine, 434–435
Dorsal respiratory groups, 144–145
Double helix, 27, *28*
Drainage, pleural, 540–541
Drinker respirator, 517–519, *518*, 533
Drug(s). See also specific drugs and drug families.
  absorption of, 416
  and respiratory depression, 148, *148*
  antimicrobial, 365–366, 366t, 430
  autonomic nervous system, 423–426
  bronchodilator, 426–430
  cardiovascular, 434–438
  cough suppressant, 433
  decongestant, 433–434
  diuretic, 438–439
  dosage of, 420
  efficacy of, 417
  for breathing control, 430–433
  half-life of, 419
  inhalational route for, 418–419
  interactions among, 420
  intramuscular route for, 418
  intravenous route for, 417–418
  intrinsic activity of, 417
  mechanism of action of, 416
  metabolism and excretion of, 416, 419–420
  mucokinetic, 420–423
  oral route for, 418
  receptor affinity for, 417
  rectal route for, 418
  redistribution of, 417
  routes of administration for, 417–419
  side effects of, 416–417
  sites of action of, 416
  structurally specific, 416
  subcutaneous route for, 418

Drug-receptor interactions, 416–417
Dry-rolling seal spirometer, 298, *300*
Ductus arteriosus, *224*, 225, *229*, 230
  closure of, 231
  patent, 232
  and persistent fetal circulation, 234
Ductus venosus, 228, *229*
Dullness, on percussion, 261, *263*
Dye dilution cardiac output determination, 291–292, *292*
Dynamic compression, 108–110, *109*
Dynamic lung compliance, measurement of, 307–308
Dyspnea, 408
  assessment of, 250
  in left ventricular failure, 193
  paroxysmal nocturnal, 250
Dyspneic index, 354
Dysrhythmias. See *Arrhythmias*.

Echocardiography, 294, *294*
Eclampsia, 174–175
Ectopic beats, drug therapy for, 436
Edema, 73–74
  in right heart failure, 199
  pulmonary, 123, 123t
Egophony, 267, *268*
Ejection fraction, 60
Elastic recoil, 102–103
  assessment of, 307–308
Electrical axis, cardiac, 277–279, *279*
Electrocardiography, 47–53, 272–284
  electrodes for, 272, *274*, *275*
  equipment for, 272–275, *273*–*277*
  for cardiac cycle, *56*, 56–58
  in exercise testing, for exertional myocardial ischemia evaluation, 353, *353*
  for heart rate, 349, *350*
  in heart block, 279–281, *280*, *281*
  in heart rate assessment, 277, 278, *279*, *280*
  in ischemic heart disease, 184, *185*
  in myocardial ischemia and infarction, *185*, 186, 283–284, 283t
  in premature contractions, 281–282, *282*
  in sinus arrhythmias, 279, *280*
  in tachyarrhythmias, *282*, 282–283
  lead systems for, 49, *50*, 272–275, *276*
  mean electrical axis in, 51–52, *52*
  normal findings on, 49–53, *51*, 275–278, *278*, *279*
  P wave on, 51, *51*
  P-R interval on, 51, *51*
  QRS complex on, *51*, 51–52
  recorders for, 275, *277*
  S-T segment on, *51*, 52–53
  T wave on, *51*, 53
  two-dimensional, 53
  vector analysis for, *85*, 48–49
  waveforms and intervals in, 275–277, *278*

Electrodes, blood gas analyzer, 325–326
  electrocardiogram, 49, *50*, 272, *274*, *275*
  in exercise testing, 349, *350*
Electrolytes, 9, 18–20, 19t, *361*, 361–362
  abnormalities in, 362
  management of, 362–363
  normal values for, 567
  plasma, 37
  replacement of, 438
Electromyography, pediatric, 404–405
Electron, 4
  octet rule for, 9
  valence, 5, 465
Electron shell, 4
Electron subshell, 4–5, 455
Electronegativity, 10, *11*
Elements, 4
  atomic mass (weight) of, 4
  atomic number of, 4
  in human body, 22–23, 23t
  mineral, 22
  periodic table of, *8*, 9
Embden-Meyerhof pathway, *30*, 30–31, 37
Embolism, and ischemic heart disease, 182
  fat, 551
  pulmonary, 195
Embolization, retrograde, in arterial catheterization, 329
Embryologic development, *220*–*224*, 220–227, *226*, *227*
Emphysema, 196, 557
  and chronic bronchitis, 203, 204t, 205–206
  subcutaneous, radiography of, 382, *383*
Emulsion, 18
Endobronchial intubation, 502–504, *503*
  radiography in, 382, *383*
Endocardial cushions, 220–221, *221*, *222*
Endocytosis, 74
Endotracheal intubation. See *Intubation*.
Energy, and work, 10–11, 11t
  cellular production of, *30*, 30–31
  conservation of, 11
  kinetic, 11
  potential, 11–12
Energy expenditure, Weir equations for, 373
Energy shell, 4
Energy sublevels, 4–5, 455
Enzymes, 22
  antiproteolytic, 205–206
  proteolytic, 205
Eosinophil, 37
Eosnophilic granuloma, 556
Ephedrine, 428
Epiglottis, 91, *91*
  in children, 239
  in laryngoscopy, 496
Epiglottitis, 240

578 INDEX

Epinephrine, 427–428
  in circulatory control, 68, 69
  in heart rate regulation, 45–46
Epistaxis, in nasotracheal intubation, 506
Equal pressure point hypothesis, 109, *109*
Equilibrium, chemical, and law of mass action, 22
Equipment and supplies, decontamination, disinfection, and sterilization of, 368–371, 370t
  disposable, 371
Ergometer, two-step, 344, *347*
Erythrocytes, 37
Erythropoiesis, in acclimatization, 170
Erythropoietin, 84
Esophageal gastric tube airway, 492–493, *493*
Esophageal obturator airway, 492–493, *493*, 493t, *494*. See also *Airway, artificial.*
Ethylene oxide, in gas sterilization, 370t, 371
Eupnea, 100
Evaporating devices, for gas humidification, 462–464, *463*
Evaporation, 17
Excitability, of cardiac cells, 44, 44–46, *45*, 47t
Excitation-contraction coupling, cardiac, 54, *54*, 55
Exercise, cardiopulmonary response to, 344, *345*
  cardiovascular response to, 158–160, *159*
  and age, 242
  pulmonary response to, 160–163, *160–163*,
  ventilatory response to, and age, 160–163, *160–163*, 245
Exercise prescription, 356
Exercise testing, 344–356
  cardiac stress test, 348, 348t
  contraindications to, 346t
  data collection in, 349–352, *350–352*
  emergency procedures for, 349, 349t
  for exercise-induced bronchospasm, 349, 349t
  measurements made in, 347–348, 347t
  modes of, 344–346, *347*
  procedures for, 346–349, 347t–349t
Exercise training, and breathing retraining, 477
Exercise-induced bronchospasm, test for, 349, 349t. See also *Exercise testing.*
Expectorants, as mucokinetics, 423
Expiration, mechanics of, 101t, 102
Expiratory reserve volume, 111, *112*
Expiratory retard, in mechanical ventilation, 527–528
Extra-alveolar vessels, 118–120, *119*, *120*
Extracellular fluid, 360
Extracorporeal membrane oxygenation, 404

Extubation, 509–510
  accidental, 508
Exudate, drainage of, 470

Face tent, 453, *454*
Fahrenheit temperature scale, 14, *14*
Fat embolism, 551
Fatty acids, 26, *28*
Fetal assessment, 400–401
Fetal circulation, 227–230, *229*, *230*
  perinatal alterations in, 230–231
  persistent, 234
Fetal development, *220–224*, 220–227, *226*, *227*
Fetal heart rate, monitoring of, 401
Fetal lung maturity, assessment of, 400–401
Fetal scalp blood monitoring, 401
Fetoprotein, in fetal assessment, 400
Fibrillation, *282*, 282–283
  atrial, 282, *282*
  ventricular, *282*, 283
Fibrosing alveolitis, 556
Fick cardiac output determination, 291, 291t
Fick principle, 353
Fick method, for cardiac output, 291, 291t
Fick's law, 16, *17*, 125–126
Filters, ventilator, 368, 369
Filtration, capillary, 72
  in respiratory system, 151
  pulmonary, 153
Fingernails, clubbing of, 257, *257*, 408
Fistula, bronchopulmonary, 553
  tracheoesophageal, 237, *237*, 405–406
Flail chest, 257
  treatment of, case presentation for, 550–553
Flatness, on percussion, 261, *263*
Fleisch pneumotachograph, 299
Flow. See also *Blood flow; Circulation.*
  laminar, 63–64, *64*, 107
  pulsatile, 65–66
  resistance to, 61–63, *63*
  transitional, 64
  turbulent, 63–64, *64*, 107
Flow meter, gas therapy, 446–447, *449*
Flow-sensing devices, 299, *301*
Flow-volume analysis, 309–310, *310*
Fluid, electrolyte composition of, *361*, 361–362
  extracellular, 360
  interstitial, 360
    buffers in, 140
  intracellular, 360
  intravascular, 360
  total body, 360, *360*
  transcellular, 360
Fluid balance, disturbances of, 360–361, 361t
  maintenance of, 360
Fluid compartments, 360, *360*
Fluid loss, insensible, 362
  third space, 362
Fluid therapy, 18, 362–363, 437–438

Fluoroscopy, 394–395
Foramen ovale, 221
  closure of, 230–231
  patent, 231
    and persistent fetal circulation, 234
Foramen primum, 221, *222*
  patent, 231
Foramen secundum, 221, *222*
Forced vital capacity, assessment of, 309, *309*
Forceps, in nasotracheal intubation, 502, *520*
Foreign body, and upper airway obstruction, 206–207
  aspiration of, 405
  bronchosopy in, 409
  prevention of, airway for, 489
  radiography in, 389–390, *391*
  sensation of, 407
Formed elements, 36
Fowler's test, *313*, 313–314
Fracture, basilar skull, and nasotracheal intubation, 506–507
  radiography of, 379
  rib, 257
    radiography of, 379
    treatment of, case presentation for, 550–553
Frank-Starling relationship, 58–60, *59*
Fremitus, tactile, 189, 261
Friction rub, 265, 267
Fructose, *26*
Functional residual capacity, 111–112, *112*
  age-related changes in, *243*, 244
  definition of, 105
  determination of, 303–307, *304–306*

Gas(es). See also *Carbon dioxide; Oxygen.*
  diagnostic and therapeutic use of, 419. See also *Medical gas therapy.*
  diffusion of, 16–17, 125–129, *128*
  ideal, 15–16
  kinetic theory of, 12
  noble, 9
  partial pressure of, 14
  pressure-volume relationships of, 12–16
  properties of, 12–17
  specific gravity of, 15, *15*
  transfer of, diffusion limitation of, 127
  perfusion limitation of, 126–127
Gas analyzers, in exercise testing, 351, *352*
Gas cylinders, 444–446, *445*, 446t, *447*
Gas exchange, respiratory, 88
Gas sterilization, 370
Gastrointestinal circulation, 81–82
Gay-Lussac's law, *13*, 13–14
Gel, 18
Glomerular filtration rate, 80
  during hemorrhage, *164*, 165
Glottis, 91–92

Glucocorticoids, as bronchodilators, 429–430
  in infant respiratory distress syndrome, 236
  structure of, 26, *29*
Glucose, molecular structure of, 24, *26*
Glutaraldehyde, as disinfectant, 370t, 371
Glycogen, structure of, 26, *28*
Glycolytic pathway, *30*, 30–31, 37
Graham's law, 16
Gram stain, 364
Granulocytes, 37
Gravity, and regional distribution of pulmonary blood flow, 121–122, *122*
Great vessels, 34–36, *36*
  transposition of, 233
Guanosine 3′, 5′-monophosphate, and bronchoconstriction, 426
Guillain-Barré syndrome, 210

Haldane effect, 135
Half-life, drug, 419
Halogens, 9
Handwashing, 368
Harris-Benedict equation, for basal energy expenditure, 373t
Head, H., paradoxical reflex of, 146
Head, positioning of, for airway obstruction relief, 490, *490*
Heart. See also under *Cardiac; Cardiopulmonary; Cardiovascular.*
  anatomy of, 34–36, *36*, 38
  as pump, 53–61
  autoregulation of, 61
  conduction pathways of, 46–47, *47*, 47t
  contraction-relaxation mechanism of, 55, 55–56
  and ventricular function, 58–60, *59*
  depolarization of, *44*, 44–47, *45*, 47t
  electrical activity of, 42–53. See also *Electrocardiography.*
  electrical axis of, 277–279, *279*
  embryologic development of, 220–221, *220–223*
  excitation-contraction coupling in, 54, *54*, *55*
  myocardial ultrastructure of, 53, *54*
  radiographic appearance of, 380, *381*, *381*
Heart block, 279–281, *280*, *281*
  pacemaker for, 284, *284*
Heart disease, congenital, 231–234
  drug therapy for, 434–437
  ischemic, 182–184, *183*
    and myocardial infarction, 184–187, *185*, *186*
    drug therapy for, 436–437
    electrocardiography in, 283–284, 283t. See also *Electrocardiography.*
Heart failure, backward, 194
  congestive, 194

Heart failure (*Continued*)
  left-sided, 180–194
    and cardiomyopathies, 180–182
    and ischemic heart disease, 182–186
    and valvular dysfunction, 189–192
    pathophysiology of, 192–194, *193*
  low-output, 180
  right-sided, 192, 195–199
Heart murmurs, 58
  and aortic stenosis, 189
  phonocardiographic assessment of, *299*, 294–295
Heart rate, abnormalities of. See *Arrhythmias.*
  and cardiac output, 74–75
  assessment of, by palpation, 258–259, *259*
  electrocardiographic. See *Electrocardiography.*
  in exercise testing, 349, *350*
  during exercise, 158, *159*, 349, *350*
  during hemorrhage, 164, *164*
  in children, 239
  in pregnancy, 173
  maximum, prediction of, 352
  regulation of, 45–46
Heart sounds, 56, 58, 189, 261
  auscultation of, *265*, 266
  phonocardiographic assessment of, *294*, 294–295
Heart tubes, 220, *220*
Height–arm span conversion table, *303*
Heimlich maneuver, 206–207, 490
Heliox therapy, 461
Helium, diagnostic and therapeutic use of, 419, 461
Helium dilution technique, for lung volume determination, 304, *304*
Helium-oxygen therapy, 461
Helix, double, 27, *28*
Hematemesis, 253–254, 254t
Hematocrit, 36
Hematology, normal values for, 567
Hemodynamic monitoring, 285–293
Hemodynamics, 39, *40*, *41*, 61–71
  physical principles of, 61–66
Hemoglobin, 37
  abnormal, oxygen affinities of, 134
  oxygen binding to, 130, 131
  oxygen saturation of, 130, 131
    measurement of. See also *Blood gas analysis.*
      by blood gas analyzer, 326–327
      by oximetry, *337*, 337–338
Hemoglobin S, oxygen affinities of, 134
Hemoptysis, assessment of, 253–254, 254t
Hemorrhage, cardiovascular response to, 163–165, *164*
  renal response to, *164*, 165
  respiratory response to, *164*, 165–166
Hemosiderosis, 556
Hemothorax, 540–541
Henderson-Hasselbalch equation, 138
Henry's law, 16, 126
Heparin, 438

Hepatic circulation, 82
Hepatic portal vein hypertension, 408
Hering-Breuer deflation reflex, 146
Hering-Breuer inflation reflex, 145–146
Hernia, diaphragmatic, 237
  case presentation for, 544–545
High-pressure nervous syndrome, 172–173
Hilus, 94
Histamine, 70, 70t, 153
  in asthma, 200, 201t
Histiocytosis X, 556
Histotoxic hypoxia, 167, 450
Hoover's sign, 202
Hot-wire anemometer, *299*, *301*
Huffing, 476
Humidification, complications of, 467
  devices for, 462–466, *463–466*
Humoral control, of blood flow, 69–70, 70t
Humoral immunity, 367, 367t
Hyaline membrane disease. See *Infant respiratory distress syndrome.*
Hydrogen ions, and acidity, 137
  ventilatory response to, 150
Hydrophilic, 18
Hydrophobic, 18
Hydroxytryptamine, 69–70, 70t
Hyoid bone, 91, *91*
Hyperalimentation, and lipogenesis, 339, 371–372, 437, 543
Hyperbaric chambers, 459, *460*
Hyperbaric conditions, cardiopulmonary response to, 170–173
Hypercapnia, in chronic bronchitis, 205
  ventilatory response to, age-related changes in, 245
  assessment of, 318–319, *319*
Hyperemia, reactive, 71
Hyperglycemia, and lipogenesis, 339, 371–372, 437, 543
Hyperinflation, periodic automatic, in mechanical ventilation, 528
  pulmonary, in asthma, 202–203
Hyperoxia, hazards of. See *Oxygen toxicity.*
Hyperresonance, on percussion, 261, *263*
Hypersensitivity reaction, 254–255, 367–368
  type I, *200*, 200–202, *201*, 201t
Hypersensitivity pneumonitis, 209, 556
Hypertension, 187–188
  drug therapy for, 437
  in toxemia of pregnancy, 174–175
  malignant, 188
  portal, 408
  pulmonary, 195–197
  renal, 187–188
Hypertonic saline, as mucokinetic, 422–423
Hyperventilation, and respiratory alkalosis, 141, 334,
Hyperventilation syndrome, 216
Hypnotics, 431

Hypocapnia, and inspiratory positive-pressure breathing, 483
Hypoperfusion hypoxia, 167, 450
Hypopharynx, 90
Hypotension, and suctioning, 479
  drug therapy for, 437
Hypoventilation, and hypoxia, 167–168
  and respiratory acidosis, 140–141, 334
  and ventilatory control disorders, 215–216
  drugs for, 432–433
  idiopathic, 216
  mechanical ventilation for. See *Mechanical ventilation*.
Hypoxemia, acute, treatment of, 332t
  and endobronchial intubation, 503
  and suctioning, 479
  evaluation of, by blood gas analysis, 331–332
  ventilatory response to, 147–148, *148*, 150, *150*
Hypoxemic hypoxia, 450
Hypoxia, 166–170
  adaptations to, 170
  and pulmonary hypertension, 196
  and pulmonary vasoconstriction, 122–123
  anemic, 167, 450
  assessment of, by arterial blood gas analysis, 331–333
  cardiopulmonary response to, 168–169
  causes of, 166–167, 166t
  cellular consequences of, 324
  effects of, 167–168
  histotoxic, 450
  hypoperfusion, 450
  hypoxemic, 450
  in chronic bronchitis, 205
  oxygen therapy for, 442–461. See also *Oxygen therapy*.
  perinatal, management of, 403–404
  monitoring for, 401–402
  physiologic response to, 450–451, 450t
  types of, 450
  ventilatory response to, 150
    age-related changes in, 245
    assessment of, *319*, 319–321
Hypoxic drive, 548
Hypoxic hypoxia, 166–167
Hysteresis, 103

I alpha cells, 145
I beta cells, 145
Iatrogenic infection, 430
Ideal gas, 15–16
Idiopathic fibrosing alveolitis, 209
Immune function, and nutritional status, 372t, 373
Immunity, cellular, 367, 367t
  humoral, 367, 367t
Immunodeficiency, 367
Immunoglobulins, 36
Immunopathology, 367–368, 367t

Incentive spirometry, *480*, 481, *481*
Incisura, 58
Incubator, 458–459
Indicator dilution technique, for cardiac output measurement, in exercise testing, 350
Indirect calorimetry, 372, 373t
Inert gas dilution tests, for functional residual capacity, *304*, 304–305, *305*
Infant respiratory distress syndrome, 234–236, *235*
  oxygen therapy in, and retrolental fibroplasia, 238, 332, 461
  radiography in, 391, *394*
Infarction, myocardial, electrocardiography in, 283–284, 283t
Infections, pulmonary. See *Pulmonary disease, infectious*.
Inferior vena cava, fetal, 228, *229*
Inflation hold, 525
Infrahyoid muscles, 91
Infrared absorption analysis, for carbon dioxide measurement, *338*, 338–339
Inhalation anesthetics, 419
Inhalation drug administration, 418–419
Innominate artery, 39, *39*
Inotropic drugs, 434–435, 437
Inspection, in physical examination, 255–258, *256*, *257*
Inspiration, mechanics of, 100–101, 101t
Inspiratory capacity, 112, *112*
Inspiratory muscle fatigue, in obstructive pulmonary disease, 202–203
Inspiratory positive-pressure breathing, 99, 481–484, *482*, 558
  artificial airway in, 489
Inspiratory reserve volume, 111, *112*
Intensive care, 545–546, 546t
Intercostal arteries, 39, *39*
Intercostal muscles, 100, 102
Intermittent mandatory ventilation, 515, 523, *524*, 558
Internal intercostal muscles, 100, 102
Internodal pathways, 46, *47*
Interstitial fluid, 360
  buffers in, 140
Interstitial hydrostatic pressure, 73
Interstitial oncotic pressure, 73
Interstitial pneumonitis, 209
Interventricular foramen, 221
Interventricular septum, 221, *221*, *222*
Intracardiac shunt, left heart catheterization in, 290
Intracellular fluid, 360
Intracranial pressure, increased, mechanical ventilation for, 516
  treatment of, case presentation for, 549–550
Intrapleural pressure, 76, *76*, 99–101
Intrapulmonary shunt, 167, 317–318
Intrathoracic pressure, elevated, and inspiratory positive-pressure breathing, 484

Intravascular fluid, 360
Intravenous drug administration, 417–418
Intravenous fluid therapy, 18, 362–363, 437–438
Intraventricular blocks, 280–281, *281*
Intubation. See also *Airway, artificial*.
  complications of, 506–509, *508*
  endobronchial, 502–504, *503*
  endotracheal, 494–502
    and mechanical ventilation, 516. See also *Mechanical ventilation*.
    cricothyroidotomy in, *504*, 504–505, *505*
    cuff pressure in, 498, 509
    difficulty in, 500–501
    emergency, 500, 504–506, *504–506*
    fiber-optic, 501
    introducer in, 500
    laryngoscopy in, *495*, 495–496, *496*, 500
    nasal, 501–502, *502*
    oral, 496–501, *497–501*
    retrograde, 501
    Sellick maneuver in, 500, *501*
    stylet in, 500–501
    tracheotomy for, 505–506, *506*
    tubes for, 496–498, *497*, 497t, *498*
      position of, radiography of, 380, 382, *383*
  equipment for, malfunction of, 508
  intrapleural, 540–541
  long-term, complications of, 508–509
  nasogastric, tube position in, radiographic appearance of, 380
  termination of, 509–511
    accidental, 508
Ion, 4, 18–19, *19*
Ionic bonds, 9
Ionic theory, 19
Ionization potential, 10
Ipratropium, 428
Irritant receptors, 146
Ischemia, exertional exercise testing for, 352–353
Ischemia response, central nervous system, 83
Ischemic heart disease, 182–184, *183*
  and myocardial infarction, 184–187, *185*, *186*
  drug therapy for, 436–437
  electrocardiography in, 283–284, 283t
Isoelectric line, 51, *51*
Isoetharine, 428
Isolation procedures, 368
Isoproterenol, 428
Isotopes, 5–7, 475
Isovolumetric contraction, *56*, 57
Isovolumetric pressure-flow curve, 110, *110*
Isovolumetric relaxation, 58

J point, 276
Jaw thrust, for airway obstruction relief, 490, *490*

INDEX 581

Jet nebulizer, 464, *464*, 465
Job-related disease, 207–208
  history-taking in, 255

K' (dissociation constant), 138
Kelvin temperature scale, 14, *14*
Ketose, 24, *26*
Kidney, circulation in, 78–80, *79*
  compensatory mechanism for acid-base imbalances in, 142–143, *143*
  in blood pressure regulation, 187–188
  in blood volume regulation, 84
  in left ventricular failure, 194
  response of to hemorrhage, *164*, 165
Kinetic energy, 11
Kinetic theory of gases, 12
Korotkoff sounds, 285
Krebs' cycle, *30*, 30–31
Kussmaul's respiration, 216
Kyphoscoliosis, 210, 406

Labor, induction of, 402
  inhibition of, pharmacologic, 401
Laboratory measurements, normal values for, 567
Lactose, 27
Lamellar bodies, 95
Laminar flow, 63–64, *64*, 107
Lanthanoid elements, 9
Laplace's law, 65, *65*
Laryngeal reflexes, after extubation, 510
Laryngopharynx, 90
Laryngoscopy, in endotracheal intubation, *495*, 495–496, *496*, 500
Laryngotracheal groove, 225
Larynx, in children, 239
  structure and function of, *91*, 91–92, *92*
Leads, electrocardiographic, 49, *50*, 272–275, *276*
Lecithin-sphingomyelin ratio, and fetal lung maturity, 400
Left atrium, 35, *36*, 38
Left bundle branch, 46, *47*
Left bundle branch block, 280–281, *281*
Left cardiac work, 293
Left heart catheterization, 290, *291*
Left ventricle, 35, *36*, 38
Left ventricular failure, and cardiomyopathies, 180–182
  and ischemic heart disease, 182–186
  and valvular dysfunction, 189–192
  pathophysiology of, 192–194, *193*
Left ventricular hypertrophy, and aortic stenosis, 189, *190*
  and mitral insufficiency, 191–192
  in aortic insufficiency, 191
Leukocytes, 37–38
Leukotriene blockers, as bronchodilators, 430
Leukotrienes, and bronchospasm, 427
Lewis dot symbol, 5, 465
Lidocaine, 436

Limb leads, electrocardiographic, 49, *50*, 272–275, *276*
Lipids, 26, 528–294
Lipogenesis, 543
Liquid, properties of, 12, 17–21
Liquid mixtures, types of, 17–18
Liver, circulation in, 81–82
  drug metabolism in, 419–420
Lobar veins, 35, *36*
Lung. See also under *Cardiopulmonary; Pulmonary; Respiratory.*
  and chest wall, mechanical interdependence of, *100*, 105–106, *106*
  blood supply of, 95, 116–123
  cancer of, 214
    case study of, 409–412
    radiography of, 390, *391*
  compliance of, 102–103
    and pressure-volume relationships, 102–106
    assessment of, 307–308
    in restrictive disease, 211–212
  contusion of, 551
  elastic recoil of, 102–103, *103*
    assessment of, 307–308
  fetal, development of, 225–227, *226*, *227*
    maturity assessment for, 400
  filtration in, 153
  granulomatous disease of, and pulmonary hypertension, 196
  hyperinflation of, in asthma, 202–203
  hypoplastic, and diaphragmatic herniation, 237
    case presentation for, 544–545
  metabolic functions of, 153
  parenchyma of, 94–95, *96–98*
  radiographic appearance of, 380, *381*
  segments of, 94, *94*, *262*, 298
  structure of, in children, 240
  volume and capacity of, 111–113, *112*
    age-related changes in, *243*, 243–244
    and airway resistance, 107–108, *108*
    and systemic vascular resistance, 118–119, *119*
    assessment of, in exercise testing, 350–351, *351*
    determination of, 298–307
    in asthma, 203
    in children, 240
    in restrictive disease, 211–212
    parameters of, 298, *299*
  zones of, 121–122, *122*
Lung bud, 225, *226*
Lung diffusing capacity, 314–316, 317t
Lung sounds, auscultation of, 264, *265*, *266–267*, *268*, 557
Lymph nodes, in head and neck, palpation for, 259–261, *261*
Lymphadenopathy, 259–261
Lymphatic system, 42
Lymphocytes, 38
Lymphoid alveolitis, 554

Machine gun cough, 476
Macrophage, alveolar, 152, *152*
Magill forceps, in nasotracheal intubation, 502, *502*
Magnetic resonance imaging, 397, *397*
Malignant hypertension, 188
Malnutrition, assessment of, 371–372, 373t, 374
  signs and symptoms of, 257–258, 258t
Maltose, 27
Mandatory minute ventilation, 534
Mandatory minute volume, 524
Mask, air-entrainment, *455*, 455–456, *456*, 456t
  nonrebreathing, 454–455, *455*, 558
  oxygen, 452–453, *453*
  partial rebreathing, 453–454, *454*, 558
  rebreathing, 455, *455*
  tracheostomy, 456, *457*
  T-tube, 456
  Venturi, *455*, 455–456, *456*, 456t, 558
Mass action law, 22
Mass spectrometry, for carbon dioxide measurement, 339
Mast cells, 37
  and bronchospasm, 426–427
Master's two-step test, 344, *347*
Matter, states of, 12
Maximum expiratory pressure, determination of, *311*, 311–312
Maximum inspiratory pressure, determination of, *311*, 311–312
Maximum oxygen consumption, measurement of, in exercise testing, 352–353
Maximum static recoil pressure, 308
Maximum ventilatory capacity, 354
Maximum voluntary ventilation, 353–354
  assessment of, 309
MCL_1 lead, electrocardiographic, 49
Mean electrical axis, 51–52, *52*, 277–279, *279*
Mechanical dead space, 558
Mechanical ventilation, aerosol therapy in, 467
  airway pressure release, 525
  and endotracheal intubation, 516. See also *Intubation, endotracheal.*
  and nosocomial infections, 368
  artificial airway in, 489. See also *Airway, artificial.*
  assist/control, 523
  assisted, 523
  bucking the ventilator in, 532
  complications of, 530–533, *531*
  controlled, 523, 523t, 558
  during transport, 539, 540t
  equipment for, decontamination, disinfection, and sterilization of, 368–370, 370t
  malfunction in, 533
  expiratory retard in, 527–528
  high frequency, 528–530, *529*, *530*
  high-pressure, patient selection for, 533

582 INDEX

Mechanical ventilation (*Continued*)
  history of, 514–515
  in chest trauma, 552–553
  in increased intracranial pressure, 550
  in neonate, 403–404, 531
    case presentation for, 544–545
  independent, 504
  indications for, 514t–516t, 515–517
  inflation hold in, 525
  inspiratory flow patterns in, 525
  intermittent mandatory, 515, 523, *524*
  mandatory minute volume in, 524
    in weaning, 534
  monitors and alarms for, 528
  negative end-expiratory pressure, 528
  negative-pressure, 517–519, *518*
    patient selection for, 533
  periodic hyperinflation in, 528
  positive end-expiratory pressure, 525–527, *526–527*
  positive-pressure, 519–528, 520t, *521*, *524*, *526*, *527*
    cycling mechanism in, 521–522, 522t
    special functions in, 525–528
    tidal volume generation in, 519
    types of, 520t
    ventilatory mode in, 522–525, 523t, *524*
  pressure support, 524–525, 534
  rate and tidal volume settings for, 533–544
  respiratory depressants in, 431
  transtracheal catheter, 504–505, *505*
  types of, 517–530
    selection of, 533–534
  ventilatory modes in, 533–534
  weaning from, 532, 534–535
Meconium aspiration, 236–237, 401, 402
Mediastinoscopy, 409
Mediastinal crunch, 557
Mediastinum, 94
  radiographic appearance of, 380, 381, *381*, 383, *385*
Medical gas therapy, 419
  carbon dioxide–oxygen, 461–462
  equipment for, *443–445*, 443–447, 446t, *447–449*
  helium-oxygen, 461
  humidification in, 462–467, *463–466*
  oxygen. See *Oxygen therapy*.
  safety systems for, 447–449, *449*
  with inspiratory positive-pressure breathing, 482
Medical history, 250–255, *251–252*
Medullary respiratory center, 144–145
Membrane. See *Cell membrane*.
Membrane diffusion, Fick's law of, 16–17, *17*
Meperidine, 431
Metabolic acidosis, 141
  causes of, 142t
  compensated, 141–143, *143*, 333–334, 333t

Metabolic acidosis (*Continued*)
  sodium bicarbonate for, 417
  uncompensated, 333t, 334
Metabolic alkalosis, 141, 142t
  causes of, 142t
  compensated, 141–143, *143*, 333t, 334
  uncompensated, 333t, 334
Metabolic autoregulation, 70–71
Metabolic complications, in mechanical ventilation, 532
Metabolic measurements, in exercise testing, 351–352, *352*
Metabolic rate, and respiratory quotient, 372, 374, 374t
  assessment of, 372, 374, 374t
Metabolism, 23
  aerobic, 324
  anaerobic, 324
  cellular, *30*, 30–31
Metaproterenol, 428
Methemoglobinemia, and oxygen transport, 134
Methylxanthines, as bronchodilators, 428–429, 429t
Metoprolol, 435
Microatelectasis, 388
Microbial control, antibiotic, *365*, 365–366, 366t
Microbial culture, specimen collection for, *363*, 363–364
  techniques for, 364–365
Microbial identification, techniques of, 364–365, *365*
Microcirculation, 39–40, *42*
  structure of, 71–72
Microorganisms, respiratory, 366–367
Microscopy, 364, *365*
Mid-arm muscle circumference, 372
Miliary atelectasis, 209
Mineral elements, 22
Minute ventilation, during exercise, *160*, 160–161, *161*
Minute volume, 113
Mitral insufficiency, 191–192, *192*
Mitral regurgitation, murmur in, *294*, 295
Mitral stenosis, and right ventricular failure, 197–198, *198*
  murmur in, *294*, 295
Mitral valve, 35, *36*, 38
Mixed acidosis, 334
Mixed alkalosis, 334–335
Mixed sleep apnea, 215, 319–321
Mixed venous blood gas analysis. See *Blood gas analysis*.
Mobitz block, type I, 280
  type II, 280, *281*
    pacemaker for, 284, *284*
Monocytes, 37–38
Monomer, 24, *27*
Monosaccharides, 24, *27*
Morphine, 431
Mountain sickness, 168
Mucociliary escalator, 94, 151
Mucokinetic agents, 420–423
  as antimicrobials, 430

Mucokinetic system, 420–422, *421*
Mucus, 420–421
  in chronic bronchitis, 204
  in cystic fibrosis, 241
  production of, 421
  retention of, causes of, 422, 422t
    management of, 422–423
  transport of, 94, 151, *421*, 421–422
  drugs for, 420–423, 430
Multibreath nitrogen washout test, 314, *315*
Murmurs, 58
  and aortic stenosis, 189
  phonocardiographic assessment of, *294*, 294–295
Murphy bevel, 497
Muscarinic receptors, 425
Muscle(s), blood flow to, during exercise, 158–160
  cardiac. See *Myocardium*.
  mid-arm, measurement of, 372
  of respiration, 97–99, *99*, *100*, *102*
    control of, 120–121
Muscle and tendon receptors, in breathing control, 147
Muscle contraction, and blood flow, 76, *76*
Muscle relaxants, 431–432
Myasthenia gravis, 210
Myocardial infarction, 184–187, *186*
  electrocardiography in, 283–284, 283t
  pain in, 253
Myocardial ischemia, drug therapy for, 436–437
  electrocardiography in, 283–284, 283t
  exertional, exercise testing for, 352–353, *353*
Myocardium, 38, 53, *54*
  contractility of, 53, *55*, 55–56, 60, *61*, *62*
  and Frank-Starling relationship, 59, *59*
  and ventricular function, 58–60, *60*, 61
  length-tension relationship for, 58–60, *59*
  ultrastructure of, 53, *54*
Myocytes, action potential of, *44*, 44–45
Myofibril, myocardial, 53, *54*, 55
Myoglobin, 171
Myosin, 53, 55, *55*

Nails, clubbing of, 257, *257*, 408
Narcotic antagonists, 432
Narcotics, 148, *148*, 431
Nasal cannula, 452, *453*
Nasal catheter, 451–452, *452*
Nasal septum, structure and function of, 89, *90*
Nasal turbinates, structure and function of, 89, *90*
Nasogastric intubation, tube position in, radiography of, 380

INDEX 583

Nasopharyngeal airway, 491–492, *492.* See also *Airway, artificial.*
Nasopharynx, structure and function of, 89–90, *90*
Nasotracheal intubation, 501–502, *502.* See also *Intubation, endotracheal.*
Nasotracheal suctioning, *478,* 478–480
Nebulization, of mucokinetics, 422–423
Nebulizers, 464–466, *464–466*
Negative end-expiratory pressure, 528
Negative-pressure breathing, 99, 558
Negative-pressure ventilation, 517–519, *518*
  patient selection for, 533
Neonate, apnea of, 237–238
  assessment of, 404–404, 402t
  blood gas analysis in, 330, 402–403
  cardiopulmonary function in, 230–231
  cardiovascular disorders in, 231–234
  intensive care of, 544, 544t
  mechanical ventilation in, 531
    case presentation for, 544–545
  mediastinal widening in, 380, 383, *385*
  pulmonary disorders in, 234–238
  resuscitation in, 403–404
  retinopathy in, oxygen-related, 238, 332, 461
  transient tachypnea in, 238
  treatment planning for, case presentation of, 545–546, *546*
Nervous system, in cardiac control, 61
  in circulatory control, 66–68, *67*
  in respiratory control, 144–147
  structure and function of, 423–425, *425,* 425t
Neurogenic hypertension, 188
Neuromuscular disorders, and restrictive lung disease, 210–211
Neurons, 424, *425*
  respiratory group, 144–145
Neurotransmitters, 424
  in heart rate regulation, 45–46
Neutron, 4
Nicotinic receptors, 425
Nitrogen balance, in nutritional assessment, 372
Nitrogen narcosis, 172
Nitrogen washout technique, for functional residual capacity determination, 304–305, *305*
Nitrous oxide, perfusion limitation of diffusion of, 127
Noble gases, 9
Nodal premature beats, 281, *282*
Nonpolar covalent bond, 10, *10*
Nonrebreathing mask, 454–455, *455,* 558
Norepinephrine, in circulatory control, 67–68, *69*
Nose, air filtration in, 151
  structure and function of, 89–91, *90*
Nosebleed, in nasotracheal intubation, 506
Nosocomial infections, 213, 366–367
  and respiratory therapy equipment, 368

Nuclear scanning, 395–396, *396*
Nucleic acids, 26–30, *29, 30*
Nucleotide, 27
Null cells, 38
Nutritional assessment, 257–258, 258t, 371–372, 373t, 374
Nutritional support, and lipogenesis, 339, 371–372, 437, 543

Obesity, and restrictive lung disease, 211
Obstructive pulmonary disease, 199–207
  chronic, 199, 557. See also *Asthma; Chronic bronchitis; Emphysema.*
  flow-volume analysis in, 309–310, *310*
  static lung volume measurements in, *306,* 307
Obstructive sleep apnea, 148, 211, 215–216
  assessment of, 319–321, *320*
Occupational lung disease, 207–208, 209
  history-taking in, 255
Octet rule, 9
Olfaction, 151
Oligosaccharide, 24–26, *27*
Ondine's curse, 216
Opiate receptors, 431, 431t
Opiates, 431
Oral drug administration, 418
Oropharyngeal airway, 490–491, *491.* See also *Airway, artificial.*
Oropharynx, structure and function of, 90, *90*
Orotracheal intubation, 496–501, *497–501.* See also *Intubation, endotracheal.*
Orotracheal suctioning, *478,* 478–480
Orthopnea, 193
  assessment of, 250
Osmosis, 18, *19*
Osmotic pressure, 18
Overhydration, 360–361, 360t
  in humidity and aerosol therapy, 466
Overnutrition, assessment of, 371–374
Overutilization hypoxia, 167
Oxidative phosphorylation, 324
Oximetry, *337,* 337–338
Oxygen, binding of to hemoglobin, 130, 131
  diffusion of, 127–129, *128*
  and hypoxia, 169
  during exercise, 129, 163
  dissolved in blood, 129–130, 131
  in alveolar gas, 113–114
  loading of in lung, 130–131
  measurement of. See *Blood gas analysis.*
  partial pressure of, 114. See also *Oxygenation.*
    age-related changes in, 244
    normal values for, 330–331
  physical properties of, 442

Oxygen (*Continued*)
  purified, preparation of, 442–443, 442t, *443*
  storage of, *443–445,* 443–446, *447*
  solubility of, 126
  toxicity of, and retrolental fibroplasia, 332
  transfer of, maternal-fetal, 228, *230*
  transport of, 129–134
    and hypoxia, 169
    during exercise, 163
  unloading of at tissues, 131–132
  ventilatory equivalents of, and anaerobic threshold, 354
Oxygen carrying capacity, 130, 131
Oxygen consumption, measurement of, in exercise testing, 352–353
Oxygen mask, 452–453, *453,* 558
Oxygen pulse, 353–354
Oxygen saturation, 129–130, 131
  measurement of. See also *Blood gas analysis.*
    by blood gas analyzer, 326–327
    by oximetry, *337,* 337–338
Oxygen tents, 457–458, *458*
Oxygen therapy, 419, 434
  administration of, 451–459
    environmental devices for, 457–459, *458–460*
    high-flow devices for, 451
    low-flow devices for, 451
  aerosol, 464–466, 464–467
  and atelectasis, 460
  and circulatory depression, 460–461
  and pulmonary damage, 462
  and respiratory depression, 459–460
  and retrolental fibroplasia, 238, 332, 462
  by mask, 452–456, *453–457*
  by nasal cannula, 452, *453*
  by nasal catheter, 451–452, *452*
  complications of, 459–461
  equipment for, *443–445,* 443–447, 446t, *447–449*
  flow meters for, 446–447, *449*
  humidification in, 462–467, *463–466*
  hyperbaric, 459, *460*
  indications for, 449–450
  oxygen preparation for, 442–443, *443*
  oxygen storage for, *443–445,* 443–446, 446t, *447*
  regulators for, 446, 446t, *448*
  safety systems for, 447–449, *449*
  suctioning during, 479
  with inspiratory positive-pressure breathing, 482
Oxygen toxicity, 172, 236
Oxygenation, arterial, assessment of, 331–333. See also *Blood gas analysis.*
  extracorporeal membrane, 404
  normal values for, 330–331
  transcutaneous, 336
  venous, evaluation of, 335–336
Oxygen–carbon dioxide therapy, 461–462
Oxygen-helium therapy, 461

Oxyhemoglobin dissociation curve, 130, *131*
  factors influencing, *132*, 132–133
  fetal, 228, *230*
Oxyhood, 458, *459*

P wave, 275
Pacemaker, cardiac, 284, *284*
  ectopic, 46
  phrenic, radiography of, 391, *394*
  sinoatrial node, *45*, 46–47, 47t
Pacemaker cells, 42
  action potential of, *45*, 45–46
Pain, chest. See also *Angina*.
  assessment of, 250–253, 408
Pain receptors, in breathing control, 147
Palatine tonsils, 90
Palpation, 258–261, *259–261*
Palpitations, 191
Paradoxical breathing, 408
Paradoxical reflex of Head, 146
Paralyzing agents, 431–432
Paranasal sinuses, 90
Parasympathetic nervous system, 424–425, 425t
  in circulatory control, 68
Parasympatholytics, as bronchodilators, 428
Parasympathomimetics, in bronchoprovocation, 312
Parenchyma, pulmonary, 94–95, *96–98*
Parenteral hyperalimentation, and lipogenesis, 339, 371–372, 437, 543
Paroxysmal nocturnal dyspnea, 250
Partial pressure, of gases, 14
Partial rebreathing mask, 453–454, *454*, 558
Pass-over humidifier, 462–464, *463*
Pasteurization, 369
Patent ductus arteriosus, 232
  and persistent fetal circulation, 234
Patent foramen ovale, 231
  and persistent fetal circulation, 234
Patent foramen primum, 231
Pathognomonic symptom, 407
Patient assessment. See also *Physical examination*.
  adult, 407–412
  integrated approach to, 400–411
  pediatric, 404–407
  perinatal, 400–404
Patient therapeutics, integrated approach to, 538–553. See also *Treatment; Treatment planning*.
Patient transport, 539
Pectoriloquy, whispered, 267
Pediatric assessment, 404–407
PEEP. See *Positive end-expiratory pressure*.
Peptide bond, 23, *25*
Percussion, diagnostic, 261, *263*, 558
  therapeutic, 475
Perfusion limitation of diffusion, 127
Perfusion scan, *396*, 397–396
Pericardial effusion, 180

Pericardial rub, 558
Pericardial tamponade, 180, *181*
Pericarditis, 180
Pericardium, 38
Perinatal assessment, 400–404, 402t. See also *Neonate*.
Periodic law, 9
Periodic table, *8*, 9
Perioperative care, 542–543
Peripheral artery catheterization, 286, 286t
Peripheral nerves, 424
pH, 20, 137. See also *Acid-base balance*.
  and oxyhemoglobin dissociation curve, *132*, 132–133
  of arterial blood, evaluation of, 332–335
  normal values for, 330
Phagocytosis, 37
Pharmacology. See *Drug(s)*.
Pharynx, structure and function of, 89–91, *90*
Phenylephrine, 434
Phenytoin, 436
Pheochromocytoma, 188
Phonation, 89
Phonocardiography, 266, *294*, 294–295
Phosphate buffer system, 139–140
Phosphate ions, in acid-base regulation, 142–143, *143*
Phosphatidylglycerol, and fetal lung maturity, 400
Phospholipids, 26, *28*
Phrenic pacemaker, radiography of, 391, *394*
Physical examination, 255–268
  auscultation in, *263–265*, 263–268, 267
  inspection in, 255–258, *256*, *257*, 258t
  palpation in, 258–261, *259–261*
  percussion in, 263
Physiologic dead space, 113, 316–317
  calculation of, 339
Physiologic pressure transducers, *286*, 286–287
Physiologic shunt, 167, 317–318
Physostigmine, 432
Pickwickian syndrome, 211
Pin Index Safety System, 448–449, *449*
Pink puffers, 203
Pitt speaking tracheostomy tube, 506
pK', 138
Placenta, 227–228, *229*
  biopsy of, 401
Plaque, atheromatous, 182, *183*
Plasma, 36–37
  replacement of, 438
Plasma cells, 38
Plasma oncotic pressure, 73
Plasma proteins, 36, 140
Plateau pressure, in mechanical ventilation, 525
Platelet, 38
Platelet-activating factor, in asthma, 201, 201t

Plethysmography, for airway resistance assessment, 310–311, *311*
  for functional residual capacity determination, 305–307, *306*
  for lung compliance determination, 307–308
Pleura, 94
Pleural drainage, 540–541
Pleural fluid, 540–541
  culture of, collection for, 364
  technique for, 364–365
  radiography of, 385–386, *386–387*
Pleural friction rub, *265*, 267, 577
Pleuritic pain, 253
Pleximeter, 261
Pneumatometry, for functional residual capacity determination, 305–307, *306*
Pneumoconiosis, 207–208, 556
  history-taking in, 255
Pneumocytes, 94–95
Pneumonia, 213
  and inspiratory positive-pressure breathing, 483
  and suctioning, 480
  causative organisms in, 366–367
  iatrogenic, 430
  nosocomial, 213, 366, 367
    and respiratory therapy equipment, 368
  prevention of, aseptic and isolation techniques for, 368
  radiography in, 390–391, *392*
Pneumonitis, 213
  hypersensitivity, 209, 556
  interstitial, 209
Pneumotaxic center, 145
Pneumothorax, 540–541
  and inspiratory positive-pressure breathing, 483
  radiography of, 386, *388*
  spontaneous, 540
  tension, 540
    radiography of, 384–385, *386*
  treatment planning for, case presentation for, 549
Pneumotachography, 299, *301*
Poiseuille's law, 63, *63*
Polar covalent bond, 10, *10*
Polarization, of pacemaker cells, 42
Poliomyelitis, 210
Polymer, 24–26, *27*
Polymorphonuclear leukocytes, 37
Polysaccharide, 24–26
Polysomnography, 215, 319–321, *320*
Pontine respiratory center, 145
Portal vein hypertension, 408
Positive airway pressure, artificial airway in, 489
Positive end-expiratory pressure, 525–527, *526–527*, 558
  during transport, 539, 540t
  in adult respiratory distress syndrome, 212–213, 212t
  in chest trauma, 552–553
  in increased intracranial pressure, 550
  weaning from, 534–535

Positive-pressure breathing, 99, 481–484
  artificial airway in, 489
Postganglionic fibers, 424, *425*
Postural drainage, 470–475, *471–474*
Potassium ions, and resting membrane potential, 42–44, *44*
Potassium levels, 361–363
Potential energy, 11–12
Potentiation, pharmacologic, 420
P-R interval, 51, *51*
P-R segment, 275–276
Precordial leads, electrocardiographic, 49, *50*, 272–275, *276*
Prednisone, as bronchodilator, 429–430
Preeclampsia, 174–175
Preganglionic fibers, 424, *425*
Pregnancy, cardiopulmonary response to, 173–175
  fetal assessment in, 400–401
  toxemia of, 174–175
Preload, 59–60
  and stroke volume, 75, 292–293
Premature contractions, 281–282, *282*
Premature ectopic beats, drug therapy for, 436
Prematurity, retinopathy of, 238, 332, 461
Pressor area, vasomotor, 66, *67*
Pressure, alveolar, 100–101, *101*
  and flow and resistance, 61–63
  capillary hydrostatic, 73
  central, 75–76
  colloid osmotic, 72, 123t
  critical opening, 120
  interstitial hydrostatic, 73
  interstitial oncotic, 73
  intrapleural, 76, *76*, 99–101
  intrathoracic, elevated, 484
  maximum respiratory, *311*, 311–312
  maximum static recoil, 308
  negative end-expiratory, 528
  osmotic, 18
  plasma oncotic, 73
  pulse, 65–66
  transpulmonary, 102, *102*
  units of measurement for, 62
  vapor, 17
  zero reference level for, 62
Pressure support, in mechanical ventilation, 524–525, 534
Pressure transducers, *286*, 286–287
Pressure ventilator, 558
Pressure-flow relationships, in breathing, 99–106
  and compliance, 102–106
Pressure-volume relationships, gas, 12–16
Primary aldosteronism, 188
Prinzmetal's angina, exercise testing for, 353, *353*
Procainamide, 436
Progesterone, for hypoventilation, 432–433
Propranolol, 435
Proprioceptors, in breathing control, 147

Prostaglandins, 70, 70t, 153
  as bronchodilators, 430
Prosthetic heart valve, radiography of, 383, *385*
Protein(s), as buffers, 140
  contractile, myocardial, 53
  fibrous, 24
  functional categories of, 24
  globular, 24
  oligomeric, *25*
  plasma, 36, 140
  serum, in nutritional assessment, 372, 374
  structure and composition of, 23–24, *24*, *25*
Proteolytic enzymes, 205
Protocols, clinical, 541
Proton, 4
Protriptyline, 433
Psychologic complications, in mechanical ventilation, 532–533
Pulmonary alveolar microlithiasis, 556
Pulmonary alveolar proteinosis, 556
Pulmonary artery angiography, 394, *395*
Pulmonary artery catheterization, 287–290, *287–290*
  for blood gas analysis, 329–330. See also *Blood gas analysis*.
Pulmonary artery pressure, in children, 239
Pulmonary artery wedge pressure, measurement of, 287–290, *287–290*
Pulmonary blood flow, regional distribution of, 121–122
Pulmonary capillaries, 34–35, *36*, 41–42, 95–97, *97–98*, 117
  recruitment and distention of, 119–120
Pulmonary circulation, 95, 117–123
  age-related changes in, 242t, 243
  anatomy of, 35, 35–36, *36*, 41–42
  and hypoxia, 169
  during anesthesia, 176
  during exercise, 162
  nonrespiratory functions of, 152–153
  vs. systemic circulation, 117, *118*
Pulmonary complications, of mechanical ventilation, 531, *531*
Pulmonary defense mechanisms, 89, 151–152, *152*
  age-related changes in, 245
Pulmonary diffusing capacity, age-related changes in, 245
Pulmonary disease, infectious, 213–214
  and inspiratory positive-pressure breathing, 484
  and suctioning, 480
  causative organisms in, 366–367
  iatrogenic, 430
  interstitial, 209, 555, 556
  nosocomial, 213, 366–367
    and respiratory therapy equipment, 368
  prevention of, aseptic and isolation precautions for, 368
  radiography in, 390–391, *392*
  sputum in, 253
  neoplastic, 214, 390, *391*, 409–412

Pulmonary disease (*Continued*)
  obstructive, 199–207
    chronic, 199, 557. See also *Asthma; Chronic bronchitis; Emphysema*.
    flow-volume analysis in, 309–310, *310*
    static lung volume measurements in, *306*, 307
  occupational, 207–208, 209
    history-taking in, 255
  restrictive, 207–212
    flow-volume analysis in, 310, *310*
    static lung volume measurements in, *306*, 307
  vascular, 195–197
Pulmonary disorders, neonatal, 234–238
Pulmonary edema, 123, 123t
Pulmonary embolism, 195
Pulmonary emphysema, 196, 557
  and chronic bronchitis, 203, 204t, 205–206
Pulmonary fibrosis, 209
Pulmonary function testing, 298–321. See also specific tests and parameters.
  for breathing control, 318–321
  for dynamic lung function, 308–312
  for lung compliance, 307–308
  for lung diffusing capacity, 298–307
  for ventilation distribution, 312–314
  for ventilation-perfusion ratio, 316–318
  in adult case study, 410, 411t
  in pediatric case study, 406, 406t
  indications for, 298t
  normal values for, 565–566
Pulmonary hemosiderosis, 556
Pulmonary histiocytosis, 556
Pulmonary hygiene. See *Bronchopulmonary hygiene*.
Pulmonary hypertension, 195–197
Pulmonary infiltrates, diffuse, 556
  radiography of, 390–391, *393–394*
Pulmonary metabolism, 89
Pulmonary parenchyma, 94–95, *96–98*
  radiography of, 390–391, *391–394*
Pulmonary resistance, 107
Pulmonary secretions. See *Mucus; Sputum*.
Pulmonary stenosis, and right ventricular failure, 197, *197*
  in tetralogy of Fallot, 233
Pulmonary surfactant, 105, 235–236
Pulmonary terms and symbols, 555–564
Pulmonary vascular disease, 195–197
Pulmonary vascular reflexes, 146
Pulmonary vascular resistance, 117–123, 293
  and control of pulmonary vascular smooth muscle, 120–121
  and hypoxic pulmonary vasoconstriction, 122–123
  and lung volume, 118–119, *119*
  and pulmonary edema, 123, 123t
  and recruitment and distensibility, *119*, 119–120

Pulmonary vascular resistance (*Continued*)
  and regional distribution of pulmonary blood flow, 121–122
  calculation of, 117, *118*
  determinants of, 117–123
  distribution of, 118
  during exercise, 162
Pulmonary vasculitis, 196
Pulmonary vasoconstriction, hypoxic, 122–123
Pulmonary veins, 117
Pulmonary veno-occlusive disease, 196
Pulmonary vessels, 34–35, *36*, 117
  embryologic development of, 225–227, *226*, *227*
  innervation of, 120–121
  occlusion of, 195–196
Pulsatile flow, 65–66
Pulse, assessment of, 258–259, *259*, *260*
  oxygen, 353–354
Pulse oximetry, *337*, 337–338
Pulse pressure, 65–66
Pulsus alternans, 259
Pulsus paradoxus, 259, 531
Purines, 27, *29*
Purkinje fibers, 46, *47*
Pursed-lip breathing, 477
  in emphysema, 206
Pyrimidines, 27, *29*

QRS complex, *51*, 51–52, 276, *278*
Q-T interval, *51*, 57
Q-T segment, 277
Quinidine, 436

R wave, 51, *51*
Racemic epinephrine, 427–428
Radiation, diagnostic, 378–379. See also *Radiography*.
  for sterilization, 369
  hazards of, 378
Radioactive isotopes, 7
Radiographic unknown, *397*, 397
Radiography, body orientation in, 379
  bony tissue appearance on, 379–380
  interpretation methods in, 379–380
  normal findings on, 379–381, *381*
  of atelectasis, 388, *389*
  of bony tissue, 379–380
  of bronchial intubation, 382, *383*
  of cardiomegaly, 382, *383*, *384*, *385*
  of diaphragm, 386–389, *389*, *390*
  of heart, 380
  of lung infiltrates, 390–391, *393*–*394*
  of lung lobes and segments, 380
  of lung masses, 390, *391*
  of mediastinum, 380, 383, *385*
  of pleural fluid, 385–386, *386*–*387*
  of pneumothorax, 384–385, 386, *386*, *388*
  of prosthetic heart valve, 383, *385*
  of soft tissue, 380

Radiography (*Continued*)
  of subcutaneous emphysema, 382, *383*
  of tension pneumothorax, 384–385, *386*
  patient rotation on, 381, *382*
  principles of, 378–379
  symmetry in, 379
Radioisotope scanning, 395–396, *396*
Radiology, 378–397. See also specific radiologic techniques.
Rales, *265*, 266, 557
Rankine temperature scale, 14, *14*
Reactive airway disease, 199
Reactive hyperemia, 71
Rebreathing mask, 455, *455*
Receptors. See also specific types; e.g., *Baroreceptors*; *Respiratory receptors*.
  drug, 416–417
Recruitment, and pulmonary vascular resistance, 120
Rectal drug administration, 418
Red cells, 37
Reflection coefficient, 73
Reflex(es), Bainbridge, 83
  cardiopulmonary, 82–84
  cough, 151–152
  diving, 171
  Head's paradoxical, 146
  Hering-Breuer deflation, 146
  Hering-Breuer inflation, 145–146
  in respiratory control, 145–147
  laryngeal, after extubation, 510
  pulmonary vascular, 146
  sneeze, 151–152
Regulator, gas cylinder, 446, 446t
Rehabilitation, 544
Renal circulation, 78–80, *79*
Renal complications, in mechanical ventilation, 532
Renal hypertension, 187–188, 408
Renin-angiotensin-aldosterone system, during hemorrhage, *164*, 165
  in blood pressure regulation, 187–188
Renovascular hypertension, 188
Repolarization, cardiac, 44, 44–47, *45*, 47t, 53
Residual volume, 111, *112*
  determination of, 303–307, *304*–*306*
Resistance, addition of, 62–63
  airways, 106–110
  and pressure and flow, 61–63, *63*
  determinants of, 63
  systemic vascular, 62
  total peripheral, 62
  vascular, 293
Resistance breathing, 477
Resonance, on percussion, 261, *263*
Respiration. See *Breathing*.
Respirator, body tank (Drinker), 517–519, *518*, 533
Respiratory acidosis, 140–141
  causes of, 142t
  compensated, 141–143, *143*, 333–334, 333t
  uncompensated, 333t, 334

Respiratory alkalosis, causes of, 142t
  compensated, 141–143, *143*, 333, 333t
  uncompensated, 333t, 334
Respiratory depressant drugs, 431, 431t
Respiratory depression, and oxygen therapy, 459–460
Respiratory distress syndrome, adult, 212–213, 212t, 461, 556
  radiography in, 390–391, *393*
  infant, 234–236, *235*, 556
  radiography in, 391, *394*
Respiratory exchange ratio, and anaerobic threshold, 356
Respiratory failure, 216–217
  definition of, 514
  ventilation in. See *Mechanical ventilation*.
Respiratory gases. See also *Carbon dioxide*; *Oxygen*.
  diagnostic and therapeutic use of, 419
  diffusion of, 125–129, *128*
  partial pressures of, 114
Respiratory group neurons, 144–145
Respiratory microorganisms, 366–367
Respiratory quotient, 339
  and metabolic rate, 373–374, 374t
Respiratory receptors, irritant, 146
  juxtapulmonary-capillary, 146
Respiratory secretions. See *Mucus*; *Sputum*.
Respiratory sinus arrhythmia, 279, *280*
Respiratory stimulant drugs, 432–433
Respiratory system. See also consituent parts of.
  age-related changes in, 242–245, 242t, *243*
  compensatory mechanisms for acid-base imbalances in, *140*, 141–142
  during anesthesia, 175–176
  during diving, 170–173
  during exercise, 160–163, *160*–*163*
  during hemorrhage, 165–166
  during hypoxia, 167–170
  during pregnancy, 174
  during surgery, 175–176
  embryologic development of, 225–227, *226*, *227*
  functions of, 88–89
  infections of. See also *Pulmonary disease, infectious*.
    and respiratory therapy equipment, 368
  nonrespiratory functions of, 150–153
  perinatal alterations in, 230
  postnatal development of, 239–240
  structure of, 89–99
Respiratory therapy, and nosocomial infections, 368
  equipment for, decontamination, disinfection, and sterilization of, 368–370, 370t
  microbiological surveillance of, 368
Resting membrane potential, 42–43
Restrictive lung disease, 207–212
  flow-volume analysis in, 310, *310*
  static lung volume measurements in, *306*, 307

Restrictive pulmonary disease, 207–212
  flow-volume analysis in, 310, *310*
Resuscitation, cardiopulmonary, 538–539
  in exercise testing, 349, 349t
  neonatal, 403–404
Resuscitator, 558
Retinopathy of prematurity, 238, 332, 461
Retractions, 408
Retrolental fibroplasia, 238, 332, 461
Reynold's number, 64
Rhonchi, *265*, 267, 557
Rib fractures, 257
  radiography of, 379
  treatment of, case presentation for, 550–553
Ribonucleic acid (RNA), 26–30, *29*, *30*
Right atrium, 34, *36*, 38
Right bundle branch, 46, *47*
Right bundle branch block, 280, *281*
Right cardiac work, 293
Right heart catheterization, 287–290, *287*–*290*
Right ventricle, 34, *36*, 38
Right ventricular failure, 192, 195–199
Right ventricular hypertrophy, causes of, 197–199
  in tetralogy of Fallot, 233
Right-to-left shunt, 167, 317–318
Ringer's lactate, 437–438
RNA, 26–30, *29*, *30*
Robertshaw endobronchial tube, 503
Rub, pericardial 558
  pleuropericardial, 558
  pleural friction, *265*, 266

S wave, 51, *51*
S1 heart sound, 58, 264, 265–268, *267*
S2 heart sound, 58, 264, 265–268, *267*
S3 heart sound, 58
S4 heart sound, 58
Saline, as mucokinetic, 422–423
  normal, 438
Sanz electrode, 325–326
Sarcoidosis, 208–209
Sarcolemma, myocardial, 53, 54, *54*
Sarcomere, myocardial, 53, *54*, *55*
Sarcoplasmic reticulum, myocardial, 54
Scalp blood sampling, fetal, 401
Scapula, radiography of, 379
Scoliosis, 210, 406
Scuba diving, 171–173
Segmental breathing, 477
Sellick maneuver, 500, *501*
Septum primum, 221, *221*
Septum secundum, 221, *222*
Serotonin, 69–70, 70t, 153
Serum, 36
Severinghaus electrode, 326
Shiley's tracheostomy tube, *506*
Shock, cardiogenic, 194
  hemorrhagic, 164–165
Shunt, and hypoxia, 167
  arteriovenous, 39–40, *42*

Shunt (*Continued*)
  intracardiac, left heart catheterization in, 290
  physiologic (right-to-left), 167, 317–318
Shunt equation, 335–336
Shunt-like states, calculation of, 317–318
Sighs, 146, 175
  in mechanical ventilation, 528
Signs and symptoms, 407–408
Silhouette sign, 390, *392*
Silicosis, 207–208
Single-breath carbon monoxide test, 315–316
Single-breath oxygen test, *313*, 313–314
Sinoatrial block, 279, *280*
Sinoatrial node, 42
  as pacemaker, *45*, 45–47, 47t
Sinus arrhythmias, 279, *280*. See also *Arrhythmias.*
Sinus venosus, 220, *220*–*222*
Sinuses, paranasal, 90
Sinusoids, hepatic, 82
Situs inversus, 381
Skeletal disorders, and restrictive lung disease, 210
Skin, blood flow to, during exercise, 160
  circulation in, 80–81
Skinfold measurement, 372
Skull fracture, basilar, and nasotracheal intubation, 506–507
Sleep apnea, 148
  assessment of, 319–321, *320*
  central, 215
  mixed, 215
  obstructive, 211, 215–216
Sliding filament theory, 53, *55*, 55–56
Slow-reacting substance of anaphylaxis, and bronchospasm, 200–201, 201t, 426–427
Smoking, and chronic bronchitis, 204
  and emphysema, 205, *206*
  history-taking for, 255
Sneezing, 151
Snogging, 476
Sodium, and myocyte action potential, *44*, 44–45
Sodium bicarbonate, as mucokinetic, 423
  for metabolic acidosis, 417
Sodium-potassium pump, 43–44, *44*
Soft tissue, radiographic appearance of, 380
Sol, 18
Solids, properties of, 12, 17–21
Solute, 17–18
Solution, 17
  dilution of, calculation of, 20–21
  quantification of, 20–21, 21t
Solvent, 17
Specific gravity, of gases, 15, *15*
Sphygmomanometry, 285–286, *286*
Spinal cord, in breathing control, 145
Spirometry, 298–303, 302t
  in exericse testing, 350–351, *351*

Spirometry (*Continued*)
  incentive, *480*, 481, *481*
  standards for, 299, 302t
  technique for, 302–303
  with flow-sensing devices, 299, *301*
  with volume-collecting devices, 298–299, *300*
Spironolactone, 439
Splanchnic circulation, 81–82
Splinting, 470
Sputum. See also *Mucus*.
  assessment of, 253
  collection of, 213, 253, *254*, *363*, 363–364
  culture of, 364–365
  staining and microscopic evaluation of, 364
Squeeze, 172
S-T segment, 52–53, 276
Stagnant hypoxia, 167
Staining, bacterial, 364
Standard limb leads, electrocardiographic, 49, *50*, 272–275, *276*
Starling equation, 72
Starling's law, 58–60, *59*
Static lung compliance, measurement of, 307, *308*
Step test, 344, *347*. See also *Exercise testing*.
Sterilization, of equipment and supplies, 368–370
Steroids, as bronchodilators, 429–430
  in infant respiratory distress syndrome, 236
  structure of, 26, *29*
Stethoscope, 262, *263*–*265*, 264, 266
Stewart-Hamilton dye dilution method, for cardiac output determination, 291, *292*
Strain gauge transducer, *286*, 287
Stress test. See also *Exercise testing*.
  cardiac, 348, 348t
  cardiopulmonary, 348–349, 349t
Stridor, 240, *265*, 267
Stroke index, 292
Stroke volume, 59, 190, 292–293
  and cardiac output, 74–75
  during exercise, 158, *159*
Stroke work, 59–60, 75, 293
Subatomic particles, 4, 475
Subclavian artery, 39, *39*
Subcutaneous drug administration, 418
Subcutaneous emphysema, radiography of, 382, *383*
Succinylcholine, 432
Sucrose, 27
Suctioning, *478*, 478–480
  during extubation, 510
  for sputum collection, 363–364
  meconium, 403
Sudden infant death syndrome, 237–238
Superior vena cava, fetal, 228, *229*
Supplies, decontamination, disinfection, and sterilization of, 368–371, 370t
  disposable, 371

Surface tension, in alveoli, 103–105, *104*
Surfactant, 105, 235–236
Surgery, cardiopulmonary monitoring in, 406–407
  cardiopulmonary response to, 175–176
Suspension, 18
Swan-Ganz catheter, 287–290, *287–290*
  radiographic appearance of, 380
Sweat test, 405
Sympathetic cholinergic fibers, 68
Sympathetic nervous system, in cardiac control, 61
  in circulatory control, 66–68
  structure and function of, 424–425, 425t
Sympathomimetics, in bronchoprovocation, 312
Symptoms, definition of, 407
  evaluation of, 407–408
  in noncardiopulmonary disease, 408
  nonspecific, 407
  pathognomonic, 407
Synapse, 424
Synergism, pharmacologic, 420
Syringe, blood gas, 327–328
Systemic circulation, 39–41, 439–435. See also *Circulation.*
Systemic vascular resistance, 62, 293
  during hemorrhage, 164–165
Systole, 56
  atrial, 38, *56*, 57
  ventricular, *56*, 57–58
Systolic murmur, phonocardiographic assessment of, *294*, 294–295

T cells, 38
T wave, 53, 276–277
Tachyarrhythmias, *282*, 282–283. See also *Arrhythmias.*
Tachycardia, 279, *280*
  drug therapy for, 435–436
  ventricular, *282*, 283
Tachypnea, 216
  transient neonatal, 238
Tactile fremitus, 189, 261
Tamponade, cardiac, 180, *181*
Teeth, dislodgement of, during intubation, 507
Temperature scales, 14, *14*
Temperature–vapor pressure relationship, for water, 17, 18t
Tendon receptors, in breathing control, 147
Tension pneumothorax, 540
  radiography of, 384–385, *386*
Tent, croup, 457–458, *458*
  face, 453, *454*
  oxygen, 457–458, *458*
Terbutaline, 428
Terminal air sacs, 225, *227*
Tetralogy of Fallot, 233
Theophylline, 428–429, 429t
Therapy. See *Treatment.*

Thermodilution cardiac output determination, 291–292, 350
Third space fluid loss, 363
Thoracentesis, 364, 540
Thoracoabdominal pump, 76, *76*
Thorpe tube, 446–447, *449*
Thrill, 189, 261
Thromboembolism. See *Embolism.*
Thymus, radiographic appearance of, 380, 383, *385*
Thyroid cartilage, 91, *91*
Tickle tube, for cough induction, 476
Tidal volume, 111, *112*
  definition of, 111
  during exercise, 161–162, *162*
  in mechanical ventilation, generation of, 519
  regulation of, 533–534
  in pregnancy, 174
Tissot spirometer, in exercise testing, 350–351, *351*
Tomography, 395
Tonsils, palatine, 90
Tooth, dislodgement of, during intubation, 507
Total lung capacity, 112, *112*
  age-related changes in, *243*, 243–244
  determination of, 303–307, *304–306*
Total peripheral resistance, 62
Toxemia of pregnancy, 174–175
T-piece weaning, from mechanical ventilation, 535
Tracheal breath sounds, 265, 266
Tracheal intubation, 494–502. See also *Intubation.*
Tracheal position, palpation of, 259, 260
Tracheal stenosis, after intubation, 509
Tracheal suctioning, *478*, 478–480
Tracheobronchial tree, embryologic development of, 225–227, *226*, *227*
  in children, 239–240
  structure and function of, 92, 93–94, *94*
Tracheoesophageal fistula, 237, *237*, 405–406
Tracheoesophageal septum, 225, *226*
Tracheostomy, 505–506, *506*
  chronic, in obstructive sleep apnea, 216
  closure of, 510
Tracheostomy mask, 456, *457*
Tracheotomy, 505–506, *506*
Tranquilizers, 431
Transcellular fluid, 360
Transcutaneous blood gas monitoring, 336
Transferrin, in nutritional assessment, 372–373, 373t
Transfusion, 438
Transitional flow, 64
Transmural pressure gradient, 65, *65*
Transpleural aspiration, 364
Transpleural biopsy, 364
Transport, patient, 539, 540t
Transposition of great vessels, 233

Transpulmonary pressure, 102, *102*
Transtracheal aspiration, 213, *363*, 363–364
Transtracheal catheter, for cough induction, 476
Transtracheal catheter ventilation, 504–505, *505*
Transverse tubules, myocardial, 54, *54*
Transpleural biopsy, 364
Treadmill, 344–346, *347*. See also *Exercise testing.*
Treatment, chronic, 544
  emergency, 538–540
  integrated approach to, 538–553
  perioperative, 542–543
  rehabilitative, 544
Treatment planning, 541–553
  algorithmic approach to, 541
  case presentations for, 545–553
  goals of, 541
Tricarboxylic acid cycle, *30*, 30–31
Tricuspid valve, 34, *36*, 38
Triglycerides, 26, *28*
Tropomyosin, 53, *55*, 55–56
Troponin, 53, *55*, 55–56
Truncus arteriosus, embryologic development of, 220, *220*, 221, *223*, *224*
  persistent, 233–234
T-tube mask, 456
T-tubules, myocardial, 54, *54*
Tube. See also *Intubation.*
  chest, 540–541
  endotracheal, 496–498, *497*, 497t, *498*
Tuberculosis, 214
Turbine flowmeter, 299, *301*
Turbulent flow, 63–64, *64*, 107
Tussive syncope, 476
Tympany, on percussion, 261, *263*

U wave, 277
Ultrasonic nebulizer, 465–466, *466*
Ultrasonography, 396–397
  fetal, 400
Umbilical blood flow, perinatal cessation of, 230
Umbilical blood gas analysis, 330, 336, 402–403
Umbilical vein, 228, *229*
Upper airway obstruction. See *Airway obstruction.*
Urinary nitrogen, in nutritional assessment, 372
Uterine contractions, and fetal heart rate, 401

Valence electrons, 5, 465
Valves, cardiac, 34–35, *36*, 38
  disorders of, and hypertension, 188
  and left heart failure, 189–192, *190–193*

Valves (*Continued*)
  cardiac, disorders of, and right heart faillure, 189–192, *190–193*, 197, 197–198, *198*
    prosthetic, radiography of, 383, *385*
  venous, 40–41, *43*
Valvular stenosis, left heart catheterization in, 290
Vapor pressure, 17
Vascular compliance, age-related changes in, 242
Vascular distensibility, age-related changes in, 242
Vascular impedance, 65
Vascular resistance, 293
Vasculitis, pulmonary, 196
Vasoactive drugs, 437
Vasomotor center, 66, *67*
Vasopressin, 69–70, 70t
  as vasoconstrictor, 437
  during hemorrhage, *164*, 165
Vector analysis, *48*, 48–49
Vectorcardiogram, 53
Vein(s), pulmonary, 35, *36*
  structure and function of, 40–41, *43*
  umbilical, 228, *229*
Venae cavae, 34, *36*
  fetal, 228, *229*
Venous admixture, 318
Venous blood gas analysis, 325. See also *Blood gas analysis.*
  interpretation of results of, 335–336
Venous congestion, in right heart failure, 198
Venous oximetry, 337
Venous return, determinants of, 75–76, *76*
Ventilation, age-related changes in, 244–245
  alveolar. See *Alveolar ventilation.*
  and hypoxia, 169
  collateral, 97
  distribution of, assessment of, 312–314, *313*, *315*
  during anesthesia, 175
  during exercise, 160–163, *160–163*
  during hemorrhage, 166
  during pregnancy, 174
  in asthma, 202–203
  in children, 240
  in chronic bronchitis, 205
  in emphysema, 206
  in restrictive disease, 212
  maximum voluntary, 353
    assessment of, 309

Ventilation (*Continued*)
  minute, during exercise, *160*, 160–161, *161*
  unilateral, intraoperative, 503–504
  wasted, 354
Ventilation-perfusion ratio, 123–125, *124*
  age-related changes in, 244–245
  determination of, 316–318
  during exercise, 162–163, *163*
  mismatched, 123–124, *124*
    and hypoxia, 167
  regional variation in, 124–125, *125*
Ventilation-perfusion scanning, 395–396, *396*
Ventilator, 558
  pressure, 558
  volume, 558
Ventilatory capacity, maximum, 354
Ventral respiratory groups, 144–145
Ventricles, 3, 35, *36*, 38
  embryologic development of, 220, *220–222*
Ventricular afterload, 59–60
  and stroke volume, 75, 292–293
Ventricular arrhythmias. See also *Arrhythmias.*
  drug therapy for, 436
Ventricular contractility, and stroke volume, 292–293
Ventricular contractions, premature, 281–282, *282*
Ventricular depolarization, 46–47, 47t
Ventricular diastole, 38
Ventricular escape rhythm, 279, *280*
Ventricular failure, left-sided, and cardiomyopathies, 180–182
  and ischemic heart disease, 182–186
  and valvular dysfunction, 189–192
  pathophysiology of, 192–194, *193*
  right-sided, 192, 195–199
Ventricular fibrillation, *282*, 283
Ventricular filling, *56*, 57, 58
Ventricular function, 58–61, *59–61*
Ventricular hypertrophy, and mitral insufficiency, 191–192
  left-sided, and aortic stenosis, 189, *190*
    and mitral insufficiency, 191–192
    in aortic insufficiency, 191
  right-sided, causes of, 197–199
    in tetralogy of Fallot, 233
Ventricular preload, 59
  and stroke volume, 75, 292–293

Ventricular repolarization, 47, 47t, 53
Ventricular septal defects, 232
  in tetralogy of Fallot, 233
Ventricular stroke work, 293
Ventricular systole, *56*, 57–58
Ventricular tachycardia, *282*, 282–283
Venturi mask, *455*, 455–456, *456*, 456t, 558
Venules, 35, *36*, 39, 40, *42*
Verapamil, 435
Vertebrae, radiography of, 379
Vesicular breath sounds, *265*, 266
Vessel(s), alveolar, 118–119, *119*, *120*
  corner, 119, *120*
  extra-alveolar, 118–119, *119*, *120*
Vibration, therapeutic, 475
Visceral pain, 253
Vital capacity, *112*, 112–113
  determination of, 298–307, *306*
  in restrictive disease, 211–212
Vocal cords, 91, *91*
Volume, compressible, 558
  rebreathing, 558
Volume ventilator, 558
Volume-pressure relationships, gas, 12–16

Wasted ventilation, 354
Water. See also under *Fluid.*
  biochemical properties of, 23
  temperature–vapor pressure relationship for, 17, 18t
Water-seal spirometer, 298, *300*
Weight, in nutritional assessment, 373t
Weir equations, for energy expenditure, 373
Wenckebach block, 280
Wetting agents, mucokinetic, 422–423
Wheezes, *265*, 267, 557
Whispered pectoriloquy, 267
White endobronchial tube, 503, *503*
Work, and energy, 10–11, 11t
Work of breathing, 110–111
  and exercise, 162
  and hypoxia, 169
  and respiratory rate, 255–257, *257*
  during diving, 171–172

X-rays, 378–379. See also *Radiography.*

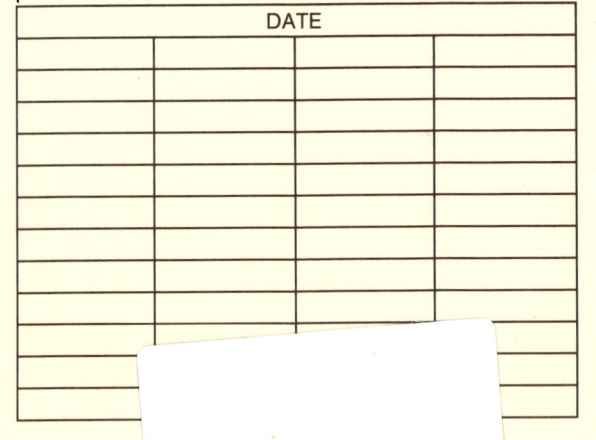